# Macular Surgery

SECOND EDITION

# Macular Surgery

## SECOND EDITION

### HUGO QUIROZ-MERCADO, M.D.

**Director of Ophthalmology**
**Denver Health Medical Center**
**Professor of Ophthalmology**
**School of Medicine, University of Colorado**
**Denver, Colorado**
**Research Consultant, Asociacion para Evitar la**
**    Ceguera en Mexico**
**Associate Professor, Universidad Nacional Autonoma**
**    de Mexico**
**Consultant, Medica Sur**
**Mexico City, Mexico**

### JOHN B. KERRISON, M.D.

**Retina Consultants of Charleston**
**Charleston, South Carolina**
**Clinical Assistant Professor**
**Storm Eye Institute**
**Medical University of South Carolina**
**Charleston, South Carolina**

### D. VIRGIL ALFARO III, M.D.

**Retina Consultants of Charleston**
**Charleston, South Carolina**

### WILLIAM F. MIELER, M.D.

**Professor and Vice-Chairman**
**Department of Ophthalmology & Visual Sciences**
**University of Illinois at Chicago**
**Chicago, Illinois**

### PETER E. LIGGETT, M.D.

**President, New England Retina Associates**
**Clinical Professor of Ophthalmology**
**Yale School of Medicine**
**Weill Cornell Medical College**
**New York, New York**

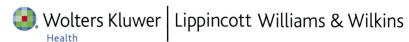

Wolters Kluwer | Lippincott Williams & Wilkins
Health

Philadelphia • Baltimore • New York • London
Buenos Aires • Hong Kong • Sydney • Tokyo

*Senior Executive Editor*: Jonathan W. Pine Jr.
*Senior Product Manager*: Emilie Moyer
*Vendor Manager*: Bridgett Dougherty
*Senior Manufacturing Manager*: Benjamin Rivera
*Marketing Manager*: Lisa Lawrence
*Creative Services Director*: Doug Smock
*Production Service*: Aptara, Inc.

**© 2011 by LIPPINCOTT WILLIAMS & WILKINS, a WOLTERS KLUWER business**
**Two Commerce Square**
**2001 Market Street**
**Philadelphia, PA 19103 USA**
**LWW.com**

First Edition copyright 2000 by Lippincott Williams & Wilkins

Printed in China

**Library of Congress Cataloging-in-Publication Data**
Macular surgery / editors, Hugo Quiroz-Mercado . . . [et al.]. – 2nd ed.
       p. ; cm.
  Includes bibliographical references and index.
  Summary: "The second edition of Macular Surgery has been completely rewritten to reflect diagnostic and therapeutic point of view. Macular surgery has been most dramatically impacted by the development of smaller instrumentation allowing surgery to be performed more rapidly and with less morbidity. The continued advancement of ocular coherence tomography has allowed the surgeon greater insight into diseases of the vitreo-macular interface including macular hole, epiretinal membrane, and vitreo-macular traction"–Provided by publisher.
  ISBN 978-0-7817-9715-3 (hardback)
  1. Macula lutea–Surgery.   I. Quiroz-Mercado, Hugo.
  [DNLM: 1. Macula Lutea–surgery.   2. Ophthalmologic Surgical Procedures–methods. 3. Retinal Diseases–surgery. WW 270]
  RE661.M3M342 2011
  617.7–dc22
                                             2011003430

To purchase additional copies of this book, call our customer service department at (800) 638-3030 or fax orders to (301) 223-2320. International customers should call (301) 223-2300.

Visit Lippincott Williams & Wilkins on the Internet: at LWW.com. Lippincott Williams & Wilkins customer service representatives are available from 8:30 am to 6 pm, EST.

10 9 8 7 6 5 4 3 2 1

CCS0411

To our patients, colleagues, and students.
To our families for their understanding and support.

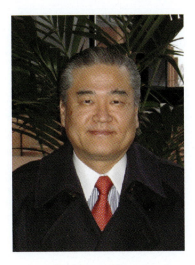

Dr. Yasuo Tano

All contributors to the second edition of *Macular Surgery* who had the opportunity to meet Dr. Yasuo Tano know the impact that he had on the field of macular surgery.

In the first edition of *Macular Surgery*, Dr. Tano proposed that his friend and mentor, Dr. Robert Machemer, write the Foreword. Dr. Machemer graciously accepted. When planning the second edition of *Macular Surgery*, Dr. Tano and our fellow editors once again were going to ask Dr. Machemer to write the Foreword.

We are saddened that neither Dr. Machemer and Dr. Tano are here to witness the publication of the second edition of *Macular Surgery*. These two pioneers left great contributions to the field of macular surgery, from the first epiretinal membrane surgery performed by Dr. Machemer to the novel design of instruments to remove macular membranes and the internal limiting membrane by Dr. Tano. Other contributions from Dr. Tano on the field of retina surgery include design of lenses used in vitrectomy, techniques of minimal invasive surgery, technology on optical coherent tomography, and artificial vision, among others. Few ophthalmologists will match Dr. Tano in the scope, number, and quality of his scientific contributions, which include peer-reviewed articles and books.

Dr. Tano's academic contribution was not confined to publishing and designing new instruments. He enjoyed sharing his ideas and knowledge to help other academic programs beyond Osaka University where he was professor for several years. He was a mainstay in many retinal courses around the world where he gave inspiring and brilliant lectures. He enjoyed demonstrating his operating room techniques to many aspiring retina surgeons. In spite of his busy academic life, he always allocated time to his family.

Yasuo Tano was popular not only for his genius and scientific work, but his great sense of humor brought friends around the world with whom he enjoyed having good times. He was genuine, kind and friendly.

As a small tribute, we dedicate *Macular Surgery*, second edition, to the memory of our good friend Yasuo who will always be remembered as a giant in the field of the ophthalmology.

**Hugo Quiroz-Mercado, MD**

**Denver, Colorado**

**Maximino Abraldes, M.D., Ph.D.** Instituto Tecnológico de Oftalmologia, Santiago de Compostela, Spain

**Anthony P. Adamis, M.D.** Vice President, Head of Ophthalmology, Genetech, Inc., Nutley, New Jersey

**D. Virgil Alfaro III, M.D.** Retina Consultants of Charleston, Charleston, South Carolina

**J. Fernando Arevalo, M.D., F.A.C.S.** Chief Professor, Department of Retina, Clinica Oftalmologica "Centro Caracas," Caracas, Venezuela

**Albert J. Augustin, M.D.** Professor and Chairman, Professor of Ophthalmology, Department of Ophthalmology, University of Mainz, Mainz, Germany; Chief, Department of Ophthalmology, Klinikum Karlsruhe, Karlsruhe, Germany

**Dolores Berger, M.D.** Retina Consultants of Charleston, Charleston Neurosciences Institute, Charleston, South Carolina

**María H. Berrocal, M.D.** Associate Professor, Department of Ophthalmology, University of Puerto Rico, San Juan, Puerto Rico

**Maria José Blanco, M.D., Ph.D.** Hospital Provincial de Conxo, Santiago de Compostela, Spain

**Mark Blumenkranz, M.D.** Chair and Ophthalmology Professor, Stanford University School of Medicine, Stanford University, San Francisco, California

**Susanne Binder, M.D.** Professor and Chair, The Ludwig Boltzmann Mit for Retinology and Biomicroscopic Laser Surgery; University Professor, M.D., Department of Ophthalmology, Rudolf Foundation Clinic, Vienna, Austria

**Antonio López Bolaños, M.D.** Vitreo and Retina Service, Institute of Ophthalmology Foundation, Universidad Nacional Autonoma de México

**Adriana Bratu, M.D.** Department of Ophthalmology, "Santa Maria delle Croci" Hospital, Ravenna, Italy

**Alexander J. Brucker, M.D.** Scheie Eye Institute, Department of Ophthalmology, University of Pennsylvania, Philadelphia, Pennsylvania

**Rafael Bueno-Garcia, M.D.** Chief of Retina Service Hospital General a "Dr. Manuel Gea Gonzalez", Mexico City, Mexico Collaborative Professor Retina Service Asociacion, Para Evitar La Ceguera en Mexico, APEC, Mexico City, Mexico

**J. Peter Campbell, M.D., M.P.H.** Wilmer Eye Institute, Johns Hopkins University School of Medicine, Baltimore, Maryland

**Luca Campi, M.D.** Institute of Ophthalmology, University of Modena and Reggio Emilia, Modena, Italy

**Antonio Capone Jr., M.D.** Co-Program Director, Vitreoretinal Fellowship, Beaumont Eye Institute, William Beaumont Hospital, Royal Oak, Michigan

**Pablo Carnota Méndez, M.D.** Centro de Ojos de La Coruña, La Coruña, Spain

**Gian Maria Cavallini, M.D.** Institute of Ophthalmology, University of Modena and Reggio Emilia, Modena, Italy

**R.V. Paul Chan, M.D., M.S.** Department of Ophthalmology, New York-Presbyterian Hospital, Weill Medical College of Cornell University, New York, New York

**Louis Chang, M.D.** Department of Ophthalmology, Columbia University, New York, New York

**Steve Charles, M.D.** Clinical Professor of Ophthalmology, Department of Ophthalmology, University of Tennessee/ Hamilton Eye Institute, Charles Retina Institute, Memphis, Tennessee

**Nauman Chaudry, M.D.** New England Retina Associates, Hamden, Connecticut

**Carl Claes, M.D.** Head of Department, Vitreo-Retinal Department, Saint-Augustinus Hospital, Wilrijk, Antwerp, Belgium

**Lucienne Collet, M.D.** Retina and Vitreous Service, Centro de Cirugia Oftalmologica (CECOF), Caracas, Venezuela

**Borja Corcostegui, M.D.** Professor of Ophthalmology, Department of Ophthalmology, Universitat Autónoma de Barcelona, Chief Director of the Ocular Microsurgery Institute (I.M.O), Barcelona, Spain

**Rafael Cortez, M.D.**   Retina and Vitreous Service, Centro de Cirugia Oftalmologica (CECOF), Caracas, Venezuela

**Donald J. D'Amico, M.D.**   Department of Ophthalmology, New York-Presbyterian Hospital, Weill Medical College of Cornell University, New York, New York

**Giuseppe Di Stefano, M.D.**   Institute of Ophthalmology, University of Trieste, Trieste, Italy

**Diana V. Do, M.D.**   Wilmer Eye Institute, Johns Hopkins University School of Medicine, Baltimore, Maryland

**Jay S. Duker, M.D.**   Tufts University, New England Medical Center, Boston, Massachusetts

**Juan V. Espinoza, M.D.**   Retina and Vitreous Service, Clínica Oftalmologica Centro Caracas, Caracas, Venezuela

**Michel E. Farah, M.D., Ph.D.**   President of the Vision Institute, Professor and Vice-Chief Department of Ophthalmology Federal University of São Paulo, São Paulo, Brazil

**Sharon Fekrat, M.D., F.A.C.S.**   Associate Professor, Department of Ophthalmology, Duke University School of Medicine, Durham, North Carolina

**Javier Ferro, M.D.**   Chief, Retina and Vitreo, Clinicas Oculsur, Spain

**Howard F. Fine, M.D., MHSc.**   The LuEsther T. Mertz Retinal Research Center, Vitreous Retina Macula Consultants, Edward S. Harkness Eye Institute, Columbia University College of Physicians and Surgeons, New York, New York

**Daniel Finkelstein, M.D.**   Professor, Department of Ophthalmology, Johns Hopkins University School of Medicine, Baltimore, Maryland

**Cesare Forlini, M.D.**   Department of Ophthalmology, "Santa Maria delle Croci" Hospital, Ravenna, Italy

**Matteo Forlini, M.D.**   Institute of Ophthalmology, University of Modena and Reggio Emilia, Modena, Italy

**Arnd Gandorfer, M.D., Ph.D.**   Associate Professor, Department of Ophthalmology, Consultant VR Surgeons, VR and Pathology Unit, Ludwig-Maximilians University, Munich, Germany

**Gerardo García-Aguirre, M.D.**   Retina Department, Asociación para Evitar la Ceguera en México, México DF, México

**Reinaldo A. Garcia Arismendi, M.D.**   Associate Professor, Department of Retina, Clinica Oftalmologica "El Viñedo," Valencia, Venezuela; Domingo Luciani Hospital, Caracas, Venezuela

**Rosa Evangelina Garnica Hayashi, M.D.**   Retina and Vitreo, San Juan Rio, Queretaro, Mexico

**Peter Gehlbach, M.D., Ph.D.**   Department of Ophthalmology, Johns Hopkins University School of Medicine, Baltimore, Maryland

**David T. Goldenberg, M.D.**   Vitreoretinal Surgery Fellow, Eye Research Institute, Oakland University, Rochester, Michigan; Beaumont Eye Institute, William Beaumont Hospital, Royal Oak, Michigan

**Francisco Gómez-Ulla, M.D., Ph.D.**   Professor of Ophthalmology, University of Santiago de Compostela, Hospital Provincial de Conxo, Instituto Tecnológico de Oftalmología, Spain

**Maximiliano Gordon, M.D.**   Medical Staff, Department of Retina, Centro de la Vision, Professor of Retina, Hospital Provincial del Centenario, Rosario, Argentina

**Michael A. Grassi, M.D., Ph.D.**   Assistant Professor, Department of Ophthalmology, University of Chicago, University of Chicago School of Medicine, Chicago, Illinois

**Craig M. Greven, M.D.**   Wake Forest University Eye Center, Medical Center Boulevard, Winston-Salem, North Carolina

**James T. Handa, M.D.**   Associate Professor, Associate Chief, Retina Division, Wilmer Eye Institute, Johns Hopkins School of Medicine, Baltimore, Maryland

**Josephine Hoh, Ph.D.**   Yale University School of Medicine, New Haven, Connecticut

**Nancy M. Holekamp, M.D.**   Partner, Barnes Retina Institute, Professor of Clinical Ophthalmology, Washington University School of Medicine, Saint Louis, Missouri

**Odette M. Houghton, M.D.**   Department of Ophthalmology, University of North Carolina School of Medicine, Chapel Hill, North Carolina

**Eric P. Jablon, M.D.**   Consultant, Retina Consultants of Charleston, Charleston, South Carolina

**Peter K. Kaiser, M.D.**   Cole Eye Institute, Cleveland Clinic Foundation, Cleveland, Ohio

**Motohiro Kamei, M.D.**   Clinical Professor, Ophthalmology, Osaka University Graduate School of Medicine, Osaka, Japan

**Anselm Kampik, M.D., Ph.D.**   Department of Ophthalmology, University Eye Hospital, Ludwig-Maximilians University, Munich, Germany

**John B. Kerrison, M.D.**   Retina Consultants of Charleston, Charleston, South Carolina, Clinical Assistant Professor, Storm Eye Institute, Medical University of South Carolina, Charleston, South Carolina

**Aziz A. Khanifar, M.D.**   Department of Ophthalmology, New York-Presbyterian Hospital, Weill Medical College of Cornell University, New York, New York

**Yunyoung Kim, M.D.**   Department of Ophthalmology, School of Medicine, Catholic University of Daegu, Daegu Republic of Korea

**Christina M. Klais, M.D.**   The LuEsther T. Mertz Retinal Research Center, New York, New York

**Ronald Klein, M.D., M.P.H.**   Department of Ophthalmology & Visual Science, University of Wisconsin School of Medicine and Public Health-Madison, Madison, Wisconsin

**Veronica Kon-Jara, M.D.**   Retina Department, Asociación para Evitar la Ceguera en México, México DF, México

**Arthur Korotkin, M.D.**   Department of Ophthalmology, University of Colorado, Denver, Colorado

**Nancy Kunjukunju, M.D.**   Retinal Fellow, Department of Ophthalmology, Ochsner Medical Center, New Orleans, Louisiana

**Baruch D. Kupperman, M.D., Ph.D.**   Professor, Department of Ophthalmology, University of California, Irvine, California

**Anna Paula R. Lafeta, M.D.**   Retina Surgeon, Vitreo-Retinal Department, Centro de Oftalmologia Avançada, Belo Horizonte, Brazil

**Eleonora Lavaque, M.D.**   Fellow de vítreo y retina, Departamento de Retina, Hospital Oftalmológico Santa Lucia, Buenos Aires, Argentina

**Hilel Lewis, M.D.**   The Cleveland Clinic, Cleveland, Ohio

**Peter Liggett, M.D.**   Clinical Professor of Ophthalmology, Cornell, New England Retina Associates, Hamden, Connecticut

**Richard C. Lin, M.D., Ph.D.**   Department of Ophthalmology and Visual Science, University of Chicago, Chicago, Illinois

**Mauricio Maia, M.D.**   Vision Institute-IPEPO, Department of Ophthalmology, Federal University of São Paulo, São Paulo, Brazil

**Naresh Mandava, M.D.**   Professor and Chairman, Department of Ophthalmology, Rocky Mountain Lions Eye Institute, University of Colorado School of Medicine, Denver, Colorado

**Travis A. Meredith, M.D.**   Department of Ophthalmology, University of North Carolina School of Medicine, Chapel Hill, North Carolina

**William F. Mieler, M.D.**   Department of Ophthalmology and Visual Science, University of Chicago, Chicago, Illinois

**Virgilio Morales-Canton, M.D.**   Assistant Professor, Department of Ophthalmology, Chief, Retina Service of Asociacion Para Evitar La Ceguera en México, Hospital Dr. Luis Sanchez Bulnes, Mexico City, Mexico

**Carlos A. Moreira, Jr., M.D.**   Professor and Chairman, Department of Ophthalmology, Universidade Federal do Parana, Brasil

**Raja Narayanan, M.D.**   Department of Ophthalmology, Tel Aviv Medical Center, Sackler Faculty of Medicine, Tel Aviv University, Tel Aviv, Israel

**Quan Dong Nguyen, M.D., M.Sc.**   Wilmer Eye Institute, Johns Hopkins University School of Medicine, Baltimore, Maryland

**Michael D. Ober, M.D.**   The LuEsther T. Mertz Retinal Research Center, New York, New York; Retinal Consultants of Michigan, Southfield, Michigan

**Masahito Ohji, M.D.**   Department of Ophthalmology, Shiga University of Medical Science, Shiga, Japan

**Scott C.N. Oliver, M.D.**   Assistant Professor, Department of Ophthalmology, Rocky Mountain Lions Eye Institute, University of Colorado School of Medicine, Denver, Colorado

**Jeffrey L. Olson, M.D.**   Associate Professor, Department of Ophthalmology, Rocky Mountain Lions Eye Institute, University of Colorado School of Medicine, Denver, Colorado

**Kirk H. Packo, MD.**   Chair, Department of Ophthalmology, Rush Medical College, Chicago, Illinois

**Chirag C. Patel, M.D.**   Fellow in Vitreoretinal Diseases and Surgery, Department of Ophthalmology, Rocky Mountain Lions Eye Institute, University of Colorado School of Medicine, Denver, Colorado

**Fabio Patelli, MD.**   Department of Ophthalmology and the Department of Statistics, Villa Tiberia Clinic, Rome, Italy, Retina Research Center, Carones Ophthalmology Center, Milan, Italy

**Lorena Patricia Pimentel, M.D.**   Vitreo-Retina Surgery Master at Ocular Microsurgery Institute, Santiago de Compostela, España

**Hugo Quiroz-Mercado, M.D.**   Chief of Ophthalmology, Denver Health Medical Center, School of Medicine, University of Colorado, Denver, Colorado

**Jawad Ahmad Qureshi, M.D., M.B.A.**   Vitreoretinal Surgery Fellow, Department of Ophthalmology, Duke University School of Medicine, Durham, North Carolina

**Gema Ramírez, M.D.**   Retina and Vitreous Service, Centro de Cirugia Oftalmologica (CECOF), Caracas, Venezuela

**Tushar M. Ranchod, M.D.**   Department of Ophthalmology, Scheie Eye Institute, University of Pennsylvania, Philadelphia, Pennsylvania

**Franco M. Recchia, M.D.** Associate Professor of Ophthalmology and Visual Sciences, Chief, Retina Division, Director, Fellowship in Vitreoretinal Diseases and Surgery, Vanderbilt University Medical Center, Nashville, Tennessee

**Carl D. Regillo, M.D.** Professor of Ophthalmology, Thomas Jefferson University; Director, Retina Research, Wills Eye Institute, Philadelphia, Pennsylvania

**Elias Reichel, M.D.** Associate Professor and Vice Chair, Department of Ophthalmology, Tufts University School of Medicine; Director, Vitreoretinal Diseases and surgery Service, Tufts/New England Medical Center, Boston, Massachusetts

**Guido Ripandelli, M.D.** Chief, Department of Vitreoretinal Surgery, IRCCS-Foundazione "G.B. Bietti" Per Lo Studio E La Nicenca in Oftalmolagia, Rome, Italy

**Eduardo B. Rodrigues, M.D.** Vision Institute-IPEPO, Department of Ophthalmology, Federal University of São Paulo, São Paulo, Brazil

**Monica Rodriguez-Fontal, M.D.** Retina Consultants of Charleston, Charleston Neuroscience Institute, Charleston, South Carolina

**Paolo Rossini, M.D.** Department of Ophthalmology, "Santa Maria delle Croci" Hospital, Ravenna, Italy

**Hirokazu Sakaguchi, M.D.** Department of Ophthalmology, Osaka University Graduate School of Medicine, Yamadaoka, Japan

**Yukihiro Sato, M.D.** Professor, Department of Ophthalmology, Toho University, Chiba, Japan

**Miki Sawa, M.D.** Associate Professor, Ophthalmologist, Department of Ophthalmology, Osaka University Medical School, Suita, Osaka, Japan

**Carol L. Shields, M.D.** Professor of Ophthalmology, Thomas Jefferson University Hospital; Codirector, Oncology Service, Wills Eye Institute, Philadelphia, Pennsylvania

**Jerry A. Shields, M.D.** Professor of Ophthalmology, Thomas Jefferson University, Director of Ocular Oncology Services, Wills Eye Hospital, Philadelphia, Pennsylvania

**Fumio Shirga, M.D.** Professor, Department of Ophthalmology, Kagawa University Faculty of Medicine, Chairman, Department of Ophthalmology, Kagawa University Hospital, Kagawa, Japan

**Rishi P. Singh, M.D.** Cole Eye Institute, Cleveland Clinic Foundation, Cleveland, Ohio

**Jason S. Slakter, M.D.** Clinical Professor of Ophthalmology, Department of Ophthalmology, New York University School of Medicine, Vitreous-Retina-Macula Consultants of New York, New York City, New York

**R. Theodore Smith, M.D.** Harkness Eye Institute, Columbia University College of Physicians and Surgeons, New York, New York

**Marc J. Spirn, M.D.** Wills Eye Institute, Philadelphia, Pennsylvania

**Einar Stefánsson, M.D., Ph.D.** Professor of Ophthalmology, Department of Ophthalmology, University of Iceland; Chief, Department of Ophthalmology, Landspitali University Hospital, Reykjavik, Iceland

**Paul Sternberg Jr., M.D.** George Weeks Hale Professor and Chair, Department of Ophthalmology and Visual Sciences, Vanderbilt University Medical Center; Director, Vanderbilt Eye Institute, Nashville, Tennessee

**Mario Stirpe, M.D.** Istituto di Ricovero e Cura a Carattere Scientifico Fondazione G. B. Bietti per lo Studio e la Ricerca in Oftalmo-logia, Rome, Italy

**Beatriz S. Takahashi, M.D.** Vitreo Retinal Specialist, Department of Ophthalmology, Medical School of the University of São Paulo, São Paulo, Brazil

**Yasuo Tano, M.D.** Former Professor and Chairman, Department of Ophthalmology, Osaka University; Chief, Department of Ophthalmology; Osaka University Hospital, Suita, Osaka, Japan*

**Hiroko Terasaki, M.D.** Department of Ophthalmology, Nagoya University School of Medicine, Nagoya, Japan

**Michael T. Trese, M.D.** Clinical Professor of Biomedical Sciences, Eye Research Institute, Oakland University, Rochester, Michigan; Chief Pediatric and Adult Vitreoretinal Surgery, Beaumont Eye Institute, William Beaumont Hospital, Royal Oak, Michigan

**Giora Treister, M.D.** Sheba Medical Center, Tel Aviv University, Tel Aviv, Israel

**Raul Velez-Montoya, M.D.** Retina Department, Asociación para Evitar la Ceguera en México, México DF, México

**Ximena Vasquez, M.D.** Hospital de Clinicas, Montevideo, Uruguay

**Juan Ignacio Verdaguer, M.D.** Department of Medicine, Clinical Hospital University of Chile, Santiago, Chile

---

*Deceased

**Juan Ignacio Verdaguer, M.D.**   Department of Medicine, Clinical Hospital University of Chile, Santiago, Chile

**Oria Veronica, M.D.**   Clinica Oftalmológica Centro Caracas, Caracas, Venezuela

**Mark K. Walsh, M.D., Ph.D.**   Vitreoretinal Fellow, Associated Retinal Consultants, William Beaumont Hospital, Royal Oak, Michigan

**Jie Jin Wang, M.Med., Ph.D.**   Associated Professor, Senior Research Fellow, Australian National Health and Medical Research Council (NHMRC), Centre for Vision Research; Department of Ophthalmology and the Westmead Millennium Institute, University of Sydney, Sydney, Australia

**David J. Wilson, M.D.**   Professor and Thiele-Petti Chair, Department of Ophthalmology, Director, Casey Eye Institute, Oregon Health and Sciences University, Portland, Oregon

**William J. Wirostko, M.D.**   The Eye Institute, Medical College of Wisconsin, Milwaukee, Wisconsin

**Andre J. Witkin, M.D.**   Clinical Associate, Department of Ophthalmology, Tufts University School of Medicine; Resident Physician, Department of Ophthalmology, Tufts/New England Medical Center, Boston, Massachusetts

**Lihteh Wu, M.D.**   Associate Surgeon, Department of Vitreoretinal, Instituto de Cirugia Ocular, San José, Costa Rica

**Wayne W. Wu, M.D., Ph.D.**   Private Practice, Eau Claire, Wisconsin

**Lawrence A. Yannuzzi, M.D.**   The LuEsther T. Mertz Retinal Research Center, Harkness Eye Institute, Columbia University College of Physicians and Surgeons, New York, New York

**Yoshihiro Yonekawa, M.D.**   Department of Ophthalmology, New York-Presbyterian Hospital, Weill Medical College of Cornell University, New York, New York

Diseases of the macula are a common and devastating cause of blindness. Visual function loss in macular disease is characterized by visual distortion and scotoma. This pattern of vision loss impairs one's ability to read and drive. It is a major cause of visual morbidity.

Age-related macular degeneration and diabetic macular disease are among the biggest challenges to retinal physicians and their patients. Both diseases are chronic and have complex pathophysiologies. Both diseases are increasing in prevalence and incidence. In both diseases, a precise anatomic understanding of a patient's pattern and extent of disease is required for therapeutic decisions that are individualized to the patient. New interventions for preserving and improving vision in patients with macular disease are needed and continue to be a dynamic area of research.

The field of macular surgery is a natural step in the evolution of vitreoretinal surgery. Vitreoretinal surgery was initially used to treat complex retinal detachment and proliferative diabetic disease. Major technological improvements in surgical microscopes, fiberoptic illumination, instruments, pharmacotherapeutics, and adjunctive tools have allowed the retinal physician to continue to use surgical intervention as a vital therapeutic tool. Macular disease as an indication for surgery continues to increase.

Since publication of the first edition of *Macular Surgery*, the field has dramatically evolved from both a diagnostic and therapeutic point of view. The second edition of *Macular Surgery* has been completely rewritten to reflect these developments. It is truly an international and collaborative work. It has more than 70 authors from 15 countries and four continents. The ability to compose such a work is a testament to the high level of expertise which characterizes the international community of retinal physicians.

At the time of publication of the first edition of *Macular Surgery*, surgical interventions for wet macular degeneration offered great promise. These treatments included submacular surgery for the removal of subretinal neovascular membranes and macular translocation in order to reposition the macular retina to areas where the underlying retinal pigment epithelium was less damaged. Such complex surgeries are no longer necessary because of effective intravitreal anti–vascular endothelial growth factor pharmacotherapies.

Since the publication of the first edition of *Macular Surgery*, macular surgery has been most dramatically impacted by the development of smaller instrumentation allowing surgery to be performed more rapidly and with less morbidity. The continued advancement of ocular coherence tomography has allowed the surgeon greater insight into diseases of the vitreomacular interface including macular hole, epiretinal membrane, and vitreomacular traction. The use of triamcinolone to stain the vitreous and dyes to stain membranes has improved intraoperative visualization of pathologies. The ability to stain and remove the internal limiting membrane has led to better surgical outcomes.

These are some of the new developments in macular surgery that are chronicled in *Macular Surgery*. Those who witnessed the evolution of cataract surgery over the last 50 years from intracapsular cataract extraction to multifocal lens implantation will recognize that macular surgery is undergoing a similar transformation. Synergism between surgical intervention and new biologic-based therapies will continue. It is a blessing to offer our patients new and effective treatments for macular disease.

**Hugo Quiroz-Mercado**

**D. Virgil Alfaro III**

**John B. Kerrison**

# CONTENTS

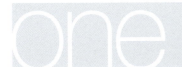
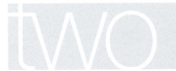

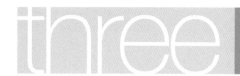

*Deceased

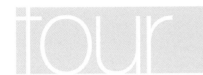

## Section 4: Diabetic Retinopathy

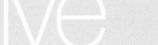

## Section 5: Macular Edema

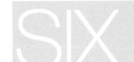

## Section 6: Vitreous Traction Maculopathies

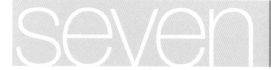

**Section 7: Macular Holes**

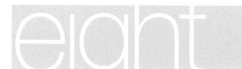

**Section 8: Choroidal Neovascularization and Age-Related Macular Degeneration**

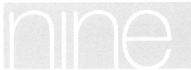

## Section 9: Infectious Diseases of the Macula, Pediatrics, and Trauma

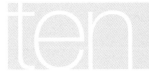

## Section 10: Miscellaneous and Tumors

## Section 11: Prevention and Treatment of Complications

## Section 12: Frontiers in Macular Surgery

one

# Anatomy and Pathophysiology of the Macula

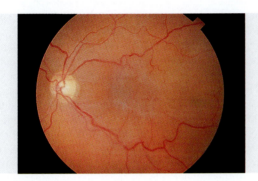

# Pathophysiology of the Vitreoretinal Interface

Yunyoung Kim ■ David J. Wilson

## ANATOMY AND PHYSIOLOGY OF THE VITREORETINAL INTERFACE

It is not surprising that the junction of the vitreous and the retina is a critical interface for both physiologic and pathologic processes. At this site, there are numerous, abrupt transitions at the molecular, biochemical, cellular, and structural level. An appreciation of the features of molecular structure, histology, and gross anatomy of this interface is critical for understanding a diverse group of states including retinal development, retinopathy of prematurity, ocular trauma, retinovascular disease, retinal detachment, macular hole development, vitreous detachment, epiretinal membrane, and others.

The vitreoretinal interface is composed of the cortical vitreous, the internal limiting membrane (ILM; lamina) of the retina, and the innermost portion of the Mueller cells. It is easiest to consider this zone of tissue by initially appreciating the structure and function of the ILM, which represents the basement membrane of the Mueller cells. One can subsequently assess how the ILM is related to the cortical vitreous and the Mueller cell in a functional and structural sense.

Basement membranes are ubiquitous extracellular protein matrices that form a border between cells and their adjacent mesenchymal tissue. These membranes have multiple functions including structural cell support and attachment, interaction with cellular receptors, storage or repository site for growth factors and cytokines, tissue compartmentalization, and functioning as a molecular sieve to exclude proteins above a certain size. The interaction with cellular receptors has effects on cell shape, gene expression, cell migration and proliferation, and programmed cell death (1).

Given the above list, it is simplistic and inaccurate to think of basement membranes as purely structural elements, but an appreciation of their structure is helpful in understanding the more dynamic aspects of this interface. The ultrastructure of the ILM contains three distinct areas: the lamina rara, the lamina densa, and the lamina rara interna (2) (Fig. 1-1). There are topographic variations in the ILM, and Foos (3) has divided these variations into three zones: basal, equatorial, and posterior. In addition to these three broad zones, there are specific features of the ILM of the fovea and the optic nerve.

In the basal zone, the ILM is uniformly thin, averaging 510 Angstroms (Å) in thickness. In this zone, the vitreous collagen fibrils have an orientation perpendicular to the surface of the ILM. The equatorial zone is characterized by a progressive and gradual thickening of the ILM, achieving an average thickness of 2600 Å. In this zone, the vitreous fibrils are oriented more tangentially to the surface of the ILM. In the posterior zone, the ILM has an average thickness of 25,000 Å, and the retinal surface is markedly uneven, corresponding to the undulating surface of the Mueller cells. In the posterior zone, the overlying vitreous fibrils continue to have an orientation tangential to the surface of the ILM.

One distinction between these three zones is the relative abundance of Mueller cell attachment plaques. These plaques represent condensations of the fibrils of the Mueller cell cytoskeleton. Attachment plaques were noted to be more

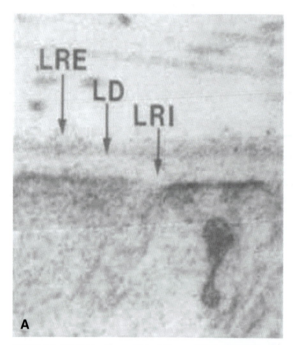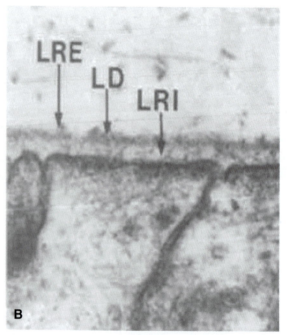

**Figure 1-1.** Electron micrographs of the medullary ray region of the rabbit eye showing the internal limiting membrane (ILM). **A:** Tissue fixed with glutaraldehyde and paraformaldehyde. The ILM is adjacent to the Mueller cell end feet and has three layers. One of these layers is electron dense (lamina densa [LD]) and is readily seen in the transmission electron micrograph (TEM). The other layers are electron transparent and are not evident in aldehyde-fixed material. The lamina rara interna (LRI) is between two electron-dense areas: the cytoplasm of the Mueller cell and the LD. The lamina rara externa (LRE) is on the vitreal face of the lamina densa and is an ill-defined layer, 5–10-nm thick. Collagen fibrils are 16-nm thick filaments without cross bands. (×96,000) **B:** Tissue fixed with Alcian blue. The LD is more electron dense after Alcian blue fixation, and material can be seen within the LRI (×62,000). (From Matsumoto B, Blanks JC, Ryan SJ. Topographic variations in the rabbit and primate internal limiting membrane. *Invest Ophthalmol Vis Sci* 1984;25:71–82, with permission.)

abundant in the basal zone and virtually absent in the posterior zone. Foos (3) attributed the topographical differences of vitreous fibril orientation and attachment plaque density to the variation in the amount of vitreous traction in the different zones.

The ILM of the fovea is distinct from the remainder of the posterior zone, in that it is much thinner, starting at the clivus, diminishing to a thickness of 200 Å at the foveola. Mueller cell attachment plaques also reappear in this same location. At the optic nerve head margin, the thick ILM of the posterior zone abruptly diminishes to a thickness of 450 Å.

The ILM, like other basement membranes, is composed of several collagens, laminins, proteoglycans, calcium-binding proteins, and other structural and adhesive proteins (1) (Table 1-1). Type IV collagen provides a highly cross-linked structural framework that maintains mechanical stability. A second network of laminins is more variable in composition between tissue and also may vary within the same tissue (1). There have been only limited studies of the specific laminin and other protein/proteoglycan content of the ILM (4–7). Studies in other tissues have implicated laminin binding sites as providing the adhesion of the basement membrane to the underlying cells (1,8), possibly through alpha-dystroglycan linkage of the basement membrane to the actin skeleton of the underlying cell. Although ultrastructural studies initially suggested the vitreous collagen inserted into the collagenous network of the ILM, more recent studies suggest that this adhesion is the result of noncovalent binding of proteoglycan moieties to the vitreous and basement membrane collagens (7). Hence, the adhesion of the vitreous to the retina is not maintained by a collagenous network but rather by noncovalent binding of laminins and proteoglycan constituents of the vitreoretinal interface. This mechanism of adhesion can be affected by various degenerative and pathologic states as we will see later in this chapter.

In addition to its mechanical and structural features, the ILM is capable of playing a dynamic role by regulation of cell binding and of the local cytokine microenvironment. Basement membranes contain multiple proteins, that when bound by cell surface receptors initiate intracellular signaling pathways that alter cellular behavior. During basement membrane remodeling, exposure of these proteins can lead to cellular activities that promote tissue repair such as recruitment of immune cells and activation of fibroblasts. ILM also is a repository for vascular endothelial growth factor (7). Following injury, or as a result of disease, vascular endothelial growth factor and other stored cytokines may impact the microenvironment for angiogenesis. Anti-angiogenic fragments of basement membrane collagen released during remodeling of the ILM (endostatin, tumstatin, and arresten) may also play a role in the angiogenic response at the vitreoretinal interface (9).

Changes that occur in the retina and the vitreous often have their clinical manifestations at the vitreoretinal interface. These changes may be on the basis of mechanical injury, metabolic processes, or age-related degeneration. Because the vitreoretinal interface is the junction between the relatively fluid vitreous and the retina, the manifestations of a wide variety of diseases occur at this location.

## Age-Related Changes in the Vitreoretinal Interface

Age-related and other degenerative changes in the vitreous commonly lead to separation of the vitreous from the ILM. The molecular basis for this degeneration has not been fully elucidated, but recent studies have found that there is fragmentation of vitreous collagen that leads to the formation of pockets of fluid within the normally homogeneous matrix of collagen separated by a proteoglycan matrix (10,11). This degeneration may be catalyzed by endogenous enzymes including plasmin and other matrix metalloproteinases (12–14).

The availability of optical coherence tomography (OCT) has provided great insight into the process of separation of the vitreous from the ILM, in particular how this separation is related to the pathophysiology of many common retinal conditions (15). Uchino and coworkers (16) have described five stages of posterior vitreous detachment (PVD) in a study of normal eyes. In Stage 0, the vitreous remains completely attached to the ILM. In Stage 1, there is perifoveal detachment of the vitreous, in as many as three quadrants around the fovea, with the vitreous remaining attached at the fovea and in one quadrant. There is a predilection for detachment of one of the superior quadrants first. In Stage 2, the vitreous has detached in all perifoveal quadrants but remains attached

## TABLE 1-1  REPRESENTATIVE BASEMENT MEMBRANE PROTEINS

| Components | $M_r$ (kDa) | Chain assembly form | Special features |
|---|---|---|---|
| Collagen IV | 550 | Heterotrimer containing two different a chains | Three isoforms<br>Network forming |
| Laminins | 400–900 | α, β, γ heterotrimers | >10 isoforms<br>Network forming |
| Perlecan | 500[a] | Monomer | Proteoglycan |
| Agrin | 250[a] | Monomer | Proteoglycan |
| Nidogen | 150 | Monomer | Network connecting |
| BM-40/SPARC[b] | 35 | Monomer | Calcium binding |
| Fibulin-1 | 90 | Monomer | Calcium binding |
| Fibulin-2 | 340 | Homodimer | Calcium binding |

[a]This value is the $M_r$ of the core proteins. The $M_r$ is about 50% larger after glycosaminoglycan attachment.
[b]Secreted protein, acidic and rich in cysteines.

at the fovea and at the optic nerve. The vitreous has detached from the fovea in Stage 3 but remains attached to the optic nerve. Stage 4 consists of detachment of the vitreous from the optic nerve to complete the PVD. Although this was not a longitudinal study, it suggested that there is a stagewise detachment of the vitreous from the posterior pole and that his process may occur over an extended period of time. This more gradual process of PVD is consistent with the time course and pathophysiology of common abnormalities of the vitreoretinal interface in the posterior pole, particularly epiretinal membrane, vitreomacular traction, and macular hole. The complete separation that occurs in transition between stages 3 and 4 is probably responsible for the more dramatic conditions of retinal tear and rhegmatogenous retinal detachment.

Once the vitreous has even partially separated from the ILM, the stage has been set for cell proliferation and traction to occur at the vitreoretinal interface; these processes are responsible for epiretinal membranes, vitreomacular traction, macular holes, retinal tears, and detachment.

## Epiretinal Membrane

In the absence of a PVD, it is very uncommon to find cells on the vitreous surface of the ILM. However, once the vitreous is even partially detached, cell migration and proliferation along the vitreous surface of the ILM may occur. It seems likely that there is some sort of inhibition of cell migration that is lost with separation of the vitreous, but the mechanism of this inhibition is not known. It is likely that the predominant cell in most age-related and degenerative epiretinal membranes is the glial cell. However, in cases of retinal tear or detachment, there is a greater abundance of retinal pigment epithelium (RPE) cells than in idiopathic epiretinal membranes. Characterization of cells on the basis of morphologic, or even morphology combined with immunohistology, features is difficult, so the exact composition by cell of origin is hard to know with certainty (17).

The changes that occur in the laminin composition of the ILM following PVD are not known. It is not known whether existing cell binding sites are exposed secondary to PVD or whether the laminin composition of the ILM changes to create new binding sites. However, once a membrane is established, the intracellular filament apparatus responsible for cell migration can result in surface traction that distorts retinal architecture, and may even result in retinal folds (Fig. 1-2).

## Vitreomacular Traction

In cases of vitreomacular traction, the vitreous remains attached to the optic nerve and to a portion of the posterior retina. In this condition, there is often an epiretinal membrane present on the portion of the ILM in which there has been vitreous detachment. This creates a situation in which there is surface traction as well as anterior posterior traction.

## Macular Hole

Few topics have elicited such a great variety of mechanistic hypotheses. With the availability of OCT, it is clear that macular hole development is the result of forces working at the vitreoretinal interface. These forces are identical to those that

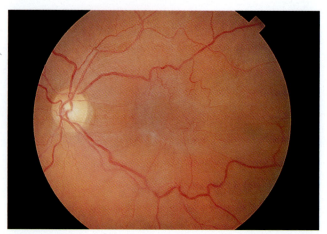

**Figure 1-2.** Severe macular pucker. Note the gray-appearing central epiretinal membrane and tortuosity of the perifoveal vessels.

occur in the course of PVD, but with incomplete separation of the vitreous from the perifoveal retinal surface, there is continued anterior–posterior and perhaps to a lesser degree tangential forces on the retina. These forces lead to the various stages of foveal elevation, schisis, and full-thickness hole formation.

## Retinal Tear

There are sites at which the vitreous is more adherent to the retinal surface, and with posterior vitreous detachment, these sites of adhesion may lead to retinal tears. The normal sites of greater vitreoretinal adhesion are the vitreous base, the retinal vessels, and the optic nerve head. Careful study of the vitreous base has found that with age there is a migration of the posterior border of the vitreous base with age. The strength of adhesion of the vitreous at this location also increases with age (18). Pathologic sites of increased adhesion also exist, such as lattice degeneration.

## Retinovascular Disease and the Vitreoretinal Interface

In the early stages of retinovascular disease, the effects of the disease are principally on the retina side of the ILM. However, changes occur at the vitreoretinal interface in these conditions that may contribute to the clinical manifestations of the diseases, including neovascularization and macular edema. However, in diabetic retinopathy, branch retinal vein occlusion and retinopathy of prematurity, retinal neovascularization may extend through the ILM to involve the vitreous.

## Diabetic Retinopathy

There are several functional and structural changes that occur at the level of the vitreoretinal interface in diabetic retinopathy. The thickness of the ILM increases in diabetic retinopathy, and there is an increase in heparan sulfate proteoglycan, fibronectin, laminin, and type I and III–V collagen (19). In addition, there is an increased incidence of cells on the vitreous surface of the ILM (19). These pathologic changes most certainly account for the greater incidence of OCT vitreoretinal interface abnormalities (20,21). The most common of these abnormalities is the incomplete separation of the vitreous from the retina. This abnormal adherence may be a contributing factor to diabetic macular edema.

In proliferative diabetic retinopathy, for the growth of new blood vessels to extend past the ILM, there needs to be active degradation of the ILM. Enzymes capable of this degradation, gelatinases (MMP-2 and -9), have been shown to be elevated in patients with proliferative diabetic retinopathy (22). With growth of new blood vessels through the ILM, the neovascular tissue becomes intimately associated with the vitreous collagen (23) (Fig. 1-3). This pathologic development predisposes the eye to preretinal hemorrhage resulting from PVD-induced traction on the neovascular tissue.

## Other Retinovascular Diseases

Although there are no substantial studies of the vitreoretinal interface changes in branch and central retinal vein occlusion

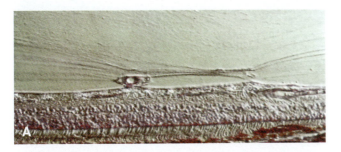
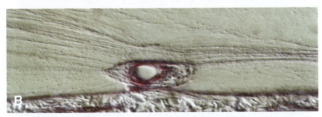
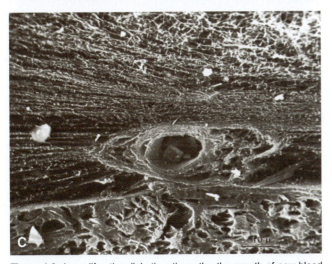

**Figure 1-3.** In proliferative diabetic retinopathy, the growth of new blood vessels to extend past the internal limiting membrane and become intimately associated with the vitreous collagen. Traction lines of vitreous lamellae converging to microproliferation: **A** celloidin paraffin, PAS, Interference Contrast, 320:1; **B** same, Interference Contrast, 800:1; **C** same microproliferation, scanning electron microscopy. (From Faulborn J, Bowald S. Microproliferations in proliferative diabetic retinopathy and their relationship to the vitreous: corresponding light and electron microscopic studies. *Graefe's Arch Clin Exp Ophthalmol* 1985;223:130–138, with permission.)

and radiation retinopathy, it seems likely that similar changes will be present in these conditions. In diseases such as retinopathy of prematurity that have a significantly different pathogenesis, there may be distinct changes at the vitreoretinal interface.

## Trauma to the Vitreoretinal Interface

At this point in time the most common type of trauma to the vitreoretinal interface is surgical trauma in peeling the ILM for macular hole. This is perhaps the only condition and tissue in which the basement membrane of a cell is purposefully stripped from the cell, with the intent to improve a healing response. Consequently, there are not similar diseases from which to extrapolate long-term effects. However, as yet, no significant, long-term clinical consequences of removing the basement membrane of the Mueller cell have been identified.

Certain features of the normal structure of the ILM are important in the removal of the ILM as part of macular hole surgery. The ILM in the posterior pole is much thicker than in other parts of the retina, and this contributes to the surgeon's ability to engage the membrane, providing sufficient strength to allow tractional "peeling" of the membrane from the underlying retina. Peeling of the ILM is often associated with microhemorrhages, so there is little doubt that removal of the ILM results in some damage to the underlying tissue. Studies have shown that with peeling of the ILM, there is removal of fragments of the Mueller cell (19,24–28). This has been shown by the presence of cellular material on the retinal side of ILM specimens (19,24,25,27,28). Experimental study of fresh, postmortem human eyes (29) has demonstrated that only a portion of the Mueller cells is affected. There was no loss of the Mueller cell bodies or nuclei, so it may be that Mueller cells are able to survive this type of trauma. Functional studies with microperimetry have failed to disclose any functional deficit specifically attributable to ILM peeling. However, electrophysiologic testing has shown a persistent reduction in the b wave following ILM peeling, when compared with eyes treated with vitrectomy only (29).

In addition to the Mueller cell injury, some of the injury from the tangential traction accompanying ILM peeling may occur in deeper retinal layers. This tangential force applied at the vitreoretinal interface may be transmitted to the photoreceptor/RPE interface and lead to damage of the photoreceptor outer segments with subsequent RPE hyperplasia (30) (Fig. 1-4).

Removal of the ILM with macular hole surgery has been reported to result in a higher rate of closure of macular holes and a reduced likelihood of subsequent re-opening of a macular hole. Surveys of vitreoretinal surgeons have indicated that ILM removal is considered to be an important adjunct to vitrectomy in the successful management of this condition. However, studies are not definitive in showing a visual acuity outcome difference between macular hole patients treated with or without removal of the ILM.

Because of difficulty in visualizing the ILM for removal, various vital dyes have been used to stain the ILM intraoperatively. By far the most frequently used of these is indocyanine green (ICG). Many publications have raised the question of whether ICG is toxic to the retina or RPE (24,25,31–33). Reports have associated atrophic RPE changes with the use of

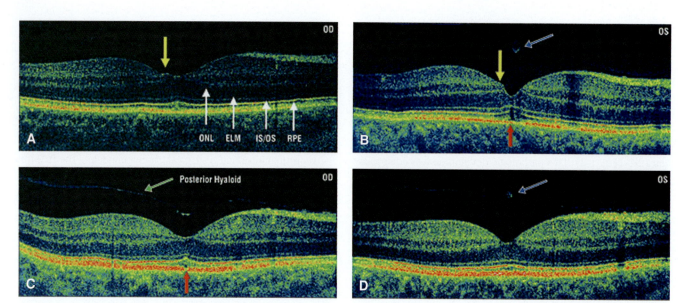

**Figure 1-4. A:** High-speed ultrahigh-resolution optical coherence tomography (UHR-OCT) image of the right eye 1 week after cataract extraction in the left eye. Note a slight irregularity in the foveal contour (*yellow arrow*). Outer retinal layers are indicated. **B:** High-speed UHR-OCT image of the left eye 1 week after cataract extraction. A pseudooperculum is present above the retina (*blue arrow*). The inner foveal contour is irregular (*yellow arrow*), and there is a disruption of the foveal inner and outer segment junction (*red arrow*). **C:** High-speed UHR-OCT image of the right eye 4 months later. The posterior hyaloid has detached from the fovea, with a return to normal inner foveal contour. A small disruption of the foveal photoreceptor outer segments is present (*red arrow*). **D:** High-speed UHR-OCT image of the left eye 4 months later. The inner foveal contour has returned to normal, and the photoreceptor outer segment disruption has disappeared. ELM, external limiting membrane; IS/OS, photoreceptor inner and outer segment junction; ONL, outer nuclear layer; and RPE, retinal pigment epithelium. (From Witkin AJ, Wojtkowski M, Reichel E, et al. Photoreceptor disruption secondary to posterior vitreous detachment as visualized using high speed ultrahigh resolution optical coherence tomography. *Arch Ophthalmol* 2007;125:1579–1580, with permission.)

ICG. In addition, there are reports that the amount of cellular material on the posterior surface of the ILM is greater when the ILM was stained with ICG than when peeling was performed without staining. Reports vary with regard to whether there are any differences in functional outcome with or without staining of the ILM with ICG.

## Pharmacologic Vitreous Detachment

Strong adherence of the vitreous to the retina makes management of some retinal conditions quite difficult. Specifically, in young patients undergoing surgery for trauma, retinopathy of prematurity (ROP), or retinal detachment repair, complete separation of the vitreous from the retina and subsequent removal may be quite difficult. Studies have shown that surgical creation of PVD in experimental animals, or in postmortem human eyes, results in identifiable injuries to the optic nerve and the retina (34). These injuries are compatible with the visual field defects that have been reported following surgically induced PVD (34). Consequently, there have been efforts to find an enzymatic mechanism that would facilitate separation of the vitreous from the retina.

It is desirable that enzymatic agents accomplish two things: liquefaction of the vitreous and separation of the vitreous from the ILM (35). Various enzymes have been investigated for their effectiveness in accomplishing these steps in creating an enzyme-induced PVD including plasmin, hyaluronidase, collagenase, chondroitinase, and dispase (35–42). Of these, plasmin and dispase, as single agents, have been shown to effect both vitreous liquefaction and separation of the vitreous from the ILM (35). This latter attribute of plasmin and dispase relates to

their ability to break down fibronectin and laminin, which appear to be involved in the vitreoretinal adhesion.

One of the stated advantages of enzymatic PVD is that it potentially leads to a more complete removal of the vitreous collagen from the surface of the ILM (37). Residual vitreous collagen has been noted in various diseases of the vitreoretinal interface and has been implicated as contributing to the growth of surface membranes (26).

At present some of these agents are undergoing evaluation in U.S. Food and Drug Administration (FDA) trials. Their widespread adoption will require that the limited toxicities observed in experimental animal studies are observed in humans and that the costs are outweighed by a substantial improvement in the ability to mechanically address diseases of the vitreoretinal interface.

## References

1. Timpl R. Macromolecular organization of basement membrane. *Curr Opin Cell Biol* 1996;8:618–624.
2. Matsumoto B, Blanks JC, Ryan SJ. Topographic variations in the rabbit and primate internal limiting membrane. *Invest Ophthalmol Vis Sci* 1984;25:71–82.
3. Foos RY. Vitreoretinal juncture: topographical variations. *Invest Ophthalmol Vis Sci* 1972;11:801–808.
4. Halfter W, Dong S, Balasubramani M, et al. Temporary disruption of the retinal basal lamina and its effect on retinal histogenesis. *Dev Biol* 2001;238:79–96.
5. Bystrom B, Virtanen I, Rousselle P, et al. Distribution of laminins in the developing human eye. *Invest Ophthalmol Vis Sci* 2006;47:777–785.
6. Kohno T, Sorgente N, Ishibashi T, et al. Immunofluorescent studies of fibronectin and laminin in the human eye. *Invest Ophthalmol Vis Sci* 1987;28:506–514.
7. Russell SR, Shepherd JD, Hageman GS. Distribution of glycoconjugates in the human retinal internal limiting membrane. *Invest Ophthalmol Vis Sci* 1991;32:1986–1995.

8. Pall EA, Bolton KM, Ervasti JM. Differential heparin inhibition of skeletal muscle alpha-dystroglycan binding to laminins. *J Biol Chem* 1996;271:3817–3821.

9. Lebleu VS, Macdonald B, Kalluri R. Structure and function of basement membranes. *Exp Biol Med* 2007;232:1121–1129.

10. Bishop PN, Holmes DF, Kadler KE, et al. Age-related change on the surface of vitreous collagen fibrils. *Invest Ophthalmol Vis Sci* 2004;45:1041–1046.

11. Los LI, van der Worp RJ, vas Lurn MJ, et al. Age-related liquefaction of the human vitreous body: LM and TEM evaluation of the role of proteoglycans and collagen. *Invest Ophthalmol Vis Sci* 2003;44:2828–2833.

12. Vaughan-Thomas A, Gilbert S, Duance V. Elevated levels of proteolytic enzymes in the aging human vitreous. *Invest Ophthalmol Vis Sci* 2004;41:3299–3304.

13. Delapaz MA, Itoh Y, Toth CA, et al. Matirx metalloproteinases and their inhibitors in human vitreous. *Invest Ophthalmol Vis Sci* 1998;39:1256–1260.

14. Brown DJ, Hamdi H, Bahri S, et al. Characterization of an endogenous metalloproteinase in human vitreous. *Curr Eye Res* 1994;13:639–647.

15. Mirza RG, Johnson MW, Jampol LM. Optical coherence tomography use in evaluation of the vitreoretinal interface: a review. *Surv Ophthalmol* 2007;52:397–421.

16. Uchino E, Uemura A, Ohba N. Initial stages of posterior vitreous detachment in healthy eyes of older persons evaluated by optical coherence tomography. *Arch Ophthalmol* 2001;119:1475–1479.

17. Vinores SA, Campochiaro PA, Conway BP. Ultrastructural and electron immunocytochemical characterization of cells in epiretinal membranes. *Invest Ophthalmol Vis Sci* 1990;31:14–28.

18. Wang J, Mclead D, Henson D, et al. Age-dependent changes in the basal retinovitreous adhesion. *Invest Ophthalmol Vis Sci* 2003;44:1793–1800.

19. Matsunaga N, Ozeki H, Hirabayashi Y, et al. Histopathologic evaluation of the internal limiting membrane surgically excised from eyes with diabetic maculopathy. *Retina* 2005;25:311–316.

20. Gaucher D, Tadayoni R, Erginay A, et al. Optical coherence tomography assessment of the vitreoretinal relationship in diabetic macular edema. *Am J Ophthalmol* 2005;139:807–813.

21. Ghazi NG, Ciralsky JB, Shah S, et al. Optical coherence tomography findings in persistent diabetic macular edema: the vitreomacular interface. *Am J Ophthalmol* 2007;144:747–754.

22. Noda K, Ishida S, Inoue M, et al. Production and activation of matrix metalloproteinase-2 in proliferative diabetic retinopathy. *Invest Ophthalmol Vis Sci* 2003;44:2163–2170.

23. Faulborn J, Bowald S. Microproliferations in proliferative diabetic retinopathy and their relationship to the vitreous: corresponding light and electron microscopic studies. *Graefe's Arch Clin Exp Ophthalmol* 1985;223:130–138.

24. Nakamura T, Murata T, Hisatomi T, et al. Ultrastructure of the vitreoretinal interface following the removal of the internal limiting membrane using indocyanine green. *Curr Eye Res* 2003;27:395–399.

25. Gandorfer A, Haritoglou C, Kampik A, et al. Ultrastructure of the vitreoretinal interface following removal of the internal limiting membrane using indocyanine green [Letter to the editor]. *Curr Eye Res* 2004;29:319–320.

26. Schumann R, Schaumberger MM, Rohleder M, et al. Ultrastructure of the vitreomacular interface in full thickness idiopathic macular holes: a consecutive analysis of 100 cases. *Am J Opthalmol* 2006;141:1112–1119.

27. Heij EC, Dieudonne SC, Mooy CM, et al. Immunohistochemical analysis of the internal limiting membrane peeled with infracyanine green. *Am J Ophthalmol* 2005;140:1123–1125.

28. Wolf S, Schnurbruch U, Wiedemann P, et al. Peeling of the basal membrane in the human retina. *Ophthalmology* 2004;111:238–243.

29. Terasaki H, Miyake Y, Nomura R, et al. Focal macular ERGs in eyes after removal of macular ILM during macular hole surgery. *Invest Ophthalmol Vis Sci* 2001;42:229–234.

30. Witkin AJ, Wojtkowski M, Reichel E, et al. Photoreceptor disruption secondary to posterior vitreous detachment as visualized using high speed ultrahigh resolution optical coherence tomography. *Arch Ophthalmol* 2007;125:1579–1580.

31. Haritoglou C, Priglinger S, Gandorfer A, et al. Histology of the vitreoretinal interface after indocyanine green staining of the ILM, with illumination using a halogen and xenon light source. *Invest Ophthalmol Vis Sci* 2005;46:1468–1472.

32. Kuhn F. Point: to peel or not to peel, that is the question. *Ophthalmology* 2002;109:9–11.

33. Hassan T, Williams G. Counterpoint: to peel or not to peel: is that the question? *Ophthalmology* 2002;109:11–12.

34. Yamamoto S, Yamamoto T, Ogata K, et al. Morphological and functional changes of the macula after vitrectomy and creation of posterior vitreous detachment in eyes with diabetic macular edema. *Doc Ophthalmol* 2004;109:249–253.

35. Sebag J. Molecular biology of pharmacologic vitreolysis. *Trans Am Ophthalmol Soc* 2005;103:473–494.

36. Hara A. Surface structure of rabbit and human retina after enzymatic separation of inner limiting membrane. *Jpn J Ophthalmol* 1994;38:375–381.

37. Gandorfer A, Putz E, Welge-Luβen U, et al. Ultrastructure of the vitreoretinal interface following plasmin assisted vitrectomy. *Br J Ophthalmol* 2001;85:6–10.

38. Uemura A, Nakamura M, Kachi S, et al. Effect of plasmin on laminin and fibronectin during plasmin-assisted vitrectomy. *Arch Ophthalmol* 2005;123:209–213.

39. Chen W, Huang X, Ma XW, et al. Enzymatic vitreolysis with recombinant microplasminogen and tissue plasminogen activator. *Eye (Lond)* 2008;22:300–307.

40. Asami T, Terasaki H, Kachi S, et al. Ultrastructure of internal limiting membrane removed during plasmin-assisted vitrectomy from eyes with diabetic macular edema. *Ophthalmology* 2004;111:231–237.

41. Tanaka M, Qui H. Pharmacological vitrectomy. *Semin Ophthalmol* 2000;15:51–61.

42. Staubach F, Nober V, Janknecht P. Enzyme-assisted vitrectomy in enucleated pig eyes: a comparison of hyaluronidase, chondroitinase, and plasmin. *Curr Eye Res* 2004;29:261–268.

# CHAPTER

## 2

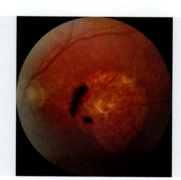

# Pathophysiology of the Retinal Pigmented Epithelium and Choroid

James T. Handa

# INTRODUCTION

The retinal pigmented epithelium (RPE)-Bruch's membrane-choroid complex is a vital structure that maintains the health of the neurosensory retina. The RPE interacts closely with the photoreceptors of the neurosensory retina, and has multiple functions including photoreceptor outer segment (POS) turnover, neutralization of photo-oxidative stress, heat dissipation, and vitamin A homeostasis. For example, the RPE processes the phagocytosis of 25,000 to 30,000 POS tips every day (1). The Bruch's membrane is a complex pentalaminar extracellular matrix composed of the RPE basement membrane, inner collagenous layer, middle elastic layer, outer collagenous layer, and the choriocapillaris basement membrane. This specialized membrane is critical for maintaining special diffusional capabilities between the RPE and choriocapillaris. The choroid is composed of three layers including the choriocapillaris, medium vessels, and large vessels. The choriocapillaris is the main oxygen source for the photoreceptors.

The health of each of these layers contributes to specific diseases of the macula. This tissue, on a histopathological basis, responds in predictable fashion that can be clinically useful. With discovery of the molecular pathogenetic causes of macular disease, a new spectrum of diseases may become amenable to surgical management. The purpose of this chapter is to describe the basic histopathologic responses of the RPE-Bruch's membrane-choroidal complex, how the overlay of aging can affect this response, and how new discoveries may influence our surgical management of the macula in the near future.

# GENERAL PATTERNS OF PATHOLOGIC CHANGE TO THE RETINAL PIGMENTED EPITHELIUM

Regardless of the stimulus, the RPE responds to a stress in several stereotypic pathologic ways that have clinical and surgical relevance. Understanding these responses will help the clinician better diagnose and manage RPE disease. In response to insult or disease, the RPE can undergo hypertrophy, metaplasia, migration, or hyperplasia. More advanced or sustained insults can result in atrophy and, ultimately, cell death. The RPE is normally a cuboidal epithelium. The apical region is rich in microvilli to help with the phagocytosis of POSs. The basal region has infoldings to increase surface area for the exchange of materials with the choriocapillaris. The RPE is packed with melanin granules to improve visual resolution and neutralize photo-oxidative stress. It is rich with mitochondria because of the high metabolic demands.

Hypertrophic RPE cells become enlarged. Melanin granules are enlarged without increasing in their number. The result is a dark, jet-black appearance to the RPE. Hyperplastic RPE cells are the result of proliferation and migration. The cell number is increased. For example, RPE cell hyperplasia can appear as "bony spicules" in a perivascular configuration when

they migrate into the neurosensory retina along retinal vasculature.

The RPE is a postmitotic simple epithelium that typically undergoes little cell division. However, in response to injury, inflammation, or another similar stimulus, it can undergo metaplasia. A classic example is during a retinal tear where RPE cells are dislodged from its monolayer and released into the vitreous cavity where they can attach to the vitreous and develop a fibroblastic phenotype. With altered cell-matrix interactions, the cell undergoes migration, metaplasia, and proliferation. Crypopexy can exaggerate this process by introducing inflammation and cellular injury that augment this response. Clinically, the consequence is an epiretinal membrane, or in severe cases, proliferative vitreoretinopathy membranes can develop on the inner and outer surface of the neurosensory retina and induce a tractional retinal detachment.

# RETINAL PIGMENTED EPITHELIUM ATROPHY AND APOPTOSIS IN AGING AND AGE-RELATED MACULAR DEGENERATION

With aging, the RPE undergoes progressive degeneration that can lead to atrophy. The RPE loses its normal cuboidal morphology to become irregular in shape and flattened, or atrophic. The atrophic cells contain fewer pigment granules than normal RPE (2–4). Clinically, this can be visualized by hypopigmentation in affected areas of the macula (Fig. 2-1).

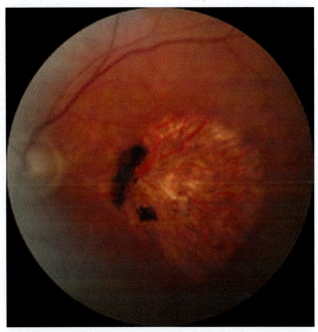

**Figure 2-1.** Fundus photograph of nonneovascular age related macular degeneration showing geographic atrophy. Note the clinical appearance of retinal pigmented epithelium (RPE) atrophy so that the large choroidal vessels are easily visualized. The nasal edge has RPE hyperplasia.

Ultrastructurally, aging atrophic RPE cells contain few pure melanin granules, and instead, are filled with melanolipofuscin and melanolysosomes (5). Many of these changes are due to the relentless accumulation of lipofuscin, or insoluble biomolecules that arise from incomplete digestion of phagocytosed POSs beginning in the first or second decade of life (6,7). Lipofuscin is contained within lysosomes. Remarkably, lipofuscin can occupy up to 19% of the RPE cell by the time the patient is 80 years of age (7). The RPE basal infoldings are fewer in number, and some RPE can be detached from the RPE basement membrane, due to the development of basal laminar deposits (BlamD) or accumulations of heterogeneous material between the RPE and its basement membrane.

With flat mount sections, the RPE cells appear hexagonal and more densely packed in the macula than in the periphery in young eyes, but they lose their hexagonal shape and resemble nonfoveal RPE with aging (8). Young macular RPE has a homogeneous cell density that becomes heterogeneous with aging (9). Overall, the number of RPE cells in the macula declines with aging and age-related macular degeneration (AMD), although this number is more variable than in young maculas. The major pathophysiologic mechanism for the cell loss is apoptosis. Del Priore et al. showed that the proportion of apoptotic human RPE cells increases significantly with age (10). The apoptotic RPE are confined mainly to the macula, and account for the preferential decrease of RPE cells in the macula. Dunaief et al. showed that RPE cell loss in AMD is due to apoptosis (11). Apoptotic cells are seen in areas of RPE atrophy at the edge of geographic atrophy. The factors that cause RPE cells to enter apoptosis are unclear, but at present include oxidative stress, photo-oxidative stress, lipid accumulation, or uncontrolled complement mediated inflammation.

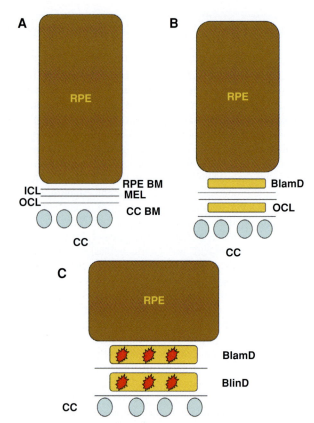

**Figure 2-2.** Cartoon of basal deposit location in Bruch membrane with aging and age related macular degeneration (AMD). **A:** Normal retinal pigmented epithelium (RPE) and Bruch membrane. **B:** Aging changes including basal laminar deposits (BlamD) and outer collagenous layer deposits (OCL). **C:** AMD changes. Basal linear deposits (BlinD) and thick BlamD contain heterogeneous deposits. RPE BM, RPE basement membrane; ICL, inner collagenous layer; MEL, middle elastic layer; OCL, outer collagenous layer; CC BM, choriocapillaris basement membrane; CC, choriocapillaris.

## CHANGES TO BRUCH'S MEMBRANE WITH AGING AND AGE-RELATED MACULAR DEGENERATION

Coincident with atrophy and potentially loss of the RPE, Bruch's membrane undergoes a series of histopathologic changes. The hallmark change of aging and AMD is the development of basal deposits, or accumulation of heterogeneous debris. The location and composition of basal deposits define whether the changes are due to aging or age-related disease (Fig. 2-2). As early as in the second decade of life, the outer collagenous layer accumulates homogenous material (12). In addition, accumulations between the RPE and its basement membrane known as BlamD also develop with aging. If the accumulations become thick and contain heterogeneous debris such as inflammatory proteins, cellular fragments, lipoproteins, and "long spacing collagen," they are a marker for AMD. The accumulation of apolipoprotein B100 containing lipoproteins within the inner collagenous layer during aging is a recent discovery of significant importance (13). Its accumulation most likely creates a "lipid" barrier restricting the normal diffusional characteristics of Bruch's membrane that can lead to injury to the RPE (14). Importantly, these lipoproteins have

been hypothesized to induce basal linear deposit (BlinD) formation, or accumulations in the inner collagenous layer. BlinDs are one of the strongest histopathological markers for AMD. Clinically, basal deposits are typically not visualized. However, a later stage change is the appearance of drusen, yellowish deposits that are the clinical hallmark of aging and AMD (15).

## CONSEQUENCES OF SUBRETINAL FLUID

Visual recovery after rhegmatogenous retinal detachment is negatively influenced by subretinal fluid under the macula. While there are direct adverse effects on the neurosensory macular retina, the subretinal fluid clearly alters the RPE, which can contribute to a poor outcome. In experimental models of rhegmatogenous retinal detachment, RPE migration and proliferation are observed within a day. The proliferation occurs at the interface between the RPE apex and photoreceptor tips (16). The RPE also undergoes morphologic alterations including retraction of apical microvilli, which are typically in contact with the photoreceptors, and a rounding of the cells at the apex (17). These proliferative and metaplastic changes to the RPE can adversely influence the recovery of the photoreceptors, and when there are changes to the RPE, the morphologic recovery of the RPE is protracted and correlates with the slow recovery of vision. Clinically this is manifested by macular pigmentary changes. Hackett et al. examined RPE migration and proliferation by adding blood-free subretinal fluid to RPE cells in culture (18). Several variables were examined for correlation with migration and proliferation, including age and sex of the patient; extent, duration, and height of the detachment; protein content of the fluid; and amount of cryopexy. They found that retinal cryopexy enhanced RPE cell migration activity in subretinal fluid, while RPE proliferative activity increased with the size and duration of detachment. While the vitreoretinal surgeon has little control over the size and duration of any retinal detachment, these results suggest that the surgeon should judiciously use cryopexy during retinal reattachment surgery.

The overlay of aging changes to the RPE on recovery from subretinal fluid or another insult can predictably impair the recovery process and restoration of visual acuity. For example, several groups have shown that advanced age negatively influences visual recovery after repair of a macula off retinal detachment (19–21).

## GENETIC DISEASES

The RPE can be the target of specific genetic diseases. Mutations in the RPE65 gene result in Leber Congenital Amaurosis. RPE65 is involved in retinoid metabolism. It catalyzes the critical step in the visual cycle converting all-trans-retinyl ester to 11-cis-retinol that permits normal photoreceptor function and vision. Its absence results in undetectable rhodopsin, rod photoreceptor dysfunction, the development of inclusions in the RPE, and subsequent retinal degeneration. 9-cis-retinal can restore visual pigmentation and function in mice. One intriguing observation is that patients with this mutation have disproportionately greater photoreceptor layer thickness than cone photoreceptor function (22). This highlights the fact that the primary abnormality lies in the RPE and is distinct from primary retinal degenerations where the photoreceptor layer is thin, consistent with lost photoreceptor function. Theoretically, it could indicate that therapeutic rescue is possible in the late stages of the disease if the photoreceptor layer remains relatively intact.

Several years ago, a genetic disease such as RPE65 deficiency would not have been an appropriate topic for a textbook on vitreoretinal surgery. However, the rapid advances in gene therapy make genetic diseases a suitable topic for discussion. Gene therapy is the use of a vector, typically a bioengineered virus, to deliver a gene of interest into target tissue to restore the normal production of the gene in the intended tissue. In 2001, Ackland et al. showed that gene therapy restored vision in a dog with RPE65 deficiency (23). The RPE65 gene was placed in a recombinant adeno-associated virus (AAV) and injected subretinally into the fundus of a dog with RPE65 deficiency. There was electroretinographic improvement in treated animals and, importantly, evidence of improved visual function using behavioral testing. Recently, AAV-RPE65 was shown to be safe after subretinal injections in nonhuman primates (22). Specifically, there were no abnormalities in ERG wave forms, or histopathologic evidence of toxicity such as loss of photoreceptor layer thickness. At the time of writing this, the first patient has been successfully subretinally injected with AAV-RPE65. If successful, this treatment strategy could open up a new avenue for treatment of other genetic diseases.

## NEW INSIGHTS INTO RETINAL PIGMENTED EPITHELIUM REGENERATION

While the past decade has seen innovations in RPE cell transplantation and various surgical techniques for retinal translocation, progress has been limited. This enigmatic cell layer has, for the most part, defied replacement strategies. Significant progress has been made with vascular repair using adult hematopoietic stem cells. A similar strategy has been discovered for the RPE. Several recent studies have demonstrated the ability of hematopoietic stem cells, when mobilized to the peripheral circulation, to relocate to focal areas of RPE injury. Li et al. have shown that hematopoietic stem cells *in vitro* can be induced to express RPE specific markers, and that when using sodium iodate to induce RPE specific injury, hematopoietic stem cells mobilized to the peripheral circulation migrated to the subretinal space and expressed RPE specific markers (24). In a mouse model of laser induced choroidal neovascularization (CNV), Chan-Ling et al. showed that hematopoietic stem cells can localize to the area of laser injury where angiogenesis develops. At the edge of the injury, stem cells homed and differentiated into RPE cells (25). At present, it is unclear whether significant function is restored to these nascent RPE cells. While it appears to have a small role in the natural healing of the RPE after any kind of injury or disease, this strategy nevertheless raises the possibility of a new way of repairing the RPE, regardless of the disease process.

## CHOROID

### General Considerations

The choroid is comprised of a vascular network and pigmented tissue that is histologically separated into three layers. The outermost layer is the suprachoroid. Here, the large choroidal vessels are attached to the sclera by an array of connective tissues, creating a space that can potentially be separated, as will be described below. The layer contains melanocytes and houses many nerves. The stroma consists of a network of blood vessels that decrease in caliber from the exterior to the interior. These large and medium vessels are not fenestrated. The choriocapillaris is a plexus of capillaries that have fenestrations. The diameter of the choriocapillaris capillaries is larger than most capillaries to allow more than a single red blood cell to pass through. The fenestrations allow passage of a number of molecules. The capillary network is configured in a lobular pattern, consisting of a central arteriole that empties into post-capillary venules. The system is designed for rapid blood flow to accommodate the high metabolic demand of the outer neurosensory retina and RPE.

The choroidal circulation has one of the highest blood flow rates in the body (26). It provides nourishment to the RPE and outer retina. Regulation of choroidal flow is under autonomic control. The high blood flow suggests that oxygen content more than meets tissue demands and provides a margin of safety. The choroid provides a vital link with the systemic circulation. This link also provides a conduit for pathologic developments, as will be summarized below.

## Choroidal Detachment and Hemorrhage

The potential space between the sclera and outer choroid can be filled with either exudative fluid or hemorrhage. When filled, the fluid/blood is bounded by the scleral spur anteriorly and the optic nerve posteriorly. In addition, the choroid is attached firmly to the sclera at the vortex vein ampullas. This attachment contributes to the classic lobular appearance seen on ophthalmoscopy. Choroidal detachment is defined by a serous effusion within the suprachoroidal space (Fig. 2-3). Hypotony and inflammation are the principal causes (27). Suprachoroidal hemorrhage associated with trauma or intraocular surgery is a well known phenomenon. Many descriptors have been used based on the size, that is, "limited," "massive," or "kissing," when the inner retinal surfaces are in apposition; or on the onset, such as "expulsive" to denote a sudden onset or "delayed"/"postoperative" when the hemorrhage occurs in the early postoperative period. Histopathologic studies indicate that a four-step process occurs: (a) choriocapillaris engorgement; (b) serous effusion into the suprachoroidal space; (c) stretching and tearing of choroidal and ciliary body vessels; and (d) hemorrhage from the choroidal/ciliary body vessels (28). The risk factors for such cases include glaucoma, increased axial length of the eye, elevated intraocular pressure (IOP), generalized atherosclerosis, advanced age, and elevated intraoperative pulse pressure (29).

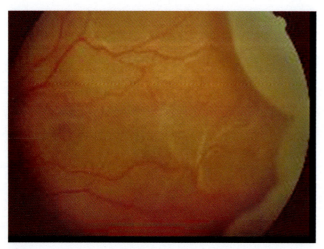

**Figure 2-3.** Fundus photograph of a serous choroidal detachment.

## Choroidal Blood Flow Changes in Age-Related Macular Degeneration

Choroidal blood flow decreases with aging (30). A more severe decline in blood flow is seen with AMD. Histopathologic studies also show changes in the choroid with AMD. Sarks et al. showed a decrease in choriocapillaris cross-section area with AMD (31). This work has been confirmed by Ramrattan et al., who found decreased density and diameter of choriocapillaris in AMD eyes (32). Choroidal perfusion abnormalities have also been identified in AMD that correlate with these histopathologic findings. For example, Chen et al. used fluorescein angiography to identify areas of delayed choroidal perfusion and associated these changes with decreased visual acuity (33). Likewise, Holz et al. found that slow choroidal filling is associated with the subsequent development of geographic atrophy (34). Prolonged choroidal filling has also been observed with indocyanine green angiography in patients with AMD (35). Recently, Grunwald et al. demonstrated a systematic decline in choroidal blood flow with increasing severity of AMD using features that are associated with CNV (36).

The association of systemic factors and AMD has been the topic of numerous epidemiologic studies. For example, some studies show an association of systemic hypertension with AMD although others have not (37–41). The Macular Photocoagulation Study found that patients with hypertension did not respond as well to laser photocoagulation for CNV, suggesting that hypertension has a negative impact on the disease process (42). Patients with AMD and systemic hypertension were recently found to have significantly lower choroidal blood flow beyond that seen in patients with AMD without hypertension (43). Hypertension has been shown to be a potential risk factor for choroidal neovascular development, and the recent work by Melelitsina et al. suggests that choroidal ischemia plays a role in CNV development (43). Ross et al. showed that CNV develops at watershed vascular filling areas (44), further supporting the contribution of relative ischemia in CNV development.

The impact of reduced choroidal blood flow at this point, however, remains unresolved. While the choroidal blood flow appears to exceed that necessary to meet the metabolic demand for oxygen, the ischemia seen with aging is hypothesized to impair diffusion of important substances across the RPE-Bruch's membrane barrier, whether nutrients are being delivered to the photoreceptor layer, or metabolic waste being exported to the choriocapillaris. The added changes of a lipid barrier to Bruch's membrane with aging and early AMD, could further compromise the necessary flow of metabolites across the RPE-Bruch's membrane complex. However, the specific factors that are lost which drive AMD progression or delayed recovery after an injury or insult with aging, have not been established.

Choroidal blood flow is under autonomic control. In response to a physiological stimulus such as increased ocular perfusion pressure, the choroidal blood flow remains constant in normal, healthy volunteers, whether they are young or elderly. In contrast, while patients with neovascular AMD typically have reduced choroidal blood flow, in response to a physiological stimulus, these same patients exhibit increased blood flow, reflecting altered responses to changes in perfusion pressure, and an inability of new blood vessels to increase their flow resistance during this stimulus (45). These changes are most likely the result of a combination of reduced sympathetic innervation to choroidal blood vessels and increased stiffness of vessels. Thus, the increased choroidal blood flow in neovascular AMD from a physiologic stimulus such as exercise could increase the exudation and bleeding that is commonly seen as in neovascular AMD.

Recent studies have highlighted the importance of genetic susceptibility to AMD. In particular, several polymorphisms in complement factors, including complement factor H, B, C2, and C, indicate the importance of the complement related inflammation during AMD development (46–51). Factor H, for example, inhibits the alternative complement system. The Y402H polymorphism in factor H is thought to prevent this inhibition from occurring, thereby leading to increased complement mediated inflammation. The choroid clearly has a role in facilitating the effects of local complement activation by the RPE. In patients harboring the Y402H factor H polymorphism, elevated levels of C-reactive protein from the circulation are deposited in the choroid, as compared to that for non-AMD patients (52). The elevated CRP indicates that increased levels of inflammation in the choroid during AMD, and CRP itself, can activate inflammatory molecules. Thus, the elevated CRP levels in susceptible patients could add to the inflammatory response.

An important response during complement mediated inflammation is the upregulation of vascular endothelial growth factor (VEGF). Complement components C3a and C5a are bioactive components present in drusen that can induce VEGF, which can induce a neovascular response (53). Other inflammatory mediators within drusen could also activate VEGF. Recently, carboxyethylpyrrole, a specific oxidatively modified product of docosahexanoic acid, a major fatty acid component of photoreceptor tips, has been identified in drusen of AMD patients. carboxyethylpyrrole (CEP) also induces angiogenesis through VEGF independent pathways (54). Thus, components within drusen may predispose patients to neovascular AMD, whether mediated through or independent of VEGF pathways. Regardless, the recent development of pegaptanib, bevacizumab, and ranibizumab has clearly had an impressive impact on salvaging and preserving vision loss associated with neovascular AMD (55–57). With greater understanding of how the RPE, Bruch's membrane, and choroid functions, additional and better targeted molecular therapy for diseases specific to these regions can be invented.

## References

1. Ershov AV, Bazan NG. Photoreceptor phagocytosis selectively activates PPARgamma expression in retinal pigment epithelial cells. *J Neurosci Res* 2000;60:328–337.
2. van der Schaft TL, Mooy CM, de Bruijn WC, et al. Histologic features of the early stages of age-related macular degeneration. A statistical analysis. *Ophthalmology* 1992;99:278–286.
3. Green WR, McDonnell PJ, Yeo JH. Pathologic features of senile macular degeneration. *Ophthalmology* 1985;92:615–627.
4. Sarks SH. Ageing and degeneration in the macular region: a clinicopathological study. *Br J Ophthalmol* 1976;60:324–341.
5. Feeney-Burns L, Burns RP, Gao CL. Age-related macular changes in humans over 90 years old. *Am J Ophthalmol* 1990;109:265–278.
6. Feeney-Burns L, Berman ER, Rothman H. Lipofuscin of human retinal pigment epithelium. *Am J Ophthalmol* 1980;90:783–791.
7. Feeney-Burns L, Hilderbrand ES, Eldridge S. Aging human RPE: morphometric analysis of macular, equatorial, and peripheral cells. *Invest Ophthalmol Vis Sci* 1984;25:195–200.
8. Watzke RC, Soldevilla JD, Trune DR. Morphometric analysis of human retinal pigment epithelium: correlation with age and location. *Curr Eye Res* 1993;12:133–142.
9. Harman AM, Fleming PA, Hoskins RV, et al. Development and aging of cell topography in the human retinal pigment epithelium. *Invest Ophthalmol Vis Sci* 1997;38:2016–2026.
10. Del Priore LV, Kuo YH, Tezel TH. Age-related changes in human RPE cell density and apoptosis proportion in situ. *Invest Ophthalmol Vis Sci* 2002;43:3312–3318.
11. Dunaief JL, Dentchev T, Ying GS, et al. The role of apoptosis in age-related macular degeneration. *Arch Ophthalmol* 2002;120:1435–1442.
12. van der Schaft TL, Mooy CM, de Bruijn WC, et al. Immunohistochemical light and electron microscopy of basal laminar deposit. *Graefes Arch Clin Exp Ophthalmol* 1994;232:40–46.
13. Li CM, Chung BH, Presley JB, et al. Lipoprotein-like particles and cholesteryl esters in human Bruch's membrane: initial characterization. *Invest Ophthalmol Vis Sci* 2005;46:2576–2586.
14. Ruberti JW, Curcio CA, Millican CL, et al. Quick-freeze/deep-etch visualization of age-related lipid accumulation in Bruch's membrane. *Invest Ophthalmol Vis Sci* 2003;44:1753–1759.
15. Abdelsalam A, Del Priore L, Zarbin MA. Drusen in age-related macular degeneration: pathogenesis, natural course, and laser photocoagulation-induced regression. *Surv Ophthalmol* 1999;44:1–29.
16. Anderson DH, Stern WH, Fisher SK, et al. The onset of pigment epithelial proliferation after retinal detachment. *Invest Ophthalmol Vis Sci* 1981;21:10–16.
17. Anderson DH, Stern WH, Fisher SK, et al. Retinal detachment in the cat: the pigment epithelial-photoreceptor interface. *Invest Ophthalmol Vis Sci* 1983;24:906–926.
18. Hackett SF, Conway BP, Campochiaro PA. Subretinal fluid stimulation of retinal pigment epithelial cell migration and proliferation is dependent on certain features of the detachment or its treatment. *Arch Ophthalmol* 1989;107:391–394.
19. Liu F, Meyer CH, Mennel S, et al. Visual recovery after scleral buckling surgery in macula-off rhegmatogenous retinal detachment. *Ophthalmologica* 2006;220:174–180.
20. Yang CH, Lin HY, Huang JS, et al. Visual outcome in primary macula-off rhegmatogenous retinal detachment treated with scleral buckling. *J Formos Med Assoc* 2004;103:212–217.
21. Koriyama M, Nishimura T, Matsubara T, et al. Prospective study comparing the effectiveness of scleral buckling to vitreous surgery for rhegmatogenous retinal detachment. *Jpn J Ophthalmol* 2007;51:360–367.
22. Jacobson SG, Boye SL, Aleman TS, et al. Safety in nonhuman primates of ocular AAV2-RPE65, a candidate treatment for blindness in Leber congenital amaurosis. *Hum Gene Ther* 2006;17:845–858.
23. Acland GM, Aguirre GD, Ray J, et al. Gene therapy restores vision in a canine model of childhood blindness. *Nat Genet* 2001;28:92–95.
24. Li Y, Atmaca-Sonmez P, Schanie CL, et al. Endogenous bone marrow derived cells express retinal pigment epithelium cell markers and migrate to focal areas of RPE damage. *Invest Ophthalmol Vis Sci* 2007;48:4321–4327.
25. Chan-Ling T, Baxter L, Afzal A, et al. Hematopoietic stem cells provide repair functions after laser-induced Bruch's membrane rupture model of choroidal neovascularization. *Am J Pathol* 2006;168:1031–1044.
26. Alm A, Bill A. Ocular and optic nerve blood flow at normal and increased intraocular pressures in monkeys (Macaca irus): a study with radioactively labeled microspheres including flow determinations in brain and some other tissues. *Exp Eye Res* 1973;15:15–29.
27. Brubaker RF, Pederson JE. Ciliochoroidal detachment. *Surv Ophthalmol* 1983;27:281–289.
28. Beyer CF, Peyman GA, Hill JM. Expulsive choroidal hemorrhage in rabbits. A histopathologic study. *Arch Ophthalmol* 1989;107:1648–1653.
29. Speaker MG, Guerriero PN, Met JA, et al. A case-control study of risk factors for intraoperative suprachoroidal expulsive hemorrhage. *Ophthalmology* 1991;98:202–209; discussion 210.
30. Grunwald JE, Hariprasad SM, DuPont J. Effect of aging on foveolar choroidal circulation. *Arch Ophthalmol* 1998;116:150–154.
31. Sarks JP, Sarks SH, Killingsworth MC. Evolution of geographic atrophy of the retinal pigment epithelium. *Eye* 1988;2(Pt 5):552–577.
32. Ramrattan RS, van der Schaft TL, Mooy CM, et al. Morphometric analysis of Bruch's membrane, the choriocapillaris, and the choroid in aging. *Invest Ophthalmol Vis Sci* 1994;35:2857–2864.
33. Chen JC, Fitzke FW, Pauleikhoff D, et al. Functional loss in age-related Bruch's membrane change with choroidal perfusion defect. *Invest Ophthalmol Vis Sci* 1992;33:334–340.
34. Holz FG, Wolfensberger TJ, Piguet B, et al. Bilateral macular drusen in age-related macular degeneration. Prognosis and risk factors. *Ophthalmology* 1994;101:1522–1528.
35. Pauleikhoff D, Spital G, Radermacher M, et al. A fluorescein and indocyanine green angiographic study of choriocapillaris in age-related macular disease. *Arch Ophthalmol* 1999;117:1353–1358.
36. Grunwald JE, Metelitsina TI, Dupont JC, et al. Reduced foveolar choroidal blood flow in eyes with increasing AMD severity. *Invest Ophthalmol Vis Sci* 2005;46:1033–1038.

37. Hyman L, Schachat AP, He Q, et al. Hypertension, cardiovascular disease, and age-related macular degeneration. Age-Related Macular Degeneration Risk Factors Study Group. *Arch Ophthalmol* 2000;118:351–358.

38. Risk factors associated with age-related macular degeneration. A case-control study in the age-related eye disease study: Age-Related Eye Disease Study Report Number 3. *Ophthalmology* 2000;107:2224–2232.

39. Klein R, Klein BE, Franke T. The relationship of cardiovascular disease and its risk factors to age-related maculopathy. The Beaver Dam Eye Study. *Ophthalmology* 1993;100:406–414.

40. Smith W, Mitchell P, Leeder SR, et al. Plasma fibrinogen levels, other cardiovascular risk factors, and age-related maculopathy: the Blue Mountains Eye Study. *Arch Ophthalmol* 1998;116:583–587.

41. Vingerling JR, Dielemans I, Bots ML, et al. Age-related macular degeneration is associated with atherosclerosis. The Rotterdam Study. *Am J Epidemiol* 1995;142:404–409.

42. Macular Photocoagulation Study Group. Laser photocoagulation for juxtafoveal choroidal neovascularization. Five-year results from randomized clinical trials. *Arch Ophthalmol* 1994;112:500–509.

43. Metelitsina TI, Grunwald JE, DuPont JC, et al. Effect of systemic hypertension on foveolar choroidal blood flow in age related macular degeneration. *Br J Ophthalmol* 2006;90:342–346.

44. Ross RD, Barofsky JM, Cohen G, et al. Presumed macular choroidal watershed vascular filling, choroidal neovascularization, and systemic vascular disease in patients with age-related macular degeneration. *Am J Ophthalmol* 1998;125:71–80.

45. Pournaras CJ, Logean E, Riva CE, et al. Regulation of subfoveal choroidal blood flow in age-related macular degeneration. *Invest Ophthalmol Vis Sci* 2006;47:1581–1586.

46. Haines JL, Hauser MA, Schmidt S, et al. Complement factor H variant increases the risk of age-related macular degeneration. *Science* 2005; 308(5720):419–421.

47. Edwards AO, Ritter Iii R, Abel KJ, et al. Complement factor H polymorphism and age-related macular degeneration. *Science* 2005;308:421–424.

48. Klein RJ, Zeiss C, Chew EY, et al. Complement factor H polymorphism in age-related macular degeneration. *Science* 2005;308(5720):385.

49. Hageman GS, Anderson DH, Johnson LV, et al. A common haplotype in the complement regulatory gene factor H (HF1/CFH) predisposes individuals to age-related macular degeneration. *Proc Natl Acad Sci U S A* 2005;102:7227–7232.

50. Zareparsi S, Branham KE, Li M, et al. Strong association of the Y402 H variant in complement factor H at 1q32 with susceptibility to age-related macular degeneration. *Am J Hum Genet* 2005;77:149–153.

51. Yates JR, Sepp T, Matharu BK, et al. Complement C3 variant and the risk of age-related macular degeneration. *N Engl J Med* 2007;357(6):553–561.

52. Johnson PT, Betts KE, Radeke MJ, et al. Individuals homozygous for the age-related macular degeneration risk-conferring variant of complement factor H have elevated levels of CRP in the choroid. *Proc Natl Acad Sci U S A* 2006;103:17456–17461.

53. Nozaki M, Raisler BJ, Sakurai E, et al. Drusen complement components C3 a and C5 a promote choroidal neovascularization. *Proc Natl Acad Sci U S A* 2006;103:2328–2333.

54. Ebrahem Q, Renganathan K, Sears J, et al. Carboxyethylpyrrole oxidative protein modifications stimulate neovascularization: Implications for age-related macular degeneration. *Proc Natl Acad Sci U S A* 2006;103:13480–13484.

55. Gragoudas ES, Adamis AP, Cunningham ET Jr, et al. Pegaptanib for neovascular age-related macular degeneration. *N Engl J Med* 2004;351:2805–2816.

56. Rich RM, Rosenfeld PJ, Puliafito CA, et al. Short-term safety and efficacy of intravitreal bevacizumab (Avastin) for neovascular age-related macular degeneration. *Retina* 2006;26:495–511.

57. Rosenfeld PJ, Brown DM, Heier JS, et al. Ranibizumab for neovascular age-related macular degeneration. *N Engl J Med* 2006;355:1419–1431.

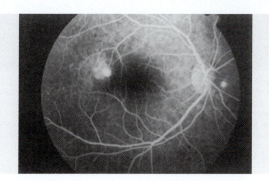

# Pathophysiology of the Blood-Retinal Barrier

Pablo Carnota ■ Rafael Bueno ■ Monica Rodriguez-Fontal ■ John B. Kerrison

## INTRODUCTION

In order to maintain the unique microenvironment needed for viability and optimal function of retinal cells, there is a system of dynamic equilibrium adjustments and regulation mechanisms. Akin to the central nervous system, homeostatic regulation is facilitated by a restrictive permeability system known as blood retinal barrier (BRB). Like blood brain barrier (BBB) in brain, BRB restricts the accessibility to the retina of circulating factors such as lipophilic compounds, blood gases, and certain molecules that depend upon active transport.

BRB is known to be disrupted in several pathological situations such as retinal microangiopathies (e.g., diabetic retinopathy), inflammatory-infectious diseases (e.g., Irvine-Gass syndrome) and other exudative conditions (e.g., age-related macular disease (ARMD) or central serous chorioretinopathy (CSC)). This breakdown leads to disturbances of tissue microenvironment, which subsequently accelerates the progression of the pathology (1,2).

## INNER VERSUS OUTER BLOOD RETINAL BARRIER

The BRB is composed of two anatomically and functionally different structures, the inner and the outer BRB. The inner BRB is formed by the endothelial cells of retinal capillaries. The outer BRB is formed by the retinal pigment epithelium (RPE).

### Inner Blood Retinal Barrier

Endothelial cells of retinal capillaries display distinctive characteristics in comparison with capillaries in other locations such as lack of fenestrations and presence of apical structures known as tight junctions or zonulae occludentes (Fig. 3-1). These structures not only confer a very restrictive permeability at the

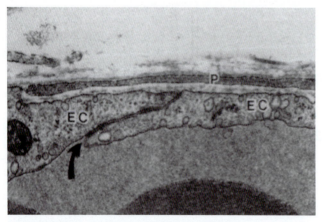

**Figure 3-1.** Electron micrograph of a control venule showing normal ultrastructural appearance of a pericyte process (P), endothelial cells (EC) and an endothelial cell junction (*curved arrow*). The space between the pericyte and endothelial cells is occupied by basal lamina. x31,000. (With permission from Shepro D, Morel N. Pericyte physiology. *FASEB J* 1993;7: 1031–1038).

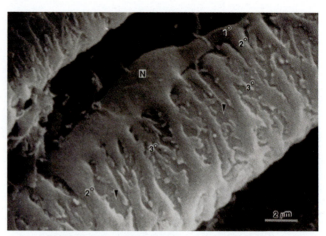

**Figure 3-2.** Scanning electron micrograph of pericytes covering the surface of an arterial capillary of the rat mirabile. Note the plump nuclear area (N), a primary process (1°) of the pericyte paralleling the long axis of the capillary, secondary processes (2°) encircling the capillary at right angles to the primary process, and branching, tertiary processes extending from the secondary process. The surface of an underlying endothelial cell can be seen at the arrowheads. x8804. (From Shepro D, Morel N. Pericyte physiology. *FASEB J* 1993;7:1031–1038.)

intercellular clefts but allow close regulation of transendothelial transport as well as maintenance of endothelial polarity. This phenotypic expression of endothelial cells is dynamic and can be altered, as discussed below, by the local extracellular matrix, soluble growth factors, and heterotypic (other) and homotypic (same) cellular interactions via intercellular junctions. The lumen (5 to 6 μm) of retinal capillaries is created by a single layer of endothelial cells surrounded by intramural pericytes and encompassed by a common basement membrane (3–5). Pericytes have several functions such as regulation of vascular tone, mechanical support of the vessel wall, production of extracellular matrix, and phagocytosis (6,7). Pericytes exhibit a 1:1 ratio with endothelial cells in normal human retinal capillaries (8), and their pseudopod-like processes encircle the retinal capillary and contain contractile proteins such as smooth muscle type alpha-actin, nonsmooth muscle actin and smooth muscle myosin (6,9) (Fig. 3-2). Additionally, pericytes release extracellular components, such as fibronectin, which provide anchorage points for mechanical force transfer during capillary lumen constriction (6).

Tight junctions are formed by a complex network of proteins that importantly can be regulated and dynamically altered by different conditions and pathologies. There are three types of transmembrane proteins within tight junctions: occludins, claudins, and junctional adhesion molecules (JAM). The transmembrane proteins bind junctional proteins in adjacent cells and create the actual barrier. Other proteins have been identified such as intracellular protein ZO-1 and cadherin, the main component of another type of junction between cells known as adherens junction.

Occludin was the first identified membrane component of tight junctions (10) (Fig. 3-3). However, subsequent studies demonstrated that occludin was not essential for the tight junction assembly and rather was involved in signal transduction of endothelial cells (11,12). Actually, other studies suggested that the main role of occludin could be the control of

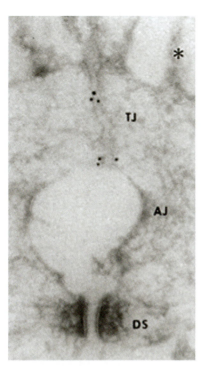

**Figure 3-3.** Ultrastructural localization of occludin. Ultrathin cryosection of formalin-fixed intestinal epithelial cells were labelled with monoclonal antibodies anti-occludin-2. Gold particles accumulated at the tight junction region (TJ), and are hardly detected in the adherens junction (AJ) and desmosome (DS) regions. AJ is artifactually opened, probably due to the formaldehyde fixation. (From Furuse M, Hirase T, Itoh M, et al. Occludin: a novel integral membrane protein localizing at tight junctions. *J Cell Biol* 1993;123:1777–1788.)

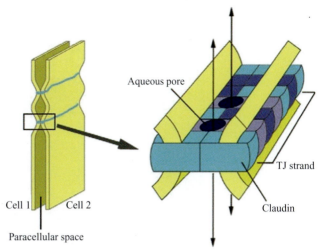

**Figure 3-4.** Model for the assembly of claudins into tight junctions (TJ) strands. A TJ strand of cell 1 associates laterally with a TJ strand in the opposing membrane of the adjacent cell 2 to constitute a paired TJ strand. Different claudin species, which are indicated in different colors, copolymerize in individual TJ strands, and associate between adjacent cells in both a heterotypic and homotypic manner. Aqueous pores are postulated to occur within paired TJ strands. (From Furuse M, Tsukita S. Claudins in occluding junctions of humans and flies. *Trends Cell Biol* 2006;16: 181–188.)

paracellular flux, mainly of ions and small organic cations (13–15). Thus, occludin contributes both structurally and as signal transducers and regulators of barrier properties. Two studies on diabetic retinas and on bovine retinal endothelial cells treated with vascular endothelial growth factor (VEGF) have revealed decreased occludin content concomitant with increased BRB permeability (16,17). Another protein, tricellulin, has recently been identified as a protein localized specifically at regions where three cells make contact (18). Together, these proteins create the final subset of known transmembrane tight junction proteins.

Later, claudins were found to be other components of tight junctions (19) (Fig. 3-4). Accumulative evidence has revealed that they are key molecules in the tight junction assembly by playing a very important role in the control of ion flux (20–25). However, the complexity of the system is only beginning to be understood. Claudins are a multigene family of more than 20 members (26–28), and the pattern of expression of different claudin family members varies among tissue types, which confers tissue-specific properties to tight junctions (20). Claudins expressed in endothelial cells of neural (and retinal) tissue are claudin-1, claudin-3, claudin-5, and claudin-12 (28–30). They are suggested to be candidate molecules responsible for structural endothelial barrier function as shown by a study of claudin-5-deficient mice that disclosed that claudin-5 is indispensable for the barrier function of neural blood vessels for small molecules (29). Alterations in claudins have been associated with a variety of disease states

(31–32). Mutations in claudin 16 exemplify the role of claudins in barrier selectivity since it has been demonstrated as the cause of familial hypomagnesemia with hypocalcemia and nephrocalcinosis (33).

Another integral membrane protein of tight junctions is JAM found at the tight junctions of epithelial and endothelial cells. The exact function of JAM is still unclear. It has been demonstrated that transfection of JAM into epithelial cells does not reconstitute tight junctions strands (34). However, it contributes to tight junctions assembly and cell-to-cell adhesion in epithelial and endothelial cells (35–38) and contributes to extravasation of monocytes through endothelial monolayers (38).

Zonula occludens or ZO proteins are intracellular proteins associated with the cytoplasmic surface of tight junctions. The first ZO protein recognized, ZO-1, is a transmembrane protein that acts as a scaffold due to its multiple binding domains; its several domains bind to transmembrane tight junction proteins occludin, claudin, and ZO-2 and to adherens junction proteins afadin and cadherin (39–46) (Fig. 3-5). ZO-1 presence can readily be observed in both retinal vascular endothelial cells and RPE. In both cell types, agents that induce permeability such as VEGF or hepatocyte growth factor induce redistribution of ZO-1 from the cell border to the cell interior (47,48). In contrast, increasing barrier properties increases ZO-1 border staining. Elevated hydrostatic pressure across bovine aortic endothelial cells first increases water and solute flux, which then decreases over the next 30 to 60 minutes, reaching a new equilibrium; ZO-1 can readily be seen to increase at plasma membrane during this adaptive response (49,50). Therefore ZO-1 acts as a central organizer of the tight junction complex.

There is another type of junction between endothelial cells called adherens junction. Adherens junctions are characterized by the expression of cadherins ($Ca^{++}$-dependent

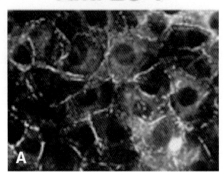

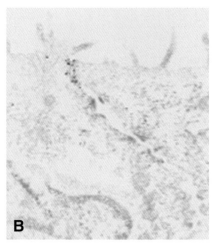

**Figure 3-5.** Localization of ZO-1. **A:** Cells stained with a monoclonal antibody against ZO-1 showing a subcellular localization of this protein. (From Imamura Y, Itoh M, Maeno Y, et al. Functional domains of alpha-catenin required for the strong state of cadherin-based cell adhesion. *J Cell Biol* 1999;144:1311–1322.) **B:** Immunoelectron micrograph of the junctional complex region in cells stained with a monoclonal antibody against ZO-1; ZO-1 labelling is exclusively concentrated in the junctional complex region. (From Yamamoto T, Harada N, Kano K, Taya et al. The Ras target AF-6 interacts with ZO-1 and serves as a peripheral component of tight junctions in epithelial cells. *J Cell Biol* 1997;139:785–795.)

transmembrane adhesion proteins) whose function consists of maintaining a space between cell membranes, while allowing homotypic cell contact (51).

Within this microenvironment several soluble vasoactive molecules have been identified as playing a more or less important role in the regulation of permeability of the inner BRB. Molecules such as nitric oxide, adenosine or $CO_2$ or hypoxia cause retinal pericytes relaxation whereas other molecules such endothelin-1, angiotensin II, ATP or hyperoxia lead to pericyte contraction.

Tissue oxygen concentration is known to influence the expression of various molecules including growth factors, cytokines, and enzymes (52). Hypoxia stimulates cellular production of erythropoietin (53), VEGF (54), tyrosine hydroxylase (55), phosphoglycerate kinase 1, and lactate dehydrogenase A (56). Many of these hypoxia-sensitive molecules are implicated in adaptive processes of organisms to hypoxic circumstances such as erythropoiesis, angiogenesis, increase in respiratory volume and conversion of the metabolism to an anaerobic state. In addition, changes in expression of certain oxygen-sensitive molecules can also trigger the progression of disease processes in patients with cerebral ischemic diseases, diabetic retinopathy and other diseases (57). Among components of tight junctions, occludin, claudin-1, claudin-3 and claudin-5 are reported to be hypoxia-sensitive molecules and promote breakdown of the neural endothelial barrier (52,58,59).

Endothelial cells synthesize nitric oxide in response to several stimuli like increased local shear force, bradykinins, insulin-like growth factor 1, acetylcholine, thrombin and various platelet products (60–62). Nitric oxide diffuses to the pericyte and smooth muscle cell surface, where it binds to guanylate cyclase, causing intracellular cGMP accumulation and vasodilation (63,64). In addition to its vasodilatory actions, nitric oxide protects vessels by inhibiting platelet aggregation, platelet granule secretion, leukocyte adhesion, and possibly smooth muscle cell proliferation (65). However, high levels of nitric oxide can induce retinal toxicity through neuronal nitric

oxide synthase, which may be important during retinal ischemia, degenerative retinal disease, and diabetic vascular dysfunction (66–71).

Endothelins are released by endothelial cells on the abluminal side of capillary and bind to receptors on adjacent pericytes and smooth muscle cells (72). Endothelins (ET1, ET2, and ET3) are the most potent vasoconstrictor agents currently known (73). ET-dependent contraction is mediated by three receptor subtypes (ETR A, B, and C) (74). Human studies have shown that vasoconstriction following intravenous injection of ET1 is mediated through ETR-A (75). In general, ETR-A mRNA is localized to pericytes and smooth muscle cells, whereas ETR-B mRNA can be found also in endothelial cells. Animal studies have shown that stimulation with ET1 on pericytes causes contraction, aggregation of actin fibers, and proliferation (76–78).

Vascular endothelium generates basal levels of superoxide anions but can be stimulated to produce deleterious amounts of these molecules during many pathologic conditions (79). Superoxide anions inactivate nitric oxide, thereby inhibiting vasodilatory capacity. This pathologic inhibition may mediate vascular changes found in hypertension, hypercholesterolemia, retinopathy of prematurity, diabetes, and ischemia/reperfusion injury (79,80). Superoxide anions may induce endothelial damage resulting in a prothrombotic state; this pathologic mechanism may contribute to diabetic retinopathy (81).

VEGF stimulates occludin phosphorylation through activation of the protein kinase C (PKC) signaling pathway. Binding of VEGF to its tyrosine kinase receptor activates PKC signal transduction pathway and this activation has been correlated to VEGF's mitogenic effects in endothelial cells (82). In a recent study on bovine retinal epithelium cells, Harhaj et al. showed that VEGF stimulates occludin phosphorylation increasing the endothelial permeability, an effect that can be inhibited using PKC inhibitors or by expressing a dominant negative PKC-bII mutant (83). However, only part of VEGF-induced permeability was prevented by classical PKC inhibitors indicating additional pathways are likely involved in the regulation of permeability.

Another regulator of vascular permeability is the renin-angiotensin system. Human and animal ocular tissues locally express the necessary components (renin, angiotensinogen and angiotensin-converting enzyme, ACE) for an intrinsic renin-angiotensin system (84–88). ACE bound to endothelial cell luminal surface rapidly converts angiotensin I to angiotensin II; ACE itself inactivates bradykinin and angiotensin II stimulates retinal vasoconstriction via smooth muscle cells and pericytes (89). Isolated porcine ophthalmic arteries vasoconstrict in response to angiotensin II and relax in response to bradykinin via a nitric oxide-dependent mechanism. ACE-inhibitors used in this model prevented angiotensin-mediated constriction and potentiated bradykinin relaxation (90).

Vascular permeability often accompanies angiogenesis, particularly in pathologies of the BBB and BRB. New evidence suggests that tight junction proteins may contribute to growth control through either activation or sequestration of signaling components, potentially linking changes in permeability with angiogenesis. However, most studies have focused on epithelial to mesenchymal transition and not on vascular endothelial cells.

## Outer Blood Retinal Barrier

The main component of outer BRB is the RPE. The RPE prevents blood components from passing freely to the subretinal space from fenestrated blood vessel of the choriocapillaris. Tight junctions between RPE cells (similar to endothelial cells in the inner barrier) are the principal mechanism involved in the barrier. However, tight junctions of RPE are more permeable than inner BRB, emphasizing the differential physiological role of the outer and inner BRB. Apical and basal RPE membranes contain a variety of selective ion channels and a variety of active and facilitative transport systems that control the movement of ions and water and the transport of metabolites, such as glucose and amino acids, from choriocapillaris to neural retina and vice versa (91). There are different channels and transporters within apical and basal surfaces, such as an electrogenic sodium-potassium pump on apical membrane and a chloride-bicarbonate exchange transporter on basal membrane. This asymmetry between apical and basal membranes is allowed by tight junctions and accounts for the development of a voltage (called the standing potential) across the RPE that results in a net movement of ions away from the subretinal space that drives the transport of water towards the choroid. Passive transport mechanisms, such as intraocular pressure against the retina and osmotic pressure from the choroid, also tend to drive fluid out of the subretinal space, but passive water movement is normally restricted by the BRB. When the RPE barrier is damaged, fluid actually leaves the subretinal space faster than under normal conditions. In other words, a normal eye will not accumulate fluid in the subretinal space just because the RPE barrier is disrupted (92). These observations have relevance for clinical disorders such as serous detachments. They show that the presence of a defect in the RPE is not by itself sufficient to cause serous detachment, even though it may be necessary (93) (see further discussion below in pathophysiology of CSC).

## IMMUNE PRIVILEGE

The eye is an immune privileged site, protected from the immune system by different mechanisms (94). At the level of posterior segment of the eye, RPE cells have a crucial role in induction and maintenance of this immune privilege (95). Failure in outer BRB leads to a breakdown of the immune privilege with subsequent development of intraocular inflammation, as happens in posterior uveitis.

Much work has been done to better understand mechanisms underlying RPE protection role, especially how these cells interact with lymphocytes. It is now evident that active processes are likely to be involved. Liverdsidge et al. first showed that RPE cells could inhibit lymphocyte proliferation (96). From then on, three main pathways have been proposed to explain this RPE immunosuppression. First, RPE cells might inhibit T-cell proliferation through secretion of inhibitory factors like prostaglandins and immunosuppressive cytokines. Among the latter, transforming growth factor b or IL-1 receptor antagonist have been proposed (95–96). Second, the apoptosis phenomenon might also contribute to RPE induced immunosuppression. Apoptosis is a programmed cell death with no inflammatory reaction commonly used by the immune system to eliminate cells (opposite to processes such as necrosis). Moreover, apoptotic body phagocytosis has been shown to downregulate proinflammatory cytokine secretion in macrophages (97). Interestingly, several studies have demonstrated that apoptosis occurs within T-cells following coincubation with RPE cells, suggesting that this could be an important mechanism in RPE immunosuppression (98,99). Finally, other studies have shown that, by lacking expression of a complete set of costimulatory molecules, RPE cells only partially activate lymphocytes and act as deviant antigen presenting cells, driving the lymphocyte to a state of hyporesponsiveness rather than activation (100–102).

Considering that human RPE cells are known as phagocytic cells, since they largely phagocytose photoreceptor outer segments, phagocytosis may also contribute to RPE immunosuppression directly by decreasing T-cell number and clearing apoptotic lymphocytes and indirectly by downregulating proinflammatory cytokine secretion such IL-1b. Therefore, they participate *in vivo* in induction and maintenance of the immune privilege of the eye, preventing the development of intraocular inflammation (100).

## PATHOPHYSIOLOGIC MECHANISMS OF BREAKDOWN OF THE BLOOD RETINAL BARRIER

### Diabetic Retinopathy

It is known that fundus changes observed in nonproliferative diabetic retinopathy are the result of pathologic changes at the level of the retinal blood vessels, but the exact mechanism that leads to the breakdown of inner BRB remains poorly understood. The choroidal vasculature is also altered in diabetic patients, but not as significantly as retinal vasculature. Disruption of inner BRB is an early phenomenon in preclinical diabetic retinopathy (PCDR). Two vascular permeability pathways may be affected: the paracellular pathway involving endothelial cell tight junctions and the endothelial transcellular pathway mediated by endocytotic vesicles (103,104). The relative contribution of both pathways to vascular permeability in PCDR is still unknown (105).

The breakdown of inner BRB is a consequence of retinal ischemia in diabetic retinopathy, and there is a hypothesis about how ischemia develops in this disease. Several histopathological changes are known to occur in diabetic retinopathy in humans and in animal models: pericytes and endothelial cell loss, capillary dropout, and basement membrane thickening. As commented above, in normal retinal vasculature, endothelial cells and intramural pericytes are distributed in a ratio of approximately 1:1. It has been shown that eyes with diabetic retinopathy demonstrate a preferential loss of microvascular pericytes (106) (Fig. 3-6). This happens even before retinopathy becomes clinically apparent. Lack of pericytes in retinal capillaries leads to loss of retinal blood flow autoregulation in response to changes in partial pressure of oxygen and to a functional alteration in endothelial cells. As retinopathy progresses, and even later than appearance of microaneurysms, diabetic retinal capillaries can become acellular (with no endothelial cells). A study by de Venecia et al. provided direct evidence that these acellular ghost capillaries are not perfused in life (107). Perhaps as a response to the retinal hypoxia caused by this capillary dropout, the adjacent capillary bed becomes dilated and hypercellular. Subsequently the lumen of these capillaries narrows and leads, along with other contributing factors such as thickening of endothelial basement membranes and blood viscosity abnormalities, to more retinal capillary closure.

The sorbitol pathway could be an explanation for the pericyte and endothelial dropout and the vascular basement membrane thickening in these patients. Under hyperglycemic conditions, aldose reductase reduces glucose to its sugar alcohol, the sorbitol, which can subsequently reach high levels in cells, and is toxic to them. Besides this, hyperglycemic retinal pericytes display blunted ability to respond to ET1, via PKC-induced downregulation of ET receptors (108–110), which leads to alteration in the retinal blood flow autoregulation. Osmotic swelling of the endothelium secondary to intracellular sorbitol accumulation could also impair blood flow through small vessels by narrowing their lumens. However, Akagi et al. found that aldose reductase is present only in pericytes but not in endothelial cells, which explains the specific loss of pericytes in diabetic retinopathy; the loss of endothelial cells, therefore, could be secondary to loss of pericytes (111). Several studies postulate that the sorbitol pathway is also the mechanism for vascular basement membrane thickening although its mechanism remains unclear (112–116). However, the role of aldose reductase inhibitors (sorbinil) in preventing these microvascular changes in animal models has been controversial and their efficacy in retarding the progression of diabetic retinopathy in humans has not yet been demonstrated (113–117).

Defects in normal tight junctions between endothelial cells may arise secondary to obstruction of adjacent vessels or from the dropout of capillary pericytes. Even before any retinopathy is demonstrable clinically, evidence of abnormal vascular permeability may be seen on fluorescein angiography as focal staining of arteriole wall. As retinopathy develops and progresses, accumulation of fluid and plasma constituents in the surrounding retina can lead to marked retinal thickening, cystoids changes in the fovea and formation of hard exudates (118). Moreover, this process could explain the link between abnormal retinal hemodynamics (such as arterial hypertension) and the prevalence of macular edema (119, 120).

Besides the paracellular pathway there is a transcellular pathway that contributes to breakdown of the inner BRB, and it has two possible anatomic explanations. One, retinal endothelial cells, normally unfenestrated, develop fenestrae similar to those in choriocapillaris, allowing fluid and plasma components to go out of capillaries (121). The other potential explanation is an increase in transport by endocytic vesicles (122), but this mechanism has not yet been reported from human or experimental animal subjects with diabetes.

There are other pathogenic mechanisms by which capillary nonperfusion occurs and that contribute to inner BRB breakdown.

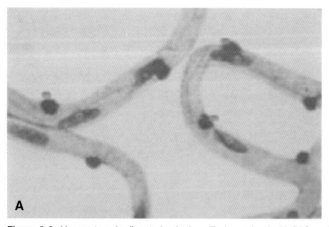
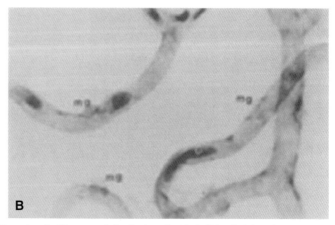

**Figure 3-6.** Human trypsin-digested retinal capillaries stained with PAS and hematoxylin. The normal distribution of endothelial cells (e) and mural cells (m) are illustrated in **(A)**, while in **(B)**, the selective loss of these mural cells (mural cell ghosts, mg) in the diabetic retina can be observed. (From Akagi Y, Kador PF, Kuwabara T et al. Aldose reductase localization in human retinal mural cells. *Invest Ophthalmol Vis Sci* 1983;24:1516–1519.)

There is growing evidence that suggests that increased leukocyte-endothelial cell adhesion and entrapment (retinal leukostasis) in retinal capillaries is an early event associated with areas of vascular nonperfusion and the development of diabetic retinopathy (123). Leukocytes possess large cell volume, high cytoplasmic rigidity, a natural tendency to adhere to vascular endothelium and a capacity to generate toxic superoxide radicals and proteolytic enzymes. In diabetes, there is increased retinal leukostasis that affects retinal endothelial function, retinal perfusion, angiogenesis, and vascular permeability. In particular, leukocytes in diabetes are less deformable, a higher proportion is activated and they may be involved in capillary nonperfusion, endothelial cell damage, and vascular leakage in the retinal microcirculation (124). Wang et al. found that dexamethasone may diminish retinal edema by inhibiting retinal leucocyte accumulation, leukostasis, and vascular permeability through its blockage on VEGF and ICAM-1 expression (125). Kim et al. showed that blockade of angiotensin II attenuates VEGF-mediated BRB breakdown in diabetic retinopathy. Inhibition of angiotensin II by perindopril (a long acting ACE inhibitor) attenuated increased vascular permeability of diabetic retina accompanied by recovery of tight junction proteins in retinal vessels. Furthermore, ACE inhibitors may have a therapeutic potential in the treatment of diabetic BRB breakdown (126).

## Pseudophakic/Aphakic Cystoid Macular Edema

Cystoid macular edema (CME) is defined as the accumulation of intraretinal fluid in the macula, with secondary formation of cystic spaces that may be identified either ophthalmoscopically or angiographically. In pseudophakic/aphakic CME (Irvine-Gass syndrome) edema mainly develops following breakdown of the inner BRB with leakage of plasma from perifoveal capillaries. Less importantly, a breakdown of the outer BRB may play a role in this entity. The pathogenesis of the BRB disruption has not been fully discerned, but five major causes have been suspected to be at the origin of it: intraocular inflammation, ultraviolet (UV) light exposure, mechanical traction by the vitreous, secondary irritation of ciliary body, and pharmacologically induced CME (127). However, Terasaki et al. studied eyes with postoperative CME by means of electroretinography (ERG), and they found that they had a reduction in oscillatory potentials amplitudes. Because peripheral retina contributes more significantly to full-field ERGs than the macula does, this suggests a functional impairment not only in the macula but also throughout the retina (128). Postoperative CME must be differentiated from CME resulting from irreversible vascular damage such as in diabetic CME or due to vein occlusions.

Inflammation is thought to be the main pathogenetic mechanism in most cases of postoperative CME. In 1977, Martin et al. found a perivascular mononuclear cell infiltration in eyes with disruption of the inner BRB (129). The inflammatory theory was supported later by the observation that prostaglandins permit the breakdown of the blood-ocular barrier by opening the normally tight junctions of iris and ciliary body vessels, leading to flare and cells in the anterior aqueous. Since there are no diffusional barriers in the vitreous, soluble mediators such as prostaglandins may be free to diffuse to the posterior segment and induce perivascular leakage from vessels in the macula by means of breaking the inner BRB (130). The most important and widely studied mediators of inflammation in CME are the prostaglandins, but there are many others mediators known to play a role in the development of CME, such as leukotrienes, bradykinins, histamine, serotonin, complement and neuropeptides. Actually, pharmacological inhibition of metabolic byproducts of the arachidonic acid pathway is the currently accepted way to manage CME. Cyclo-oxygenase inhibitors such as non-steroidal anti-inflammatory drugs (NSAIDs) prevent the formation of thromboxane, prostaglandins and prostacyclin (131); diclofenac also affects lipo-oxygenase, preventing the synthesis of leukotrienes; and corticosteroids block phospholipase A2, inhibiting the transformation of membrane lipids in arachidonic acid.

The role of UV light in the development of CME is controversial. It is known that UV light has the ability to generate activated forms of oxygen free radicals in the retina, which may cause lipid peroxidation of tissues and contribute to the synthesis of prostaglandins (132). However, the site of lipid peroxidation by oxygen free radicals in the retina is the photoreceptor outer segments, which is not the site of structural changes seen in CME. There are two UV light sources: microscope light during the surgery and postoperative UV light exposure. The first one was studied by Byrnes et al., who concluded that intraoperative exposure to UV light was not associated with CME (133,124). Komatsu et al. compared the incidence of CME in patients who had an UV-absorbing intraocular lens in one eye and a non-UV-absorbing intraocular lens in the other eye and found that there was no statistically significant difference in visual acuity or in the incidence of CME between both groups (134).

Another factor purported to contribute to postoperative CME is vitreous traction. Some recent studies have demonstrated that vitreous and posterior hyaloid removal leads to resolution of postoperative CME with visual acuity improvement in most of cases (135), but factors that relate vitreous traction to the development of CME are still unknown. This was first theorized in 1971, when it was observed that intracapsular cataract extraction (ICCE) was often associated with disruption of the anterior hyaloid face and secondary herniation of vitreous gel into the anterior chamber. The normal physiologic pupillary constriction and dilation produced a tugging on fibrils of vitreous protruding through the pupil, causing tension to be transmitted to the vitreous base and subsequently to the macula (136). Later, in another study of patients with post-ICCE CME who underwent vitrectomy, less than 5% of eyes had vitreous strands attached to the macula at the time of surgery. Therefore investigators proposed that the more likely causal mechanism was chronic inflammation resulting from irritated anterior uveal structures after ICCE (137). This could explain the cases of CME following noncomplicated extracapsular cataract extraction. However, some authors still theorize that vitreous traction could cause irritation in Müller's cells, releasing local mediators that facilitate vascular leakage (138).

## Central Serous Chorioretinopathy

The pathophysiology of CSC is still not completely understood, but it is well known that a breakdown in the outer BRB is necessary, although not sufficient, for the development of CSC. As commented above, the asymmetric electric configuration of RPE cells leads to active transport mechanisms through them, resulting in a net movement of ions away from subretinal space. However, the balance of tissue osmotic and hydrostatic pressures causes fluid flow from the retina toward the choroid faster. Marmor and Negi carried several studies that showed that experimental destruction or injury of RPE speeded the resorption of subretinal fluid, what suggests that a simple defect of integrity of the RPE alone cannot explain the findings seen in CSC (139–141). The most accepted theory about the pathophysiology of CSC combines this fact with the clinical and angiographic findings observed in these patients.

Fluorescein and indocyanine green (ICG) angiography is not only a test that aids ophthalmologists in the diagnosis of CSC but also a tool to help clarify the disease pathophysiology. Fluorescein angiography usually shows one or more leak points at the level of RPE but, more importantly, ICG angiogram reveals multifocal areas with choroidal vascular hyperpermeability. Excessive tissue hydrostatic pressure within the choroid from vascular hyperpermeability may lead to mechanical disruption of the tight junctions, damage of RPE cells and abnormal egress of fluid under the retina (by changing the direction of passive flow). Functional loss of contiguous RPE cells may allow fluid to accumulate in the subretinal space, causing a neurosensory detachment. It has been shown that leaks at the level of the RPE seen on fluorescein angiography (breaks at the tight junctions) are contiguous with areas of choroidal vascular hyperpermeability in ICG angiography (142) (Fig. 3-7), but most areas of choroidal hyperpermeability are not associated with fluorescein leaks.

It is hypothesized that these areas of hyperpermeability without leaks may not be clinically silent: increased tissue hydrostatic pressure within the choroid could affect the ability of the overlying RPE to pump fluid from the retina to the choroid. This would potentially limit the absorption of subretinal fluid and contribute to size, shape and chronicity of the overlying neurosensory detachment. Moreover, the choroidal hyperpermeability could also explain the occult (with no clinical effect) serous pigment epithelium detachments (PED) seen in ICG videoangiography in most cases of CSC.

There are two molecular factors that have been related to CSC: epinephrine and cortisol. The effects of endogenous circulating adrenergic effectors and sympathetic innervations combine to produce vasoconstriction and alteration of blood flow in the choroidal vessels, which may lead to choroidal hyperpermeability. This could explain the association of CSC with a preceding stressful event (143) and type A personality (144). The relationship between CSC and cortisol has been studied for a long time, and it is known that there is a higher incidence of CSC in patients with Cushing's disease (145), patients who have had organ transplants and are being treated with corticosteroids to prevent rejections (146,147) and pregnant women (a state with increased level of free circulating endogenous cortisol) (148,139). Corticosteroids reduce the production of nitric oxide, increase capillary fragility, and hyperpermeability and may cause delayed healing of RPE defects (149–151). By suppressing synthesis of extracellular matrix components and inhibiting fibroblastic activity, corticosteroids may also directly damage RPE cells or their tight junctions, delaying the reparative process in damaged cells. Steroids also directly affect ion transport and thus may reverse the polarity of RPE cells, resulting in secretion of ions into the subretinal space. This would change the osmotic pressure gradient to favor fluid flow from the choroid to the retina, resulting in a neurosensory detachment.

To summarize, a disturbance in the microcirculation of the choriocapillaris leads to leakage of fluid into the sub-RPE space. Initially RPE cells are able to maintain their integrity and pump fluid in the retinal-choroidal direction. However, prolonged stress ultimately causes pump failure and loss of function. A combination of choroidal hyperpermeability and impaired RPE function leads to pooling of fluid in the sub-RPE space with eventual leakage through the RPE (juxtacellularly and transcellularly) into the subretinal space. This theory provides an explanation for some of the clinical characteristics of CSC but some others, such as the spontaneous healing or the recurrent character of the disease, still remain unexplained.

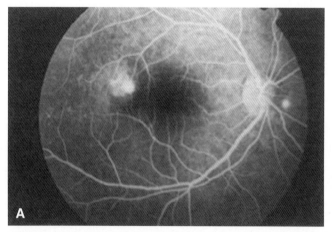 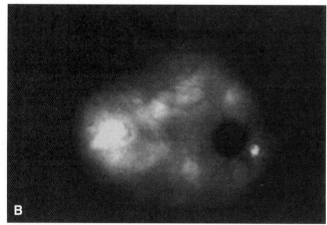

**Figure 3-7. A:** The fluorescein angiogram of a patient with central serous chorioretinopathy reveals two leakage points. One point is superotemporal to the macula and the other is nasal to the optic disc. **B:** The indocyanine green angiogram demonstrates the diffuse nature of this disease and the increased hyperpermeability in areas away from focal leaks that may not be appreciated with fluorescein angiography. (From Guyer DR, Yannuzzi LA, Slakter JS et al. Digital indocyanine green videoangiography of central serous chorioretinopathy. *Arch Ophthalmol* 1994;112:1057–1062.)

## Neovascular Age-Related Macular Degeneration

The main site of disturbance in neovascular age-related macular degeneration (ARMD) is Bruch's membrane. Bruch's membrane provides a semipermeable filtration barrier through which major metabolic exchange takes place. Nutrients pass from choriocapillaris to photoreceptors and RPE, and cellular breakdown products travel in the opposite direction (152). Alteration in extracellular matrix and biophysical properties of Bruch's membrane would lead to altered nutrition and consequent abnormal functioning of the RPE and photoreceptors. It has been suggested that these changes in Bruch's membrane have a major influence on the development and subsequent outcome of disease (153). However, the changes in Bruch's membrane that predispose to neovascularization are unclear. It is likely that inward growth of choroidal new vessels through Bruch's membrane is suppressed by the metabolic environment of Bruch's membrane, which may be influenced by diffusible agents produced by the RPE (154,155). New vessel formation is thought to occur as a consequence of an imbalance in the stimulating and inhibiting influences of growth factors and any disruption to their diffusion through Bruch's membrane to choroid could alter this balance (156,157).

All these changes in Bruch's membrane could lead to functional disturbance in RPE cells. In the other hand, some aging changes in RPE also develop independently which actually can lead to disturbance in Bruch's membrane. Among them are included lipofuscin accumulation, RPE basement membrane thickening, and increasing intracellular residual body content. Therefore this could explain the presence of characteristic features of neovascular ARMD that are due to a breakdown in outer BRB, such as CME, neurosensory detachment, subretinal/intraretinal hemorrhages, serous PED and RPE tears.

There are three types of PED associated with ARMD: drusenoid, serous and fibrovascular. Drusenoid PED is a confluence of several soft drusen. Fibrovascular PED is a form of occult choroidal neovascularization. Serous PED is not exactly a breakdown in outer BRB. It seems to develop from a dysfunction in the complex RPE cells – Bruch's membrane. In 1986 it was suggested that in serous PED, sub-RPE fluid is derived from the RPE rather than from the choroid (153). Fluid moves from the retina into Bruch's membrane as a result of active movement of ions by the RPE cells. If Bruch's membrane became hydrophobic, resistance to water flow could cause fluid to collect between RPE and Bruch's membrane (158–161).

Sometimes a shallow neurosensory detachment may occur as a result of breakdown of physiologic RPE pump or from disruption of tight junctions between adjacent RPE cells. This can happen even in the absence of choroidal neovascularization (CNV). For the same reason, some fluid could accumulate within the layers of the neurosensory retina, leading to a CME. An inflammatory hypothesis has been proposed: debris derived from compromised RPE cells constitutes a chronic inflammatory stimulus. This would release a variety of inflammatory mediators that could contribute to damage to RPE cells and breakdown of inner and outer BRB (162).

In RPE tears, tear occurs at the junction of attached and detached RPE, perhaps when the PED can no longer resist the stretching forces from the fluid in the sub-RPE space emanating from the underlying occult CNV or from the contractile forces of the underlying fibrovascular tissue that may be intimately associated or entwined with the overlying RPE. When the RPE tears, the free edge of the RPE retracts and rolls toward the mound of fibrovascular tissue. Acutely, a serous detachment of the sensory retina may be caused by the leaking of fluid from the exposed choriocapillaris.

## SUMMARY

In conclusion, the BRB maintains the unique tissue milieu needed for viability and optimal function of retinal cells. Many retinal diseases may be viewed as a disturbance or "breakdown" of the BRB. This breakdown leads to disturbances of tissue microenvironment, which subsequently accelerate the progression of the pathology.

### References

1. Del Zoppo GJ, Mabuchi T. Cerebral microvessel responses to focal ischemia. *J Cereb Blood Flow Metab* 2003;23:879–894.
2. Frank RN. Diabetic retinopathy. *N Engl J Med* 2004;350:48–58.
3. Antonelli-Orlidge A, Smith S, D'Amore P. Influence of pericytes on capillary endothelial cell growth. *Am Rev Respir Dis* 1989;140:1129–1131.
4. Kuwabara T, Cogan DG. Retinal vascular patterns: IV. Mural cells of the retinal capillaries. *Arch Ophthalmol* 1963;69:492–502.
5. Tilton R, Kilo C, Williamson J et al. Differences in pericyte contractile function in rat cardiac and skeletal muscle microvasculatures. *Microvasc Res* 1979;18:336–352.
6. Shepro D, Morel N. Pericyte physiology. *FASEB J* 1993;7:1031–1038.
7. Sims D. Recent advances in pericyte biology – implications for health and disease. *Can J Cardiol* 1991;7:431–443.
8. Maeda J. Electron microscopy of the retinal vessels report I. Human retina. *Jpn J Ophthalmol* 1959;3:37–46.
9. Tilton R. Capillary pericytes: perspectives and future trends. *J Electron Microscopy Tech* 1991;19:327–344.
10. Furuse M, Hirase T, Itoh M, et al. Occludin: A novel integral membrane protein localizing at tight junctions. *J Cell Biol* 1993;123:1777–1788.
11. Saitou M, Furuse M, Sasaki H, et al. Complex phenotype of mice lacking occludin, a component of tight junction strands. *Mol Biol Cell* 2000;11:4131–4142.
12. Saitou M, Fujimoto K, Doi Y, et al. Occludin-deficient embryonic stem cells can differentiate into polarized epithelial cells bearing tight junctions. *J Cell Biol* 1998;141:397–408.
13. Yu ASL, McCarthy KM, Francis SA, et al. Knockdown of occludin expression leads to diverse phenotypic alterations in epithelial cells. *Am J Physiol Cell Physiol* 2005;288:C1231–C1241.
14. Balda M, Whitney J, Flores C, et al. Functional dissociation of paracellular permeability and transepithelial electrical resistance and disruption of the apical- basolateral intramembrane diffusion barrier by expression of a mutant tight junction membrane protein. *J Cell Biol* 1996;134:1031–1049.
15. McCarthy K, Skare I, Stankewich M, et al. Occludin is a functional component of the tight junction. *J Cell Sci* 1996;109:2287–2298.
16. Barber AJ, Antonetti DA. Mapping the blood vessels with paracellular permeability in the retinas of diabetic rats. *Invest Ophthalmol Vis Sci* 2003;44:5410–5416.
17. Antonetti D, Barber A, Khin S, et al. Vascular permeability in experimental diabetes is associated with reduced endothelial occludin content: vascular endothelial growth factor decreases occludin in retinal endothelial cells. Penn State Retina Research Group. *Diabetes* 1998;47:1953–1959.
18. Ikenouchi J, Furuse M, Furuse K, et al. Tricellulin constitutes a novel barrier at tricellular contacts of epithelial cells. *J Cell Biol* 2005;171:939–945.
19. Furuse M, Fujita K, Hiiragi T, et al. Claudin-1 and -2: novel integral membrane proteins localizing at tight junctions with no sequence similarity to occludin. *J Cell Biol* 1998;141:1539–1550
20. Gonzalez-Mariscal L, Betanzos A, Nava P, et al. Tight junction proteins. *Prog Biophys Mol Biol* 2003;81:1–44.
21. Furuse M, Tsukita S. Claudins in occluding junctions of humans and flies. *Trends Cell Biol* 2006;16:181–188.

22. Van Itallie CM, Anderson JM. Claudins and epithelial paracellular transport. *Annu Rev Physiol* 2006;68:403–429.

23. Furuse M, Sasaki H, Fujimoto K, et al. A single gene product, claudin-1 or -2, reconstitutes tight junction strands and recruits occludin in fibroblasts. *J Cell Biol* 1998;143:391–401.

24. Tsukita S, Furuse M. Occludin and claudins in tight-junction strands: leading or supporting players? *Trends Cell Biol* 1999;9:268–273.

25. Morita K, Furuse M, Fujimoto K, et al. Claudin multigene family encoding four-transmembrane domain protein components of tight junction strands. *PNAS* 1999;96:511–516.

26. Tsukita S, Furuse M, Itoh M. Multifunctional strands in tight junctions. *Nat Rev Mol Cell Biol* 2001;2:285–293.

27. Turksen K, Troy T-C. Barriers built on claudins. *J Cell Sci* 2004;117:2435–2447.

28. Morita K, Sasaki H, Furuse M, et al. Endothelial claudin: claudin-5/TMVCF constitutes tight junction strands in endothelial cells. *J Cell Biol* 1999, 147:185–194.

29. Nitta T, Hata M, Gotoh S, et al. Size-selective loosening of the blood-brain barrier in claudin-5-deficient mice. *J Cell Biol* 2003;161:653–660.

30. Wolburg H, Wolburg-Buchholz K, Kraus J, et al. Localization of claudin-3 in tight junctions of the blood-brain barrier is selectively lost during experimental autoimmune encephalomyelitis and human glioblastoma multiforme. *Acta Neuropathol (Berl)* 2003;105:586–592.

31. Landau D. Epithelial paracellular proteins in health and disease. *Curr Opin Nephrol Hypertens* 2006;15:425–429.

32. Mazzon E, Puzzolo D, Caputi AP, et al. Role of IL-10 in hepatocyte tight junction alteration in mouse model of experimental colitis. *Mol Med* 2002;8:353–366.

33. Kausalya PJ, Amasheh S, Gunzel D, et al. Disease-associated mutations affect intracellular traffic and paracellular Mg2+ transport function of Claudin-16. *J Clin Invest* 2006;116:878–891.

34. Itoh M, Sasaki H, Furuse M, et al. Junctional adhesion molecule (JAM) binds to PAR-3: a possible mechanism for the recruitment of PAR-3 to tight junctions. *J Cell Biol* 2001;154:491–498.

35. Bazzoni G, Martinez-Estrada OM, Mueller F, et al. Homophilic Interaction of junctional adhesion molecule. *J Biol Chem* 2000;275:30970–30976.

36. Liu Y, Nusrat A, Schnell F, et al. Human junction adhesion molecule regulates tight junction resealing in epithelia. *J Cell Sci* 2000;113:2363–2374.

37. Palmeri D, van Zante A, Huang C-C, et al. Vascular endothelial junction-associated molecule, a novel member of the immunoglobulin superfamily, is localized to intercellular boundaries of endothelial cells. *J Biol Chem* 2000;275:19139–19145.

38. Saitou M, Ando-Akatsuka Y, Itoh M, et al. Mammalian occludin in epithelial cells: its expression and subcellular distribution. *Eur J Cell Biol* 1997;73:222–231.

39. Itoh M, Furuse M, Morita K, et al. Direct binding of three tight junction-associated MAGUKs, ZO-1, ZO-2, and ZO-3, with the COOH termini of claudins. *J Cell Biol* 1999;147:1351–1363.

40. Fanning AS, Jameson BJ, Jesaitis LA, et al. The tight junction protein ZO-1 establishes a link between the transmembrane protein occludin and the actin cytoskeleton. *J Biol Chem* 1998;273:29745–29753.

41. Itoh M, Morita K, Tsukita S. Characterization of ZO-2 as a MAGUK family member associated with tight as well as adherens junctions with a binding affinity to occluding and alpha-catenin. *J Biol Chem* 1999;274:5981–5986.

42. Schmidt A, Utepbergenov DI, Mueller SL, et al. Occludin binds to the SH3-hinge-GuK unit of zonula occludens protein 1: potential mechanism of tight junction regulation. *Cell Mol Life Sci* 2004;61:1354–1365.

43. Imamura Y, Itoh M, Maeno Y, et al. Functional domains of alpha-catenin required for the strong state of cadherin-based cell adhesion. *J Cell Biol* 1999;144:1311–1322.

44. Yamamoto T, Harada N, Kano K, et al. The Ras target AF-6 interacts with ZO-1 and serves as a peripheral component of tight junctions in epithelial cells. *J Cell Biol* 1997;139:785–795.

45. Itoh M, Nagafuchi A, Moroi S, et al. Involvement of ZO-1 in cadherin-based cell adhesion through Its direct binding to alpha-catenin and actin filaments. *J Cell Biol* 1997;138:181–192.

46. Muller SL, Portwich M, Schmidt A, et al. The tight junction protein occludin and the adherens junction protein [alpha]-catenin share a common interaction mechanism with ZO-1. *J Biol Chem* 2005;280:3747–3756.

47. Fischer S, Wobben M, Marti HH, et al. Hypoxia-Induced hyperpermeability in brain microvessel endothelial cells involves VEGF-mediated changes in the expression of zonula occludens-1. *Microvascular Res* 2002;63:70–80.

48. Jin M, Barron E, He S, et al. Regulation of RPE intercellular junction integrity and function by hepatocyte growth factor. *Invest Ophthalmol Vis Sci* 2002;43:2782–2790.

49. DeMaio L, Chang YS, Gardner TW, et al. Shear stress regulates occludin content and phosphorylation. *Am J Physiol Heart Circ Physiol* 2001;281:H105–H113.

50. Sill HW, Chang YS, Artman JR, et al. Shear stress increases hydraulic conductivity of cultured endothelial monolayers. *Am J Physiol Heart Circ Physiol* 1995;268:H535–H54351.

51. Geiger B, Ayalon O. Cadherins. *Ann Rev Cell Biol* 1992;8:307–332.

52. Scheurer SB, Rybak JN, Rosli C, et al. Modulation of gene expression by hypoxia in human umbilical cord vein endothelial cells: a transcriptomic and proteomic study. *Proteomics* 2004;4:1737–1760.

53. Krantz SB. Erythropoietin. *Blood* 1991;77:419–434.

54. Ikeda E, Achen MG, Breier G, et al. Hypoxia-induced transcriptional activation and increased mRNA stability of vascular endothelial growth factor in C6 glioma cells. *J Biol Chem* 1995;270:19761–19766.

55. Czyzyk-Krzeska MF, Furnari BA, Lawson EE, et al. Hypoxia increases rate of transcription and stability of tyrosine hydroxylase mRNA in pheochromocytoma (PC12) cells. *J Biol Chem* 1994;269:760–764.

56. Firth JD, Ebert BL, Pugh CW, et al. Oxygen-regulated control elements in the phosphoglycerate kinase 1 and lactate dehydrogenase A genes: similarities with the erythropoietin 3_ enhancer. *Proc Natl Acad Sci USA* 1994;91:6496–6500.

57. Ikeda E. Cellular response to tissue hypoxia and its involvement in disease progression. *Pathol Int* 2005;55:603–610.

58. Mark KS, Davis TP. Cerebral microvascular changes in permeability and tight junctions induced by hypoxia-reoxygenation. *Am J Physiol Heart Circ Physiol* 2002;282:H1485–H1494.

59. Brown RC, Mark KS, Egleton RD, et al. Protection against hypoxia-induced increase in blood-brain barrier permeability: role of tight junction proteins and NFkappaB. *J Cell Sci* 2003;116:693–700.

60. Anderson T, Meredith I, Ganz P, et al. Nitric oxide and nitrovasodilators: similarities, differences and potential interactions. *J Am Coll Cardiol* 1994;24:555–566.

61. Meidell R. Endothelial dysfunction and vascular disease. *Southwest Intern Med Conference* 1994;307:378–389.

62. Tsukahara H, Gordienko D, Tonshoff B, et al. Direct demonstration of insulin-like growth factor-I-induced nitric oxide$^{Rx}$ production by endothelial cells. *Kidney Intern* 1994;45:598–604.

63. Oku H, Yamaguchi H, Sugiyama T, et al. Retinal toxicity of nitric oxide released by administration of a nitric oxide donor in the albino rabbit. *Invest Ophthalmol Vis Sci* 1997;38:2540–2544.

64. Vane JR, Anggard EE, Botting R. Regulatory function of the vascular endothelium. *New Eng J Med* 1990;323:27–36.

65. Harrison D. The endothelial cell. *Heart Dis Stroke* 1992;14:95–99.

66. Corbett J, Tilton R, Williamson J. Aminoguanidine, a novel inhibitor of nitric oxide formation, prevents diabetic vascular dysfunction. *Diabetes* 1992;41:552–556.

67. Geyer O, Almog J, Lupu-Meiri M, et al. Nitric oxide synthase inhibitors protect rat retina against ischemic injury. *FEBS Lett* 1995;374:399–402.

68. Haefliger I, Flammer J, Luschert T. Heterogeneity of endothelium-dependent regulation in ophthalmic and ciliary arteries. *Invest Ophthalmol Vis Sci* 1993;34:1722–1730.

69. Kulkarni P, Joshua IG, Roberts AM, et al. A novel method to assess reactivities of retinal microcirculation. *Microvasc Res* 1994;48:39–49.

70. Tilton R, Williamson J. Prevention of diabetic vascular dysfunction by guanidines inhibition of nitric oxide synthase versus advanced glycation end-product formation. *Diabetes* 1993;42:221–232.

71. Vorwerk CK, Hyman BT, Miller JW, et al. The role of neuronal and endothelial nitric oxide synthase in retinal excitotoxicity. *Invest Ophthalmol Vis Sci* 1997;38:2038–2044.

72. Ramachandran E, Frank R, Kennedy A. Effects of endothelin on cultured bovine retinal microvascular pericytes. *Invest Ophthalmol Vis Sci* 1993;34:586–595.

73. Rubanyi G, Polokoff M. Endothelins: molecular biology, biochemistry, pharmacology, physiology, and pathophysiology. *Pharmacol Rev* 1994;46:325–415.

74. Sakurai T, Yanagisawa M, Masaki T. Molecular characteristics of endothelin receptors. *Trends Pharmacol Sci* 1992;13:103–108.

75. Wenzel R, Noll G, Luscher T. Endothelin receptor antagonists inhibit endothelin in human skin. *Microcirc Hypertens* 1994;23:581–586.

76. Chakravarthy U, Gardiner T, Anderson P, et al. The effect of endothelin 1 on the retinal microvascular pericyte. *Microvasc Res* 1992;43:241–254.

77. Higgins R, Hendricks-Munoz K, Gerrets R, et al. Modulation of hyperoxia induced endothelin-1 secretion from retinal endothelial cells by captopril and nifedipine. *Invest Ophthalmol Vis Sci* 1995;36:S67.

78. McDonald DM, Bailie JR, Archer DB. Characterization of endothelin A (ET A) and Endothelin B (ET B) receptors in cultured bovine retinal pericytes. *Invest Ophthalmol Vis Sci* 1995;36:1088–1094.

79. Haefliger IO, Meyer P, Flammer J, et al. The vascular endothelium as a regulator of the ocular circulation: a new concept in ophthalmology? *Surv Ophthalmol* 1994;39:123–132.

80. Harrison D. The endothelial cell. *Heart Dis Stroke* 1992;14:95–99.

81. Merimee TJ. Diabetic retinopathy: a synthesis of perspectives. *New Eng J Med* 1990;322:978–983.

82. Xia P, Aiello LP, Ishii H, et al. Characterization of vascular endothelial growth factor's effect on the activation of protein kinase C, it isoforms, and endothelial cell growth. *The J Clinic Inves* 1996;98:2018–2026.

83. Harhaj NS, Felinski EA, Wolpert EB, et al. VEGF activation of protein kinase C stimulates occludin phosphorylation and contributes to endothelial permeability. *Invest Ophthalmol Vis Sci* 2006;47:5106–5115.

84. Danser AHJ, van den Dorpel MA, Deimum J, et al. Renin, prorenin, and immunoreactive renin in vitreous fluid from eyes with and without diabetic retinopathy. *J Clin Endo Metab* 1989;68:106–167.
85. Danser AHJ, Derkx FHM, Admiraal PJJ, et al. Angiotensin levels in the eye. *Invest Ophthalmol Vis Sci* 1994;35:1008–1018.
86. Ferrari-Dileo G, Davis EB, Anderson DR. Angiotensin binding sites in bovine and human retinal blood vessels. *Invest Ophthalmol Vis Sci* 1987;28:1747–1751.
87. Ferrari-Dileo G, Davis EB, Anderson DR. Angiotensin II binding receptors in retinal and optic nerve head blood vessels. *Invest Ophthalmol Vis Sci* 1991;32:21–32.
88. Ferrari-Dileo G, Ryan JW, Rockwood EJ et al. Angiotensin-converting enzyme in bovine, feline, and human ocular tissues. *Invest Ophthalmol Vis Sci* 1988;29:876–881.
89. Ferrari-Dileo G, Davis EB, Anderson DR. Glaucoma, capillaries, and pericytes. 3. Peptide hormone binding and influence on pericytes. *Opthalmologica* 1996;210:269–275.
90. Meyer P, Flammer J, Lüscher TF. Local action of the renin angiotensin system in the porcine ophthalmic circulation: effects of ACE-inhibitors and angiotensin receptor antagonists. *Invest Ophthalmol Vis Sci* 1995;36:555–562.
91. Hughes BA, Gallemore RP, Miller SS. Transport mechanisms in the RPE. In: Marmor MF, Wolfensberger TJ (eds). *The retinal pigment epithelium: function and disease.* New York: Oxford University Press, 1998.
92. Negi A, Marmor MF. Experimental serous retinal detachment and focal pigment epithelium damage. *Arch Ophthalmol* 1984;102:445–449.
93. Marmor MF. On the cause of serous detachments and central serous chorioretinopathy. *Br J Ophthalmol* 1997;81:812–813.
94. Streilein JW. Peripheral tolerance induction: lessons from immune privileged sites and tissues. *Transplant Proc* 1996;28:2066–2070.
95. Wenkel H, Sreilein JW. Analysis of immune deviation elicited by antigens injected into the subretinal space. *Invest Ophthalmol Vis Sci* 1998;39:1823–1834.
96. Liversidge J, McKay D, Mullen G, et al. Retinal pigment epithelial cells modulate lymphocyte function at the blood-retina barrier by autocrine PGE2 and membrane-bound mechanisms. *Cell Immunol* 1993;149:315–30.
97. Holtkamp G, De Vos A, Peek R, et al. Analysis of the secretion pattern of monocyte chemotactic 1 (MCP-1) and transforming growth factor-beta2 (TGF-beta2) by human retinal pigment epithelial cells. *Clin Exp Immunol* 1999;118:35–40.
98. Holtkamp G, de Vos A, Kijlstra A, et al. Expression of multiple forms of IL-1 receptor antagonist by human retinal pigment epithelial cells: identification of a new IL-ra exon. *Eur J Immunol* 1999;29:215–224.
99. Fadok V, Bratton D, Konowal A, et al. Macrophages that have ingested apoptotic cells in vitro inhibit proinflammatory cytokine production through autocrine/paracrine mechanisms involving TGF-beta, PGE2, and PAF. *J Clin Invest* 1998;101:890–898.
100. Willermain F, Caspers-Velu L, Nowak B, et al. Retinal pigment epithelial cell phagocytosis of T lymphocytes: possible implication in the immune privilege of the eye. *Br J Ophthalmol* 2002;86:1417–1421.
101. Jorgensen A, Wiencke A, la Cour M, et al. Human retinal pigment epithelial cell-induced apoptosis in activated T cells. *Invest Ophthalmol Vis Sci* 1998;39:1590–1599.
102. Rezai K, Semnani R, Farrokh Siar L, et al. Human fetal retinal pigment epithelial cells induce apoptosis in allogenic T-cells in a Fas ligand and PGE2 independent pathway. *Curr Eye Res* 1999;18:430–439.
103. Essner E. Role of vesicular transport in breakdown of the blood-retinal barrier. *Lab Invest* 1987;56:457–460.
104. Essner E, Pino RM, Griewski RA. Breakdown of blood retinal barrier in RCS rats with inherited retinal degeneration. *Lab Invest* 1980;43:418–426.
105. Klaassen I, Hughes JM, Vogels IM, et al. Altered expression of genes related to blood-retinal barrier disruption in streptozotocin-induced diabetes. *Exp Eye Res* 2009;89(1):4–15.
106. Cogan DG, Toussaint D, Kubawara T. Retinal vascular patterns. IV. Diabetic retinopathy. *Arch Ophthalmol* 1961;66:366–378.
107. De Venecia G, Davis M, Engerman R. Clinicopathologic correlations in diabetic retinopathy. I. Histology and fluorescein angiography of microaneurysms. *Arch Ophthalmol* 1976;94:1766–1773.
108. De La Rubia G, Oliver F, Inoguchi T, et al. Induction of resistance to endothelin-1's biochemical actions by elevated glucose levels in retinal pericytes. *Diabetes* 1992;41:1533–1539.
109. Awazu M, Parker RE, Harvie BR, et al. Down-regulation of endothelin-1 receptors by protein kinase C in streptozotocin diabetic rats. *J Cardiovasc Pharmacol* 1991;17:S500–S502.
110. Chakravarthy U, Hayes RC, Stitt AW, et al. Endothelin expression in ocular tissues of diabetic and insulin-treated rats. *Invest Ophthalmol Vis Sci* 1997;38:2144–2151.
111. Akagi Y, Kador PF, Kuwabara T, et al. Aldose reductase localization in human retinal mural cells. *Invest Ophthalmol Vis Sci* 1983;24:1516–1519.

112. Robison WG Jr, Laver NM, Lou MF. The role of aldose reductase in diabetic retinopathy: Prevention and intervention studies. In: Osborne NN, Chader GJ (eds)., *Progress in retinal and eye research.* Oxford: Pergamon Press, 1995;14:593–640.
113. Robison WG Jr, Kador PF, Kinoshita JH. Retinal capillaries: basement membrane thickening by galactosemia prevented with aldose reductase inhibitor. *Science* 1983;221:1177–1179.
114. Frank RN, Keirn RJ, Kennedy A, et al. Galactose-induced retinal capillary basement membrane thickening: prevention by sorbinil. *Invest Ophthalmol Vis Sci* 1983;24:1519–1524.
115. Das A, Frank RN, Zhang NL, et al. Increases in collagen type IV and laminin in galactose-induced retinal capillary basement membrane thickening – prevention by an aldose reductase inhibitor. *Exp Eye Res* 1990;50:269–280.
116. Robison WG Jr, Kador PF, Akagi Y, et al. Prevention of basement membrane thickening in retinal capillaries by a novel inhibitor of aldose reductase, tolrestat. *Diabetes* 1986;35:295–299.
117. Sorbinil Retinopathy Trial Research Group: a randomized trial of sorbinil, an aldose reductase inhibitor, in diabetic retinopathy. *Arch Ophthalmol* 1990;108:1234–1244.
118. Kim JW, Ai E. Diabetic retinopathy. In: Regillo CD, Brown GC, Flynn HW Jr (eds). *Vitreoretinal disease: the essentials.* Thieme Medical Publishers: New York, 1999.
119. Arend O, Wolf S, Harris A, et al. The relationship of macular microcirculation to visual acuity in diabetic patients. *Arch Ophthalmol* 1995;113:610–614.
120. Klein R, et al. The Wisconsin Epidemiologic Study of Diabetic Retinopathy. IV. Diabetic macular edema. *Ophthalmology* 1984;91:1464–1474.
121. Sorbinil Retinopathy Trial Research Group. A randomized trial of sorbinil, an aldose reductase inhibitor, in diabetic retinopathy. *Arch Ophthalmol* 1990;108:1234–1244.
122. Essner E. Role of vesicular transport in breakdown of the blood-retinal barrier. *Lab Invest* 1987;56:457–460.
123. Chibber R, Ben-Mahmud BM, Chibber S, et al. Leukocytes in diabetic retinopathy. *Curr Diabetes Rev* 2007;3 (1):3–14.
124. Miyamoto K, Ogura Y. Pathogenetic potential of leukocytes in diabetic retinopathy. *Semin Ophthalmol* 1999;14:233–239.
125. Wang K, Wang Y, Gao L, et al. Dexamethasone inhibits leukocyte accumulation and vascular permeability in retina of streptozocin-induced diabetic rats via reducing vascular endothelial growth factor and intercellular adhesion molecule-1 expression. *Biol Pharm Bull* 2008;31(8):1541–1546.
126. Kim JH, Kim JH, Yu YS, et al. Blockade of angiotensin II attenuates VEGF-mediated blood-retinal barrier breakdown in diabetic retinopathy. *J Cereb Blood Flow Metab* 2009;29(3):621–628.
127. Guex-Crosier Y. The pathogenesis and clinical presentation of macular edema in inflammatory diseases. *Doc Ophthalmol* 1999;97(3–4):297–309.
128. Terasaki H, Miyake K, Miyake Y. Reduced oscillatory potentials of the full-field electroretinogram of eyes with aphakic or pseudophakic cystoids macular edema. *Am J Ophthalmol.* 2003;135(4):477–82.
129. Martin NF, Green WR, Martin LW. Retinal phlebitis in the Irvine-Gass syndrome. *Am J Ophthalmol* 1977;83:377–386.
130. Vinores SA, Amin A, Derevjanik NL, et al. Immunohistochemical localization of blood-retinal barrier breakdown sites associated with post-surgical edema. *Histochemistry* 1994;26:655–665.
131. Flach AJ. Cyclo-oxygenase inhibitors in ophthalmology. *Surv Ophthalmol* 1992;36(4):259–284.
132. Jampol LM. Aphakic cystoids macular edema: a hypothesis. *Arch Ophthalmol* 1985;103:1134–1135.
133. Byrnes GA, Chang B, Loose I, et al. Prospective incidence of photic maculopathy after cataract surgery. *Am J Ophthalmology* 1995;119:231–232.
134. Komatsu M, Kanagami S, Shimizu K. Ultraviolet-absorbing intraocular lens versus non-UV-absorbing intraocular lens: comparison of angiographic cystoid macular edema. *J Cataract Refract Surg* 1989;15(6):654–657.
135. Kumagai K, Ogino N, Furukawa M, et al. Vitrectomy for pseudophakic cystoids macular edema. *Nippon Ganka Gakkai Zasshi* 2002;106(5):297–303.
136. Iliff CE. Treatment of the vitreous-tug syndrome. *Am J Ophthalmol* 1971;62:856–859.
137. Kraff MC, Saunders DR, Jampol LM, et al. Prophylaxis of pseudophakic cystoids macular edema with topical indomethacin. *Ophthalmology* 1982;89:885–890.
138. Schubert HD. Cystoid macular edema: the apparent role of mechanical factors. *Prog Clin Biol Res* 1989;312:277–291.
139. Negi A, Marmor MF. The resorption of subretinal fluid after diffuse damage of the retinal pigment epithelium. *Invest Ophthalmol Vis Sci* 1983;24:1475–1479.
140. Negi A, Marmor MF. Experimental serous retinal detachment and focal pigment epithelium damage. *Arch Ophthalmol* 1984;102:445–449.
141. Marmor MF. New hypotheses on the pathogenesis and treatment of serous retinal detachment. *Graefes Arch Clin Exp Ophthalmol* 1988;226:548–552.

142. Guyer DR, Yannuzzi LA, Slakter JS, et al. Digital indocyanine green videoangiography of central serous chorioretinopathy. *Arch Ophthalmol* 1994;112:1057–1062.
143. Gelber GS, Schatz H. Loss of vision due to central serous chorioretinopathy following psychological stress. *Am J Psychiatry* 1987;144:46–50.
144. Yannuzzi LA. Type-A behavior and central serous chorioretinopathy. *Retina* 1987;7:111–130.
145. Garg SP, Dada T, Talwar D, et al. Endogenous cortisol profile in patients with central serous chorioretinopathy. *Br J Ophthalmol* 1997;81:962–964.
146. Gass JDM, Little HL. Bilateral bullous exudative retinal detachment complicating idiopathic central serous chorioretinopathy during systemic corticosteroid therapy. *Ophthalmology* 1995;102:737–747.
147. Friberg TR, Eller AW. Serous retinal detachment resembling central serous chorioretinopathy following organ transplantation. *Graefes Arch Clin Exp Ophthalmol* 1990;288:305–309.
148. Gass JDM. Central serous chorioretinopathy and white subretinal exudation during pregnancy. *Arch Ophthalmol* 1991;109:677–681.
149. Warren JB, Loi RK, Coughlan ML. Involvement of nitric oxide[Rx] in the delayed vasodilator response to ultraviolet light irradiation of rat skin in vivo. *Br J Pharmacol* 1993;109:802–806.
150. Chrousos GP, Gold PW. The concepts of stress and stress system disorders. Overview of physical and behavioral homeostatsis. *JAMA* 1992;267:1244–1252.
151. Gill GN. Adrenal gland. In: West JB (ed). *Best and Taylor's physiological basis of medical practice*. Baltimore, MD: Williams & Wilkins, 1990:820–830.
152. Bok D. Retinal photoreceptor-pigment epithelium interactions. *Invest Ophthalmol Vis Sci* 1985;26:1659–1694.
153. Bird AC, Marshall J. Retinal pigment epithelial detachments in the elderly. *Trans Ophthalmol Soc UK* 1986;105:674–682.
154. Killingsworth MC, Sarks JP, Sarks SH. Macrophages related to Bruch's membrane in age-related macular degeneration. *Eye* 1990;4:613–621.
155. Penfold PL, Killingsworth MC, Sarks SH. Senile macular degeneration: the involvement of giant cells in atrophy of the retinal pigment epithelium. *Invest Ophthalmol Vis Sci* 1986;27:364–371.
156. Glaser BM. Extracellular modulating factors and the control of intraocular neovascularization. *Arch Ophthalmol* 1988;106:603–610.
157. Glaser BM, Campochiaro PA, Davis JL, et al. Retinal pigment epithelial cells release an inhibitor to neovascularization. *Arch Ophthalmol* 1985;103:1870–1875.
158. Pauleikhoff D, Zuels S, Sheraidah G, et al. Correlation between biochemical composition and fluorescein binding of deposits in Bruch's membrane. *Ophthalmology* 1993;99:1548–1553.
159. Schoeppner G, Chuang EL, Bird AC. The risk of fellow eye visual loss with unilateral retinal pigment epithelial tears. *Am J Ophthalmol* 1989;108:683–685.
160. Chuang EL, Bird AC. The pathogenesis of tears of the retinal pigment epithelium. *Am J Ophthalmol* 1988;105:285–290.
161. Barondes MJ, Pagliarini S, Chisholm IH et al. Controlled trial of laser photocoagulation of pigment epithelial detachments in the elderly: a four-year review. *Br J Ophthalmol* 1992;76:5–7.
162. Anderson DH, Mullins RF, Hageman GS, et al. A role for local inflammation in the formation of drusen in the ageing eye. *Am J Ophthalmol* 2002;134:411–431.

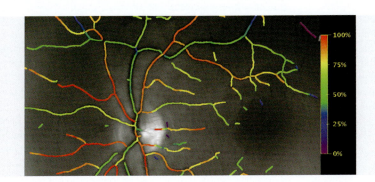

# Macular Oxygenation and Edema

Einar Stefánsson

## INTRODUCTION

The supply of nutrition and oxygenation of the eye is unlike that for any other tissues in the body. In most other tissues, oxygen and nutrients are supplied to the cells from adjacent capillaries by diffusion over a concentration gradient that spans 50 to 100 micrometers at most. The eye on the other hand is mostly avascular, and cells must survive in areas where the nearest capillary is far away. The cornea receives oxygen in part from the atmosphere. The lens relies on nutrition and oxygen dissolved in the aqueous and vitreous humor. The cells in the vitreous humor also must rely on diffusion that carries oxygen and nutrients over almost a centimeter from the nearest capillaries in the retina.

It is obvious why the eye must be avascular. Visible light is absorbed by hemoglobin, and blood in the visual pathway impairs vision. A vascularized crystalline lens or vitreous humor (as in fetal stage) would render the eye virtually blind. The blood vessels in these tissues regress before birth and allow vision to develop unhindered. The visible light that we see must pass not only through the cornea, lens, and vitreous humor, but also through the retina itself. Fortunately, the retina is mostly transparent to visible light, with the notable exception of hemoglobin in the retinal blood vessels. While neural mechanisms mostly hide the presence of these vessels from our vision, we are able to visualize them in some conditions, such as when induced by blue light in the entoptic phenomenon.

The retinal circulation is in the pathway of light. In some species it is absent (guinea pig), partial and out of the way (rabbit), or minimal in extent (man). In the human, the retinal circulation only involves the inner retina, leaving the outer retina avascular and reliant on the choriocapillaris. The choriocapillaris supplies about 80% of the oxygen used by the retina. In addition, the inner retinal circulation is reduced to about 50% of the blood flow that a comparable volume of brain tissue would enjoy. The retina extracts more than 40% of the oxygen from the blood in the retinal circulation, whereas the average extraction for the brain and the body in general is 20% (Fig. 4-1). If the retina were vascularized in the same fashion as regular brain tissue, the amount of blood vessels and volume of blood would be about 10 times greater than it is. This would reduce the quality of vision considerably.

While the pattern of vascularization is very helpful for acute vision, it creates vulnerabilities. First, the inner retina normally has a very low oxygen tension, only about 20 mm Hg partial pressure, which is necessary for the extraction of 40%

to 50% of the hemoglobin bound oxygen. It is operating on the edge in terms of oxygen tension and must employ a sophisticated autoregulation system to adapt to changes in oxygen supply or demand. Second, since the outer retina depends on oxygen and nutrients from the choriocapillaris, it is very sensitive to anything that disturbs or lengthens the diffusion path, including retinal detachment and subretinal hemorrhage.

## DOUBLE OXYGENATION

The retina receives oxygen from two sources, the retinal circulation and the choriocapillaris. The retinal circulation supplies the inner part of the retina and the choroid the avascular outer retina, including the photoreceptors. The blood flow in the retinal circulation is carefully regulated by a control mechanism known as "the autoregulation" and disturbances in inner retinal oxygenation generally result from occlusions of blood vessels, arterioles, capillaries or venules. On the other hand, disturbance in the oxygenation from the choroid are the result of an increased distance from the choriocapillaris to the retina or, less frequently, vascular occlusions in the choroid.

The blood flow in the choroid is relatively large. Whereas the retinal circulation loses about 40% to 50% of the available oxygen, the choroid only gives up about 4% of the available oxygen (1,2). This has led to some confusion about the role of the choroidal blood flow in the eye. Some have suggested that the main role of the choroid is to maintain temperature control in the fundus. While the choroid may contribute in this way, it is clear that the high blood flow is necessary to maintain a high enough oxygen tension in the choriocapillaris so that the oxygen tension gradient from the choriocapillaris to the mitochondria in the inner segments of the photoreceptors is steep enough to maintain the oxygen flux required. If the choroidal blood flow were so low that more hemoglobin dissociation would take place, the oxygen tension in the choroid and the oxygen flux to the photoreceptors would not meet the need of the rods and cones (Fig. 4-2).

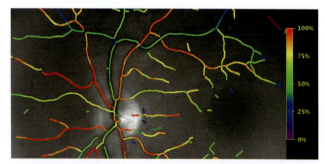

**Figure 4-1.** A color-coded map of hemoglobin oxygen saturation in the human retina. The map is generated automatically by a retinal oximeter.

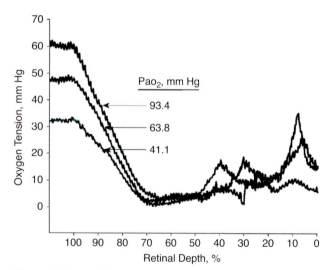

**Figure 4-2.** Intraretinal oxygen profiles recorded in dark during normoxia and hypoxemia. From *The Journal of General Physiology* 1992;99:177–197, with permission from The Rockefeller University Press.

## DISTURBANCE IN CHOROIDAL OXYGEN SUPPLY

Stefánsson (3) presented a mathematical model of the oxygenation of the retina. The model is based on Fick's law, $J = -D \, dC/dx$, where $J$ is the flux of oxygen, $D$ the diffusion coefficient, and $dC/dx$ the concentration gradient. If the distance between the retina and choriocapillaris is increased ($dx$ is bigger), then the concentration gradient becomes flatter and the oxygen flux is decreased. Obviously, this takes place when a retinal detachment is present (3). Subretinal fluid in any form of retinal detachment, rhegmatogenous, exudative, or tractional, will decrease the oxygen flux from the choroid to the retina, and the same will be true if this distance is increased by pigment epithelial detachment, extensive drusen, or subretinal hemorrhage. Recent studies have shown the role of oxygen in retinal detachments (4).

Hyperoxia has been shown to improve photoreceptor survival in the detached retina (5,6). Wang and Linsenmeier (7) showed that hyperoxia is protective because it allows more photoreceptor oxygen consumption.

## AUTOREGULATION

Ocular blood flow follows the rule of Hagen-Poiseuille:

blood flow = perfusion pressure/vascular resistance
$$F = (OAP-IOP)/R$$

The autoregulation influences vascular resistance (R) and thereby affects blood flow (F). OAP is the ophthalmic artery pressure and IOP the intraocular pressure. If metabolic requirements are constant, the autoregulation tries to keep blood flow constant. However, if metabolic requirements change, it changes the blood flow accordingly. The autoregulation does not primarily aim to maintain a constant rate of blood flow in the retina and optic nerve. It tries to maintain a constant chemical environment in the tissue. Blood flow is highly variable in normal retina. One example of this is that retinal blood flow varies with different $O_2$ levels in breathing mixture (Fig. 4-3) (8).

Retinal blood flow also changes if the oxygen consumption of the retina is changed. Feke et al. (9) showed that human retinal blood flow is 40% to 70% lower in light than in dark. The change in retinal blood flow provides the appropriate change of available oxygen for the inner retinal tissue to compensate for increased oxygen consumption in the dark by the photoreceptor-RPE complex. The same group (10) showed that optic atrophy reduces retinal blood flow in humans. They found that blood flow in the temporal retinal arteries of the affected eyes, measured by the laser Doppler technique, was 48% +/− 20% lower than in the fellow eyes (four patients). Arterio-venous $O_2$ saturation difference for temporal and nasal vascular segments of the affected eyes, evaluated by retinal vessel oximetry, was 12% +/− 9% higher than in the fellow eyes. The combination of these results indicated a 40% +/− 29% reduction in $O_2$ delivery in the affected eyes, thereby

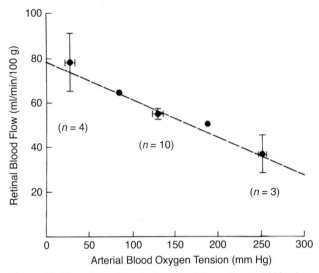

**Figure 4-3.** The relationship of retinal blood flow with arterial blood oxygen tension, measured in cats. (From Stefansson E, Wagner HG, Seida M. Retinal blood flow and its autoregulation measured by intraocular hydrogen clearance. *Exp Eye Res* 1988;47:669–678, with permission).

quantifying the decrease in retinal metabolism that resulted from inner retinal degeneration.

Naturally, if the metabolic demand is constant, the retinal autoregulation will try to keep blood flow and the chemical environment constant. If the IOP is changed (and the OAP is constant), the perfusion pressure will change. In this case the autoregulation will dilate the arterioles, decrease the resistance (R) and maintain constant blood flow. Figure 4-4 (11,12) shows the oxygen tension over the optic nerve in pigs, where the IOP is stepwise changed. With moderate changes in IOP the oxygen tension does not change, as the autoregulation keeps it constant. However, a large change in IOP overwhelms the autoregulation and oxygen tension falls.

## STARLING'S LAW AND MACULAR EDEMA

Ernest Henry Starling (1866–1927) stated in 1896: "There must be a balance between the hydrostatic pressure of the blood in the capillaries and the osmotic attraction of the blood for the surrounding fluids…. and whereas capillary pressure determines transudation, the osmotic pressure of the proteins of the serum determines absorption." In other words, the hydrostatic pressure forcing fluids from the vessel into the tissue must be balanced by the osmotic pressure, generated by the colloidal protein solutions in the capillary, forcing absorption of the fluid from the tissues (13).

Starling's four forces that govern the transport of water between the vascular compartment and the tissue compartment are the following: (a) Hydrostatic pressure in the capillary (Pc). (b) Hydrostatic pressure in the interstitium (Pi), which in the eye equals the intraocular pressure, IOP. (c) Osmotic (oncotic) pressure exerted by plasma proteins in the capillary (Qc). (d) Osmotic pressure exerted by proteins in the interstitial fluid (Qi).

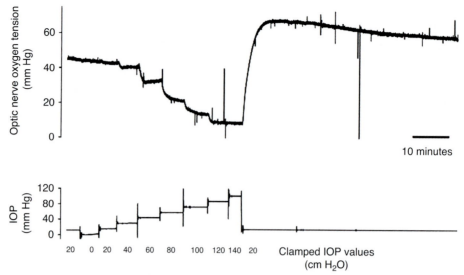

**Figure 4-4.** Optic nerve oxygen tension measured with a polarographic oxygen electrode placed in the vitreous approximately 0.5 mm above the optic nerve head in a pig. The intraocular pressure (IOP) was controlled by means of a canula placed in the anterior chamber and connected to a saline reservoir. Intraocular pressure was continuously regulated and optic nerve oxygen tension measured continuously at the same time. (From la Cour M, Kiilgaard JF, Eysteinsson T, et al. Optic nerve oxygen tension: effects of intraocular pressure and dorzolamide. *Br J Ophthalmol* 2000;84:1045–1049, with permission.)

The balance of these forces allows the calculation of the net driving pressure for filtration

$$\text{Net Driving Pressure} = (Pc - Pi) - (Qc - Qi)$$

The hydrostatic pressure, which originates in the heart, is higher in the vessel than in the tissue and this drives water from the vessel into the tissue. The hydrostatic pressure gradient, $\Delta P$, must be balanced by the osmotic pressure gradient, $\Delta Q$, where the osmotic pressure is higher in the blood than in the interstitial fluid and pulls water back into the blood vessel. If the hydrostatic pressure gradient and the osmotic pressure gradient are equal, no net transport of water takes place and edema is neither formed nor resolved. Starling's law is frequently shown in this form as

$$\Delta P - \Delta Q = 0$$

describing the steady state of the equal and opposing hydrostatic, $\Delta P$, and osmotic pressure, $\Delta Q$, gradients (13).

Starling's law has been generally accepted in medicine and physiology for more than a century as the fundamental rule governing the formation and disappearance of edema in the body. It is reasonable to believe that the ocular tissues follow the same general laws of physiology and physics as the rest of the body, and those who believe otherwise should be burdened with the duty of disproving Starling's law in the eye.

## EDEMA

Edema is the swelling of soft tissues due to an abnormal accumulation of fluid, that is, water. Edema may be cytotoxic or vasogenic in origin. In cytotoxic or ischemic edema the abnormal water accumulation and swelling occurs within cells (14), whereas in vasogenic edema the water accumulates in the interstitial space between cells. While retinal edema may be either cytotoxic or vasogenic, Starling's law applies to the vasogenic edema, which presumably is the most frequent and important form of edema in vascular retinopathies.

With abnormal accumulation of water in the retina the tissue volume increases and the retina thickens. The thickening may be measured with ocular coherent tomography (OCT). At the same time the specific gravity of the tissue is decreased proportionally with the increased water content (15).

## WHAT CREATES EDEMA?

According to Starling's law, edema will form if the hydrostatic pressure gradient between vessel and tissue is increased or the osmotic pressure gradient is decreased. The hydrostatic gradient increases if the blood pressure in the microcirculation rises or the tissue pressure decreases. The osmotic pressure gradient decreases if proteins accumulate in the interstitium to increase the osmotic pressure in the tissue, and also if the osmotic pressure in blood goes down.

### Increased Hydrostatic Pressure Gradient

The hydrostatic pressure in the microcirculation, capillaries, and venules is a function of the work of the heart, arterial blood pressure, and the resistance and pressure fall in the arterioles. Arterial hypertension tends to increase the hydrostatic pressure in the capillaries and is a well-known risk factor for diabetic macular edema (16–21). Diabetic macular edema tends to improve if arterial hypertension is successfully treated (17,18).

The resistance in the retinal arterioles and thereby the pressure drop in the arterioles is a function of the diameter of

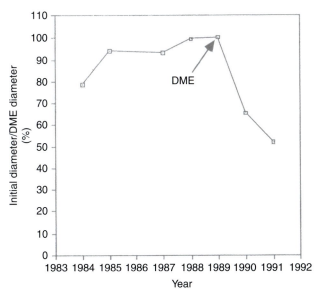

**Figure 4-5.** Arteriolar diameter in a temporal arteriole in a diabetic woman, who developed diabetic macular edema in 1989 and received argon grid laser photocoagulation at that time. The vessel diameter is measured each year from color fundus photographs and is typical of changes seen in a group of diabetic persons who developed macular edema. (From Kristinsson JK, Gottfredsdottir MS, Stefansson E. Retinal vessel dilatation and elongation precedes diabetic macular oedema. *Br J Ophthalmol* 1997;81:274–278, with permission.)

the arterioles. The resistance to flow is described by the Hagen-Poiseuille law, where the resistance is inversely related to the fourth power of the vessel radius (13). If the arterioles dilate, as they do in hypoxia, the resistance in the arterioles decreases and the hydrostatic pressure in the capillary bed rises (22–24). This is also seen in diabetic retinopathy, where progressive dilatation of the retinal blood vessels has been observed during the development of diabetic macular edema (Fig. 4-5) (25).

The hydrostatic pressure gradient between vessel and tissue is the difference between the hydrostatic pressure in the microcirculation and the intraocular pressure. In ocular hypotony where the intraocular pressure is low, the hydrostatic pressure gradient in Starling's law will increase (22). Ocular hypotony is associated with retinal edema, which may improve if the intraocular pressure increases (26,27).

The hydrostatic pressure in the tissue will also decrease if there is traction on the retina, which relieves some of the tissue pressure, according to Newton's second law. Relieving such traction will restore the tissue pressure to normal and decrease the hydrostatic pressure gradient between the vessel and tissue (28–30).

## Decreasing Osmotic Pressure Gradient

The traditional example of a decrease in the osmotic pressure in blood is in hypoalbuminemia, which may be seen in nephrotic syndrome or starvation with severe generalized edema. A more frequent cause of decreased osmotic pressure gradients between vessel and tissue comes from capillary leakage, where plasma proteins may leak from the capillaries and venules into the tissue. The accumulation of plasma proteins in the tissue will increase the osmotic pressure in the tissue and thereby decrease the osmotic pressure difference between the vessel

and the tissue compartment. The reduction of this osmotic pressure gradient will facilitate fluid movement from the vessel into the tissue and thereby result in edema formation (22). Funatsu et al. (31) demonstrated the close correlation between macular edema and vascular endothelial growth factor (VEGF), which is a potent stimulator of capillary leakage (32).

Retinal edema, such as in diabetic retinopathy and branch retinal vein occlusion, is significantly associated with retinal capillary leakage. Fluorescein angiography and fluorophotometry have shown a close association between retinal and macular edema formation and fluorescein leakage. This has indeed been one of the most frequently used clinical tools to access retinal edema (33–38). It is the leakage of plasma proteins that is important due to the effect they have on osmotic pressure. The leakage of fluorescein is naturally not involved in the pathophysiology of edema and the vessels are naturally "leaky" to water, in their healthy state also.

It is important to realize that Starling's law takes into account both the osmotic pressure gradient and the hydrostatic pressure gradient. It is the balance between the two that governs water movement and the formation and disappearance of edema.

## HOW DO WE TREAT EDEMA?

It should be obvious from the previous discussion that, according to Starling's law, retinal edema may be treated either by decreasing the hydrostatic pressure gradient between vessel and tissue or increasing/restoring the osmotic pressure gradient between vessel and tissue.

## Decreasing Hydrostatic Pressure Gradient

Treatment of arterial hypertension is a well established method for treating diabetic macular edema and is certainly beneficial in some cases (17,18).

Another way to reduce the hydrostatic pressure in the microcirculation is to constrict the arterioles. This may be done simply by breathing oxygen enriched air which has been shown to reduce diabetic macular edema (39,40). Retinal oxygenation may also be improved by scattered laser treatment which destroys a part of the retina and thereby reduces its oxygen consumption (22,24,41–46). The laser treatment destroys some of the photoreceptors and allows oxygen to diffuse from the choroid through the laser scars into the inner retina where it improves retinal oxygen tension and leads to constriction of retinal blood vessels (9,47–49). Retinal vessel constriction has been shown with oxygen breathing and laser treatment, and the vasoconstriction goes hand in hand with the resolution of retinal edema both in diabetic retinopathy and branch retinal vein occlusion (47,48). Vitrectomy also improves the oxygenation of the retina by increasing the diffusion of oxygen within the vitreous cavity (50) and allowing transport of oxygen from well perfused areas of the retina to those that are hypoxic (23,51–53).

Retinal vein occlusions are an obvious case of high hydrostatic pressure due to the occlusion of the central retinal vein or a branch retinal venule. The high hydrostatic pressure in

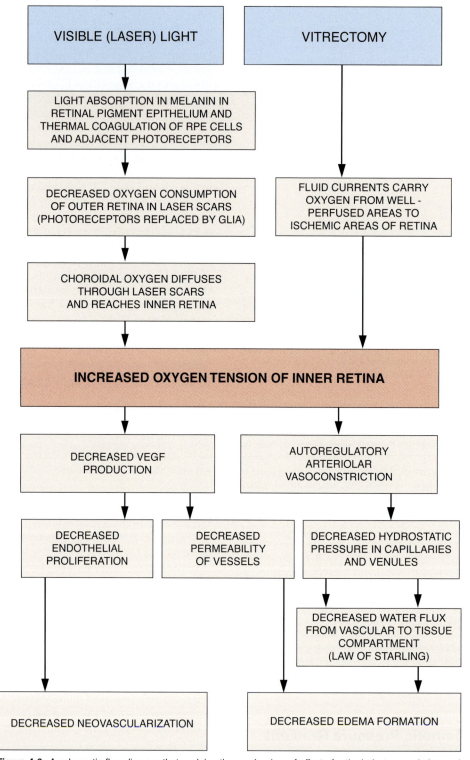

**Figure 4-6.** A schematic flow diagram that explains the mechanism of effect of retinal photocoagulation and vitrectomy on retinal neovascularization and macular edema in diabetic retinopathy and other ischemic retinopathies.

the venule is obvious from the dilatation and tortuosity which reflects the increased transmural pressure difference according to the law of Laplace (54–56). Laser treatment has been shown to reduce the vessel diameter in branch retinal vein occlusion and resolve the macular edema at the same time

(47,48). It may be presumed that other methods to relieve the high vascular pressure such as the creation of shunt vessels or resolution of the occlusion would have the same effect.

Since the hydrostatic pressure gradient is the difference between the blood pressure in the microcirculation and the intraocular pressure, this will increase in ocular hypotony which may be associated with retinal edema as was previously mentioned. Such edema may be successfully treated simply by raising the intraocular pressure (57). It is less clear whether intraocular pressure changes have a function when the intraocular pressure is in the normal range and whether the intraocular pressure should be considered in patients with macular edema and normal or high intraocular pressure.

It may not be intuitively obvious that relief of retinal traction (28–30) fits into Starling's law. However, the tractional force exerted on the retina by vitreous traction will inevitably decrease the tissue pressure in the tissue, as predicted by Isaac Newton, who stated that forces must remain opposite and equal at any point.

## Increasing Osmotic Pressure Gradient

Leaking capillaries and venules in the retina are closely associated with retinal and macular edema (33–38). Fluorescein leakage has been used for diagnostic purposes in macular edema. The leaky blood vessels presumably leak plasma proteins from blood into the interstitial tissue compartment thus decreasing the osmotic pressure gradient between the two compartments. The protein leakage may be influenced by administering drugs that reduce VEGF, which is one of the most powerful agents known to induce capillary leakage (58,59).

Corticosteroids such as triamcinolone and dexamethasone also stabilize capillaries and tend to reduce capillary leakage (60–63). These treatment modalities will decrease the leakage of proteins into the interstitial tissue compartment and help to re-establish the osmotic gradient between blood and tissue compartments. This will resolve edema formation according to Starling's law (Fig. 4-6).

The physiological way to reduce VEGF production is to relieve hypoxia, which is the main stimulator for VEGF production.

## THE CENTRAL ROLE OF OXYGEN

Oxygen places an important role in influencing both the hydrostatic and the osmotic forms of Starling's equation. On one hand, oxygen controls the diameter of retinal arterioles and thereby the hydrostatic pressure in the microcirculation. On the other hand, oxygen controls the production of VEGF and other hypoxia induced growth factors and exerts influence on capillary leakage. VEGF is produced in hypoxia and oxygen is the natural anti-VEGF factor (64).

Retinal oxygenation may be improved by breathing oxygen. Retinal photocoagulation as well as vitreous surgery improve retinal oxygenation (22,23,51,52). The mechanism by which retinal oxygenation improves retinal oxygenation has recently been reviewed (22,23), and the reader is referred to these review papers as well as reports from a number of laboratories (24,41–46).

Retinal photocoagulation and vitreous surgery improve oxygenation and thereby influence the hemodynamic consequences of hypoxia, as well as the hypoxia induced production of growth and permeability factors such as VEGF. If the hypoxia is still not controlled, it is possible to decrease the effect of the hypoxia induced growth/permeability factor with anti-VEGF drugs, and with corticosteroids, which decrease the permeability effect of VEGF. All these actions are easily understood in light of Starling's law, keeping in mind the hydrodynamic and osmotic arms of the law (Fig. 4-6).

## References

1. Alm A, Bill A. Blood flow and oxygen extraction in the cat uvea at normal and high intraocular pressures. *Acta Physiol Scand* 1970;80:19–28.
2. Alm A, Bill A. Ocular and optic nerve blood flow at normal and increased intraocular pressures in monkeys (Macaca irus): a study with radioactively labelled microspheres including flow determinations in brain and some other tissues. *Exp Eye Res* 1973;15:15–29.
3. Stefansson E. *Ocular oxygenation and neovascularization*. Durham, North Carolina: Duke University, 1981.
4. Roos MW. Theoretical estimation of retinal oxygenation during retinal detachment. *Comput Biol Med* 2007;37:890–896.
5. Mervin K, Valter K, Maslim J, et al. Limiting photoreceptor death and deconstruction during experimental retinal detachment: the value of oxygen supplementation. *Am J Ophthalmol* 1999;128:155–164.
6. Sakai T, Lewis GP, Linberg KA, et al. The ability of hyperoxia to limit the effects of experimental detachment in cone-dominated retina. *Invest Ophthalmol Vis Sci* 2001;42:3264–3273.
7. Wang S, Linsenmeier RA. Hyperoxia improves oxygen consumption in the detached feline retina. *Invest Ophthalmol Vis Sci* 2007;48:1335–1341.
8. Stefansson E, Wagner HG, Seida M. Retinal blood flow and its autoregulation measured by intraocular hydrogen clearance. *Exp Eye Res* 1988;47: 669–678.
9. Feke GT, Zuckerman R, Green GJ, et al. Response of human retinal blood flow to light and dark. *Invest Ophthalmol Vis Sci* 1983;24:136–141.
10. Sebag J, Delori FC, Feke GT, et al. Effects of optic atrophy on retinal blood flow and oxygen saturation in humans. *Arch Ophthalmol* 1989;107: 222–226.
11. la Cour M, Kiilgaard JF, Eysteinsson T, et al. Optic nerve oxygen tension: effects of intraocular pressure and dorzolamide. *Br J Ophthalmol* 2000;84:1045–1049.
12. Stefansson E, Pedersen DB, Jensen PK, et al. Optic nerve oxygenation. *Prog Retin Eye Res* 2005;24:307–332.
13. Pocock G, Richards CD. *Human physiology. The basis of medicine*, 2nd ed. New York: Oxford University Press Inc., 2004.
14. Bringmann A, Uckermann O, Pannicke T, et al. Neuronal versus glial cell swelling in the ischaemic retina. *Acta Ophthalmol Scand* 2005;83:528–538.
15. Stefansson E, Wilson CA, Lightman SL, et al. Quantitative measurements of retinal edema by specific gravity determinations. *Invest Ophthalmol Vis Sci* 1987;28:1281–1289.
16. Kohner EM, Aldington SJ, Stratton IM, et al. United Kingdom Prospective Diabetes Study, 30: diabetic retinopathy at diagnosis of non-insulin-dependent diabetes mellitus and associated risk factors. *Arch Ophthalmol* 1998;116:297–303.
17. Matthews DR, Stratton IM, Aldington SJ, et al. Risks of progression of retinopathy and vision loss related to tight blood pressure control in type 2 diabetes mellitus: UKPDS 69. *Arch Ophthalmol* 2004;122:1631–1640.
18. Stratton IM, Kohner EM, Aldington SJ, et al. UKPDS 50: risk factors for incidence and progression of retinopathy in Type II diabetes over 6 years from diagnosis. *Diabetologia* 2001;44:156–163.
19. UKPDS-Group. Cost effectiveness analysis of improved blood pressure control in hypertensive patients with type 2 diabetes: UKPDS 40. UK Prospective Diabetes Study Group. *BMJ* 1998;317:720–726.
20. UKPDS-Group. Efficacy of atenolol and captopril in reducing risk of macrovascular and microvascular complications in type 2 diabetes: UKPDS 39. UK Prospective Diabetes Study Group. *BMJ* 1998;317:713–720.
21. UKPDS-Group. Tight blood pressure control and risk of macrovascular and microvascular complications in type 2 diabetes: UKPDS 38. UK Prospective Diabetes Study Group. *BMJ* 1998;317:703–713.
22. Stefansson E. Ocular oxygenation and the treatment of diabetic retinopathy. *Surv Ophthalmol* 2006;51:364–380.
23. Stefansson E. The therapeutic effects of retinal laser treatment and vitrectomy. A theory based on oxygen and vascular physiology. *Acta Ophthalmol Scand* 2001;79:435–440.
24. Stefansson E, Landers MB 3rd, Wolbarsht ML. Increased retinal oxygen supply following pan-retinal photocoagulation and vitrectomy and lensectomy. *Trans Am Ophthalmol Soc* 1981;79:307–334.
25. Kristinsson JK, Gottfredsdottir MS, Stefansson E. Retinal vessel dilatation and elongation precedes diabetic macular oedema. *Br J Ophthalmol* 1997;81:274–278.

26. Kokame GT, de Leon MD, Tanji T. Serous retinal detachment and cystoid macular edema in hypotony maculopathy. *Am J Ophthalmol* 2001;131:384–386.

27. Schubert HD. Postsurgical hypotony: relationship to fistulization, inflammation, chorioretinal lesions, and the vitreous. *Surv Ophthalmol* 1996;41:97–125.

28. Kaiser PK, Riemann CD, Sears JE, et al. Macular traction detachment and diabetic macular edema associated with posterior hyaloidal traction. *Am J Ophthalmol* 2001;131:44–49.

29. Lewis H. The role of vitrectomy in the treatment of diabetic macular edema. *Am J Ophthalmol* 2001;131:123–125.

30. Lewis H, Abrams GW, Blumenkranz MS, et al. Vitrectomy for diabetic macular traction and edema associated with posterior hyaloidal traction. *Ophthalmology* 1992;99:753–759.

31. Funatsu H, Yamashita H, Nakamura S, et al. Vitreous levels of pigment epithelium-derived factor and vascular endothelial growth factor are related to diabetic macular edema. *Ophthalmology* 2006;113:294–301.

32. Patel JI, Tombran-Tink J, Hykin PG, et al. Vitreous and aqueous concentrations of proangiogenic, antiangiogenic factors and other cytokines in diabetic retinopathy patients with macular edema: Implications for structural differences in macular profiles. *Exp Eye Res* 2006;82:798–806.

33. Cunha-Vaz JG. Vitreous fluorophotometry recordings in posterior segment disease. *Graefes Arch Clin Exp Ophthalmol* 1985;222:241–247.

34. Krogsaa B, Lund-Andersen H, Mehlsen J, et al. Blood-retinal barrier permeability versus diabetes duration and retinal morphology in insulin dependent diabetic patients. *Acta Ophthalmol (Copenh)* 1987;65:686–692.

35. Phillips RP, Ross PG, Sharp PF, et al. Use of temporal information to quantify vascular leakage in fluorescein angiography of the retina. *Clin Phys Physiol Meas* 1990;11(Suppl A):81–85.

36. Ring K, Larsen M, Dalgaard P, et al. Fluorophotometric evaluation of ocular barriers and of the vitreous body in the aphakic eye. *Acta Ophthalmol Suppl* 1987;182:160–162.

37. Sander B, Larsen M, Moldow B, et al. Diabetic macular edema: passive and active transport of fluorescein through the blood-retina barrier. *Invest Ophthalmol Vis Sci* 2001;42:433–438.

38. Smith RT, Lee CM, Charles HC, et al. Quantification of diabetic macular edema. *Arch Ophthalmol* 1987;105:218–222.

39. Averous K, Erginay A, Timsit J, et al. Resolution of diabetic macular oedema following high altitude exercise. *Acta Ophthalmol Scand* 2006;84:830–831.

40. Nguyen QD, Shah SM, Van Anden E, et al. Supplemental oxygen improves diabetic macular edema: a pilot study. *Invest Ophthalmol Vis Sci* 2004;45:617–624.

41. Maeda N, Tano Y. Intraocular oxygen tension in eyes with proliferative diabetic retinopathy with and without vitreous. *Graefes Arch Clin Exp Ophthalmol* 1996;234(Suppl 1):S66–S69.

42. Molnar I, Poitry S, Tsacopoulos M, et al. Effect of laser photocoagulation on oxygenation of the retina in miniature pigs. *Invest Ophthalmol Vis Sci* 1985;26:1410–1414.

43. Novack RL, Stefansson E, Hatchell DL. Intraocular pressure effects on optic nerve-head oxidative metabolism measured in vivo. *Graefes Arch Clin Exp Ophthalmol* 1990;228:128–133.

44. Pournaras CJ. Retinal oxygen distribution. Its role in the physiopathology of vasoproliferative microangiopathies. *Retina* 1995;15:332–347.

45. Stefansson E, Hatchell DL, Fisher BL, et al. Panretinal photocoagulation and retinal oxygenation in normal and diabetic cats. *Am J Ophthalmol* 1986;101:657–664.

46. Stefansson E, Machemer R, de Juan E Jr, et al. Retinal oxygenation and laser treatment in patients with diabetic retinopathy. *Am J Ophthalmol* 1992;113:36–38.

47. Arnarsson A, Stefansson E. Laser treatment and the mechanism of edema reduction in branch retinal vein occlusion. *Invest Ophthalmol Vis Sci* 2000;41:877–879.

48. Gottfredsdottir MS, Stefansson E, Jonasson F, et al. Retinal vasoconstriction after laser treatment for diabetic macular edema. *Am J Ophthalmol* 1993;115:64–67.

49. Wilson CA, Stefansson E, Klombers L, et al. Optic disk neovascularization and retinal vessel diameter in diabetic retinopathy. *Am J Ophthalmol* 1988;106:131–134.

50. Stefansson E, Loftsson T. The Stokes-Einstein equation and the physiological effects of vitreous surgery. *Acta Ophthalmol Scand* 2006;84:718–719.

51. Holekamp NM, Shui YB, Beebe D. Lower intraocular oxygen tension in diabetic patients: possible contribution to decreased incidence of nuclear sclerotic cataract. *Am J Ophthalmol* 2006;141:1027–1032.

52. Holekamp NM, Shui YB, Beebe DC. Vitrectomy surgery increases oxygen exposure to the lens: a possible mechanism for nuclear cataract formation. *Am J Ophthalmol* 2005;139:302–310.

53. Stefansson E, Novack RL, Hatchell DL. Vitrectomy prevents retinal hypoxia in branch retinal vein occlusion. *Invest Ophthalmol Vis Sci* 1990;31:284–289.

54. Kylstra JA, Wierzbicki T, Wolbarsht ML, et al. The relationship between retinal vessel tortuosity, diameter, and transmural pressure. *Graefes Arch Clin Exp Ophthalmol* 1986;224:477–480.

55. Larsen M. Unilateral macular oedema secondary to retinal venous congestion without occlusion in patients with diabetes mellitus. *Acta Ophthalmol Scand* 2005;83:428–435.

56. Stefansson E, Landers MB 3rd, Wolbarsht ML. Oxygenation and vasodilatation in relation to diabetic and other proliferative retinopathies. *Ophthalmic Surg* 1983;14:209–226.

57. Karasheva G, Goebel W, Klink T, et al. Changes in macular thickness and depth of anterior chamber in patients after filtration surgery. *Graefes Arch Clin Exp Ophthalmol* 2003;241:170–175.

58. Iturralde D, Spaide RF, Meyerle CB, et al. Intravitreal bevacizumab (Avastin) treatment of macular edema in central retinal vein occlusion: a short-term study. *Retina* 2006;26:279–284.

59. Mason JO 3rd, Albert MA Jr, Vail R. Intravitreal bevacizumab (Avastin) for refractory pseudophakic cystoid macular edema. *Retina* 2006;26:356–357.

60. Audren F, Erginay A, Haouchine B, et al. Intravitreal triamcinolone acetonide for diffuse diabetic macular oedema: 6-month results of a prospective controlled trial. *Acta Ophthalmol Scand* 2006;84:624–630.

61. Edelman JL, Lutz D, Castro MR. Corticosteroids inhibit VEGF-induced vascular leakage in a rabbit model of blood-retinal and blood-aqueous barrier breakdown. *Exp Eye Res* 2005;80:249–258.

62. Jonas JB. Intravitreal triamcinolone acetonide for treatment of intraocular oedematous and neovascular diseases. *Acta Ophthalmol Scand* 2005;83:645–663.

63. Sorensen TL, Haamann P, Villumsen J, et al. Intravitreal triamcinolone for macular oedema: efficacy in relation to aetiology. *Acta Ophthalmol Scand* 2005;83:67–70.

64. Vinores SA, Xiao WH, Aslam S, et al. Implication of the hypoxia response element of the VEGF promoter in mouse models of retinal and choroidal neovascularization, but not retinal vascular development. *J Cell Physiol* 2006;206:749–758.

# Imaging of the Macula

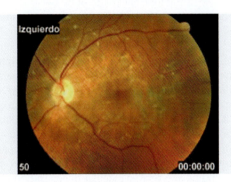

# Fluorescein Angiography of the Ocular Fundus

Eleonora Lavaque ■ D. Virgil Alfaro, III ■ John B. Kerrison

## INTRODUCTION

Over the past thirty years, fluorescein angiography has been technically refined and continues to be a vital tool in the evaluation, diagnosis, and follow-up of patients with retinal and choroidal disease. The principles of fluorescein angiography were first described in 1960 by Angus McLean and Edward Maumenee. In its initial usage, fluorescein was given by intravenous injection followed by angioscopy at the slit lamp using a cobalt blue filter without photographic documentation (1). Later Novotny and Alvis presented the first human fluorescein angiogram, what they called "a method of photographing fluorescein circulating in blood vessels" (2).

Currently, two intravascular dyes are in use, sodium fluorescein and indocyanine green. They produce a different angiographic pattern because of their physical and chemical properties. By far, fluorescein angiography is more commonly used than indocyanine green angiography because it is inexpensive, easy to use, and diagnostically useful for a wide range of retinal diseases, many of them illustrated in this chapter. Indocyanine green angiography is selected for cases that require visualization of the choroidal vasculature or the imaging of structures blocked by hemorrhage, melanin, xanthophyll pigment, lipid exudates, retinal pigment epithelial detachment, or serosanguinous fluid (3).

## PRINCIPLES

Luminescence is the emission of light in the visible spectrum from any source that has been stimulated by electromagnetic radiation. It occurs when energy in the form of electromagnetic radiation is absorbed at a shorter wavelength, shifted, and re-emitted at a longer visible wavelength. The process involves decay from a wavelength of higher energy to a wavelength at a lower energy state. Fluorescence is the luminescence maintained in response to continuous excitation. Therefore, fluorescence is present only if the excitation is present.

Retinal angiography is possible because of the chemical and physical properties of sodium fluorescein. It is a water-soluble, yellow-red hydrocarbon ($C_{20}H_{12}O_5Na$) that is highly fluorescent, nontoxic, and inexpensive. It absorbs blue light energy between 465 and 490 nm and emits yellow-green light at a wavelength of 520 to 530 nm. In other words, if a blue light is projected as an exciting light from a camera into the eye, the sodium fluorescein circulating inside the eye will absorb and discharge a green-yellow re-emission or responder light that will come towards the camera. Eighty percent of intravenously injected sodium fluorescein is bound by serum proteins while 20% is unbound or free. Only the 20% of sodium fluorescein not bound to protein will fluoresce.

Two filters are placed in a camera for angiography: a blue filter and a green-yellow filter. The projector filter is a blue filter that allows only the blue wavelengths of the color spectrum to pass and reach the eye. The receptor filter is a green-yellow filter that allows only re-emitted green-yellow wavelengths to pass back towards the camera without residual blue light reflected. A mismatch of these two filters allows part of the reflected blue light from the fundus to come back through the system. This will make nonfluorescent objects appear to fluoresce. In other words, pseudofluorescence occurs when the two filters are overlapped. For example if a blue filter overlaps the green one, both blue and green light will pass. This phenomenon creates a decrease in contrast, increased background illumination, and loss of photographic detail (4).

*Autofluorescence* is the emission of fluorescent light from the ocular fundus in the absence of sodium fluorescein. Conditions that cause autofluorescence are optic nerve drusen and astrocytic hamartomata. More recently, other autofluorescent substances in the ocular fundus have been recognized using imaging techniques that give more information than obtained by conventional methods, such as fundus photography and fluorescein angiography (5). These techniques have permitted topographic mapping of lipofuscin distribution in the retinal pigment epithelium (RPE) as well as of other fluorophores occurring in the outer retina and subretinal space. Excessive accumulation of lipofuscin granules in the lysosomal compartment of RPE cells represents a common downstream pathogenetic pathway in various hereditary and complex retinal diseases, including age-related macular degeneration (5).

## EQUIPMENT

Immediately after the injection of dye, photographs are taken. Cameras must be able to take rapid sequence images to ensure a high quality angiogram. Photographs may be film based or digital based. Digital fluorescein angiography stores information in an electronic record that allows immediate study of the angiogram and modification of illumination. This allows evaluation and adjustment of the quality of a study while it is still in progress. However, good stereoscopic images are best obtained in film-based photographs.

## DYE ADMINISTRATION

Before the angiogram, the patient should be informed about the nature and side effects of the study. After signing a consent form, the patient is seated in front of the camera with one forearm extended. Color and red-free photographs are taken. An antecubital, forearm, or hand vein is cannulated. Prior to injecting a bolus of fluorescein, it is important to administer a small test dose injection in order to ensure that the dye is properly flowing into the vein. Ensuring proper flow will allow one to avoid painful extravasation with bolus injection that may occur if the intravenous cannulation site is infiltrated. Then, 5 to 10 milliliters of fluorescein dye is injected intravenously. The injection is given rapidly in order to ensure quality images.

There are few immediate side effects associated with fluorescein injection, particularly nausea and vomiting. Later effects include temporary tan or yellow skin color, fluorescent urine, and photosensitivity for 24 hours. Severe reactions are rare and include hives, asthmatic symptoms, and laryngeal edema. These can usually be managed by intravenous administration of cortisone. Syncope, anaphylactic reaction, myocardial infarction, and respiratory or cardiac arrest are very rare events.

Fluorescein is a safe drug. It is advisable to have equipment and plans necessary to manage serious reactions. Such reactions typically appear in the first minutes following the intravenous injection, although it takes 24 hours for the liver and the kidney to eliminate fluorescein completely. Fluorescein angiography will interfere with laboratory testing that utilizes fluorescent-based methods.

## ANATOMIC AND PHYSIOLOGIC CONSIDERATIONS

In comparison with ophthalmoscopy or color photography, blood vessels appear larger with fluorescein angiography. With angiography it is possible to see the entire caliber of the vessel, as compared to ophthalmoscopy or color photography, where it is only possible to see the central blood column and not the outer clear plasma layer.

The pattern of fluorescence is influenced by the size of the sodium fluorescein molecules and anatomic considerations. Sodium fluorescein does not cross intact retinal endothelial tight junctions (the inner blood-retinal barrier) or zonula occludens of the RPE (the outer blood-retinal barrier). However, it leaks freely through the porelike fenestrations of the choriocapillaris.

The macula is an oval area measuring 3.5 disc diameters between the vascular arcades and appears dark on fluorescein angiography. It is characterized by a high concentration of cone photoreceptors, the thickest ganglion cell layer, and the tallest RPE cells with high concentrations of lipofuscin and melanin. These characteristics block fluorescence emanating from the choriocapillaris beneath the macula, giving its dark appearance on fluorescein angiography.

The fovea, the center of the macula, is even darker due to the absence of retinal vessels. The fovea contains xanthophyll pigment, a progressive thinning of the inner retinal layers, and no retinal vessels. The foveal avascular zone, referred to as the FAZ, is approximately 400 to 500 um in diameter and is the darkest area at the center of the macula on an angiogram.

In a normal angiogram, fluorescein leaks from the porelike fenestrated choriocapillaris and is absorbed by the sclera. If there is chorioretinal atrophy, the fluorescence of the sclera may be observed. Bruch's membrane allows the transmission of fluorescent light from the dye in the choriocapillaris as well as passage of the dye itself. As the dye continues to diffuse toward the retina from the choriocapillaris, the close apposition of the RPE cells prevents the dye from diffusing further into the subretinal space and retina.

In a normal angiogram, the optic disc fluoresces primarily due to fluorescein that has diffused into it from the surrounding permeable choriocapillaris.

## NORMAL FLUORESCEIN ANGIOGRAM

A normal angiogram must be well understood and interpreted in order to provide a basis for comparison to abnormal angiograms. An angiogram will be interpreted as abnormal in terms of the amount of fluorescence, whether increased or decreased, in a specific area.

Prior to injection, color and red-free photographs are taken (Fig. 5-1). They are useful for correlation with pathologic areas found in an angiogram. No fluorescence should be evident at this stage. If there is fluorescence prior to injection of fluorescein, it is due to suboptimal matching of the two filters, pseudofluorescence, or less commonly a pathologic structure that is autofluorescent, such as optic nerve drusen. The most common autofluorescent structures of the fundus are flecks from fundus flavimaculatus, Best vitelliform lesions, and optic nerve drusen (Fig. 5-2) (6).

A normal angiogram has classically been divided into progressive phases: prearterial, arterial, arteriovenous, venous, and recirculation. The prearterial phase is the first phase, where fluorescein fills the choroid and choriocapillaris, occurring one

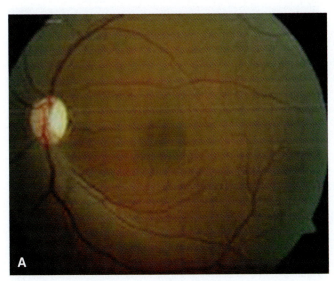 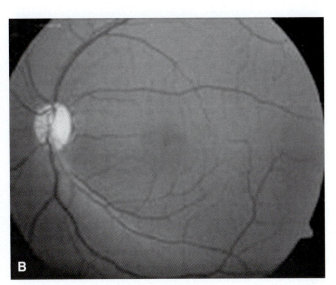

**Figure 5-1.** Color **(A)** and red free **(B)** photos of the ocular fundus.

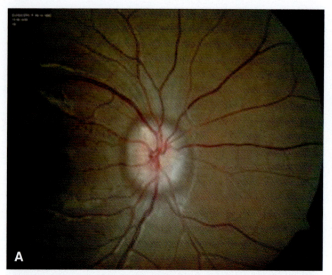

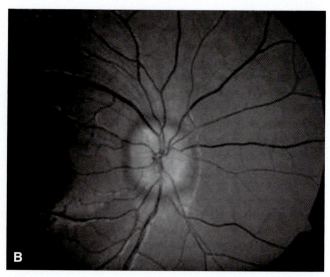

**Figure 5-2.** Color **(A)** and red free **(B)** photos of optic disc drusen.

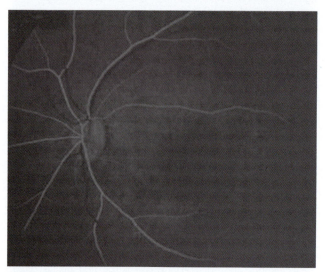

**Figure 5-3.** The arterial phase progress and ends when the arteries are completely filled.

second before the retinal arterial circulation. It has a distinct pattern that is patchy and variable even in normal angiograms. The arterial phase progresses and ends when the arteries are completely filled (Fig. 5-3). The arteriovenous phase follows and is a transition phase with filling of the arteries and the veins (Fig. 5-4). The venous phase begins with laminar venous flow and persists until they are filled (Fig. 5-5).

The normal time between the artery filling and the complete vein filling is 8 to 12 seconds. The juxtafoveal capillaries are maximally fluorescent during this phase (Fig. 5-6). The recirculation phase starts when the venous phase has finished and with the return of fluorescein from the kidney and liver passage. It begins 30 seconds after the dye has been injected and lasts about 2 minutes and 30 seconds. It has little contrast and is not useful unless a pathologic structure leaks progressively during this phase (Fig. 5-7).

Due to the retinal pigment epithelial barrier and the rapid leakage of fluorescein from the choriocapillaris, the choroidal anatomy is not clearly seen in the angiogram. Cilioretinal vessels fill simultaneously with the choroidal vasculature,

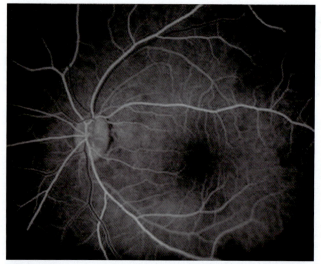

**Figure 5-4.** The arteriovenous phase is a transition phase that begins with the appearance of laminar flow in the veins.

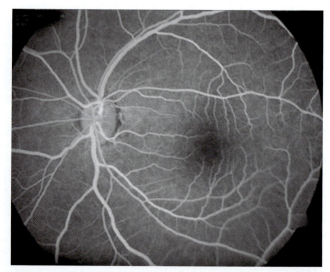

**Figure 5-5.** The venous phase begins with laminar venous flow and persists until they are filled.

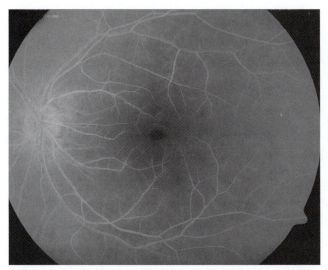

**Figure 5-6.** The normal time between the artery filling and the complete vein filling is 8 to 12 seconds. The juxtafoveal capillaries are maximally fluorescent during this phase.

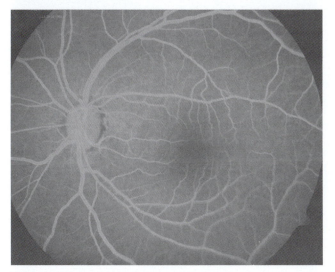

**Figure 5-7.** The recirculation phase starts when the venous phase has finished and with the return of fluorescein from kidney and liver passage. It begins 30 seconds after the dye has been injected and lasts 2 to 3 minutes. It has little contrast but may show pathologic structures that increasingly leak as the study progresses.

1 second before the retinal vessels. A cilioretinal artery is present in 32% of patients (Fig. 5-8) (7). Pathologic vessels giving rise to choroidal neovascular membranes are derived from the choroid and are also filled before the retinal vessels. The choroidal and the retinal phase, as they are separated from 0.5 to 1 second, usually overlap.

## ABNORMAL FLUORESCEIN ANGIOGRAM

A pathological angiogram is characterized by structures that are hypofluorescent or hyperfluorescent in comparison with normal.

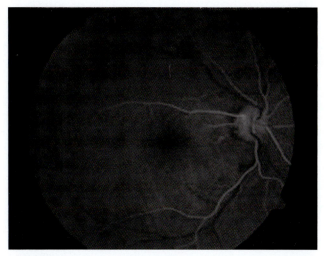

**Figure 5-8.** The cilioretinal vessels fluoresce with the choroidal vessels, filling 1 second before the retinal vessels.

## HYPOFLUORESCENCE

Hypofluorescence is caused by blockage of the underlying fluorescence or by a vascular filling defect. Blockage occurs when an overlying opaque substance covers the underlying fluorescence (Table 5-1). Common examples are melanin

### TABLE 5-1   CAUSES OF BLOCKED HYPOFLUORESCENCE

| Causes | Examples |
| --- | --- |
| Congenital | Grouped pigmentation<br>Congenital hypertrophy of the retinal pigment epithelium<br>Choroidal nevus |
| Inborn errors of metabolism | Primary hyperoxaluria |
| Infiltrative | Leopard-spot pattern after treatment of ocular lymphomas |
| Inflammatory | Hyperpigmented chorioretinal scars |
| Infectious | Rubella retinopathy (salt-and-pepper pigmentary changes) |
| Trauma | Pigmented epiretinal membranes |
| Degenerative | Pigmentary clumping in age-related macular degeneration |
| Hemorrhage | |
| Vitreous | Proliferative diabetic retinopathy<br>Proliferative sickle cell retinopathy<br>Retinal arterial macroaneurysm |
| Retinal | Background diabetic retinopathy<br>Retinal arterial macroaneurysm |
| Subretinal | Choroidal neovascularization<br>Retinal arterial macroaneurysm |

From Spaide RF. Fluorescein angiography. In: *Diseases of the vitreous and retina*. Philadelphia: WB Saunders, 1999, with permission.

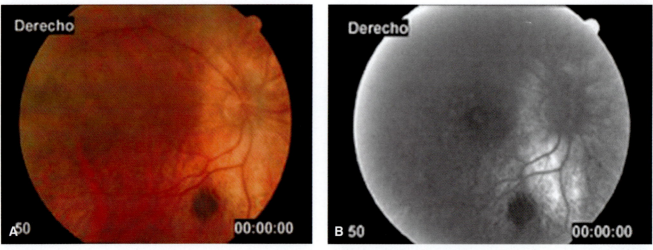

**Figure 5-9.** Choroidal nevus **(A)**. Note the blockage of the underlying fluorescence by the choroidal melanin **(B)**.

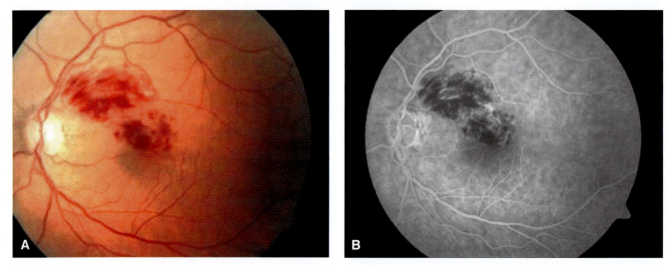

**Figure 5-10.** Retinal flame shaped hemorrhages from a branch vein occlusion **(A)**. Note the blockage of the underlying choroidal fluorescence from the blood located in the nerve fiber layer **(B)**.

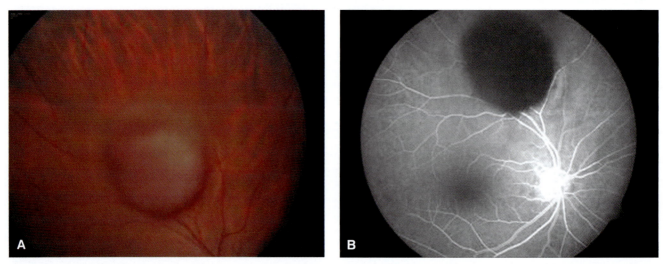

**Figure 5-11.** Retinal subhyaloid hemorrhage from valsalva maculopathy **(A)**. Note the blockage of the underlying fluorescence of the retinal vessels **(B)**.

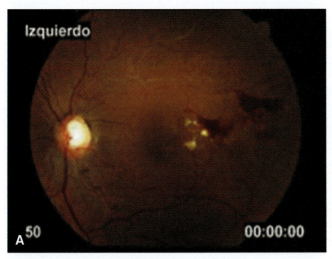
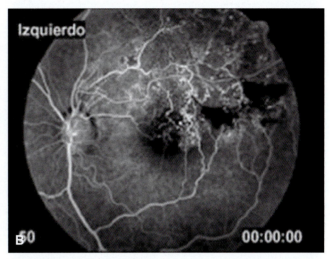

**Figure 5-12.** Color photograph of a superior and temporal branch vein obstruction **(A)**. Note the hypofluorescence due to the nonperfused capillary bed and blocked fluorescence by intraretinal hemorrhage **(B)**. Also, hyperfluorescent vessels are present due to slow blood drainage through collaterals.

(Fig. 5-9) and blood (Figs. 5-10 and 5-11). Blockage may also be caused by lipofuscin or inflammatory cells. The goal of interpretation is to determine the anatomic location and the nature of the blocking substance. It is useful to note the relationship of retinal vessels relative to the blocking substance in determining the anatomic location of the blocking substance.

Vascular filling defects may be present in the retinal and choroidal vessels. A retinal arterial occlusion will produce hypofluorescence of the vessels occluded as well as in their corresponding area of perfusion. On the other hand, a retinal vein occlusion can produce hypofluorescence because of closure of large areas of the capillary bed or hyperfluorescence because of slow blood drainage (Fig. 5-12).

## HYPERFLUORESCENCE

Hyperfluorescence is caused by increased intensity over the normal fluorescence or by fluorescence in areas that normally do not fluoresce. An increase in intensity over normal fluorescence occurs in the absence of the blocking pigment from the RPE. This is referred to as a window defect (Table 5-2). Hyperfluorescence also occurs from progressive and abnormal dye leakage from pathologies that cause breakdown of the blood ocular barrier (Table 5-3).

Window defects may be observed in age-related macular degeneration with geographic atrophy (Fig. 5-13), drusen (Fig. 5-14), and multifocal choroiditis (Fig. 5-15). Hyperfluorescence from dye leakage occurs in cystoid macular edema from Irvine Gass Syndrome and uveitis. Cystoid spaces are formed from incompetent perifoveal capillaries at the plexiform layer resulting in a petaloidlike pattern of hyperfluorescence (Fig. 5-16). Other examples of retinal vascular leakage are microaneurysms in diabetic patients and vasculitis

| TABLE 5-2 | CAUSES OF HYPERFLUORESCENCE FROM TRANSMISSION DEFECTS | |
|---|---|
| **Type of Transmission Detect** | **Examples** |
| Congenital | Ocular albinism<br>Cone dystrophy<br>Stargardt's disease |
| Infiltrative | Leopard-spot pattern after treatment of ocular lymphomas |
| Inflammatory | Healed areas after resolution of acute multifocal posterior placoid pigment epitheliopathy (AMPPPE) |
| Infectious | Myiasis tracks |
| Radiation | Retinal pigment epithelial atrophy after photic maculopathy |
| Toxic | Chloroquine |
| Trauma | Choroidal rupture<br>Macular holes |
| Degenerative | Retinal pigment epithelial rips<br>Retinal pigment epithelial rarefaction over drusen<br>Geographic atrophy<br>Lacquer cracks in degenerative myopia |

From Spaide RF. Fluorescein angiography. In: *Diseases of the vitreous and retina*. Philadelphia: WB Saunders, 1999, with permission.

(Fig. 5-17). Neovascularization, as occurs in proliferative diabetic retinopathy, produces hyperfluorescence that becomes greater with the progression of the angiogram due to incompetent vessels (Fig. 5-18).

## TABLE 5-3   CAUSES OF HYPERFLUORESCENCE FROM ABNORMAL LEAKAGE OF FLUORESCEIN DYE

| Types of Causes of Breakdown of Blood–Ocular Barrier | Inner Blood–Retinal Barrier (Retinal Vessels) | Outer Blood–Retinal Barrier (Retinal Pigment Epithelium) |
|---|---|---|
| Congenital | Coat's disease<br>Parafoveal telangiectasis | |
| Ischemic | Ocular ischemia syndrome<br>Venous occlusive disease | Thrombotic thrombocytopenic purpura<br>Malignant hypertension |
| Inflammatory | Retinal vasculitis | Vgot–Koyanagi–Harada disease<br>Posterior scleritis |
| Radiation | Radiation retinopathy | Photic maculopathy |
| Infiltrative | Lymphoma | Lymphoma |
| Infectious | Viral retinitis | Tuberculosis |
| Traction | Epimacular membrane | |
| Degenerative | Retinal vascular leakage in chronic detachments | Retinal pigment epithelial ooze over occult choroidal neovascularization |
| Neovascularization | Proliferative diabetic retinopathy<br>Sickle retinopathy | Choroidal neovascularization |
| Excessive hydrostatic pressure | Carotid cavernous sinus fistula | Central serous chorioretinopathy |

From Spaide RF. Fluorescein angiography. In: *Diseases of the vitreous and retina*. Philadelphia: WB Saunders, 1999, with permission.

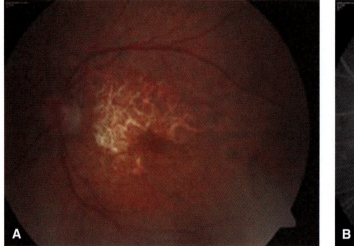
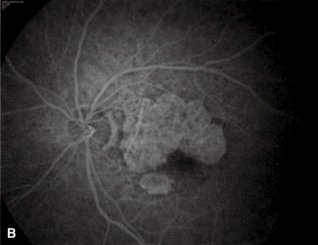

**Figure 5-13.** Geographic atrophy **(A)**. The circumscribed area of RPE atrophy appears as a window defect on the angiogram **(B)**.

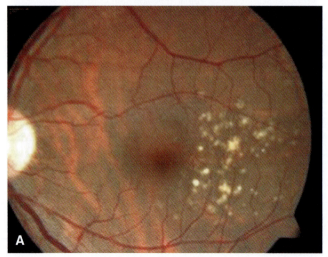
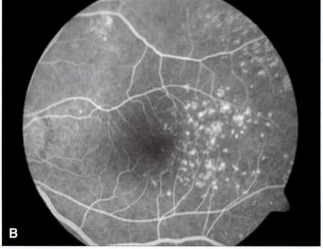

**Figure 5-14.** Drusen **(A)**. Multiple discrete soft drusen hyperfluoresce on the angiogram **(B)**.

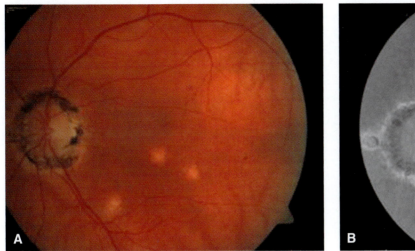
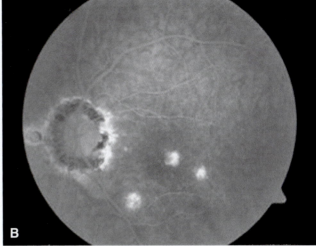

**Figure 5-15.** Multifocal choroiditis fundus **(A)**. Hyperfluorescence from macula spots and peripapillary chorioretinal atrophy **(B)**.

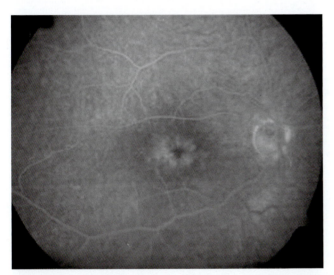

**Figure 5-16.** Late phase fluorescein angiogram of a cystoid macular edema. Note its classic petaloid pattern.

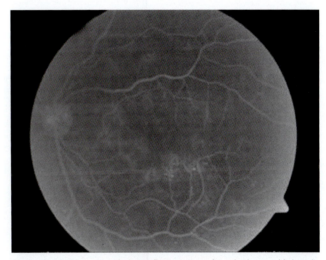

**Figure 5-18.** New vessels hyperfluorescence from leakage with breakdown of the blood retinal barrier.

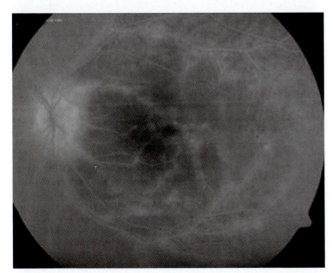

**Figure 5-17.** Perivascular hyperfluorescence from vascular leakage.

Hyperfluorescence from leakage into the subretinal space has a different pattern. Central serous retinopathy, characterized by a localized neurosensory detachment, will *slowly* accumulate and pool dye in the subretinal space as it as it passes from the choriocapillaris through a small retinal pigment defect (Fig. 5-19). On the other hand, choroidal neovascular membranes associated with subretinal fluid display a *rapid* pooling because of breakdown of the outer blood-retinal barrier (Fig. 5-20).

Staining with fluorescein can also be found with normal and abnormal structures of the ocular fundus, both a chorioretinal scar (Fig. 5-21) and a damaged Bruch's membrane stain (Fig. 5-22). Scleral staining is seen in pathologies reduce the blockage effect of the retinal pigment epithelium like albinism and highly myopic fundus (Fig. 5-23).

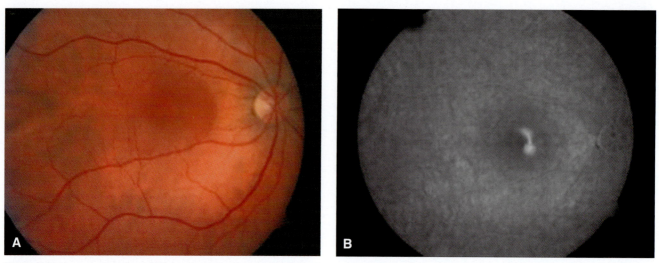

**Figure 5-19.** A serous macular detachment in central serous retinopathy fundus **(A)**. Late phase angiogram shows hyperfluorescence from leakage with a pinpoint focus and the characteristic "smokestack" **(B)**.

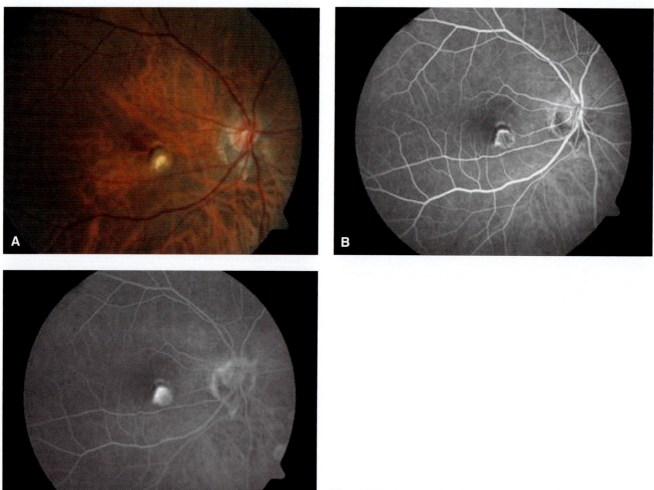

**Figure 5-20.** A classic choroidal neovascular membrane **(A)**. Note the hyperfluorescence in the early phase of the angiogram **(B)** and pooling in the late phase of the angiogram **(C)**.

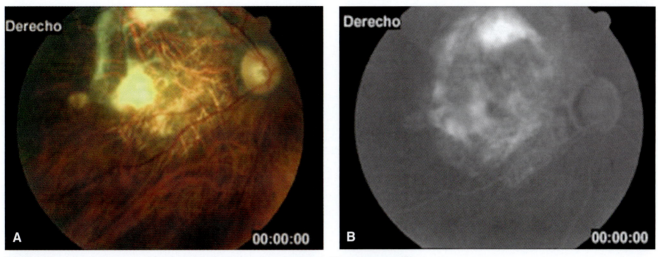

**Figure 5-21.** A chorioretinal scar **(A)**. Hyperfluorescence in the late phase of the angiogram **(B)**.

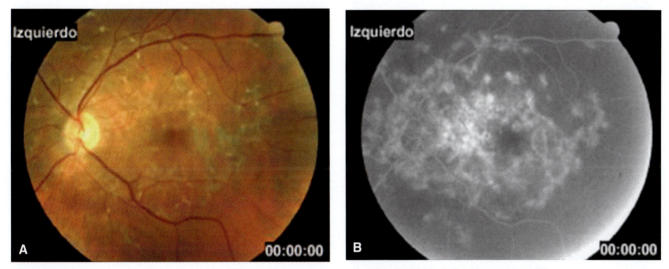

**Figure 5-22.** Angioid streaks of the ocular fundus **(A)**. Hyperfluorescence corresponds to the cracks in Bruch's membrane **(B)**.

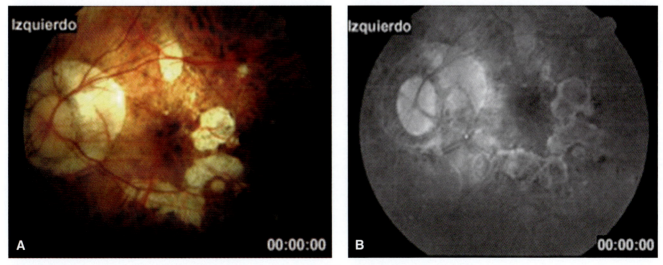

**Figure 5-23.** High myopia fundus **(A)**. Hyperfluorescence due to atrophy of the retinal pigment epithelium **(B)**.

## SUMMARY

Fluorescein angiography continues to be germane to the identification, diagnosis and treatment of various macular diseases. Not only does it provide anatomic information but also functional information on the status of the blood retinal barrier.

### References

1. Maclean AL, Maumenee AE. Hemangioma of the choroid. *Am J Ophthalmol* 1960;50:3–11.

2. Novotny HR, Alvis DL. A method of photographing fluorescence in circulating blood in the human retina. *Circulation* 1961;24:82–86.
3. Arevalo JF, Fuenmayor-Rivera D, Giral A, et al. Aspectos Grales e interpretación de la angiografía con verde de Indocianina. In: *Retina médica*. Caracas, Venezuela: Amolca, 1997;3:40–52.
4. Johnson R, McDonald HR, Ai E, et al. Fluorescein angiography: basic principles and interpretation. In: Ryan, SJ (ed), *Retina*. Philadelphia: Elsevier, 2006;51:874–916.
5. Schmitz-Valckenberg S, Holz FG, Bird AC, et al. Fundus autofluorescence imaging: review and perspectives. *Retina* 2008;28(3):385–409.
6. Miler SA. Fluorescence in Best's viteliform dystrophy, lipofuscin and fundus flavimatulatus. *Br J Ophthalmol* 1978;62:256–260.
7. Justice J, Lehmann RP. Cilioretinal Arteries. *Arch Ophthalmol* 1976;94: 1355–1358.

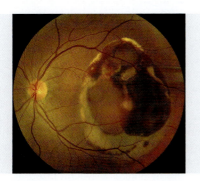

# Indocyanine Green Angiography of the Ocular Fundus

Michael D. Ober ■ Howard F. Fine ■ Louis Chang ■ Christina M. Klais
■ Lawrence A. Yannuzzi

Fluorescein angiography (FA) has revolutionized the diagnosis, classification, and management of retinal diseases. It allows visualization of the retinal circulation and the integrity of the blood retinal barrier. Although the resolution of the retina provided by FA is unparalleled, it has limited transmission through the retinal pigment epithelium (RPE), restricting its ability to image the choroidal circulation (1). Furthermore, relatively small amounts of blood, lipid, pigment, or serosanguineous fluid can significantly impair the penetration of fluorescence.

Indocyanine green (ICG) angiography functions best in several areas where FA has limited utility, such as imaging the choroidal vasculature or through hemorrhage. The recognition of the role of the choroid in retinal diseases as well as the wide availability of digital angiography has increased interest in ICG angiography. The applications for ICG angiography continue to expand, particularly in differential diagnosis, disease management, targeting of therapy, and furthering our understanding of the etiopathogenesis of various diseases.

## PHYSICAL AND CHEMICAL PROPERTIES

ICG is a water-soluble tricarbocyanine dye. It contains sodium iodide (less than 5%), which increases solubility in blood. It comes supplied with an aqueous solvent which yields a solution with a pH between 5.5 and 6.5. ICG will precipitate at high concentration or when mixed in normal saline. Once mixed with the supplied solvent, it tends to decay at a rate of approximately 10% over 10 hours and should be used within this time.

ICG shows peak absorption at 605 nm and maximal fluorescence at 835 nm, which are both in the near-infrared portion of the electromagnetic spectrum. These wavelengths permit superior penetration of ocular tissues allowing detection through pigmented barriers such as the RPE and hemorrhage. ICG is rapidly and nearly completely bound to plasma proteins (98%) which help to retain the dye within vascular spaces. This property aids in delineation of the choriocapillaris, which is difficult to image with fluorescein because of rapid extravasation into the extravascular space (2).

ICG is excreted exclusively by the liver where is to secreted unaltered in bile. There is negligible renal, respiratory, or cerebrospinal uptake, and ICG does not cross the placenta (2). These properties are likely due to its strong binding to plasma proteins.

## HISTORY OF MEDICAL USE

ICG was first used in medicine in 1956 to record dilution in whole blood (3). It was injected in a single bolus and samples of blood were removed at set time periods to analyze for ICG concentration. This technique was soon applied to determine cardiac output (4). Once it was established that ICG is excreted exclusively by the liver, the rate of concentration decrease was used to measure hepatic blood flood and function (5,6).

Kogure and Choromokos were the first to attempt ocular ICG angiography in dogs (7,8). After discussing their findings with David, they together performed the first ICG angiogram in monkeys (9). Later, David et al. published a discussion of the first human ICG angiogram in 1969 via an intracarotid injection (10). Flower and Hochheimer performed the first human intravenous ICG angiogram in 1972, which successfully imaged the choroidal circulation (11,12). Through the next several years, Flower, Patz, Hochheimer, and their colleagues refined the procedure and published reports detailing normal and pathological states of the choroidal circulation (12–15).

Videoangiography with ICG was introduced in 1984 by Tokoro (16) who worked along with Hayashi et al. to subsequently make adjustments to the excitation and barrier filters (17–19). This new system provided an excellent movie format of the choroidal circulation, but individual images suffered from poor resolution and the halogen bulb risked retinal toxicity when used for extended periods. The progression to digital ICG videoangiography was pioneered by Guyer et al. who were the first to display their results immediately on a high-resolution monitor (20). Yannuzzi et al. further modified an ICG video angiographic system, by adding a synchronized flash rather than the continuous illumination in previous renditions, which reduced overall light exposure and allowed later images to be captured (21). This system was the first to show the characteristics of late phase ICG angiography which have become familiar today.

## TOXICITY

ICG is a relatively safe dye and considered to have fewer adverse reactions than fluorescein (22). A classification system has been published by Hope-Ross et al., dividing adverse reactions into three categories (23). Mild reactions, which are defined as transient and resolve without treatment, occur in approximately 0.15% of patients. These include nausea, vomiting, extravasation, sneezing and pruritus. Moderate reactions occur in 0.02% and may require medical treatment although complete recovery occurs without severe sequelae. These include urticaria, syncope, fever, nerve palsy, and local tissue necrosis. Severe reactions occur in 0.05% of patients and exhibit prolonged effects requiring treatment with variable recovery including bronchospasm, laryngospasm, cardiac events, seizures, and anaphylaxis. At least three deaths attributed to ICG administration can be found in the literature (23–25), although none of them occurred during ocular angiography.

Adverse reactions do not appear to be related to the dose injected (26). There also does not seem to be a significant correlation to previous allergies to ICG or other medications (23). There is, however, a relation to adverse reactions and renal failure (27,28). While impaired renal function should not change the excretion of ICG, patients undergoing hemodialysis may be hypersensitive due to many factors (28).

ICG does contain iodine and therefore should be used with caution, if at all, in those with sensitivity to iodine. Other high-risk groups for adverse reactions include those with hepatic disease. Overall, adverse reactions to ICG angiography are very rare and it generally is a safe diagnostic test.

## PHOTOGRAPHIC TECHNIQUE

To obtain ICG angiographic images using a digital fundus camera, typically color, red-free, and/or green-free images are taken in the area of interest. ICG angiography can be performed before or after FA because the barrier filters for each study will exclude the dye from the other. For eyes receiving combined FA/ICG angiography, the transit phase is typically shot using FA, unless identification of feeder vessels is required. When possible, images are taken immediately after injection of the dye to demonstrate the early phase of choroidal filling. Note that should the photographer wait until the dye is first noted on the alignment and focus monitor, the early phase of the study may be missed. Images are obtained in a rapid, sequential manner at approximately 1-second intervals until the retinal and choroidal circulations are at maximum brightness. There is no direct viewing of the fundus; therefore, the image exposure must be continuously adjusted by altering the flash illumination control or gain setting based upon the image displayed on a high-resolution monitor. Initially, the gain must be set high to compensate for low fluorescence levels during the early choroidal filling phase, but a reduction must be made immediately to compensate for the rapid influx of dye during the early retinal and later recirculation phases.

Once the point of maximal brightness has been captured, images are taken at 1-minute intervals until 5 minutes into the study. Thereafter, images are obtained at 3- to 5- minute intervals until satisfactory late images are available. Late ICG images are characterized by optic nerve and dark retinal vessels silhouetted against the relatively hyperfluorescent diffuse gray background of the choroid. Throughout the course of the study, the liver continuously removes ICG from circulation resulting in a gradual decrease of the fluorescence which requires a corresponding increase in the intensity of the flash illumination to maintain uniform images.

## INTERPRETATION

The interpretation of ICG angiographic images is more complex than that of FA. It is based on the same principles, which include classification into areas of relative hyper- and hypofluorescence during specific phases of the angiogram. The early phase of the ICG angiogram shows the larger choroidal vessels individually. Over time the choriocapillaris continues to emit a diffuse hyperfluorescence while dye is removed from the intravascular circulation making the individual choroidal vessels indistinguishable. The degree of relative fluorescence in ICG is dependent on many variables, the most important of which is often the internal structure of the lesion itself, but also upon the intensity of the exciting light source, concentration of dye, the particular technique used (scanning

laser ophthalmoscope versus digital fundus camera), as well as location and quality of the barrier and excitation filters.

Hyperfluorescence can occur for several reasons. Defects in the RPE yield areas of transmitted fluorescence (window defect) which are hyperfluorescent in early phases. The late phase appearance depends on the status of the choriocapillaris. When it is intact, the area becomes hyperfluorescent. In areas with choriocapillaris loss (from atrophy or other), however, hypofluorescence in the late phases predominates. Abnormal vessels are also a source of hyperfluorescence that can be distinguished from leakage, which occurs in later frames of the angiogram and increases in size and relative intensity over time. Autofluorescence can also occur, although it is much more uncommon than with FA. For example, certain blood breakdown products have fluorescent properties that overlap with ICG yielding hyperfluorescence prior to dye injection in some patients with subretinal hemorrhage.

Hypofluorescence in early phases typically occurs secondary to blocked fluorescence or vascular abnormalities. Blocked fluorescence is seen secondary to many conditions such as increased pigmentation, hemorrhage, myelination, exudation, and/or fluid, among others. Choroidal vascular abnormalities are emphasized over retinal circulatory conditions in ICG. Choriocapillaris atrophy, physiologic filling defects, choroidal ischemia, or infarctions, among others, will yield hypofluorescent areas in the early phases.

The terms used to describe FA images do not always apply directly to ICG angiography; therefore, several terms specific to ICG have been developed. A "hot spot" is an area of focal hyperfluorescence less than one disc diameter in size that is usually associated with an area of active neovascularization seen most commonly with retinal angiomatous proliferation (RAP), polypoidal choroidal vasculopathy (PCV), or focal occult choroidal neovascularization (CNV). Plaques are defined as areas of hyperfluorescence greater than one disc diameter in size seen on late phases of the angiogram. Plaques occur most commonly in areas of quiescent neovascularization and can be seen with an adjacent hot spot indicating a zone of activity.

There is a wide range of variation in normal ICG angiograms which can make interpretation complex. It is best used in combination with clinical examination and other ancillary tests including color/red free photos, FA, and/or optical coherence tomography (OCT).

## CLINICAL ENTITIES

ICG angiography can be useful in aiding the diagnosis and treatment of a wide variety of retinal disorders; however, ICG is especially valuable in several specific clinical entities which we will briefly review below.

### Central Serous Chorioretinopathy

Central serous chorioretinopathy (CSC) is a disorder characterized by serous neurosensory detachment of the retina. ICG

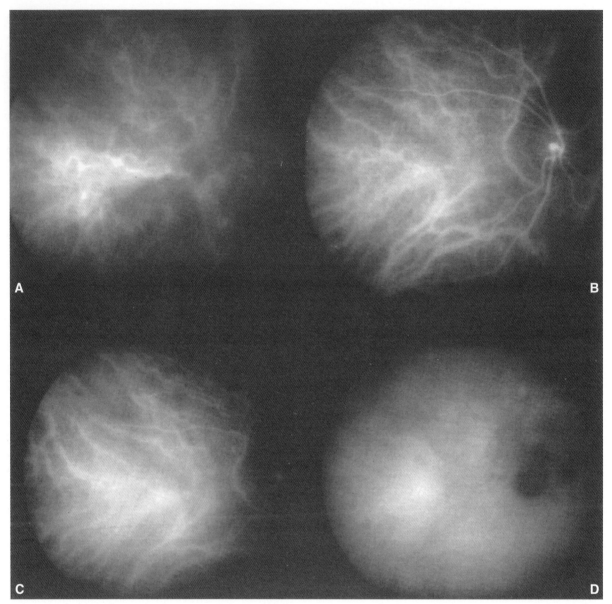

**Figure 6-1.** Indocyanine green angiographic phases in a normal patient. **A:** Choroidal arteriolar filling phase. **B:** Choroidal venous filling phase. **C:** Mid phase demonstrating the gradual fading of the choroidal vessels. The background fluorescence becomes more uniform as a result of the progressive leakage of the dye through the fenestrated walls of the choriocapillaris. In this phase the veins are more evident than the arteries. **D:** Late phase showing the hypoflourescent optic disc and the relatively hypoflourescent larger choroidal veins, which have become devoid of dye. The uniform background fluorescence is the result of the indocyanine green staining of the extrachoroidal space.

angiography has greatly expanded the understanding of the pathogenesis as well as the treatment options for CSC.

ICG angiography reveals multiple hyperfluorescent areas in the mid phases which are believed to correspond to zones of choroidal hyperpermeability (Fig. 6-1). These hyperpermeable regions not only surround active neurosensory detachments, but are also found in areas which are otherwise quiet clinically and on FA. This characteristic finding is not known to occur with other disorders and therefore can be helpful in solidifying the diagnosis of CSC.

ICG-guided photodynamic therapy (PDT) is becoming the standard of care for recalcitrant, chronic CSC (Figs. 6-2 and 6-3).

Yannuzzi et al. described the technique in several early cases that showed rapid resolution of subretinal fluid and improvement in vision (29). In chronic CSC, the FA often reveals mottled fluorescence without evidence of a focal leak at the level of the RPE secondary to pigmentary changes common with chronic neurosensory detachment. This does not reveal the specific location for application of PDT. ICG angiography divulges the underlying hyperpermeable zone at the level of the inner choroid, which is the optimal target for PDT. Several other studies have since confirmed the efficacy of this technique (30–34). ICG guided PDT has also been successfully applied to acute central serous with focal leaks at the level of the RPE (35,36).

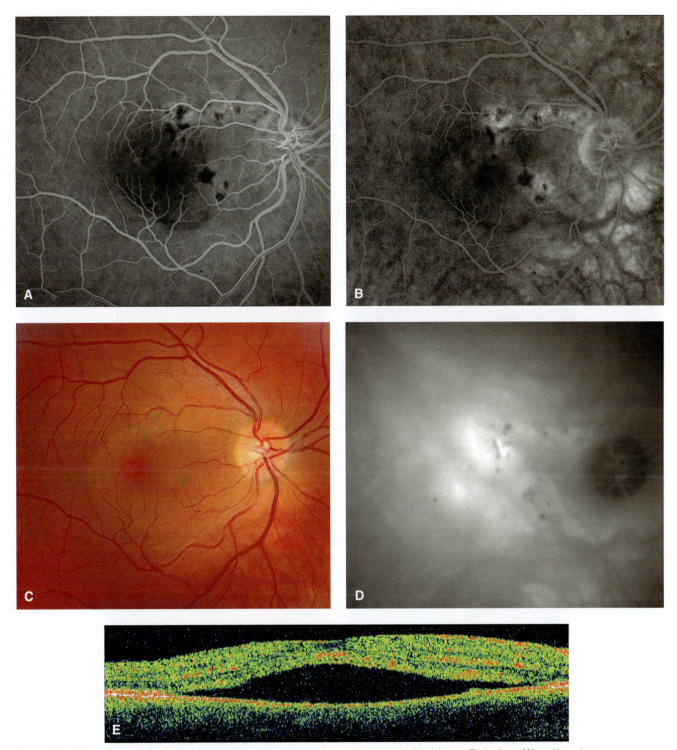

**Figure 6-2.** A 34-year-old female presented with 20/40 vision and complaints of distortion in the right eye. Early phase **(A)** and late phase **(B)** fluorescein angiogram (FA) reveals areas of hyper and hypofluorescence without obvious focal leakage. The color fundus photograph **(C)** shows a macular neurosensory detachment with pigmentary change. The mid phase indocyanine green angiogram **(D)** shows a region of hyperfluorescence believed to represent choriocapillaris hyperpermeability in the central macula. The optical coherence tomography **(E)** confirms the neurosensory detachment including the fovea.

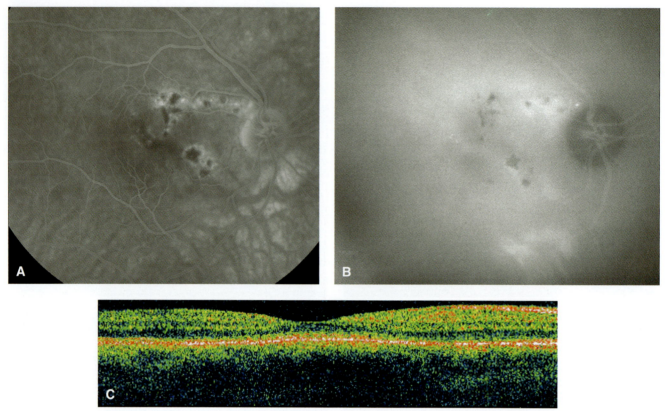

**Figure 6-3.** The patient from Figure 2 returned 3 months following indocyanine green (ICG) angiography guided photodynamic therapy to the right eye with improvement in vision to 20/25+ and reduction in metamorphopsia. Late phase fluorescein angiogram **(A)** reveals areas of hyper- and hypofluorescence without an apparent change from the images in central serous chorioretinopathy (CSC), Figure 1. The mid phase ICG angiogram **(B)**, however, shows a significant reduction in hyperfluorescence of the central macula indicating a localized reduction in choriocapillaris hyperpemeability and an excellent treatment response. Optical coherence tomography **(C)** confirms resolution of the neurosensory detachment with restoration of normal foveal architecture.

## Age-Related Macular Degeneration

ICG angiography can be very helpful in analyzing patients with age-related macular degeneration (ARMD), especially those classified with occult CNV on FA or pigment epithelial detachments (PEDs). Occult CNV represents the vast majority of newly diagnosed wet ARMD. ICG angiography in these patients can vary widely but will help to differentiate cases of PCV and RAP, which have different natural histories and responses to treatment or late leakage of undetermined origin. While the majority of PCV and RAP display characteristics of occult CNV on FA, they can rarely present as classic CNV (Fig. 6-4).

PEDs are differentiated into two categories by ICG. A serous PED displays a circular or oval area of hypofluorescence with relatively distinct borders where underlying choroidal vascular fluorescence is obstructed in early and mid phases. This is in contrast to the fluorescein findings, which show relatively uniform hyperfluorescence in the same area. A vascularized PED (Fig. 6-5) has similar features, except that hot spots develop in mid to late phases. The hot spot does not show on FA because the entire PED is hyperfluorescent. Certain cases respond well to selected focal treatment of the hot spot, which again allows ICG identify treatable components of relatively unresponsive lesions to (37).

## Polypoidal Choroidal Vasculopathy

PCV is a choroidal vascular disorder characterized by aneurysmal polyplike structures in the inner choroid which can leak fluid, blood, and/or lipid in active stages (Figs. 6-6 and 6-7). ICG angiography is integral to making the diagnosis of PCV. Early phases show a distinct hyperfluorescent network of enlarged choroidal vessels that are characteristic of the disorder. Active areas may remain hyperfluorescent or even leak in late phases, while the majority of the polypoidal lesions become hypofluorescent as the dye is removed from vascular channels (38–41).

## Retinal Angiomatous Proliferation

RAP is a distinct subdivision of neovascular macular degeneration where the neovascularization begins within the retina and progresses to form anastamoses between the retinal and choroidal circulation (Fig. 6-5). The development of retinal-retinal anastamoses and chorioretinal anastamoses leads to a clinical presentation with intra- and subretinal hemorrhage, PEDs, and exudates. There is some evidence that RAP lesions may also begin with the choroidal circulation. Because of the degree of hyperfluorescence seen with FA, individual components of

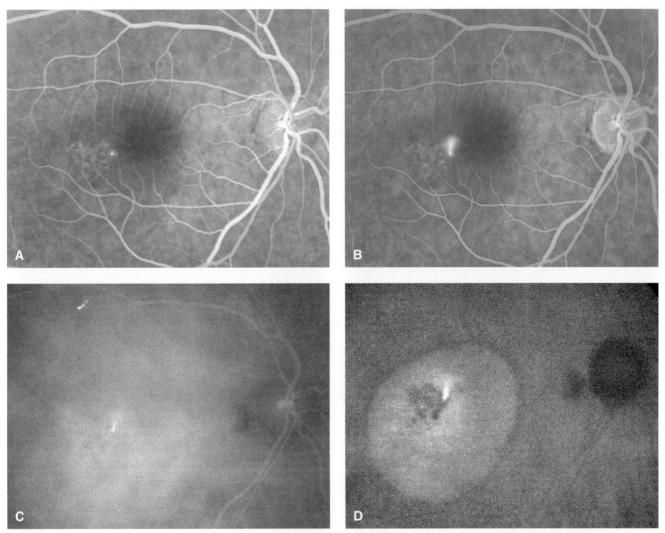

**Figure 6-4.** A 33-year-old male with a neurosensory detachment in the right eye presented complaining of decreased vision. Early **(A)** phase fluorescein angiography (FA) shows a focal leak at the level of the retinal pigment epithelium **(B)** with a smokestack pattern. Indocyanine green (ICG) angiography reveals a focal area of hyperfluorescence in mid phase **(C)** which leaks in a smokestack pattern in late phase **(D)** corresponding to that seen on FA. The neurosensory detachment itself becomes hyperfluorescent in the late phase of the ICG angiogram (D).

RAP lesions are difficult to identify. As a larger, more heavily protein bound molecule, ICG more easily demonstrates vascular anastamoses and hot spots that characterize these lesions (42–44).

## Inflammatory Diseases

ICG can be helpful in evaluating patients with inflammatory conditions that affect the choroid (45). In general, areas of active inflammation produce hypofluorescent areas with ICG angiography in all phases of the study becoming most apparent in the late phase. ICG hyperfluorescence is rare with these disorders and often signifies the presence of secondary neovascularization. Frequently, the number and distribution of hypofluorescent lesions are greater with ICG than on clinical exam or FA (43,46). This phenomenon has been documented for many inflammatory diseases including multiple evanescent white dot syndrome (MEWDS) (43), birdshot chorioretinopathy

(Fig. 6-8) (47), and multifocal choroiditis (48) among others (Fig. 6-9). ICG can be helpful in diagnosis, but mainly serves to gauge the clinical course and response to treatment by monitoring changes to hypofluorescent spots (46).

## Intraocular Tumors

ICG angiography offers a unique view of the vascular pattern of intraocular tumors. Because ICG remains within vessels walls better than fluorescein, it yields less early leakage and is superior to FA in demonstrating the microvascular pattern of intraocular tumors (49,50). For this reason, ICG is very helpful in differentiating and evaluating tumors with intrinsic vasculature (51). A dense network of vessels is often present in tumors such as hemangiomas (Fig. 6-10) and melanomas and quite variable in others such as metastases and inflammatory lesions, which makes ICG potentially useful to distinguish such lesions.

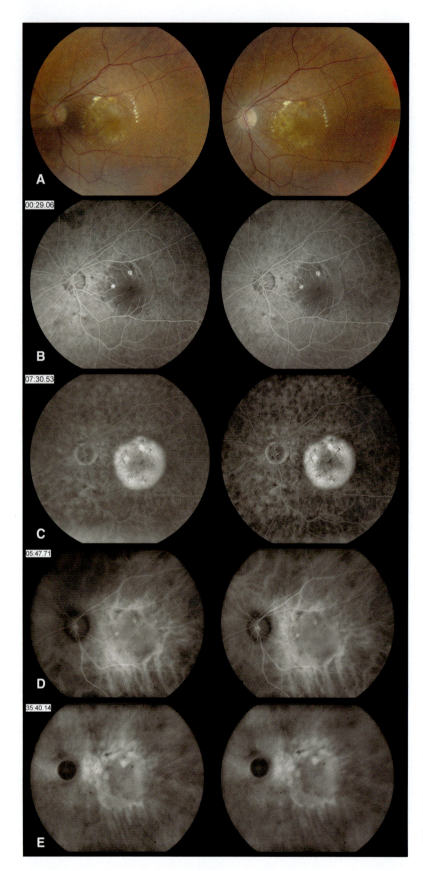

**Figure 6-5.** A 77-year-old female presented with complaints of decreased vision in the left eye. These images are best viewed using a stereo viewer. Color fundus photographs **(A)** show a central macular neurosensory detachment with intraretinal hemorrhages, fibrin, and lipid exudates. The early phase fluorescein angiogram (FA) **(B)** reveals two well defined intraretinal hyperfluorescent areas within the neurosensory elevation that contain retinal-retinal anastamoses. Late phase FA **(C)** shows intense hyperfluorescence of the entire neurosensory elevation with blocking defects from the hemorrhages and pigmentation. Mid phase indocyanine green (ICG) angiographic images **(D)** reveal small hyperfluorescent spots emanating from within the retina in the region of the retinal-retinal anastamosis which persist as hot spots in late phases **(E)**.

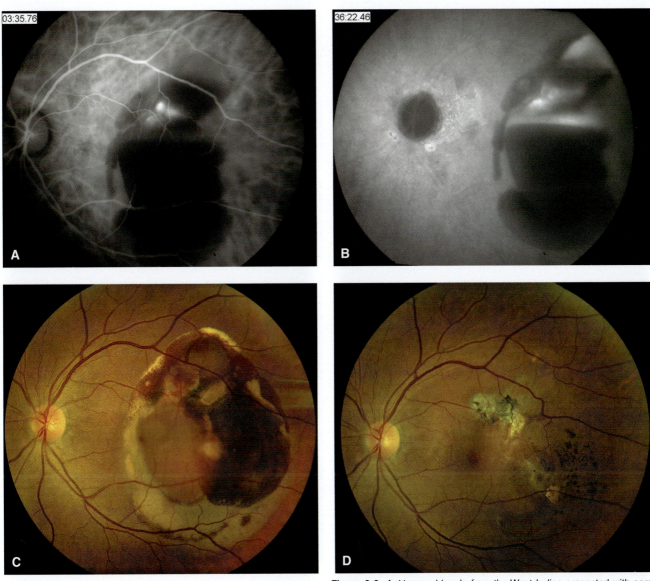

**Figure 6-6.** A 41-year-old male from the West Indies presented with complaints of vision loss in the left eye. Mid phase indocyanine green (ICG) angiogram **(A)** shows a lobulated area of hyperfluorescence in the inner choroid overlying and superior to a large blocking defect consistent with polypoidal choroidal vasculopathy. Late phase **(B)** shows intense hyperfluorescence adjacent in the superior macula with persistent blocking defect. The color photo on presentation **(C)** confirms a large subretinal elevation with areas of fluid as well as both old (dehemoglobinized) and new blood. The patient was treated with ICG guided thermal laser to the hyperfluorescent areas seen in early phases (A) which lead to involution of the polypoidal vessels and resorption of the hemorrhage and fluid **(D)**.

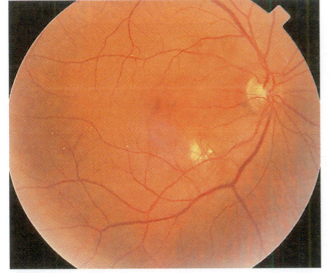

**Figure 6-7.** Polypoidal choroidal neovascularization. Color fundus photograph demonstrating tortuous vascular branches in the inner choroid, polypoid lesions of varying sizes, a larger neovascular complex within a serous pigment epithelial detachment, and serous and hemorrhagic detachment of the retinal pigment epithelium temporally. Flourescein study showing fine vessels within the larger polypoidal structure. Blocked fluorescence from blood can be seen.

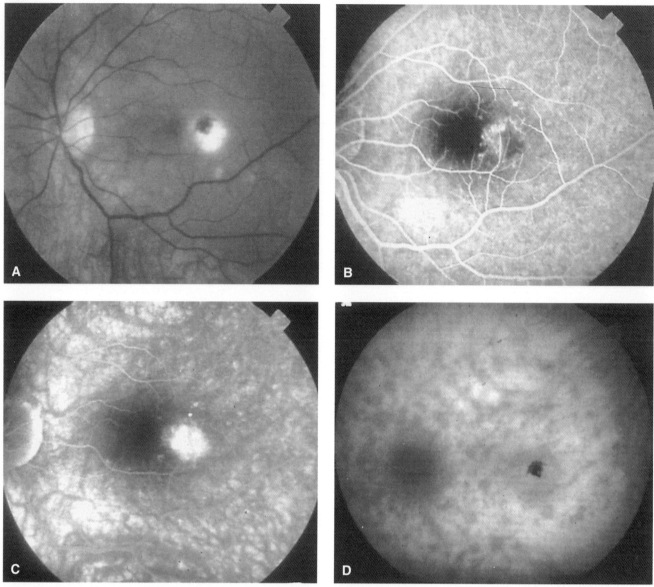

**Figure 6-8.** Multifocal choroiditis. **A:** Color fundus photograph of a myopic patient demonstrating an atrophic chorioretinal scar from previous laser photocoagulation of a choroidal neovascularization and scattered white spots. An enlarged blind spot was seen on visual field testing. **B:** Early phase fluorescein angiogram demonstrating an atrophic chorioretinal scar and white spots in the temporal macula. **C:** Late phase fluorescein study showing staining for the scar and focal hyperflourescent macular spots. **D:** Late phase indocyanine green study revealing multiple large hypoflourescent spots throughout the posterior pole and mid periphery. The confluence of the spots around the optic nerve could explain the enlarged blind spot.

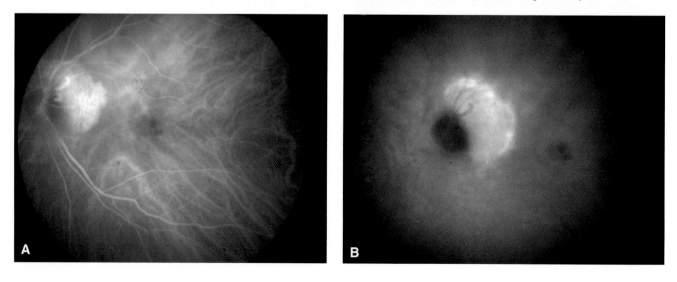

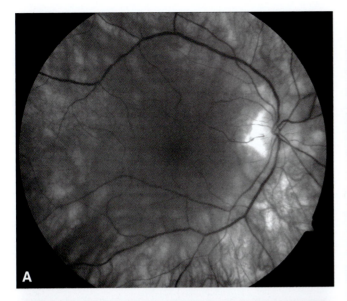

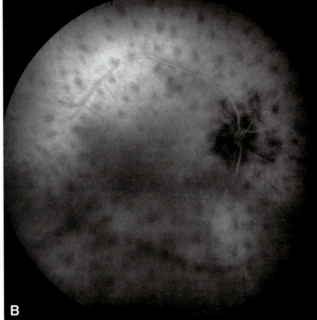

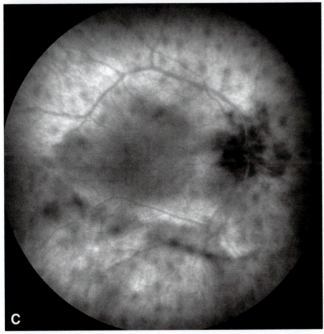

**Figure 6-10.** A 45-year-old woman with complaints of persistent photopsias was diagnosed with birdshot chorioretinopathy confirmed by the presence of HLA-B27. Red-free **(A)** photograph reveals multiple light flecks in the outer macula and periphery. Mid phase indocyanine green (ICG) angiogram **(B)** shows multiple hypofluorescent areas which persist on late frames **(C)** and are more numerous than those seen clinically.

**Figure 6-9.** A 68-year-old man with an acquired retinal capillary hemangioma adjacent to the optic nerve in the left eye. Early phase indocyanine green (ICG) angiogram **(A)** shows intense hyperfluorescence with enlarged feeding and draining vessels. Late phase ICG angiogram **(B)** reveals persistent hyperfluorescence of the lesion itself with overlying silhouetted vessels.

## CONCLUSION

The role of ICG angiography in ophthalmology continues to grow. It has proven vital to understanding the pathophysiology of several retinal disorders including CSC, PCV, and RAP, among others. Its unique properties reveal a perspective on retinal pathology that other techniques cannot replicate. As the technology becomes more widely available and used, the spectrum of disorders in which it plays a fundamental role will greatly expand.

### References

1. Archer D, Krill AE, Newell FW. Fluorescein studies of normal choroidal circulation. *Am J Ophthalmol* 1970;69(4):543–554.
2. Cherrick GR, Stein SW, Leevy CM, et al. Indocyanine green: observations on its physical properties, plasma decay, and hepatic extraction. *J Clin Invest* 1960;39:592–600.
3. Flower RW, Yannuzzi LA, Slakter JS. History of indocyanine green dye choroidal angiography. In: Yannuzzi LA, Flower RW, Slakter, JS (eds). *Indocyanine green angiography*. St. Louis: Mosby, 1997.
4. Fox IJ, Brooker LG, Heseltine DW, et al. A tricarbocyanine dye for continuous recording of dilution curves in whole blood independent of variations in blood oxygen saturation. *Mayo Clin Proc* 1957;32(18):478–484.

5. Wiegand BD, Ketterer SG, Rapaport E. The use of indocyanine green for the evaluation of hepatic function and blood flow in man. *Am J Dig Dis* 1960;5:427–436.

6. Caesar J, Shaldon S, Chiandussi L, et al. The use of indocyanine green in the measurement of hepatic blood flow and as a test of hepatic function. *Clin Sci* 1961;21:43–57.

7. Kogure K, Choromokos E. Infrared absorption angiography. *J Appl Physiol* 1969;26(1):154–157.

8. Choromokos E, Kogure K, David NJ. Infrared absorption angiography. *J Biol Photogr Assoc* 1969;37(2):100–104.

9. Kogure K, David NJ, Yamanouchi U, et al. Infrared absorption angiography of the fundus circulation. *Arch Ophthalmol* 1970;83(2):209–214.

10. David N. Infrared absorption angiography. In: Proceedings of the International Symposium on Fluorescein Angiography: Albi, Basel: Karger, 1969.

11. Flower RW, Hochheimer BF. Clinical infrared absorption angiography of the choroid. *Am J Ophthalmol* 1972;73(3):458–459.

12. Flower RW. Infrared absorption angiography of the choroid and some observations on the effects of high intraocular pressures. *Am J Ophthalmol* 1972;74(4):600–614.

13. Patz A, Klein ML. Clinical applications of indocyanine green angiography. *Doc Ophthalmol Proc Series* 1976;9:245–251.

14. Flower RW, Hochheimer BF. A clinical technique and apparatus for simultaneous angiography of the separate retinal and choroidal circulations. *Invest Ophthalmol* 1973;12(4):248–261.

15. Flower RW, Hochheimer BF. Indocyanine green dye fluorescence and infrared absorption choroidal angiography performed simultaneously with fluorescein angiography. *Johns Hopkins Med J* 1976;138(2):33–42.

16. Tokoro T. Recording ICG angiograms by means of an infrared sensitive video camera. In: Proceedings of the workshop on clinical choroidal angiography held in conjunction with the 1984 meeting of the International Congress on Eye Research. Alcante, Spain: APL Press, 1984.

17. Hayashi K, Hasegawa Y, Tazawa Y, et al. Clinical application of indocyanine green angiography to choroidal neovascularization. *Jpn J Ophthalmol* 1989;33(1):57–65.

18. Hayashi K, de Laey JJ. Indocyanine green angiography of choroidal neovascular membranes. *Ophthalmologica* 1985;190(1):30–39.

19. Hayashi K, de Laey JJ. Indocyanine green angiography of submacular choroidal vessels in the human eye. *Ophthalmologica* 1985;190(1):20–29.

20. Guyer DR, Puliafito CA, Mones JM, et al. Digital indocyanine-green angiography in chorioretinal disorders. *Ophthalmology* 1992;99(2):287–291.

21. Yannuzzi LA, Slakter JS, Sorenson JA, et al. Digital indocyanine green videoangiography and choroidal neovascularization. *Retina* 1992;12(3):191–223.

22. Bischoff PM, Flower RW. Ten years experience with choroidal angiography using indocyanine green dye: a new routine examination or an epilogue? *Doc Ophthalmol* 1985;60(3):235–291.

23. Hope-Ross M, Yannuzzi LA, Gragoudas ES, et al. Adverse reactions due to indocyanine green. *Ophthalmology* 1994;101(3):529–533.

24. Garski TR, Staller BJ, Hepner G, et al. Adverse reactions after administration of indocyanine green. *JAMA* 1978;240(7):635.

25. Hope-Ross MW. ICG dye: physical and pharmacologic properties. In: Yannuzzi LA, Flower RW, Slakter JS, (eds). *Indocyanine green angiography*. St. Louis: Mosby, 1997.

26. Benya R, Quintana J, Brundage B. Adverse reactions to indocyanine green: a case report and a review of the literature. *Cathet Cardiovasc Diagn* 1989;17(4):231–233.

27. Michie DD, Wombolt DG, Carretta RF, et al. Adverse reactions associated with the administration of a tricarbocyanine dye (Cardio-Green) to uremic patients. *J Allergy Clin Immunol* 1971;48(4):235–239.

28. Iseki K, Onoyama K, Fujimi S, et al. Shock caused by indocyanine green dye in chronic hemodialysis patients. *Clin Nephrol* 1980;14(4):210.

29. Yannuzzi LA, Slakter JS, Gross NE, et al. Indocyanine green angiography-guided photodynamic therapy for treatment of chronic central serous chorioretinopathy: a pilot study. *Retina* 2003;23(3):288–298.

30. Chan WM, Lam DS, Lai TY, et al. Choroidal vascular remodeling in central serous chorioretinopathy after indocyanine green guided photodynamic therapy with verteporfin: a novel treatment at the primary disease level. *Br J Ophthalmol* 2003;87(12):1453–1458.

31. Azad RV, Rani A, Pal N, et al. Current and future role of photodynamic therapy in chronic central serous chorioretinopathy. *Am J Ophthalmol* 2005;139(2):393–394; author reply 4.

32. Cardillo Piccolino F, Eandi CM, Ventre L, et al. Photodynamic therapy for chronic central serous chorioretinopathy. *Retina* 2003;23(6):752–763.

33. Chan WM, Lai TY, Lai RY, et al. Safety enhanced photodynamic therapy for chronic central serous chorioretinopathy: one-year results of a prospective study. *Retina* 2008;28(1):85–93.

34. Lai TY, Chan WM, Li H, et al. Safety enhanced photodynamic therapy with half dose verteporfin for chronic central serous chorioretinopathy: a short term pilot study. *Br J Ophthalmol* 2006;90(7):869–874.

35. Ober MD, Yannuzzi LA, Do DV, et al. Photodynamic therapy for focal retinal pigment epithelial leaks secondary to central serous chorioretinopathy. *Ophthalmology* 2005;112(12):2088–2094.

36. Chan WM, Lai TY, Lai RY, et al. Half-dose verteporfin photodynamic therapy for acute central serous chorioretinopathy one-year results of a randomized controlled trial. *Ophthalmology* 2008;115(10):1756–1765.

37. Eandi CM, Ober MD, Freund KB, et al. Selective photodynamic therapy for neovascular age-related macular degeneration with polypoidal choroidal neovascularization. *Retina* 2007;27(7):825–831.

38. Yannuzzi LA, Wong DW, Sforzolini BS, et al. Polypoidal choroidal vasculopathy and neovascularized age-related macular degeneration. *Arch Ophthalmol* 1999;117(11):1503–1510.

39. Yannuzzi LA, Ciardella A, Spaide RF, et al. The expanding clinical spectrum of idiopathic polypoidal choroidal vasculopathy. *Arch Ophthalmol* 1997;115(4):478–485.

40. Spaide RF, Yannuzzi LA, Slakter JS, et al. Indocyanine green videoangiography of idiopathic polypoidal choroidal vasculopathy. *Retina* 1995;15(2):100–110.

41. Ciardella AP, Donsoff IM, Huang SJ, et al. Polypoidal choroidal vasculopathy. *Surv Ophthalmol* 2004;49(1):25–37.

42. Freund KB, Ho IV, Barbazetto IA, et al. Type 3 neovascularization: the expanded spectrum of retinal angiomatous proliferation. *Retina* 2008;28(2):201–211.

43. Gross NE, Yannuzzi LA, Freund KB, et al. Multiple evanescent white dot syndrome. *Arch Ophthalmol* 2006;124(4):493–500.

44. Yannuzzi LA, Negrao S, Iida T, et al. Retinal angiomatous proliferation in age-related macular degeneration. *Retina* 2001;21(5):416–434.

45. Ciardella AP, Borodoker N, Costa DL, et al. Imaging the posterior segment in uveitis. *Ophthalmol Clin North Am* 2002;15(3):281–296.

46. Cimino L, Auer C, Herbort CP. Sensitivity of indocyanine green angiography for the follow-up of active inflammatory choriocapillaropathies. *Ocul Immunol Inflamm* 2000;8(4):275–283.

47. Fardeau C, Herbort CP, Kullmann N, et al. Indocyanine green angiography in birdshot chorioretinopathy. *Ophthalmology* 1999;106(10):1928–1934.

48. Slakter JS, Giovannini A, Yannuzzi LA, et al. Indocyanine green angiography of multifocal choroiditis. *Ophthalmology* 1997;104(11):1813–1819.

49. Mueller AJ, Freeman WR, Folberg R, et al. Evaluation of microvascularization pattern visibility in human choroidal melanomas: comparison of confocal fluorescein with indocyanine green angiography. *Graefes Arch Clin Exp Ophthalmol* 1999;237(6):448–456.

50. Sallet G, Amoaku WM, Lafaut BA, et al. Indocyanine green angiography of choroidal tumors. *Graefes Arch Clin Exp Ophthalmol* 1995;233(11):677–689.

51. Shields CL, Shields JA, De Potter P. Patterns of indocyanine green videoangiography of choroidal tumours. *Br J Ophthalmol* 1995;79(3):237–245.

CHAPTER

7

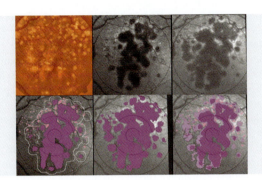

# Fundus Autofluorescence

Miki Sawa ■ R. Theodore Smith ■ Lawrence A. Yannuzzi

Retinal pigment epithelium (RPE) cells are essential to maintain normal photoreceptor function. The RPE has the important task of phagocytosing spent photoreceptor outer segment discs. However, *in vivo* imaging of the RPE is difficult due to low contrast and strong absorption by melanin pigments. Indirect information about the RPE cell layer can be obtained using fluorescein and indocyanine green angiography. However, functional assessment of the RPE is incomplete even if these techniques are performed. Recently, fundus autofluorescence (FAF) has been studied as a noninvasive test of RPE function based on the fluorescence characteristics of a curious waste material, lipofuscin, which deposits in the RPE over time (1–9).

*In vivo* recording of FAF was described by Delori (1), who showed that FAF arose from lipofuscin in the RPE. Lipofuscin is derived in large part from phagocytosis of outer segment discs containing bisretinoid byproducts of light absorption. A number of retinoid-derived lipofuscin pigments have now been described (2,3,7,9), a major one being the molecule A2E (3), that is formed through a series of chemical reactions from two molecules of all-*trans*-retinal and one molecule of phosphatidylethanolamine. Precursors of A2E, specifically dihydroA2PE and A2PE, all of which are autofluorescent, form in the outer segments prior to phagocytosis by the RPE (4,7,9). A2E and its precursors are potentially susceptible to oxidative damage and capable of entering into photo-oxidative reactions with neighboring molecules (8). RPE in the macula contains a higher concentration of lipofuscin than nonmacular RPE (5). With aging, lipofuscin accumulates normally in the lysosomal compartment (1,5). It is also known to accumulate abnormally in various monogenetic and complex retinal diseases and is associated with photoreceptor degeneration (10). Lipofuscin is photoreactive and can produce a variety of reactive oxygen species and other radicals, may induce apoptosis of the RPE, and mediates blue light-induced RPE apoptosis (3,8).

The emission of lipofuscin has a broad band ranging from 500 nm to 750 nm (1). The optimal excitation is 630 nm. The intensity of FAF parallels the amount and distribution of lipofuscin (1). The confocal scanning laser ophthalmoscope using the excitation wavelength 488 nm and a barrier filter of 500 nm is able to provide FAF imaging demonstrating AF distribution *in vivo* (10,11). Spaide et al. demonstrated FAF photography using a fundus camera-based system with a band pass filter for the excitation light of 580 nm and a barrier filter of 695 nm to avoid autofluorescence (AF) from the crystalline lens (12).

In the normal FAF pattern, diffuse AF is most intense between 5 degrees and 15 degrees from the fovea. The optic disc and retinal blood vessels have a low (dark) autofluorescent signal. Abnormal AF is classified into increased FAF (hyperautofluorescence) or decreased FAF (hypoautofluorescence) in comparison to the normal AF distribution or to the surrounding autofluorescent pattern. Decreased FAF is thought to indicate low lipofuscin concentration and can be due to RPE atrophy or RPE cell loss, or blocking effect due to overlying material such as hemorrhage. Increased FAF is thought to indicate excessive lipofuscin (Fig. 7-1). This manifestation of abnormal metabolism may result from high turnover of photoreceptor outer segments or an intrinsic defect in the ability of the RPE to recycle metabolites (10).

## SPECIFIC DISEASES

### Age-related Macular Degeneration, Geographic Atrophy, and Choroidal Neovascularization

The sub-RPE deposits known as drusen and accumulation of debris in Bruch's membrane are believed to play an important

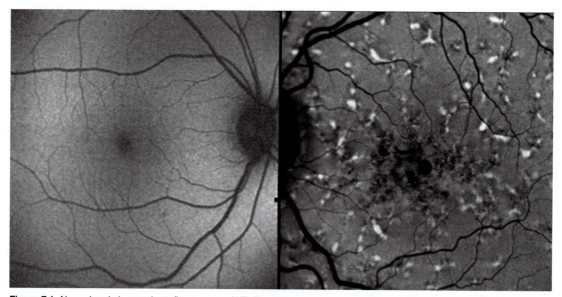

**Figure 7-1.** Normal and abnormal autofluorescence (AF). The left image is a normal AF scan. Note the hypoautofluorescence of the optic disc and vessels. The foveal area is darker due to blocking of blue light by luteal pigment. Autofluorescence is normally most intense in a band between 5-degrees and 15-degrees from the fovea. The image on the right is an abnormal AF image. There are multiple areas of hypoautofluorescence centrally due to retinal pigment epithelial damage; surrounding the center are multiple focal sources of hyperautofluorescence that represent abnormal lipofuscin deposits.

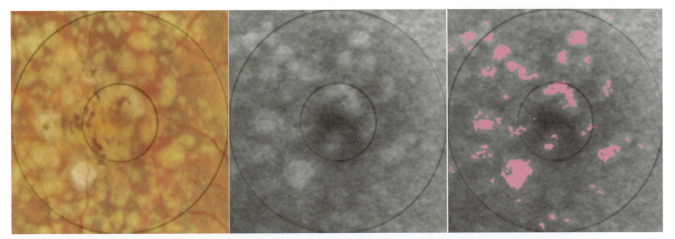

**Figure 7-2.** Drusen. The first image is a color photo of a central macula that is laden with large soft drusen. The second image is the corresponding autofluorescence (AF) scan. In the third image, areas of focally increased AF (FIAF, greater than 2 standard deviations greater than the image mean) have been labeled in pink. These areas of FIAF are seen to lie almost entirely over the large soft drusen. However, many of the drusen have a weaker or no FIAF signal and are not labeled.

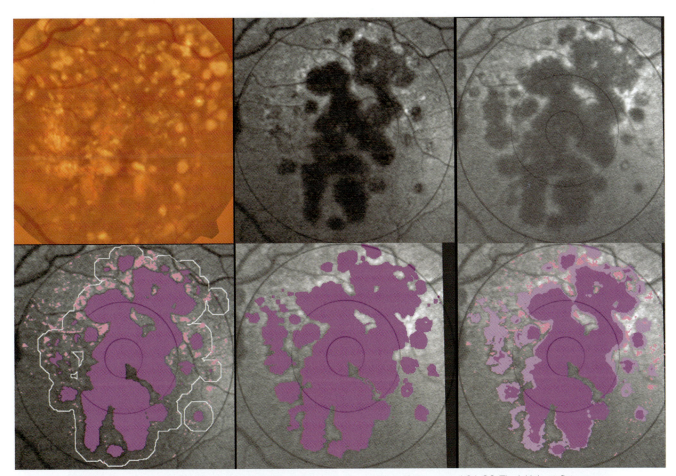

**Figure 7-3.** Geographic atrophy (GA). Top (Original images). The color photo shows large soft drusen and GA OS. The initial autofluorescence (AF) image outlines the GA very well as hypoautofluorescent multilobed structures. Surrounding the GA there are focal areas of focally increased autofluorescence (FIAF). There are also such rings around a few of the soft drusen. The final AF image shows the progression of the GA in 2 years. Bottom (image analysis). The initial AF has been segmented into GA (*purple*) and FIAF (*pink*). The white line outlines the 250 micron border zone around the GA. Next, the final AF image has had its GA also segmented (*purple*). To see the relationships between all these structures, the last panel has divided the final GA into the initial GA (*purple*) and new GA (*light purple*). In addition, the initial FIAF has been superimposed on the final GA image to see which areas with FIAF became atrophic over the 2 years. There are areas of GA growth superiorly, which are associated with initial FIAF, but there are also large areas of GA growth inferiorly, which had no preceding FIAF.

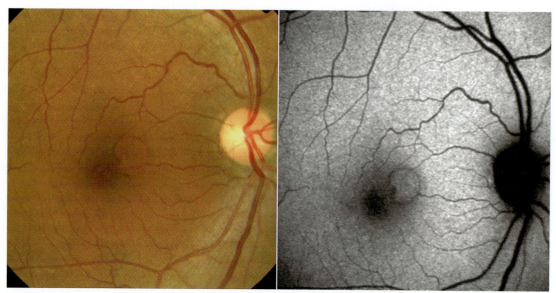

**Figure 7-4.** Retinal Pigment Epithelial Detachment (RPED). The color photo shows a well-defined RPED. The autofluorescence scan shows corresponding mild focally increased autofluorescence with a well-defined darker border.

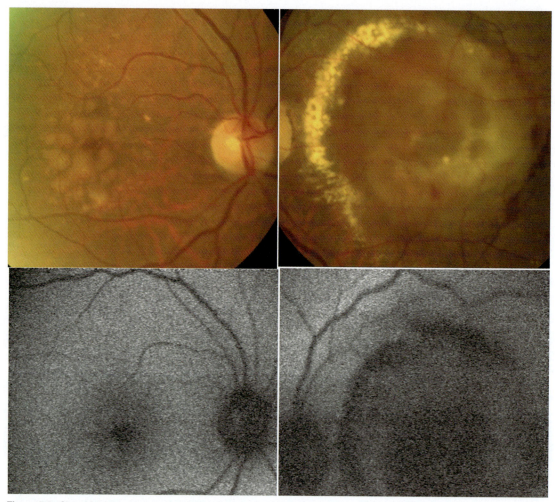

**Figure 7-5.** Choroidal neovascularization (CNV). The top row (color photographs) shows large soft drusen in the right eye and massive exudation from CNV in the left eye. The bottom row (autofluorescence [AF] scans) shows faint focally increased autofluorescence in the right eye and large areas of hypoautofluorescence signifying widespread retinal pigment epithelium damage in the left eye. This demonstrates that the fellow eye, right eye in this case, of a CNV eye with massive AF abnormalities, can have a nearly normal AF scan.

role in the pathogenesis of age-related macular degeneration (AMD). Drusen are a representative clinical manifestation of early AMD (13). In the earlier stages of the disease, large soft drusen and focally increased AF (FIAF) are spatially closely linked (See Fig. 7-2) (14–16). With progression to the atrophic stage of the disease, it is common to see thinning of the RPE overlying large drusen, with a diminished AF signal, while adjacent to the base there are relatively thicker RPE cells and/or dispersed lipofuscin causing a ring of FIAF.

In geographic atrophy, atrophic lesions are seen as well-defined dark areas indicating loss of RPE cells with subsequent atrophy of the overlying retina and the underlying choriocapillaris. Geographic atrophy (GA) regions are surrounded by various patterns of increased AF, such as banded, patchy, focal and diffuse patterns (11). It has been theorized that these patterns may reflect heterogeneity on the molecular level, and may represent different disease entities with specific genetic or environmental factors. It has also been suggested that the hyper AF regions in the border zone are at higher risk for future atrophy than the normofluorescent regions (17–20), but quantitative analysis of exactly superimposed serial AF images of GA patients has failed to support this (See Fig. 7-3) (21). It is therefore uncertain whether these areas of increased lipofuscin in the AMD/GA process are specifically signs of new RPE stress or have accumulated by other mechanisms (RPE reduplication, lipofuscin dispersal, etc.).

Areas of retinal pigment epithelial detachment show a mild diffuse increased AF corresponding exactly with the detached area (Fig. 7-4). In the eyes with choroidal neovascularization (CNV), FAF is irregular with regions of greater and lesser

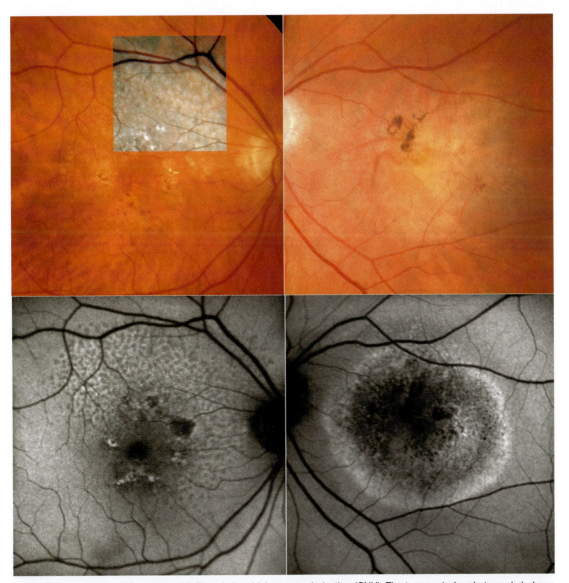

**Figure 7-6.** Reticular autofluorescence (AF) and choroidal neovascularization (CNV). The top row (color photographs) shows large soft drusen centrally and reticular pseudodrusen (enhanced for visualization) along the superotemporal arcade in the right eye. There is scarring from CNV in the right eye. The bottom row (AF scans) shows typical focal hyper- and hypoautofluorescence centrally and reticular autofluorescence superotemporally in the right eye. The pox-like pattern of reticular AF, which covers the same area as the reticular pseudodrusen, is more easily visualized than the reticular pseudodrusen, and can be seen to extend into the papillo-macular bundle. There is central hypoautofluorescence in the left eye surrounded by a ring of hyperautofluorescence signifying lipofuscin dispersal from damaged retinal pigment epithelium.

fluorescence than the background (Fig. 7-5) (14). The AF distribution changes over time, and focal regions of increased AF may develop into regions of decreased AF (14). Thus, AF over disciform scars is less than background. AF photography has been used to evaluate fellow eyes with CNV. In one study, fellow eyes of exudative AMD had larger amounts of AF than the eyes of patients without AMD of a similar age (12). However, most authors now agree that fellow eyes of CNV do not generally show patterns of increased lipofuscin. In one study, increased AF was rarely seen in eyes with CNV and in fellow eyes, suggesting that increased AF, and thus, RPE- lipofuscin, may not play an essential role in CNV formation (Fig. 7-5) (15). In fact, in another study the most common AF marker for such eyes was a pattern known as reticular AF (RAF), which is a speckled pattern of *decreased* FAF (16). This pattern was also found to be highly correlated reticular pseudodrusen (RPD) on fundus photography (Fig. 7-6). In this study, 36% of 55 fellow eyes of CNV eyes showed either RAF or RPD (16). An independent study that used blue light fundus photography confirmed that characteristic RPD had a high prevalence among AMD patients with newly diagnosed CNV (24% of cases) (17). The etiology of these lesions is unknown, but their pattern of distribution has suggested an inflammatory etiology. If so, this inflammation may also be an activator of the complement factor H pathway that has been strongly implicated in the genetics of AMD (18,19).

## INHERITED RETINAL DISORDERS

In macular and retinal dystrophies, various changes in FAF have been described (10). In early Best disease, adult vitelliform

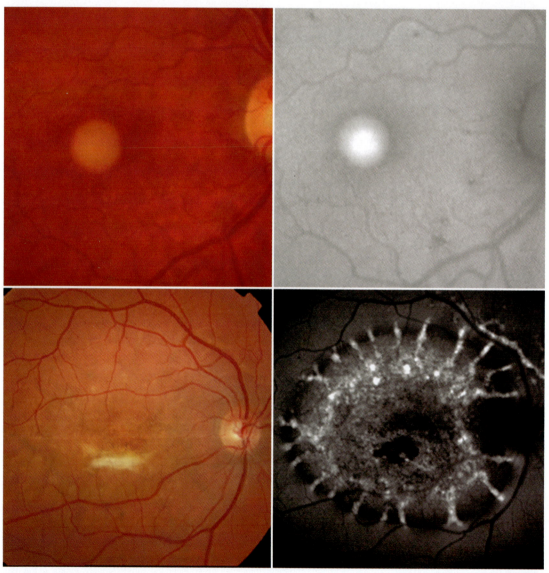

**Figure 7-7.** Best disease. The first color photo shows the typical "egg yolk" appearance of a central Best lesion of the right eye. The autofluorescence (AF) scan shows corresponding marked focally increased AF (FIAF) emanating from the subretinal lipofuscin deposits. The second color photo shows a late stage or "scrambled yolk" appearance of another Best patient's right eye. The AF scan shows central hypoautofluorescence corresponding to damaged retinal pigment epithelium that has lost most of its lipofuscin, surrounded by radiating lines of FIAF which may correspond to tracks of the dispersed lipofuscin.

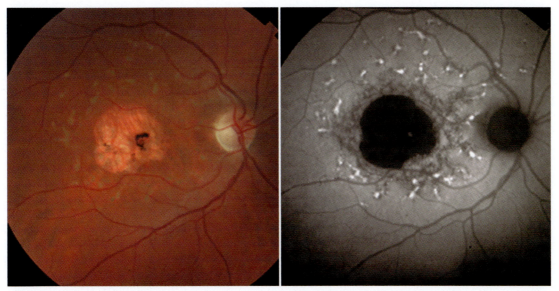

**Figure 7-8.** Stargardt Disease (SGTD). The color photo of the right eye shows the central geographic atrophic atrophy surrounded by pisciform pale flecks at the level of the retinal pigment epithelium of a classic case of STGD. The autofluorescence (AF) scan shows marked hypoautofluorescence corresponding to the area of geographic atrophy (GA), and marked focally increased AF (FIAF) corresponding to the lipofuscin in the visible flecks. The AF scan also shows spotty hypoautofluorescence around the central GA, suggesting that the GA may progress further.

macular dystrophy, and fundus flavimaculatus, yellowish-pale deposits at the level of RPE and Bruch's membrane are associated with a markedly increased FAF signal. In later Best disease, with loss of lipofuscin centrally and dispersal peripherally, the pattern changes dramatically (Fig. 7-7) (1). In Stargardt disease, focal flecks typically show bright, increased FAF, which may fade as atrophy develops (22,23). These flecks are abnormal regions of RPE engorged with lipofuscin. The central macula characteristically develops geographic atrophy (Fig. 7-8).

Retinitis pigmentosa (RP) causes a gradual loss of photoreceptors and then RPE cells that consequently cause

decreased FAF (24,25). However, a ring of increased FAF ("bull's eye") may occur in many forms of RP. The location of this ring is typically at 4 to 5 degrees eccentricity from the fovea, but can vary from 1.5 to 9 degrees eccentricity. The location of this ring correlates well with the classic decrease in retinal function in RP as measurements are made from the macula towards the retinal periphery by electroretinography and perimetry (24,25). Thus, the ring of increased FAF appears to represent the border between functional (macular) and dysfunctional (extramacular) retina (Fig. 7-9).

Areas of preserved RPE retain AF. Thus, in those types of RP with functional loss out of proportion to photoreceptor

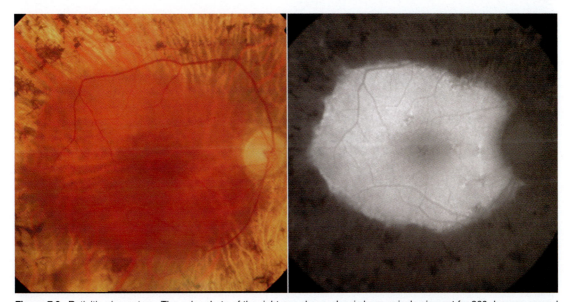

**Figure 7-9.** Retinitis pigmentosa. The color photo of the right eye shows classic bone spicule pigment for 360 degrees around the macula, arteriolar narrowing and waxy pallor of the disc. The macula itself is spared. The autofluorescence scan shows a bright ring of hyperautofluorescence centrally whose border corresponds to the border between functional and diseased retina.

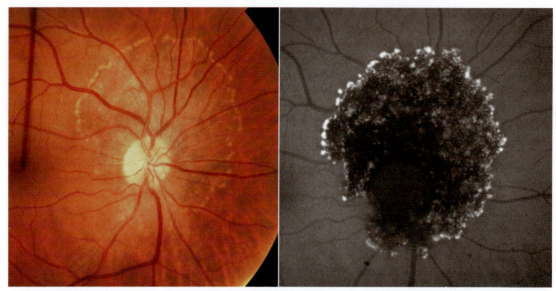

**Figure 7-10.** Acute zonal occult outer retinopathy (AZOOR). The color photo of the right eye shows a slightly opacified neural retina in a fan-like distribution around the optic nerve. The borders of the lesion are well-demarcated by pale yellow deposits. The autofluorescence (AF) scan demonstrates markedly and irregularly decreased AF throughout this expanding lesion with increased AF at the outer border that corresponds to the yellow lesions seen in the color photo. The hypoautofluorescence findings suggest significant damage to the retinal pigment epithelium, i.e., that more than the outer retina is involved in AZOOR.

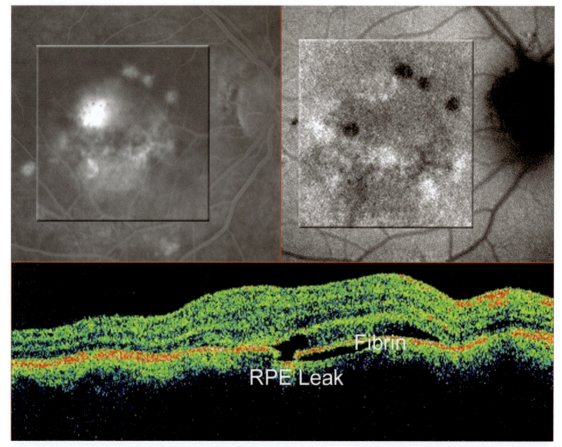

**Figure 7-11.** Central serous chorioretinopathy (CSR). The first image is a fluorescein angiogram, right eye, of an eye with multifocal CSR. The embossed inset shows magnified detail of the central macula with several areas of dye leakage. The next image is the autofluorescence (AF) scan of the same eye, also with an embossed inset showing magnified detail of the central macula. There are several distinct hypoautofluorescent foci corresponding to areas of dye leakage on the angiogram. The optical coherence tomography (OCT) scan demonstrates the reason behind this correspondence of the FA and AF images: the retinal pigment epithelium is actually missing at the sites of dye leakage; hence there is no AF signal at these points. The OCT also shows fibrin in the subretinal space.

loss, the photoreceptors have a near normal complement of rhodopsin, and the FAF would be maintained. However, when there is outer segment loss early (in proportion to visual loss), the RPE would have correspondingly reduced FAF.

## INFLAMMATORY DISORDERS

Acute zonal occult outer retinopathy (AZOOR) has shown a unique autofluorescent finding of absent AF in the center of the expanding lesion with increased AF at the outer border (Fig. 7-10) (26). The outer border cells with increased AF appear to proceed to atrophy in this disease. The AF findings also suggest that more than the outer retina is involved in AZOOR.

## CENTRAL SEROUS CHORIORETINOPATHY

Focal leakage on a fluorescein angiogram in central serous chorioretinopathy (CSR) is accompanied by corresponding foci of hypoautofluorescence on the AF scan, due to defects in the RPE at these points. These RPE defects can be demonstrated on an optical coherence tomography (OCT) scan. Increased AF develops a few months after the onset of serous retinal detachment (27). In an eye with persistent serous retinal detachment (so-called chronic CSR), decreased FAF (RPE atrophy) can also be demonstrated, for example, as in the center of a chronic serous tract. On the other hand, with increasing duration of the detachment, material located by OCT in the outer retina shows increasing FAF (28). (Fig. 7-11)

## CONCLUSION

In conclusion, FAF imaging is a non-invasive new technique of retinal imaging that demonstrates disease activity most specifically at the level of the RPE. Characteristic patterns of increased and decreased FAF have already been documented that aid in the diagnosis and prognosis of macular diseases as diverse as AMD, RP, and CSR. This knowledge base is growing rapidly. In the future, we expect that functional measurements such as microperimetry and multifocal electroretinography (ERG) will be combined with FAF to enhance our understanding of these diseases.

### References

1. Delori FC, Dorey CK, Staurenghi G, et al. In vivo fluorescence of the ocular fundus exhibits retinal pigment epithelium lipofuscin characteristics. *Invest Ophthalmol Vis Sci* 1995;36:718–729.
2. Parish CA, Hashimoto M, Nakanishi K, et al. Isolation and one-step preparation of A2E and iso-A2E, fluorophores from human retinal pigment epithelium. *Proc Natl Acad Sci USA* 1998;95(25):14609–14613.
3. Sparrow JR, Parish CA, Hashimoto M, et al. A2E, a lipofuscin fluorophore, in human retinal pigmented epithelial cells in culture. *Invest Ophthalmol Vis Sci* 1999;40:2988–2995.
4. Liu J, Itagaki Y, Ben-Shabat S, et al. The biosynthesis of A2E, a fluorophore of aging retina, involves the formation of the precursor, A2-PE, in the photoreceptor outer segment membrane. *J Biol Chem* 2000;275:29354–29360.
5. Feeney-Burns L, Berman ER, Rothman H. Lipofuscin of human retinal pigment epithelium. *Am J Ophthalmol* 1980;90:783–791.
6. Eldred GE, Lasky MR. Retinal age pigments generated by self-assembling lysosomotropic detergents. *Nature* 1993;361:724–726.
7. Fishkin N, Sparrow JR, Allikmets R, et al. Isolation and characterization of a retinal pigment epithelial cell fluorophore: an all-trans-retinal dimer conjugate. *Proc Natl Acad Sci USA* 2005;102(20):7091–7096.
8. Sparrow JR, Parish CA, Nakanishi K. The lipofuscin fluorophore A2E mediates blue-light induced damage to retinal pigmented epithelial cells. *Invest Ophthalmol Vis Sci* 2000;41:1981–1989.
9. Fishkin N, Jang YP, Itagaki Y, et al. A2-rhodopsin: a new fluorophore isolated from photoreceptor outer segments. *Org Biomol Chem* 2003;1:1101–1105.
10. von Ruckmann A, Fitzke FW, Bird AC. In vivo fundus autofluorescence in macular dystrophies. *Arch Ophthalmol* 1997;115:609–615.
11. Holz FG, Bellmann C, Margaritidis M, et al. Patterns of increased in vivo fundus autofluorescence in the junctional zone of geographic atrophy of the retinal pigment epithelium associated with age-related macular degeneration. *Graefes Arch Clin Exp Ophthalmol* 1999;237:145–152.
12. Spaide RF. Fundus autofluorescence and age-related macular degeneration. *Ophthalmology* 2003;110:392–399.
13. Pauleikhoff D, Barondes MJ, Minassian D, et al. Drusen as risk factors in age-related macular disease. *Am J Ophthalmol* 1990;109:38–43.
14. Dandekar SS, Jenkins SA, Peto T, et al. Autofluorescence imaging of choroidal neovascularization due to age-related macular degeneration. *Arch Ophthalmol.* 2005;123:1507–1513.
15. McBain J, Townend J, Lois N. Fundus autofluorescence in exudative age-related macular degeneration. *Br J Ophthalmol* 2007;91:491–496.
16. Smith RT, Chan JK, Busuoic M, et al. Autofluorescence characteristics of early, atrophic and high risk fellow eyes in age-related macular degeneration. *Invest Ophthalmol Vis Sci* 2006;47:5495–5504.
17. Cohen SY, Dubois L, Tadayoni R, et al. Prevalence of reticular pseudodrusen in age-related macular degeneration with newly diagnosed choroidal neovascularization. *B J Ophthalmol* 2007;91:354–359.
18. Hageman GS, Anderson DH, Johnson LV, et al. A common haplotype in the complement regulatory gene, factor H (*HF1/CFH*), predisposes individuals to age-related macular degeneration. *Proc Nat Acad Sci USA* 2005;102:7227–7232.
19. Gold B, Merriam JE, Zernant J. Variation in factor B (BF) and complement component 2 (C2) genes is associated with age-related macular degeneration. *Nature Genetics* 2006;38(4):458–462.
20. Holz FG, Bellman C, Staudt S, et al. Fundus autofluorescence and development of geographic atrophy in age-related macular degeneration. *Invest Ophthalmol Vis Sci* 2001;42:1051–1056.
21. Hwang JC, Chan J, Chang S, et al. Predictive value of fundus autofluorescence for development of geographic atrophy in age-related macular degeneration. *Invest Ophthalmol Vis Sci* 2006;47:2655–2661.
22. Delori FC, Staurenghi G, Arend O, et al. In vivo measurement of lipofuscin in Stargardt's disease–Fundus flavimaculatus. *Invest Ophthalmol Vis Sci* 1995;36:2327–2331.
23. von Ruckmann A, Fitzke FW, Bird AC. Distribution of pigment epithelium autofluorescence in retinal disease state recorded in vivo and its change over time. *Graefes Arch Clin Exp Ophthalmol* 1999;237:1–9.
24. Robson AG, El-Amir A, Bailey C, et al. Pattern ERG correlates of abnormal fundus autofluorescence in patients with retinitis pigmentosa and normal visual acuity. *Invest Ophthalmol Vis Sci* 2003;44:3544–3550.
25. Popovic P, Jarc-Vidmar M, Hawlina M. Abnormal fundus autofluorescence in relation to retinal function in patients with retinitis pigmentosa. *Graefes Arch Clin Exp Ophthalmol* 2005;243:1018–1027.
26. Spaide RF. Collateral damage in acute zonal occult outer retinopathy. *Am J Ophthalmol* 2004;138:887–889.
27. von Ruckmann A, Fitzke FW, Fan J, et al. Abnormalities of fundus autofluorescence in central serous retinopathy. *Am J Ophthalmol* 2002;133:780–786.
28. Spaide RF, Klancnik JM, Jr. Fundus autofluorescence and central serous chorioretinopathy. *Ophthalmology* 2005;112:825–833.

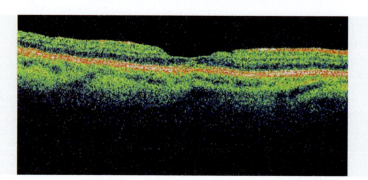

# Retinal Imaging: Optical Coherence Tomography

Andre J. Witkin ■ Jay S. Duker ■ Elias Reichel

Optical coherence tomography (OCT) is a high-resolution cross-sectional imaging technique that has become a standard in ophthalmology. Initially developed as a research tool in 1991, it was soon recognized that OCT could be utilized to image the retina with an unprecedented spatial resolution of approximately 10 microns, allowing visualization of intraretinal layers as well as accurate measurement of retinal and intraretinal thicknesses. Since the development of commercial OCT models in 1996, advancements in software and equipment have allowed it to become a powerful clinical tool for the diagnosis and management of macular disease and glaucoma. OCT imaging systems can be used to take multiple images through a given point on the fundus, automatically measure retinal or intraretinal thicknesses, and, by combining images, create retinal thickness maps. The abilities to obtain high-resolution images and highly accurate retinal thickness measurements allow detailed analysis of retinal anatomy at consecutive visits, providing a useful assessment of the efficacy of treatments over time.

## OPTICAL COHERENCE TOMOGRAPHY INSTRUMENTATION

The most widely used model to date has been the OCT3 or Stratus OCT, developed in 2002 by Carl Zeiss Meditec, Inc. This model has imaging software protocols used to scan the macula and optic nerve head. For macular applications, the most useful scanning modes are the retinal thickness mapping and fast retinal thickness mapping modes. These scanning modes acquire six linear images centered at the point of fixation, spaced 30 degrees apart and typically 6 mm in length. The retinal thickness mapping protocol obtains six high pixel density images acquired individually. Each image

in this mode can be examined separately to assess macular anatomy, or the images can be combined and measured using the standard computer software to obtain a topographic thickness map of the macula. A second protocol, the fast retinal thickness mapping mode, acquires six lower pixel density OCT images at once, and is usually used to create a topographic map only. Individual images as well as topographic thickness maps have been shown to be useful in a variety of retinal diseases.

OCT is based on the principle of low-coherence interferometry. In this technique, the distances and sizes of different structures in the eye are determined by measuring the "echo" time it takes for light to be backscattered from different structures at various axial distances. This is analogous to A-mode ultrasound, in which the axial length of the eye is measured using sound rather than light (1,2). When successive axial measurements at different transverse points are combined, a tomographic or cross-sectional image of tissue is obtained, similar to B-mode ultrasound. In StratusOCT, a normal 6 mm macular image is created using 512 A-lines. Further details of OCT principles and operation are beyond the scope of this text.

## NORMAL RETINA

In order to detect abnormalities in OCT images, it is important for the clinician to be familiar with normal macular anatomy. The vitreoretinal interface is noted by the contrast between the nonreflective vitreous and the reflective surface of the retina. The foveal center demonstrates a characteristic depression in its contour. The retinal nerve fiber layer, inner plexiform layer, outer plexiform layer, photoreceptor layer, retinal pigment epithelium (RPE), and choroid all are well delineated (Fig. 8-1). The high contrast between the outer reflective layers and the outer nuclear layer in OCT images provides a clear

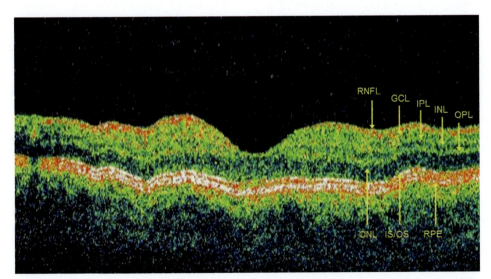

**Figure 8-1.** Optical coherence tomography image of the normal retina. Note the normal depression of the retinal contour at the fovea. Waviness of the image is due to slight axial motion of the patient during image capture (axial motion artifact). Retinal layers are labeled: RNFL, retinal nerve fiber layer; GCL, ganglion cell layer; IPL, inner plexiform layer; INL, inner nuclear layer; OPL, outer plexiform layer; ONL, outer nuclear layer; IS/OS, inner segment/outer segment junction; RPE, retinal pigment epithelium.

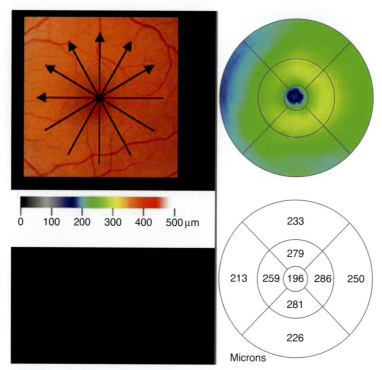

**Figure 8-2.** Example of a macular map created from six 6 mm optical coherence tomography (OCT) images through the macula. OCT software calculates a false color map as well as a numerical map with 9 thickness zones. The central foveal circle is the most accurate calculation, as it is a mean of 512 a-scans. Foveal thickness of this patient is 196 microns.

boundary in the computation of retinal thicknesses using computer segmentation algorithms.

OCT offers an objective test for serial quantitative evaluations of retinal thickness (3). Macular mapping algorithms calculate a number of different thicknesses. Six radial scans are combined to create a retinal thickness map with nine zones, as well as a central foveal thickness measurement at the point of intersection of the six scans (Fig. 8-2). The central foveal circle on the macular map is calculated as a mean of 512 data points in the macular mapping protocol and 128 data points in the fast macular mapping protocol. This central foveal circle measurement is probably the most clinically relevant, as it includes the highest number of data points from six separate scans. Mean central foveal circle thickness measurements in normal subjects are around 212 ± 20 microns (4). Fast macular mapping thickness measurements have been found to be comparable to the regular mapping protocol, but individual cross-sectional images of 128 lines are much poorer quality than the 512-line scans obtained with the regular macular mapping protocol (5).

## MACULAR EDEMA

Many retinal disease processes can result in an increase in macular thickness due to an accumulation of intraretinal fluid. This fluid widens the distance between the well-delineated anterior and posterior boundaries of the retina, which are easily detected using OCT thickness measurement software. Because of the high axial resolution of OCT, retinal thickness can be measured accurately and reproducibly to within 10 microns and followed serially. OCT has been shown to be a more sensitive method of detecting macular edema than dilated fundus examination using a 78-diopter lens (6) and has been shown to be equally effective as fluorescein angiography (FA) in detecting macular edema (7).

Macular edema typically has one of three appearances on OCT: diffuse retinal thickening, subretinal fluid, or cystoid macular edema. These three appearances are not mutually exclusive and are not pathognomonic of the underlying cause. Cystoid macular edema is characterized by fluid accumulation in intraretinal cystic spaces (Fig. 8-3A). OCT images demonstrate cystic areas of decreased reflectivity within the retina. The ability to quantify the extent of thickening is particularly useful in assessing the response to a variety of treatment modalities (Figs. 8-3A and 8-3B).

For example, in diabetes, OCT can be used to follow the clinical response to focal laser treatment for clinically significant macular edema. Intravitreal corticosteroid injections have also been used in the treatment of macular edema. OCT has been shown to be a sensitive method to measure changes in macular thickness following intravitreal triamcinolone treatment, and it may be useful in directing retreatment with intravitreal corticosteroids (8).

In exudative age-related macular degeneration (AMD), changes in macular thickness can be followed over time. OCT has been used to follow patient responses to photodynamic therapy and anti-vascular endothelial growth factor (anti-VEGF) therapy and to guide retreatment decisions, as the presence of increased macular thickness implies an actively leaking choroidal

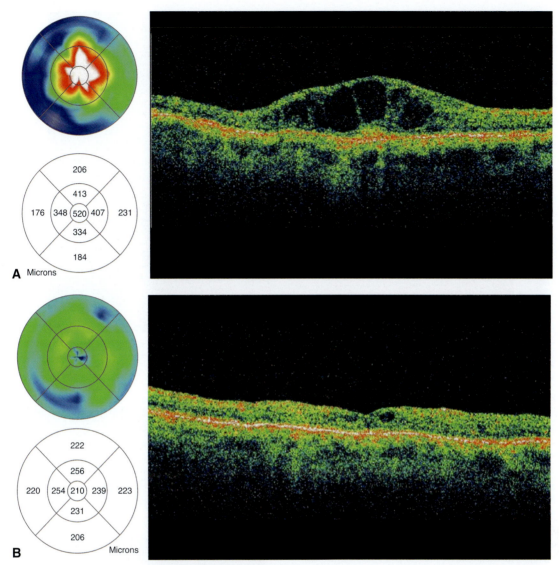

**Figure 8-3  A:** Example of an optical coherence tomography (OCT) image and macular map from a patient with cystoid macular edema. Note the optically clear zones of fluid within the neural retina. **B:** Optical coherence tomography (OCT) images from the same patient, 2 months after treatment with intravitreal kenalog. Note the drastic reduction in macular thickness as well as resolution of most of the cystic spaces within the retina.

neovascularization (CNV) (9). Although FA remains the gold standard to diagnose patients with choroidal neovascularization, differentiating scar tissue from active CNV may be difficult on FA. By its ability to measure macular edema and thickness in a quick and noninvasive manner, OCT has become a standard in the management of previously diagnosed CNV in many clinics.

## CHOROIDAL NEOVASCULARIZATION

OCT is able to localize a choroidal neovascular membrane to the subretinal or sub-RPE space. Thus, OCT may have utility in defining surgically approachable membranes in AMD as well as from other causes of CNV. Figure 8-4 shows a choroidal neovascular membrane that has penetrated the RPE to lie primarily

in the subretinal space. In exudative AMD, OCT may be able to distinguish between occult versus classic forms of CNV by identifying whether the lesion is subretinal or sub-RPE (10,11). CNV membranes that are small and classic or primarily classic, such as in Figure 8-5, are typically the best candidates for submacular surgery (12). With the advent of anti-VEGF therapy, submacular surgery for CNV has become a less widely used form of therapy.

## MACULAR HOLES

As OCT was developed for clinical use in ophthalmology, it was immediately recognized that the technology could be used to image the vitreomacular interface with exquisite detail. One of the earliest applications of OCT was in imaging macular holes.

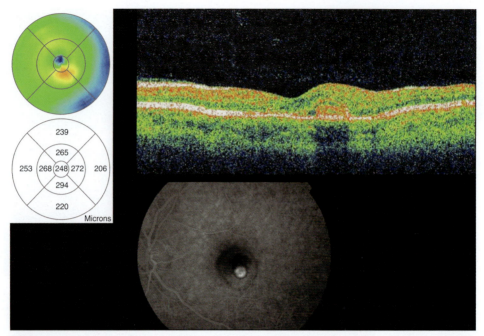

**Figure 8-4.** Example of a classic choroidal neovascular membrane. In the optical coherence tomography (OCT) image, there is a highly reflective neovascular lesion clearly seen above the retinal pigment epithelium.

OCT is able to measure macular hole size and depth, identify epiretinal and posterior hyaloid membranes, and differentiate full-thickness holes from pseudoholes and lamellar holes, making it a useful classification and staging tool prior to surgery.

Using OCT, stage I holes appear as a foveal pseudocyst within the inner retina (13,14). In a stage II hole, an anvil- or flask-shaped full-thickness retinal defect is present, usually with an anterior flap of attached retina (Fig. 8-5A). In contrast, OCT images through stage III holes demonstrate an anvil- or flask-shaped defect without an anterior retinal flap. In stage IV macular holes, a full-thickness retinal defect is noted in addition to complete separation of the posterior hyaloid face from the retina (Fig. 8-5B).

Successful hole closure after surgery also may be documented using OCT (Fig. 8-6). A variety of postoperative OCT appearances are correlated with visual acuity following macular hole repair, including foveal thickness and foveal contour (15–19). In many patients with normal fundus examinations who continue to have decreased visual acuity following macular hole repair, OCT reveals small foveal abnormalities, usually seen as a small cystic space at the level of the photoreceptors (20,21).

Lamellar macular holes, in which a separation of inner retinal tissue occurs without the formation of a full-thickness hole, are also clearly imaged by OCT (Fig. 8-7). Although macular surgery may be attempted in the case of lamellar holes, published results following repair of lamellar holes are sparse and visual results mixed (22,23).

Finally, periodic OCT examination of fellow eyes may be performed to identify impending macular holes, as patients with unilateral idiopathic macular holes are at risk for bilateral disease. Early stages of partial vitreous detachment have been demonstrated on OCT in fellow eyes of macular holes. In these patients, partial vitreous detachment with continued foveal

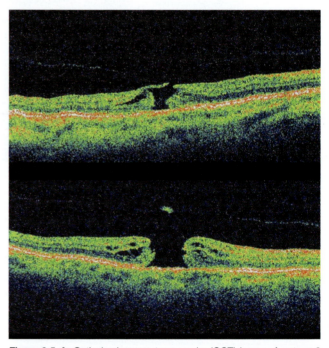

**Figure 8-5 A:** Optical coherence tomography (OCT) image of a stage 2 macular hole. The posterior hyaloid is seen as a reflective line anterior to the retina, partially detached from the retina but inserting at the site of the macular hole. An anterior flap of tissue is covering part of the retinal defect. **B:** Optical coherence tomography (OCT) image of a stage 4 macular hole. The posterior hyaloid is completely detached from the macula, with an operculum or pseudo-operculum visualized. Note the cystic spaces within the neural retina lining the edge of the macular hole.

hyaloid attachment was termed a "stage 0" macular hole, and was a significant risk factor for the development of full-thickness macular holes (Fig. 8-8) (24).

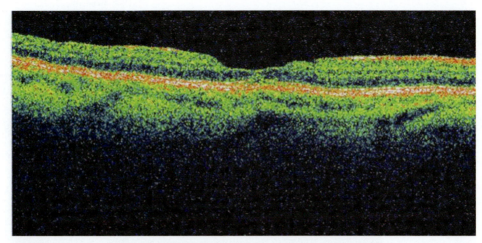

**Figure 8-6.** Optical coherence tomography image of the same patient as in Figure 6-6A, 6 months after surgical repair of the macular hole. The retinal contour is close to normal, with some irregularity of the inner retina and a small defect of the inner segment/outer segment junction at the fovea. This patient's visual acuity returned to 20/40.

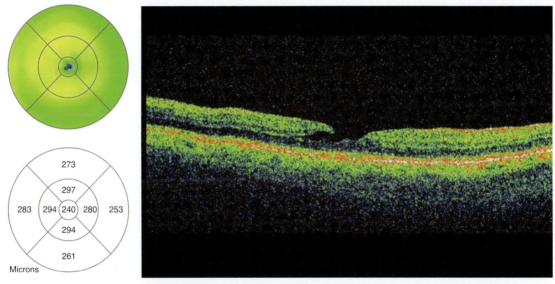

**Figure 8-7.** Example of a lamellar hole. There is a separation between the inner and outer retinal layers. Macular thickness remains nearly normal, as there is no intraretinal fluid present.

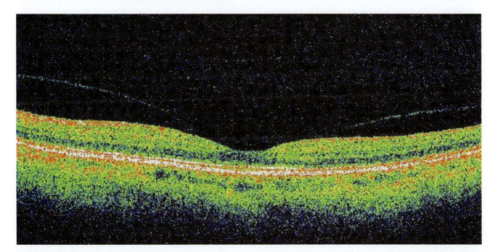

**Figure 8-8.** Optical coherence tomography image of a stage 0 macular hole. This is the fellow eye of a patient with a full-thickness macular hole. Note the partial separation of the posterior hyaloid with persistent attachment of the hyaloid at the fovea.

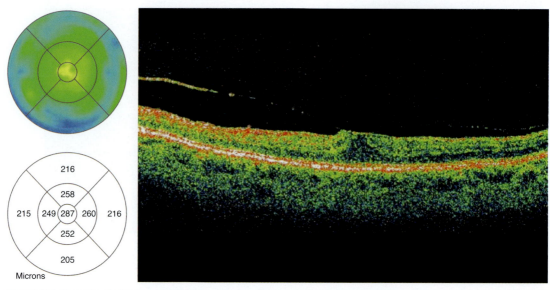

**Figure 8-9.** Example of vitreomacular traction syndrome. The posterior hyaloid is partially separated from the macula, with persistent attachment at the fovea causing distortion of the foveal contour and subsequent thickening of the macula, which may be visualized on the macular thickness map.

## VITREOMACULAR TRACTION

With OCT, the posterior hyaloid becomes clearly visible as a thin band when it separates from the retina. Early stages of vitreous detachment may be detected on OCT while invisible biomicroscopically (25). Occasionally, partial vitreous detachment may result in persistent vitreomacular traction, causing a distortion in the foveal contour; this condition is termed "vitreomacular traction syndrome," and OCT has proven beneficial in its diagnosis (Fig. 8-9). OCT demonstrates vitreomacular traction syndrome in some cases of macular edema in which the cause is not clinically evident. The visualization of vitreomacular traction is important, because vitrectomy surgery to relieve traction may be performed (26,27). In many cases, an additional epiretinal membrane can be visualized on OCT, which can help when planning surgery. It has been suggested that vitreomacular traction patients with persistent attachment of the posterior hyaloid nasal to the fovea may not fare as well as patients with both nasal and temporal vitreous detachment as visualized with OCT (28). Postoperatively, intra- and subretinal fluid sometimes persists for months after surgery, which may be accurately documented with serial OCT imaging (28).

## EPIRETINAL MEMBRANES

Epiretinal membranes (ERM) from a variety of causes may be imaged clearly using OCT (29). Epiretinal membranes appear as a band of moderate to high reflectivity anterior to the retinal surface (Fig. 8-10). In some cases, epiretinal membranes that are barely detectable clinically are well detailed on OCT images. In addition to direct visualization of the epiretinal membrane, secondary retinal thickening from membrane contraction can be accurately measured.

OCT imaging of epiretinal membranes is useful in several respects. Longitudinal observation can help the clinician with the timing of surgery (in cases where serial OCT images demonstrate progressive retinal thickening) (30). Macular pseudohole from an epiretinal membrane sometimes can be difficult to differentiate from a true macular hole on ophthalmoscopic examination alone. Macular pseudohole appears as a thickened band of moderate reflectivity on the retinal surface, with a steepened foveal pit contour but without loss of foveal tissue. OCT may also be helpful in following patients after vitrectomy and ERM peeling. As with vitreomacular traction syndrome, macular thickening may persist after vitrectomy and prevent return of visual acuity (31,32).

## LIMITATIONS AND ARTIFACTS

There are a few limitations of OCT, which include the inability to obtain high quality images through media opacities, requirement of substantial cooperation with the patient, motion and blink artifacts, and algorithmic failure of thickness measurement software. Due to the complexity of OCT equipment, a high level of operator training is necessary. The penetration depth of OCT is limited to around 1.5 mm due to scattering of signal. OCT may be obscured by anterior opacities such as cataract or vitreous hemorrhage. The patient is required to fixate on a point for ~1.3 seconds. Image quality may be degraded by axial or transverse motion and blink artifacts (33). Additionally, computer algorithms to detect retinal thickness may fail, particularly in cases of retinal distortion, low OCT signal, posterior hyaloid detachment, and RPE distortion or abnormalities (34). For example, in some patients with posterior vitreous detachment, the computer will incorrectly detect the posterior hyaloid as the inner boundary of the retina. Failure of the computer algorithm can often be seen as an artificial

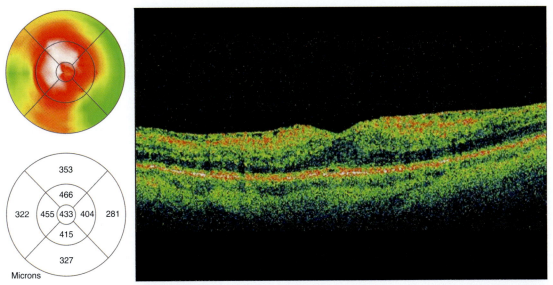

Microns

**Figure 8-10.** Optical coherence tomography of an epiretinal membrane. The membrane may be seen as a thin highly reflective band anterior to the retinal nerve fiber layer. Although the retinal contour appears normal, the macular map clearly demonstrates an increase in macular thickness.

spokelike pattern in the retinal thickness map (35). Despite these limitations, OCT has been shown to be highly accurate and reproducible (36,37).

## FUTURE DIRECTIONS

The abilities of OCT have been expanded through research over the past few years. Broader bandwidth light sources have enabled ultrahigh resolution OCT with axial resolutions as high as 3 microns (38). Adaptive optics may be employed to correct for natural optical aberrations of the human eye, improving transverse resolutions to around 5 microns (39). OCT has been combined with scanning laser ophthalmoscopy to create en-face (c-scan) OCT images (40). Most recently, new methods in signal detection, termed "spectral domain" or "frequency domain" OCT, are being employed to increase the imaging speed of OCT 50 to 100 times, allowing for high pixel density imaging as well as three-dimensional OCT imaging (41). Several spectral domain OCT systems are now available on the commercial market. These new systems may become a new standard in macular imaging for surgical and postsurgical decision making.

## CONCLUSION

OCT is useful in planning treatment for macular disease as well as following macular anatomy after treatment. Serial OCT measurements can help visualize retinal and vitreoretinal anatomy, and can accurately measure changes in retinal thickness. OCT is particularly helpful in following macular thickness before and after treatment and in detailing the contour of the vitreoretinal interface. OCT is also helpful in a number of other macular diseases not included in this chapter, such as central

serous chorioretinopathy and retinal detachment, as well as in glaucoma management (42–44). As OCT has become more widely available, it has proven to be a valuable tool to the retinal surgeon.

## References

1. Hee MR, Izatt JA, Swanson EA, et al. Optical coherence tomography of the human retina. *Arch Ophthalmol* 1995;113:325–332.
2. Huang D, Swanson EA, Lin CP, et al. Optical coherence tomography. *Science* 1991;254:1178–1181.
3. Hee MR, Puliafito CA, Wong C, et al. Quantitative assessment of macular edema with optical coherence tomography. *Arch Ophthalmol* 1995;113:1019–1029.
4. Chan A, Duker JS, Ko TH, et al. Normal macular thickness measurements in healthy eyes using stratus optical coherence tomography. *Arch Ophthalmol* 2006;124(2):193–198.
5. Polito A, Del Borrello M, Isola M, et al. Repeatability and reproducibility of fast macular thickness mapping with stratus optical coherence tomography. *Arch Ophthalmol* 2005;123(10):1330–1337.
6. Browning DJ, McOwen MD, Bowen RM Jr, et al. Comparison of the clinical diagnosis of diabetic macular edema with diagnosis by optical coherence tomography. *Ophthalmology* 2004;111:712–715.
7. Antcliff RJ, Stanford MR, Chauhan DS, et al. Comparison between optical coherence tomography and fundus fluorescein angiography for the detection of cystoid macular edema in patients with uveitis. *Ophthalmology* 2000;107:593–599.
8. Sutter FK, Simpson JM, Gillies MC. Intravitreal triamcinolone for diabetic macular edema that persists after laser treatment: three-month efficacy and safety results of a prospective, randomized, double-masked, placebo-controlled clinical trial. *Ophthalmology* 2004;111:2044–2049.
9. Rogers AH, Martidis A, Greenberg PB, et al. Optical coherence tomography findings following photodynamic therapy of choroidal neovascularization. *Am J Ophthalmol* 2002;134:566–576.
10. Hee MR, Baumal CR, Puliafito CA, et al. Optical coherence tomography of age-related macular degeneration and choroidal neovascularization. *Ophthalmology* 1996;103(8):1260–1270.
11. Hughes EH, Khan J, Patel N, et al. In vivo demonstration of the anatomic differences between classic and occult choroidal neovascularization using optical coherence tomography. *Am J Ophthalmol* 2005;139:344–346.
12. Shimada H, Fujita K, Matsumoto Y, et al. Preoperative factors influencing visual outcome following surgical excision of subfoveal choroidal membranes. *Eur J Ophthalmol* 2006;16(2):287–294.
13. Gaudric A, Haouchine B, Massin P, et al. Macular hole formation: new data provided by optical coherence tomography. *Arch Ophthalmol* 1999;117:744–751.
14. Haouchine B, Massin P, Gaudric A. Foveal pseudocyst as the first step in macular hole formation: a prospective study by optical coherence tomography. *Ophthalmology* 2001;108:15–22.

15. Ullrich S, Haritoglou C, Gass C, et al. Macular hole size as a prognostic factor in macular hole surgery. *Br J Ophthalmol* 2002;86:390–393.

16. Ip MS, Baker BJ, Duker JS, et al. Anatomical outcomes of surgery for idiopathic macular hole as determined by optical coherence tomography. *Arch Ophthalmol* 2002;120:29–35.

17. Kang SW, Ahn K, Ham DI. Types of macular hole closure and their clinical implications. *Br J Ophthalmol* 2003;87:1015–1019.

18. Desai VN, Hee MR, Puliafito CA. Optical coherence tomography of macular holes. In: Madreperla SA, McCuen BW (eds). *Macular hole: Pathogenesis, diagnosis and treatment.* Oxford: Butterworth-Heinemann, 1999:37–47.

19. Imai M, Iijima H, Gotoh T, et al. Optical coherence tomography of successfully repaired idiopathic macular holes. *Am J Ophthalmol* 1999;128:621–627.

20. Kitaya N, Hikichi T, Kagokawa H, et al. Irregularity of photoreceptor layer after successful macular hole surgery prevents visual acuity improvement. *Am J Ophthalmol* 2004;138:308–310.

21. Villate N, Lee JE, Venkatraman A, et al. Photoreceptor layer features in eyes with closed macular holes: optical coherence tomography findings and correlation with visual outcomes. *Am J Ophthalmol* 2005;139:280–289.

22. Haouchine B, Massin P, Tadayoni R, et al. Diagnosis of macular pseudoholes and lamellar macular holes by optical coherence tomography. *Am J Ophthalmol* 2004;138:732–739.

23. Witkin AJ, Ko TH, Fujimoto JG, et al. Redefining lamellar holes and the vitreomacular interface: an ultrahigh-resolution optical coherence tomography study. *Ophthalmology* 2006;113:388–397.

24. Chan A, Duker JS, Schuman JS, et al. Stage 0 macular holes: observations by optical coherence tomography. *Ophthalmology* 2004;111:2027–2032.

25. Uchino E, Uemura A, Ohba N. Initial stages of posterior vitreous detachment in healthy eyes of older persons evaluated by optical coherence tomography. *Arch Ophthalmol* 2001;119:1475–1479.

26. Munuera JM, Garcia-Layana A, Maldonado MJ, et al. Optical coherence tomography in successful surgery of vitreomacular traction syndrome. *Arch Ophthalmol* 1998;116:1388–1389.

27. Gallemore RP, Jumper JM, McCuen BW II, et al. Diagnosis of vitreoretinal adhesions in macular disease with optical coherence tomography. *Retina* 2000;20:115–120.

28. Yamada N, Kishi S. Tomographic features and surgical outcomes of vitreomacular traction syndrome. *Am J Ophthalmol* 2005;139(1):112–117.

29. Wilkins JR, Puliafito CA, Hee MR, et al. Characterization of epiretinal membranes using optical coherence tomography. *Ophthalmology* 1996;103:2142–2151.

30. Massin P, Allouch C, Haouchine B, et al. Optical coherence tomography of idiopathic macular epiretinal membranes before and after surgery. *Am J Ophthalmol* 2000;130:732–739.

31. Hillenkamp J, Saikia P, Gora F, et al. Macular function and morphology after peeling of idiopathic epiretinal membrane with and without the assistance of indocyanine green. *Br J Ophthalmol* 2005;89(4):437–443.

32. Niwa T, Terasaki H, Kondo M, et al. Function and morphology of macula before and after removal of idiopathic epiretinal membrane. *Invest Ophthalmol Vis Sci* 2003;44(4):1652–1656.

33. Hee MR. Artifacts in optical coherence tomography topographic maps. *Am J Ophthalmol* 2005;139:154–155.

34. Ray R, Stinnett SS, Jaffe GJ. Evaluation of image artifact produced by optical coherence tomography of retinal pathology. *Am J Ophthalmol* 2005;139:18–29.

35. Jaffe GJ, Caprioli J. Optical coherence tomography to detect and manage retinal disease and glaucoma. *Am J Ophthalmol* 2004;137:156–169.

36. Massin P, Vicaut E, Haouchine B, et al. Reproducibility of retinal mapping using optical coherence tomography. *Arch Ophthalmol* 2001;119:1135–1142.

37. Muscat S, Parks S, Kemp E, et al. Repeatability and reproducibility of macular thickness measurements with the Humphrey OCT system. *Invest Ophthalmol Vis Sci* 2002;43:490–495.

38. Ko TH, Fujimoto JG, Duker JS, et al. Comparison of ultrahigh- and standard-resolution optical coherence tomography for imaging macular hole pathology and repair. *Ophthalmology* 2004;111:2033–2043.

39. Hermann B, Fernandez EJ, Unterhuber A, et al. Adaptive-optics ultrahigh-resolution optical coherence tomography. *Opt Lett* 2004;29:2142–2144.

40. Podoleanu AG, Dobre GM, Cucu RG, et al. Combined multiplanar optical coherence tomography and confocal scanning ophthalmoscopy. *J Biomed Opt* 2004;9:86–93.

41. Wojtkowski M, Bajraszewski T, Gorczynska I, et al. Ophthalmic imaging by spectral optical coherence tomography. *Am J Ophthalmol* 2004;138:412–419.

42. Hee MR, Puliafito CA, Wong C, et al. Optical coherence tomography of central serous chorioretinopathy. *Am J Ophthalmol* 1995;120:65–74.

43. Schocket LS, Witkin AJ, Fujimoto JG, et al. Ultrahigh-resolution optical coherence tomography in patients with decreased visual acuity after retinal detachment repair. *Ophthalmology* 2006;113(4):666–672.

44. Schuman JS, Hee MR, Puliafito CA, et al. Quantification of nerve fiber layer thickness in normal and glaucomatous eyes using optical coherence tomography. *Arch Ophthalmol* 1995;113:586–596.

# Surgical Techniques

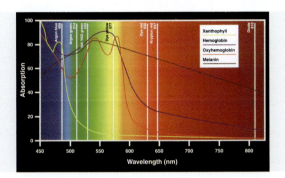

# Principles of Macular Laser Surgery

Alexander J. Brucker  ■  Tushar M. Ranchod

Lasers have diverse applications in the treatment of posterior segment disease. All of these applications rely on the common characteristics of laser light: monochromatism, coherence, and directionality (1). Laser is an acronym for Light Amplification by Stimulated Emission of Radiation, a name which succinctly describes the mechanism of action.

Light is produced by the release of photons in one of two ways. An unexcited atom may be stimulated to an excited state and then spontaneously release a photon as it decays to the lower energy level (spontaneous emission). In lasers, however, a single photon strikes an excited atom to stimulate the release of a second photon (stimulated emission). This stimulated emission results in two photons with uniform frequency and phase (coherence). A chain reaction of stimulated emission requires population inversion, in which the rate of excitation to a higher energy state exceeds the rate of decay to a lower energy state. The released energy (in the form of photons) is amplified by enclosing the system within mirrors. Light is reflected back and forth within the laser, and a partial reflector at one end of the instrument allows a fraction of the light to leave in a single direction (limited divergence). Figure 9-1 illustrates a simple laser.

## WAVELENGTH SELECTION

The specific wavelength of light produced by a laser depends on the choice of lasing medium. Media used in ophthalmic lasers include solid-state materials (i.e., neodymium-Yag), gases (i.e., argon, krypton), organic dyes, combinations of reactive and inert gases (i.e., excimer), and semiconductors (i.e., diode) (2–4). Laser wavelength determines absorption by anatomic structures and pigments as well as scatter by media opacities.

Choice of wavelength during macular laser surgery must account for retinal pigments and their absorptive characteristics

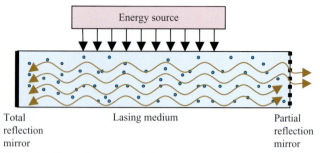

**Figure 9-1.** Illustration of a simple laser.

with respect to therapeutic goals. Melanin, located in the retinal pigment epithelium (RPE) and choroidal melanocytes, has a broad spectrum of absorption and generally does not influence wavelength choice (5). By contrast, hemoglobin in arterial and venous blood, and xanthophylls in the inner and outer plexiform layers possess narrower spectra of absorption. In general, laser light is not well absorbed by pigments of a similar color wavelength (6). For example, the yellow pigment xanthophyll absorbs yellow laser light poorly while hemoglobin absorbs red laser light poorly but absorbs yellow wavelengths well. For this reason, yellow wavelengths are useful for focal macular treatment both to avoid uptake in the fovea, where xanthophyll is most concentrated, and to focus concentration on vascular lesions such as micro-aneurysms. Blue wavelengths are not widely used any longer due to absorption by xanthophylls causing undesired inner segment damage, as well as greater scatter than other visible wavelengths (5).

Longer wavelengths such as red tend to penetrate more deeply than shorter wavelengths such as green, and longer wavelengths are scattered less by media opacities such as cataract. Figure 9-2 illustrates the absorption properties of various ophthalmic lasers by retinal pigments.

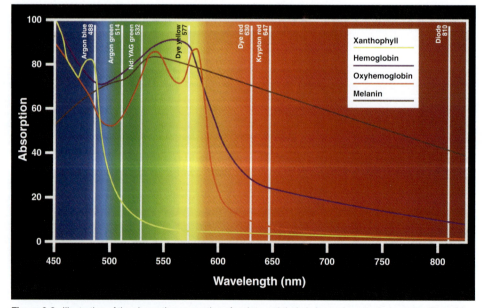

**Figure 9-2.** Illustration of the absorption properties of various ophthalmic lasers by retinal pigments. (From *laser surgery of the posterior segment* Bloom SM, Brucker AJ, 1997, 2nd ed, Lippincott Raven. Figure 1-3 Absorption characteristics of the major ocular pigments for the wavelengths current used for posterior segment photocoagulation, reprinted with permission)

## TISSUE EFFECTS

The combination of wavelength and power determines a laser's effect on tissue. These effects can be classified as photocoagulative, photodisruptive, photoablative, or photochemical. Photocoagulation results when tissue pigments absorb laser energy and tissue temperature rises enough to cause protein denaturation. Panretinal photocoagulation (PRP) with an argon laser is an example of photocoagulation. Photodisruption occurs when concentrated power delivery creates a shock wave that disrupts tissue bonds. The Nd:Yag laser's photodisruptive properties allow for the creation of iridotomies and capsulotomies and can be used to disrupt the posterior hyaloid face, for example in cases of premacular hemorrhage (3,7). Photoablation results when laser energy elevates the temperature of water to the point of vaporization. Excimer lasers use photoablation to reshape the cornea in procedures such as laser in situ keratomileusis, and excessive burns during retinal photocoagulation may result in photoablation of posterior segment tissues (8). Photochemical reactions, also known as photoactivation, occur when laser energy alters chemical bonds in order to activate a target compound (1). Photodynamic therapy with verteporfin is an example of photochemical activation, in which a 489 nm nonthermal diode laser is used to locally activate intravenously injected verteporfin within a treatment zone, thereby resulting in occlusion of a neovascular membrane (9).

## DELIVERY MODALITIES

Laser treatments to the posterior segment can be delivered using a variety of modalities. A slit lamp-mounted laser may be used in combination with a variety of lenses, discussed later in this chapter. A laser fitted to an indirect ophthalmoscope allows treatment with less accuracy but more flexibility than a slit lamp-mounted laser; this setup is often useful for patients who cannot sit comfortably or safely in a chair, or when treatment must be delivered to the far periphery. Laser treatments may also be delivered intraoperatively using an endoscopic laser probe, thereby bypassing anterior segment media opacities (10,11).

A surgeon may choose from a wide variety of lenses when delivering laser treatment to the posterior segment (12). A contact lens is generally used at the slit lamp, with the benefit of stabilizing the globe and ensuring an uninterrupted view during treatment. Contact lenses may provide direct views (virtual, upright image) or indirect views (real, inverted image) at a variety of magnifications (13). Lower image magnification is used for treatments over wide areas, such as panretinal photocoagulation, while higher image magnification is used for macular treatments. Laser spot size magnification is inversely related to angular image magnification, so that lenses which magnify the surgeon's fundus view will proportionately minify the laser spot size (13). Table 9-1 provides a list of commonly used contact lenses along with their image and laser magnification characteristics.

| TABLE 9-1 | COMMON CONTACT LENSES WITH MAGNIFICATION CHARACTERISTICS | |
|---|---|---|
| **Direct contact lenses** | **Image magnification** | **Laser magnification** |
| Haag-Streit | 0.98x | 1.02x |
| Goldman 3-mirror | 0.94x | 1.06x |
| Volk Fundus | 0.8x | 1.25x |
| Indirect contact lenses | | |
| SuperQuad 160 | 2.0x | 0.5x |
| Rodenstock | 1.6x | 0.63x |
| Volk PDT | 1.5x | 0.67x |
| TransEquator | 1.44x | 0.69x |
| Mainster | 1.0x | 1.0x |
| Area Centralis | 0.94x | 1.06x |

Noncontact lenses can be used at the slit lamp or with the indirect headset. Noncontact lenses are helpful at the slit lamp when corneal contact is undesirable, as in the case of a corneal erosion or wound. The condensing lenses used are generally the same as those used for clinical examination. As with contact lenses, laser spot size is minified as an inverse function of retinal image magnification. Image and laser spot magnification depend in part upon the diopteric power of the condensing lens, with lower power lenses providing greater image magnification and spot size minification. Treatment with the indirect headset introduces further complexity to spot size determination, since the degree of image and laser spot magnification varies with the surgeon's working distance from both the condensing lens and patient (14). The real inverted fundus image, located between the surgeon and lens, can be magnified in the surgeon's view by decreasing the distance between surgeon and patient and by moving the lens towards the surgeon to maintain focus (15). The laser spot size at the fundus image plane varies separately with the surgeon's distance from the image plane, since the indirect laser beam is focused rather than collimated. The laser spot size is minimized when the laser focal point meets the fundus image, and increases slightly if the surgeon moves closer or farther from the fundus image. Given the multiple factors influencing laser spot size during indirect treatment, comparing spot size to retinal landmarks may assist the surgeon in achieving a desired spot size. In addition, the surgeon may deliberately adjust the working distance to fine-tune burn size and intensity, in combination with adjustments to the laser power settings.

Most treatment lenses, both contact and indirect, include antireflective coatings to reduce glare from incident white light as well as reduce reflection of the treatment beam into the surgeon's eyes (12). Treatment beam exposure to the surgeon's eyes is further reduced by a filter incorporated into the laser apparatus, whether indirect headset or slit lamp-based. The filter, which necessarily degrades the surgeon's view, may be present constantly, as is the case with most indirect headset systems, or the filter may be integrated into a shutter which drops only when treatment is applied, as with many slit lamp systems (14).

## LASER SETTINGS

Most lasers used for posterior segment treatment display power in watts rather than joules. Watts measure power per unit time, while joules measure total power.

1 watt = 1 joule per second, and 1 joule = 1 watt × 1 second

For a given power displayed in watts, an increase in duration will increase the total power delivered per shot fired. The total power delivered per shot (in joules) is distributed across the surface of the treatment spot. Therefore, for a given total power, a smaller spot size will increase the concentration of laser energy in the target tissue.

Laser settings are titrated based on the desired tissue effect (16,17). Light treatment (barely visible blanching) is desired when treatment aims to stimulate RPE function without causing photocoagulative destruction of the overlying neurosensory retina, as in the case of grid laser for macular edema. Mild treatment (faint retinal whitening) allows destruction of small retinal lesions while minimizing destruction of surrounding retina, as in the case of focal treatment to macular microaneurysms. Moderate to heavy treatment (more intense retinal whitening or grey discoloration of the RPE) allows for more significant destruction of structures adjacent to the RPE, as in the cases of panretinal photocoagulation or thermal laser for choroidal neovascular membranes.

Full thickness coagulation of the neurosensory retina overlying the RPE results in delayed adhesion between these layers. Laser retinopexy of a retinal tear or detachment takes advantage of this adhesion, but the neurosensory retina must remain intact against the RPE after laser delivery since adhesion does not occur instantly, and adhesive forces increase over a period of days to weeks (18).

Several characteristics of a patient's eye may affect laser light vergence, fluence, and scatter. Media opacities such as cataract or vitreous hemorrhage may absorb or scatter incoming laser light, thereby increasing the power required to achieve a retinal burn. Longer wavelengths such as argon red are less subject to scatter and are therefore preferable in patients with dense cataract or vitreous hemorrhage. Intraocular lenses may cause some attenuation of laser output, particularly tinted lenses (19).

Laser treatment through a gas-fluid interface, as in the case of gas pneumoretinopexy, introduces the problem of reflection at the interface (20). Treatment should be delivered entirely through the bubble or entirely around the bubble rather than through the periphery of a bubble or through a collection of small bubbles. Treating perpendicular to the gas-fluid interface minimizes the possibility of laser reflections resulting in burns at unintended sites.

## COMPLICATIONS

Anterior segment complications are relatively uncommon during posterior segment laser surgery. Corneal abrasions may occur due to contact lens trauma, particularly in diabetics with compromised corneal epithelial basement membranes.

Iatrogenic laser burns to the cornea, iris and crystalline lens have been reported, as have corneal edema, hypoesthesia, and endothelial loss without edema (21–26). Thermal damage to intraocular lens implants and unintended posterior capsulotomy have been reported with indirect laser, particularly at higher power settings (27,28). Intraocular pressure elevation may occur following retinal photocoagulation, with angle closure occurring in a minority of these cases, possibly due to transient ciliochoroidal effusions (29,30).

Neurologic complications of posterior segment laser may take the form of internal ophthalmoplegia, pain, or more rarely generalized seizures. The suprachoroidal space contains parasympathetic nerves governing pupillary miosis and accommodation. Laser-induced damage to these nerves may cause internal ophthalmoplegia with sectoral iris palsies, light-near dissociations, pilocarpine hypersensitivity, and accommodative paresis (25,31–33). The suprachoroidal space also contains ciliary nerves, particularly in the horizontal meridian. Patients tend to experience greater pain during retinal laser treatments in the horizontal meridian and more anterior retinal zones. Generalized seizure has been reported following panretinal photocoagulation, possibly induced by the oculocardiac reflex or rhythmic photic stimulation.

Retinal complications of posterior segment photocoagulation may occur by various means. Macular edema following PRP occurs commonly, although usually transiently (34). Direct damage to retinal blood vessels may result in preretinal, intraretinal or subretinal hemorrhage. Intraoperative hemorrhage may be dampened by application of pressure to the globe using a contact lens, thereby elevating intraocular pressure to provide a tamponade effect. Laser photocoagulation may be applied if hemorrhage fails to stop with manual pressure alone. Green and yellow wavelengths with large spot size and long duration burns are particularly effective for this purpose. Laser-induced inflammation may cause a retinal vasculitis that is either clinically evident or subclinical with vessel wall staining and leakage on fluorescein angiogram. Branch artery and vein occlusions have been reported in the setting of panretinal photocoagulation; some surgeons prefer to avoid direct treatment of large retinal vessels for this reason. Epiretinal membranes presumably occur after photocoagulation by an inflammatory mechanism, as does subretinal fibrosis, which may occur in conjunction with laser scar enlargement or independent of scar progression (35). Papillitis may occur when photocoagulation is delivered adjacent to the optic disc, and direct application of thermal laser to the nerve head was abandoned due to observations of presumed ischemic or thermal damage (36).

Laser scar enlargement, also known as atrophic creep, is well documented and particularly concerning when photocoagulation is delivered to the macula (37). Macular scars necessarily produce scotomas, and scar enlargement over time may contribute to diminution of the central visual field. Atrophic creep may occur more extensively in the posterior pole compared to the periphery, particularly in high myopes (38). Scar enlargement may occur over months or years and may result in extrafoveal burns extending into the fovea with resultant decrease in central visual acuity (38,39).

Macular photocoagulation must be delivered with great care, particularly when treating near the fovea. Off-target burns produce unnecessary scotomas, and the surgeon must remain constantly alert to the laser spot location relative to the fovea. Unexpected patient movement may result in foveal burns, and retrobulbar anesthesia may assist the surgeon by paralyzing ocular movement during macular laser surgery.

Heavy photocoagulation can damage the RPE and Bruch's membrane, producing both short term and long-term complications. Perforation of the RPE and Bruch's membrane may cause exudative retinal detachment, particularly during treatment of choroidal vascular lesions. Injury to subretinal layers may also result in longer-term development of choroidal neovascularization (CNV), with laser-induced injury providing an entry point for neovascularization to enter the sub-RPE or subretinal space (40). Burns of short duration and higher power are more likely to perforate the RPE and Bruch's membrane (14). Even subthreshold burns may contribute to the risk of CNV in patients with drusen, as demonstrated in the Prophylactic Treatment of Age-Related Macular Degeneration (PTAMD) trial, and risk of CNV appears to increase with higher intensity laser application (41,42).

Posterior segment manipulation can theoretically cause rips in the pigment epithelium when a pigment epithelial detachment is present, and RPE rips have been documented following macular laser surgery (43–45).

## References

1. Marshall J. Lasers in ophthalmology: the basic principles. *Eye* 1988;2(Suppl):S98–S112.
2. Balles MW, Puliafito CA. Semiconductor diode lasers: a new laser light source in ophthalmology. *Int Ophthalmol Clin* 1990;30:77–83.
3. Mainster MA, Ho PC, Mainster KJ. Nd: YAG laser photodisruptors. *Ophthalmology* 1983(Suppl):45–47.
4. Mainster MA, Ho PC, Mainster KJ. Argon and krypton laser photocoagulators. *Ophthalmology* 1983(Suppl);90:48–54.
5. Mainster MA. Wavelength selection in macular photocoagulation. Tissue optics, thermal effects, and laser systems. *Ophthalmology* 1986;93:952–958.
6. Trempe CL, Mainster MA, Pomerantzeff O, et al. Macular photocoagulation. Optimal wavelength selection. *Ophthalmology* 1982;89:721–728.
7. Aralikatti AK, Haridas AS, Smith JM. Delayed Nd:YAG laser membranotomy for traumatic premacular hemorrhage. *Arch Ophthalmol* 2006;124:1503.
8. Trokel SL, Srinivasan R, Braren B. Excimer laser surgery of the cornea. *Am J Ophthalmol.* 1983;96:710–715.
9. Schlotzer-Schrehardt U, Viestenz A, Naumann GO, et al. Dose-related structural effects of photodynamic therapy on choroidal and retinal structures of human eyes. *Graefes Arch Clin Exp Ophthalmol* 2002;240:748–757.
10. Charles S. Endophotocoagulation. *Retina.* 1981;1:117–120.
11. Peyman GA, Salzano TC, Green JL Jr. Argon endolaser. *Arch Ophthalmol* 1981;99:2037–2038.
12. Dieckert JP, Mainster MA, Ho PC. Contact lenses for laser applications. *Ophthalmology* 1983(Suppl):55–62.
13. Mainster MA, Crossman JL, Erickson PJ, et al. Retinal laser lenses: magnification, spot size, and field of view. *Br J Ophthalmol* 1990;74:177–179.
14. Friberg TR. Principles of photocoagulation using binocular indirect ophthalmoscope laser delivery systems. *Int Ophthalmol Clin* 1990;30:89–94.
15. Rubin ML. The Optics of Indirect Ophthalmoscopy. *Surv Ophthalmol* 1964;146:459–464.
16. Bresnick GH. Diabetic maculopathy. A critical review highlighting diffuse macular edema. *Ophthalmology* 1983;90:1301–1317.

17. Wallow IH. Repair of the pigment epithelial barrier following photocoagulation. *Arch Ophthalmol* 1984;102:126–135.
18. Zauberman H. Tensile strength of chorioretinal lesions produced by photocoagulation, diathermy, and cryopexy. *Br J Ophthalmol* 1969;53:749–752.
19. Kawai K, Sakanishi K. The correlation between various types of intraocular lens and laser wavelength. *Am J Ophthalmol* 2003;135:902–903.
20. Whitacre MM, Mainster MA. Hazards of laser beam reflections in eyes containing gas. *Am J Ophthalmol* 1990;110:33–38.
21. Christiansen SP, Bradford JD. Cataract in infants treated with argon laser photocoagulation for threshold retinopathy of prematurity. *Am J Ophthalmol* 1995;119:175–180.
22. Irvine WD, Smiddy WE, Nicholson DH. Corneal and iris burns with the laser indirect ophthalmoscope. *Am J Ophthalmol* 1990;110:311–313.
23. Lakhanpal V, Husain D, Schocket SS. Posterior capsulotomy as a complication of indirect laser photocoagulation. *Am J Ophthalmol* 1992;114:600–602.
24. Pfister RR, Schepens CL, Lemp MA, et al. Photocoagulation keratopathy. Report of a case. *Arch Ophthalmol* 1971;86:94–96.
25. Schiodte SN. Effects on choroidal nerves after panretinal xenon arc and argon laser photocoagulation. *Acta Ophthalmol (Copenh)* 1984;62:244–255.
26. Zweng HC, Little HL, Hammond AH. Complications of argon laser photocoagulation. *Trans Am Acad Ophthalmol Otolaryngol* 1974;78:OP195–OP204.
27. Morley MG, Frederick AR Jr. Melted haptic as a complication of the indirect ophthalmic laser delivery system. *Am J Ophthalmol* 1992;114:259–261.
28. Whitacre MM, Rupani MK. Argon laser melting of a polymethylmethacrylate intraocular lens. *Am J Ophthalmol* 1994;117:259–261.
29. Blondeau P, Pavan PR, Phelps CD. Acute pressure elevation following panretinal photocoagulation. *Arch Ophthalmol* 1981;99:1239–1241.
30. Gentile RC, Stegman Z, Liebmann JM, et al. Risk for ciliochoroidal effusion after panretinal photocoagulation. *Ophthalmology* 1996;103:827–832.
31. Braun CI, Benson WE, Remaley NA, et al. Accommodative amplitudes in the Early Treatment Diabetic Retinopathy Study. *Retina* 1995;15:275–281.
32. Dellaporta A. Laser application and accommodation paralysis. *Arch Ophthalmol* 1980;98:1133–1134.
33. Lobes LA Jr. Bourgon P. Pupillary abnormalities induced by argon laser photocoagulation. *Ophthalmology* 1985;92:234–236.
34. McDonald HR, Schatz H. Macular edema following panretinal photocoagulation. *Retina* 1985;5:5–10.
35. Guyer DR, D'Amico DJ, Smith CW. Subretinal fibrosis after laser photocoagulation for diabetic macular edema. *Am J Ophthalmol* 1992;113:652–656.
36. Bloom SM. Thermal papillitis after dye red photocoagulation of a peripapillary choroidal neovascular membrane. *Retina* 1990;10:261–264.
37. Dastgheib K, Bressler SB, Green WR. Clinicopathologic correlation of laser lesion expansion after treatment of choroidal neovascularization. *Retina* 1993;13:345–352.
38. Maeshima K, Utsugi-Sutoh N, Otani T, et al. Progressive enlargement of scattered photocoagulation scars in diabetic retinopathy. *Retina* 2004;24:507–511.
39. Morgan CM, Schatz H. Atrophic creep of the retinal pigment epithelium after focal macular photocoagulation. *Ophthalmology* 1989;96:96–103.
40. Miller H, Miller B, Ishibashi T, et al. Pathogenesis of laser-induced choroidal subretinal neovascularization. *Invest Ophthalmol Vis Sci* 1990;31:899–908.
41. Friberg TR, Musch DC, Lim JI, et al. Prophylactic treatment of age-related macular degeneration report number 1: 810-nanometer laser to eyes with drusen. Unilaterally eligible patients. *Ophthalmology* 2006;113:612–622.
42. Kaiser RS, Berger JW, Maguire MG, et al. Laser burn intensity and the risk for choroidal neovascularization in the CNVPT Fellow Eye Study. *Arch Ophthalmol* 2001;119:826–832.
43. Gass JD. Retinal pigment epithelial rip during krypton red laser photocoagulation. *Am J Ophthalmol* 1984;98:700–706.
44. Goldstein M, Heilweil G, Barak A, et al. Retinal pigment epithelial tear following photodynamic therapy for choroidal neovascularization secondary to AMD. *Eye* 2005;19:1315–1324.
45. Thompson JT. Retinal pigment epithelial tear after transpupillary thermotherapy for choroidal neovascularization. *Am J Ophthalmol* 2001;131:662–664.

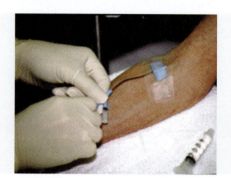

# Photodynamic Therapy

Lucienne Collet ■ Gema Ramírez ■ Rafael Cortez
D. Virgil Alfaro III ■ John B. Kerrison ■ Monica Rodriguez-Fontal

# INTRODUCTION

Age-related macular degeneration (AMD) is the leading cause of legal blindness or severe vision loss in patients older than 60 years in developed countries (1). The management of AMD differs depending on whether it is exudative or nonexudative. The only proven treatment for the nonexudative type, comprising 85% of cases, is an antioxidant/mineral supplement which can slow the progression of the disease by 25% over 5 years (2). For the remaining 15% of the cases, laser treatment, thermal laser photocoagulation, submacular surgery, photodynamic therapy (PDT), and pharmacologic therapy are considered as treatment options.

In 1982, the Macular Photocoagulation Study (MPS) Group demonstrated the effectiveness of laser treatment for choroidal neovascularization (CNV), showing decreased risk of vision loss in these patients (3). Treatment failure occurred in at least 50% of cases resulting from the development of recurrent or CNV on the foveal edge of the laser scar (4). In 1995, the MPS reported that treatment of subfoveal CNV composed of both classic and occult neovascularization was not beneficial with respect to visual acuity and recurrent neovascularization (5).

PDT was first used in ophthalmology in 1994 (6). In 1996, several multicenter randomized clinical trials of PDT with verteporfin were initiated to evaluate its safety and efficacy in treating subfoveal CNV secondary to AMD. Today, the management of exudative AMD is constantly changing with new antiangiogenic therapies.

# MECHANISM OF ACTION AND PHARMACOLOGY OF PHOTODYNAMIC THERAPY

PDT uses an intravenously injected photosensitizing drug that reaches the target tissue through the bloodstream. The photosensitizer is activated by low-intensity laser light and causes damage to choroidal neovascular tissue through a photochemical reaction. The maximum absorption spectrum of the photosensitizer determines the wavelength of the radiation. The light-dye interaction elevates the photosensitizer from its electronic ground state to a higher-level excited triplet state. The photosensitizer quickly returns to the ground state and transfers energy to other molecules, such as oxygen. Singlet oxygen and free radicals are formed and react with proteins, nucleic acids, and lipid membranes. The effective penetration depth of PDT is dependent upon the wavelength of the light. At 630 nm the effective penetration depth is 2 to 3 mm and increases to 5 to 7 mm at 700 to 800 nm (7).

The reactions that follow the formation of intravascular free radicals are classified as cellular, vascular, and immunologic (8). At the cellular level, the free radicals develop a cytotoxic effect by interacting with mitochondria, lysosomes, and other intracellular organelles (9), leading to apoptosis. At the vascular level, which is believed to be the main mechanism, the free radicals lead to destruction of the vascular endothelium. When the vascular endothelium is destroyed, the basal membrane is exposed and it interacts with blood and its components, triggering a platelet aggregation (9). After platelet activation, diverse mediators of inflammation such as thromboxane and histamine are released, thus leading to thrombosis of the vascular lumen and a closing of the vessels limited to the CNV with slight effect on the surrounding microcirculation (10–12). The effectiveness and selectivity of PDT depends on the photosensitizer and the laser used. The ideal wavelength must coincide with the peak light absorption of the photosensitizer used (13). The photosensitizer diffuses into the bloodstream and adheres to the plasmatic low-density lipoproteins. These lipoproteins have abundant receptors in the cytoplasmic membranes of tumoral cells and vascular endothelium. After the photosensitizer associates with LDL, this complex is incorporated into the cell by endocytosis, and then it can be activated by a laser with the appropriate wavelength (14).

# VERTEPORFIN

Verteporfin (Visudyne) is a tetrapyrrole derived from the benzoporphyrin, also called benzoporphyrin derivative monoacid ring A (BPD-MA). It is a potent second-generation light-activated drug. It is a chlorin-type molecule and exists as an equal mixture of two regioisomers, each of which consists of an enantiomeric pair that demonstrate similar pharmacologic activity *in vitro* and *in vivo* (15,16). Verteporfin has a molecular formula of $C_{41}H_{42}N_4O_8$ and a relative molecular weight of 718.81. Nowadays, it is the only photosensitizer approved by the U.S. Food and Drug Administration (FDA) for the treatment of CNV secondary to AMD and subfoveal CNV secondary to pathologic myopia.

Verteporfin has a long absorption wavelength with a strong absorption peak at 680 to 695 nm (15). It absorbs light efficiently at a wavelength of 689 nm (red light), which can penetrate a thin layer of blood, melanin, or fibrotic tissue. Light at this wavelength is not absorbed strongly by naturally present substances (17). The strongest absorption peak of verteporfin is at approximately 400 nm (blue light), but this wavelength is not clinically useful for treatment of CNV because it is the same as the absorption peak of oxyhemoglobin (17). The most suitable light source for use in Visudyne therapy is a nonthermal diode laser, operating at a wavelength of 689 ± 3 nm (17).

The regimen of Visudyne therapy established by the phase I/II studies and investigated in phase III placebo-controlled studies is as follows:

Visudyne dose: 6 mg/m$^2$ body surface area (BSA)
Infusion rate: 3 mL/min
Duration of infusion: 10 min
Light application interval after start of Visudyne infusion: 15 min
Wavelength: 689 nm
Dose: 50 J/cm$^2$
Intensity: 600 mW/cm$^2$
Resulting duration of light application: 83 seconds

Closure of abnormal, leaking blood vessels occurs for approximately 6 to 12 weeks in most patients. Reperfusion is common and multiple treatments are often required.

## INFLUENCE OF TREATMENT PARAMETERS ON SELECTIVITY OF VERTEPORFIN

Studies have been conducted to test the effect of changing dosimetry in order to avoid damage to the surrounding tissue (18). It has been observed that there is a significant photodynamic effect on the choroidal circulation with 50 J/cm$^2$. This parameter was established as a guideline under treatment of age-related macular degeneration with photodynamic therapy (TAP) (19–23). It has been demonstrated by indocyanine green (ICG) angiography that the TAP regimen regularly results in damage to the physiologic choroid, showing early and often persistent nonperfusion of the surrounding choroid (19,20). Histopathologic studies show a dose-dependent thrombosis of the choriocapillaris (21) and immunostaining reveals a reactive upregulation of vascular endothelial growth factor (VEGF) (22). Modification of treatment parameters with reduced fluence to 25 J/cm$^2$ allows selective closure of the CNV and reduces the impact on the physiologic choroidal vasculature (18).

## CLINICOPATHOLOGICAL FINDINGS AFTER PHOTODYNAMIC THERAPY

Histopathological findings of CNV 2 weeks to 3 months after PDT in neovascular AMD have been published (24–26). In these studies, endothelial damage of the CNV was noted. Schnurrbusch, in an electron microscopic study of surgically extracted CNV, showed occluded vessels with thrombotic masses and ultrastructural damage of the neovascular endothelium 3 months after PDT (24). Ghazi also reported endothelial cell degeneration with platelet aggregation and thrombus formation on removed CNV specimens 4 weeks after PDT (25). In a more recent study, the histopathological examination of the excised CNV membranes was done 3 days after PDT (24). It revealed fibrovascular tissue with swollen and disintegrated endothelium. However, neither a red blood cell nor a platelet/fibrin clot was observed (24). Other studies have also reported a uniform occlusion of the healthy choriocapillaris 1 week following PDT in enucleated human eyes (27). The occlusion of the choriocapillaris, perhaps, is the explanation for the nonperfusion of CNV membranes in 3 days following verteporfin PDT.

Whether PDT-induced ischemia of the choriocapillaris influences the reactivation of the CNV by increasing the expression of factors contributing to new vessel formation is not known. The absence of thrombosis in the CNV by light microscopic examination, in the presence of fluorescein angiographically proven nonperfusion of the entire treated area, suggests that choroidal ischemia induces the closure of the CNV vessels in the early period following PDT. The disintegration of the endothelium of the CNV vessels may result in thrombosis in the weeks following treatment (28). Additionally, Tatar et al. studied 50 eyes that underwent removal of choroidal neovascular membranes, 20 of them having received PDT prior to removal. The study histologically revealed many collapsed vessels, damaged endothelial cells, and an occluded choriocapillary layer within the spot produced by the laser. There was intense VEGF synthesis especially prominent in retinal pigment epithelium (RPE) cells induced by hypoxia after PDT (29–33). There was prominent inflammatory activity described in post PDT CNV (34). These findings seem to be an important angiogenic stimulus that may lead to increased vascular leakage and development of recurrent CNV (35).

## IMMUNOHISTOLOGICAL EVALUATION OF CHOROIDAL NEOVASCULARIZATION POST PHOTODYNAMIC THERAPY

Analysis of vascularization and proliferative activity of surgically extracted CNV following PDT by immunodetection of characteristic markers (CD 34, CD 105, and Ki-67) showed that there is a neoangiogenetic mechanism that leads to the formation of new vessels observed in CNV even after 37 days post PDT (36). However, Schnurrbusch (24) and Moshfeghi (37) reported that new vessel formation does not occur until a minimum of 63 days after such an event.

## ANGIOGRAPHIC FINDINGS AFTER PHOTODYNAMIC THERAPY

Fluorescein angiography in animal studies, early after PDT, demonstrated hypofluorescence with perfusion of retinal vessels. Also, ICG angiography demonstrated hypofluorescence in the area treated with PDT, although larger choroidal vessels were perfused. In animal studies, this hypofluorescence on ICG angiography resolved to some extent with follow-up but was still evident at 5 to 8 weeks after PDT. The hypofluorescence may be caused by PDT-induced choriocapillaris occlusion or retinal pigment swelling leading to blocked fluorescence. Follow-up at 2 to 5 weeks after PDT demonstrated staining of the irradiated CNV by ICG angiography and may represent staining of the remaining fibrovascular tissue (29).

## OCT AFTER PHOTODYNAMIC THERAPY

Rogers et al. (38) studied the optical coherence tomography (OCT) characteristics following PDT in eyes treated for CNV secondary to AMD. They correlated it to fluorescein angiography findings and proposed an OCT classification system as follows:

In Stage I there is evidence of acute inflammatory response, confirmed at 1 hour and up to 1 week following PDT.

Fluorescein angiography revealed hyperfluorescence of both the CNV and treatment area, with later frames of the angiogram demonstrating increased leakage of fluorescein in the treatment zone. The OCT demonstrated increased accumulation of intraretinal fluid in a circular distribution delineating the treatment spot.

In Stage II there is resolution of subretinal fluid with choroidal hypoperfusion. Approximately 1 to 2 weeks following treatment, there is hypoperfusion of the CNV and choriocapillaris with a well-delineated area of hypofluorescence corresponding to the treatment spot on fluorescein angiography (FA). OCT exhibits resolution of subretinal fluid in the treatment area with the reestablishment of a normal appearing foveal contour. Stage II typically lasts up to 4 weeks or whenever choroidal reperfusion occurs.

In Stage III, there is reaccumulation of subretinal fluid with subretinal fibrosis. They observed that after the fourth week of treatment, reperfusion of the CNV is typically present on FA with variable degrees of leakage. The treatment spot is less visible on angiography, as the choriocapillaris is rapidly perfused. Intraretinal and subretinal fluid reaccumulates and early subretinal fibrosis becomes evident on OCT between the retina and underlying RPE. They propose that Stage III is subdivided into two separate stages: stage IIIa and IIIb, depending on the ratio of fluid to fibrosis on OCT. In stage IIIa retinal fluid to fibrosis ratio is higher, representing a more active neovascular process. In stage IIIb, the fibrotic component of the CNV is prominent with minimal intraretinal fluid on OCT. Stage IIIb lesions are relatively inactive due to the predominance of subretinal fibrosis with minimal intraretinal fluid, which still leak on fluorescein angiography.

In Stage IV, there is subretinal fibrosis with cystoid macular edema (CME). On FA, the borders of the lesion remain relatively fixed with staining of the fibrotic CNV. However, a component of active leakage in FA is present, which is defined on OCT as CME. The cysts are represented by hyporeflective black circular spaces in the retina. The involuting CNV is represented on the OCT as a highly reflective band merging with RPE/choriocapillaris layer (38).

## ELECTRO-OCULOGRAPHY AFTER PHOTODYNAMIC THERAPY

Osner et al. found that the Arden ratio of the electro-oculogram (EOG) decreased 1 week after PDT and the differences were statistically significant. The decrease in Arden ratio persisted at the first month, as assessed by EOG recordings. PDT may affect the interaction between RPE and photoreceptors (39).

## CLINICAL TRIALS

There are numerous controlled studies that employ PDT. They can be divided into Phase I/II dose-finding studies, where the dose parameters are established, and Phase III placebo-controlled studies that include TAP, verteporfin in

photodynamic therapy (VIP), and verteporfin in the ocular histoplasmosis (VOH).

In order to determine an effective treatment regimen as well as the safety and efficacy of Visudyne therapy, a total of 1236 patients were included: 142 in the phase I/II dose-finding study, 609 in the TAP investigation, 459 in the VIP trial, and 26 in the VOH syndrome study.

## DOSE-FINDING STUDY (PHASE I/II)

### Dose Determination

Some experiments with thermal laser-induced neovascularization in primate eyes were conducted in order to determine the optimal parameters for effective closure of CNV with Visudyne therapy (14,23,30,40–57). Maximal closure of CNV was achieved using Visudyne 0.375 mg/kg with light application 20 to 50 minutes after Visudyne injection at a light dose of $150 \text{ J/cm}^2$ (light intensity $600 \text{ mW/cm}^2$) (56). Lower doses of Visudyne were more selective for CNV, reduced damage to surrounding tissues, and permitted a shorter time interval between Visudyne infusion and light application (56). Light intensities of 300 or $600 \text{ mW/cm}^2$ enabled shorter, more practical treatment times and were not accompanied by any apparent adverse effects (57). Light doses of 50 to $600 \text{ J/cm}^2$ stopped fluorescein leakage from CNV, but doses of $\geq 400 \text{ J/cm}^2$ were associated with unacceptable toxicity in normal retinal tissues (52). These parameters formed the basis for phase I/II dose-finding studies in patients with CNV.

Phase I/II dose-finding study was carried out in patients with subfoveal CNV (30–32). It was a nonrandomized, dose-finding study that was conducted at a total of four centers in Europe and North America. It included 142 patients with subfoveal CNV secondary to AMD ($n = 128$), pathologic myopia ($n = 10$), ocular histoplasmosis syndrome (OHS) ($n = 1$), angioid streaks ($n = 1$), and idiopathic causes ($n = 1$). All of them had evidence of classic CNV and were not eligible for laser photocoagulation.

All patients received one of five treatment regimens and were monitored for 12 weeks. Within each regimen, light at 689 nm (intensity $600 \text{ mW/cm}^2$) was increased up to a maximum of $150 \text{ J/cm}^2$; each light dose was tested on three patients, and the dose was only increased if these patients did not experience adverse events. The maximum tolerated light dose was below $150 \text{ J/cm}^2$ and the minimum effective light dose was greater than $25 \text{ J/cm}^2$ (30). At $150 \text{ J/cm}^2$, nonselective effects on the retinal vasculature and loss of visual acuity were observed, and little evidence of effect on neovascular tissue was seen at light doses of $25 \text{ J/cm}^2$ (30).

## PLACEBO-CONTROLLED STUDIES (PHASE III)

In order to study the efficacy of Visudyne therapy in terms of visual function and angiographic outcomes, in patients with

CNV, the following phase III clinical trials in patients with CNV were conducted:

– Treatment of AMD with Photodynamic therapy (TAP) Investigation (23,40)
– Verteporfin in Photodynamic therapy (VIP) Trial (41,42)

## TREATMENT OF AGE-RELATED MACULAR DEGENERATION WITH PHOTODYNAMIC THERAPY INVESTIGATION (PHASE III)

The TAP Investigation (23,40) included two clinical trials, designed to determine if PDT with Visudyne significantly reduced the risk of vision loss compared with placebo in patients with subfoveal CNV secondary to AMD. It was a 2-year study that was conducted in 22 centers in North America and Europe, and the enrollment was completed in 1997. Patients were randomized in a ratio of 2:1 to receive either Visudyne ($n = 402$) or placebo (dextrose in water) ($n = 207$) in a double-masked fashion.

The inclusion criteria were as follows: patients over 50 years of age with new or recurrent subfoveal CNV secondary to AMD; the lesion had to have classic CNV (although the presence of occult CNV was permitted) with evidence that either classic or occult CNV involved the geometric center of the foveal avascular zone; the combined area of classic CNV had to occupy at least 50% of the total CNV; the greatest linear dimension could not exceed the diameter of a circle measuring 9 MPS disc areas (approximately 5400 μm); and the treatment eye had to have a best-corrected visual acuity score of at least 34 and not more than 73 letters (Snellen equivalent: 20/200 – 20/40). The characteristics of the treatment groups were balanced, except that there were more women assigned to placebo than Visudyne ($p = 0.025$) and more lesions with blood assigned to placebo ($p = 0.028$). The follow-up examinations were scheduled every 3 months. The treating physician considered retreatment if there was leakage from CNV on the fluorescein angiogram. All randomized patients received treatment at the baseline visit, and the final treatment was given at month 21, with follow-up at month 24. From month 6 through month 21, re-treatments were required by 12% to 20% fewer patients treated with Visudyne than placebo (40). The mean number of treatments administered per patient through the 2 years of the TAP Investigation was 5.6 in the Visudyne group and 6.5 in the placebo group. In the second year, fewer treatments were required (mean 2.1) than in the first year (mean 3.4) in the group treated with Visudyne (40).

TAP Report 5 (42) is an open label extension of selected patients from TAP trial where patients were followed beyond 2 years. The purpose was to describe the visual outcomes between the month 24 and month 36 for verteporfin-treated patients who had a predominantly classic lesion at baseline. The results show little change from the two-year findings for patients with lesions that were composed of predominantly classic CNV and assigned to verteporfin therapy at baseline. The results provide evidence that the benefits of this therapy continued through 3 years in patients with subfoveal CNV caused by AMD (42).

## VERTEPORFIN IN PHOTODYNAMIC THERAPY TRIAL (PHASE IIIB)

The VIP Trial (41) was designed to investigate the efficacy of PDT with Visudyne in a wider range of patients compared to the TAP trial. The study included patients with AMD with better visual acuity (70 letters or better, approximate Snellen equivalent better than 20/40), patients with occult CNV with no classic CNV, and patients with CNV secondary to pathologic myopia. It was a 2-year study involving 28 centers in North America and Europe. The enrollment was completed in 1998. Patients were stratified according to the cause of CNV and randomized in the ratio of 2:1 to either Visudyne ($n = 306$) or placebo ($n = 153$).

The inclusion criteria were as follows: patients with new or recurrent subfoveal CNV secondary to AMD or pathologic myopia; patients at least 50 years of age whose CNV was secondary to AMD; the area of classic CNV plus occult CNV had to occupy at least 50% of the total lesion; the greatest linear dimension of the lesion could not exceed the diameter of a circle measuring 9 MPS disc areas (approximately 5400 μm); and the treatment eye had to have a best-corrected visual acuity score of at least 50 letters (20/100 or better), except for eyes with lesions containing classic CNV secondary to AMD, which had to have a best-corrected visual acuity score or better than 70 letters (20/40 or better). Lesions with occult CNV and no classic CNV either had to contain blood or show progression of disease within the 3 months preceding randomization to treatment (defined as either a loss of at least six letters of visual acuity or growth of at least 10% of the lesion's greatest linear dimension within 3 months). If the subfoveal CNV was secondary to pathologic myopia, the spherical equivalent had to be equal to or more negative than –6 diopters, or the axial length had to be at least 26.5 mm. Only 22% of eyes had classic CNV at the baseline examination; 68% had occult CNV with no evidence of classic CNV (41). The majority of lesions were predominantly classic (83%), and only 14% of eyes had evidence of occult CNV at the baseline examination (43). In patients with AMD, the mean treatment rate was 3.1 in the Visudyne group and 3.6 in the placebo group (43). In patients with pathologic myopia, the mean treatment rate was 3.4 in the Visudyne group and 3.2 in the placebo group.

## OTHER STUDIES

### Japanese Age-Related Macular Degeneration Trial Study Group

Japanese Age-Related Macular Degeneration Trial (JAT) reported 1-year results of PDT with verteporfin in Japanese patients with subfoveal CNV secondary to AMD (44). After

1 year of follow-up, 50% and 77% of verteporfin-treated patients demonstrated no leakage from classic or occult CNV, respectively.

## VOH STUDY (PHASE I/II) (45,46)

The VOH Study is an open-label, three-center, 1-year study of 26 patients with OHS (45). The patients included in this study had OHS with subfoveal CNV lesions no larger than 5400 μm in greatest linear dimension with classic or occult CNV extending under the geometric center of the foveal avascular zone and best-corrected visual acuity letter score of 73 to 34 (approximate Snellen equivalent 20/40 to 20/200). The patients received verteporfin (6 mg/m2) with the same regimen of Visudyne therapy used in the TAP and VIP Trial. At 3-month follow-up examinations, retreatment with the same regimen was given if angiography showed fluorescein leakage.

By month 12, patients had received an average of 2.9 treatments of a maximum of four possible treatments. The month 12 median improvement from baseline in visual acuity of the remaining 25 patients was seven letters, and median contrast sensitivity improved by two letters. At the month 12 examination, 14 (56%) patients gained seven or more letters of visual acuity from baseline, whereas four (16%) patients lost eight or more letters, of which two (8%) lost 15 or more letters. No serious systemic or ocular adverse events were reported. They concluded that the median visual acuity improved after verteporfin therapy for at least 1 year (45).

The VOH Study published 2-year results (46) of an open-label, 3-center, uncontrolled clinical study. At 24-month examination, which was completed in 84% of the participants, median improvement from baseline in visual acuity was six letters; median contrast sensitivity improved by 3.5 letters. Ten patients (45%) gained seven or more letters of visual acuity from baseline, whereas four patients (18%) lost eight or more letters. There was absence of fluorescein angiographic leakage from classic CNV in 17 of the 20 evaluable lesions (85%). They concluded that the median visual acuity improved and fluorescein angiographic leakage decreased after verteporfin therapy in OHS patients (46).

## SAFETY OF PHOTODYNAMIC THERAPY WITH VERTEPORFIN

The systemic and ocular safety of Visudyne therapy has been evaluated in three studies in patients with CNV secondary to AMD, pathologic myopia, and OHS. A total of 1094 patients were included in the TAP, VIP Trial, and the VOH Study (23,41,45). Systemic adverse events and ocular adverse events affecting the treated eye were recorded during each study. Other evaluations included measurement of vital signs, physical examinations, electrocardiograms, and laboratory assessments of hematology, serum chemistry, and urinalysis. Visudyne therapy is considered well tolerated. In fact, the withdrawal rate due to adverse events is low (3.8%). Serious

adverse events related to treatment occurred in 3.5% of patients treated with verteporfin and 1.4% of placebo patients. In fact, photosensitivity reactions occurred in fewer than 3% of Visudyne-treated patients; injection-site adverse events occurred more frequently with Visudyne therapy (11.2%) than placebo (4.4%). The only reports of infusion-related back pain (2.0%) were in AMD patients treated with Visudyne therapy. All the cases were transient and resolved by the end of the infusion.

## SERIOUS ADVERSE EVENTS

In the first year of TAP (23), the incidence of injection-site events was 11.9% in Visudyne treated patients and 1.9% in those who received placebo. In the second year of TAP (40), it increased to 14.4% and 4.8%, respectively. The total incidence of treatment-related serious adverse events was 3.5% for Visudyne-treated patients compared with 1.4% for patients who received placebo. No treatment-related deaths occurred in any of the ocular studies. The total rate of withdrawal from the ocular studies due to adverse events was low: 3.8% for Visudyne-treated patients compared with 0.3% for patients who received placebo.

In the TAP trial, three Visudyne-treated patients were withdrawn because of serious verteporfin-related adverse events, such as gastrointestinal bleeding, right-sided body pain with shortness of breath, high blood pressure, and suprachoroidal hemorrhage. An additional three patients were withdrawn due to nonserious treatment-related events, such as severe injection-site pain, skin rash, and infusion-related back pain. Additionally, in the AMD arm of the VIP trial, six verteporfin-treated patients were withdrawn because of adverse events, such as decrease in vision. Seven verteporfin patients (3.1%) had adverse events but were not withdrawn from the trial; their adverse events were central scotoma, vitreous hemorrhage, subretinal hemorrhage, vision loss in two cases, anemia, and knee infection. Four placebo patients had serious adverse events that were considered to be related to therapy (subretinal hemorrhage, vitreous hemorrhage, submacular hemorrhage, and hyponatremia).

In the myopia arm of the VIP trial, the treatment was discontinued in one Visudyne-treated patient who complained of dyspnea and flushing during the second minute of the first infusion. The infusion was discontinued and the dyspnea resolved within 15 minutes of treatment with intravenous (IV) steroids. Treatment was not discontinued in the VOH Study.

## OCULAR ADVERSE EVENTS

Clinically significant ocular events were defined in the study protocols of TAP and VIP as serious adverse events including severe vision decrease, defined as vision decrease of at least four lines occurring within 7 days of treatment, arteriolar or venular nonperfusion, retinal capillary nonperfusion of at least 1 MPS disc area, or vitreous hemorrhage.

These ocular events occurred in a total of 24 (3.3%) verteporfin-treated patients and six (1.7%) patients who received placebo. They occurred in patients with AMD and in patients with minimally classic or no classic lesions at baseline (21 of 24 Visudyne patients and four of six placebo patients). There were no clinically significant ocular events in patients with pathologic myopia or OHS. In the three trials, 13 patients there were reported to have an acute severe decrease in vision (1.8%) treated with verteporfin. Four episodes of severe vision decrease were reported in three (0.7%) verteporfin-treated patients within 9 days of treatment in the TAP trial. Two of these patients improved their vision (>5 letters) at the next 3-month visit. Ten patients in the AMD arm of the VIP Trial experienced a severe decrease in vision. No clinically significant ocular adverse events occurred in either treatment group in patients with pathologic myopia.

## PHOTOSENSITIVITY REACTIONS

In the TAP trial of 2 years (23) and VIP 1-year trial (43), the photosensitivity reactions reported were 2.2%, seen in patients treated with Visudyne therapy. The photosensitivity reactions were transient and mild to moderate secondary to direct exposure to sunlight within 3 days of treatment and resolved within 1 week. Such reactions can be prevented, and patients should take precautions such as avoiding exposure to direct sunlight or bright indoor lighting, wearing dark sunglasses outdoors during the first 48 hours, and avoiding exposure to powerful operating lights.

## ABSORPTION AND BIODISTRIBUTION OF VERTEPORFIN

The pharmacokinetics of verteporfin have been studied in animal models. The apparent volume of distribution at steady state (VSS) in mice, rats, and dogs ranged from 0.26 to 0.94 L/kg depending on the dose and animal studied (47). Dose-dependent variables, such as area under the plasma concentration–time curve and maximum measured plasma concentration (Cmax) demonstrated dose proportionality and were similar under single and multiple dosing, suggesting that there was no accumulation of verteporfin with multiple dosing (47). Verteporfin rapidly distributes in the liver, spleen, and kidneys. Maximal concentrations were observed in all tissues within 3 hours of administration but decreased within 24 hours. Verteporfin reached higher levels in tumors than in normal tissues other than liver, spleen, and kidney, and elimination from tumor tissue was slower than from other tissues, resulting in a higher tumor-to-tissue concentration ratio 24 hours after administration.

Biodistribution studies show that verteporfin accumulates within 5 minutes in vascular structures in the eye, such as the choroid and ciliary body (48). Verteporfin accumulates less in avascular structures such as the cornea, lens, and vitreous. However, it accumulates within 5 minutes in RPE cells. Two hours after administration, it is no longer detectable in the choroid or photoreceptors and reduced in the RPE. Verteporfin is selectively taken up and retained more by malignant, rapidly dividing cells than by normal or resting cells (49). Verteporfin selectively accumulates in neovasculature such as the proliferating vasculature within tumors (50). Also, *in vivo* studies have indicated that verteporfin is taken up rapidly and selectively by ocular neovascular endothelial cells (14). After verteporfin is administered intravenously it associates almost exclusively with plasma lipoproteins (47).

Studies of human plasma have shown that 6% of verteporfin is associated with albumin, and 91% is distributed equally among the high-density, low-density, and very low-density lipoprotein fractions (51); thus, it makes verteporfin available to rapidly dividing endothelial cells of the neovasculature through LDL receptor-mediated pathway and possibly via direct diffusion (47). This enhanced delivery is due to high levels of expression of LDL receptors on endothelial cells of the neovasculature.

## METABOLISM AND ELIMINATION

Verteporfin is metabolized primarily in the liver, and in the plasma, by esterases (52). The main metabolite is a less active diacid form of verteporfin, but this accounts for only 5% to 10% of the total exposure and is also rapidly eliminated. This biotransformation of verteporfin to a nonphotosensitive product could account for the rapid disappearance of photosensitivity in tissues such as the skin (53). Verteporfin is eliminated rapidly from plasma and exhibits multicomponent kinetics consisting of an initial rapid phase during the first 30 minutes after administration, a second slightly slower elimination rate lasting 8 hours, and a third more prolonged phase (52). Elimination is through the biliary route and less than 0.01% is recovered in urine. The mean plasma half-life of verteporfin is 2 to 5 hours after intravenous doses of 0.5 to 2.0 mg/kg (52).

## CLINICAL PHARMACOKINETICS

After a 10-minute infusion of Visudyne 6 mg/m$^2$ BSA the following variables were determined (54):

- Maximum plasma concentration (Cmax) of 1.1 to 1.3 µg/mL
- Area under the plasma concentration–time curve (AUC0-t) of 1.5 to 1.7 µg·h/mL
- Apparent volume of distribution (vss) of 0.45 to 0.6 L/kg
- Plasma elimination half-life (t1/2) of 5 to 6 h
- Total body clearance (CL) of 90 to 110 mL/h/kg

Less than 0.01% of the dose is excreted in the urine (54). Dose alterations are therefore unnecessary in patients with renal impairment. The pharmacokinetics of verteporfin are altered in patients with mild hepatic dysfunction (54). The effect is a

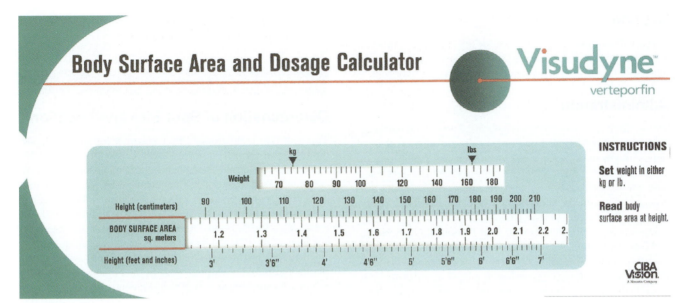

**Figure 10-1.** Dose meter for Visudyne (vertporfin).

reduction in plasma clearance, which is predictable because biliary clearance is the main route of verteporfin elimination, and this decreased clearance is not associated with increased skin photosensitivity. Dosage adjustments are therefore not necessary in patients with mild hepatic impairment (Fig. 10-1).

With regard to verteporfin and other drug interactions, it is possible that the concomitant use of other photosensitizing agents (tetracyclines, sulfonamides, phenothiazines, sulfonylurea hypoglycemic agents, thiazide diuretics, and griseofulvin) may increase the potential for photosensitivity reactions. Other possible interactions are with calcium channel blockers, polymyxin B, or radiation therapy, because they could enhance the rate of verteporfin uptake by the neovascular endothelium. Additionally, compounds that trap active oxygen species or free radicals (e.g., dimethyl sulfoxide, β-carotene, ethanol, formate, and mannitol) may decrease the photodynamic activity of Visudyne therapy. Also, the efficacy of verteporfin may be decreased by thromboxane A2 inhibitors, which decrease platelet aggregation, clot formation, and vasoconstriction.

## ADMINISTRATION AND LASER APPLICATION

### Preparation

Visudyne is designed for IV use. It is supplied in 15 mg vials as a sterile, lyophilized powder and requires reconstitution with sterile water and dilution with 5% dextrose solution before administration.

### Reconstitution

For a total volume of 7.5 ml of reconstituted drug, 7.0 ml of sterile water for injection has to be injected into the Visudyne

vial, which should then be gently agitated until it is completely dissolved. The reconstituted solution must be used within 4 hours. Saline solution must not be used because Visudyne precipitates in saline (Fig. 10-2).

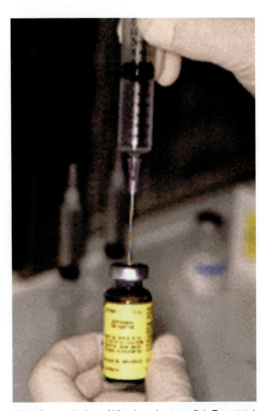

**Figure 10-2.** Reconstitution of Visudyne (verteporfin). For a total volume of 7.5 ml of reconstituted drug, 7.0 ml of sterile water for injection has to be injected into the Visudyne vial, which should then be gently agitated until it is completely dissolved. The reconstituted solution must be used within 4 hours. Saline solution must not be used because Visudyne precipitates in saline.

## Dilution

Further dilution with 5% dextrose for injection is required to achieve a drug dose of 6 mg/m² BSA and a total infusion volume of 30 mL. BSA is determined using a graphic algorithm.

## Administration

The solution is infused intravenously at a rate of 3 ml/min over 10 minutes. Precautions must be taken to prevent extravasation. The standard precautions include careful monitoring of the IV line throughout the 10-minute infusion. It is recommended that the largest vein possible in the arm be used, preferably antecubital, for infusion because of the possible fragility of vein walls in some elderly patients (Fig. 10-3). If Visudyne extravasates, it can cause severe pain, inflammation, swelling, and discoloration of the injection site. Analgesics may be necessary to relieve the pain. If the patient experiences discomfort or pain at or near the infusion site or if extravasation occurs, the infusion must be stopped immediately. In cases when less than half of the solution is estimated to have been administered intravenously, it is recommended to obtain better venous access as soon as possible and restart the infusion. Laser application should be done 15 minutes after the second start of the infusion. If venous access cannot be obtained, patients can be retreated after 24 hours. In the case that more than half of the solution is estimated to have been administered intravenously, the infusion is discontinued. Light application can be carried out 15 minutes after the start of the infusion, even if the duration of the infusion is shorter than 10 minutes. If extravasation has occurred, the infusion should be discontinued. Immediate application of cold compresses or ice is recommended, and the patient's arm should be elevated for 1 day when possible. Warm compresses can be used 24 hours after the event. To avoid severe local reactions, the site of extravasation must be protected from direct light for a minimum of 2 days after the infusion or for as long as swelling and discoloration of the skin is visible. If venous access cannot be obtained and treatment is not given, the patient should be retreated after 7 days. If venous access is achieved and the treatment is given, the patient should return for the routine follow-up examination after 3 months.

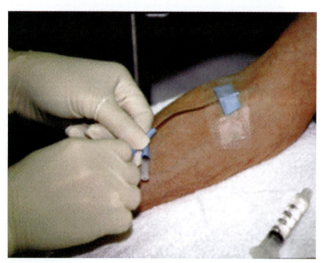

**Figure 10-3.** Care must be taken to avoid extravasation of Visudyne (verteporfin).

## LASER APPLICATION

### Determination of Spot Size and Location

The spot size is determined by measuring the greatest linear dimension of the lesion, including all classic and occult CNV, blood, and/or blocked fluorescence. This measurement can be estimated using a transparent millimeter ruler placed on a fluorescein angiogram obtained with a fundus camera or measured with digital software on the digital picture. An additional 1000 μm is added to the value to allow a 500 μm margin to ensure full coverage of the lesion and to allow for small eye movements.

The laser spot covering the lesion should be no closer than 200 μm to the temporal edge of the optic disc, even if the lesion is located closer to it. If the lesion or the proposed treatment area extends closer than 200 μm to the optic disc, that portion of the lesion should be left untreated.

### Laser Application

Laser light of 689 nm is delivered with an intensity of 600 mW/cm² by a nonthermal diode laser. It should begin 15 minutes after the start of the 10-minute Visudyne infusion. A laser dose of 50 J/cm² is delivered to the lesion as a circular spot using the slit lamp and a specially designed ophthalmic magnification lens. The time to deliver laser dose is 83 seconds (Fig. 10-4).

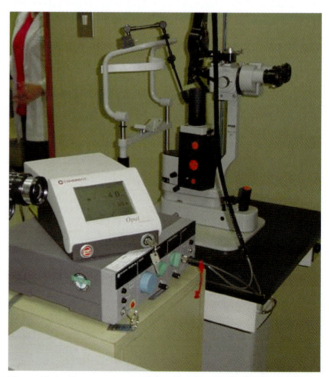

**Figure 10-4.** Photodynamic therapy laser. Laser light of 689 nm is delivered with an intensity of 600 mW/cm² by a nonthermal diode laser. It should begin 15 minutes after the start of the 10-minute Visudyne infusion. The laser dose of 50 J/cm² is delivered to the lesion as a circular spot using the slit lamp and a special designed ophthalmic magnification lens. The time to deliver the laser dose is 83 seconds.

## Retreatment

Patients should be followed every 3 months after any initial or subsequent treatment. Patients are retreated if there is evidence of leakage from CNV on the fluorescein angiogram. Patients who experience severe vision loss of four lines or more within 1 week of treatment should not be retreated until their vision has returned to pretreatment levels.

## INDICATIONS OF PHOTODYNAMIC THERAPY

PDT is indicated in cases of subfoveal or juxtafoveal CNV caused by AMD, OHS, angioid streaks, or pathological myopia (23,32,41,58); choroidal hemangioma; and central serous chorioretinopathy (56).

## CONTRAINDICATIONS

Visudyne therapy is contraindicated in patients with known hypersensitivity to verteporfin or any other component of the lipid-based formulation, porphyria, and in patients with severe hepatic impairment.

## TREATMENT COMBINATIONS

The potential and success of verteporfin PDT, however, is considerably compromised by a recurrence rate of about 90% within 3 months and a mean visual acuity loss of two Early Treatment Diabetic Retinopathy Study (ETDRS) lines within 6 months (17,23). Also, the number of re-treatments necessary for persistent CNV closure was found to be as high as 5.6 over 2 years in a study of classic subfoveal CNV (41). Even, results from patients with occult CNV larger than four disc areas and good visual acuity appeared less favorable (40), and the reason could be the damage of choriocapillaris and RPE after PDT (37,59,60). The associated damage results in retinal edema and release of angiogenesis factors like VEGF (22,38). Therefore, it is important to identify agents that might increase the efficacy of PDT in the treatment of CNV. Combining verteporfin therapy with antiangiogenic and anti-inflammatory therapies is currently under discussion.

Nowadays, the agents considered for combination therapy are steroids and anti- VEGF agents. Steroids have a number of antiangiogenic, antifibrotic, and antipermeability properties that can contribute to the stabilization of the blood–retina barrier, resorption of exudation, and downregulation of inflammatory stimuli. Triamcinolone acetonide has demonstrated to have potent antiangiogenic properties and can inhibit angiogenesis growth factors that decrease release of cytokines, affect interendothelial cell tight junctions, and cell proliferation and migration (61,62). However, clinical studies using intravitreal triamcinolone acetonide (IVTA) alone in treating CNV secondary to AMD have failed to confirm the beneficial

visual outcome (63,64). Therefore, a combination therapy of PDT with intravitreal triamcinolone might have adjuvant effects to improve the outcome of PDT.

New pharmacological therapies that target VEGF-A have significantly enhanced the treatment of AMD by limiting the progression of the disease, and sometimes improving vision. This combination therapy of PDT and antiangiogenic therapies are discussed in another chapter.

## PHOTODYNAMIC THERAPY AND TRIAMCINOLONE

Several studies have been conducted using a combination therapy of PDT and triamcinolone. The results appear favorable as combined therapy is associated with lower retreatment rates and patients having visual improvements (65–68). Combined PDT with IVTA appears to have better results than PDT alone (69). In several studies, researchers have found that patients in the combined treatment group have significantly better visual outcome in terms of lines of best-corrected visual acuity changes (69). Spaide et al. showed a mean improvement of 2.4 lines after PDT with IVTA (68). Additionally, the mean number of treatments needed during a mean follow-up period of 43 weeks was a low: 1.21 (70) versus 5.6 over 2 years (41). The combination is well tolerated. There are treatable adverse effects such as cataract progression in 48% (70) and a transient increase in intraocular pressure (IOP) in 25% of the patients (70). Results of using a combination of PDT and IVTA suggest the potential to improve visual outcomes while reducing treatment rates.

PDT alone used to treat CNV associated with AMD necessitates retreatment at month 3 in 90.8% patients and slightly fewer patients at month 6, with an average of 3.3 sessions in the first year of therapy (23). In a study conducted by Ruiz-Moreno 71) in which patients were treated with a combination of PDT and high dose of IVTA (20 mg), 93% of 15 eyes were retreated at month 3, 67% at month 6, 47% at month 9, and 33% at month 12. The average number of sessions in the first year was 1.6. After two years, the researchers reported that a reduction in the number of PDT sessions needed to stop CNV growth was statistically significant during the first year, but it was not during the second year of the study.

## TRIPLE THERAPY

New therapies are available to treat CNV secondary to AMD. However, there is no single treatment that addresses the multifactorial pathogenesis of the disease. It has been recognized that the genetic variation in the complement regulatory gene factor H (HF1/CFH) predisposes individuals to AMD. CFH has been identified as a key regulator of the complement system of innate immunity. This contributes to the hypothesis that AMD is the result of an aberrant inflammatory process that includes inappropriate complement activation (71–74). The ideal treatment for CNV is one that eradicates the CNV, reduces inflammation, and decreases VEGF expression to prevent further

CNV growth. There are no treatments that demonstrate all these functions, and this has led to the development of combination therapy.

Triple therapy is the combination of verteporfin PDT, intravitreal anti-VEGF agents, and intravitreal steroids. The rationale for their use is based on their different mechanisms of action and promising preliminary combination study results (75). Verteporfin PDT has an angio-occlusive effect, and it selectively damages the endothelial cells of new vessels, leading to their occlusion. The reaction to this CNV occlusion is an inflammatory response and upregulation of VEGF and other growth factors (22).

In a study by Augustin et al. (76) after one cycle of triple therapy (verteporfin PDT, plus bevacizumab and dexamethasone) mean visual acuity (VA) significantly improved by 1.8 lines in 104 patients with CNV caused by AMD. Until now, the mean follow-up time is 40 weeks. In 18 patients the triple therapy was complemented by an additional intravitreal injection of bevacizumab. The safety of triple therapy was good, and no IOP increases were observed. Recurrence of the CNV was seen in five patients. The authors propose that the sustained VA improvement observed is due to termination of CNV by verteporfin PDT combined with inhibition of inflammation by dexamethasone and blockage of continued neovascularization due to VEGF by bevacizumab.

## REDUCED AND STANDARD LIGHT APPLICATION

Current PDT treatment for AMD uses a standard radiant exposure of 50 J/cm$^2$ at an irradiance of 600 mW/cm$^2$ (23). Nichols and Foster emphasized the importance of photochemical oxygen depletion in limiting the effectiveness of PDT with relatively high irradiation fluence rates (77,78). Thus, there is a problem with unusually high irradiance used to treat CNV: the rate of photochemical production of singlet oxygen may be limited by insufficiently oxygenized neovascular tissue (77). It is likely that PDT treatment for AMD would be more effective and selective in terms of sparing photoreceptors using lower laser intensity. Framme et al. (77) evaluated the efficacy of verteporfin photoactivation to induce thrombosis of choriocapillaris in experimentally induced corneal neovascularizations in rabbits by varying irradiance and retinal radiant exposure. They concluded that fluorescein angiography performed 1 h after irradiation revealed vessel closure determined by hypofluorescence at radiant exposures of 20 J/cm$^2$. Additionally, there were indications of higher effectiveness for irradiation with 100 mW/cm$^2$ rather than with 600 mW/cm$^2$. Thrombosis and damage were seen at lower radiant exposures of 100 rather than with 600 mW/cm$^2$ irradiation. Also, with 100 mW/cm$^2$ irradiation, the area of angiographic hypofluorescence was greater than that with irradiation of 600 mW/cm$^2$. They concluded that low-intensity PDT seems to enhance the PDT effects because of vessel occlusion at lower damage thresholds and possibly higher selectivity in sparing RPE and photoreceptors. Further studies should be done to determine the selectivity of low intensity PDT as well as the best treatment parameters.

## CONCLUSION

AMD is the leading cause of legal blindness in patients older than 60 years, and its management is constantly changing with new therapeutic approaches. After thermal laser photocoagulation, PDT became the only therapeutic weapon used for the treatment of CNV. With the introduction of antiangiogenic therapeutics, their use alone or in combination with PDT is offering new options for the treatment for exudative AMD or CNV secondary to other nosologic entities.

### References

1. National Institute for Neurological Diseases and Blindness, Section on Blindness Statistics. Statistics on blindness in the model reporting area, 1969–1970. DHEW publication no. (NIH) 73–427. US Department of Health, Education, and Welfare. Washington, DC: US Government Printing Office, 1973.
2. Age-Related Eye Disease Study Research Group. A randomized, placebo-controlled, clinical trial of high-dose supplementation with vitamins C and E, beta carotene, and zinc for age-related macular degeneration and vision loss: AREDS report no. 8. *Arch Ophthalmol* 2001;119:1417–1436.
3. Macular Photocoagulation Study Group. Argon laser photocoagulation for senile macular degeneration: results of a randomized clinical trial. *Arch Ophthalmol* 1982;100:912–918.
4. Macular Photocoagulation Study Group. Recurrent choroidal neovascularization after argon laser photocoagulation for neovascular maculopathy. *Arch Ophthalmol* 1986;104:503–512.
5. Macular Photocoagulation Study Group. Occult choroidal neovascularization. Influence on visual outcome in patients with age-related macular degeneration. *Arch Ophthalmol* 1995;114:400–412.
6. Schmidt-Erfurth U, Hasan T, Flotte T. Photodynamic therapy of experimental intraocular tumors with benzoporphyrin-lipoprotein. *Ophthalmology* 1994;91:348–356.
7. Arias L, Monés J, Lavaque A, et al. *Age related macular degeneration.* Philadelphia: Lippincott Williams and Wilkins, 2006.
8. Henderson BW, Dougherty TJ. How does PDT work? *Photochem Photobiol* 1992;55:145–157.
9. Jori G, Reddi E. The role of lipoproteins in the delivery of tumor targeting photosensitizers. *Int J Biochem* 1993;25:1369–1375.
10. Schmidt-Erfurth U, Bauman W, Gragoudas ES, et al. Photodynamic therapy of experimental choroidal melanoma using lipoprotein-delivered benzoporphyrin. *Ophthalmology* 1994;101:89–99.
11. Fingar VH. Vascular effects of PDT. *J Clin Laser Med Surg* 1996;14:323–328.
12. Fingar VH, Kik PK, Haydon PS, et al. Analysis of acute vascular damage alter PDT using benzoporphyrin derivative. *Br J Cancer* 1999;79:1702–1708.
13. Svaasand LO, Gomer CJ, Morinelli E. On the physical rationale of photodynamic therapy. Future directions and applications in photodynamic therapy. *SPIE Institute Series* 1990;IS6:233–248.
14. Kramer M, Kenney AG, Delori F, et al. Imaging of experimental CNV using liposomal benzoporphyrin derivative mono-acid angiography. *Invest Ophthalmol Vis Sci* 1995;36:S236.
15. Aveline B, Hasan T, Redmond RW. Photophysical and photosensitizing properties of benzoporphyrin derivative monoacid ring A (BPD-MA). *Photochem Photobiol* 1994;59:328–335.
16. Richter AM, Yip S, Meadows H, et al. Photosensitizing potencies of the structural analogues of benzoporphyrin derivative in different biological test systems. *J Clin Laser Med Surg* 1996;14:335–341.
17. Schmidt-Erfurth U, Hasan T. Mechanisms of action of photodynamic therapy with verteporfin for the treatment of age-related macular degeneration. *Surv Ophthalmol* 2000;45:195–214.
18. Michels S, Hansmann F, Geitzenauer W, et al. Influence of treatment parameters on selectivity of verteporfin therapy. *Invest Ophthalmol Vis Sci* 2006;47:371–376. doi:10.1167/iovs.05–0354.
19. Michels S, Schmidt-Erfurth U. Sequence of early vascular events after photodynamic therapy. *Invest Ophthalmol Vis Sci* 2003;44:2147–2154.
20. Schlotzer-Schrehardt U, Viestenz A, Naumann GO, et al. Dose related structural effects of photodynamic therapy on choroidal and retinal structures of human eyes. *Graefes Arch Clin Exp Ophthalmol* 2002;240:748–757.
21. Schmidt-Erfurth U, Michels S, Barbazetto I, et al. Photodynamic effects on choroidal neovascularization and physiological choroid. *Invest Ophthalmol Vis Sci* 2002;43:830–841.
22. Schmidt-Erfurth U, Schloetzer-Schrehard U, Cursiefen C, et al. Influence of photodynamic therapy on expression of vascular endothelial growth factor (VEGF), VEGF receptor 3, and pigment epithelium-derived factor. *Invest Ophthalmol Vis Sci* 2003;44:4473–4480.

23. Treatment of Age-Related Macular Degeneration with Photodynamic Therapy (TAP) Study Group. Photodynamic therapy of subfoveal choroidal neovascularization in age-related macular degeneration with verteporfin. One-year results of 2 randomized clinical trials – TAP Report 1. *Arch Ophthalmol* 1999;117:1329–1345.

24. Schnurrbusch UEK, Welt K, Horn LC, et al. Histological findings of surgically excised choroidal neovascular membranes after photodynamic therapy. *Br J Ophthalmol* 2001;85:1086–1091.

25. Ghazi NG, Jabbour NM, De la Cruz ZC, et al. Clinicopathologic studies of age-related macular degeneration with classic subfoveal choroidal neovascularization treated with photodynamic therapy. *Retina* 2001;21:478–486.

26. Grossniklaus HE, Brooks HL, Sippy BD, et al. Retinal translocation and photodynamic therapy for age-related macular degeneration with classic choroidal neovascularization: a clinicopathologic case report. *Retina* 2002;22:818–824.

27. Schmidt-Erfurth U, Laqua H, Schloetzer-Schrehard U, et al. Histopathological changes following photodynamic therapy in human eyes. *Arch Ophthalmol* 2002;120:835–843.

28. Gelisken F, Lafaut BA, Inhoffen W, et al. Clinicopathological findings of choroidal neovascularization following verteporfin photodynamic therapy *Br J Ophthalmol* 2004;88:207–211. doi: n10.1136/bjo.2003.018754.

29. Husain D, Kramer M, Kenny A, et al. Effects of photodynamic therapy using verteporfin on experimental choroidal neovascularization and normal retina and choroid up to 7 weeks after treatment. *Invest Ophthalmol Vis Sci* 1999;40:2322–2331.

30. Miller JW, Schmidt-Erfurth U, Sickenberg M, et al. Photodynamic therapy with verteporfin for choroidal neovascularization caused by age-related macular degeneration: results of a single treatment in a phase 1 and 2 study. *Arch Ophthalmol* 1999;117:1161–1173.

31. Schmidt-Erfurth U, Miller JW, Sickenberg M, et al. Photodynamic therapy with verteporfin for choroidal neovascularization caused by age-related macular degeneration: results of retreatments in a phase 1 and 2 study. *Arch Ophthalmol* 1999;117:1177–1187.

32. Sickenberg M, Schmidt-Erfurth U, Miller JW, et al. A preliminary study of photodynamic therapy using verteporfin for choroidal neovascularization in pathologic myopia, ocular histoplasmosis syndrome, angioid streaks, and idiopathic causes. *Arch Ophthalmol* 2000;118:327–336.

33. Tatar O, Kaiserling E, Adam A, et al. Consequences of verteporfin photodynamic therapy on choroidal neovascular membranes. *Arch Ophthalmol* 2006;124:815–823.

34. Bula DV, Iliaki E, Gragoudas E, et al. Pigment epithelium–derived factor, angiopoietin-1, and VEGF expression in human choroidal neovascular membranes treated with photodynamic therapy [ARVO abstract]. *Invest Ophthalmol Vis Sci* 2004;45:E-abstract 1787. http://www.iovs.org. Accessed February 15, 2005.

35. Spilsbury K, Garrett KL, Shen WY, et al. Overexpression of vascular endothelial growth factor (VEGF) in the retinal. *J Pathol* 2000;157:135–144.

36. Grisanti S, Tatar O, Canbek S, et al. Immunohistopathologic evaluation of choroidal neovascular membranes following verteporfin-photodynamic therapy. *Am J Ophthalmol* 2004;137:914–923.

37. Moshfeghi DM, Kaiser PK, Grossniklaus HE, et al. Clinicopathologic study after submacular removal of choroidal neovascular membranes treated with verteporfin ocular photodynamic therapy. *Am J Ophthalmol* 2003;135:343–350.

38. Rogers A, Martidis A, Greenberg P, et al. Optical coherence tomography findings following photodynamic therapy of choroidal neovascularization. *Am J Ophthalmol* 2002;134:566–576.

39. Oner A, Karakucuk S, Mirza E, et al. Electrooculography after photodynamic therapy. *Doc Ophthalmol* 2005;111:83–86.

40. Treatment of Age-Related Macular Degeneration with Photodynamic Therapy (TAP) Study Group. Photodynamic therapy of subfoveal choroidal neovascularization in age-related macular degeneration with verteporfin. Two-year results of 2 randomized clinical trials – TAP Report 2. *Arch Ophthalmol* 2001;119:198–207.

41. Verteporfin In Photodynamic Therapy (VIP) Study Group. Verteporfin therapy of subfoveal choroidal neovascularization in age-related macular degeneration: 2-year results of a randomized clinical trial including lesions with occult with no classic choroidal neovascularization – VIP Report #2. *Am J Ophthalmol* 2001;131:541–560.

42. Verteporfin Therapy for subfoveal CNV in AMD. Three-year results of an open label extension of two randomized clinical trials—TAP Report 5. *Arch Ophthalmol* 2002;120:1307–1314.

43. Verteporfin in Photodynamic Therapy (VIP) Study Group. Photodynamic therapy of subfoveal choroidal neovascularization in pathologic myopia with verteporfin: 1-year results of a randomized clinical trial – VIP Report #1. *Ophthalmology* 2001;108:841–853.

44. Japanese age-related macular degeneration trial: 1-year results of photodynamic therapy with verteporfin in Japanese patients with subfoveal choroidal neovascularization secondary to age-related macular degeneration. *Am J Ophthalmol* 2003;136:1049–1061.

45. Saperstein D, Rosenfeld P, Bressler N, et al. Photodynamic therapy of subfoveal choroidal neovascularization with verteporfin in the ocular histoplasmosis syndrome. *Ophthalmology* 2002;109:1499–1505.

46. Rosenfeld P, Saperstein D, Bressler N, et al. Photodynamic therapy with verteporfin in ocular histoplasmosis: uncontrolled, open-label 2-year study. *Ophthalmology* 2004;111:1725–1733.

47. QLT PhotoTherapeutics Inc. Nonclinical pharmacology and toxicology. *NDA* 1999;Section 5:21–119.

48. Haimovici R, Kramer M, Miller JW, et al. Localization of lipoprotein-delivered benzoporphyrin derivative in the rabbit eye. *Curr Eye Res* 1997;16:83–90.

49. Richter AM, Cerruti-Sola S, Sternberg ED, et al. Biodistribution of tritiated benzoporphyrin derivative (3 H-BPD-MA), a new potent photosensitizer, in normal and tumor-bearing mice. *J Photochem Photobiol B* 1990;5:231–244.

50. Roberts WG, Hasan T. Role of neovasculature and vascular permeability on the tumor retention of photodynamic agents. *Cancer Res* 1992;52:924–930.

51. Richter AM, Waterfield E, Jain AK, et al. Liposomal delivery of a photosensitizer, benzoporphyrin derivative monoacid ring A (BPD), to tumor tissue in a mouse tumor model. *Photochem Photobiol* 1993;57:1000–1006.

52. QLT PhotoTherapeutics Inc. Clinical Investigator's Brochure. BPD-MA (verteporfin) 1996.

53. Wolford ST, Novicki DL, Kelly B. Comparative skin phototoxicity in mice with two photosensitizing drugs: benzoporphyrin derivative monoacid ring A and porfimer sodium (Photofrin). *Fundam Appl Toxicol* 1995;24:52–56.

54. Houle J, Bain S, Azab M, et al. Clinical pharmacokinetics of verteporfin in healthy volunteers and patients with CNV. *Invest Ophthalmol Vis Sci* 2001;42:S437.

55. Husain D, Miller JW, Michaud N, et al. Intravenous infusion of liposomal benzoporphyrin derivative for photodynamic therapy of experimental choroidal neovascularization. *Arch Ophthalmol* 1996;114:978–985.

56. Kramer M, Miller JW, Michaud N, et al. Liposomal benzoporphyrin derivative verteporfin photodynamic therapy. Selective treatment of choroidal neovascularization in monkeys. *Ophthalmology* 1996;103:427–438.

57. Miller JW, Walsh AW, Kramer M, et al. Photodynamic therapy of experimental choroidal neovascularization using lipoprotein-delivered benzoporphyrin. *Arch Ophthalmol* 1995;113:810–818.

58. Jurklies B, Bornfeld N, Schilling H. Photodynamic therapy using verteporfin for choroidal neovascularization associated with angioid streaks – long-term effects. *Ophthalmic Res* 2006;38:209–221.

59. Flower RW, von Kerczek C, Zhu L, et al. Theoretical investigation of the role of choriocapillaris blood flow in the treatment of subfoveal choroidal neovascularization associated with age-related macular degeneration. *Am J Ophthalmol* 2001;132:85–93.

60. Wachtlin J, Behme T, Heimann H, et al. Concentric retinal pigment epithelium atrophy after a single photodynamic therapy. *Graefes Arch Clin Exp Ophthalmol* 2003;241:518–521.

61. Ishibashi T, Miki K, Sorgente N, et al. Effects of intravitreal administration of steroids on experimental subretinal neovascularization in subhuman primate. *Arch Ophthalmol* 1985;103:708–711.

62. Antoszyk AN, Gottlieb JL, Machemer R, et al. The effects of intravitreal triamcinolone acetonide on experimental pre-retinal neovascularization. *Graefes Arch Clin Exp Ophthalmol* 1993;231:34–40.

63. Challa JK, Gillies MC, Penfold PL, et al. Exudative macular degeneration and intravitreal triamcinolone: 18 month follow up. *Aust N Z J Ophthalmol* 1998;26:277–281.

64. Danis RP, Ciulla TA, Pratt LM, et al. Intravitreal triamcinolone acetonide inexudative age-related macular degeneration. *Retina* 2000;20:244–250.

65. Gillies MC, Simpson JM, Billson FA, et al. Safety of an intravitreal injection of triamcinolone: results from a randomized clinical trial. *Arch Ophthalmol* 2004;122:336–340.

66. Spaide RF, Sorenson J, Maranan L. Combined photodynamic therapy with verteporfin and intravitreal triamcinolone acetonide for choroidal neovascularization. *Ophthalmology* 2003;110:1517–1525.

67. Rechtman E, Danis RP, Pratt LM, et al. Intravitreal triamcinolone with photodynamic therapy for subfoveal choroidal neovascularization in age related macular degeneration. *Br J Ophthalmol* 2004;88:344–347.

68. Spaide RF, Sorenson J, Maranan L. Photodynamic therapy with verteporfin combined with intravitreal injection of triamcinolone acetonide for choroidal neovascularization. *Ophthalmology* 2005;112:301–304.

69. Chan WM, Lai TYY, Wong AL, et al. Age related macular degeneration: a comparative study subfoveal choroidal neovascularization in age triamcinolone injection for the treatment of combined photodynamic therapy and intravitreal. *BJO* 2006;90:337–341.

70. Augustin AJ, Schmidt-Erfurth U. Verteporfin therapy combined with intravitreal triamcinolone in all types of choroidal neovascularization due to age-related macular degeneration. *Ophthalmology* 2006;113:14–22.

71. Ruiz-Moreno JM, Montero JA, Zarbin MA. Photodynamic therapy and high-dose intravitreal triamcinolone to treat exudative age-related macular degeneration 1-year outcome. *Retina* 2006;26:602–612.

72. Ruiz-Moreno JM, Montero JA, Zarbin MA. Photodynamic therapy and high-dose intravitreal triamcinolone to treat exudative age-related macular degeneration 2-year outcome. *Retina* 2007;27:458–461.

73. Haines JL, Hauser MA, Schmidt S, et al. Complement factor h variant increases the risk of age-related macular degeneration. *Science* 2005;308:419–421.

74. Edwards AO, Ritter R 3rd, Abel KJ, et al. Complement factor h polymorphism and age related macular degeneration. *Science* 2005;308:421–424.

75. Augustin AJ. Change of treatment paradigms for wet age related macular degeneration. *Business Briefing: European Pharmacotherapy* 2006:30–33.

76. Augustin A, Puls S, Offermann I. Triple therapy for choroidal neovascularization due to age related macular degeneration verteporfin PDT, bevacizumab and dexamethasone. *Retina* 2007;27:133–140.

77. Framme C, Flucke B, Birngruber R. Comparison of reduced and standard light application in photodynamic therapy of the eye in two rabbit models. *Graefes Arch Clin Exp Ophthalmol* 2006;244:773–781.

78. Nichols MG, Foster TH. Oxygen diffusion and reaction kinetics in photodynamic therapy of multicell tumor spheroids. *Phys Med Biol* 1994;39:2161–2181.

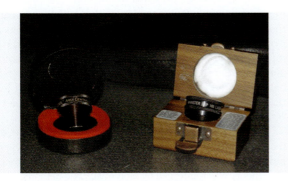

# Pattern Scan Laser (PASCAL) Photocoagulation

Raul Velez-Montoya ■ Gerardo García-Aguirre ■ Mark Blumenkranz ■ Hugo Quiroz-Mercado

## INTRODUCTION

Thirty years ago, in the 1970s, the Diabetic Retinopathy Study (DRS) established the foundation of modern panretinal photocoagulation (PRP). The study results demonstrated a benefit from the application of laser photocoagulation to the retina by reducing the risk of severe visual loss in patients with proliferative diabetic retinopathy (PDR) by 50% (1). Later, the Early Treatment Diabetic Retinopathy Study (ETDRS) likewise showed similar results by decreasing the risk of moderate visual loss in patients with nonproliferative diabetic retinopathy from 16.3% to 6.4%, and up to 50% in patients with diabetic macular edema (2). Since then, the treatment of the retina with laser photocoagulation has become a fundamental part of the everyday medical practice for ophthalmologists and is the treatment of choice for ischemic and neovascular diseases (1–4).

Panretinal, direct focal, and macular grid photocoagulation have been the leading techniques of laser treatment to the retina for nearly 40 years. In ischemic diseases, patients usually receive 1200 to 1800 laser burns, divided into two to four sessions, each one separated at intervals of 2 to 4 weeks and with each session lasting 10 to 15 minutes. This treatment scheme has remained virtually unchanged for over 20 years (5–7).

Since solar and xenon arc lamp photocoagulation were introduced in the late 1950s by Meyer-Schwickerath as a therapeutic method in ophthalmology, the indications for their use as well as the equipment used for their administration have evolved. The first device, successfully used in clinical practice, was the xenon arc lamp (8). This light source had the disadvantage of being composed of a polychromatic wavelength. This made it very inefficient in terms of the amount of energy absorbed by the tissue, and unpredictable in terms of tissue interaction. With the next generation of laser photocoagulators, more efficient equipment appeared, providing monochromatic wavelength (e.g., the ruby, argon, and krypton laser). Since then, advances in technology have focused on designing devices more convenient for the physician than for the patient. The emergence of systems with air-cooling modules and the advent of fiber optic allowed companies to significantly reduce the size of the equipment. However, despite the fact that today we have more compact and efficient solid-state lasers, the way in which the treatment is administered remains unchanged since the mid-1970s (8). In short, the procedure is tedious for the patient and physician and varies between uncomfortable and painful for the patient, occasionally requiring the administration of retrobulbar anesthetic injections.

## LASER MECHANISM OF ACTION

The mechanism through which the laser exerts its therapeutic action is still undetermined. When photocoagulation was applied for the first time in PDR, it was thought that the mechanism of action was the photocoagulation and destruction of areas of neovascularization, thus preventing vitreous hemorrhage and tractional retinal detachment. In later observations, it was clear that the clinical effect of photocoagulation seemed to depend more on applying laser to healthy retina than to areas of neovascularization (9).

The first theory about the effectiveness of laser was based on the initial observation by Michaelson, in which he proposed the existence of a "growth factor X," responsible for neovascularization of the hypoxic retina (10). Patz et al. took up this idea and suggested that the therapeutic effect of laser was exercised by destroying sick and hypoxic tissue. In such a way, the source of production of the "factor X" was destroyed and hence its intraocular levels were lowered. The problem with this theory was, in the case of PDR, that hypoxia is located in the inner retinal layers, being primarily a problem of microangiopathy and occlusion of the microcirculation, while the outer retinal layers remain apparently normal. Histological evidence demonstrated that mild to moderate laser burns destroy the outer layers and the retinal pigment epithelium (RPE), leaving the inner layers intact, which was the alleged source of the "growth factor X" (9,10).

Another theory, based on histological observations, stated that laser destruction of RPE cells produces the release of protective factors that slows the process of neovascularization. This theory was reinforced by Mori et al., who demonstrated the protection that a platelet-derived factor produced on delaying neovascularization of the retina and choroid. However, a direct relationship between the application of laser and the release of these factors has never been proven conclusively (9,11).

The oxygen theory suggested that photocoagulation destroys the photoreceptors, decreasing oxygen demands of the outer retina and improving oxygenation of the inner layers. This, in turn, decreases the production of growth factors and alters retinal hemodynamics. The acceptance of this theory is based in the fact that it explains the effect of laser not only in proliferative diseases but also on macular edema (9,12).

Under normal circumstances, oxygen and nutrients diffuse through the choriocapillaris to the retina to be consumed by photoreceptors, which have a high number of mitochondria and hence a high level of oxygen consumption. After a laser burn, the photoreceptor layer is replaced by glial tissue. This tissue then has fewer mitochondria and therefore lowers the overall oxygen demand (9,12). This means that laser injuries serve as "windows" in the outer retina, where oxygen consumption is low and may spread further to the inner retina, increasing the oxygen tension in this space (Fig. 11-1). Besides lowering the total consumption of oxygen, laser photocoagulation also decreases the production of growth factors (e.g., vascular endothelial growth factor [VEGF]) by destroying hypoxic tissue. Aiello et al. and Agustin et al. published that levels of VEGF were significantly elevated in the vitreous of patients with PDR and that these decreased significantly after laser treatment (13).

An important proof that laser treatment improves the effects of hypoxia in the retina is the observed changes in the vascular diameter. Under conditions of low oxygen tension, the arterioles are dilated, which increases local blood flow and thus the hydrostatic pressure within capillaries. When oxygen levels return to normal, the arterioles contract. This in turn decreases the blood flow and the hydrostatic pressure. In the ETDRS, fundus photographs were taken of all patients before and after the laser treatment. The analysis of this material

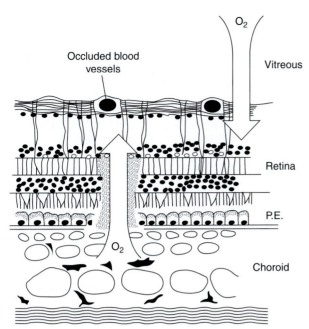

**Figure 11-1.** Laser burns serve as a "window" for oxygen diffusion, allowing the molecule to pass directly from the choroid to the inner retina and vitreous, without being consumed by highly active cells like retinal pigment epithelium cells and photoreceptors. (Reprinted with permission from Blackwell Publishing. Stefánsson E. *Acta Ophthalmol. Scand* 2001;79:435–440.)

proved that blood vessel caliber decreased 10% to 15% after laser treatment with xenon arc or argon laser photocoagulation (9,14).

Vasoconstriction, secondary to the increased oxygen tension, in turn, reduces the distention of capillary endothelial cells, which can reduce their growth potential. This is due to a decreased captation of thymidine and VEGF by the endothelial cell, limiting cell proliferation. In summary, laser diminishes neovascularization through two pathways: (a) by decreasing the production of VEGF secondary to hypoxia and (b) through contraction of capillaries, which limits their growth potential (12).

In the case of macular edema, laser therapy produces a therapeutic effect through two different mechanisms. Arteriolar vasoconstriction decreases the hydrostatic pressure in capillaries and venules, while the oncotic pressure remains constant. According to Starling's law, this reverses the flow of fluid toward the capillary lumen. Alternatively, the correction of hypoxia reduces VEGF production by retinal tissues, reducing capillary permeability (15).

## PATTERN SCAN LASER PHOTOCOAGULATOR PRINCIPLES

The first attempt to make photocoagulation a completely automated procedure involved a series of complex robotic equipment, image recognition software, and special tracking devices (16). This allowed the production of retinal burns in real time, based on laser shots of 100 ms duration. These systems had the disadvantage of requiring a previous retinal image as well as a shot calibration system, to establish the proper depth of

the lesion (17). The complexity of these systems prevented their commercial introduction (16–18).

The pattern scan laser photocoagulator (PASCAL, OptiMedica Corp. Santa Clara, CA) is a semiautomatic system based on a frequency-doubled Nd:YAG laser, with a wavelength of 532 nm, which can apply from a single burn (single or continuously), up to 56 burns per second, with depression of the foot pedal (Figs. 11-2 and 11-3) (8). The system has an automated table, which allows height adjustment; the slit lamp has magnification factors of 7x, 12x, and 20x. The control of

| Pattern | System capabilities | | Retinal image |
|---|---|---|---|
| 1 × 1 | Spot: | 60–400 µm | |
| | Exposition: | 10–1000 ms | |
| | Intervals: | 1.0–8.0 Hz | |
| | Power: | 100–2000 mW | |
| | Fluence: | 35–159 J/cm² | |
| 2 × 2 | Spot: | 100–400 µm | |
| | Exposition: | 20 & 30 ms | |
| | Space between burns: | 0.25–3.0 ∅ | |
| | Power: | 100–2000 mW | |
| | Fluence: | 25–573 J/cm² | |
| 3 × 3 | Spot: | 100–400 µm | |
| | Exposition: | 20 & 30 ms | |
| | Space between burns: | 0.25–3.0 ∅ | |
| | Power: | 100–2000 mW | |
| | Fluence: | 25–573 J/cm² | |
| 4 × 4 | Spot: | 100–400 µm | |
| | Exposition: | 20 & 30 ms | |
| | Space between burns: | 0.25–3.0 ∅ | |
| | Power: | 100–2000 mW | |
| | Fluence: | 25–573 J/cm² | |
| 5 × 5 | Spot: | 100–400 µm | |
| | Exposition: | 20 & 30 ms | |
| | Space between burns: | 0.25–3.0 ∅ | |
| | Power: | 100–2000 mW | |
| | Fluence: | 25–573 J/cm² | |
| Lg Arc (single-row) | Shots: | 6–42 Hz | |
| | Areas: | 7–8 section | |
| | Spot: | 200 & 400 µm | |
| | Radius: | 800–4100 µm | |
| | Power: | 100–2000 mW | |
| | Space between burns: | 0.25–3.0 ∅ | |
| | Exposition: | 20 ms | |
| | Fluence: | 2–127 J/cm² | |
| Lg Arc, Arc (triple-row) | Shots: | 3–50 Hz | |
| | Areas: | 180–360° | |
| | Spot: | 200 & 400 µm | |
| | Radius: | 800–2000 µm | |
| | Power: | 100–2000 mW | |
| | Space between burns: | 0.25–3.0 ∅ | |
| | Exposition: | 20 ms | |
| | Fluence: | 2–127 J/cm² | |

**Figure 11-2.** Peripheral patterns: system capabilities. For most treatments, we use a combination of patterns and parameters, as reported in Figure 11-1. The figure also shows a representation of the patterns imaged on the retina. The arc pattern is formed by a triple row of laser shots.

| Patern | System capability | | Image |
|---|---|---|---|
| Mac A & B | Shots: | 56 | |
| | Treatment area: | Macula | |
| | Spot: | 100 & 200 μm | |
| | Power: | 100–200 mW | |
| | Space between burns: | 0.25–2.0 ⌀ | |
| | Exposition: | 10 ms | |
| | Fluence: | 3–191 J/cm² | |
| Mac Oct A, B, A+B | Shots: | 28 & 56 Hz | |
| | Treatment area: | Macula | |
| | Spot: | 100 & 200 μm | |
| | Power: | 100–200 mW | |
| | Space between burns: | 0.25–2.0 ⌀ | |
| | Exposition: | 10 ms | |
| | Fluence: | 3–191 J/cm² | |

**Figure 11-3.** Macular patterns: system capabilities. The macular octant is composed of two different patterns offset by one clock hour and can each be used as a single treatment or combined. The retina images depicted in Figure 11-2 are approximations.

laser parameters is performed by means of a touch screen graphic user interface, facilitating navigation among the different patterns of photocoagulation. Control of power can be achieved in two ways: through the display or through a small knob that is located at the side of the ocular arm of the slit lamp. This control allows changes in 50 mW steps, allowing the adjustment of the intensity of the shots without the need to shift the clinician's gaze from the patient to the display. The laser is activated by depressing the foot pedal. It is necessary to keep the pedal depressed until the entire pattern is completed, in a manner similar to the way in which an excimer laser is activated. If a complication occurs, the physician can deactivate the foot pedal, and the laser will stop. The application of the laser is made via contact lens for laser treatment (Figs. 11-4A to D and 11-5).

The PRP patterns allow the application of laser energy in the peripheral retina, placing 1 to 25 shots per activation of the foot pedal. The authors recommend the use of large patterns (4 × 4 and 5 × 5) for mid periphery and smaller ones (2 × 2 and 3 × 3) for more anterior treatment. As the ora serrata is approached, the retina becomes thinner and the radius of

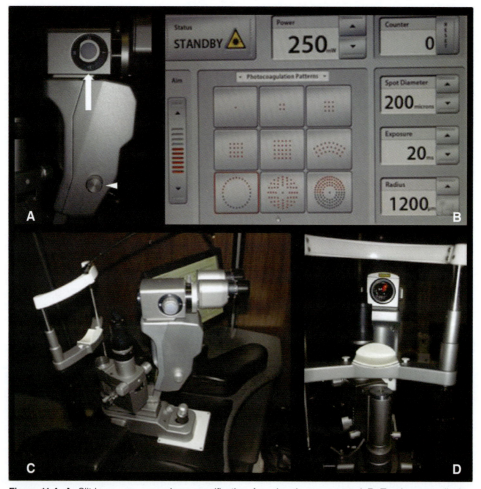

**Figure 11-4. A:** Slit lamp arm, arrow: lens magnification. Arrowhead: power control. **B:** Touch screen display, showing all the available patterns and mains controls. **C:** Top view of the device; notice the arm rest, which is very comfortable for the patient. **D:** Patients' view of the device.

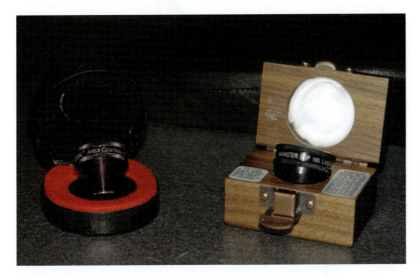

**Figure 11-5.** Posterior pole lenses for laser treatment. **A:** Lens for macular patterns: *Area Centralis,* Field of view: 70/84°, Image magnification: 1.06x, Retina spot size: 0.94x (Volk Optical Inc. Mentor, OH). **B:** Lens for periphery patterns: Mainster PRP 165, Field of view: 165/180°, Image magnification: 0.51x, Retina spot size: 1.96x (Ocular Instruments, Bellevue, Washington USA). Even though these are the lenses commonly used in our practice, the device can operate with any kind and brands of lenses, irrespective of the field of view, magnification, or real spot size.

curvature of the eye changes, making it more difficult to maintain focus of the entire pattern and maintain the proper power density. Smaller patterns with short pulses are more easily focused anteriorly on a curved surface (Fig. 11-6A). There is a special pattern called "triple arc," specially designed for the far periphery. This pattern consists of 6 to 24 burns per second (depending on the size and separation) per each foot pedal depression. It is made up of three rows of concentric arcs that allow quick and safe photocoagulation of lattice degeneration or retinal tears (Fig. 11-6B). A shortcoming of this pattern lies in the fact that the eye is not a perfect sphere; therefore, controlling the radius of curvature with no correction for inclination angle can make it difficult to place the patterns in the correct position.

The circular pattern is designed for the photocoagulation of small holes and other predisposing lesions. It consists of the application of laser in a circular pattern with a variable radius of curvature, which allows for rapid treatment of lesions. This pattern requires, in addition to a cooperative patient, an experienced ophthalmologist in order to achieve perfectly concentric lesions (Fig. 11-6C).

The patterns for macular photocoagulation allow for the placement of macular grids from 28 to 56 shots in a single activation of the foot pedal, leaving a central space of about 2000 µm. This allows safe laser application without the risk of damage to the foveal avascular zone. The pattern has a central fixation light to facilitate the patient to fixation. Usually, when performing macular grids with subthreshold powers, the burns

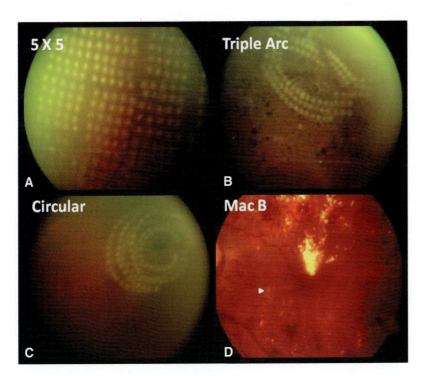

**Figure 11-6.** Retinal laser burns. **A:** Fundus photograph of a right eye which shows an example of the 5 × 5 pattern. **B:** Lattice lesion of a right eye with a previous history of retinal detachment in the contralateral eye and retinitis pigmentosa, treated with a combination of the Lg Arc and the 3 × 3 pattern. **C:** Retinal tear treated with Lg Arc Arc patterns, using a combination of complete circles and 180° arcs. **D:** Fundus photograph of an eye with macular edema treated with the macular pattern Mac B. Arrow head shows one of the laser burns.

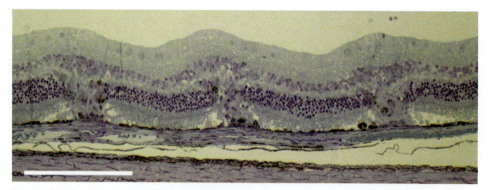

**Figure 11-7.** Histologic section of a rabbit retina, treated with a pattern scanning laser, with exposition time of 10 ms. There are three similar burns; the boundary between treated and untreated tissue is well defined and the inner retina looks unaffected. The eye was enucleated 1 week after the treatment (toluidine blue staining; original magnification, x10). (Reprinted with permission from Ophthalmic Communications Society. WK Health, LWW. *Retina* 2006;26(3):370–376.)

are very difficult to visualize. Using the grid with a preconfigured pattern avoids the need to "remember" the location of the macula that was already treated and avoids double applications (Fig. 11-6D).

## SPECIAL FEATURES

One of the greatest innovations of the PASCAL system is that it uses different parameters (shorter duration, increased power) than those used for traditional photocoagulation. Shortening pulse duration from 10 to 30 ms allows for placement of a greater amount of burns in the same time it would take to make single burns of 100 ms, thus completing the programmed patterns in an acceptable time and shortening the treatment time (8).

Theoretically, using a preconfigured pattern of 5 × 5 and shorter exposure times could reduce the treatment time by a factor of approximately 15 compared with single shot photocoagulation delivered in repetition mode at 2.0 Hz (8). In our experience, focusing the patterns correctly in the retina, calculating the power required to produce useful burns, and navigating between the different screens are also time-consuming procedures. Therefore, in clinical practice, treatment time is shortened approximately by a factor of 10.

With a reduction in exposure time from 100 ms to 10 or 20 ms, it requires 1.5 to 3 times the power normally required to produce a clinically visible burn (17). However, the pulse energy is much lower compared with conventional photocoagulation. A histological examination of animal retina shows more uniform and well-defined lesions, with preservation of the inner nuclear layer, inner plexiform layer, and nerve fiber layer (Fig. 11-7). Another important feature is that by using exposure time shorter than 50 ms, the damage to the RPE is basically mechanic and nonthermal, due to the vapor microbubbles that are formed around the melanosomes (19,20).

The final retinal scar size has less progression and is less dependent on the power used during treatment and posterior pole pigmentation. This results in photocoagulation lesions without thermal expansion and much less scarring or progressive RPE atrophy (20).

One of the drawbacks of laser photocoagulation is that the patient's experience may negatively influence compliance.

Based on our experience, the use of shortened pulses produces a subjective sensation of pain up to 4.5 lower than conventional parameters. This is likely the result of two factors: less diffusion of heat energy which in turn decreases the production of prostaglandins and proinflammatory cytokines (18,21). In addition, there is less flow of heat energy to pain receptors located in the deeper choroid. Although the pain produced by each laser pulse depends on many factors (fundus pigmentation, laser power, number of previous treatments, sector of the retina to be treated, patient anxiety), we have observed that the delivery of shots with short exposure time (20 ms) proved to be significantly less painful to the patient ($p < 0.001$), while maintaining the same level of efficacy observed in long term follow-up (18).

In summary, the pattern scan laser system is an innovative device that makes treatment with laser more efficient with less pain and less damage to neighboring tissue. Other unproven advantages include less inflammation after treatment, which may be reflected as less postlaser macular edema; less alteration of the visual field; and preservation of the a-wave and b-wave in the electroretinogram, which may be reflected as better contrast sensitivity after treatment (22–24).

### References

1. Rema M, Sujatha P, Pradeepa R. Visual outcomes of pan-retinal photocoagulation in diabetic retinopathy at one-year follow-up and associated risk factors. *Indian J Ophthalmol* 2005;53:93–99.
2. Early Treatment Diabetic Retinopathy Study Research Group. Early photocoagulation for diabetic retinopathy. ETDRS report number 9. *Ophthalmology* 1991;98:766–785.
3. Stratton IM, Cull CA, Adler AI, et al. Additive effects of glycaemia and blood pressure exposure on risk of complications in type 2 diabetes: a prospective observational study (UKPDS 75). *Diabetologia* 2006;49:1761–1769.
4. Mohamed Q, Gillies MC, Wong TY. Management of diabetic retinopathy: a systematic review. *JAMA* 2007;298:902–916.
5. Dodson PM. Diabetic retinopathy: treatment and prevention. *Diab Vasc Dis Res* 2007;4:S9–S11.
6. Photocoagulation treatment of proliferative diabetic retinopathy: the second report of diabetic retinopathy study findings. *Ophthalmology* 1978;85:82–106.
7. The Diabetic Retinopathy Study Research Group. Photocoagulation treatment of proliferative diabetic retinopathy. Clinical application of Diabetic Retinopathy Study (DRS) findings, DRS report number 8. *Ophthalmology* 1981;88:583–600.
8. Blumenkranz MS, Yellachich D, Andersen DE, et al. Semiautomated patterned scanning laser for retinal photocoagulation. *Retina* 2006;26:370–376.
9. Stefánsson E. Ocular oxygenation and the treatment of diabetic retinopathy. *Surv Ophthalmol* 2006;51:364–380.
10. Michaelson IC. The mode of development of the vascular system of the retina with some observations of its significance for certain retinal disease. *Trans Ophthalmol Soc UK* 1948;68:137–180.

11. Mori K, Duh E, Gehlbach P, et al. Pigment epithelium-derived factor inhibits retinal and choroidal neovascularization. *J Cell Physiol* 2001;188: 253–263.
12. Stefánsson E. The therapeutic effects of retinal laser treatment and vitrectomy. A theory based on oxygen and vascular physiology. *Acta Ophthalmol Scand* 2001;79:435–440.
13. Aiello LP, Avery RL, Arrigg PG, et al. Vascular endothelial growth factor in ocular fluid of patients with diabetic retinopathy and other retinal disorders. *N Eng J Med* 1994;331:1519–1520.
14. Wilson CA, Stefánsson E, Klombers L, et al. Optic disk neovascularization and retinal vessel diameter in diabetic retinopathy. *Am J Ophthalmol* 1988;106:131–134.
15. Gottfredsdóttir MS, Stefánsson E, Jónasson F, et al. Retinal vasoconstriction after laser treatment for diabetic macular edema. *Am J Ophthalmol* 1993;115:64–67.
16. Barrett SF, Wright CH, Oberg ED, et al. Development of an integrated automated retinal surgical laser system. *Biomed Sci Instrum* 1996;32:215–224.
17. Barrett SF, de Graaf PW, Wright CH. Hybrid tracking system for retinal photocoagulation prototype II. *Biomed Sci Instrum* 1999;35:259–264.
18. Al-Hussainy S, Dodson PM, Gibson JM. Pain response and follow-up of patients undergoing panretinal laser photocoagulation with reduced exposure times. *Eye* 2008;22:96–99.
19. Schuele G, Rumohr M, Huettmann G, et al. RPE damage thresholds and mechanisms for laser exposure in the microsecond-to-millisecond time regimen. *Invest Ophthalmol Vis Sci* 2005;46:714–719.
20. Jain A, Blumenkranz MS, Paulus Y, et al. Effect of pulse duration on size and character of the lesion in retinal photocoagulation. *Arch Ophthalmol* 2008;126:78–85.
21. Nonaka A, Kiryu J, Tsujikawa A, et al. Inflammatory response after scatter laser photocoagulation in nonphotocoagulated retina. *Invest Ophthalmol Vis Sci* 2002;43:1204–1209.
22. Perlman I, Gdal-On M, Miller B, et al. Retinal function of the diabetic retina after argon laser photocoagulation assessed electroretinographically. *Br J Ophthalmol* 1985;69:240–246.
23. Lövestam-Adrian M, Svendenius N, Agardh E. Contrast sensitivity and visual recovery time in diabetic patients treated with panretinal photocoagulation. *Acta Ophthalmol Scand* 2000;78:672–676.
24. Greenstein VC, Chen H, Hood DC, et al. Retinal function in diabetic macular edema after focal laser photocoagulation. *Invest Ophthalmol Vis Sci* 2000;41:3655–3664.

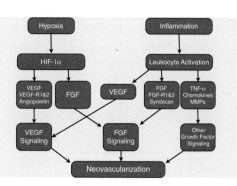

# New and Future Antiangiogenic Therapy

Rishi P. Singh ■ Peter K. Kaiser

# INTRODUCTION

Blood vessel development is termed either vasculogenesis or angiogenesis. Vasculogenesis is the process of normal blood vessel formation during development. Angiogenesis occurs when pre-existing vascular beds sprout new vessels in response to stimuli. Angiogenesis in adulthood is primarily seen in pathologic situations and is a highly complex process requiring the coordinated action of growth factors and cellular events. The process is controlled by a balance of pro- and antiangiogenic factors. Although there are several potential regulators of angiogenesis, reports have suggested that vascular endothelial growth factor (VEGF) may be one of the most important regulators of vascular development and differentiation seen in age-related macular degeneration (AMD), perhaps because it is the most specific growth factor for the vascular endothelium. This hypothesis was verified with major breakthroughs in molecules that suppress VEGF including pegaptanib (Macugen™, OSI-Eyetech, New York, NY), bevacizumab (Avastin™, Genentech, South San Francisco, CA), and ranibizumab (Lucentis™, Genentech, South San Francisco, CA), and they have helped in achieving significant success in the treatment of AMD (1,2).

Despite the impressive gains in vision seen with anti-VEGF therapy, not all patients exhibit improvement after treatment. In the MARINA trial of ranibizumab for AMD, 10% of patients suffered three lines of visual loss despite receiving monthly injections for 24 months. One possible explanation for this is that anti-VEGF therapy only addresses one of multiple pathways of pathogenesis. Another explanation is that as vessels mature, they lose their VEGF sensitivity and thus other pathways are required to treat these patients. Furthermore, anti-VEGF therapies are very costly and often require monthly intravitreal injections. Thus, there is a prevailing clinical need for pharmacotherapeutics that are less costly, less invasive, and require less frequent administration either through combination therapy or different delivery methods in monotherapy. Finally, studies with ranibizumab have elucidated that anti-VEGF drugs are not without safety issues including a risk of stroke in patients with prior history of stroke (3). This has led to the development of alternative antiangiogenesis therapies to improve the results of anti-VEGF therapy.

When examining potential future targets for angiogenesis, researchers have returned to the root causes of AMD. There is increasing evidence that suggests that AMD is not strictly a vascular disease, but instead is a more complex process. The process of choroidal neovascular membrane coroidal neovascularization (CNV) formation is a multifaceted interplay between genetic predisposition, hypoxia, inflammation, oxidative stress, and other factors. CNV was once thought to be only a vascular disease; however, lately nonvascular components including myofibroblasts, macrophages, and other inflammatory cells have been found in AMD specimens. In addition, disregulation and mutations in complement factor 3 and other mutations in the alternate complement pathway have also been causally related to an increased risk of development choroidal neovascularization in AMD, leading to researchers looking at the inflammatory cascade as a potential target. Finally, drusen accumulation has been shown to lead to localized tissue hypoxia

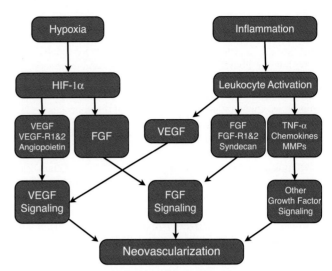

**Figure 12-1.** Mechanisms leading to choroidal neovascularization. VEGF, vascular endothelial growth factor; FGF, fibroblast growth factor; MMP, matrix metalloproteinase.

as it impairs nutrient transport from the choriocapillaris to outer retinal tissues. These factors lead to modification of the upstream and downstream regulators of VEGF that are proangiogenic and promotion of antiangiogenic molecules such as pigment epithelium derived factor (PEDF) as the potential targets (Fig. 12-1). The purpose of this chapter is to describe new therapies for pathologic angiogenesis currently under development. The majority of targets discussed have never appeared in the ophthalmic literature but have shown significant promise in other fields of medicine.

# HYPOXIA-INDUCED FACTORS IN AGE-RELATED MACULAR DEGENERATION

Hypoxia has been established as a major contributor to tumor growth. However, only recently has it also been identified as a risk factor in the formation of choroidal neovascularization in AMD. Studies have established that relative hypoxia is caused by disturbance of the limited blood supply in the macula and the high oxygen demand of the photoreceptors over time. Alterations in choroidal blood flow have been previously described in patients with AMD (4). With age, Bruch's membrane undergoes an accumulation of incompletely degraded cellular debris (lipofuscin) that leads to the formation of drusen. This change in Bruch's membrane has a pronounced impact on the metabolic transfer leading to localized hypoxia.

The regulation of angiogenesis by hypoxia is mediated by hypoxia-inducible factor (HIF-1). This factor switches on a series of genes participating in compensatory mechanisms that support cell survival. In particular, the α subunit stimulates neovascularization by activating the transcription of over 60 genes including the activation and release of erythropoietin, hemo-oxygenase (mediates oxygen binding to heme), VEGF, and inducible nitric oxide synthase, which participates in local blood vessel dilation (5–8). The increased vascular permeability seen in angiogenesis, which is largely mediated by VEGF, leads to the extravasation of plasma proteins such as fibrin, inflammatory mediators, and numerous growth factors (fibroblast growth factor, FGF; insulinlike growth factor, IGF-1). Growth factor liberation in turn causes increased expression of integrins, which are cellular adhesion molecules that interact with the extracellular matrix (ECM), and proteinases that breakdown the surrounding ECM. Both of these processes are essential for cellular migration and tubule formation. Therefore, the inhibition of HIF-1α could be a potential therapeutic target in AMD.

One example of such an inhibitor is RTP801i (Quark Biotech, Inc./Pfizer). This molecule uses RNA interference to block the production of RTP801 which is upstream of HIF-1α, leading to direct transcriptional inhibition of HIF-1α. RTP801i has been shown to be effective in animal models of ischemic disease. For example, a study using RTP801 knockout mice revealed a significant reduction in retinal neovascularization (9). In animal models of ischemic stroke, RTP801 is significantly upregulated, and its inhibition results in decreased neovascularization (10). RTP801i is in phase 2 testing for exudative AMD.

## mTOR INHIBITION AS AN INHIBITOR OF ANGIOGENESIS

Rapamycin is produced by *Streptomyces hygroscopicus* and was first isolated from soil samples taken from Easter Island (11). It was initially used as an antifungal and potent immunosuppressant (12,13). It was not until much later that the downstream target of rapamycin, mTOR (mammalian target of rapamycin), was identified as a serine/threonine kinase in budding yeast *Saccharomyces cervisiae* (14). mTOR functions to control cellular growth by regulating the cell-cycle dependent polarization of the actin cytoskeleton.

Recent studies have shown that HIF-1α transcription is dependent on mTOR activation. Thus, rapamycin inhibitors would indirectly cause HIF-1α inhibition and lead to decreased angiogenesis and choroidal neovascularization. Current rapalogs in clinical trials for nonocular diseases include rapamycin/sirolimus (Wyeth), RAD-001/everolimus (Novartis), and A23573 (Ariad). Each of these molecular structures differs only slightly from each other in solubility and stability (15). Rapamycin and its analogs form a ternary complex with FK-506 binding protein and mTOR resulting in a potent inhibition of mTOR signaling.

Systemic rapamycin has been shown to inhibit retinal and choroidal neovascularization in animal models of disease. Adult mice that underwent laser-induced CNV formation and treatment with rapamycin showed significant reduction in CNV size and extent compared to controls. The impact on retinal neovascularization by rapamycin was studied using the ROP hyperoxia/hypoxia model in mice. Again, a significant reduction in retinal neovascularization in rapamycin-treated animals over placebo was observed. Increases in VEGF were seen in both studies suggesting that rapamycin was acting in a pathway different from the VEGF pathway for inhibition (16).

Sirolimus (Macusight) is an ocular rapalog being tested in phase 1 study in AMD.

## INTEGRINS

Integrins are receptors on the cell surface that have been shown to be critical in a wide variety of cellular events including adhesion, migration, invasion, proliferation, cell survival, and apoptosis. Integrins also serve as receptors on cell surfaces allowing for adhesion of cells to ECM proteins such as vitronectin, fibronectin, laminin, collagen, and fibrinogen. Integrins are obligate heterodimers containing two distinct membrane spanning chains, called the α (alpha) and β (beta) subunits. In mammals, 19 α and 8 β subunits have been characterized. The subunits span through the cellular membrane, and in general have very short cytoplasmic domains of about 40 to 70 amino acids. Recent studies have also demonstrated that growth factors such as bFGF and VEGF isoforms (189, 165, but not soluble VEGF 121) can directly bind to $\alpha_5\beta_3$ (17–19). The binding of integrins to ECM proteins causes intracellular signal transduction leading to the activation of intracellular tyrosine kinases and transcription factors.

Initial observations regarding the role played by integrins in angiogenesis came from tumor vasculature studies. Brooks and then Friedlander were the first to identify that integrin blockade can lead to inhibition of the angiogenic response seen in tumors and in retinal neovascularization (20–23). In particular, the $\alpha_5\beta_3$ and $\alpha_5\beta_1$ integrins are found on proliferating endothelial cells. However, the presence of these integrins is dependent on the tissue studied. Only $\alpha_5\beta_3$ was found in choroidal neovascular membrane specimens. However, both sets of integrins are found on retinal neovascular specimens from proliferative diabetic retinopathy (21,24). Blockade of $\alpha_5\beta_3$ or $\alpha_5\beta_1$ function by an antibody or peptide antagonists prevents blood vessel formation in numerous preclinical models of angiogenesis including chick chorioallantoic membrane, rabbit cornea, and mouse retina (20,22,25).

The process of integrins-induced angiogenesis is still being elucidated and several potential mechanisms are hypothesized. Overall, integrins are required for the transmission of the initial signals leading to the activation of the angiogenesis cascade and are subsequently altered to allow for invasion and remodeling of the ECM. Crosstalk between integrins and other growth factor receptors has been demonstrated and are thought to play a critical role in angiogenesis. Reynolds et al. found that inhibition of $\alpha_5\beta_3$ downregulates VEGF receptor 2 (VEGF R2) in endothelial cells (26). Functional blocking antibodies against integrins block endothelial tube formation *in vitro*. Integrins also bind directly to matrix metalloproteinases and may shed light on how integrins and proteases function in a coordinated manner to promote cell invasion during angiogenesis (27). Finally, integrins are also thought to be regulators of apoptosis through various pathways such as the PI3 Kinase-AKT and caspase pathways (28,29). Endothelial cells undergo apoptosis when denied integrin mediated attachment to cytoskeletal elements. Therefore, depending on the integrin subtypes, integrin presence is necessary for endothelial cell survival, or alternatively integrin-induced apoptosis of endothelial cells can then lead to the angiogenic stimulus for neovascularization.

The external location of the receptors makes it an excellent target for inhibitors, and several studies have validated the idea that inhibition of integrins leads to inhibition of angiogenesis in various *in-vitro* and *in-vivo* assays. Inhibition of $\alpha_5$ integrins with antibodies decreases solid tumors and is associated with downregulation of VEGF (23,27). Systemic administration of a $\alpha_5\beta_1$ integrin antagonist in mice leads to suppression and regression of choroidal neovascularization (30). In rats with laser induced CNV, a cyclic $\alpha_5\beta_3$ antagonist inhibits progression of the lesion (31). These promising study results will likely lead to the development of potential therapeutics.

Significant recent publications have supported the use of integrin inhibitors. In particular, $\alpha_5\beta_1$ and $\alpha_5\beta_3$ have shown significant *in-vitro* efficacy. In studies of an orally bioavailable $\alpha_5$ inhibitor, significant reductions in retinal neovascularization in an ROP model and changes in retinal vascular permeability in diabetic-induced rats were reported (32). Endothelial cell migration and tubule formation using a HUVEC migration platform were reduced with the use of an integrin $\alpha_5\beta_1$ interfering molecule (33). Similar studies by Campochiaro et al. demonstrate significant regression of neovascularization and induction of apoptosis of cultured vascular endothelial cells when treated with this inhibitor (30). Antibodies against $\alpha_5\beta_1$, volociximab, (Ophthotech), a small molecule inhibitor against $\alpha_5\beta_1$, JSM 6427 (Jerini), and a small molecule $\alpha_5\beta_3$ antagonist (AngioQuest) are all in preclinical or phase 1 development for exudative AMD.

## TYROSINE KINASE INHIBITORS

After VEGF binds to its cell surface receptors (VEGFR1 and VEGFR2), a variety of intracellular downstream kinase pathways are activated. Binding to only VEGFR1 leads to weak activation of tyrosine kinase phosphorylation, and it is thought that this receptor may function as a decoy receptor to regulate the amount of free extracellular VEGF that can bind VEGFR2 (34). In comparison, VEGFR2 causes phosphorylation of several tyrosine kinases pathways including RAf-Mek-Erk pathway, PI-3 kinase-AKT, Src, and protein kinase C (PKC) which includes alpha, beta, and delta isoforms. VEGF mediates its mitogenic effects predominantly through the PKC beta and Raf pathways. The PI-3 pathway leads to transcription of anti-apoptotic genes that protect endothelial cells in a nascent vessel in embryonic and pathologic conditions (35). Other growth factors such as platelet-derived growth factor (PDGF) and FGF have their own receptor tyrosine kinases that add another dimension to the complexity of the angiogenesis activation process (36–38).

Current pharmacologic approaches have been directed toward blocking tyrosine kinases specifically activated by VEGF or broad spectrum intracellular kinase inhibition (39). Since multiple kinase cascades are activated in ocular neovascular disease, broad spectrum kinase deactivation may be more desirable since this would also inhibit the other growth factors involved in the process. A series of studies have been performed on kinase inhibitors from many companies to treat choroidal neovascularization caused by AMD in preclinical models and phase 1 studies (Fig. 12-2).

## COMPLEMENT INHIBITORS

The complement system consists of a family of enzymes and regulators of innate immunity that are derived from the liver and extrahepatic cells such as monocytes, endothelial cells, and epithelial cells. Three principle pathways have been identified and they all converge with activation of C3 complement (Figs. 12-3 and 12-4). The cascade then results in the activation and dimerization of the C5b-9 complex into a membrane attack complex (MAC) that inserts into cell walls and promotes cell lysis and the release of proinflammatory cytokines such as C3a, C4a, and C5a, which further amplify the response.

Numerous basic science and clinical studies have implicated complement activation in the pathogenesis of AMD. Primates who underwent laser-induced CNV formation demonstrated significant levels of C3 and C5 to C9 in the neovascular complex (40). Biochemical examinations of drusen have shown that several components of the complement cascade including C3 fragments, C4, and C5b to C9 have been identified (41,42). Anatomical studies have provided initial evidence for the role of inflammation in CNV formation (43–45). Activated leukocytes, macrophages, and other inflammatory cells secrete enzymes and degrade and damage Bruch's membrane fostering CNV growth.

The most compelling evidence of complement's role in AMD involves complement factor H (CFH). CFH's main role is in the alternative complement pathway where it inhibits activation of C3 to C3a and C3b. It also directly binds to C3b preventing further downstream activation. Smoking, an established risk factor for AMD, decreases plasma CFH levels (46,47). CFH is produced by retinal pigment epithelial (RPE) cells and accumulates within drusen, and recent studies show that it may play a significant role in the pathogenesis of AMD (48–51). The identification of CFH in the pathogenesis of AMD first came from linkage studies and gene screenings of AMD patients that identified the locus of CFH (Chromosome 1q25–32) (52–54). With one particular allele for CFH (tyrosine-histidine substitution at amino acid 402), heterozygosity confers a two-to four- fold increase in developing AMD, and homozygosity confers a five- to seven-fold increased risk. Thus, complement inhibitors represent a novel pathway for management of both dry and wet AMD. First, inhibitors of complement could be given prior to choroidal neovascularization as a means of prevention. Second, inhibitors can be given along with current therapies as an alternative pathway. Numerous companies are in preclinical and early phase 1 testing including a C3 inhibitor,

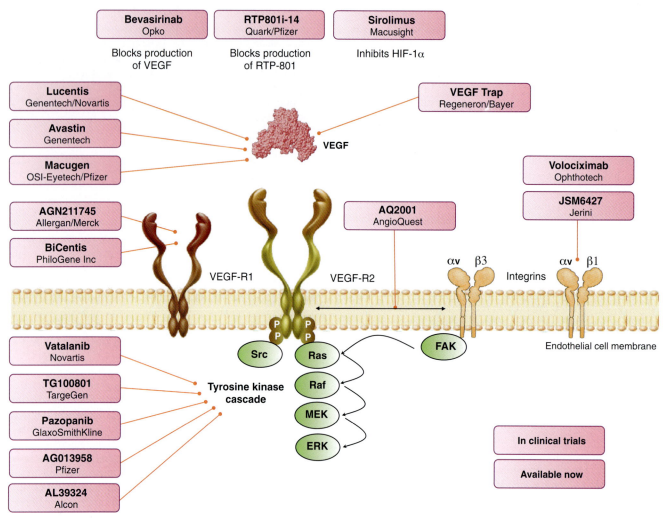

**Figure 12-2.** A series of studies have been conducted on kinase inhibitors from many companies to treat choroidal neovascularization caused by AMD in preclinical models and phase 1 studies. VEGF, vascular endothelial growth factor.

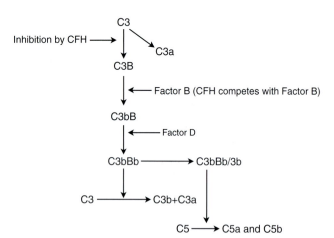

**Figure 12-3.** Three principle pathways have been identified and they all converge with activation of C3 complement. CFH, complement factor H.

compstatin or POT-4 (Potentia Pharmaceuticals), TA106a Fab fragment of a monoclonal antibody which inhibits complement factor B (Taligen Therapeutics), a small molecule peptidomimetic that inhibits the C5a receptor, JPE1375 (Jerini), an antibody that inhibits C5 (Alexion), and a C5 inhibiting aptamer, ARC1905 (Ophthotech).

## PIGMENT EPITHELIUM DERIVED FACTOR

PEDF is one of the most potent antiangiogenic factors expressed in adult retina and choroid (55). Adenoviral vectors that express PEDF in animal studies have been shown to induce the regression of choroidal neovascularization (56). In human AMD studies, PEDF expression is significantly reduced in RPE cells, Bruch's membrane, choriocapillaris, and vitreous compared to age-matched controls (57,58). This was also confirmed in a retrospective review of excised CNV specimens which demonstrated reduced PEDF expression (59). In a phase I clinical trial of adenoviral vectors with PEDF for CNV, AdPEDF (GenVec), the antiangiogenic activity persisted for several months following a single intravitreal dose of at least $10^8$ particle units. There were no significant adverse events or dose-limiting toxicity in the patients

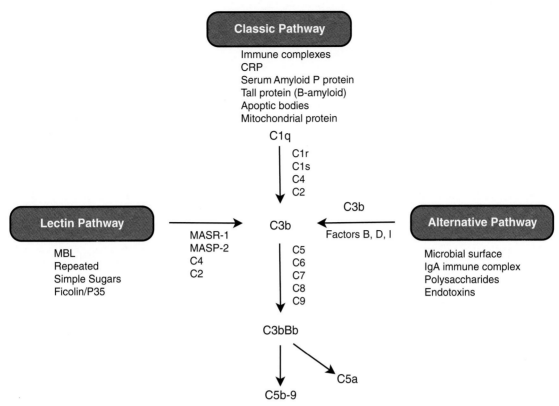

**Figure 12-4.** Three principle pathways have been identified and they all converge with activation of C3 complement. CRP, C-reactive protein; MBL, mannose binding lectin.

studied (60,61). Thus, PEDF may be a potential therapeutic agent for CNV caused by AMD.

## CONCLUSION

Current antiangiogenic drugs target only a small, albeit an important component of the entire pathway leading to choroidal neovascularization. Future antiangiogenics will focus on upstream and downstream pathways in order to hopefully reduce lesion size, decrease treatment frequency, and improve clinical outcomes. Although some of the drugs discussed here may not become first line pharmacotherapeutics, certainly the pathways that they utilize may be the targets of more effective agents.

### References

1. Brown DM, Kaiser PK, Michels M, et al. Ranibizumab versus verteporfin for neovascular age-related macular degeneration. *N Engl J Med* 2006;355:1432–1444.
2. Rosenfeld PJ, Brown DM, Heier JS, et al. Ranibizumab for neovascular age-related macular degeneration. *N Engl J Med* 2006;355:1419–1431.
3. Genentech. November 7th, 2005 press release. Available at http://www.gene.com/gene/news/press-releases/display.do?method=detail&id=9087.
4. Grunwald JE, Hariprasad SM, DuPont J, et al. Foveolar choroidal blood flow in age-related macular degeneration. *Invest Ophthalmol Vis Sci* 1998;39:385–390.
5. Ozaki H, Yu AY, Della N, et al. Hypoxia inducible factor-1alpha is increased in ischemic retina: temporal and spatial correlation with VEGF expression. *Invest Ophthalmol Vis Sci* 1999;40:182–189.
6. Lee PJ, Alam J, Wiegand GW, et al. Overexpression of heme oxygenase-1 in human pulmonary epithelial cells results in cell growth arrest and increased resistance to hyperoxia. *Proc Natl Acad Sci USA* 1996;93:10393–10398.
7. Levy AP, Levy NS, Wegner S, et al. Transcriptional regulation of the rat vascular endothelial growth factor gene by hypoxia. *J Biol Chem* 1995;270:13333–13340.
8. Liu Y, Cox SR, Morita T, et al. Hypoxia regulates vascular endothelial growth factor gene expression in endothelial cells. Identification of a 5' enhancer. *Circ Res* 1995;77:638–643.
9. Brafman A, Mett I, Shafir M, et al. Inhibition of oxygen-induced retinopathy in RTP801-deficient mice. *Invest Ophthalmol Vis Sci* 2004;45:3796–3805.
10. Corradetti MN, Inoki K, Guan KL. The stress-inducted proteins RTP801 and RTP801L are negative regulators of the mammalian target of rapamycin pathway. *J Biol Chem* 2005;280:9769–9772.
11. Vezina C, Kudelski A, Sehgal SN. Rapamycin (AY-22,989), a new antifungal antibiotic. I. Taxonomy of the producing streptomycete and isolation of the active principle. *J Antibiot (Tokyo)* 1975;28:721–726.
12. Baker H, Sidorowicz A, Sehgal SN, et al. Rapamycin (AY-22,989), a new antifungal antibiotic. III. In vitro and in vivo evaluation. *J Antibiot (Tokyo)* 1978;31:539–545.
13. Martel RR, Klicius J, Galet S. Inhibition of the immune response by rapamycin, a new antifungal antibiotic. *Can J Physiol Pharmacol* 1977;55:48–51.
14. Heitman J, Movva NR, Hall MN. Targets for cell cycle arrest by the immunosuppressant rapamycin in yeast. *Science* 1991;253:905–909.
15. Easton JB, Houghton PJ. mTOR and cancer therapy. *Oncogene* 2006;25:6436–6446.
16. Dejneka NS, Kuroki AM, Fosnot J, et al. Systemic rapamycin inhibits retinal and choroidal neovascularization in mice. *Mol Vis* 2004;10:964–972.
17. Rusnati M, Tanghetti E, Dell'Era P, et al. Alphavbeta3 integrin mediates the cell-adhesive capacity and biological activity of basic fibroblast growth factor (FGF-2) in cultured endothelial cells. *Mol Biol Cell* 1997;8:2449–2461.
18. Tanghetti E, Ria R, Dell'Era P, et al. Biological activity of substrate-bound basic fibroblast growth factor (FGF2): recruitment of FGF receptor-1 in endothelial cell adhesion contacts. *Oncogene* 2002;21:3889–3897.
19. Hutchings H, Ortega N, Plouet J. Extracellular matrix-bound vascular endothelial growth factor promotes endothelial cell adhesion, migration, and survival through integrin ligation. *FASEB J* 2003;17:1520–1522.
20. Hammes HP, Brownlee M, Jonczyk A, et al. Subcutaneous injection of a cyclic peptide antagonist of vitronectin receptor-type integrins inhibits retinal neovascularization. *Nat Med* 1996;2:529–533.
21. Friedlander M, Theesfeld CL, Sugita M, et al. Involvement of integrins alpha v beta 3 and alpha v beta 5 in ocular neovascular diseases. *Proc Natl Acad Sci USA* 1996;93:9764–9769.
22. Friedlander M, Brooks PC, Shaffer RW, et al. Definition of two angiogenic pathways by distinct alpha v integrins. *Science* 1995;270:1500–1502.

23. Brooks PC, Montgomery AM, Rosenfeld M, et al. Integrin alpha v beta 3 antagonists promote tumor regression by inducing apoptosis of angiogenic blood vessels. *Cell* 1994;79:1157–1164.

24. Ljubimov AV, Burgeson RE, Butkowski RJ, et al. Basement membrane abnormalities in human eyes with diabetic retinopathy. *J Histochem Cytochem* 1996;44:1469–1479.

25. Drake CJ, Cheresh DA, Little CD. An antagonist of integrin alpha v beta 3 prevents maturation of blood vessels during embryonic neovascularization. *J Cell Sci* 1995;108 (Pt 7):2655–2661.

26. Reynolds LE, Wyder L, Lively JC, et al. Enhanced pathological angiogenesis in mice lacking beta3 integrin or beta3 and beta5 integrins. *Nat Med* 2002;8:27–34.

27. Brooks PC, Stromblad S, Sanders LC, et al. Localization of matrix metalloproteinase MMP-2 to the surface of invasive cells by interaction with integrin alpha v beta 3. *Cell* 1996;85:683–693.

28. Buckley CD, Pilling D, Henriquez NV, et al. RGD peptides induce apoptosis by direct caspase-3 activation. *Nature* 1999;397:534–539.

29. Adderley SR, Fitzgerald DJ. Glycoprotein IIb/IIIa antagonists induce apoptosis in rat cardiomyocytes by caspase-3 activation. *J Biol Chem* 2000;275:5760–5766.

30. Umeda N, Kachi S, Akiyama H, et al. Suppression and regression of choroidal neovascularization by systemic administration of an alpha5beta1 integrin antagonist. *Mol Pharmacol* 2006;69:1820–1828.

31. Yasukawa T, Hoffmann S, Eichler W, et al. Inhibition of experimental choroidal neovascularization in rats by an alpha(v)-integrin antagonist. *Curr Eye Res* 2004;28:359–366.

32. Santulli RJ, Kinney WA, Ghosh S, et al. Studies with an orally bioavailable {alpha}V integrin antagonist in animal models of ocular vasculopathy: retinal neovascularization in mice and retinal vascular permeability in diabetic rats. *J Pharmacol Exp Ther* 2008; 324(3):894–901.

33. Maier AK, Kociok N, Zahn G, et al. Modulation of hypoxia-induced neovascularization by JSM6427, an integrin alpha5beta1 inhibiting molecule. *Curr Eye Res* 2007;32:801–812.

34. Waltenberger J, Claesson-Welsh L, Siegbahn A, et al. Different signal transduction properties of KDR and Flt1, two receptors for vascular endothelial growth factor. *J Biol Chem* 1994;269:26988–26995.

35. Ferrara N. Role of vascular endothelial growth factor in regulation of physiological angiogenesis. *Am J Physiol Cell Physiol* 2001;280:C1358–C1366.

36. Jain RK. Molecular regulation of vessel maturation. *Nat Med* 2003;9:685–693.

37. Cristofanilli M, Charnsangavej C, Hortobagyi GN. Angiogenesis modulation in cancer research: novel clinical approaches. *Nat Rev Drug Discov* 2002;1:415–426.

38. Bikfalvi A, Bicknell R. Recent advances in angiogenesis, anti-angiogenesis and vascular targeting. *Trends Pharmacol Sci* 2002;23:576–582.

39. Erber R, Thurnher A, Katsen AD, et al. Combined inhibition of VEGF and PDGF signaling enforces tumor vessel regression by interfering with pericyte-mediated endothelial cell survival mechanisms. *FASEB J* 2004;18:338–340.

40. Bora PS, Sohn JH, Cruz JM, et al. Role of complement and complement membrane attack complex in laser-induced choroidal neovascularization. *J Immunol* 2005;174:491–497.

41. Johnson LV, Leitner WP, Staples MK, et al. Complement activation and inflammatory processes in drusen formation and age related macular degeneration. *Exp Eye Res* 2001;73:887–896.

42. Crabb JW, Miyagi M, Gu X, et al. Drusen proteome analysis: an approach to the etiology of age-related macular degeneration. *Proc Natl Acad Sci USA* 2002;99:14682–14687.

43. Grindle CF, Marshall J. Ageing changes in Bruch's membrane and their functional implications. *Trans Ophthalmol Soc UK* 1978;98:172–175.

44. Penfold PL, Provis JM, Billson FA. Age-related macular degeneration: Ultrastructural studies of the relationship of leucocytes to angiogenesis. *Graefes Arch Clin Exp Ophthalmol* 1987;225:70–76.

45. Penfold PL, Gyory JF, Hunyor AB, et al. Exudative macular degeneration and intravitreal triamcinolone. A pilot study. *Aust N Z J Ophthalmol* 1995;23:293–298.

46. Male DA, Ormsby RJ, Ranganathan S, et al. Complement factor H: Sequence analysis of 221 kb of human genomic DNA containing the entire fH, fHR-1 and fHR-3 genes. *Mol Immunol* 2000;37:41–52.

47. Esparza-Gordillo J, Soria JM, Buil A, et al. Genetic and environmental factors influencing the human factor H plasma levels. *Immunogenetics* 2004;56:77–82.

48. Zareparsi S, Branham KE, Li M, et al. Strong association of the Y402H variant in complement factor H at 1q32 with susceptibility to age-related macular degeneration. *Am J Hum Genet* 2005;77:149–153.

49. Edwards AO, Ritter R, 3rd, Abel KJ, et al. Complement factor H polymorphism and age-related macular degeneration. *Science* 2005;308:421–424.

50. Haines JL, Hauser MA, Schmidt S, et al. Complement factor H variant increases the risk of age-related macular degeneration. *Science* 2005;308:419–421.

51. Hageman GS, Anderson DH, Johnson LV, et al. A common haplotype in the complement regulatory gene factor H (HF1/CFH) predisposes individuals to age-related macular degeneration. *Proc Natl Acad Sci USA* 2005;102:7227–7232.

52. Weeks DE, Conley YP, Tsai HJ, et al. Age-related maculopathy: an expanded genome-wide scan with evidence of susceptibility loci within the 1q31 and 17q25 regions. *Am J Ophthalmol* 2001;132:682–692.

53. Schick JH, Iyengar SK, Klein BE, et al. A whole-genome screen of a quantitative trait of age-related maculopathy in sibships from the beaver dam eye study. *Am J Hum Genet* 2003;72:1412–1424.

54. Seddon JM, Santangelo SL, Book K, et al. A genomewide scan for age-related macular degeneration provides evidence for linkage to several chromosomal regions. *Am J Hum Genet* 2003;73:780–790.

55. Bhutto IA, McLeod DS, Hasegawa T, et al. Pigment epithelium-derived factor (PEDF) and vascular endothelial growth factor (VEGF) in aged human choroid and eyes with age-related macular degeneration. *Exp Eye Res* 2006;82:99–110.

56. Mori K, Gehlbach P, Ando A, et al. Regression of ocular neovascularization in response to increased expression of pigment epithelium-derived factor. *Invest Ophthalmol Vis Sci* 2002;43:2428–2434.

57. Renno RZ, Youssri AI, Michaud N, et al. Expression of pigment epithelium-derived factor in experimental choroidal neovascularization. *Invest Ophthalmol Vis Sci* 2002;43:1574–1580.

58. Holekamp NM, Bouck N, Volpert O. Pigment epithelium-derived factor is deficient in the vitreous of patients with choroidal neovascularization due to age-related macular degeneration. *Am J Ophthalmol* 2002;134:220–227.

59. Tatar O, Adam A, Shinoda K, et al. Expression of VEGF and PEDF in choroidal neovascular membranes following verteporfin photodynamic therapy. *Am J Ophthalmol* 2006;142:95–104.

60. Rasmussen H, Chu KW, Campochiaro P, et al. Clinical protocol. An open-label, phase I, single administration, dose-escalation study of ADGVPEDF.11D (ADPEDF) in neovascular age-related macular degeneration (AMD). *Hum Gene Ther* 2001;12:2029–2032.

61. Campochiaro PA, Nguyen QD, Shah SM, et al. Adenoviral vector-delivered pigment epithelium-derived factor for neovascular age-related macular degeneration: results of a phase I clinical trial. *Hum Gene Ther* 2006;17:167–176.

# 13

# Pharmacologic Vitreolysis

Raja Narayanan ■ Baruch D. Kuppermann

The importance of vitreous in the pathogenesis of various retinal disorders has been well recognized, and currently vitreous can only be dealt with surgically. Anomalous posterior vitreous detachment (PVD), which is a condition where the vitreous liquefies without vitreoretinal dehiscence (1), can worsen diabetic retinopathy and cause retinal tears, detachment, macular pucker, macular hole, or vitreous hemorrhage (2). Vitreous hemorrhage is a major cause of vision loss. The most common cause of vitreous hemorrhage is diabetic retinopathy, which can also lead to tractional retinal detachment (3). Various enzymes have been investigated to dissolve the vitreous hemorrhage or modify the structural characteristics of the vitreous to allow diffusion of blood out of the visual axis. Enzymatic vitreolysis has several advantages over conventional surgery, including the ability to treat the hemorrhage earlier, in an office setting, and with lower costs. With pharmacologic vitreolysis, complications of surgery such as cataract, endophthalmitis, retinal hemorrhage, tear or detachment, and anesthesia-related complications can be avoided. A number of vitreolytic enzymes have been investigated, including hyaluronidase, plasmin, dispase, tissue plasminogen activator, and chondroitinase, with varying effects. Such pharmacologic therapies rely upon a good understanding of the biochemical composition and organization of the vitreous.

Ultrastructural studies have shown that the adult human vitreous contains fine, parallel fibers of collagen coursing in an anteroposterior direction (4,5). Although several agents have been investigated in animal models, only a few have been employed in humans. Autologous plasmin enzyme (APE) has been used in some patients but has never been subjected to the rigors of a controlled clinical trial. Chondroitinase and hyaluronidase have been tested in clinical trials, but the former never entered Phase II testing. Hyaluronidase (Vitrase) failed a Phase III U.S. Food and Drug Administration (FDA) trial conducted in the United States. The Vitrase clinical trial results will be discussed in more detail later in this chapter.

## HYALURONAN

Hyaluronan is a major macromolecule of the vitreous (5). Hyaluronan is a long, unbranched polymer of repeating disaccharide (glucuronic acid $\beta$ [1,3]-$N$-acetylglucosamine) moieties linked by $\beta$ 1–4 bonds. It is a linear, left-handed, threefold helix with a rise per disaccharide on the helix axis of 0.98 nm. The sodium salt of hyaluronan has a molecular weight of 3 to $4.5 \times 10^6$ in the normal human vitreous. Hyaluronan is not normally a free polymer *in vivo*, but it is covalently linked to a protein core to form a proteoglycan. Hyaluronan plays a pivotal role in stabilizing the vitreous gel.

## COLLAGEN

Studies have shown that the vitreous contains collagen type II, a hybrid of types V/XI, and type IX collagen in a molar ratio of 75:10:15, respectively (6). Vitreous collagens are organized into fibrils with types V/XI residing in the core, type II collagen surrounding the core, and type IX collagen on the surface of the fibril. The fibrils are 7 to 28 nm in diameter, but their length in situ is unknown.

## SUPRAMOLECULAR ORGANIZATION

Vitreous is a dilute meshwork of collagen fibrils interspersed with extensive arrays of hyaluronan molecules. The collagen fibrils provide a scaffoldlike structure that is "inflated" by the hydrophilic hyaluronan. If collagen is removed, the remaining hyaluronan forms a viscous solution. However, if hyaluronan is removed, the gel shrinks but is not destroyed. Electrostatic binding occurs between the negatively charged hyaluronan and the positively charged collagen in the vitreous (7).

Studies have shown that the chondroitin sulfate chains of type IX collagen bridge between adjacent collagen fibrils in a ladderlike configuration spacing them apart (8). Such spacing is necessary for vitreous transparency, because keeping vitreous collagen fibrils separated by at least one wavelength of incident light minimizes light scattering, allowing the unhindered transmission of light to the retina for photoreception. Bishop (6) proposed that the leucine-rich repeat protein opticin is the predominant structural protein responsible for short-range spacing of collagen fibrils.

Numerous changes occur in the structure of the vitreous with age. There is a significant decrease in the gel volume and an increase in the liquid volume of the human vitreous. Derangement of the normal hyaluronan/collagen association results in the simultaneous formation of liquid vitreous and aggregation of collagen fibrils into bundles of parallel fibrils seen macroscopically as large fibers (9). In the posterior vitreous, such age-related changes form large pockets of liquid vitreous.

Vitreoretinal adhesion at the posterior pole is more fascial than focal (at the disc, fovea, and along retinal blood vessels), consistent with the concept that the two tissues are held together by an extracellular matrix tissue (10). With age, there is weakening of vitreoretinal adhesion, most likely due to biochemical alterations in the extracellular matrix tissue at the vitreoretinal interface. Studies using lectin probes have identified that one component of the extracellular matrix at the vitreoretinal interface [galactose $\beta$ (1,3)-$N$-acetylglucosamine] is present in youth but absent in adults (11). This difference and others may play a role in the observed weakening of the vitreoretinal interface during aging.

## POSTERIOR VITREOUS DETACHMENT

PVD results from weakening of the adhesion between the posterior vitreous cortex and the retina, in conjunction with liquefaction within the vitreous body. Weakening of the posterior vitreous cortex/retinal adhesion at the posterior pole allows liquid vitreous to enter the retrocortical space via the prepapillary hole and perhaps the premacular vitreous cortex as well. Volume displacement from the central vitreous to the preretinal space causes the observed collapse of the vitreous body.

For PVD to occur without complications, two different processes must occur concurrently and to a similar extent: weakening of vitreoretinal adhesion and vitreous liquefaction. There must be sufficient weakening of vitreoretinal adherence so that when the critical amount of liquefied gel has accumulated, the collapsing vitreous separates away from the retina and PVD occurs without untoward effects.

## ANOMALOUS POSTERIOR VITREOUS DETACHMENT

Anomalous PVD results when the extent of vitreous liquefaction exceeds the degree of vitreoretinal interface weakening, resulting in traction exerted at the vitreoretinal interface (12). There can be various untoward effects of anomalous PVD. Effects on the retina include hemorrhage, retinal tears and detachment, vitreomacular traction syndromes, and some cases of diffuse diabetic macular edema. Proliferative diabetic retinopathy can be greatly aggravated by anomalous PVD. Effects on the vitreous involve posterior vitreoschisis, where splitting of the posterior vitreous cortex and forward displacement of the vitreous body leaves the outer layer of the split posterior vitreous cortex still attached to the retina. This can result in macular pucker, contribute to macular holes, or complicate proliferative diabetic retinopathy.

## PHARMACOLOGIC VITREOLYSIS

Various pharmacologic vitreolysis agents including hyaluronidase, urea, plasmin, dispase, tissue plasminogen activator, and chondroitinase have been tested to date (13), but little is known about the exact mechanism of action of these substances, and so far none have met with sufficient success to result in widespread use.

Plasmin is a broad spectrum proteolytic enzyme which can lyse fibrinogen, fibrin and most proteins in the extracellular matrix. Plasmin has been used only in limited series of uncontrolled clinical testing (two published series of nine and seven cases), chondroitinase was used only on 20 patients in a Phase I FDA trial, and hyaluronidase failed a Phase III FDA trial.

Previous studies have suggested that plasmin from a variety of sources may be useful for pharmacologic vitreolysis. APE was reported to induce vitreoretinal separation in rabbits, but there were no studies on its molecular effects. These laboratory investigations were followed by treatment in small series of patients undergoing vitrectomy for macular holes (n = 9) and diabetic retinopathy (n = 7) (14,15). However, to date, no controlled clinical trials have been undertaken with APE. The methods employed to extract APE from the patient's blood preoperatively have inherent variability, making dosing and quality control difficult. Human recombinant microplasmin, which is much smaller than plasmin and is manufactured in a standardized manner that provides quality control and standardized dosing, is being developed for pharmacologic vitreolysis. Microplasmin is a direct-acting thrombolytic agent that contains the protease domain but lacks the five "kringle" domains of plasmin, making it a much smaller molecule than plasmin. Recent studies found that microplasmin is able to detach the posterior vitreous cortex in pigs and cats and postmortem human eyes. However, as in the case of APE, there are no studies on the molecular effects of microplasmin on the vitreous gel.

Microplasmin and collagenase have been studied in *ex vivo* eyes and have been shown to liquefy the vitreous in a dose-dependent manner.

## DISPASE

An *in vitro* study on porcine and human cadaver eyes using dispase has shown that PVD was induced with 5 IU per ml of the enzyme incubated for 15 minutes. Microscopy demonstrated that the attachment of the posterior hyaloid to the internal limiting membrane was cleaved without structural damage to the inner retina (16).

## UREA (VITREOSOLVE)

Vitreosolve is a potential drug for intra-ocular use that is being studied in a Phase II/III trial. It has the potential to induce PVD in most patients within a week after a single intravitreal injection. This may help prevent progression of retinopathy in patients with diabetes and can also make vitreoretinal surgery easier in difficult cases such as pediatric retinal detachments and proliferative vitreoretinopathy. Vitreosolve may also have some neuroprotective role, and it has been shown to be safe in preclinical and Phase I/II studies.

## HYALURONIDASE

Hyaluronidase cleaves glycosidic bonds of hyaluronic acid and, to a variable degree, other acid mucopolysaccharides of the connective tissue. Dissolution of the hyaluronic acid and collagen complex results in decreased viscosity of the extracellular matrix. This in turn increases the diffusion rate of erythrocytes and exudates along with phagocytes through the vitreous and facilitates red blood cell lysis and phagocytosis.

### Vitrase (hyaluronidase)

Vitrase was studied in a large, multicenter, randomized controlled trial (17). A total of 1,125 patients with persistent vitreous hemorrhage were randomized to 55 IU (n = 365), 75 IU (n = 377), and saline (n = 383). The percentage of patients reaching primary efficacy by month 1 in the 55 IU, 75 IU, and saline groups was 13.2%, 10.6%, and 5.5% ($p = .001$ and $p = .010$), respectively. By month 3, 32.9%, 30.5%, and 25.6% of patients treated with 55 IU, 75 IU, and saline, respectively, reached the primary efficacy endpoint ($p = .025$, $p = .144$). A statistically significant improvement in best corrected visual acuity (BCVA) was observed. By month 3, 44.9% and 43.5% of patients in the 55 IU and 75 IU treatment groups, respectively, had at least a 3-line improvement in BCVA compared with 34.5% of patients in the saline group ($p = .004$ and $p = .011$). The analysis of the investigator-graded reduction in vitreous hemorrhage density also showed statistical significance in the 55 IU and 75 IU dose groups compared with saline by months 1, 2, and 3. In the analysis of the clinical assessment of therapeutic utility (clearance of the hemorrhage sufficient to diagnose the underlying pathology), there was a significant difference for patients in the 55 IU and 75 IU treatment groups compared with saline-treated patients by months 1, 2, and 3. By month 3, 40.8% and 39.3% of patients in the 55 IU ($p = .001$) and 75 IU ($p = .002$) groups, respectively, reached this endpoint compared with 28.5% of patients in the saline group.

In summary, data from the Phase III clinical trials demonstrated that intravitreous injection of ovine hyaluronidase was efficacious and had a favorable safety profile. The primary ocular adverse event associated with the use of ovine hyaluronidase was acute, self-limited anterior uveitis. This iritis was resolved with or without treatment, and without sequelae. Additionally, clinical experience has demonstrated that these injections do not prohibit or complicate subsequent vitrectomies when they are required.

## References

1. Sebag J, Ansari RR, Suh KI. Pharmacologic vitreolysis with microplasmin increases vitreous diffusion coefficients. *Graefe's Arch Clin Exp Ophthalmol* 2007;245:576–580.
2. Sebag J. Pharmacologic vitreolysis. *Retina* 1998;18:1–3.
3. Spraul CW, Grossniklaus HE. Vitreous hemorrhage. *Surv Ophthalmol* 1997;42(1):3–39.
4. Sebag J, Balazs EA. Pathogenesis of CME: anatomic considerations of vitreoretinal adhesions. *Surv Opthalmol* 1984;28:493–498.
5. Sebag J. Molecular biology of pharmacologic vitreolysis. *Trans Am Ophthalmol Soc* 2005;103:473–494.
6. Bishop PN. Structural macromolecules and supramolecular organization of the vitreous gel. *Prog Ret Eye Res* 2000;19:323–344.
7. Comper WD, Laurent TC. Physiological functions of connective tissue polysaccharides. *Physiol Rev* 1978;58:255–315.
8. Scott JE, Chen Y, Brass A. Secondary and tertiary structures involving chondroitin and chondroitin sulphate in solution, investigated by rotary shadowing electron microscopy and computer simulation. *Eur J Biochem* 1992;209:675–680.
9. Sebag J, Balazs EA. Morphology and ultrastructure of human vitreous fibers. *Invest Ophthalmol Vis Sci* 1989;30:1867–1871.
10. Sebag J. Age-related differences at the human vitreo-retinal interface. *Arch Ophthalmol* 1991;109:966–971.
11. Russell SR, Shepherd JD, Hageman GS. Distribution of glycoconjugates in the human internal limiting membrane. *Invest Ophthalmol Vis Sci* 1991;32:1986–1995.
12. Sebag J. Anomalous PVD—a unifying concept in vitreo-retinal disease. *Graefe's Arch Clin Exp Ophthalmol* 2004;242:690–698.
13. Bhisitkul RB. Anticipation for enzymatic vitreolysis. *Br J Ophthalmol* 2001;85:1–2.
14. Trese MT, Williams GA, Hartzer MK. A new approach to stage 3 macular holes. *Ophthalmology* 2000;107:1607–1611.
15. Williams KG, Trese MT, Williams GA, et al. Autologous plasmin enzyme in the surgical management of diabetic retinopathy. *Ophthalmology* 2001;108:1902–1905.
16. Tezel TH, Del Priore LV, Kaplan HJ. Posterior vitreous detachment with dispase. *Retina* 1998;18:7–15.
17. Kuppermann BD, Thomas EL, de Smet M, et al. Pooled efficacy results from two multinational randomized controlled trials of a single intravitreous injection of highly purified ovine hyaluronidase for the management of vitreous hemorrhage. *Am J Ophthalmol* 2005;140:573–584.

# 14

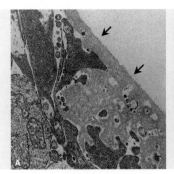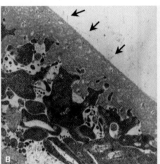

# Microplasmin and Vitreoretinal Surgery

David Goldenberg ■ Anselm Kampik ■ Arnd Gandorfer ■ Michael Trese

## INTRODUCTION

The vitreoretinal interface plays an important role in the pathogenesis of many retinal disorders. It is a common belief that traction at this interface contributes to the retinal pathology observed in proliferative diabetic retinopathy, proliferative vitreoretinopathy, macular pucker, diabetic macular edema, vitreomacular traction, macular holes, and retinal detachments. Traction is believed to be mediated by the vitreous cortex and by fibrocellular proliferation, and therefore complete removal of the cortical hyaloid is often a principal goal of vitreoretinal surgery (1). The surgical management of these disorders often targets this interface by separating the posterior hyaloid from the internal limiting membrane (ILM), thereby creating a posterior vitreous detachment (PVD). Mechanical separation of the vitreoretinal interface with vitrectomy may not remove all of the vitreous or completely separate the vitreoretinal junction (2), as cortical vitreous fibrils are left behind on the ILM (3). In addition, incomplete removal of the vitreous may result in surgical failure (4).

Vitrectomy with peeling of the ILM necessitates direct mechanical manipulation of the macula, and although it is generally safe, it can potentially result in trauma to the retina (5,6). Mechanical separation of the posterior hyaloid from the retina in adult primates demonstrates incomplete vitreoretinal separation and frequently causes damage to the macula and optic disc, including partial or full thickness foveal tears, damage to the optic nerve, separation of the ILM from the retina, and avulsion of the ganglion cells and other retina layers (2). Therefore, the development of a pharmacologic agent that can aid in vitreous liquefaction and PVD creation may facilitate surgical separation of the posterior hyaloid, thus reducing intraoperative time and potential complications. Pharmacologic vitreous liquefaction may help to reduce vitreous viscosity, thereby facilitating removal during vitrectomy and reducing surgical time, especially when using smaller gauge instruments such as 25-gauge and 23-gauge vitrectors.

Intraocular enzymatic agents have been discussed for many years, one of the earliest being alpha-chymotrypsin and its effect on zonular proteins during intracapsular cataract extraction. The search for an appropriate agent to manipulate the vitreous has included several enzymes, most of which are autologous enzymes that activate other endogenous enzymes. Unfortunately, many of the earliest studied agents were fraught with failure due to lack of efficacy, retinal toxicity, or difficult preparation. Microplasmin is a recombinant human enzyme that appears to be a promising agent for pharmacologic manipulation of the vitreous. It has recently been shown to cause vitreous liquefaction and cleavage of the vitreoretinal interface with a single intravitreal injection (7–10). Pharmacologic alteration of the vitreous with microplasmin and other agents is an evolving modality that will likely be used more frequently for therapy and preventative measures (11).

## ANATOMICAL CONSIDERATIONS

In the past, the vitreous was considered unimportant in the development of vitreoretinal pathology (7). With recent advancements in biochemistry and vitreous anatomy, we are now able to appreciate the complex arrangement of the vitreous gel and its influence on retinal diseases. The vitreous is a clear, semisolid gel containing hyaluronic acid interspersed in a framework of parallel collagen fibrils coursing in an anteroposterior direction (7). Posterior to the pars plana, the concentration of collagen and hyaluronic acid is greatest in the vitreous cortex, which lies along the inner retinal surface (12). The collagen fibrils, which are condensed to form an outer layer of the vitreous cortex, are adherent to the ILM of the retina (12). Glycoproteins such as laminin and fibronectin are located at the vitreoretinal junction (13) and are believed to contribute to the adhesion of the posterior vitreous cortex to the ILM.

## POSTERIOR VITREOUS DETACHMENT

As the human vitreous ages, syneresis and liquefaction of the gel occur with the development of pools of fluid usually in the premacular region or in the central part of the vitreous cavity. Foos and Wheeler (14) found a strong correlation between increasing amounts of vitreous syneresis and the prevalence of PVD. This suggests that the human vitreous gel can tolerate only a certain amount of liquefaction and instability before PVD occurs. Age-related PVD usually occurs as an acute event. A tear in the posterior cortical vitreous allows fluid from the central part of the liquefied vitreous gel to then pass through the break in the vitreous cortex and separate the surrounding cortical vitreous from the retina.

Similar to the development of an endogenous age-related PVD, the success of pharmacologic vitreolysis depends on simultaneous vitreous liquefaction and separation of the vitreoretinal interface. Sebag (7,15) has used the term "anomalous PVD" to describe the situation in which these two processes are uncoupled, whereby the extent of vitreous liquefaction exceeds the degree of vitreoretinal interface weakening. Anomalous PVD may lead to traction at the vitreoretinal interface and subsequent pathologic conditions including vitreomacular traction syndrome, macular holes, and retinal tears (15).

## HISTORICAL CONSIDERATIONS

Prior to the advent of microplasmin, multiple other pharmacologic agents have been developed for enzymatic manipulation of the vitreous. Enzymes such as dispase, chondroitinase, hyaluronidase, tissue plasminogen activator (tPA), and plasmin have had variable success (7,16). Dispase was initially believed to be a good candidate for pharmacologic vitreolysis due to its ability to hydrolyze several proteins including type IV collagen and fibronectin. In fact, dispase can lead to the creation of a PVD (17,18); however, it causes anterior chamber and vitreous inflammation, epiretinal membranes, preretinal and intraretinal hemorrhages, cataract, electroretinogram (ERG) amplitude reductions, and ultrastructural damage to the retina (17–19). This intraocular toxicity has limited its clinical utility. Chondroitinase lyses the proteoglycan chondroitin sulfate, which is associated with the vitreoretinal interface (20). A recent masked, placebo-controlled, *in vivo* study concluded that chondroitinase failed to produce a PVD (21).

Hyaluronidase (Vitrase) is a highly purified ovine enzyme that primarily digests the proteoglycan hyaluronan, which constitutes a large component of the vitreous body. Hyaluronidase has been suggested as an agent to liquefy the central vitreous with the assumption that it may also lead to a PVD after an extended period of time. Hyaluronidase was originally targeted toward patients with dense vitreous hemorrhages in the hope of causing vitreous liquefaction (and settling of blood) to allow for laser photocoagulation in cases of proliferative diabetic retinopathy. A recent prospective, double-masked phase III trial concluded that hyaluronidase is more effective than placebo injections in clearing vitreous hemorrhages (22). Although it has been shown to decrease vitreous macromolecule size suggesting a role for vitreous liquefaction (7), other reports have concluded that intravitreal injection of hyaluronidase cannot induce a PVD in animal models (10,23,24). As mentioned earlier, vitreous liquefaction without simultaneous separation of the vitreoretinal interface may induce untoward effects, including vitreomacular traction syndrome, macular holes, and retinal tears (7,15). Nevertheless, a recent phase III trial concluded that there were no serious safety issues and the incidence of retinal detachment was not statistically different between hyaluronidase and controls (25).

Plasmin enzyme is a nonspecific protease capable of hydrolyzing glycoproteins such as laminin and fibronectin (26,27), which bridge and bind vitreous collagen fibers between the posterior vitreous cortex and the ILM (13). The liquefaction of vitreous gel by plasmin enzyme is based on its activity on collagenases (16). Unlike dispase, plasmin enzyme spares type IV collagenase, leaving the ILM intact but causing liquefaction in a dose-dependent fashion in the central vitreous cavity (16,28). tPA has worked through a similar pathway as plasmin enzyme, by activating endogenous plasminogen. The endogenous plasminogen then converts to plasmin enzyme and works on the vitreoretinal junction. Gandorfer et al. (28) reported that a single injection of plasmin enzyme is able to cleave the vitreoretinal junction without causing morphological changes to the retina in postmortem porcine eyes. The authors concluded that the degree of vitreoretinal separation depends on the concentration and length of exposure to plasmin. Plasmin enzyme reaches its peak activity in 15 to 30 minutes and remains at this peak for approximately 90 minutes (29). This activity then falls off over the next several hours to an immeasurable level (29).

Encouraging results with animal studies prompted the desire to pursue human trials. Autologous plasmin enzyme (APE), which can be isolated from the patient's serum, has been studied extensively in humans. Multiple reports have confirmed that a concentration of 0.4 to 1.2 U of APE can cause vitreous liquefaction and induce a PVD in humans (30–35). Wang et al. (18) evaluated the safety of intravitreal plasmin injections in rabbit eyes. At a concentration that was ten times (4 U) the amount required for PVD formation (0.4 U), they found transient mild intraocular inflammation without ERG changes or morphologic changes to the ILM and retina.

Plasmin-assisted vitrectomy in cadaver eyes demonstrates a smooth retinal surface with only sparse collagen fibrils (3). Human pilot trials with APE-assisted vitrectomy in traumatic macular holes, idiopathic macular holes, and diabetic eyes have been reported (30,32–35). In these eyes, plasmin enzyme has been shown to allow the vitreous gel to be easier to peel than expected or spontaneously separated in the majority of eyes. The use of plasmin enzyme in diabetics may facilitate membrane peeling by acting on the extracellular matrix fibrin between the cellular pegs of the epiretinal membrane and neurosensory retina, allowing improved exposure and access to the pegs and making them easier to divide (16,32).

## MICROPLASMIN BIOCHEMISTRY

Microplasmin (ThromboGenics Ltd., Dublin, Ireland) is a recombinant protein containing one active protease site of human plasmin but lacking many of the remaining "kringle" domains (36). It functions as a direct-acting thrombolytic agent, and it is a much smaller molecule (29 kD) than human plasmin (88 kD) (36). It has been proposed that the smaller size of microplasmin enables the molecule to penetrate the epiretinal tissue more effectively than plasmin (8). Because it is a recombinant protein, it can be prepared and manufactured in large quantities in limited time. Thus, the venipuncture and labor-intensive preparation that is needed for plasmin can be avoided.

Microplasmin is also in development as a neuroprotective agent with thrombolytic potential for the treatment of ischemic stroke (37). It has been shown to reduce ischemic brain damage and improve neurologic dysfunction in a rat stroke model (38). Microplasmin is currently being investigated in clinical trials for the treatment of acute ischemic strokes and deep vein thromboses.

## MICROPLASMIN EFFICACY

In order for pharmacologic vitreolysis to be beneficial, two successful components are necessary: (a) vitreous liquefaction and (b) complete vitreoretinal interface separation (PVD). Sebag (7) has indicated a dose-dependent reduction in the size of porcine vitreous macromolecules (hyaluronan and collagen) after injection with microplasmin. Using dynamic light scattering, the highest dose of microplasmin (0.8 mg) demonstrated an overall reduction in size of about 85% after just 30 minutes. These results suggest that significant vitreous liquefaction is achieved with microplasmin after a relatively brief period of time (7).

Gandorfer et al. (8) injected postmortem human eyes and *in vivo* feline eyes with microplasmin or saline and confirmed the presence or absence of a PVD with scanning and transmission electron microscopy. The microplasmin-injected eyes demonstrated complete vitreoretinal separation in a dose- and time-dependent fashion in both species (Fig. 14-1). The authors suggested that the effect of microplasmin continues beyond 24 hours. Nevertheless, they concluded that complete

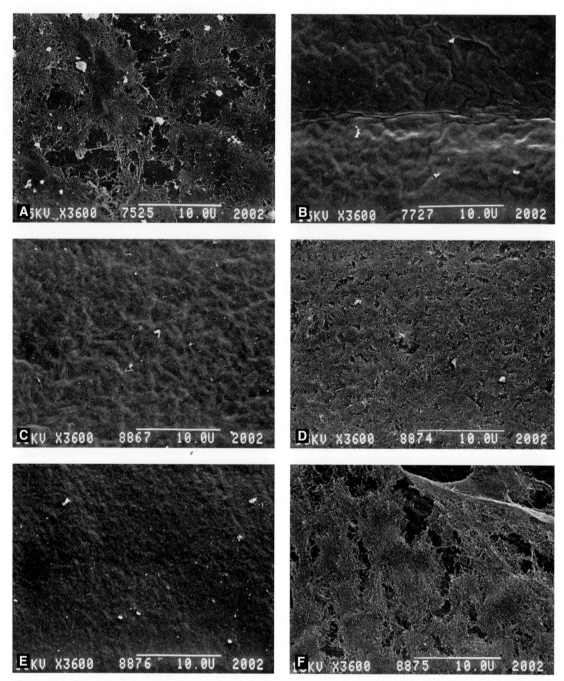

**Figure 14-1.** Scanning electron micrographs of the vitreoretinal interface in human postmortem eyes. **A:** Intravitreal injection of 62.5 μg of microplasmin resulted in remnants of collagen fibrils covering the internal limiting membrane (ILM). **B:** 125 μg and **C:** 188 μg of microplasmin produced complete posterior vitreous detachment (PVD) and a bare ILM. **D:** Compression of collagen fibrils toward the ILM in an eye treated with 62.5 μg microplasmin and gas. **E:** Complete PVD following treatment with 125 μg microplasmin and gas. **F:** Dense network of collagen fibrils in control eye. Magnification 3600x. (From Gandorfer A, Rohleder M, Sethi C, et al. Posterior vitreous detachment induced by microplasmin. *Invest Ophthalmol Vis Sci.* 2004;45:641–647, reprinted with permission.)

vitreoretinal separation can be induced within 30 minutes after injection (Fig. 14-2). Subsequent reports (9,10) have confirmed the dose dependency of microplasmin and successful PVD induction with microplasmin in animal models using rabbits, guinea pigs, rats, and cats. Thus, microplasmin can successfully induce both vitreous liquefaction and PVD induction in animal studies. These results prompted the idea that

microplasmin may be effective in inducing a prophylactic PVD (7). To date, no human pilot trials with microplasmin have been reported; however, clinical trials are underway in Europe and the United States.

It has been suggested that complete posterior vitreous separation allows for resolution of diabetic macular edema (32). In addition, a complete PVD is a strong negative risk

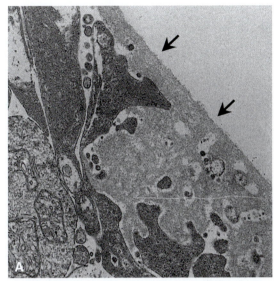 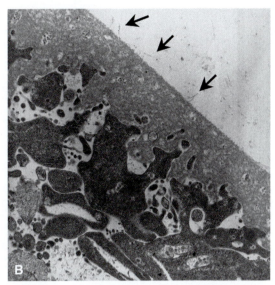

**Figure 14-2.** Transmission electron micrographs of the internal limiting membrane (ILM) in human postmortem eyes. **A:** Microplasmin-treated eye. Note the absence of collagen fibrils (*arrows*) on the ILM. Magnification: 13600x. **B:** Control eye. Collagen fibrils are still present (*arrows*). Magnification: 6800x. (From Gandorfer A, Rohleder M, Sethi C, et al. Posterior vitreous detachment induced by microplasmin. *Invest Ophthalmol Vis Sci* 2004;45:641–647, reprinted with permission.)

factor for the progression of diabetic retinopathy (39). Multiple growth factors, including vascular endothelial growth factor (VEGF), have been implicated in the pathogenesis of diabetic macular edema and neovascularization (40–42). It is possible that a PVD may alter the flux of molecules in the vitreous cavity and influence the concentration of vitreal growth factors. Quiram et al. (10) have recently demonstrated that the creation of a microplasmin-assisted PVD increases vitreal oxygen and the rate of oxygen exchange within the vitreous cavity in animal models. Other studies have suggested that an injection of microplasmin increases the vitreous diffusion coefficient in porcine eyes using dynamic light scattering (11). Preliminary data from cat models have indicated that microplasmin-induced PVD leads to decreased levels of vitreal VEGF (43). It is possible that a microplasmin-induced PVD increases vitreous oxygenation, thereby decreasing retinal ischemia and altering growth factor production. If so, this may have profound implications for the management of diabetic retinopathy. Microplasmin may be able to delay the progression of diabetic retinopathy and diabetic macular edema by inducing a prophylactic PVD. A specific relationship between a PVD and vitreous growth factor levels remains unclear. Prospective clinical trials will be required to address this theory.

The ability of microplasmin to induce a complete PVD in only 30 minutes is significant. This brief period of time seems to be an acceptable amount of delay for pharmacologic vitreolysis to have a clinical effect. Microplasmin could feasibly be injected in the operating room as an adjunct to surgery or in the clinic as prophylaxis.

In the operating room, this injection would not cause an insurmountable delay prior to beginning a vitrectomy; in the clinic setting, it would not be unheard of for a patient to wait 30 minutes for a possible repeat examination in order to ensure the agent's efficacy and to identify potential complications.

## MICROPLASMIN SAFETY

As previously stated, pharmacologic vitreolysis is a technique in which a chemical agent (i.e., microplasmin) is injected into the mid-vitreous in order to digest specific components of the extracellular matrix proteins in the vitreoretinal interface and in the vitreous gel without disrupting retinal structure and function. Obvious concerns arise regarding the safety and potential toxicity of injected agents. Gandorfer et al. (8) used light and transmission electron microscopy to evaluate the cytoarchitecture of the retina after microplasmin injection in postmortem human and *in vivo* feline eyes. They reported that the ultrastructure of the inner retina and the ILM were normal for both microplasmin-treated eyes and control eyes. In addition, electron microscopy and laser confocal microscopy did not show any evidence of inflammatory cellular infiltration of the retina after the microplasmin injection.

In a similar study designed to specifically address the safety of microplasmin injections in rabbit eyes, Sakuma et al. (9) used ERG to evaluate retinal toxicity. A transient decrease in a- and b-wave amplitudes was observed in all eyes injected with microplasmin. At 14 days after injection, a- and b-wave amplitudes fully recovered in the eyes receiving 125 μg or less microplasmin (the lowest dose needed for complete PVD in the study). Animals injected with the highest dose of 250 μg showed ERG changes even 90 days after the injection. In addition, a mild transient inflammatory reaction was present in the vitreous and anterior chamber, which completely resolved by day five. Light microscopy and transmission electron microscopy confirmed normal ILM and retinal histologic findings. The authors concluded that microplasmin was not toxic to the rabbit retina if using 125 μg or less.

It has been suggested that Müller cells have a high reactivity to any form of surgical trauma, including peeling of the ILM, which leads to protein up-regulation and gliosis (8). Gandorfer et al. (8) used antibodies specific for Müller cell reactivity and observed no difference between microplasmin-treated eyes and control eyes. The quiescent state of Müller cells provides additional experimental evidence for the safety of microplasmin in inducing a PVD.

Pharmacologic manipulation of the vitreoretinal interface presents the inherent risk of causing a retinal tear or detachment. Although no reports to date have specifically addressed this concern, a retinal tear is an intrinsic risk during PVD creation, especially in patients with abnormal vitreoretinal adhesions such as lattice degeneration. The development of a retinal tear following a microplasmin injection would only lend more support for its ability to successfully induce a PVD. Nevertheless, closely monitoring patients following administration of a microplasmin injection in the practitioner's office would be prudent in order to identify retinal tears early and avoid subsequent retinal detachment. Fortunately, clinical efficacy of microplasmin occurs within 30 minutes, which allows for an examination after the injection in a reasonable amount of time.

## FUTURE DIRECTIONS

Encouraging results with microplasmin in animal models and postmortem human eyes have prompted several clinical trials. A Phase IIb, multicenter, randomized, placebo-controlled, dose-ranging clinical trial designed to evaluate the safety and efficacy of microplasmin intravitreal injection prior to vitrectomy is currently underway in the United States. The results of this trial are expected to allow dose selection for subsequent clinical development. In parallel with this, Phase IIb trial is a European study evaluating microplasmin injection for the nonsurgical treatment of diabetic macular edema.

The ability to induce vitreous liquefaction and a complete PVD with a single intravitreal injection has potentially significant implications for the management of multiple vitreoretinopathies. If used as a surgical adjunct, it has the potential to facilitate more complete removal of the vitreous gel, decrease surgical time, and reduce intra-operative complications. If used as prophylactic therapy, its uses may include vitreomacular traction syndrome, proliferative diabetic retinopathy, and macular holes. If successful, it may even replace surgical intervention for select cases.

## References

1. Gandorfer A, Rohleder M, Kampik A. Epiretinal pathology of vitreomacular traction syndrome. *Br J Ophthalmol* 2002;86:902–909.
2. Russell SR, Hageman GS. Optic disc, foveal, and extrafoveal damage due to surgical separation of the vitreous. *Arch Ophthalmol* 2001;119:153–1658.
3. Gandorfer A, Ulbig M, Kampik A. Plasmin-assisted vitrectomy eliminates cortical vitreous remnants. *Eye* 2002;16:95–97.
4. Sebag J. Diabetic vitreopathy. *Ophthalmology* 1996;103:205–206.
5. Gandorfer A, Haritoglou C, Gandorfer A, et al. Retinal damage from indocyanine green in experimental macular surgery. *Invest Ophthalmol Vis Sci* 2003;44:2722–2729.
6. Haritoglou C, Gass CA, Schaumberger M, et al. Long-term follow-up after macular hole surgery with internal limiting membrane peeling. *Am J Ophthalmol* 2002;134:661–666.
7. Sebag J. Molecular biology of pharmacologic vitreolysis. *Trans Am Ophthalmol Soc* 2005;103:473–494.
8. Gandorfer A, Rohleder M, Sethi C, et al. Posterior vitreous detachment induced by microplasmin. *Invest Ophthalmol Vis Sci* 2004;45:641–647.
9. Sakuma T, Tanaka M, Mitzota A, et al. Safety of in vivo pharmacologic vitreolysis with recombinant microplasmin in rabbit eyes. *Invest Ophthalmol Vis Sci* 2005;46:3295–3299.
10. Quiram PA, Leverenz VA, Baker RM, et al. Microplasmi-induced posterior vitreous detachment affects vitreous oxygen levels. *Retina* 2007;27:1090–1096.
11. Sebag J, Ansari RR, Suh KI. Pharmacologic vitreolysis with microplasminin increases vitreous diffusion coefficients. *Graefe's Arch Clin Exp Ophthalmol* 2007;245:576–580.
12. Gass JD. *Stereoscopic atlas of macular diseases: diagnosis and treatment*. St. Louis: Mosby, Inc. 1997.
13. Kohno T, Sorgente N, Ishibashi T, et al. Immunofluorescent studies of fibronectin and laminin in the human eye. *Invest Ophthalmol Vis Sci* 1987;28:506–514.
14. Foos RY, Wheeler NC. Vitreoretinal juncture. Synchysis senilis and posterior vitreous detachment. *Ophthalmology* 1982;89:1502–1512.
15. Sebag J. Pharmacologic vitreolysis. *Retina* 1998;18:1–3.
16. Trese MT. Enzymatic-assisted vitrectomy. *Eye* 2002;16:365–368.
17. Zhu D, Chen H, Xu X. Effects of intravitreal dispase on vitreoretinal interface in rabbits. *Curr Eye Res* 2006;31:935–946.
18. Wang F, Wang Z, Sun X, et al. Safety and efficacy of dispase and plasmin in pharmacologic vitreolysis. *Invest Ophthalmol Vis Sci* 2004;45:3286–3290.
19. Jorge R, Oyamaguchi EK, Cardillo JA, et al. Intravitreal injection of dispase causes retinal hemorrhages in rabbit and human eyes. *Curr Eye Res* 2003;26:107–112.
20. Hagemann GS, Russell SR. Chondroitinase-mediated disinsertion of the primate vitreous body. *Invest Ophthalmol Vis Sci* 1994;35(suppl):28.
21. Hermel M, Schrage NF. Efficacy of plasmin enzymes and chondroitinase ABC in creating posterior vitreous separation in the pig: a masked, placebo-controlled *in vivo* study. *Grafes Arch Clin Exp Ophthalmol* 2007;245:399–406.
22. Kuppermann BD, Thomas EL, De Smet MD, et al. Pooled efficacy results from two multinational randomized controlled clinical trials of a single intravitreous injection of highly purified ovine hyaluronidase (Vitrase) for the management of vitreous hemorrhage. *Am J Ophthalmol* 2005;140:573–584.
23. Wang Z, Zhang X, Xu X, et al. PVD following plasmin but not hyaluronidase: implications for combination pharmacologic vitreolysis therapy. *Retina* 2005;25:38–43.
24. Hikichi T, Kado M, Yoshida A. Intravitreal injection of hyaluronidase cannot induce posterior vitreous detachment in the rabbit. *Retina* 2000;20:195–198.
25. Kuppermann BD, Thomas EL, De Smet MD, et al. Safety results of two phase III trials of an intravitreous injection of highly purified ovine hyaluronidase (Vitrase) for the management of vitreous hemorrhage. *Am J Ophthalmol* 2005;140:585–597.
26. Liotta LA, Goldfarb RH, Brundage R, et al. Effect of plasminogen activator (urokinase), plasmin, and thrombin on glycoprotein and collagenous components of basement membrane. *Cancer Res* 1981;41:4629–4636.
27. Uemura A, Nakamura M, Kachi S, et al. Effect of plasmin on laminin and fibronectin during plasmin-assisted vitrectomy. *Arch Ophthalmol* 2005;123:209–213.
28. Gandorfer A, Putz E, Welge-Luben U, et al. Ultrastructure of the vitreoretinal interface following plasmin assisted vitrectomy. *Br J Ophthalmol* 2001;85:6–10.
29. Verstraeten TC, Chapman C, Hartzer M, et al. Pharmacologic induction of posterior vitreous detachment in the rabbit. *Arch Ophthalmol* 1993;111:849–854.
30. Asami T, Terasaki H, Kachi S, et al. Ultrastructure of internal limiting membrane removed during plasmin-assisted vitrectomy from eyes with diabetic macular edema. *Ophthalmology* 2004;111:231–237.
31. Rizzo S, Pellegrini G, Benocci F, et al. Autologous plasmin for pharmacologic vitreolysis prepared 1 hour before surgery. *Retina* 2006;26:792–796.
32. Williams JG, Trese MT, Williams GS, et al. Autologous plasmin enzyme in the surgical management of diabetic retinopathy. *Ophthalmology* 2001;108:1902–1905.
33. Trese MT, Williams GA, Hartzer MK. A new approach to stage 3 macular holes. *Ophthalmology* 2000;107:1607–1611.
34. Azzolini C, D'Angelo A, Maestranzi G, et al. Intrasurgical plasmin enzyme in diabetic macular edema. *Am J Ophthalmol* 2004;138:560–566.
35. Margherio AR, Margherio RR, Hartzer M, et al. Plasmin enzyme-assisted vitrectomy in traumatic pediatric macular holes. *Ophthalmology* 1998;105:1617–1620.
36. Nagai N, Demarsin E, Van Hoef B, et al. Recombinant human microplasmin: production and potential therapeutic properties. *Thromb Haemost* 2003;1:307–313.
37. Lapchak PA, Araujo DM, Pakola S, et al. Microplasmin: a novel thrombolytic that improves behavioral outcome after embolic stroke in rabbits. *Stroke* 2002;33:2279–2284.
38. Suzuki Y, Chen F, Ni Y, et al. Microplasmin reduces ischemic brain damage and improves neurologic function in a rat stroke model monitored with MRI. *Stroke* 2004;35:2402–2406.

39. Ono R, Kakehashi A, Yamagami H, et al. Prospective assessment of proliferative diabetic retinopathy with observations of posterior vitreous detachment. *Int Ophthalmol* 2005;26:15–19.
40. Paques M, Massin P, Gaudric A. Growth factors and diabetic retinopathy. *Diabetes and Metabolism* 1997;23:125–130.
41. Patel JI, Tombran-Tink J, Hykin PG, et al. Vitreous and aqueous concentrations of proangiogenic, antiangiogenic factors and other cytokines in diabetic retinopathy patients with macular edema: implications for structural differences in macular profiles. *Exp Eye Res* 2006;82:798–806.
42. Boulton M, Gregor Z, McLeod D, et al. Intravitreal growth factors in proliferative diabetic retinopathy: correlation with neovascular activity and glycaemic management. *Br J Ophthalmol* 1997;81:228–233.
43. Quiram PA, Leverenz V, Baker R, et al. Enzymatic induction of a posterior vitreous detachment alters molecular vitreodynamics in animal models. [ARVO Abstract]. *Invest Ophthalmol Vis Sci* 2007; Abstract nr 83.

15

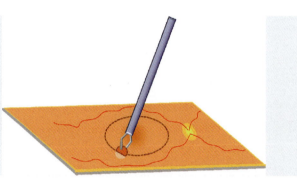

# Principles and Techniques of Macular Surgery

Gerardo García-Aguirre ■ Raúl Velez-Montoya ■ Hugo Quiroz-Mercado

## HISTORY

Since its inception in the early sixties (1,2), vitrectomy procedures have been performed in order to treat diverse vitreoretinal diseases. At the beginning, when the technique was at its infant stages (when it was performed as "open sky" vitrectomy), its purpose was mainly to treat abnormal vitreous conditions, most of the times with disappointing results. It was not until the seventies that Dr. Robert Machemer (3,4) developed a pars plana approach using specialized instruments introduced through small incisions, while maintaining an adequate intraocular pressure and thus limiting damage to the anterior segment while allowing for maneuvers in the posterior segment. This surgical advance offered vitreoretinal surgeons a whole new array of tools and techniques for the treatment of several vitreoretinal pathologies.

During its early phases, pars plana vitrectomy was performed for nonclearing vitreous hemorrhages or complicated cases of retinal detachment. It was in 1978 when Dr. Machemer (5) again reported the first case of vitrectomy and epiretinal membrane peeling, thus giving birth to macular surgery. In 1991, Drs. Kelly and Wendel (6) provided another breakthrough in macular surgery, when they published the results of a pilot study of vitreous surgery for idiopathic macular holes. Ever since, an increasing number of surgeons have adopted vitrectomy as the treatment of choice for diverse macular pathologies and refined its instruments and methods, broadening the indications for vitrectomy and improving anatomic and visual results.

## PREOPERATIVE CONSIDERATIONS

In order to improve the surgical outcome on a patient who will undergo macular surgery, a careful surgical plan must be elaborated, based on a thorough preoperative evaluation that should include a complete eye examination. Other factors, such as the general medical condition of the patient, must be considered. Before surgery, the patient must be informed about the potential risks and benefits expected from the procedure as well as the anticipated outcome based on the severity of the disease being treated.

## OPERATIVE CONSIDERATIONS

### Preoperative Instrument Check

Before administering anesthesia, a preoperative instrument check must be performed. The microscope must be inspected for adequate lighting, pedal function, and X-Y mobility. The vitrectomy console must have sufficient gas pressure. The cut-suction probe must be checked for adequate cutting rate and suction. Tamponade agents such as gas or silicone oil must be available. Foot pedals should be placed so that the surgeon can sit comfortably while maintaining balance.

## ANESTHESIA

For most vitrectomy procedures, local anesthesia (retrobulbar or peribulbar) with monitored anesthetic care is preferred. However, general anesthesia is indicated in some cases (such as performing procedures in children or in extremely anxious patients). Peribulbar or retrobulbar block is performed with a 50:50 mixture of 2% lidocaine and 0.75% bupivacaine, delivering 3 to 4 ml of anesthetic in the retrobulbar/peribulbar space, in order to achieve adequate anesthesia and akinesia. Facial block may be performed, according to the preference of the surgeon.

## OPERATIVE FIELD PREPARATION

After the patient is comfortably placed in the operative chair or table, the head is positioned with the face directed toward the ceiling. Air and/or supplemental oxygen can be delivered through a nasal cannula. The periocular skin and lids are then prepped with 5% povidone-iodine. Care must be taken so that povidone-iodine enters the conjunctival cul-de-sac, thereby contacting the ocular surface.

A forehead drape should be placed around the head and another should cover the inferior part of the face and the rest of the body. Then, a plastic adhesive drape is placed over the eye, covering the eyelids and keeping the eyelashes out of the field as much as possible. A plastic bag is placed in the temporal side of the adhesive drape in order to collect fluids. A lid speculum is then placed.

## SCLERAL INCISIONS

If using conventional 20-gauge pars plana vitrectomy, fornix-based conjunctival flaps should be created, exposing the sclera at the inferotemporal, superotemporal, and superonasal sectors. An incision is then performed with an microvitreo retinal (MVR) blade in the inferotemporal quadrant. The distance from the corneoscleral limbus varies: 4 mm in phakic patients, 3.5 mm in pseudophakic patients or patients with planned simultaneous cataract extraction, and 3 mm in aphakic patients. A single- or double-bite 6- or 7-0 Vicryl suture is placed, and an infusion cannula is inserted and secured with the preplaced suture. The superotemporal and superonasal sclerotomies are performed with an MVR blade, just superior to the meridians of the horizontal rectus insertions, in order to serve as ports for the diverse intraocular instruments that will be used during the procedure.

If using 23-gauge or 25-gauge instruments, trocars are placed transconjunctivally in an oblique fashion in order to improve wound closure. The inferotemporal trocar should be placed first and the infusion cannula must be connected to it. Superotemporal and superonasal trocars are placed after the infusion is set.

## CORE VITRECTOMY

Removal of the central vitreous is the first step in every macular procedure. The specifications of microscopes, viewing systems, and instruments necessary for vitrectomy are reviewed in the additional chapters of this section. It is of critical importance that the tip of the infusion cannula be visualized through the pupil inside the vitreous cavity before opening the infusion. After the infusion has been opened, the tip of the cut-suction probe is placed at the center of the vitreous cavity and the pedal is activated. A relatively low cutting rate (800 to 1200 cuts per minute) and a vacuum of 100 to 150 mm Hg are recommended at this time for quicker vitreous aspiration (higher vacuum is recommended for 23-gauge and 25-gauge vitrectomy). The port of the suction probe should be directed toward the vitreous to be cut. If the vitreous is free of traction, it will readily engage the port. If the vitreous is under traction, the port must be placed in contact with the vitreous to be cut. If a vitreous band is present, it must be engaged directly.

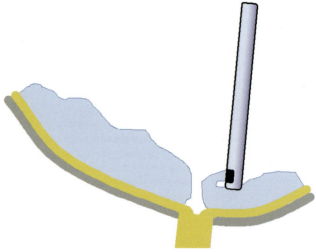

**Figure 15-1.** Posterior hyaloid removal using the cut-suction probe. The port of the cut-suction probe is placed near the nasal side of the optic disc and with the cutter off, and the cortical vitreous is aspirated. As the port becomes plugged with vitreous, the probe is pulled anteriorly, and the posterior hyaloid becomes separated from the border of the optic disc and the retina.

## POSTERIOR HYALOID REMOVAL

After core vitrectomy has been performed, the next important step is posterior hyaloid separation and removal. The posterior hyaloid is more firmly adhered around the optic disc at the foveola and over retinal blood vessels (7). Its removal is of key importance because if left attached, it may provide a surface for cellular proliferation or contribute to remaining postsurgical vitreoretinal traction. The posterior hyaloid may be removed using the cut-suction probe or using a silicone tip cannula, although other methods have been advocated.

## SILICONE TIP CANNULA

Another common and effective technique for posterior hyaloid detachment involves a silicone tip cannula connected to active suction. The cannula is inserted through a sclerotomy, and its tip is also placed above the optic disc. When suction is applied with a vacuum of 150 to 300 mm Hg, the silicone tube will bend when the membrane plugs the tip (fish stroke sign) (Fig. 15-2). The cannula then should be pulled anteriorly, until the posterior hyaloid becomes detached (9).

## CUT-SUCTION PROBE

Posterior hyaloid removal using the cut-suction probe is recommended, mainly because there is no need to change the instrument used in the previous step (core vitrectomy). The mode is set to suction only, with a vacuum of 150 to 200 mm Hg. The infusion pressure may need to be elevated in order to avoid hypotony. The tip of the probe is then positioned just above the optic disc on the nasal side, and suction is applied (Fig. 15-1). The probe is then pulled anteriorly, away from the optic disc (8). If the maneuver is successful, it will break the attachments of the posterior hyaloid to the area around the optic disc. This in turn will allow the passage of fluid to the retrohyaloidal space and facilitate the dissection. The detachment of the posterior hyaloid usually is visualized as a dark circle or shadow at the surface of the retina. After the posterior hyaloid has been detached, the mode is set to cut suction, and the remaining vitreous can be cut and aspirated.

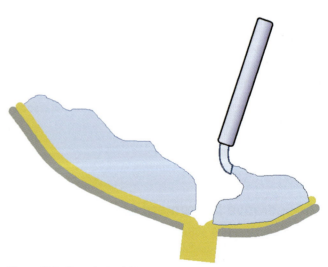

**Figure 15-2.** Posterior hyaloid removal using the silicone-tipped cannula. A soft silicone-tipped canula is connected to the aspiration tubing of the cut-suction probe. The tip of the probe is approached to the nasal side of the optic disc, and suction is applied. If there are remnants of cortical vitreous, the tip of the cannula will bend when moved (the so-called fish stroke sign). With the suction active, the cannula is pulled anteriorly, and the posterior hyaloid becomes separated from the border of the optic disc and the retina.

## OTHER TECHNIQUES

Another technique, described by Vander (10), involves removing the central and cortical vitreous and inserting a coaxial diathermy instrument into the vitreous cavity. The tip of the instrument is held approximately 1 mm above the retina on the nasal side of the optic disc. Diathermy is then applied with the power set to half the power required to cauterize episcleral vessels, creating a small hole in the posterior vitreous as the tissue contracts. An instrument can be inserted through this hole, and an extensive posterior hyaloid detachment can then be created.

Perfluorocarbon liquids can also be used to facilitate a posterior hyaloid detachment and simultaneously stabilize the retina (11). If a Weiss ring is visible, it is slightly pulled anteriorly with a pick or the cut-suction probe, and then perfluorocarbon liquid is infused through the Weiss ring into the retrohyaloidal space, facilitating the dissection. This technique is especially useful in cases of tractional or rhegmatogenous retinal detachment, although it should be avoided in cases where the retina is taut because the creation of a retinotomy may lead to the passage of perfluorocarbon liquid into the subretinal space.

The use of triamcinolone acetonide has been advocated for the facilitation of posterior hyaloid detachment (12–14). Triamcinolone crystals adhere to vitreous fibers, allowing for better visualization of the remaining vitreous. In most cases, injecting 4 to 8 mg in 0.1 to 0.2 ml after core vitrectomy is sufficient. Matsumoto et al. (14) published a study of 38 eyes of 37 patients in which vitrectomy with posterior hyaloid removal and internal limiting membrane (ILM) peeling was performed. In 14 of the 38 eyes, intravitreal triamcinolone acetonide was used prior to posterior hyaloid removal. The ILM obtained in all cases was then analyzed by transmission electron microscopy, showing less remaining posterior vitreous hyaloid in cases where triamcinolone was used, as compared to controls. Care must be taken because elevated intraocular pressure and cataract formation or progression are reported complications from the use of intravitreal triamcinolone (15).

## COMPLICATIONS

In some cases, the posterior hyaloid is firmly adhered to the retina, retinal vessels, or areas of fibrovascular proliferation. The surgeon must perform the posterior hyaloid detachment carefully, because excessive traction may lead to bleeding if the posterior hyaloid is attached to a retinal vessel or fibrovascular proliferation. In these cases, the attachment must be severed with either scissors or the cut-suction probe before completing the posterior hyaloid detachment.

Care must also be taken because traction to the posterior hyaloid may cause retinal tears at the vitreous base. Careful inspection of the retinal periphery using scleral indentation must be performed after completing the vitrectomy to detect inadvertent iatrogenic retinal tears, and treat them if necessary.

## INTERNAL LIMITING MEMBRANE PEELING

The ILM is the innermost layer of the retina and is the inner basement membrane of the Müller cells. It is believed to play a role in the pathogenesis of macular holes, creating the tangential traction from which they originate (16). It has been reported that the removal of the ILM in the macular area during surgery for stage 3 and 4 macular holes improves the rate of hole closure (17,18), although other reports state that there is no added benefit from this maneuver (19). Furthermore, some authors have reported that vitrectomy, posterior hyaloid removal, and peeling of the ILM are useful for the treatment of diabetic macular edema refractory to treatment (20–22).

## TECHNIQUE

In order to access the ILM, a posterior hyaloid detachment is mandatory, as has been explained previously. Once this step has been successfully performed, the surgeon may choose to stain the ILM for better visualization. Stains and staining techniques are described in-depth in Intraocular Dyes for Vitreoretinal Surgery in Section 8. Internal limiting membrane peeling (also called "limitorhexis") may begin by puncturing it with a sharp-tipped dissecting needle in the superior macula, about 2 or 3 mm from the foveola (Fig. 15-3A), grasping the border with ILM forceps and tearing the ILM in a circular fashion around the foveola (Fig. 15-3B). Some experienced surgeons, however, choose to directly tear and grab the ILM with forceps, without using a dissecting needle.

## COMPLICATIONS

Bleeding from the retinal capillaries may be observed at the time of puncturing the ILM with the needle or grasping it with the forceps, if the puncture is deeper than intended, which may in turn complicate ILM identification.

If the puncture is too deep or the retina is torn when pulling the ILM with forceps, a full-thickness eccentric macular hole may be created. No additional intervention is necessary in these cases, since these holes rarely cause complications.

## POSTERIOR RETINOTOMY

Performing a posterior retinotomy is sometimes indicated in cases when removal of material from under the macula is required, such as choroidal neovascular membranes (23–29), submacular hemorrhage (30–32), parasites (33–35), or hard exudates (36). It can also be indicated to implant material under the macula, such as retinal pigment epithelial cells (37–39) or subretinal chips.

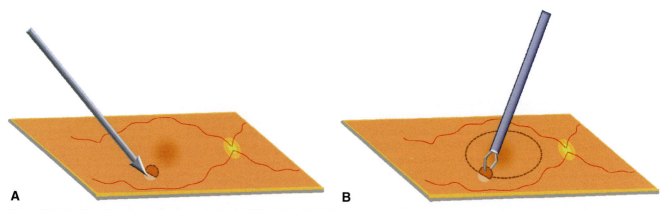

**A**                                                                          **B**

**Figure 15-3.** Peeling of the internal limiting membrane (ILM). **A:** The MVR blade or a sharp pick may be used to puncture the ILM and lift the border, in order to facilitate grasping. **B:** The border of the ILM is grasped with vitreoretinal forceps, and a tear is created in a circular fashion around the fovea in order to perform the limitorhexis.

To create a posterior retinotomy, a complete vitrectomy with posterior hyaloid detachment and removal must be performed first. A 36-gauge angled subretinal pick is then used to create a retinotomy. Balanced saline solution is then injected through the retinotomy using a 33-gauge angled cannula to create a limited neurosensory retinal detachment. An alternative is to use a 39-gauge translocation cannula connected to a viscous fluid infusor, directly injecting balanced saline solution under the retina and creating the retinal detachment (Fig. 15-4A).

The retinotomy may be enlarged as required for the procedure using vertical vitreoretinal scissors (Fig. 15-4B). It is of outmost importance that if the retinotomy is enlarged, it should follow the path of the nerve fiber layer, to avoid cutting ganglion cell axons and producing large visual field defects.

After the subretinal maneuvers are completed, a fluid/air exchange should be performed in order to aspirate the subretinal fluid and reattach the retina. Unless special circumstances indicate it (large retinotomy, extensive subretinal blood), the retinotomy site should not be treated with laser photocoagulation since the posterior hyaloid has been removed and no tractional forces remain (40).

## INSPECTION OF THE RETINAL PERIPHERY

Before concluding the procedure, a thorough inspection of the peripheral retina with scleral depression must be performed, in order to ascertain that no retinal tears occurred as a result of vitrectomy. Retinal breaks have been reported in 5.5% of cases (41). Special attention must be paid to the areas of the retina posterior to the sclerotomy sites. If retinal tears are found, they should be treated with retinal cryopexy or laser photocoagulation.

## CONCLUSION

With current vitreoretinal surgical instrumentation and procedures, a wide array of retinal diseases is now amenable to treatment. With the proper technique, visual acuity may stabilize or improve if patient selection has been adequate.

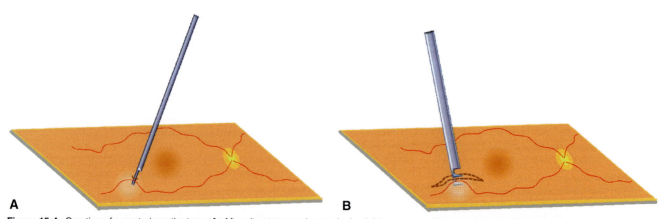

**A**                                                                          **B**

**Figure 15-4.** Creation of a posterior retinotomy. **A:** After vitrectomy and posterior hyaloid removal, a 39-gauge translocation cannula is connected to a viscous fluid infusor, and balanced saline solution is injected under the retina in order to create a retinal detachment. **B:** The retinotomy may be enlarged as needed for the procedure using vertical vitreoretinal scissors. The retinotomy must be enlarged following the path of the nerve fibers in order to avoid large visual field defects.

# References

1. Freeman HM, Anastopoulou A, Schepens CL, et al. Vitreous surgery: 1. an experimental study. *Arch Ophthalmol* 1967;77:677–680.
2. Kasner D. Vitrectomy: a new approach to the management of vitreous. *Highlights Ophthalmol* 1969;11:304–329.
3. Machemer R, Buettner H, Norton EWD, et al. Vitrectomy: a pars plana approach. *Trans Am Acad Ophthalmol Otolaryngol* 1971;75:813–820.
4. Machemer R. A new concept for vitreous surgery: 11. Surgical technique and complications. *Am J Ophthalmol* 1972;74:1022–1033.
5. Machemer R. The surgical removal of epiretinal macular membranes (macular pucker). *German Klin Manatsbl-Augenheilkd* 1978;173:36–42.
6. Kelly NE, Wendel RT. Vitreous surgery for idiopathic macular holes: results of a pilot study. *Arch Ophthalmol* 1991;109:654–659.
7. Greve MDJ. Vitreoretinal surgical anatomy. In: Peyman GA, Meffert SA, Conway MD, Chou F (eds). *Vitreoretinal surgical techniques*. London, UK: Martin Dunitz; 2001:3–9.
8. Ruby AJ, Williams GA. Simple vitrectomy. In: Peyman GA, Meffert SA, Conway MD, Chou F (eds). *Vitreoretinal surgical techniques*. London, UK: Martin Dunitz; 2001:125–135.
9. Han DP, Abrams GW, Aaberg TM. Surgical excision of the attached posterior hyaloid. *Arch Ophthalmol* 1988;106:998–1000.
10. Vander JF, Kleiner R. A method for induction of posterior vitreous detachment during vitrectomy. *Retina* 1992;12:172–173.
11. Quiroz-Mercado H, Guerrero-Naranjo H, Agurto-Rivera R, et al. Perfluorocarbon-perfused vitrectomy: a new method for vitrectomy—a safety and feasibility study. *Graefes Arch Clin Exp Ophthamol* 2005;243(6):551–562.
12. Enaida H, Hata Y, Ueno A, et al. Possible benefits of triamcinolone-assisted pars plana vitrectomy for retinal diseases. *Retina* 2003;23:764–770.
13. Furino C, Ferrari TM, Boscia F, et al. Triamcinolone-assisted pars plana vitrectomy for proliferative vitreoretinopathy. *Retina* 2003;23:771–776.
14. Matsumoto H, Yamanaka I, Hisatomi T, et al. Triamcinolone acetonide-assisted pars plana vitrectomy improves residual posterior vitreous hyaloid removal. *Retina* 2007;27:174–179.
15. Ozkiris A, Erkilic K. Complications of intravitreal injection of triamcinolone acetonide. *Can J Ophthalmol* 2005;40:63–68.
16. Yoshida M, Kishi S. Pathogenesis of macular hole recurrence and its prevention by internal limiting membrane peeling. *Retina* 2007;27:169–173.
17. Brooks HL Jr. Macular hole surgery with and without internal limiting membrane peeling. *Ophthalmology* 2000;107:1939–1948.
18. Mester V, Kuhn F. Internal limiting membrane removal in the management of full-thickness macular holes. *Am J Ophthalmol* 2000;129:769–777.
19. Margherio RR, Margherio AR, Williams GA, et al. Effect of perifoveal tissue dissection in the management of acute idiopathic full-thickness macular holes. *Arch Ophthalmol* 2000;118:495–498.
20. Recchia FM, Ruby AJ, Carvalho Recchia CA. Pars plana vitrectomy with removal of the internal limiting membrane in the treatment of persistent macular edema. *Am J Ophthalmol* 2005;139:447–454.
21. Kimura T, Kiryu J, Nishiwaki H, et al. Efficacy of surgical removal of the internal limiting membrane in diabetic cystoids macular edema. *Retina* 2005;25:454–461.
22. Patel JI, Hykin PG, Schadt M, et al. Pars plana vitrectomy with and without peeling of the inner limiting membrane for diabetic macular edema. *Retina* 2006;26:5–13.
23. Rubinstein A, Bates R, Benjamin L, et al. Iatrogenic eccentric full thickness macular holes following vitrectomy with ILM peeling for idiopathic macular holes. *Eye* 2005;19:1333–1335.
24. Adelberg DA, Del Priore LV, Kaplan HJ. Surgery for subfoveal membranes in myopia, angioid streaks, and other disorders. *Retina* 1995;15:198–205.
25. Berger AS, Conway M, Del Priore LV, et al. Submacular surgery for subfoveal choroidal neovascular membranes in patients with presumed ocular histoplasmosis. *Arch Ophthalmol* 1997;115:991–996.
26. Thomas MA, Grand MG, Williams DF, et al. Surgical management of subfoveal choroidal neovascularization. *Ophthalmology* 1992;99:952–968.
27. Lambert HM, Capone A Jr, Aaberg TM, et al. Surgical excision of subfoveal neovascular membranes in age-related macular degeneration. *Am J Ophthalmol* 1992;113:257–262.
28. Holekamp NM, Thomas MA, Dickinson JD, et al. Surgical removal of subfoveal choroidal neovascularization in presumed ocular histoplasmosis: stability of early visual results. *Ophthalmology* 1997;104:22–26.
29. Lit ES, Kim RY, D'Amico DJ. Surgical removal of subfoveal choroidal neovascularization without removal of posterior hyaloid. *Retina* 2001;21:317–323.
30. Dellaporta AN. Evacuation of subretinal hemorrhage. *Int Ophthalmol* 1994;18:25.
31. Wade EC, Flynn HW Jr., Olsen KR, et al. Subretinal hemorrhage management by pars plana vitrectomy and internal drainage. *Arch Ophthalmol* 1990;108:973–978.
32. Lewis H. Intraoperative fibrinolysis of submacular hemorrhage with tissue plasminogen activator and surgical drainage. *Am J Ophthalmol* 1994;118:559.
33. Steinmetz RL, Masket S, Sidikaro Y. The successful removal of a subretinal cysticercus by pars plana vitrectomy. *Retina* 1989;9:276–280.
34. Luger MH, Stilma JS, Ringens PJ, et al. In-toto removal of a subretinal Cysticercus cellulosae by pars plana vitrectomy. *Br J Ophthalmol* 1991;75:561–563.
35. Sharma T, Sinha S, Shah N, et al. Intraocular cysticercosis: clinical characteristics and visual outcome after vitreoretinal surgery. *Ophthalmology* 2003;110:996–1004.
36. Avci R, Inan UU, Kaderli B. Long-term results of excision of plaque-like foveal hard exudates in patients with chronic diabetic macular oedema. *Eye* 2008;22:1099–1104.
37. Joussen AM, Joeres S, Fawzy N, et al. Autologous translocation of the choroid and retinal pigment epithelium in patients with geographic atrophy. *Ophthalmology* 2007;114:551–560.
38. MacLaren RE, Uppal GS, Balaggan KS, et al. Autologous transplantation of the retinal pigment epithelium and choroid in the treatment of neovascular age-related macular degeneration. *Ophthalmology* 2007;114:561–570.
39. Binder S, Stanzel BV, Krebs I, et al. Transplantation of the RPE in AMD. *Prog Retin Eye Res* 2007;26:516–554.
40. Cooper BA, Thomas MA, Holekamp NM. Open retinotomy after submacular surgery. *Am J Ophthalmol* 2000;130:838–839.
41. Sjaarda RN, Glaser BM, Thompson JT, et al. Distribution of iatrogenic retinal breaks in macular hole surgery. *Ophthalmology* 1995;102:1387–1392.

# 16

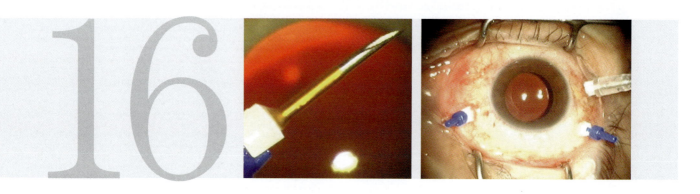

# Instrumentation and Surgical Adjunctive Techniques for Macular Surgery

Masahito Ohji ■ Yasuo Tano

## INTRODUCTION

Instrumentation and techniques, key elements in vitreous surgery, have been developed and modified over the years. As a result of improvements in instrumentation and techniques, better results are being achieved and indications for vitreous surgery have expanded. Moreover, there have been numerous developments in instrumentation and adjunctive techniques since the publication of the first edition of "Macular Surgery" in 2000. For example, the 25-gauge or 23-gauge transconjunctival sutureless vitrectomy systems combined with a bright illumination system with a xenon light source are the biggest breakthroughs in vitreous surgery in the last decade. Adjunctives have also been developed, including various dyes for staining the internal limiting membrane (ILM) and antivascular endothelial growth factor (VEGF) medications. In this chapter, we describe new instrumentations and adjunctive techniques.

## INSTRUMENTATION

### Sutureless Transconjunctival Vitrectomy

The small 25-gauge and 23-gauge transconjunctival vitreous surgery systems are among the biggest innovations in the history of vitreous surgery. The specific features of small-gauge vitreous surgery include small instruments, the transconjunctival trocar system, and the absence of suture placement at the end of the vitreous surgery.

### 25-Gauge Vitrectomy System

Various kinds of instruments have been developed since Fujii et al. (1) introduced 25-gauge vitrectomy. Trocars, light pipes, and the vitreous cutter are the essential instruments in every surgery. Other instruments including the diathermy probe, laser probes, extendable curved pick, aspirating pick, various

forceps, vertical scissors, curved scissors, and silicone-tipped brush back-flush needles have become available (2).

### Trocars

Trocars (Fig. 16-1) are essential for the 25-gauge sutureless transconjunctival vitrectomy system; some surgeons have used trocars even in the 20-gauge system. It is difficult to insert and remove instruments through both the conjunctiva and the sclera without the trocar system. Trocars also minimize damage to the wound, which is essential to prevent fluid leakage from the wound at the end of surgery.

### Vitreous Cutters

There are two different kinds of vitreous cutters (Fig. 16-2). One is the pneumatic cutter driven by air pressure and the other is motor driven. Each has advantages and disadvantages. The pneumatic cutter is light and has minimum vibrations, while the motor-driven cutter allows more precise control of the blade motions. The performance of the pneumatic vitreous cutter has been improved, and the maximum cutting speed reaches as high as 2,500 per minute as in the 20-gauge system. A new generation of vitreous machines will be available soon with a vitreous cutter with a maximum cutting speed of 5,000 per minute. Because of the narrow aperture of the vitreous cutter, the aspiration rate is smaller than that of the 20-gauge cutter. Therefore, the aspiration vacuum is usually set to 500 to 600 mm Hg instead of 200 mm Hg to achieve sufficient aspirating flow (1).

### 23-Gauge Vitrectomy System

Eckardt (3) developed the 23-gauge vitrectomy system (Fig. 16-3), which has several similarities to the 25-gauge system and some differences. The 23-gauge steel trocars can be reused; disposable trocars are also available. The trocars in the 23-gauge system are inserted obliquely following the use of the MVR blade, while a one-step insertion system is also available (Fig. 16-4). In each system, an oblique wound pathway is

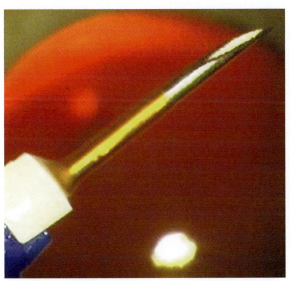

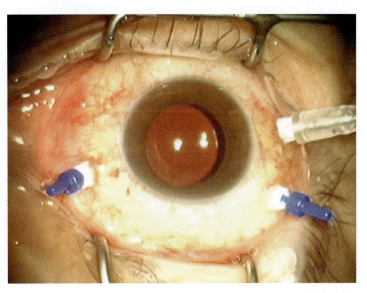

**Figure 16-1.** Trocars.

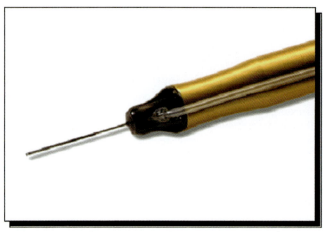
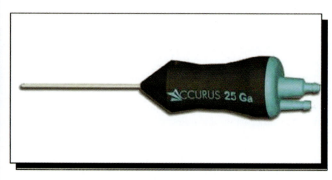

**Figure 16-2.** A 25-gauge vitreous cutter driven by motor (**left**) and 25-gauge vitreous cutter driven by air pressure (**right**).

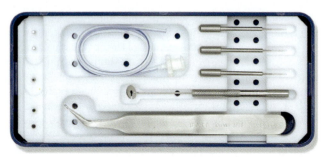

**Figure 16-3.** A 23-gauge trocar-cannula system and pressure plate.

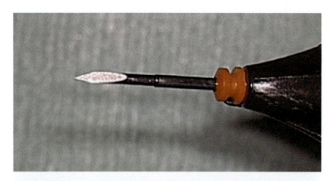

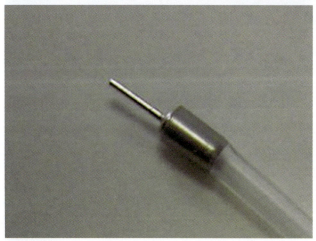

**Figure 16-4.** A 23-gauge disposable one-step trocar-cannula. The irrigation cannula (**below**) inserts easily through the trocar (**above**).

essential to prevent fluid leakage, because the scleral and conjunctival wound is obviously larger in the 23-gauge than in the 25-gauge system. The infusion rate and the aspiration rate are higher in the 23-gauge system than in the 25-gauge system. There is a considerable amount of balanced saline solution (BSS)/air flow through the trocars when the instruments are removed. Therefore, a plug or a valve attached to the trocars should be frequently used to prevent large consumption of BSS that might increase inflammation and prevent retinal damage by vigorous air flow (Fig. 16-5). The shafts of the 23-gauge instruments are much stiffer and can be used just like the 20-gauge instruments.

## Other 25- or 23-gauge Instruments

Many other instruments including the diathermy probe, laser probes with and without illumination, extendable curved pick, aspirating pick, various forceps, vertical scissors, curved scissors, and silicone-tipped brush back-flush needles have become

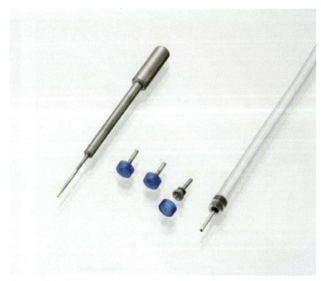

**Figure 16-5.** Closure valve for 23-gauge cannula to prevent leakage.

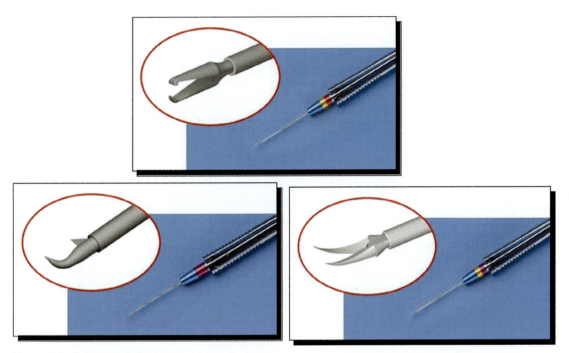

**Figure 16-6.** Forceps, vertical scissors, and curved scissors.

available (Figs. 16-6 and 16-7) (2). These instruments expand the indications for the 25-gauge sutureless vitrectomy.

The pressure plate developed by Eckardt (3) displaces the conjunctiva and allows the trocars to be inserted into the appropriate position (Fig. 16-3). A pressure plate was developed for the 23-gauge system; however, it is also useful with the 25-gauge system. The forceps have two scale marks on the top surface and on the serrated undersurface of the tip, and can be used in a similar fashion (Fig. 16-8) (4). The distance between the two scale marks is 4 mm. The scale marks can be used for accurate measurement and the serrated undersurface is useful to pull the conjunctiva.

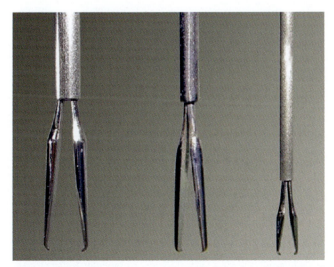

**Figure 16-7.** Comparison of 20-gauge (**left**), 23-gauge (**center**), and 25-gauge forceps (**right**).

## Bright Light Source

Endoillumination is one of the most important instruments used during vitreous surgery, and very bright endoillumination without light toxicity is extremely important. The light pipe in the 25-gauge vitrectomy system is narrower than that in the 20-gauge vitrectomy system, and the 25-gauge light pipe connected to the regular illumination source offers dim illumination and does not allow visualization of the details of the fundus lesions. A bright illumination system using a xenon light source or mercury vapor light source has been developed (Fig. 16-9).

The xenon light source combined with a good reflector can provide much brighter light than a regular halogen light source. The xenon light system provides very bright illumination even through a narrow 25-gauge light pipe that facilitates visualization of the details of the fundus lesions. A xenon light source can provide brighter light than the regular halogen light source; however, the xenon light provided contains more blue components than the halogen light. Surgical fields illuminated by the xenon light appear whiter or pale compared to the halogen light. In addition, the light toxicity associated with the blue component of the light is a consideration. Light wavelengths shorter than 550 nm are hazardous to the retina; therefore, the blue components of a wavelength shorter than 550 nm have to be filtered. By filtering the blue components of a wavelength shorter than 550 nm, the retinal safety is dramatically improved by approximately eight times (Table 16-1).

A xenon light source allows sufficient illumination through the narrow 25-gauge light pipe; however, the flexibility of the 25-gauge light pipe is still problematic. A shorter light pipe was

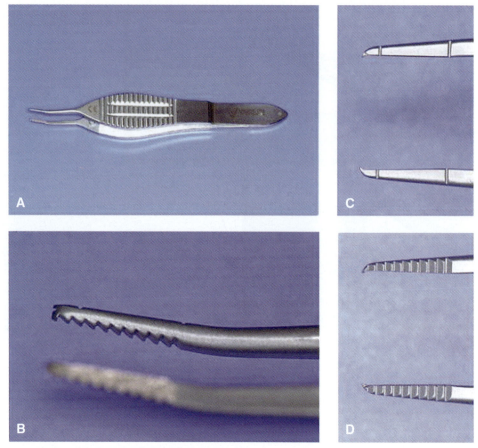

**Figure 16-8.** Forceps with scale marks.

designed as a solution (5) (Fig. 16-10). Sufficient illumination can be provided through the shorter 25-gauge light pipe and it would be safer than the regular light pipe with respect to light toxicity and mechanical damage.

Mercury vapor is another light source alternative to provide brighter illumination than xenon light (Fig. 16-9). Brighter illumination is superior during surgery; however, light toxicity is also an important consideration. It has a filter system that reduces light toxicity and provides green light.

The 25-gauge vitrectomy system might not have been widely accepted without the bright illumination, because vitrectomy under dim illumination through a narrow 25-gauge light pipe with a halogen light source is not efficient or safe. The improvement in illumination made the 25- and 23-gauge vitrectomy systems easier, more efficient, safer, and expanded the indications for small-gauge vitrectomy.

The chandelier system has been available for a long time; however, its usefulness was limited because of insufficient illumination. The 25-gauge chandelier illumination system is another instrument that became useful after the introduction of the bright xenon light source (Fig. 16-11). The system allows surgeons to remove peripheral vitreous or to apply laser to the peripheral retina with scleral indentation by themselves when the chandelier is inserted into the trocar in the 25-gauge system. Recently, a 27-gauge chandelier system with a 29-gauge light fiber became available, which provides sufficient

illumination without fluid leakage from the scleral wound at the end of surgery (6) (Fig. 16-11). The illuminated cannula also becomes useful when connected to the xenon light source or mercury vapor light source, although the illuminated cannula without a bright light source with dim illumination is available (Fig. 16-12).

In addition to its usefulness with the small-gauge vitrectomy system, the new light source is also useful in the 20-gauge system. The chandelier illumination, used as the fourth port, allows surgeons to perform bimanual techniques with standard 20-gauge instruments. The bimanual technique is useful and almost essential for treating complicated cases including severe proliferative diabetic retinopathy (PDR) or severe proliferative vitreoretinopathy (PVR); however, the bimanual technique required additional instruments including illuminated forceps and illuminated scissors. The 25/27-gauge chandelier illumination system allows surgeons to use hundreds of standard 20-gauge instruments including forceps, scissors, diathermy, aspiration needle, and laser probes.

## Wide-Angle Viewing System

A wide-angle viewing system using a binocular indirect ophthalmomicroscope (BIOM) or contact lens has become popular because surgeons can see a wider fundus area simultaneously

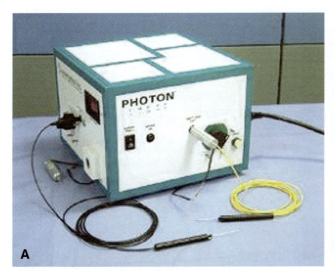
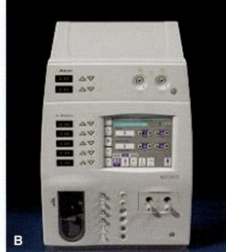
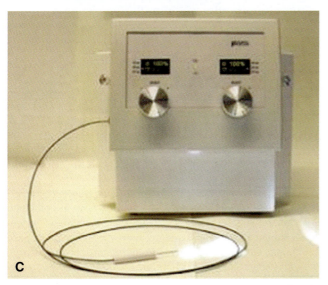
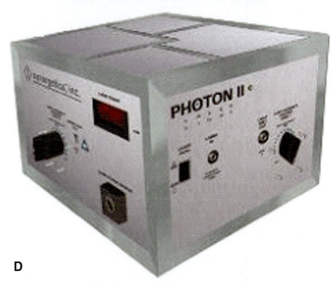

**Figure 16-9.** Xenon light source and mercury vapor light source. Each light source provides sufficient illumination for detailed observation using the 25-gauge system.

(7) (Fig. 16-13), which allows them to recognize fundus pathology better and treat lesions more safely and efficiently. A wide-angle viewing system becomes more important along with the increasing popularity of the small-gauge vitrectomy system because it is difficult to rotate the eyeball and indent the sclera during vitrectomy. The focus of the new BIOM

system can be adjusted by the surgeon using the foot pedal in contrast using a handle to adjust the focus in the old BIOM model. A new contact lens (ClariVit, Volk) for the wide-angle

| TABLE 16-1 | HAZARD EFFICACY (LUMENS/ HAZARD WATT)[a] |
|---|---|
| Light | Hazard efficacy Lm/hazard watt |
| Xenon | 1913 |
| Xenon with Yellow Filter | 16568 |
| Halogen | 1920 |
| Metal halide | 1343 |

[a] Higher numbers indicate greater safety.

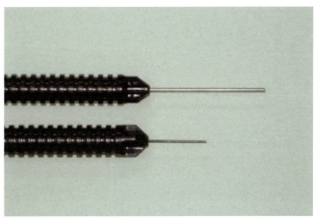

**Figure 16-10.** A shorter light pipe. A light pipe shorter (**below**) than the a light pipe of conventional length (**above**) may offer illumination but less toxicity.

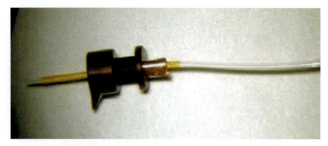

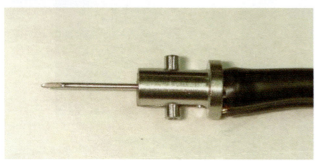

**Figure 16-11.** A 25-gauge chandelier illumination (**above**) and 27-gauge chandelier illumination with 29-gauge fiber (**below**).

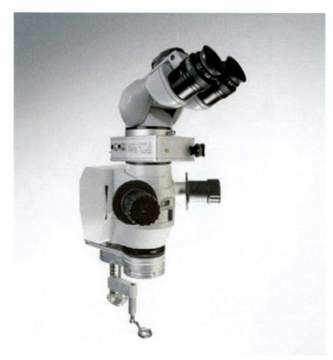

**Figure 16-13.** A binocular indirect ophthalmomicroscope (BIOM).

viewing system has a smaller diameter (8) (Fig. 16-14), making it possible to visualize the scleral port directly so that the surgical instruments can be inserted through the scleral port without problems.

An optical fiber-free intravitreal surgery system (OFFISS) is another non-contact wide-angle viewing system combined with a surgical microscope (9) (Fig. 16-15). The new system looks similar to the BIOM system; however, surgeons can see the fundus with illumination incorporated into the microscope without using a light pipe. Therefore, it allows surgeons to perform bimanual techniques using the standard instruments. Moreover, surgeons can adjust the focus using the foot pedal of the microscope, while another foot pedal different from the foot pedal of the microscope is required to adjust the focus in the BIOM.

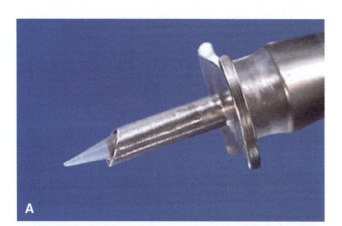

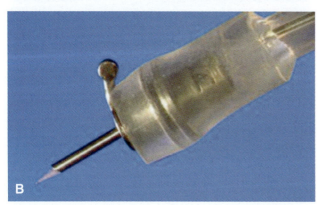

**Figure 16-12.** A 20-gauge (**top**) and 25-gauge (**bottom**) illuminated infusion cannula. The diameters of the light fiber are 500 μm and 380 μm, respectively.

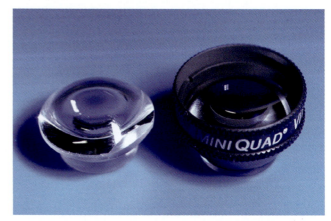

**Figure 16-14.** ClariVit, a new wide angle viewing contact lens with a smaller diameter (**left**) than the regular wide-angle viewing contact lens (**right**).

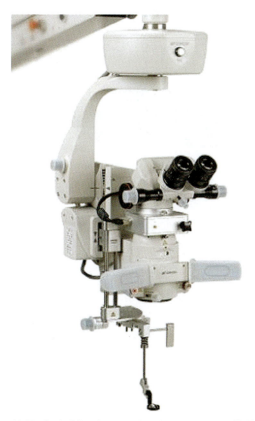

**Figure 16-15.** Optical fiber-free intravitreal surgery system (OFFISS).

Another noncontact wide-angle viewing system is the Wessels-Peyman-Landers wide-angle viewing system (10) (Fig. 16-16). The area that surgeons can see is slightly narrower than that with the BIOM or a contact lens system; however, surgeons do not require an inverter because of a prismatic system inside the system that provides a direct image.

An inverter is usually essential when a wide-angle viewing system, including the BIOM or the contact lens, is used. The Invertertube™, a new inverter incorporated into the Zeiss

microscope (Fig. 16-17), is advantageous because of the shorter working distance between the eyes and the hands compared with the previous inverter and the superior quality of the inverted images. The Invertertube™ requires only one switchable prism to invert images, while more than one prism is required to invert images in previous generation inverters. The simple mechanism produces superior inverted images.

## ADJUNCTIVE TECHNIQUES

### Internal Limiting Membrane Staining with Indocyanine Green

Brooks (11) reported the technique of ILM peeling for macular hole surgery in 1995 and the subsequent improvement in the anatomic and functional results. ILM peeling had not been widely performed, however, because it was technically difficult due to poor visibility of the ILM. Staining of the ILM with indocyanine green (ICG) makes ILM peeling much easier and more complete (12,13).

A number of studies have reported favorable results after ICG-assisted ILM peeling. Meta-analysis of these reports revealed a 96% macular hole closure rate after the initial surgery and improved visual acuity in 79% of cases (13–17). However, unfavorable results also have been reported (18–20). Visual field defects is one of the postoperative complications following ICG-assisted ILM peeling for macular holes or epiretinal membranes (13,20). Kanda et al. (21) discovered that visual field defects are strongly associated with the ICG concentration. When the ILMs were stained with 0.5% ICG for 3 minutes during macular hole surgery, visual field defects developed in all 12 eyes. The authors modified their technique to inject 0.5% ICG followed by immediate aspiration of ICG. This resulted in visual field defects in one of four eyes. When the investigators further diluted ICG and used 0.25% with immediate aspiration, no visual field defects developed. Indocyanine green is potentially toxic; however, the toxicity can be prevented or minimized by lowering its concentration.

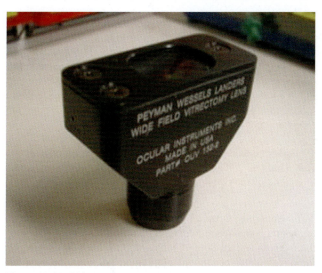

**Figure 16-16.** Wessels-Peyman-Landers wide-angle viewing system.

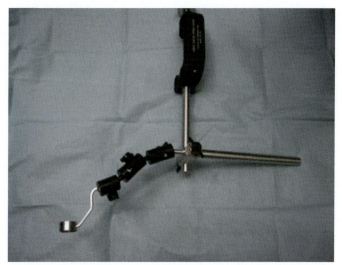

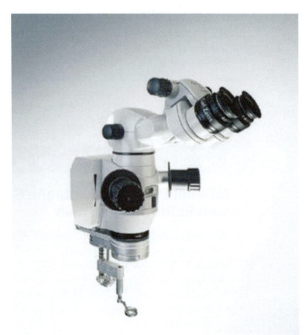
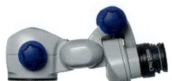

**Figure 16-17.** Invertertube, a new inverter system incorporated into the microscope.

## OTHER DYES FOR INTERNAL LIMITING MEMBRANE STAINING

There are several alternatives to ICG. Trypan blue (0.3%) can be used; however, the staining effect is weaker than ICG and the proliferative membranes are stained as well (22,23).

Triamcinolone acetonide (TA), a corticosteroid, is currently used to visualize the vitreous during vitrectomy (24,25), because it is almost impossible to detect the thin layer of the vitreous cortex, especially in highly myopic eyes. It also can be used to visualize the ILM (26). It does not stain the ILM but sits on it and allow surgeons to visualize it. Therefore, surgeons might overlook small pieces of the ILM that remain on the retina.

Brilliant blue G (BBG), also known as acid blue 90 and Coomassie BBG, is a blue dye and a candidate for ILM staining. It does not stain the epiretinal membrane well but does stain the ILM well (27). The safety of the use of BBG for staining the ILM was evaluated in rats and humans using electroretinography, TUNEL staining, and light and electron microscopy (28). A subretinal injection of BBG up to 0.25 mg per ml was not toxic (29).

## BEVACIZUMAB

Bevacizumab (Avastin, Genentech, South San Francisco, CA) is a humanized recombinant antibody that binds all isoforms of VEGF (30). The drug has been approved to treat metastatic colorectal cancer in many countries (31). Intravitreal injection of bevacizumab has been used as an off-label treatment for age-related macular degeneration and macular edema due to diabetic retinopathy and retinal vein occlusion (32–35). After administering a bevacizumab injection (1.25 mg/0.05 ml), the leakage diminished and the neovascularization appeared to resolve, although a lower dose might be sufficient to achieve the same effect (35). The drug also has been used as an off-label preoperative adjunctive treatment for vitrectomy for PDR and retinopathy of prematurity (36,37). Preoperative intravitreal bevacizumab injection seems to facilitate vitrectomy by reducing the intraoperative bleeding and surgical time (36), although progression of tractional detachment may occur after injection (38).

## MICROPLASMIN

Plasmin is an enzyme that may be useful for pharmacologic vitrectomy. It has been used for vitrectomy in traumatic pediatric macular holes and diabetic retinopathy (39–41). Plasmin also seems to help separate the vitreous hyaloid from the ILM surface in patients with diabetic retinopathy (39). Microplasmin, a fragment of plasmin, may be useful for pharmacologic vitrectomy (42).

## PERFLUOROCARBON LIQUID AND HEAVY SILICONE OIL

Perfluorocarbon liquid (PFCL), which is heavier than water, has been used to reattach the retina during surgery. It is crucial to treat retinal detachment resulting from giant tears or complicated vitreoretinopathy and macular translocation (43–45). Perfluorocarbon liquids cannot be used as a tamponade for the long term and must be removed at the end of surgery, because long-term tamponade causes severe retinal damage.

Perfluorohexyloctane is a semifluorinated alkane with gravity of 1.35 g per cm$^3$. A mixture of 30% perfluorohexyloctane and 70% silicone oil may be useful for PVR. It is slightly heavier than water, which has a gravity of 1.06 g per cm$^3$, and has been used in Europe as a tamponade for eyes with retinal detachment caused by an inferior break (46,47).

## References

1. Fujii GY, de Juan E, Humayun MS, et al. Initial experience using the transconjunctival sutureless vitrectomy system for vitreoretinal surgery. *Ophthalmology* 2002;109:1814–1820.
2. Fujii GY, de Juan E, Humayun MS, et al. A new 25-gauge instrument system for transconjunctival sutureless vitrectomy surgery. *Ophthalmology* 2002;109:1807–1813.
3. Eckardt C. Transconjunctival sutureless 23-gauge vitrectomy. *Retina* 2005;25:208–211.
4. Ohji M, Sakaguchi H, Tano Y. Forceps with scale marks for transconjunctival sutureless vitrectomy system. *Retina* 2006;26(5):583–585.
5. Ohji M, Tano Y. A stiffer and safer light pipe for 25-gauge vitrectomy. *Arch Ophthalmol* 2007;125:1415–1416.
6. Oshima Y, Chow DR, Awh CC, et al. Novel mercury vapor illuminator combined with a 27/29-gauge chandelier light fiber for vitreous surgery. *Retina* 2008;28:171–173.
7. Spitznas M. A binocular indirect ophthalmomicroscope (BIOM) for non-contact wide-angle vitreous surgery. *Graefes Arch Clin Exp Ophthalmol* 1987;225:13–15.
8. Nakata K, Ohji M, Ikuno Y, et al. Wide-angle viewing lens for vitrectomy. *Am J Ophthalmol* 2004;137:760–762.
9. Horiguchi M, Kojima Y, Shima Y. Removal of lens material dropped into the vitreous cavity during cataract surgery using an optical fiber-free intravitreal surgery system. *J Cataract Refract Surg* 2003;29:1256–1259.
10. Landers MB, Peyman GA, Wessels IF, et al. A new, non-contact wide field viewing system for vitreous surgery. *Am J Ophthalmol* 2003;136:199–201.
11. Brooks HL. ILM peeling in full thickness macular hole surgery. *Vitreoretinal Surg Technol* 1995;7:2.
12. Burk SE, Da Mata AP, Snyder ME, et al. Indocyanine green-assisted peeling of the retinal internal limiting membrane. *Ophthalmology*. 2000;107:2010–2014.
13. Kadonosono K, Itoh N, Uchio E, et al. Staining of internal limiting membrane in macular hole surgery. *Arch Ophthalmol* 2000;118:1116–1118.
14. Kwok AK, Lai TY, Man-Chan W, et al. Indocyanine green assisted retinal internal limiting membrane removal in stage 3 or 4 macular hole surgery. *Br J Ophthalmol* 2003;87:71–74.
15. Wolf S, Reichel MB, Wiedemann P, et al. Clinical findings in macular hole surgery with indocyanine green-assisted peeling of the internal limiting membrane. *Graefes Arch Clin Exp Ophthalmol* 2003;241:589–592.
16. Sheidow TG, Blinder KJ, Holekamp N, et al. Outcome results in macular hole surgery: an evaluation of internal limiting membrane peeling with and without indocyanine green. *Ophthalmology* 2003;110:1697–1701.
17. Da Mata AP, Burk SE, Foster RE, et al. Long-term follow-up of indocyanine green-assisted peeling of the retinal internal limiting membrane during vitrectomy surgery for idiopathic macular hole repair. *Ophthalmology* 2004;111:2246–2253.
18. Engelbrecht NE, Freeman J, Sternberg P Jr, et al. Retinal pigment epithelial changes after macular hole surgery with indocyanine green-assisted internal limiting membrane peeling. *Am J Ophthalmol* 2002;133:89–94.
19. Haritoglou C, Gandorfer A, Gass CA, et al. Indocyanine green-assisted peeling of the internal limiting membrane in macular hole surgery affects visual outcome: a clinicopathologic correlation. *Am J Ophthalmol* 2002;134:836–841.
20. Ando F, Sasano K, Suzuki F, et al. Indocyanine green-assisted ILM peeling in macular hole surgery revisited. *Am J Ophthalmol* 2004;138:886–887.
21. Kanda S, Uemura A, Yamashita T, et al. Visual field defects after intravitreous administration of indocyanine green in macular hole surgery. *Arch Ophthalmol* 2004;122:1447–1451.
22. Feron EJ, Veckeneer M, Parys-Van Ginderdeuren R, et al. Trypan blue staining of epiretinal membranes in proliferative vitreoretinopathy. *Arch Ophthalmol* 2002;120:141–144.
23. Li K, Wong D, Hiscott P, et al. Trypan blue staining of internal limiting membrane and epiretinal membrane during vitrectomy: visual results and histopathological findings. *Br J Ophthalmol* 2003;87:216–219.
24. Peyman GA, Cheema R, Conway MD, et al. Triamcinolone acetonide as an aid to visualization of the vitreous and the posterior hyaloid during pars plana vitrectomy. *Retina* 2000;20:554–555.
25. Sakamoto T, Miyazaki M, Hisatomi T, et al. Triamcinolone-assisted pars plana vitrectomy improves the surgical procedures and decreases the postoperative blood-ocular barrier breakdown. *Graefes Arch Clin Exp Ophthalmol* 2002;240:423–429.
26. Kimura H, Kuroda S, Nagata M. Triamcinolone acetonide-assisted peeling of the internal limiting membrane. *Am J Ophthalmol* 2004;137:172–173.
27. Enaida H, Hiasatomi T, Hatano Y, et al. Brilliant blue G selectively stains the internal limiting membrane/brilliant blue G-assisted membrane peeling. *Retina* 2006;26:631–636.
28. Enaida H, Hiasatomi T, Goto Y, et al. Preclinical investigation of internal limiting membrane staining and peeling using intravitreal brilliant blue G. *Retina* 2006;26:623–630.
29. Ueno A, Hiasatomi T, Enaida H, et al. Biocompatibility of brilliant blue G in a rat model of subretinal injection. *Retina* 2007;27:499–504.
30. Ferrara N. Vascular endothelial growth factor: basic science and clinical progress. *Endocr Rev* 2004;25:581–611.
31. Hurwitz H, Fehrenbacher L, Novotny W, et al. Bevacizumab plus irinotecan, fluorouracil, and leucovorin for metastatic colorectal cancer. *N Engl J Med* 2004;350:2335–2342.
32. Avery RL, Pieramici DJ, Rabena MD, et al. Intravitreal bevacizumab (Avastin) for neovascular age-related macular degeneration. *Ophthalmology* 2006;113:363–372.
33. Haritoglou C, Kook D, Neubauer A, et al. Intravitreal bevacizumab (Avastin) therapy for persistent diffuse diabetic macular edema. *Retina* 2006;26:999–1005.
34. Rosenfeld PJ, Fung AE, Puliafito CA. Optical coherence tomography findings after an intravitreal injection of bevacizumab (avastin) for macular edema from central retinal vein occlusion. *Ophthalmic Surg and Lasers Imaging* 2005;36:336–339.
35. Avery RL, Pearlman J, Pieramici DJ, et al. Intravitreal bevacizumab (Avastin) in the treatment of proliferative diabetic retinopathy. *Ophthalmology* 2006;113:1695.
36. Rizzo S, Genoveci-Ebert F, Di Bartolo E, et al. Injection of intravitreal bevacizumab (Avastin) as a preoperative adjunct before vitrectomy surgery in the treatment of severe proliferative diabetic retinopathy (PDR). *Graefes Arch Clin Exp Ophthalmol* 2008;246:837–842.
37. Kusaka S, Chima C, Shimojyo H, et al. Efficacy of intravitreal injection of bevacizumab for severe retinopathy of prematurity: a pilot study. *Br J Ophthalmol* 2008;92(11):1450–1455.
38. Arevalo JF, Maia M, Flynn HW Jr, et al. Tractional retinal detachment following intravitreal bevacizumab (Avastin) in patients with severe proliferative diabetic retinopathy. *Br J Ophthalmol* 2008;92:213–216.
39. Asami T, Terasaki H, Kachi S, et al. Ultrastructure of internal limiting membrane removed during plasmin-assisted vitrectomy from eyes with diabetic macular edema. *Ophthalmology* 2004;111:231–237.
40. Williams JG, Trese MT, Williams GA, et al. Autologous plasmin enzyme in the surgical management of diabetic retinopathy. *Ophthalmology* 2001;108:1902–1905.
41. Margherio AR, Margherio RR, Hartzer M, et al. Plasmin enzyme-assisted vitrectomy in traumatic pediatric macular holes. *Ophthalmology* 1998;105:1617–1620.
42. Sakuma T, Tanaka M, Mizota A, et al. Safety of in vivo pharmacologic vitreolysis with recombinant microplasmin in rabbit eyes. *Invest Ophthalmol Vis Sci* 2005;46:3295–3299.
43. Chang S. Low viscosity liquid fluorochemicals in vitreous surgery. *Am J Ophthalmol* 1987;103:38–43.
44. Coll GE, Change S, Sun J, et al. Perfluorocarbon liquid in the management of retinal detachment with proliferative vitreoretinopathy. *Ophthalmology* 1995;102:630–638.
45. Machemer R, Steinhorst UH. Retinal separation, retinotomy, and macular relocation: II. A surgical approach for age-related macular degeneration? *Graefes Arch Clin Exp Ophthalmol* 1993;231:635–641.
46. Wong D, Van Meurs JC, Stappler T, et al. A pilot study on the use of perfluorohexyloctane/silicone oil solution as a heavier-than-water internal tamponade agent. *Br J Ophthalmol* 2005;89:649–650.
47. Romano MR, Stappler T, Marticorena J, et al. Primary vitrectomy with Densiron-68 for rhegmatogenous retinal detachment. *Graefes Arch Clin Exp Ophthalmol* 2008;246(11):1541–1546.

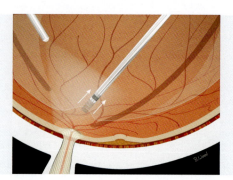

# 25-Gauge Vitrectomy for Macular Surgery

Steve Charles

Sutureless, 25-gauge (25G) vitrectomy was initially utilized by most surgeons for epimacular membranes, macular holes, and vitreomacular traction syndromes, as well as for procedures now shown to be ineffective: branch vein decompression and radial optic neurotomy. Virtually all techniques utilized for 20-gauge (20G) vitrectomy can be utilized with 25G vitrectomy (1–18) using new tools and technique modifications discussed in this chapter. Some techniques to be discussed are applicable to 25G surgery and selected 23-gauge (23G) and 20G procedures as well.

## ADVANTAGES OF 25G VITRECTOMY

There are many advantages to eliminating both scleral and conjunctival sutures, including reduced discomfort, photophobia, tearing, squeezing, conjunctival hyperemia, and bleeding. Faster visual recovery occurs because astigmatism from the sclerotomy sutures is eliminated and the ocular surface suffers less trauma. Although faster visual improvement does not translate into better long-term visual outcomes, it is important if there is impaired vision in the other eye. Elimination of sutures and conjunctival incisions greatly reduces damage to the conjunctiva, Tenon's capsule, and episclera, which is crucial for eyes with a glaucoma filtering procedure and eyes likely to have glaucoma surgery in the future. Reduced conjunctival damage is also advantageous for patients with ocular surface disorders.

It was initially thought that 25G fluidics would be limiting but this has not proven to be the case. As will be discussed later in this chapter, 25G fluidics are safer than 20G or 23G fluidics.

The new series of 25+™ (25 Plus) instruments from Alcon allows complex surgical maneuvers such as membrane peeling using cutter rather than a forceps, avoiding the use of scissors. The high cut rate (up to 5000 cpm), strong aspiration and escellent IOP control of the Constelation® system allows shaving the vitreous base with negligible traction to the surrounding tissues and retina. In the 25+™ vitrectomy probe design, the tip has been redesigned to place the port closer to the distal end of the probe, allowing vitreous shaving closer to the retina.

The port size has also been enlarged to increase aspiration rate, And the shaft has been stiffened to reduce flexure and improve control (Figs. 17-1 and 17-2).

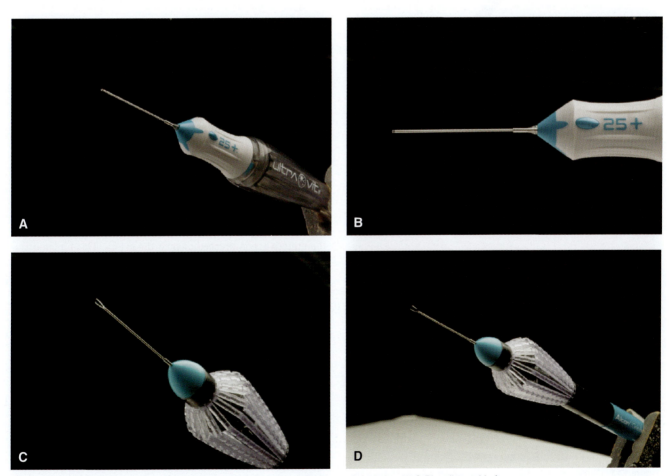

**Figure 17-1. A** and **B:** Shows new vitrctomy probe 25-G Plus. **C** and **D:** Shows Grieshaber 25-G Plus disposable forceps.

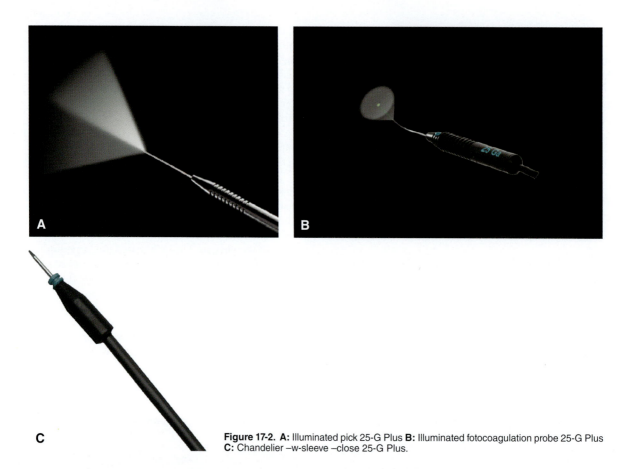

**Figure 17-2. A:** Illuminated pick 25-G Plus **B:** Illuminated fotocoagulation probe 25-G Plus **C:** Chandelier –w-sleeve –close 25-G Plus.

## WOUND CONSTRUCTION

Displacement of the conjunctival wound relative to the sclerotomy site before insertion of the trocar cannula ensures that conjunctiva will cover the self-sealed sclerotomy (Fig. 17-3). Although the author initially utilized straight-in sclerotomies

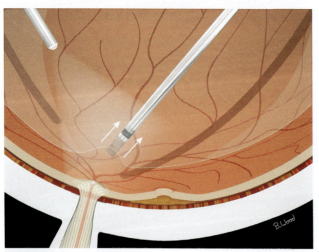

**Figure 17-3.** Displacement of the conjunctival wound relative to the sclerotomy site before insertion of the trocar-cannula ensures that conjunctiva will cover the self-sealed sclerotomy.

supplemented with fluid-air exchange, experimental leak pressure data from Kupperman and histological data from Kaiser made it clear that angulated wound construction was safer. Angulated (oblique, near-tangential) sclerotomies are not biplanar, although the motion of the trocar cannula needed to construct these incisions suggests this. The trocar should be inserted nearly tangential to the sclera until the polyimide cannula contacts the conjunctiva; the trocar should then be tilted up until closer to perpendicular to the scleral surface; and the insertion should be continued until the hub is flush with the conjunctiva, compressed against the sclera. This biplanar trajectory approach ensures creation of a scleral tunnel while preventing damage to the retina and choroid, especially in soft eyes and eyes with retinal detachments or choroidals.

Sclerotomy placement is an often overlooked detail; the superotemporal site should be on a virtual line extending from the lowest point of the supraorbital rim to the center of the pupil. The superonasal site should be on a virtual line extending from the lowest point of the bridge of the nose to the center of the pupil. This approach reduces tool flex, especially when accessing the periphery and viewing with the binocular indirect ophthalmomicroscope (BIOM). The inferotemporal infusion site should be placed just inferior to the 3 or 9 o'clock position to prevent contact with the lower lid. Pathology-specific pre- and intraoperative head positioning facilitates surgical access and reduces tool flex as well.

At the end of the case, the cannulas should be removed in a tangential manner with the intraocular pressure (IOP) at

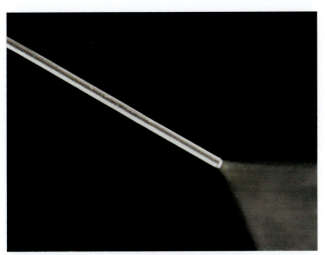

**Figure 17-4 .** At the end of the case, the cannulas should be removed in tangential manner with the intraocular pressure (IOP) at approximately 20 mm Hg while pressing on the wound with the smooth, rounded back of the plug forceps to ensure tight apposition of the inside and outside scleral tunnel layers.

approximately 20 mm Hg, while pressing on the wound with the smooth, rounded back of the plug forceps to ensure tight apposition of the inside and outside scleral tunnel layers (Fig. 17-4). Every effort must be made to reduce vitreous in the sclerotomies to reduce postoperative vitreous collagen contraction resulting in peripheral retinal breaks. Vitreous wick is a major risk factor in postoperative endophthalmitis; intentionally leaving vitreous in the wound to reduce wound leaks is a dangerous idea. Always use subconjunctival antibiotics. Cataract surgeons operate in the anterior chamber and where topical antibiotics are effective, but topical antibiotics do not produce minimum inhibitory concentrations (MICs) in the vitreous cavity of phakic or pseudophakic eyes. Antibiotics should be injected well away from the sclerotomies to prevent reflux into the vitreous cavity and retina damage. Povidone iodine (Betadine) prep is essential to reduce the risk of endophthalmitis. Vitreous wicks are a far more important risk factor for endophthalmitis than wound leaks.

## FLUIDICS AND CUTTING RATES

High cutting rates create resistance at the port because of frequent interruption of flow. Smaller lumens also restrict flow because resistance is proportional to the 4th power of the diameter of the lumen. The author coined the term "port-based flow limiting" to describe the effects of higher resistance at the port. Port-based flow limiting decreases pulsatile traction on attached retina. High cutting rates also decrease uncut collagen fiber travel, thereby reducing the likelihood of iatrogenic retinal breaks. Vitreoretinal traction is also reduced by moving the cutter to the vitreous, rather than sucking vitreous to port, an approach termed "continuous engage and advance vitrectomy." Vitreoretinal traction is the result if the cutter is pulled back while cutting; it should always be advanced while suction force is applied. Many surgeons inappropriately use lower cutting rates during core vitrectomy; the best practice is to always

use the highest setting and increase proportional vacuum until vitreous removal begins, with the port applied to the vitreous-infusion fluid interface.

## NECESSITY OF CORE VITRECTOMY

Core vitrectomy should not be omitted because patients complain bitterly about floaters if the vitreous is not removed. Although the author developed the approach of performing macular surgery without core vitrectomy this was abandoned because it was not shown to reduce postoperative retinal detachment or cataract. Nuclear sclerosis progression is almost certainly due to higher oxygen tension after vitrectomy, as shown independently by Holekamp and Chang.

## MACULAR HOLE SURGERY

25G vitrectomy is ideal for macular hole surgery. Core vitrectomy should be performed with the highest possible cutting rate and by moving the port to the vitreous, not sucking the vitreous to the port.

Posterior vitreous detachment (PVD) creation using an anteroposterior motion of the cutter without cutter activation at the superior, inferior, and nasal disk margins, (Fig. 17-5), not over the cup, theoretically reduces the risk of peripheral retinal breaks compared to lateral motion of the soft-tip cannula. PVD creation never presents a problem with 25G cutters when using anterior motion at the disk margins.

The specific mechanism of macular hole formation is not well understood but is related in some way to PVD formation. The Gass classification system is of minimal clinical value,

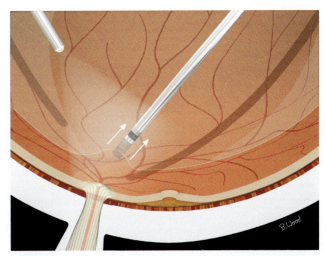

**Figure 17-5.** Posterior vitreous detachment (PVD) creation using antero-posterior motion of cutter without cutter activation at the superior, inferior and nasal disk margins, not over the cup, theoretically reduces the risk of peripheral retinal breaks compared to lateral motion of the soft-tip cannula.

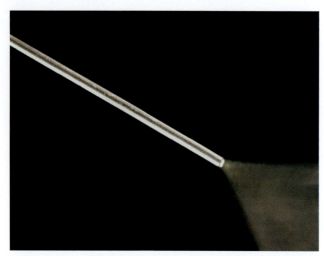

**Figure 17-6.** The Tornambe Torpedo and other chandeliers provide diffuse illumination which makes visualization of the internal limiting membrane more difficult; focal illumination with a standard Alcon 25G, 78 degree endoilluminator is preferred by the author.

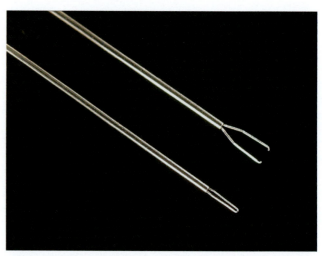

**Figure 17-7.** The Alcon DSP forceps (internal limiting membrane or ILM type) are preferred by the author for peeling residual posterior vitreous cortex, epiretinal membranes, and ILM.

while the ocular coherence tomography (OCT) is essential to determine if the hole is of full or partial thickness. It is clear that peeling of residual vitreous cortex, epiretinal membranes, and the internal limiting membrane (ILM) increase success rates. The author recommends ILM peeling in all cases, but believes that indocyanine green (ICG) increases the risk of toxicity and phototoxicity and is unnecessary when using end-opening forceps peeling of the ILM. There are an increasing number of reports suggesting that ICG is toxic and its use is decreasing. The BIOM and other wide-angle systems decrease axial and lateral resolution and are probably a factor in the use of ICG, trypan blue, and triamcinolone to improve ILM visualization. There are anecdotal reports that triamcinolone reduces closure rates in macular hole surgery. The flat contact lens provides far superior resolution and should be used for all macular surgery. The Tornambe Torpedo and other chandeliers provide diffuse illumination, which makes visualization of ILM more difficult; focal illumination with a standard Alcon 25G, 78-degree endoilluminator (Fig. 17-6) is preferred by the author.

The Alcon DSP forceps (ILM type) (Fig. 17-7), are preferred by the author for peeling residual posterior vitreous cortex, epiretinal membranes, and ILM. Either the disposable handle or QuikLok Sutherland, squeeze, and Revolution handles can be used; the author prefers the disposable handle or the QuikLok Sutherland type.

Closure mechanisms have traditionally been said to be "removal of tangential traction" and "tamponade"; both terms require clarification. Gas bubbles produce surface tension, which is a tangential, not a perpendicular force, as emphasized by Reppucci, and closes the hole immediately. The author utilized C3F8 for 16 years but recently converted to SF6 after making the observation, as Reppucci and others have, that holes that are not usually closed in a few days never close. The gas bubble also stops transhole flow, which is called "tamponade." Gas bubble surface tension also, as pointed out by the author, stops transretinal flow (uveal scleral outflow), which

addresses the Tornambe hydration hypothesis. The author has also emphasized that the gas bubble also produces retinal drying which stimulates modified astrocytes to permanently heal the hole initially closed by surface tension.

Combined procedures, meaning phaco combined with vitrectomy, have been utilized by many surgeons, but the author does not advise this approach in most instances. If phaco is performed at the beginning of pars plana vitrectomy (PPV), visualization of the ILM may be impaired; if phaco is done after PPV and ILM peeling, the vitreous cavity must be reentered for fluid-air exchange and air-gas exchange. If the preoperative view is adequate to perform macular surgery, cataract surgery can be performed 1 to 2 months after PPV, which allows more accurate A-scan data and better refractive outcomes than combined surgery. If the view is inadequate to perform macular surgery, phaco and intraocular lens (IOL) implantation can be done 2 to 4 weeks before PPV.

## EPIMACULAR MEMBRANE SURGERY

As emphasized earlier, it is inadvisable to omit core vitrectomy when performing epimacular membrane (EMM) surgery. Using fine, end-grasping forceps eliminates the need for pics, diamond dusted membrane scrapers, ICG staining, or the bent microvitreoretinal (MVR) blade. The Alcon DSP forceps (ILM type) are preferred by the author for peeling epiretinal membranes and ILM. ILM peeling should be performed after EMM peeling because it reduces EMM recurrences and residual striae, as pointed out by Kampnik and Gandorfer. The end-grasping forceps should be used in an inside-out direction starting at the EMM epicenter, not outside-in, which requires dangerous "edge" finding using pics or MVR blades. Striae often point to the epicenter. Triamcinolone is unnecessary in these cases as they virtually always have PVD. ICG is potentially toxic and unnecessary as discussed above.

## VITREOMACULAR TRACTION SYNDROME

Vitreomacular traction syndrome may result from traction due to hypocellular contraction of the posterior vitreous cortex combined with residual adherence to the umbo or even the foveola. Scissors section of posterior vitreous cortex just anterior to the retina reduces the chance of foveal avulsion from core vitrectomy induced traction. ILM peeling is necessary if striae are seen after the posterior vitreous cortex is removed. Extreme care must be taken to avoid avulsing foveal tissue.

## MACULAR EDEMA

There are several potential mechanisms by which vitrectomy can improve diabetic macular edema as well as edema from central retinal vein occlusion (CRVO) and branch vein occlusion (BRVO). Elimination of vitreomacular traction due to a taut, adherent posterior cortex, as first reported by Hilel Lewis, is very effective in eliminating macular edema as well as associated submacular fluid, because the retina is brought back into contact with the retinal pigment epithelium (RPE) pump. Ogura and others have shown that vitrectomy alone improves diabetic macular edema. Similarly, Hassan and others have shown that vitrectomy without sheathotomy improves edema in BRVO cases as well CRVO cases without performing radial optic neurotomy (RON). Increased macular oxygenation may result in less vascular endothelial growth factor (VEGF) release and edema, as shown independently by Holekamp, Chang, and Steffanson. The author has postulated that removal of the vitreous gel, as well as possibly the ILM, may reduce the concentration of VEGF in the macula, resulting in reduction of the edema.

ILM peeling probably produces better outcomes in macular edema cases, presumably because it guarantees that all traction has been removed.

The author recommends combining focal and light panretinal photocoagulation (PRP) endolaser with PPV in diabetic macular edema (DME) cases to reduce leakage from microaneurysms and intraretinal microvascular abnormality (IRMA), which may reduce the need for steroids, and decrease progression of proliferative retinopathy. Bevacizumab (Avastin) is injected at the end of all vitrectomy for DME cases to reduce rebound leakage.

## SUBMACULAR MEMBRANE SURGERY

Anti-VEGF agents (bevacizumab and ranibizumab) have dramatically reduced the need for submacular surgery, but it still an excellent procedure for non-leaking choroidal neovascular membranes between the retina and the RPE. Age-related macular degeneration (AMD) membranes are usually under the RPE and for that reason should not be operated. Surgery may be indicated for selected recent, inactive, subfoveal choroidal neovascularization (CNV) membranes: idiopathic, presumed ocular histoplasmosis, severe myopic macular, and trauma cases with intact underlying RPE.

Balanced salt solution (BSS) injection under the retina is never required and should be avoided because it may cause an acute macular hole as well as shear photoreceptor outer segments by creating an unnecessary posterior retinal detachment. It is important to separate the nerve fiber layer, not transect fibers to create the retinotomy. Neither diathermy nor laser should be used as they are unnecessary and increase the risk of recurrent CNV. It is useful to make a radial retinotomy in the papillomacular bundle if the CNV is between the fovea and the disk. Placing pics under the membrane should be avoided as this technique increases the likelihood of RPE avulsion and RPE rip. The nerve fiber should be separated by opening the blades of the forceps in the retinotomy. The author recommends using 25G Alcon DSP ILM forceps positioned over the outer margin of the CNV as far away from the fovea as possible. Both blades of the end-grasping forceps are used to grasp the top surface of the membrane; forceps blades should never be placed under the membrane. The membrane can then be mobilized and rolled like a foldable IOL to allow it be slowly removed from the subretinal space with minimal enlargement of the retinotomy. The membrane in the forceps can then be used to gently push the retinotomy back together and fluid-air exchange performed.

## SUMMARY

25G sutureless vitrectomy is applicable to all macular surgery indications, minimal technique modifications are required, and outcomes are equal or better than 20G or 23G vitrectomy surgery. Meticulous attention to scleral tunnel wound construction, making certain that there is no vitreous wick, and use of subconjunctival antibiotics is essential to minimize complications associated with small gauge sutureless surgery. As in all vitrectomy surgery, the highest cutting rate should be used with continuous engage and advance technique. Inside-out, end-grasping forceps membrane peeling technique without pics, MVR blades, membrane scrapers, or ICG staining is the preferred technique for peeling adherent posterior vitreous cortex, epiretinal membrane, and ILM.

### References

1. Patelli F, Radice P, Zumbo G, et al. 25-Gauge Macular Surgery: results and Complications. *Retina* 2007;27(6):750–754.
2. Faia LJ, McCannel CA, Pulido JS, et al. Outcomes following 25-gauge vitrectomies. *Eye* 2008;22(8):1024–1028.
3. Valmaggia C. Pars plana vitrectomy with 25-gauge instruments in the treatment of idiopathic epiretinal membranes. *Klin Monatsbl Augenheilkd* 2007;224(4):292–296.
4. Chen E. 25-Gauge transconjunctival sutureless vitrectomy. *Curr Opin Ophthalmol* 2007;18(3):188–193.
5. Jabbour J, Jabbour NM, Villers A, et al. 25-gauge vitrectomy. *Ophthalmology* 2007;114(4):827.
6. Amato JE, Akduman L. Incidence of complications in 25-gauge transconjunctival sutureless vitrectomy based on the surgical indications. *Ophthalmic Surg Lasers Imaging* 2007;38(2):100–102.

7. Rizzo S, Belting C, Cresti F, et al. Sutureless 25-gauge vitrectomy for idiopathic macular hole repair. *Graefes Arch Clin Exp Ophthalmol* 2007;245(10):1437–1440.
8. Kellner L, Wimpissinger B, Stolba U, et al. 25-gauge vs 20-gauge system for pars plana vitrectomy: a prospective randomized clinical trial. *Br J Ophthalmol* 2007;91(7):945–948.
9. Scartozzi R, Bessa AS, Gupta OP, et al. Intraoperative sclerotomy-related retinal breaks for macular surgery, 20- vs 25-gauge vitrectomy systems. *Am J Ophthalmol* 2007;143(1):155–156.
10. Romero P, Salvat M, Almena M, et al. Experience with 25-gauge transconjunctival vitrectomy compared to a 20-gauge system. Analysis of 132 cases. *J Fr Ophtalmol* 2006;29(9):1025–1032.
11. Shimada H, Nakashizuka H, Mori R, et al. 25-gauge scleral tunnel transconjunctival vitrectomy. *Am J Ophthalmol* 2006;142(5):871–873.
12. López-Guajardo L, Pareja-Esteban J, Teus-Guezala MA. Oblique sclerotomy technique for prevention of incompetent wound closure in transconjunctival 25-gauge vitrectomy. *Am J Ophthalmol* 2006;141(6):1154–1156.
13. Oshima Y, Ohji M, Tano Y. Surgical outcomes of 25-gauge transconjunctival vitrectomy combined with cataract surgery for vitreoretinal diseases. *Ann Acad Med Singapore* 2006;35(3):175–180.
14. Yanyali A, Celik E, Horozoglu F, et al. 25-Gauge transconjunctival sutureless pars plana vitrectomy. *Eur J Ophthalmol* 2006;16(1):141–147.
15. Yoon YH, Kim DS, Kim JG, et al. Sutureless vitreoretinal surgery using a new 25-gauge transconjunctival system. *Ophthalmic Surg Lasers Imaging* 2006;37(1):12–19.
16. Rizzo S, Genovesi-Ebert F, Murri S, et al. 25-gauge, sutureless vitrectomy and standard 20-gauge pars plana vitrectomy in idiopathic epiretinal membrane surgery: a comparative pilot study. *Graefes Arch Clin Exp Ophthalmol* 2006;244(4):472–479.
17. Lakhanpal RR, Humayun MS, de Juan E, et al. Outcomes of 140 consecutive cases of 25-gauge transconjunctival surgery for posterior segment disease. *Ophthalmology* 2005;112(5):817–824.
18. Ibarra MS, Hermel M, Prenner JL, et al. Longer-term outcomes of transconjunctival sutureless 25-gauge vitrectomy. *Am J Ophthalmol* 2005;139(5):831–836.

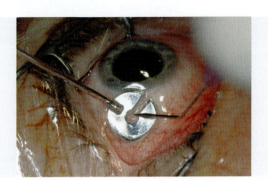

# 23-Gauge Vitrectomy

Veronica Kon-Jara ■ Hugo Quiroz-Mercado ■ Fabio Patelli ■ Kirk H. Packo

After introduction by Fujii et al. (1) of 25-gauge vitreoretinal surgical advances in recent years, Eckardt et al. (2) had shown that transconjunctival sutureless vitrectomy with 23 gauge is a newer, safer, and more effective procedure developed to improve on the reported shortcomings of 25-gauge vitrectomy vis-à-vis conventional 20-gauge vitrectomy, such as too high flexibility and poorer efficiency of the instruments as well as the associated occasional early postoperative ocular hypotony.

Tornambe considered that 23 gauge is "the Goldilocks gauge: not too big, not too small, just right" (3).

As a minimally invasive surgery, three microcannulas are inserted transconjunctivally in pars plana and after their removal from the scleral incisions, the tunnel-like wounds are so small that they self-seal; there is no surgical trauma to the conjunctiva and fewer changes in corneal topography, and rehabilitation time required is less than usual (4).

Although almost all kinds of vitreoretinal surgery can be done with 23 gauge, there are some cases in which retinal surgeons still prefer 20 gauge, such as for severe proliferative vitreoretinopathy, severe tractional diabetic retinal detachment, trauma, intraocular foreign body, or lens fragmentation (5).

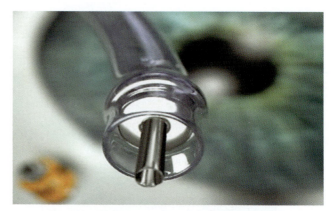

**Figure 18-1.** Microcannula.

## INSTRUMENTATION

Currently, a complete stock of vitreoretinal instruments (disposable or autoclavable) is available to perform 23-gauge surgery, that includes:

- *Microcannulas.* They have a length of 4 mm (infusion cannula) or 4.5 mm (instruments cannula), with an internal diameter of 0.65 mm and external diameter of 0.75 mm. They are made of metal (steel) vs polyamide (Fig. 18-1).
- *Cannula forceps.* They are designed for insertion and removal of cannula system (Fig. 18-2).
- *Cannula infusion line.* Infusion lines are designed to fit all microcannulas. DORC (Zuidland, Holland) has a cannula with a valve that controls or prevents the loss of intraocular fluid.
- *Vitrectome.* Two options available are:

  *Pneumatic vitrectome.* Increased stiffness and optimized flow with 2500 cuts per minute, the 23-gauge vitreous cutter

is a little bit slower than a 20-gauge cutter, but their slight flexibility is useful to performing difficult tasks in peripheral retina. The port of the 23-gauge vitrectome is 30% larger than 25 gauge and 50% closer to tip than 20 and 25 gauge. This is helpful to control and peeling membranes where close shaving is required (6) (Fig. 18-3).

*Electromagnetic vitreous cutter.*

- *Endoillumination probe.* Three types of illumination:

  *Standard.* They have a typical triple-port connector.

  *Wide angle (Total view).* Adjustable fiber/light intensity, triple-port connector with a spatula pic tip and combined endoillumination tip (standard and total view) are available.

  *Spaide Total view.* Combine direct (focused) and diffuse wide field illumination.

- *Chandelier light.* These are available for broad illumination of the fundus.
- *Backflush needle.* A blunt needle is used for passive aspiration.
- *Brush backflush needle.* A brush needle is used for active aspiration.
- *Plugs.* They are made with titanium or steel.
- *Intraocular scissors.* The radius of curvature for intraocular scissors is wider for 23-gauge scissors than 20-gauge scissors because bore size of the microcannula (3).

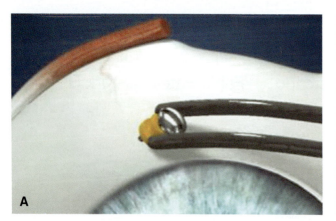

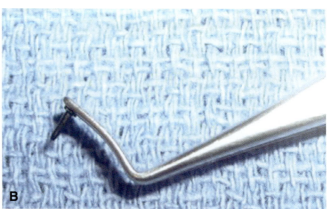

**Figure 18-2.** Cannula forceps are designed to easily grip and manipulate the microcannulas.

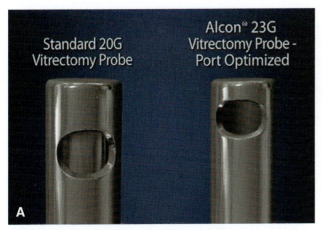
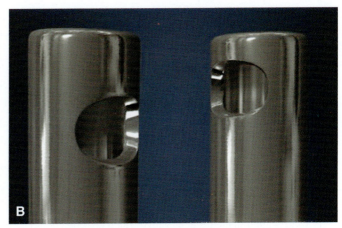

**Figure 18-3.** Pneumatic Vitrectome (Vitreous cutter).

*Curved scissors.* Sharp tipped scissors with a radius of curvature of 12 mm allows one to follow the contour of the retina for cutting membranes adherent to the retinal surface.

*Straight scissors.*

*Vertical scissors.*

■ *Forceps*

*End-gripping.* Multifunctional forceps is useful for internal limiting membrane (ILM) peeling and other macular-hexis procedures. The tip is the same length as 20-gauge instrument.

*Serrated jaws.*

*ILM forceps.* Specially created for peeling of ILM in macular surgery, with smaller tips which facilitate the peeling (Fig. 18-4).

■ *Membrane pic.* This pic is angled at 100 degrees with a sharp point. Vitreoretinal surgeons use pics to raise and dissect epiretinal membranes.

■ *Endolaser Probe.*

■ *Tano scraper.* (Fig. 18-5)

■ *Endodiathermy Probe.*

■ *Microvitreoretinal (MVR) blade.* The MVR blade is angled at 45 degrees with a width: 0.72 mm.

■ *Pressure plate.* This is used to fixate the conjunctiva at the sclera during incision and insertion technique. A 1 mm diameter opening at the center of the plate ends laterally in a slit. The outer edge of the plate's underside is equipped with small teeth to prevent slippage. The pressure plate performs three functions. First, it is used to press the conjunctiva firmly against the sclera to prevent it from moving as the scleral tunnel incision is made and following insertion of the microcannulas. This facilitates subsequent identification of the conjunctival and scleral incisions. Second, it is used to move the globe during the sclerotomy. Third, it aids in measuring the distance between the sclerotomy and the corneoscleral limbus. Placed directly on the corneoscleral limbus, the distance to the middle of the central opening in the plate is 3.5 mm.

■ *Hem-stopper.*

■ *Flute needle.*

■ *RON-knife.*

These 23-gauge instruments are very similar in design and utility to standard 20-gauge instruments.

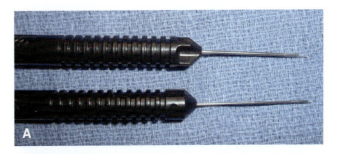
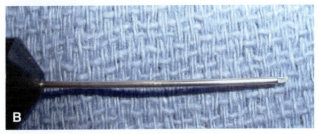

**Figure 18-5. A.** Tano scraper (20 gauge (top); 23 gauge (bottom). **B.** Note the diamond dusted silicone tip.

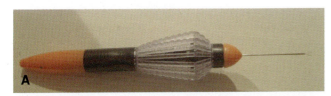
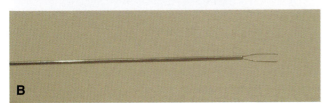

**Figure 18-4.** Internal limiting membrane forceps.

## ADVANTAGES OF 23-GAUGE VITRECTOMY OVER 20- AND 25-GAUGE VITRECTOMY

- *Flexibility.* 23-gauge vitrectomy instruments are not as flexible as 25 gauge and maintain sturdiness similar to 20 gauge allowing one to perform complicated maneuvers in vitreous cavity and eye rotation.
- *Illumination.* Illumination with 23-gauge vitrectomy is better than 20-gauge vitrectomy with uniform dispersion and a 78-degree angle of illumination.
- *Lumen.* It is well known that the standard wall thickness between 23 and 25 gauge is the same, but their difference is a wider inner diameter in 23 gauge which provides better flow and probably more stiffness. 23 gauge is narrower than 20 gauge with adequate fluidics during surgery and flow rates similar to 20 gauge.
- *Difficult cases.* Many surgeons advocate that 23 gauge could manage a broad case selection, including difficult cases of rhegmatogenous retinal detachment or proliferative diabetic retinopathy with tractional retinal detachment.
- *Sutureless.* Patients feel excellent because their rehabilitation and comfort improve, and there is no residual astigmatism (4).
- *Scleral closure.* With newer microcannula insertion technique (angled entry), there is less hypotony than had been seen in 23-gauge cases.
- *Learning curve.* It is faster in transition between 20 to 23 gauge.
- *Recovery.* Faster recovery could be related to less ocular surface inflammation.

## INCISION TECHNIQUE WITH 23-GAUGE VITRECTOMY SYSTEM

The first step to getting a clean and comfortable incision site is holding the eye firmly with a special pressure plate (Dutch Ophthalmic Research Center [DORC], Zuidland, Holland), a Thornton ring, or cotton tipped applicator; and pushing the conjunctiva laterally 1 or 2 mm (Fig. 18-6).

One can choose between two different systems to insert the microcannulas. At the initial description of the procedure (two-step entry), a 23-gauge stiletto blade was inserted at an angle of 30 to 40 degrees, 3.5 mm (pseudophakic, aphakic) or 4 mm (phakic) from the corneoscleral limbus in three directions: posterior-anterior (7), anterior-posterior (8) or parallel to the corneoscleral limbus in the superonasal, superotemporal, and inferotemporal quadrants (7,9). If the tunnel incisions ran an anterior-posterior course there was a risk that the tunnel's interior opening could lie too close to the ora serrata; this risk could be lowered by locating the exterior opening closer to the corneoscleral limbus. Since the conjunctiva

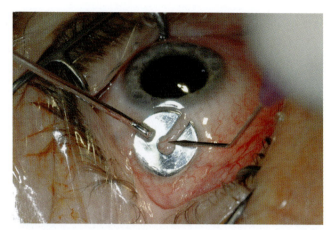

**Figure 18-6.** A pressure plate (DORC) is used to stabilize the eye for incision with a 23-gauge stiletto blade.

in this area can be displaced scarcely or not at all, the result would be a scleral incision lying directly under the conjunctival incision; so this possible shortcoming of a tunnel running parallel to the limbus is offset by the advantage of an anterior-posterior tunnel whose course runs parallel to the scleral fibers, requiring that the fibers need only be separated without cutting, facilitating postoperative closure of the sclerotomy (10,11).

The scleral tunnel-like incisions are 0.72–0.74 mm wide and the pressure applied against them has to be constant to prevent slippage of the conjunctiva. Then the microcannulas are inserted through the conjunctiva and sclera with a special blunt inserter (DORC, Zuidland, Holland) and, subsequently, the instruments through them (2). Since the tangential position of the inserter causes the globe to rotate under pressure, pressure must be applied in the direction of the apex of the orbit. To do this, the inserter must be moved from its original tangential position to a position perpendicular to the sclera, where the resistance caused by the introduction of the microcannula can be easily overcome. Before the microcannula is inserted all the way into the sclerotomy, the pressure plate is

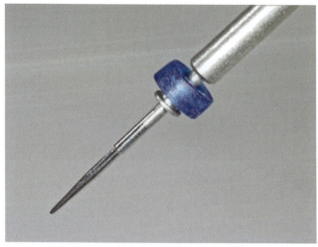

**Figure 18-7.** Microcannulas are inserted through the conjunctiva and sclera with a special blunt inserter (DORC).

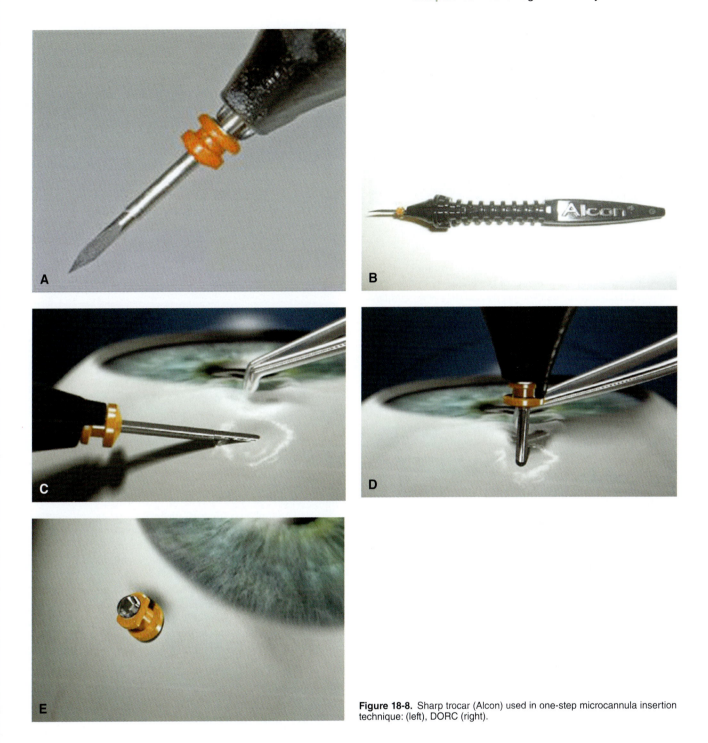

**Figure 18-8.** Sharp trocar (Alcon) used in one-step microcannula insertion technique: (left), DORC (right).

removed. As the inserter is withdrawn from the microcannula, the cannula must be held firmly in place in the sclerotomy using a special forceps (DORC). Normally, the infusion microcannula is first placed in the inferotemporal quadrant and the adequate angle of entry allows better friction to control the cannula in place; however, there is no difference depending on whether the trocar is inserted with the bevel down or up (10) (Fig. 18-7).

Currently, this technique has been modified by an easier and quicker one (single-step entry) that has been developed by Alcon (cannula-trocar system) (11,12) (Fig. 18-8). In the one-step technique, microcannulas are not inserted with a blunt inserter as in the two-step technique but with a sharp trocar. The width of the resulting scleral incision is somewhat less than that produced by a 23-gauge stiletto knife. It may be necessary to apply slightly higher pressure for insertion of the

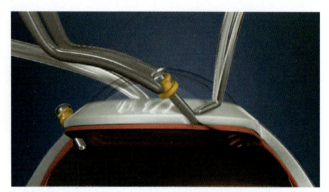

**Figure 18-9.** Beveled incision.

microcannula, occasionally causing lateral rotation of the globe. This possible shortcoming of the one-step technique is compensated for by the quicker insertion of the microcannulas. Moreover, because no stiletto knife is used, the one-step technique is also less expensive.

At the end of the procedure, cannulas are closed with plugs and intraocular pressure (IOP) maintained at 20 mm Hg (infusion turned on). The cannulas and their plugs are withdrawn one after the other in the direction of the scleral tunnels, using special cannula forceps, the infusion cannula being removed last. During removal, it is critical to follow the wound axis (2). The cannulas are withdrawn slowly through the scleral tunnels with cotton tip applicators holding pressure for 30 to 60 seconds and occasionally even longer, supporting the eye wall and pushing away the conjunctival incision from the scleral incision. A beveled angled entry is crucial to proper closure. If correctly done, scleral incisions close well and provide great transmural wall strength around the incision (Fig. 18-9).

Packo described in Retinal Physician magazine (November/December 2006) another technique that he learned from David Boyer. When the eye is pressurized, a light pipe is inserted into the infusion cannula like a plug; it is then slowly backed out, first the cannula and after few seconds, the light pipe.

If both phacoemulsification and vitrectomy are scheduled, the three cannulas have to be in place before cataract surgery. During phacoemulsification, the openings are sealed with plugs (2). Kim et al. reported that this maneuver is not necessary and cannula placement could wait until after phacoemulsification (5).

In summary, there are three requirements that every single incision should respect: beveled entry, conjunctival displacement, and globe stabilization.

## ILLUMINATION

The 23-gauge system allows a stronger light source that could combine directed or focused light, halogen or xenon, and a variety of probes:

A focused probe is the best instrument to see the vitreous and retinal surface. It offers good illumination but minimal panretinal view and increased risk of raising phototoxicity. With this probe, the only way to perform bimanual surgery is having picks on the probe, but it is very useful for epiretinal membrane peeling or shaving the vitreous base.

A nonfocused probe is a good option for panretinal viewing with lower risks of phototoxicity. It is not easy to visualize retinal topography and vitreous if it is not stained.

Chandelier illumination is the best choice for bimanual surgery, especially in complicated cases because it is safer than using endoillumination probes and the chandeliers can be easily inserted. Its advantages are a wide field of view and lower phototoxicity, although view of unstained vitreous, retinal highlights, and the vitreous base may be difficult (3).

There are two options of chandeliers: Tornambe Torpedo minilight (Insigh Instruments, Inc. Stuart, FLA) and Neptune (DORC).

## BENEFITS OF 23-GAUGE CANNULA SYSTEM

With this system proposed by Eckardt, it is easier to get in and out of the vitreous cavity, resulting in less trauma to the vitreous base. The beveled incision may reduce the risk of endophthalmitis (2,3).

Even though cannula insertion could be more difficult in reoperations because of fibrosis at scleral incision site, transconjunctival sutureless surgery provides easy access to the vitreous cavity. Charles suggests not removing silicone oil in reoperations because every single maneuver can be done under silicone oil (13).

Many surgeons suggest placement of microcannulas before cataract surgery in combined procedures; if it is done after the cataract surgery, insertion of the microcannulas with the requisite pressure could cause intraocular fluid to escape from the cornea wound. Since this cannot always be avoided even by suture closure, at least one of the three microcannulas, the infusion cannula, should be placed at the outset of the procedure. Otherwise, Kim et al. showed that there is no problem placing 23-gauge microcannulas (5).

## INFUSION

There are four options for infusion (2,3):

- The blunt, nondisposable, self-retaining cannula (DORC, *Zuidland, Holland*) that needs a previous 23-gauge sclerotomy.
- The Eckardt System.
- The sharp, self-retaining, disposable cannula can be inserted directly like a thumbtack. It can be combined with other gauge sclerotomies (14).
- The blunt-tipped, self-retaining, reusable side port infusion, which has notches on the hub of cannula and directs air or fluid flow sideways reducing risk of scotomas. It does need a 23-gauge sclerotomy.

## VITRECTORS

Alcon, Bausch & Lomb, and DORC have on the market 23-gauge vitreous cutters allowing the use of smaller ports and safe vitrectomy procedures. The DORC handpiece can be used with an Alcon pneumatic vitrectomy unit without any problem.

## FLUIDIC DYNAMICS IN 23-GAUGE SYSTEM

Poiseuille's law states that flow rates are equal to the fourth power of the radius of a cylindrical tube, and any small increase in its diameter causes a large increase in the flow rates (3). A controversial issue is that lower flow rates could be safer but may increase operating times. Since the initial promotion of high-speed cutters, a mistaken understanding of efficacy of cutting has been acknowledged; the real advantage is port-based flow limiting, a term defined by Steve Charles (13).

Port-based flow limiting is inherently produced by smaller lumens reducing pulse flow, which is the volume of fluid that goes through the port with each open-close cycle. Decreasing pulse flow increases fluidic stability and eliminates motion of detached retina making possible removal of peripheral vitreoretinal traction and easier delamination of diabetic traction without risk of iatrogenic breaks. Because of port-based flow, 23 gauge at 2500 cpm and 25 gauge at 1500 com have the same flow rate. However, it is important to use the maximum cutting rate. To get the same port-base flow limit for 23 gauge and 20 gauge, the latter has to achieve 6000 to 7000 cpm. In conclusion, port size and port location of 23-gauge probe allow an "effective flow."

The average infusion rate of the 23-gauge cannula is 1.7 and 2.8 fold greater than 20- and 25-gauge cannulas, respectively. The aspiration rate is 3.2 fold smaller than 20 gauge (15). Nevertheless, surgeons can perform hybrid surgery using a 23- or 25-gauge infusion cannula during a 20-gauge surgery (14). In such cases, surgeons should maintain higher pressures to avoid hypotony with 20-gauge vitreous cutter rates (13).

There are three kinds of duty cycles: parabolic incomplete (pneumatic), sinusoid (electric), and trapezoid (partial rotation). In the DORC 23-gauge system at 1500 cpm and 500 mm Hg, vitreous flow was low (0.0001 ml/sec). The percentage of vitreous flow rate/Balanced Salt Solution (BSS) flow rate showed an ascending curve for all instrumentation (15). Millennium 23-gauge system employs the pneumatic drive and a cut rate of 750 cpm, slower than the 25-gauge system.

The average operation time for 23-gauge cases may vary between 7 and 14 minutes (determined with a 2500 cpm cutter).

## WOUND CLOSURE

It seems that the length or size of incisions is not as important for closure of the sclerotomies as the angle of the incision. Many wound related problems have been described in 23-gauge surgery, including leakage and significant subconjunctival hemorrhage.

With regard to wound leakage, most surgeons suggest it could be related to a scleral tunnel being too short or too long. Other reasons for this complication include a perpendicular scleral tunnel, extensive peeling of vitreous base that reduces healing process and eliminates vitreous reflux that blocks inner wall of sclera, gas tamponade that could decrease unity of scleral tunnel edges, or younger patients (16,17). Other authors consider that vitreous incarceration increases risk for endophthalmitis, but pushing conjunctiva 1 or 2 mm laterally reduces entry of microorganisms (2,18).

In patients who have undergone surgery, no stitch technique produces milder inflammatory reaction and faster rehabilitation time (1).

Boker and Spitznas published the anatomic ultrasound biomicroscopy study of sclerotomy sites after vitreoretinal surgery (17). Koch et al. have shown with endoscopic studies that 23-gauge produces more vitreous reflux and incarceration in the cannula than 25 gauge (19). After numerous trials on eyes from eye banks, we concluded that the best closure can be achieved when the tunnel is made with a blade and not with a trocar.

## INDICATIONS

- Macular hole
- Retinal detachment with or without proliferative vitreoretinopathy.
- Tractional or mixed diabetic retinal detachment.
- Vitreous hemorrhage
- Lens fragmentation can be done with 23 gauge except in cases with a dense nucleus that need to convert technique to a 20-gauge system.

## PARAMETERS

### Standard 23 gauge

- Infusion: 35 mm Hg
- Vacuum: 400 to 450 mm Hg
- Cutting rate: 1500 cpm

## TAMPONADES

- *Balanced salt solution.* It is used in noncomplicated retinal surgeries, such as vitreous hemorrhage.
- *Gas: SF6 or C3F8.* Steven Charles proposed a 1/3 fluid-air exchange to get the interfacial tension of the air bubble sealing scleral incision until its healing (13). This technique had been followed by many surgeons resulting in a low incidence of hypotony, but there are still some surgeons that don't use fluid-air exchange without higher rates of hypotony as a complication.
- *Silicone oil.* Bruno et al reported 20 patients that underwent vitrectomy with silicone oil tamponade, which is

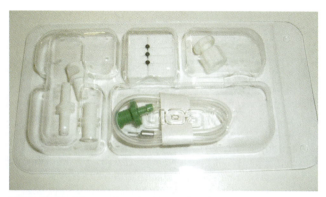

**Figure 18-10.** Silicone oil may be injected into the eye through an infusion cannula. The silicone oil tube is affixed to the head of the cannula and neither 1000 cst nor 5000 cst silicone oil causes the tube to detach from the cannula.

infused through infusion line. For this purpose the infusion tube on the head of the microcannula is exchanged for a tube filled with silicone oil and attached to a syringe. The silicone oil tube is affixed to the head of the cannula and neither 1000 cst nor 5000 cst silicone oil causes the tube to detach from the cannula.

But some considerations have to be followed to avoid silicone oil leakage, just as a real self-sealing incision (slightly longer tunnel) and lesser manipulation of tunnel-like sclerotomies (parallel inferior direction minimize scleral stretching). For removal, 1000 cst silicone oil is most rapidly removed by the application of pressure not by suction. The two instrument cannulas for drainage of the oil are left open so that the high pressure applied by the infusion solution will force the silicone oil out within a few minutes. This technique is not suitable for 5000 cst silicone oil whose higher viscosity requires a 20-gauge sclerotomy (20–26) (Fig. 18-10).

## DRAWBACKS AND SHORTCOMINGS

For some 23-gauge instruments, the smaller lumen is occasionally disadvantageous. A 23-gauge vitreous cutter for simple vitrectomy, for example, requires about 30% more time than does a 20-gauge cutter. The situation is similar for removal of a nonclotting intravitreal hemorrhage using a flute needle. For all other instruments we have experienced no appreciable difference in their efficacy versus 20-gauge instruments. This is true, for example, of the endoillumination probe and the endolaser probe, as well as for the various scissors and forceps whose handling, function, and size are wholly adequate for even the most difficult surgical procedures. Although by nature somewhat less stable than 20-gauge instruments, they have no appreciable drawbacks when used. Almost all techniques associated with 20-gauge vitrectomy, such as work on the periphery using scleral indentation or extreme lateral rotation of the globe, can be performed equally well with 23-gauge instruments.

For scleral indentation itself, however, transconjunctival vitrectomy sometimes only allows a minimal indentation in the nasal quadrants due to the anatomic situation of the conjunctiva. Scleral indentation posterior to the equator, as performed in conventional vitrectomy with large conjunctival opening, is therefore not at all or only limitedly possible. Also not feasible are techniques requiring special instruments not yet available in 23-gauge, such as endofragmentation needles or endocryocoagulation probes.

## COMPLICATIONS

Complications are similar to those found in 20-gauge surgery (18). Retinal detachment may occur after iatrogenic breaks while performing the surgery (19). Ibarra et al. reported postoperative retinal detachment in one out of 45 eyes after 25-gauge vitrectomy, determining that the incidence is not higher than that for 20 gauge (21). Lackanpal et al. (25 gauge) and Kim et al. (23 gauge) did not observe retinal detachment cases in their series (14,22). With regard to iatrogenic breaks during retinal detachment repair, 23 gauge is safer as slower flow rates and smaller ports can achieve a lower risk of snagging of the retina.

Other complications include cataract progression, postoperative vitreous hemorrhage, and creation of a new macular hole. Endophthalmitis may be reduced by conjunctival displacement and correcting angling of the microcannulas hub.

Hypotony is a recognized risk of sutureless surgery. Cases with transient hypotony showed increased risk for dangerous complications including retinal incarceration, suprachoroidal hemorrhage, and endophthalmitis (16,22,24,25). Fine et al. described an incidence of hypotony of 2.8% in their series (27). In 23-gauge vitrectomy, hypotony exists immediately after removal of the microcannulas regardless of whether or not a gas tamponade was performed. In our experience, the pressure returns to normal in only a few hours. In 30 consecutive patients, we measured the IOP between 5 and 7 hours after surgery, and only two eyes had an IOP below 10 mm Hg (6 and 8 mm Hg). In all other eyes, the pressure varied between 10 and 16 mm Hg. On the first postoperative day, all eyes had normal pressure. It is unclear whether the temporary hypotony immediately postoperative and/or the delayed sclerotomy closure are associated with a higher risk of intraocular hemorrhage and/or endophthalmitis. Only a large comparative study can provide the answer. Our experience does not suggest a higher incidence of hemorrhage. Of the more than 1800 eyes we operated on using the 23-gauge technique in 2006 and 2007, fewer than 1% had hypotony on the first day postoperative. Postoperative endophthalmitis was noted in none of these eyes.

## CONCLUSION

Twenty-three gauge is a "middle of the road" strategy because it can avoid the drawbacks related with smaller gauge surgery while still delivering the benefits of a minimally invasive technique. For many surgeons, this is the future. It allows performance of any surgery that 20 gauge does, with some advantages.

The question still lacks a definitive answer, but most vitreoretinal surgeons think that 23 gauge is going to replace 20-gauge surgery since complicated cases must often undergo multiple interventions; the best possible preservation of the conjunctiva and sclera beginning with the very first operation is therefore of inestimable value for all subsequent interventions.

## References

1. Fujii GY, de Juan E Jr, Humayun MS, et al. A new 23-gauge instrument system for transconjunctival sutureless vitrectomy surgery. *Ophthalmology* 2002;109:1807–1813.
2. Eckardt C. Transconjunctival sutureless 23-gauge vitrectomy. *Retina* 2005;25(2):209–211.
3. Roe R, Fu A. Small gauge vitrectomy: the future is now. *Retinal Physician* 2007;14(6).
4. Okamoto F, Sakata N, Hiratsuka K, et al. Changes in corneal topography following 25-gauge transconjunctival sutureless vitrectomy and 20-gauge standard vitrectomy. *Invest Ophthalmol Vis Sci* 2004;45:E-Abstract 2862.
5. Kim MJ, Park KH, Hwang JM, et al. The safety and efficacy of transconjunctival sutureless 23-gauge vitrectomy. *Korean J Ophthalmol* 2007;21(4):201–207.
6. Williams G. The evolution of 23 gauge surgery. Presentation. Beaumont Eye Institute. Royal Oak, MI 2007.
7. Kwok AK, Tham CC, Lam DS, et al. Modified sutureless sclerotomies in pars plana vitrectomy. *Am J Ophthalmol* 1999;127:731–733.
8. Assi AC, Scott RAH, Charteries DG. Reversed self-sealing pars plana sclerotomies. *Retina* 2000;20:689–692.
9. Theelen T, Verbeek A, Tilanus M, et al. A novel technique for self-sealing wedge-shaped pars plana sclerotomies and its features in ultrasound biomicroscopy and clinical outcome. *Am J Ophthalmol* 2003;136c:1085–1092.
10. Garg S, Hagemann LF, Zacharias LC, et al. Comparison of leakage pressures in bevel down versus bevel up sclerotomy incisions using 23 gauge vitrectomy trochar system. *ARVO 2007 Meeting Abstract.* Poster 2230/B839.
11. Rizzo S, Genovesi-Ebert F, Vento A, et al. A new "Single Step Entry" system for 23 gauge vitrectomy. *ARVO 2007 Meeting Abstract.* Poster 2217/B826.
12. Ho AC, Regillo CD, Kaiser PK, et al. Microincision 23 g Pars Plana Vitrectomy: Surgical results. *ARVO 2007 Meeting Abstract.* Poster 2251/B860.
13. Charles S. Debating the pros and cons of 23 g vs 25 g surgery. *Retinal Physician.* 2006;3:24–25.
14. Hubschman JP, Gonzales CR, Bourla DH, et al. Combined 25 and 23 gauge surgery: a new sutureless vitrectomy technique. *Ophthalmic Surg Lasers Imagig* 2007;38(4):345–348.
15. Magalhaes O Jr, Chong L, DeBoer C, et al. Vitreous dynamics: the new solid development concept. Vitreous flow analysis in 20, 23 and 25 gauge cutters. *ARVO 2007 Meeting Abstract.* Poster 2243/B852.
16. Tewari A, Shah GK, Fang A, et al. Visual outcomes with 23-gauge transconjunctival sutureless vitrectomy. *ARVO 2007 Meeting Abstract.* Poster 2219/B828.
17. Hagemann LF, Zacharias LC, Garg S, et al. Comparison of Leakage pressures in tunnel versus straight sclerotomy incisions using 23 gauge vitrectomy trocar system. *ARVO 2007 Meeting Abstract.* Poster 2226/B835.
18. Boker T, Spitznas M. Ultrasound biomicroscopy for examination of the sclerotomy sites after parsplana vitrectomy. *Am J Ophthalmol* 1994;118:813–815.
19. Koch FH, Luloh KP, Singh P, et al. "Mini-gauge" pars plana vitrectomy: "inside-out view" with the GRIN solid rod endoscope. *Ophthalmologica* 2007;221(5):356–362.
20. Territo C, Gieser JP, Wilson CA, et al. Influence of the cannulated vitrectomy system on the occurrence of iatrogenic sclerotomy retinal tears. *Retina* 1997;17(5):430–433.
21. Ibarra MS, Hermel M, Prenner JL, et al. Longer-term outcomes of transconjunctival sutureless 25-gauge vitrectomy. *Am J Ophthalmol* 2005;139:831–836.
22. Lackanpal RR, Humayun MS, de Juan E Jr, et al. Outcomes of 140 consecutive cases of 25-gauge transconjunctival surgery for posterior segment disease. *Ophthalmology* 2005;112:817–824.
23. Davis BL, Dyer DS. Vitrectomy time and fluid dynamics in 23 gauge and 25 gauge micro-incision vitrectomy surgery. *ARVO 2007 Meeting Abstract.* Poster 2245/B854.
24. Meyer CH, Rodrigues EB, Schmidt JC, et al. Sutureless vitrectomy surgery. *Ophthalmolog* 2003;110(12):2427–2428.
25. Lam DS, Yuen CY, Tam BS, et al. Sutureless vitrectomy surgery. *Ophthalmology* 2003;110(12):2428.
26. Bruno-Oliveira L, Costa-Reis P. Silicone oil tamponade in 23-gauge transconjunctival sutureless vitrectomy. *Retina* 2007;27:1054–1058.
27. Fine H, Iranmanesh R, Iturralde D, et al. Outcomes of 77 consecutive cases of 23-gauge transconjunctival vitrectomy surgery for posterior segment disease. *Ophthalmology* 2007;114:1197–1200.

# 19

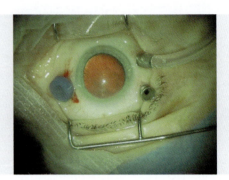

# 20-Gauge Sutureless Vitrectomy

Carl Claes ■ Anna Paula R. Lafeta

# INTRODUCTION

Sutureless pars plana vitrectomy was first proposed by Chen (1), and it was based on 20-gauge (20G) self-sealing scleral tunnels. Many complications were reported and other authors have described modifications for this technique to avoid problems such as wound leakage, dehiscence, hemorrhage, incarceration of vitreous and/or retina, retinal tears, and dialyses (2–7).

The use of trocars for sutureless vitrectomy was first described by Fugii et al. (8,9). A scleral perpendicular 25-gauge incision was used, and they suggested that the holes would be closed because they were small and the conjunctiva would also cover them, serving as a protection. However, in minimal surgery, the closure of the sclerotomies is essentially made by the peripheral vitreous, possibly increasing the risk of incarceration and secondary retinal detachment. If this peripheral vitreous were removed in order to avoid this complication, it would increase the possibility of wound leakage and hypotony.

Although the 25-gauge system seemed to be very attractive, reducing surgical time, minimizing trauma, and hastening postoperative recovery, some problems such as flexibility and fragility (10) of the instruments, low infusion and aspiration rates (8) and, of course, higher costs, have limited its use. Since then, many attempts have been made to improve sutureless vitreoretinal surgery.

Eckardt (11) presented, as an alternative to the 25-gauge, a new method using a 23-gauge system. He has used a 30 to 40 degree tunnel incision made with a stiletto and inserted the cannulas using a blunt inserter. This system offers the advantages of a sutureless surgery, but it requires a completely different set of instruments. These instruments are flexible, increasing surgery costs and limiting indications. To avoid the leakage mentioned before in the 25-gauge surgeries, Lópes-Guajardo (12) proposed that the sclerotomies should be done in the same way Eckardt (4) described for 23-gauge surgery, creating scleral tunnels with displacement of the conjunctiva.

We introduced a new 20G transconjunctival trocar system (Dutch Ophthalmic Research Corporation [DORC], Zuidland, Holland) that allows the use of the conventional 20G vitrectomy in sutureless surgeries. It is analogous to the 23-gauge approach. A tangential tunnel is made with a bent stiletto, and the trocars are introduced with a blunt inserter in a two-step technique.

# METHODS

The first generation trocars were designed 3 years ago. A set (Fig. 19-1) includes: one infusion inserter (measures 11.5 mm), one infusion trocar (measures 8.5 mm with a 4.0 mm intraocular extension), and two blunt trocar-inserters (measuring 10.0 mm with a 4.0 mm intraocular extension). The blunt trocar-inserters are used to place the 6.5 mm trocars. The external diameter for the infusion and trocars is 1.0 mm, and the internal diameter is 0.9 mm. However, the intense leakage of infusion fluids through gaping 20G ports caused hypotony at various moments during the surgery. To solve this problem, different types of disposable valves were developed (Fig. 19-2). They keep the eye sealed after retraction of the instruments

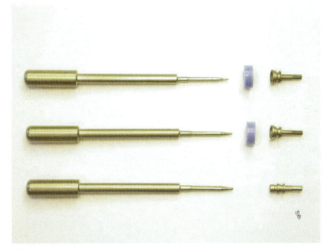

**Figure 19-1.** A complete set.

and allow the surgeon to have complete control of the intraocular pressure. Also they reduce the consumption of infusion fluids. The valves fit the distal trocar tip and are easily removable (Figs. 19-3 and 19-4). Indentation can be executed without difficulty and the periphery is easily accessible. The trocars protect the entry sites from erosion, and plugs are not needed when using this system.

The procedure is initiated using a 20-gauge bent stiletto (45-degree angle; 0.9 mm; Blumenthal; BD Visitec) that is inserted at a 10-degree angle through the conjunctiva, without displacement (Fig. 19-5), to create a 3.5 mm scleral tunnel (Fig. 19-6). Incisions are radially made at 3 mm from the limbus and tunnels are made limbus-parallel (Figs. 19-5 and 19-6). The infusion trocar is first placed into the inferotemporal tunnel (Fig. 19-7), and trocars are placed at the superior quadrants (Fig. 19-8). The two-step procedure is thus characterized by using a stiletto to create tunnels followed by trocar placement. It is felt to be relatively atraumatic and is preferred. This approach creates better sclerotomy configurations and is considered decisive for good wound closure at the end of the procedure.

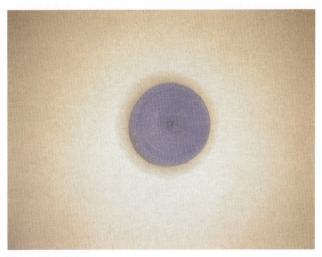

**Figure 19-2.** Valve.

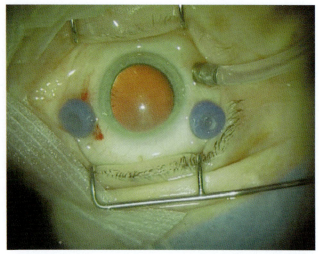

**Figure 19-3.** Trocars in place with valves.

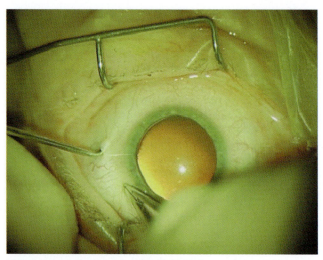

**Figure 19-6.** Scleral tunnel made with stiletto.

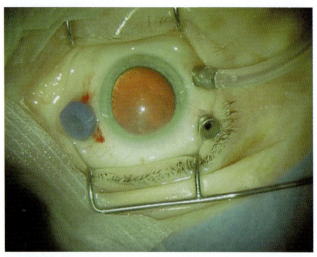

**Figure 19-4.** Trocars in place without one valve.

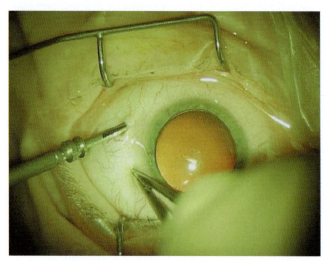

**Figure 19-7.** Placement of the infusion trocar.

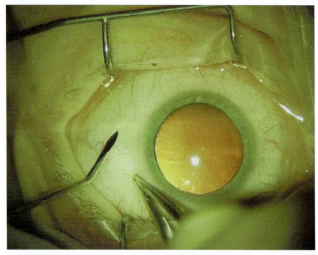

**Figure 19-5.** Incision made with 20-gauge stiletto at a 10-degree angle through the conjunctiva.

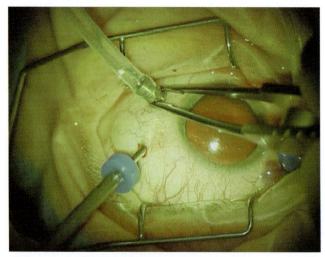

**Figure 19-8.** Placement of the valved trocar.

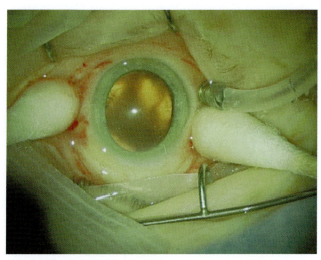

**Figure 19-9.** Massage at entry ports.

The surgery is performed using the regular straight or adapted curved 20G instruments. At the end, the eye is pressurized at 20 mm Hg, and the infusion is closed before removing the two trocars from the superior quadrants. Then, the infusion is reopened, increasing the eye pressure for a few seconds with simultaneous cotton tip massage at the entry ports in order to close the tunnels (Fig. 19-9). The massaging is continued until the absence of leakage is noted. The infusion trocar is then removed, simultaneously pressurizing its entry port with the cotton tip. Longer tunnels tend to have better closure. In case of hypotony, after the trocar's removal, air is injected through the pars plana using a 3 cc syringe and a 30-gauge needle. Additional diathermy can be applied to close conjunctival buttonholes.

## DISCUSSION

The 20G system presents advantages over the 25/23 gauges without their inconveniences. It shortens the procedure by using a larger vitrectome while being transconjunctival and sutureless. Thus, it has the advantages of fast healing and minimal postoperative inflammation, like other existing trocar systems. The 20G trocars allow the use of high-speed cutters with high infusion/aspiration rates, faster vitreous removal with easier clearance of organized vitreous, and reduced iatrogenic traction. The higher infusion volume reduces intraoperative hypotony, giving more control to the surgeon. It is also very easy to work with silicone oil, unlike with the smaller gauge systems.

The learning curve is short since the instruments are basically the same as existing 20G conventional vitrectomy probes, scissors, forceps, and others. Curved instruments that can pass through the trocars have been developed. The system can be used in almost all vitreoretinal surgeries because it provides easy access to the entire periphery with nonflexible instrumentation. Also, this system comes with a new coated phacofragmentation needle, allowing aspiration of the hardest cataracts from the posterior pole.

Another advantage of the larger size trocars is excellent visualization in scotopic conditions from 20G illumination and easy accessibility for the instruments, without damaging the sclera during each passage. The valves keep the eye closed when removing the instruments, maintaining it pressurized. Since a complete vitrectomy with careful shaving of the vitreous base is made in all patients, there is no vitreous to plug the sclerotomies. After the removal of the first two trocars, the closure of the tunnels is done by the apposition of its walls when the infusion pressure is raised. Using 10 degree incisions, we create longer tunnels, which are easier to close. The infusion tunnel is closed with local massaging.

Superior postoperative patient comfort and less eye inflammation are provided by the sutureless technique. Small conjunctival hemorrhage caused by the grasping forceps used to hold the eye during the insertion of the trocars does not cause any discomfort to the patients.

## RESULTS

With experience in over 400 cases using this technique, the indications have grown tremendously. Starting out with straightforward vitrectomies to demonstrate the feasibility of the technique and the absence of major complications, it has slowly improved. At first one feels a reduced liberty in moving the instruments inside the eye. However by getting used to the system, this minor discomfort completely disappears and is replaced by a preference for this system.

At this time we will not hesitate to deal with advanced stages of proliferative vitreoretinopathy (PVR), proliferative diabetic retinopathy (PDR), and even macular translocation using this technique. With further instrumentation development (illuminated, curved instruments, fragmentation needle) more difficult cases can be dealt with. In all our cases, we were able to close the eye and finish the surgery without placing a single suture. The technique has been used in combination with air-tamponade, gas, Balanced Salt Solution (BSS) and silicone oil tamponade.

In one case of hypotony (5 mm Hg) we injected 0.5 cc of $SF^6$ at postoperative day one. This happened during the early learning curve phase. The most severe complication was a postoperative endophthalmitis at one week postoperative. During the reintervention we could observe perfectly closed and almost invisible previous trocar sclerotomies, suggesting that leakage would not be the cause of endophthalmitis.

## CONCLUSION

In this era of sutureless surgeries, this 20G trocar system with valves is a safe, comfortable, and less expensive alternative to conventional 25- and 23-gauge vitrectomy.

Furthermore, it offers a complete set of instrumentation, like the conventional 20G vitrectomy, allowing the surgeon to deal with all kinds of pathologies, even dropped nucleus and macular translocation. In our experience, the only exclusion criterion is scleromalacia at the pars plana.

## References

1. Chen JC. Sutureless pars plana vitrectomy through self-sealing sclerotomies. *Arch Ophthalmol* 1996;114:1273–1275.
2. Milibak T, Suveges I. Complications of sutureless pars plana vitrectomy through self-sealing sclerotomies. *Arch Ophthmol* 1998;116:119.
3. Kwok AK, Tham CC, Lam DS, et al. Modified sutureless sclerotomies in pars plana vitrectomy. *Am J Ophthalmol* 1999;127:731–733.
4. Schmidt J, Nietgen GW, Briedan S. Selbstverchliessende, nahtlose SKlerotomie zur Pars-plana-Vitrektomie. *Klin Monatsbl Augenheilkd* 1999;215:247–251.
5. Jackson T. Modified sutureless sclerotomies in pars plana vitrectomy. *Am J Ophthalmol* 2000;129:116–117.
6. Assi AC, Scott RAH, Charteris DG. Reversed self-sealing pars plana sclerotomies. *Retina* 2000;689–692.
7. Rahman R, Rosen PH, Riddell C, et al. Self-sealing sclerotomies for sutureless pars plana vitrectomy. *Ophthalmic Surg Lasers* 2000;31:462–466.
8. Fugii GY, de Juan E Jr, Humayun MS, et al. A new 25-gauge instrument system for transconjunctival sutureless vitrectomy surgery. *Ophthalmology* 2002;109:1807–1812.
9. Fugii GY, de Juan E Jr, Humayun MS, et al. Initial experience using the transconjunctival sutureless vitrectomy system for vitreoretinal surgery. *Ophthalmology* 2002;109:1814–1820.
10. Inoue M, Noda K, Ishida S, et al. Intra-operative breakage of a 25-gauge vitreous cutter. *Am J Ophthalmol* 2004;138(5):867–869.
11. Eckardt C. Transconjunctival sutureless 23-gauge vitrectomy. *Retina* 2005;25:208–211.
12. Lópes-Guajardo L, Pareja-Esteban J, Teus-Guezala M. Oblique sclerotomy for prevention of incompetent wound closure in transconjunctival 25-gauge vitrectomy. *Am J Ophthalmol* 2006;141:1154–1156.

four

# Diabetic Retinopathy

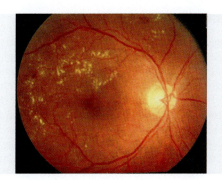

# Pharmacotherapy of Diabetic Retinopathy

Yoshihiro Yonekawa ■ Aziz A. Khanifar ■ Donald J. D'Amico ■ R.V. Paul Chan

Diabetes mellitus (DM) is a major cause of morbidity and mortality throughout the world. Over 170 million people are currently affected, and the prevalence is projected to more than double by 2030 (1). Diabetic retinopathy (DR) is the leading cause of blindness among working-age adults in the United States, and annually blinds over 12,000 patients (2). Similar to diabetic nephropathy and neuropathy, DR is a microvascular complication of both type 1 and type 2 diabetes. After 20 years of diagnosis, nearly all patients with type 1 and approximately 60% with type 2 DM have some degree of DR (3,4). DR is broadly categorized into either nonproliferative (NPDR) or proliferative DR (PDR) (5), depending on the presence of retinal fibrovascular proliferation.

Historically, the mainstays of DR treatment are glucose, blood pressure, and cholesterol control, combined with photocoagulation and/or vitrectomy as necessary. However, recent advances in our understanding of the molecular mechanisms behind the pathogenesis of DR have catalyzed the development of pharmacologic therapies such as intravitreal corticosteroids and antivascular endothelial growth factor (VEGF) agents. Many other exciting pharmacological developments have taken place as well.

## PATHOPHYSIOLOGY

Vascular basement membrane thickening, an early morphologic feature of DR (6), may cause both filtration defects and dysfunction of cell proliferation and differentiation (7,8). The loss of intramural capillary pericytes is another early histologic hallmark (9,10). Pericyte loss is thought to weaken the capillary wall, leading to microaneurysms, which are often the first clinically visible signs of DR.

Microaneurysms are hypercellular saccular outpouchings of the capillary wall (11), and an increase in their number is associated with progression of retinopathy (12,13). Microaneurysms cause disruption of the blood-retinal barrier, leading to capillary permeability, resulting in intraretinal and subretinal fluid accumulation. The fluid tends to collect in the macular area, causing diabetic macular edema (DME). Increased expression of VEGF in regions with relative hypoxia and inflammatory factors also play a role in the development of DME in addition to fibrovascular proliferative disease. Severity of retinopathy is directly correlated with the likelihood of developing DME and retinal neovascularization.

DME can be focal or diffuse, and the pathophysiology, clinical appearance, and treatment modalities are different. Hard exudates are common findings in DME that correlate with serum lipid levels (14–17). The Early Treatment Diabetic Retinopathy Study (ETDRS) defined clinically significant macular edema (CSME) as thickening of the retina within 500 μm of the center of the fovea, hard exudates within 500 μm of the fovea associated with thickening of the adjacent retina, or retinal thickening of at least one disc diameter in size, within one disc diameter of the foveal center (18).

Retinal capillary occlusion causes increasing ischemia, which can lead to the development of cotton-wool spots, retinal hemorrhages, venous beading, and intraretinal microvascular abnormalities (IRMA). Retinal ischemia upregulates signaling molecules such as VEGF that promote fibrovascular proliferation, leading to PDR, which can cause significant visual loss by vitreous hemorrhage and/or tractional or combined tractional-rhegmatogenous retinal detachment. Neovascularization of the iris (NVI) may also occur as a result of retinal ischemia.

## METABOLIC CONTROL

### Insulin and Hypoglycemic Agents

Pharmacologic primary and secondary interventions are essential in lowering the systemic risk factors for developing DR. Currently, the most effective method of preventing and slowing the progression of diabetic retinopathy is tight glycemic control. The Diabetes Control and Complications Trial (DCCT) (19–36) showed that in comparison to conventional insulin therapy, intensive glucose monitoring and aggressive insulin therapy to maintain strict glycemic control lowered the risk of developing DR in type 1 diabetics with no baseline retinopathy by 76% (95% confidence interval or CI, 62 to 85). Notably, intensive therapy lowered the risks of nephropathy and neuropathy as well. The DCCT cohort was followed by the Epidemiology of Diabetes Interventions and Complications (EDIC) study (20), which showed that former tight glucose control provided continued benefits after seven years.

The U.K. Prospective Diabetes Study (UKPDS) (21) demonstrated that in type 2 diabetics, intensive treatment with sulfonylureas (chlorpropamide, glibenclamide, or glipizide) or insulin had a protective relative risk of 0.79 ($p = 0.015$) for progression of DR, and 0.71 ($p = 0.0031$) for requiring retinal photocoagulation.

The American Diabetes Association currently recommends maintaining a hemoglobin A1c of <7.0%, preprandial capillary plasma glucose of 70 to 130 mg/dL, and peak postprandial capillary plasma glucose of <180 mg/dL for nonpregnant adult diabetics (22).The main concern of intensive glycemic control is hypoglycemic episodes, which were more common in the intensive treatment arms of both the DCCT and UKPDS.

## ANTIHYPERTENSIVES

Hypertension is associated with the development and progression of DR. The UKPDS randomized 3867 type 2 diabetics to tight (aiming for <150/85), or milder blood pressure control (<180/105) with captopril or atenolol (23). The tight control group had a 34% (99% CI, 11 to 50) risk reduction of DR progression, and a 47% (99% CI, 7 to 70) risk reduction of visual acuity deterioration by three lines. Deaths related to diabetes and stroke were also reduced (24).

In 2008, the Diabetic Retinopathy Candesartan Trials (DIRECT) reported that although candesartan reduced the incidence of new DR by 18% ($p = 0.051$) in type 1 diabetics, there was no effect on DR progression for those with baseline retinopathy (25). However, the Renin-Angiotensin System

Study (RASS) published in July of 2009 indicated that enalapril and losartan reduced the odds of early DR progression in type 1 diabetics by 65% ($p = 0.02$) and 70% ($p = 0.008$), respectively (26). These effects appear to be independent of blood pressure changes (26,27).

## ANTILIPIDS

The Wisconsin Epidemiologic Study of Diabetic Retinopathy (WESDR) (14) and the ETDRS (15) both found associations between serum lipid levels and retinal hard exudates. Lipid control may be beneficial in DR because visual acuity loss correlates with the degree of hard exudates, and permanent retinal damage can be caused by subretinal fibrosis (28).

Preliminary studies suggested the use of clofibrate to be beneficial (16,17). The Fenofibrate Intervention and Event Lowering in Diabetes (FIELD) study (29) recently demonstrated that fenofibrate reduces the rate of first laser therapy for DR or DME, from 4.9% of patients on placebo to 3.4% of patients on fenofibrate ($p = 0.0002$), but without an overall effect on the progression of DR (30). Statins have also been shown to improve DME in preliminary studies (31–33). Randomized clinical trials (RCTs) that are underway include the Atorvastatin Study for Prevention of Coronary Heart Disease Endpoints in Non-Insulin-Dependent Diabetes Mellitus (ASPEN) (34), and the Action to Control Cardiovascular Risk in Diabetes Eye (ACCORD-EYE) studies (35).

## ANTIPLATELETS

Platelet microthrombi have been identified in retinal capillaries of diabetics, and have been proposed to be a possible mechanism for the capillary occlusions resulting in retinal ischemia (36,37). The Dipyridamole Aspirin Microangiopathy of Diabetes (DAMAD) study randomized patients with mild DR to aspirin alone, aspirin combined with dipyridamole, or placebo. The treatment arms developed fewer microaneurysms on fluorescein angiograms, but there was little difference in visual acuity and ophthalmoscopy endpoints (38). Similarly, the Ticlopidine Microangiopathy of Diabetes study (TIMAD) showed that while ticlopidine slowed the formation of microaneurysms, there were no clinical benefits (39). The ETDRS concluded that aspirin therapy does not have clinical effects in DR (40), but there are no ocular contraindications (41) to taking aspirin for cardiovascular or other conditions (42).

The Steno-2 study examined the effects of multifactorial intensive therapy consisting of tight glucose control combined with renin-angiotensin system blockers, lipid-lowering drugs, and aspirin (43). There was a 43% risk reduction of DR progression ($p = 0.01$), and a 55% risk reduction in requiring laser treatment for PDR or DME ($p = 0.02$). However, multifactorial treatment of systemic risk factors was still insufficient to prevent DR progression in many patients. This highlights the importance of targeted therapies, discussed below, to be administered in conjunction with optimal metabolic control and current ophthalmic therapies.

## ALTERATION OF BIOCHEMICAL PATHWAYS

### Aldose Reductase

Several biochemical mechanisms have been proposed as links between hyperglycemia and diabetic microvascular complications (19,44). Aldose reductase is the first enzyme in the polyol pathway that catalyzes the nicotinamide adenine dinucleotide phosphate (NADPH) – dependent reduction of aldose sugars into sugar alcohols. Hyperglycemia activates the pathway and glucose becomes reduced to sorbitol, which is thought to cause osmotic stress. Aldose reductase's NADPH-consuming reactions also may cause oxidative damage by decreasing the NADPH available for glutathione reductase (45).

Clinical trials of aldose reductase inhibitors (ARIs), however, have not been promising. Data from the Sorbinil Retinopathy Trial (SRT) (46), a Phase III RCT of 497 insulin-dependent diabetics, showed no significant difference in the progression of retinopathy between subjects randomized to sorbinil or placebo. Subsequent trials of other ARIs such as zenarestat, tolrestat, and lidorestat, were prematurely halted due to toxicities (47–49).

## NONENZYMATIC GLYCATION

Advanced glycation end-products (AGEs) are found in retinal vessels (50) and renal glomeruli of diabetic patients (51). Glycation of proteins alters their functions, causing them to bind to AGE receptors on endothelial cells and macrophages, which induces receptor mediated production of reactive oxygen species, proinflammatory and procoagulative molecules, growth factors, and transcription factors that cause pathologic gene expression (45). Studies suggest that AGE receptors also promote capillary wall hyperpermeability by inducing VEGF expression (52).

Aminoguanidine (Pimagedine) is a hydrazine derivative that binds AGE precursors to decrease AGE formation (53). The efficacy and safety of aminoguanidine against DR is currently controversial (54,55). Another anti-AGE drug, alagebrium chloride (ALT-711), is being investigated in diabetic macrovascular disease (56–58).

### Protein Kinase C

Protein Kinase C (PKC) is a family of serine-threonine kinases (59) that appear to mediate vascular contractility, hemodynamics, and cellular proliferation to modulate diabetic microvascular disease (60,61). Hyperglycemia induces the synthesis of diacylglycerol (DAG), which in turn activates PKC. The β isoform has been linked most strongly with diabetes. Animal models have demonstrated that PKC-β increases retinal vascular permeability and neovascularization (62–64), most likely by involving VEGF (64,65).

Staurosporin (PKC412) is a nonselective PKC inhibitor that also inhibits VEGF receptors 1 and 2, the Platlet-derived Growth Factor (PDGF) receptor, and stem cell factor receptor.

In a Phase I/II RCT of 141 patients with DME, oral staurosporin decreased retinal thickening ($p = 0.032$) and slightly improved (4.36 letters; $p = 0.007$) visual acuity at 3 months (66), but further studies were abandoned due to gastrointestinal side effects and hepatotoxicity.

Ruboxistaurin (RBX/LY333531) is a selective inhibitor of PKC-β (61). The PKC-β Inhibitor Diabetic Retinopathy Study (PKC-DRS) randomized 252 subjects with moderately severe to severe NPDR to placebo or RBX (67). Doubling of the visual angle was delayed with 32 mg/day of RBX ($p = 0.012$), but there was no difference in the progression of NPDR to PDR. In PKC-DRS 2 (68), the follow up Phase III study with 685 subjects and 36 to 42 months of follow-up, the relative risk reduction of moderate visual loss was 40% compared to placebo ($p = 0.034$). RBX reduced initial photocoagulation in eyes that had not received laser treatment before baseline ($p = 0.008$), and decreased the progression of DME to the center-involved stage ($p = 0.003$), but there was no difference in the composite end point of DR progression. Notably, unlike staurosporin, RBX had minimal side effects.

The PKC-DME study was another Phase III RCT with 686 subjects, and examined RBX with DME progression or requirement of laser treatment as primary end points, but found no composite benefit (69). The US FDA approval of RBX for DME is currently pending on the results of further trials (70,71).

## CORTICOSTEROIDS

### Intravitreal Triamcinolone

Laser treatment is currently the first line therapy for DME, and can halve the risk for visual loss in eyes with focal DME (19,21,72). However, the results for diffuse DME have been less promising (18); perhaps this is because photocoagulation does not address the underlying cause of the edema. Increasing evidence suggests that the microvascular changes in DR and DME are at least in part secondary to inflammation (73). Leukocytes migrate and adhere to retinal vasculature in experimental models of diabetes (74,75), which has been shown to cause premature endothelial cell death, capillary ischemia, and breakdown of the blood-retinal barrier (76–78).

Intravitreal corticosteroids bypass the blood-retinal barrier and can achieve intraocular therapeutic levels while minimizing systemic toxicities. Dexamethasone was initially investigated, but was limited by its short half-life in the vitreous (79). Attention shifted to triamcinolone acetonide, which is less potent but has a longer half-life due to its minimal solubility in water (80). For example, a 4 mg dose remains measurable in the eye for approximately three months (81), and a 25 mg dose for nine months (82). It is also well tolerated (83,84). Other delivery methods, such as peribulbar triamcinolone, was recently shown to be ineffective in a Phase II RCT (85).

A number of small RCTs suggested the efficacy of intravitreal triamcinolone (IVTA) in treating advanced DME (86–90), but most studies lacked power and follow-up. The Diabetic Retinopathy Clinical Research Network (DRCR.net) was formed in 2002 as a collaborative network of sites in the United States (US) to facilitate multicenter trials.

The optimal dose of IVTA is unclear, but 4 mg is generally used in the US (80). The DRCR.net found no functional or anatomical outcome differences between 1 mg and 4 mg IVTA doses, while 4 mg had more side effects, suggesting that lower doses may be acceptable (91). Timing of reinjection is another uncertainty, because peak concentration and half-life may be heterogenous between patients (81). A study using optical coherence tomography (OCT) to monitor central macular thickness showed that recurrence of diffuse DME after one IVTA injection occurs around 24 weeks (90).

A recent Phase III DRCR.net trial of 840 eyes demonstrated that IVTA is not as effective as focal/grid photocoagulation, and is associated with cataract formation and ocular hypertension (91). At 4 months, the mean visual acuity was best in the 4 mg IVTA group ($p \leq 0.001$), but by one year, there was no difference, and at two years, visual acuity in the laser group was better than the 1 mg ($p = 0.02$) and 4 mg IVTA groups ($p = 0.002$). OCT analysis of macular thickness also paralleled the visual acuity results. Outcome measures were comparable at three years (92), suggesting that photocoagulation should remain the gold standard to compare other therapies. A Phase III DRCR.net trial is now evaluating a combined photocoagulation-IVTA regimen, in comparison to laser alone, intravitreal ranibizumab plus laser, and intravitreal ranibizumab plus deferred laser (93).

The role of IVTA in PDR is less defined. Although large scale studies are lacking, IVTA appears at least in the short term to be well tolerated (94–97). Some surgeons also use intraoperative triamcinolone to improve visualization of the posterior hyaloid face. A Phase III DRCR.net study scheduled to enroll 381 subjects will be evaluating the adjunctive use of IVTA and ranibizumab following panretinal photocoagulation (PRP) for the treatment of PDR (98).

## CORTICOSTEROID IMPLANTS

Intravitreal and retinal implant devices are being developed to allow sustained drug delivery to avoid the repeated injections of local steroids. Retisert (Bausche & Lomb, Rochester, New York) is a surgically implanted fluocinolone acetonide releasing intravitreal device that is US Food and Drug Administration (FDA) approved to treat chronic non-infectious posterior segment uveitis (99). A Phase II/III RCT with 197 subjects and 3 years of follow up found that 58% of implanted eyes compared to 30% of eyes treated with laser/observation had resolution of DME ($p < 0.001$) (100). However, of the implanted eyes, 95% of phakic eyes required cataract extraction, 35% developed ocular hypertension, and 5% necessitated implant removal to control intraocular pressure (100). Medidur is a nonsurgically implantable fluocinolone acetonide releasing device that is currently undergoing Phase II and III trials (101).

Ozurdex (Allergan, Irvine, California) is an injectable, biodegradable intravitreal dexamethasone drug delivery system (DDS). In June of 2009, the US FDA approved its use for treatment of macular edema secondary to retinal vein occlusions (RVO) (102). Data from two parallel Phase III studies demonstrated that the time to achieve $\geq 15$ letters improvement in best corrected visual acuity was faster in eyes treated with 700 ug of Ozurdex ($p < 0.01$) (103). During the first 6 months of follow up, intraocular pressure elevation and cataract formation occurred in 25% and 4% of treated eyes, respectively. The preapproval Phase II RCT showed comparable effects between eyes with RVO and DME, suggesting that Ozurdex may be an effective and relatively safe DME treatment (104).

## ANTI-VEGF THERAPIES

### Basic Science of VEGF

VEGF is a key regulator of angiogenesis and has been implicated in the pathogenesis of neovascular diseases including DR, neovascular age-related macular degeneration (AMD), retinopathy of prematurity, and retinal vein occlusion. In diabetes, VEGF gene expression is upregulated in response to several factors including hypoxia, growth factors, PKC, AGEs, and reactive oxygen species (52,105,106). VEGF levels have been found to correlate with disease severity (107–109). It is produced by retinal pigment epithelial cells, glial cells, capillary pericytes, endothelial cells, Müller cells, and ganglion cells (110).

The VEGF family includes VEGF-A, -B, -C, -D, -E and placenta growth factor (PIGF)-1 and -2. VEGF-A (hereinafter referred to as VEGF) has been most frequently implicated in pathologic neovascularization. Through alternative splicing of VEGF's eight exons, isoforms with 121, 145, 165, 183, 189, and 206 amino acids are created (111). VEGF165 is thought to be one of the key pathologic isoforms (112,113).

The VEGF family exerts their functions via membrane-bound tyrosine kinase receptors VEGFR-1, -2, and -3. VEGFR-2 appears to be the major mediator of VEGF's angiogenic properties. Soluble VEGFR-1 (sFlt-1) has also been identified as a decoy receptor that sequesters VEGF and has been shown to play a role in preventing corneal vascularization (114,115). Its levels have been found to be lower in eyes with PDR (116). Gene delivery of sFlt-1 for the treatment of DR and DME is currently under investigation (117,118).

VEGF is an attractive target for potential therapies not only because of its role in neovascularization as seen in PDR, but due to its proinflammatory and capillary permeability properties (119–121) that have been linked to the development and progression of DME. In fact, most anti-VEGF clinical research has focused on DME treatment.

### Pegaptanib (Macugen)

Pegaptanib (Macugen, Eyetech, New York) is a pegylated neutralizing RNA aptamer, which selectively binds VEGF165. Data from a Phase II RCT of 172 patients with DME randomized to repeated intravitreal pegaptanib or sham injections showed that at 36 weeks, eyes treated with pegaptanib had better visual acuity ($p = 0.03$); mean improvement was +4.7 letters with 34% improving 10 letters or more (122). Pegaptanib also reduced central retinal thickness ($p = 0.02$), and further photocoagulation ($p = 0.04$). Retrospective subgroup analysis of eyes with PDR at baseline showed that pegaptanib promoted

regression of neovascularization and/or fluorescein leakage from neovascularization in eight of 13 (62%) eyes, compared to 0 of seven fellow, nonstudy eyes or those that received sham injections (123).

### Ranibizumab (Lucentis)

Ranibizumab (Lucentis, Genentech, South San Francisco, California) and bevacizumab (Avastin, Genentech, South San Francisco, California) are both molecules that inhibit all VEGF-A isoforms. Bevacizumab is a monoclonal antibody against VEGF-A, while ranibizumab is the Fab fragment of the same antibody that has been affinity matured to provide greater affinity to VEGF. Ranibizumab was developed to treat neovascular AMD (124–126), but increasing evidence suggests that it is also useful for DR and DME (127,128). The DRCR.net (93), RESOLVE (129), READ-2 (130), and the RISE and RIDE (131) studies are several upcoming Phase II and III RCTs that are evaluating the effects of ranibizumab in DME.

### Bevacizumab (Avastin)

Bevacizumab is ranibizumab's parent molecule. It is US FDA approved for treatment of metastatic colon cancer but is being used off-label as an anti-VEGF agent for ocular diseases such as neovascular AMD and DME (Fig. 20-1). It is unknown if bevacizumab and ranibizumab have similar efficacy and safety, but some practitioners prefer bevacizumab due to its lower cost. An upcoming National Eye Institute study will be comparing the two drugs head-to-head in the treatment for AMD (132).

In Haritoglou et al's prospective case series of 51 eyes with diffuse DME, 1.25 mg of intravitreal bevacizumab reduced macular thickness at 12 weeks ($p = 0.001$). Visual acuity improvement was noted at 6 weeks ($p = 0.02$), but the improvement was not sustained at 12 weeks (133). Their follow-up study of continuous injections for chronic diffuse DME resulted in improved anatomic ($p < 0.001$) and visual ($p = 0.025$) outcomes at 12 months (134).

The Pan-American Collaborative Retina Study Group (PACORES) reported a retrospective study of 78 eyes with DME and treated with at least one injection of 1.25 mg or 2.5 mg of intravitreal bevacizumab. Improvements in best-corrected visual acuity (BCVA) ($p < 0.0001$) and central macular thickness ($p < 0.0001$) were noted at 6 months (135), and the benefits continued at 12 months (136).

The DRCR.net conducted a Phase II multi-center trial of 121 eyes with DME randomized to focal photocoagulation, intravitreal bevacizumab, or both (137). At 12 weeks, eyes treated with intravitreal injections of 1.25 mg or 2.5 mg of bevacizumab had better visual acuity outcomes compared to laser treatment ($p = 0.01$, 0.003, respectively). Central subfield thickness also decreased, but the benefit disappeared after 3 weeks. Combined bevacizumab-focal photocoagulation resulted in no apparent benefit. However, larger trials are necessary to make clinically meaningful conclusions on safety and effectiveness.

In regard to intravitreal bevacizumab for the treatment of PDR (138–145) and NVI (146,147), the efficacy of bevacizumab alone or in conjunction with PRP and/or vitrectomy have also been demonstrated by small, mostly retrospective studies.

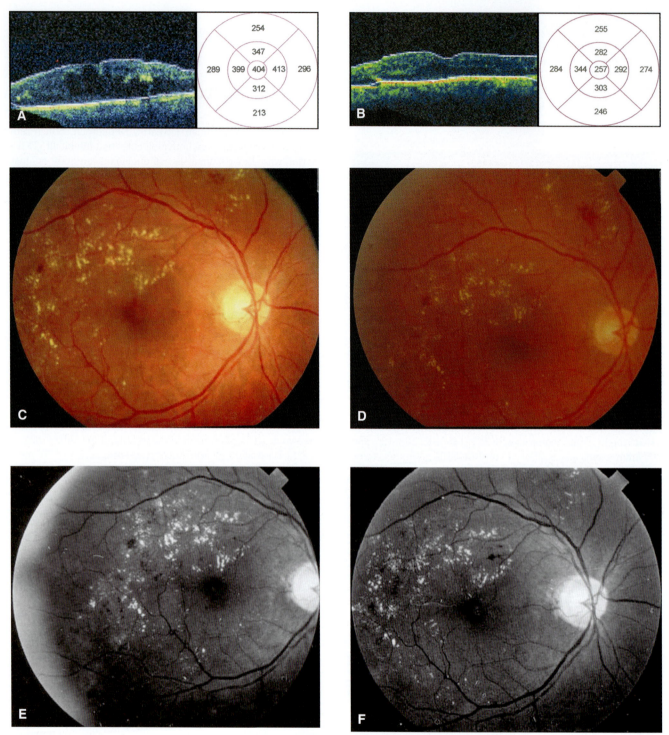

**Figure 20-1. A:** Stratus™ optical coherence tomography (OCT) of a diabetic patient's right eye, consistent with marked diabetic macular edema (DME) with large cystoid spaces. **B:** Repeat OCT of the same eye 4 weeks after injection of intravitreal bevacizumab shows decrease of DME with return of the foveal contour. The patient's visual acuity improved by 3 lines on the Early Treatment Diabetic Retinopathy Study visual acuity chart. **C:** Color fundus photograph of the same eye demonstrating several hard exudates and macular edema. **D:** Color fundus photograph following bevacizumab injection, demonstrating less exudates and edema. **E, G, I:** Early, mid, and late-frame fluorescein angiographs (FAs) of the same eye showing significant leakage from microaneurysms. **F, H, J:** Early, mid, and late-frame FAs following bevacizumab injection. Although the light exposure is different on this visit, a decreased amount of leakage can be appreciated.

*(continued)*

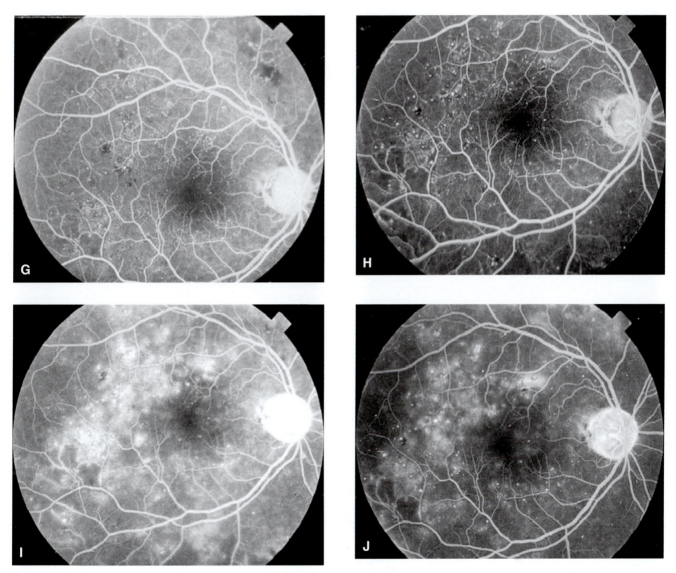

**Figure 20-1.** *(continued)*

## Aflibercept (VEGF Trap-Eye)

Aflibercept (VEGF Trap-Eye, Regeneron Pharmaceuticals, Tarrytown, New York) is a 115 kDa soluble recombinant fusion protein that blocks all members of the VEGF family by acting as a decoy receptor. It consists of the ligand-binding elements of VEGFR-1 and -2, which are fused to the Fc portion of human IgG1 (148). Mouse models have shown that it can inhibit choroidal neovascularization and VEGF-induced breakdown of the blood-retinal barrier (149). VEGF Trap-Eye has a higher binding constant for VEGF than ranibizumab and bevacizumab and even native VEGF receptors, so theoretically, the stronger affinity translates into greater activity at lower biological levels and a longer duration of action (150). A Phase I study by Do and colleagues showed good short-term results and safety in treating eyes with DME

(151). Regeneron is planning to conduct further trials (152).

## OTHER DRUG THERAPIES

Enzymatic vitreolysis has been proposed to accelerate the clearance of vitreous hemorrhage secondary to PDR by liquefying the vitreous to allow red blood cell lysis and phagocytosis. Intravitreal purified ovine hyaluronidase (Vitrase, ISTA Pharmaceuticals, Irvine, California) has been shown to be effective and safe in a Phase III double masked RCT with 1125 patients, although all primary end points were not met (153,154). Vitrase is currently not US FDA approved for DR.

# CONCLUSION

Promising new pharmacologic treatments for diabetic retinopathy have been developed and tested in recent years. In addition to the drugs discussed in this chapter, numerous potential treatments are in preclinical and early clinical stages of development. Although optimal metabolic control and photocoagulation remain time-tested first-line treatments, off-label second-line and adjuvant treatment with newer pharmacotherapies such as IVTA and anti-VEGF agents should be judiciously considered in order to reduce vision loss in the increasing number patients with diabetes. The role of pharmacotherapy will become more evident as we accumulate data from upcoming clinical trials.

## References

1. Wild S, Roglic G, Green A, et al. Global prevalence of diabetes: estimates for the year 2000 and projections for 2030. *Diabetes Care* 2004;27(5):1047–1053.
2. Centers for Disease Control and Prevention. *National diabetes fact sheet: general information and national estimates on diabetes in the United States, 2007.* Atlanta, GA: U.S. Department of Health and Human Services, Centers for Disease Control and Prevention, 2008.
3. Klein R, Klein BE, Moss SE, et al. The Wisconsin epidemiologic study of diabetic retinopathy. II. Prevalence and risk of diabetic retinopathy when age at diagnosis is less than 30 years. *Arch Ophthalmol* 1984;102(4):520–526.
4. Klein R, Klein BE, Moss SE, et al. The Wisconsin epidemiologic study of diabetic retinopathy. III. Prevalence and risk of diabetic retinopathy when age at diagnosis is 30 or more years. *Arch Ophthalmol* 1984;102(4):527–532.
5. Wilkinson CP, Ferris FL, Klein RE, et al. Proposed international clinical diabetic retinopathy and diabetic macular edema disease severity scales. *Ophthalmology* 2003;110(9):1677–1682.
6. Robison WG, Kador PF, Kinoshita JH. Retinal capillaries: basement membrane thickening by galactosemia prevented with aldose reductase inhibitor. *Science* 1983;221(4616):1177–1179.
7. Ingber DE, Folkman J. How does extracellular matrix control capillary morphogenesis? *Cell* 1989;58(5):803–805.
8. Folkman J, Klagsbrun M, Sasse J, et al. A heparin-binding angiogenic protein–basic fibroblast growth factor–is stored within basement membrane. *Am J Pathol* 1988;130(2):393–400.
9. Cogan DG, Toussaint D, Kuwabara T. Retinal vascular patterns. IV. Diabetic retinopathy. *Arch Ophthalmol* 1961;66:366–378.
10. Kuwabara T, Cogan DG. Retinal vascular patterns. VI. Mural cells of the retinal capillaries. *Arch Ophthalmol* 1963;69:492–502.
11. Kuwabara T, Cogan DG. Studies of retinal vascular patterns. I. Normal architecture. *Arch Ophthalmol* 1960;64:904–911.
12. Klein R, Meuer SM, Moss SE, et al. The relationship of retinal microaneurysm counts to the 4-year progression of diabetic retinopathy. *Arch Ophthalmol* 1989;107(12):1780–1785.
13. Klein R, Meuer SM, Moss SE, et al. Retinal microaneurysm counts and 10-year progression of diabetic retinopathy. *Arch Ophthalmol* 1995;113(11):1386–1391.
14. Klein BE, Moss SE, Klein R, et al. The Wisconsin Epidemiologic Study of Diabetic Retinopathy. XIII. Relationship of serum cholesterol to retinopathy and hard exudate. *Ophthalmology* 1991;98(8):1261–1265.
15. Chew EY, Klein ML, Ferris FL, et al. Association of elevated serum lipid levels with retinal hard exudate in diabetic retinopathy. Early Treatment Diabetic Retinopathy Study (ETDRS) Report 22. *Arch Ophthalmol* 1996;114(9):1079–1084.
16. Harrold BP, Marmion VJ, Gough KR. A double-blind controlled trial of clofibrate in the treatment of diabetic retinopathy. *Diabetes* 1969;18(5):285–291.
17. Cullen JF, Town SM, Campbell CJ. Double-blind trial of Atromid-S in exudative diabetic retinopathy. *Trans Ophthalmol Soc U K* 1974;94(2):554–562.
18. Early Treatment Diabetic Retinopathy Study research group. Photocoagulation for diabetic macular edema. Early Treatment Diabetic Retinopathy Study report number 1. *Arch Ophthalmol* 1985;103(12):1796–1806.
19. The Diabetes Control and Complications Trial Research Group. The effect of intensive treatment of diabetes on the development and progression of long-term complications in insulin-dependent diabetes mellitus. *N Engl J Med* 1993;329(14):977–986.
20. The Writing Team for the Diabetes Control and Complications Trial/Epidemiology of Diabetes Interventions and Complications Research Group. Effect of intensive therapy on the microvascular complications of type 1 diabetes mellitus. *JAMA* 2002;287(19):2563–2569.
21. UK Prospective Diabetes Study (UKPDS) Group. Intensive blood-glucose control with sulphonylureas or insulin compared with conventional treatment and risk of complications in patients with type 2 diabetes (UKPDS 33). *Lancet* 1998;352(9131):837–853.
22. American Diabetes Association. Standards of medical care in diabetes–2009. *Diabetes Care* 2009;32(Suppl 1):S13–S61.
23. UK Prospective Diabetes Study Group. Tight blood pressure control and risk of macrovascular and microvascular complications in type 2 diabetes: UKPDS 38. *BMJ* 1998;317(7160):703–713.
24. UK Prospective Diabetes Study Group. Efficacy of atenolol and captopril in reducing risk of macrovascular and microvascular complications in type 2 diabetes: UKPDS 39. *BMJ* 1998;317(7160):713–720.
25. Chaturvedi N, Porta M, Klein R, et al. Effect of candesartan on prevention (DIRECT-Prevent 1) and progression (DIRECT-Protect 1) of retinopathy in type 1 diabetes: randomised, placebo-controlled trials. *Lancet* 2008;372(9647):1394–1402.
26. Mauer M, Zinman B, Gardiner R, et al. Renal and retinal effects of enalapril and losartan in type 1 diabetes. *N. Engl. J. Med* 2009;361(1):40–51.
27. Perkins BA, Aiello LP, Krolewski AS. Diabetes complications and the renin-angiotensin system. *N. Engl. J. Med* 2009;361(1):83–85.
28. Fong DS, Segal PP, Myers F, et al. Subretinal fibrosis in diabetic macular edema. ETDRS report 23. Early Treatment Diabetic Retinopathy Study Research Group. *Arch Ophthalmol* 1997;115(7):873–877.
29. Keech A, Simes RJ, Barter P, et al. Effects of long-term fenofibrate therapy on cardiovascular events in 9795 people with type 2 diabetes mellitus (the FIELD study): randomised controlled trial. *Lancet* 2005;366(9500):1849–1861.
30. Keech AC, Mitchell P, Summanen PA, et al. Effect of fenofibrate on the need for laser treatment for diabetic retinopathy (FIELD study): a randomised controlled trial. *Lancet* 2007;370(9600):1687–1697.
31. Sen K, Misra A, Kumar A, et al. Simvastatin retards progression of retinopathy in diabetic patients with hypercholesterolemia. *Diabetes Res Clin Pract* 2002;56(1):1–11.
32. Gupta A, Gupta V, Thapar S, et al. Lipid-lowering drug atorvastatin as an adjunct in the management of diabetic macular edema. *Am J Ophthalmol* 2004;137(4):675–682.
33. Gordon B, Chang S, Kavanagh M, et al. The effects of lipid lowering on diabetic retinopathy. *Am J Ophthalmol* 1991;112(4):385–391.
34. Knopp RH, d'Emden M, Smilde JG, et al. Efficacy and safety of atorvastatin in the prevention of cardiovascular end points in subjects with type 2 diabetes: the Atorvastatin Study for Prevention of Coronary Heart Disease Endpoints in non-insulin-dependent diabetes mellitus (ASPEN). *Diabetes Care* 2006;29(7):1478–1485.
35. Chew EY, Ambrosius WT, Howard LT, et al. Rationale, design, and methods of the Action to Control Cardiovascular Risk in Diabetes Eye Study (ACCORD-EYE). *Am J Cardiol* 2007;99(12A):103i-111i.
36. Pope CH. Retinal capillary microaneurysms: a concept of pathogenesis. *Diabetes* 1960;9:9–13.
37. Boeri D, Maiello M, Lorenzi M. Increased prevalence of microthromboses in retinal capillaries of diabetic individuals. *Diabetes* 2001;50(6):1432–1439.
38. The DAMAD Study Group. Effect of aspirin alone and aspirin plus dipyridamole in early diabetic retinopathy. A multicenter randomized controlled clinical trial. *Diabetes* 1989;38(4):491–498.
39. The TIMAD Study Group. Ticlopidine treatment reduces the progression of nonproliferative diabetic retinopathy. *Arch Ophthalmol* 1990;108(11):1577–1583.
40. Early Treatment Diabetic Retinopathy Study Research Group. Effects of aspirin treatment on diabetic retinopathy. ETDRS report number 8. Early Treatment Diabetic Retinopathy Study Research Group. *Ophthalmology* 1991;98(5 Suppl):757–765.
41. Chew EY, Klein ML, Murphy RP, et al. Effects of aspirin on vitreous/preretinal hemorrhage in patients with diabetes mellitus. Early Treatment Diabetic Retinopathy Study report no. 20. *Arch Ophthalmol* 1995;113(1):52–55.
42. Early Treatment Diabetic Retinopathy Study Investigators. Aspirin effects on mortality and morbidity in patients with diabetes mellitus. Early Treatment Diabetic Retinopathy Study report 14. *JAMA* 1992;268(10):1292–1300.
43. Gaede P, Lund-Andersen H, Parving H, et al. Effect of a multifactorial intervention on mortality in type 2 diabetes. *N Engl J Med* 2008;358(6):580–591.
44. Diabetes Control and Complications Trial Research Group. Progression of retinopathy with intensive versus conventional treatment in the Diabetes Control and Complications Trial. *Ophthalmology* 1995;102(4):647–661.
45. Brownlee M. Biochemistry and molecular cell biology of diabetic complications. *Nature* 2001;414(6865):813–820.
46. Sorbinil Retinopathy Trial Research Group. A randomized trial of sorbinil, an aldose reductase inhibitor, in diabetic retinopathy. *Arch Ophthalmol* 1990;108(9):1234–1244.

47. Brown MJ, Bird SJ, Watling S, et al. Natural progression of diabetic peripheral neuropathy in the Zenarestat study population. *Diabetes Care* 2004;27(5):1153–1159.
48. Foppiano M, Lombardo G. Worldwide pharmacovigilance systems and tolrestat withdrawal. *Lancet* 1997;349(9049):399–400.
49. Greene DA, Arezzo JC, Brown MB. Zenarestat Study Group. Effect of aldose reductase inhibition on nerve conduction and morphometry in diabetic neuropathy. *Neurology* 1999;53(3):580–591.
50. Stitt AW, Li YM, Gardiner TA, et al. Advanced glycation end products (AGEs) co-localize with AGE receptors in the retinal vasculature of diabetic and of AGE-infused rats. *Am J Pathol* 1997;150(2):523–531.
51. Horie K, Miyata T, Maeda K, et al. Immunohistochemical colocalization of glycoxidation products and lipid peroxidation products in diabetic renal glomerular lesions. Implication for glycoxidative stress in the pathogenesis of diabetic nephropathy. *J Clin Invest* 1997;100(12):2995–3004.
52. Lu M, Kuroki M, Amano S, et al. Advanced glycation end products increase retinal vascular endothelial growth factor expression. *J Clin Invest* 1998;101(6):1219–1224.
53. Thornalley PJ. Use of aminoguanidine (Pimagedine) to prevent the formation of advanced glycation end products. *Arch Biochem Biophys* 2003;419(1):31–40.
54. Bolton WK, Cattran DC, Williams ME, et al. Randomized trial of an inhibitor of formation of advanced glycation end products in diabetic nephropathy. *Am J Nephrol* 2004;24(1):32–40.
55. Freedman BI, Wuerth JP, Cartwright K, et al. Design and baseline characteristics for the aminoguanidine Clinical Trial in Overt Type 2 Diabetic Nephropathy (ACTION II). *Control Clin Trials* 1999;20(5):493–510.
56. Little WC, Zile MR, Kitzman DW, et al. The effect of alagebrium chloride (ALT-711), a novel glucose cross-link breaker, in the treatment of elderly patients with diastolic heart failure. *J Card Fail* 2005;11(3):191–195.
57. Zieman SJ, Melenovsky V, Clattenburg L, et al. Advanced glycation end product crosslink breaker (alagebrium) improves endothelial function in patients with isolated systolic hypertension. *J Hypertens* 2007;25(3):577–583.
58. Kass DA, Shapiro EP, Kawaguchi M, et al. Improved arterial compliance by a novel advanced glycation end-product crosslink breaker. *Circulation* 2001;104(13):1464–1470.
59. Mellor H, Parker PJ. The extended protein kinase C superfamily. *Biochem J* 1998;332(Pt 2):281–292.
60. Sheetz MJ, King GL. Molecular understanding of hyperglycemia's adverse effects for diabetic complications. *JAMA* 2002;288(20):2579–2588.
61. Ishii H, Jirousek MR, Koya D, et al. Amelioration of vascular dysfunctions in diabetic rats by an oral PKC beta inhibitor. *Science* 1996;272(5262):728–731.
62. Xu X, Zhu Q, Xia X, et al. Blood-retinal barrier breakdown induced by activation of protein kinase C via vascular endothelial growth factor in streptozotocin-induced diabetic rats. *Curr Eye Res* 2004;28(4):251–256.
63. Danis RP, Bingaman DP, Jirousek M, et al. Inhibition of intraocular neovascularization caused by retinal ischemia in pigs by PKCbeta inhibition with LY333531. *Invest Ophthalmol Vis Sci* 1998;39(1):171–179.
64. Aiello LP, Bursell SE, Clermont A, et al. Vascular endothelial growth factor-induced retinal permeability is mediated by protein kinase C in vivo and suppressed by an orally effective beta-isoform-selective inhibitor. *Diabetes* 1997;46(9):1473–1480.
65. Xia P, Aiello LP, Ishii H, et al. Characterization of vascular endothelial growth factor's effect on the activation of protein kinase C, its isoforms, and endothelial cell growth. *J Clin Invest* 1996;98(9):2018–2026.
66. Campochiaro PA. Reduction of diabetic macular edema by oral administration of the kinase inhibitor PKC412. *Invest Ophthalmol Vis Sci* 2004;45(3):922–931.
67. PKC-DRS Study Group. The effect of ruboxistaurin on visual loss in patients with moderately severe to very severe nonproliferative diabetic retinopathy: initial results of the Protein Kinase C beta Inhibitor Diabetic Retinopathy Study (PKC-DRS) multicenter randomized clinical trial. *Diabetes* 2005;54(7):2188–2197.
68. Aiello LP, Davis MD, Girach A, et al. Effect of ruboxistaurin on visual loss in patients with diabetic retinopathy. *Ophthalmology* 2006;113(12):2221–2230.
69. The PKC-DMES Study Group. Effect of ruboxistaurin in patients with diabetic macular edema: thirty-month results of the randomized PKC-DMES clinical trial. *Arch Ophthalmol* 2007;125(3):318–324.
70. Eli Lilly and Company. Reduction in the occurrence of center-involved diabetic macular edema. http://clinicaltrials.gov. Accessed March 22, 2009.
71. Eli Lilly and Company. Effect of Ruboxistaurin on Clinically Significant Macular Edema. http://clinicaltrials.gov. Accessed March 22, 2009.
72. Photocoagulation treatment of proliferative diabetic retinopathy: the second report of diabetic retinopathy study findings. *Ophthalmology* 1978;85(1):82–106.
73. Funatsu H, Noma H, Mimura T, et al. Association of vitreous inflammatory factors with diabetic macular edema. *Ophthalmology* 2009;116(1):73–79.
74. Miyamoto K, Khosrof S, Bursell SE, et al. Prevention of leukostasis and vascular leakage in streptozotocin-induced diabetic retinopathy via intercellular adhesion molecule-1 inhibition. *Proc Natl Acad Sci U S A* 1999;96(19):10836–10841.

75. Barouch FC, Miyamoto K, Allport JR, et al. Integrin-mediated neutrophil adhesion and retinal leukostasis in diabetes. *Invest Ophthalmol Vis Sci* 2000;41(5):1153–1158.
76. Joussen AM, Murata T, Tsujikawa A, et al. Leukocyte-mediated endothelial cell injury and death in the diabetic retina. *Am J Pathol* 2001;158(1):147–152.
77. Xu Q, Qaum T, Adamis AP. Sensitive blood-retinal barrier breakdown quantitation using Evans blue. *Invest Ophthalmol Vis Sci* 2001;42(3):789–794.
78. Miyamoto K, Hiroshiba N, Tsujikawa A, et al. In vivo demonstration of increased leukocyte entrapment in retinal microcirculation of diabetic rats. *Invest Ophthalmol Vis Sci* 1998;39(11):2190–2194.
79. Graham RO, Peyman GA. Intravitreal injection of dexamethasone. Treatment of experimentally induced endophthalmitis. *Arch Ophthalmol* 1974;92(2):149–154.
80. Sobrin L, D'Amico DJ. Controversies in intravitreal triamcinolone acetonide use. *Int Ophthalmol Clin* 2005;45(4):133–141.
81. Beer PM, Bakri SJ, Singh RJ, et al. Intraocular concentration and pharmacokinetics of triamcinolone acetonide after a single intravitreal injection. *Ophthalmology* 2003;110(4):681–686.
82. Jonas JB. Intravitreal triamcinolone acetonide for diabetic retinopathy. *Dev Ophthalmol* 2007;39:96–110.
83. McCuen BW, Bessler M, Tano Y, et al. The lack of toxicity of intravitreally administered triamcinolone acetonide. *Am J Ophthalmol* 1981;91(6):785–788.
84. Gillies MC, Simpson JM, Billson FA, et al. Safety of an intravitreal injection of triamcinolone: results from a randomized clinical trial. *Arch Ophthalmol* 2004;122(3):336–340.
85. Chew E, Strauber S, Beck R, et al. Randomized trial of peribulbar triamcinolone acetonide with and without focal photocoagulation for mild diabetic macular edema: a pilot study. *Ophthalmology* 2007;114(6):1190–1196.
86. Avitabile T, Longo A, Reibaldi A. Intravitreal triamcinolone compared with macular laser grid photocoagulation for the treatment of cystoid macular edema. *Am J Ophthalmol* 2005;140(4):695–702.
87. Sutter FKP, Simpson JM, Gillies MC. Intravitreal triamcinolone for diabetic macular edema that persists after laser treatment: three-month efficacy and safety results of a prospective, randomized, double-masked, placebo-controlled clinical trial. *Ophthalmology* 2004;111(11):2044–2049.
88. Jonas JB, Söfker A. Intraocular injection of crystalline cortisone as adjunctive treatment of diabetic macular edema. *Am J Ophthalmol* 2001;132(3):425–427.
89. Gillies MC, Sutter FKP, Simpson JM, et al. Intravitreal triamcinolone for refractory diabetic macular edema: two-year results of a double-masked, placebo-controlled, randomized clinical trial. *Ophthalmology* 2006;113(9):1533–1538.
90. Massin P, Audren F, Haouchine B, et al. Intravitreal triamcinolone acetonide for diabetic diffuse macular edema: preliminary results of a prospective controlled trial. *Ophthalmology* 2004;111(2):218–224; discussion 224–225.
91. Diabetic Retinopathy Clinical Research Network. A randomized trial comparing intravitreal triamcinolone acetonide and focal/grid photocoagulation for diabetic macular edema. *Ophthalmology* 2008;115(9):1447–1449, 1449.e1–1449.e10.
92. Beck RW, Edwards AR, Aiello LP, et al. Three-year follow-up of a randomized trial comparing focal/grid photocoagulation and intravitreal triamcinolone for diabetic macular edema. *Arch Ophthalmol* 2009;127(3):245–251.
93. Diabetic Retinopathy Clinical Research Network. Intravitreal ranibizumab or triamcinolone acetonide in combination with laser photocoagulation for diabetic macular edema. http://public.drcr.net/DRCRnetstudies/studies/ProtocolI_lrtdme/ProtIInfo.html. Accessed March 23, 2009.
94. Zacks DN, Johnson MW. Combined intravitreal injection of triamcinolone acetonide and panretinal photocoagulation for concomitant diabetic macular edema and proliferative diabetic retinopathy. *Retina* 2005;25(2):135–140.
95. Zein WM, Noureddin BN, Jurdi FA, et al. Panretinal photocoagulation and intravitreal triamcinolone acetonide for the management of proliferative diabetic retinopathy with macular edema. *Retina* 2006;26(2):137–142.
96. Bandello F, Polito A, Pognuz DR, et al. Triamcinolone as adjunctive treatment to laser panretinal photocoagulation for proliferative diabetic retinopathy. *Arch Ophthalmol* 2006;124(5):643–650.
97. Jonas JB, Söfker A, Degenring R. Intravitreal triamcinolone acetonide as an additional tool in pars plana vitrectomy for proliferative diabetic retinopathy. *Eur J Ophthalmol* 2003;13(5):468–473.
98. National Eye Institute (NEI). Laser-Ranibizumab-Triamcinolone for Proliferative Diabetic Retinopathy – Full Text View – ClinicalTrials.gov. http://clinicaltrials.gov. Accessed April 15, 2009.
99. Jaffe GJ, Martin D, Callanan D, et al. Fluocinolone acetonide implant (Retisert) for noninfectious posterior uveitis: thirty-four-week results of a multicenter randomized clinical study. *Ophthalmology* 2006;113(6):1020–1027.
100. Pearson P, Levy B, Comstock T. Fluocinolone Acetonide Implant Study Group. fluocinolone acetonide intravitreal implant to treat diabetic macular edema: 3-year results of a multi-center clinical trial. *Invest. Ophthalmol. Vis. Sci* 2006;47:E-Abstract 5442.
101. Johns Hopkins University. The MAP Study: FA/Medidur(TM) for AMD Pilot. http://clinicaltrials.gov. Accessed April 12, 2009.

102. U. S. Food and Drug Administration. Drugs @ FDA: FDA approved drug products. http://www.accessdata.fda.gov/Scripts/cder/DrugsatFDA/index.cfm?fuseaction = Search.Label_ApprovalHistory#apphist. Accessed July 15, 2009.

103. Allergan, Inc. Ozurdez TM (dexamethasone intravitreal implaint) 0.7 mg. http://www.allergan.com/products/eye_care/ozurdex.htm. Accessed July 15, 2009.

104. Kuppermann BD, Blumenkranz MS, Haller JA, et al. Randomized controlled study of an intravitreous dexamethasone drug delivery system in patients with persistent macular edema. *Arch Ophthalmol* 2007;125(3):309–317.

105. Pandya NM, Dhalla NS, Santani DD. Angiogenesis–a new target for future therapy. *Vascul Pharmacol* 2006;44(5):265–274.

106. Kuroki M, Voest EE, Amano S, et al. Reactive oxygen intermediates increase vascular endothelial growth factor expression in vitro and in vivo. *J Clin Invest* 1996;98(7):1667–1675.

107. Adamis AP, Miller JW, Bernal MT, et al. Increased vascular endothelial growth factor levels in the vitreous of eyes with proliferative diabetic retinopathy. *Am J Ophthalmol* 1994;118(4):445–450.

108. Malecaze F, Clamens S, Simorre-Pinatel V, et al. Detection of vascular endothelial growth factor messenger RNA and vascular endothelial growth factor-like activity in proliferative diabetic retinopathy. *Arch Ophthalmol* 1994;112(11):1476–1482.

109. Aiello LP, Avery RL, Arrigg PG, et al. Vascular endothelial growth factor in ocular fluid of patients with diabetic retinopathy and other retinal disorders. *N Engl J Med* 1994;331(22):1480–1487.

110. Duh E, Aiello LP. Vascular endothelial growth factor and diabetes: the agonist versus antagonist paradox. *Diabetes* 1999;48(10):1899–1906.

111. Robinson CJ, Stringer SE. The splice variants of vascular endothelial growth factor (VEGF) and their receptors. *J Cell Sci* 2001;114(Pt 5):853–865.

112. Ferrara N. Vascular endothelial growth factor: basic science and clinical progress. *Endocr Rev* 2004;25(4):581–611.

113. Ishida S, Usui T, Yamashiro K, et al. VEGF164-mediated inflammation is required for pathological, but not physiological, ischemia-induced retinal neovascularization. *J Exp Med* 2003;198(3):483–489.

114. Adler EM, Gough NR, Ray LB. 2006: signaling breakthroughs of the year. *Sci STKE* 2007;2007(367):eg1.

115. Ambati BK, Nozaki M, Singh N, et al. Corneal avascularity is due to soluble VEGF receptor-1. *Nature* 2006;443(7114):993–997.

116. Patel JI, Tombran-Tink J, Hykin PG, et al. Vitreous and aqueous concentrations of proangiogenic, antiangiogenic factors and other cytokines in diabetic retinopathy patients with macular edema: Implications for structural differences in macular profiles. *Exp Eye Res* 2006;82(5):798–806.

117. Bainbridge JWB, Mistry A, De Alwis M, et al. Inhibition of retinal neovascularisation by gene transfer of soluble VEGF receptor sFlt-1. *Gene Ther* 2002;9(5):320–326.

118. Gehlbach P, Demetriades AM, Yamamoto S, et al. Periocular gene transfer of sFlt-1 suppresses ocular neovascularization and vascular endothelial growth factor-induced breakdown of the blood-retinal barrier. *Hum Gene Ther* 2003;14(2):129–141.

119. Miyamoto K, Khosrof S, Bursell SE, et al. Vascular endothelial growth factor (VEGF)-induced retinal vascular permeability is mediated by intercellular adhesion molecule-1 (ICAM-1). *Am J Pathol* 2000;156(5):1733–1739.

120. Qaum T, Xu Q, Joussen AM, et al. VEGF-initiated blood-retinal barrier breakdown in early diabetes. *Invest Ophthalmol Vis Sci* 2001;42(10):2408–2413.

121. Melder RJ, Koenig GC, Witwer BP, et al. During angiogenesis, vascular endothelial growth factor and basic fibroblast growth factor regulate natural killer cell adhesion to tumor endothelium. *Nat Med* 1996;2(9):992–997.

122. Cunningham ET, Adamis AP, Altaweel M, et al. A phase II randomized double-masked trial of pegaptanib, an anti-vascular endothelial growth factor aptamer, for diabetic macular edema. *Ophthalmology* 2005;112(10):1747–1757.

123. Adamis AP, Altaweel M, Bressler NM, et al. Changes in retinal neovascularization after pegaptanib (Macugen) therapy in diabetic individuals. *Ophthalmology* 2006;113(1):23–28.

124. Rosenfeld PJ, Brown DM, Heier JS, et al. Ranibizumab for neovascular age-related macular degeneration. *N Engl J Med* 2006;355(14):1419–1431.

125. Brown DM, Kaiser PK, Michels M, et al. Ranibizumab versus verteporfin for neovascular age-related macular degeneration. *N Engl J Med* 2006;355(14):1432–1444.

126. Brown DM, Michels M, Kaiser PK, et al. Ranibizumab versus verteporfin photodynamic therapy for neovascular age-related macular degeneration: Two-year results of the ANCHOR study. *Ophthalmology* 2009;116(1):57–65.e5.

127. Chun DW, Heier JS, Topping TM, et al. A pilot study of multiple intravitreal injections of ranibizumab in patients with center-involving clinically significant diabetic macular edema. *Ophthalmology* 2006;113(10):1706–1712.

128. Nguyen QD, Tatlipinar S, Shah SM, et al. Vascular endothelial growth factor is a critical stimulus for diabetic macular edema. *Am J Ophthalmol* 2006;142(6):961–969.

129. Novartis. RESOLVE: Safety and Efficacy of Ranibizumab in Diabetic Macular Edema With Center Involvement. http://clinicaltrials.gov. Accessed March 24, 2009.

130. Johns Hopkins University. The READ-2 Study: Ranibizumab for Edema of the Macula in Diabetes. http://clinicaltrials.gov. Accessed April 5, 2009.

131. Genentech. A Study of Ranibizumab Injection in Subjects With Clinically Significant Macular Edema With Center Involvement Secondary to Diabetes Mellitus (RISE). http://clinicaltrials.gov. Accessed April 5, 2009.

132. National Eye Institute. Comparison of AMD Treatments Trials (CATT): Lucentis – Avastin Trial. http://www.nei.nih.gov/catt/. Accessed April 5, 2009.

133. Haritoglou C, Kook D, Neubauer A, et al. Intravitreal bevacizumab (Avastin) therapy for persistent diffuse diabetic macular edema. *Retina* 2006;26(9):999–1005.

134. Kook D, Wolf A, Kreutzer T, et al. Long-term effect of intravitreal bevacizumab (avastin) in patients with chronic diffuse diabetic macular edema. *Retina* 2008;28(8):1053–1060.

135. Arevalo JF, Fromow-Guerra J, Quiroz-Mercado H, et al. Primary intravitreal bevacizumab (Avastin) for diabetic macular edema: results from the Pan-American Collaborative Retina Study Group at 6-month follow-up. *Ophthalmology* 2007;114(4):743–750.

136. Arevalo JF, Sanchez JG, Fromow-Guerra J, et al. Comparison of two doses of primary intravitreal bevacizumab (Avastin) for diffuse diabetic macular edema: results from the Pan-American Collaborative Retina Study Group (PACORES) at 12-month follow-up. *Graefes Arch. Clin. Exp. Ophthalmol* 2009;247(6):735–743.

137. Scott IU, Edwards AR, Beck RW, et al. A phase II randomized clinical trial of intravitreal bevacizumab for diabetic macular edema. *Ophthalmology* 2007;114(10):1860–1867.

138. Avery RL, Pearlman J, Pieramici DJ, et al. Intravitreal bevacizumab (Avastin) in the treatment of proliferative diabetic retinopathy. *Ophthalmology* 2006;113(10):1695.e1–1695.e15.

139. Spaide RF, Fisher YL. Intravitreal bevacizumab (Avastin) treatment of proliferative diabetic retinopathy complicated by vitreous hemorrhage. *Retina* 2006;26(3):275–278.

140. Arevalo JF, Wu L, Sanchez JG, et al. Intravitreal bevacizumab (Avastin) for proliferative diabetic retinopathy: 6-months follow-up. *Eye* 2009;23(1):117–123.

141. Minnella AM, Savastano CM, Ziccardi L, et al. Intravitreal bevacizumab (Avastin) in proliferative diabetic retinopathy. *Acta Ophthalmol* 2008;86(6):683–687.

142. Cho W, Oh S, Moon J, et al. Panretinal photocoagulation combined with intravitreal bevacizumab in high-risk proliferative diabetic retinopathy. *Retina* 2009. http://www.ncbi.nlm.nih.gov/pubmed/19262436. Accessed April 5, 2009.

143. Mason J, Yunker J, Vail R, et al. Intravitreal bevacizumab (Avastin) prevention of panretinal photocoagulation-induced complications in patients with severe proliferative diabetic retinopathy. *Retina* 2008;28(9):1319–1324.

144. Tonello M, Costa RA, Almeida FPP, et al. Panretinal photocoagulation versus PRP plus intravitreal bevacizumab for high-risk proliferative diabetic retinopathy (IBeHi study). *Acta Ophthalmol* 2008;86(4):385–389.

145. Jorge R, Costa RA, Calucci D, et al. Intravitreal bevacizumab (Avastin) for persistent new vessels in diabetic retinopathy (IBEPE study). *Retina* 26(9):1006–1013.

146. Oshima Y, Sakaguchi H, Gomi F, et al. Regression of iris neovascularization after intravitreal injection of bevacizumab in patients with proliferative diabetic retinopathy. *Am J Ophthalmol* 2006;142(1):155–158.

147. Wakabayashi T, Oshima Y, Sakaguchi H, et al. Intravitreal bevacizumab to treat iris neovascularization and neovascular glaucoma secondary to ischemic retinal diseases in 41 consecutive cases. *Ophthalmology* 2008;115(9):1571–1580, 1580.e1–1580.e3.

148. Holash J, Davis S, Papadopoulos N, et al. VEGF-Trap: a VEGF blocker with potent antitumor effects. *Proc Natl Acad Sci U S A* 2002;99(17):11393–11398.

149. Saishin Y, Saishin Y, Takahashi K, et al. VEGF-TRAP(R1R2) suppresses choroidal neovascularization and VEGF-induced breakdown of the blood-retinal barrier. *J Cell Physiol* 2003;195(2):241–248.

150. Stewart MW, Rosenfeld PJ. Predicted biological activity of intravitreal VEGF Trap. *Br J Ophthalmol* 2008;92(5):667–668.

151. Do DV, Nguyen QD, Shah SM, et al. An exploratory study of the safety, tolerability and bioactivity of a single intravitreal injection of vascular endothelial growth factor Trap-Eye in patients with diabetic macular oedema. *Br J Ophthalmol* 2009;93(2):144–149.

152. Adis International Limited. Aflibercept: AVE 0005, AVE 005, AVE0005, VEGF Trap – Regeneron, VEGF Trap (R1R2), VEGF Trap-Eye. *Drugs R D* 2008;9(4):261–269.

153. Kuppermann BD, Thomas EL, de Smet MD, et al. Pooled efficacy results from two multinational randomized controlled clinical trials of a single intravitreous injection of highly purified ovine hyaluronidase (Vitrase) for the management of vitreous hemorrhage. *Am J Ophthalmol* 2005;140(4):573–584.

154. Kuppermann BD, Thomas EL, de Smet MD, et al. Safety results of two phase III trials of an intravitreous injection of highly purified ovine hyaluronidase (Vitrase) for the management of vitreous hemorrhage. *Am J Ophthalmol* 2005;140(4):585–597.

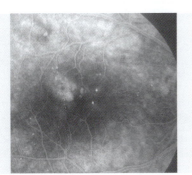

# Laser Treatment for Diabetic Retinopathy (Clinically Significant and Diffuse Macular Edema: Fundamentals of the Early Treatment Diabetic Retinopathy Study)

Yukihiro Sato

Macular edema is the most common cause of vision loss in patients with diabetic retinopathy. There are several reports of randomized clinical trials of photocoagulation for diabetic macular edema (1–6). Among these trials, the Early Treatment Diabetic Retinopathy Study (ETDRS) (5,6) included by far the largest number of patients. The ETDRS was designed to address three major questions in the management of patients with nonproliferative or early proliferative diabetic retinopathy:

■ When in the course of diabetic retinopathy is it most effective to initiate panretinal photocoagulation?
■ Is photocoagulation effective in the treatment of diabetic macular edema?
■ Is aspirin treatment effective in altering the course of diabetic retinopathy?

Because the purpose of this chapter is to clarify the efficacy of macular surgery in diabetic retinopathy, only the answer to the second question is summarized and discussed.

Data from the ETDRS shows that focal photocoagulation for "clinically significant" macular edema (CSME) in diabetic retinopathy substantially reduces the risk of moderate visual loss. Focal treatment also increased the chance of visual improvement, decreases the frequency of persistent macular edema, and causes only minor visual-field losses. The beneficial effects of treatment demonstrated in this trial suggested that all eyes with CSME should be considered for focal photocoagulation, even if visual acuity is not yet reduced. CSME includes not only focal but also diffuse macular edema (5,6). However, the beneficial effects of focal photocoagulation for diffuse macular edema are not clear, given that these eyes respond poorly to treatment as compared to eyes with focal macular edema (3).

## CLASSIFICATION OF DIABETIC MACULAR EDEMA

Bresnick (7,8) classified diabetic macular edema into focal macular edema and diffuse macular edema (Table 21-1). Focal macular edema is characterized by focal leakage mainly from microaneurysms but occasionally from dilated capillaries. This

### TABLE 21-1 CLASSIFICATION OF DIABETIC MACULAR EDEMA

I. Focal leakage
  A. Focal hard exudate rings
  B. Multifocal edema
  C. Perifoveolar edema and exudate
II. Diffuse leakage
  A. Diffuse edema (cystoid)
  B. Systemic factors
    1. Fluid retention (cardiac, renal)
    2. Severe hypertension
    3. Pregnancy
  C. Cystoid macular edema following panretinal photocoagulation

From Bresnick GH. Diabetic macular edema: a review. *Ophthalmology* 1986;93:989–997.

leakage can be demonstrated clearly by intravenous fluorescein angiography. Often there is associated accumulation of extravascular lipoprotein exudate deposition in a circinate pattern (Fig. 21-1). In contrast, diffuse macular edema is characterized by diffuse leakage from retinal vessels in and around the macular area, often accompanied by cystoid macular changes (Fig. 21-2). Bresnick (7) stated that diffuse macular edema may result from not only a breakdown of the inner blood–retinal barrier (*e.g.*, microaneurysms, retinal capillaries, and even arterioles) but also a breakdown of the outer blood–retinal barrier (*i.e.*, retinal pigment epithelium).

## DEFINITION OF CLINICALLY SIGNIFICANT MACULAR EDEMA

The ETDRS (5) defined CSME as the presence of one or more of the following criteria:

■ Thickening of the retina at or within 500 mm of the center of the macula (Fig. 21-3A,B).
■ Hard exudates at or within 500 mm of the center of the macula, if associated with thickening of adjacent retina (not residual hard exudates remaining after disappearance of retinal thickening) (Fig. 21-3C).
■ A zone or zones of retinal thickening one disc area or larger, any part of which is within one disc diameter of the center of the macula (Fig. 21-3D).

## STUDY DESIGN AND TREATMENT METHODS OF THE EARLY TREATMENT DIABETIC RETINOPATHY STUDY

The ETDRS had a somewhat complex randomization scheme (Figs. 21-4–21-6). First, eyes with macular edema were subdivided into two groups: eyes with *less* severe retinopathy (mild-to-moderate nonproliferative retinopathy), and eyes with *more* severe retinopathy (severe nonproliferative or early proliferative retinopathy). Then each subgroup was further randomly assigned to "early (immediate) photocoagulation" or "deferral of photocoagulation" until high-risk proliferative retinopathy developed. High-risk proliferative retinopathy has been previously defined by the Diabetic Retinopathy Study (9) as retinopathy with moderate or severe optic nerve neovascularization or any neovascularization with hemorrhage.

For focal treatment of macular edema, a pretreatment fluorescein angiogram was used during photocoagulation to identify "treatable lesions" (Table 21-2). Treatment was prescribed for all such lesions located within two disc diameters of the center of the macula. Treatment of lesions closer than 500 mm to the macula was not required initially. If vision was less than 20/40, however, and the retinal edema and leakage persisted, treatment of lesions up to 300 mm from the center was recommended. For focal macular edema, microaneurysms and other focal leakage sites received photocoagulation. Areas of diffuse leakage were treated in a grid pattern.

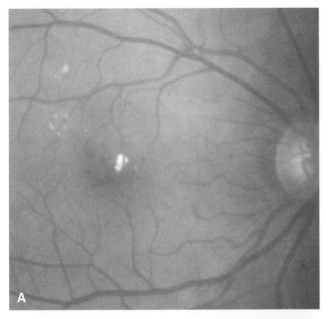

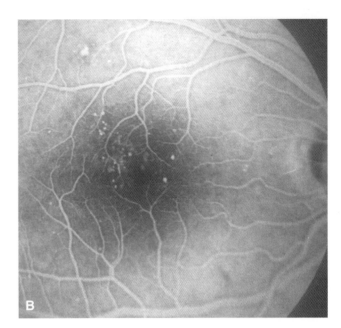

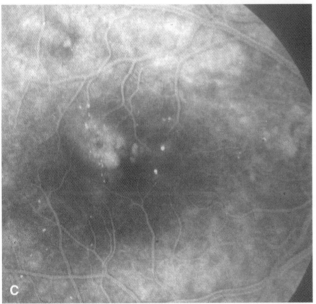

**Figure 21-1.** Focal macular edema. **A:** Right eye. Macular edema with central involvement, multiple microaneurysms scattered around the posterior pole, and hard exudates deposited in the macular and upper temporal area of the posterior pole (visual acuity 20/30). **B:** Early phase of fluorescein angiogram shows clusters of microaneurysms. **C:** Late phase of angiogram shows leakage from microaneurysms.

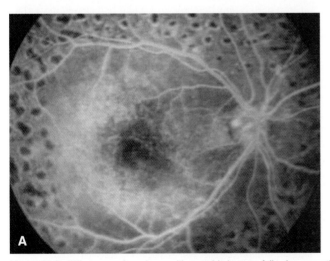

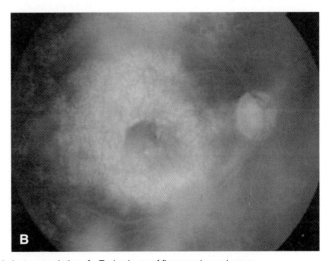

**Figure 21-2.** Diffuse macular edema with cystoid changes following panretinal photocoagulation. **A:** Early phase of fluorescein angiogram shows widespread capillary dilation and leakage in the posterior pole. **B:** Late phase of angiogram shows extensive pooling of dye in cystoid spaces in not only the macular area but also in other areas of the posterior pole (visual acuity 20/60).

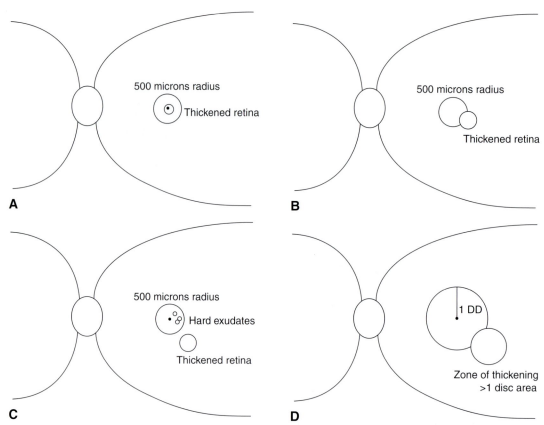

**Figure 21-3.** Definition of clinically significant macular edema. **A:** Thickening of the retina at the center of the macula. **B:** Thickening of the retina within 500 mm of the center of the macula. **C:** Hard exudates at or within 500 mm of the center of the macula with thickening of adjacent retina. **D:** A zone of retinal thickening one disc area or larger, located less than one disc diameter from the center of the macula.

For scatter (panretinal) photocoagulation, eyes were further randomized to either "mild" scatter (400–650 burns) or "full" scatter (1200–1600 burns).

## EYES WITH MACULAR EDEMA AND LESS SEVERE RETINOPATHY

Early (immediate) photocoagulation for eyes with macular edema and less severe retinopathy consisted of 1) immediate focal macular photocoagulation, with delayed scatter photocoagulation (mild or full) added if more severe retinopathy developed during follow-up; and 2) immediate scatter photocoagulation (mild or full), with focal macular photocoagulation delayed at least 4 months.

## RESULTS OF EARLY TREATMENT DIABETIC RETINOPATHY STUDY REPORT NUMBER 1

The first ETDRS report (5) compared the results of immediate focal macular photocoagulation (754 eyes) with the results of deferred photocoagulation (1490 eyes) (Fig. 21-4). The results of the comparison were as follows:

- At 3-year follow-up, 12% of the eyes undergoing immediate treatment and 24% of those undergoing deferred treatment had significant loss of visual acuity.
- Of eyes with a pretreatment visual acuity of 20/40 or worse, 40% of those undergoing immediate treatment and 20% of those undergoing deferred treatment had gained more than one line of visual improvement on the ETDRS visual acuity chart after 2 years' follow-up. Improvement of three or

| TABLE 21-2   CHARACTERISTICS OF TREATABLE LESIONS |
| --- |

1. Discrete points of retinal hyperfluorescence or leakage (most of these are microaneurysms)
2. Areas of diffuse leakage within the retina
   Microaneurysms
   Intraretinal microvascular abnormalities
   Diffuse leaking retinal capillary bed
3. Retinal avascular zones

From Early Treatment Diabetic Retinopathy Study Research Group. Photocoagulation for diabetic macular edema: Early Treatment Diabetic Retinopathy Study report number 1. *Arch Ophthalmol* 1985;103: 1746–1806.

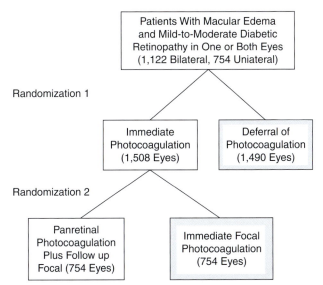

**Figure 21-4.** The Early Treatment Diabetic Retinopathy Study treatment schedule for patients with macular edema and less severe retinopathy in one or both eyes. Randomization 1: All study patients had one eye randomly assigned to immediate photocoagulation, and the other eye to deferral of photocoagulation. Randomization 2: Eyes assigned to immediate photocoagulation were further randomized to either a combination of initial panretinal photocoagulation and follow-up focal macular photocoagulation or immediate focal photocoagulation. Hatched boxes indicate those groups compared in this report. (From Early Treatment Diabetic Retinopathy Study Research Group. Photocoagulation for diabetic macular edema: Early Treatment Diabetic Retinopathy Study report number 1. *Arch Ophthalmol* 1985;103:1796–1806).

more lines, however, was uncommon (<3%) in either group.

■ The beneficial effect of immediate treatment was clearly demonstrated in eyes with CSME. In these eyes, the difference in rate of visual loss between the eyes undergoing immediate treatment and the eyes undergoing deferred treatment was statistically significant at the 8-month follow-up visit and thereafter. In contrast, eyes without CSME did not show a significant treatment effect during the first 2 years.

■ Among eyes with CSME, eyes with involvement of the center of the macula showed a more profound treatment effect compared with eyes without involvement of the center of the macula.

■ If eyes were classified into four groups by severity of retinopathy—1) mild nonproliferative retinopathy; 2) moderate nonproliferative retinopathy of level 1 (at least one of the following was present: soft exudates, intraretinal microvascular abnormalities, or venous beading); 3) moderate nonproliferative retinopathy of level 2 (at least two of those lesions were present); and 4) severe nonproliferative or early proliferative retinopathy—the treatment effect was similar in all four groups. The treatment effect was statistically significant, however, only in the two moderate nonproliferative retinopathy groups.

■ Only minor adverse effects (not statistically significant) on central visual field and no adverse effect on color vision resulting from focal photocoagulation were observed.

Based on these results, the ETDRS report suggested that eyes with CSME should be considered for prompt photo-

coagulation for macular edema, even if visual acuity is not yet reduced, to stabilize visual acuity. In contrast, eyes with macular edema that is not clinically significant can be followed without treatment unless CSME develops.

## RESULTS OF EARLY TREATMENT DIABETIC RETINOPATHY STUDY REPORT NUMBER 9

The ETDRS report number 9 (6) reported the results of photocoagulation for eyes with macular edema and less severe retinopathy, dividing eyes into four subgroups (Fig. 21-5): 1) immediate focal macular photocoagulation, with delayed mild-scatter photocoagulation added if more severe retinopathy developed during follow-up; 2) immediate mild-scatter photocoagulation, with delayed focal photocoagulation after at least 4 months; 3) immediate focal photocoagulation with delayed full-scatter photocoagulation; and 4) immediate full-scatter photocoagulation with delayed focal photocoagulation.

The results of the comparison were as follows:

■ In eyes that did not receive scatter photocoagulation initially, delayed scatter photocoagulation was performed in 10% of eyes after 1 year, in 30% after 3 years, and in 40% after 5 years. Delayed scatter photocoagulation was because of progression to more severe retinopathy in 57% and because of development of high-risk proliferative retinopathy in 43%.

■ In eyes assigned to immediate focal and delayed scatter photocoagulation, the beneficial effect of reducing the overall risk of moderate visual loss was observed from the 1-year follow-up.

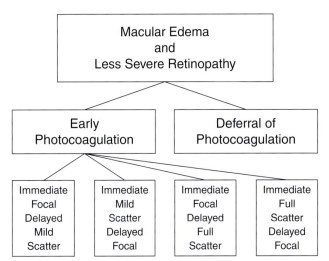

**Figure 21-5.** The Early Treatment Diabetic Retinopathy Study treatment schedule for patients with macular edema and less severe retinopathy. Eyes were assigned randomly to early photocoagulation or to deferral of photocoagulation. Eyes assigned to early photocoagulation were further randomized to either mild- or full-scatter photocoagulation, and to either immediate focal or delayed focal treatment. (From Early Treatment Diabetic Retinopathy Study Research Group. Early photocoagulation for diabetic retinopathy: Early Treatment Diabetic Retinopathy Study report number 9. *Ophthalmology* 1991;98:766–785).

■ Visual loss resulting from scatter photocoagulation was observed at both the 6-week and 4-month visits in eyes assigned to immediate scatter and delayed focal photocoagulation. These harmful effects were more severe for full scatter than mild scatter.

■ The rate of development of retinal thickening at the center of the macula was slower in eyes assigned to immediate focal and delayed scatter photocoagulation than in eyes assigned to immediate scatter and delayed focal photocoagulation.

Based on these results, it was concluded that immediate focal and delayed scatter photocoagulation was the best strategy in eyes with macular edema and less severe retinopathy.

## EYES WITH MACULAR EDEMA AND MORE SEVERE RETINOPATHY

For eyes with macular edema and more severe retinopathy, an increased rate of progression to high-risk proliferative retinopathy was expected compared with that in eyes with less severe retinopathy. Thus, early (immediate) photocoagulation for this group consisted of (a) immediate scatter photocoagulation (mild or full), with immediate focal macular photocoagulation, or (b) immediate scatter photocoagulation (mild or full), with focal photocoagulation delayed at least 4 months (Fig. 21-6).

Basically, the results in this group were similar to those in eyes with less severe retinopathy (6). However, the "pure" effects of immediate focal macular photocoagulation in this

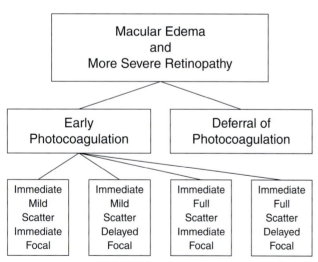

**Figure 21-6.** The Early Treatment Diabetic Retinopathy Study treatment schedule for patients with macular edema and more severe retinopathy. Eyes were assigned randomly to early photocoagulation or to deferral of photocoagulation. Eyes assigned to early photocoagulation were further randomized to either mild- or full-scatter photocoagulation, and to either immediate focal treatment or deferral of focal treatment. (From Early Treatment Diabetic Retinopathy Study Research Group. Early photocoagulation for diabetic retinopathy: Early Treatment Diabetic Retinopathy Study report number 9. *Ophthalmology* 1991;98:766–785).

group could not be identified because all eyes also received immediate scatter photocoagulation (8).

The results of the comparison were as follows:

■ There was a statistically significant adverse effect at 6 weeks with both strategies for immediate mild- or full-scatter photocoagulation. This adverse effect was more severe for full scatter than mild scatter.

■ The beneficial effect of immediate focal treatment to reduce the overall risk of moderate visual loss was observed. This beneficial effect occurred later, however, compared with that in eyes with less severe retinopathy.

■ The rate of development of retinal thickening at the center of the macula was slowest in the eyes assigned to immediate mild scatter and immediate focal photocoagulation.

Thus, it was recommended that immediate mild scatter accompanied by immediate focal photocoagulation was the best strategy in eyes with macular edema and more severe retinopathy.

## IS GRID PATTERN PHOTOCOAGULATION SUFFICIENTLY EFFECTIVE FOR DIFFUSE MACULAR EDEMA?

As mentioned previously, data from ETDRS showed that focal photocoagulation for CSME substantially reduced the risk of moderate visual loss, increased the chance of visual improvement, and decreased the frequency of persistent macular edema. The visual prognosis of photocoagulation for diffuse macular edema, however, may be worse than for focal macular edema (3). Because CSME includes not only focal macular edema but also diffuse macular edema (*i.e.*, the ETDRS did not differentiate these two types of macular edema in its reports), the beneficial effects of focal photocoagulation for diffuse macular edema are not clear.

Grid pattern photocoagulation for diffuse macular edema was first reported by Whitelocke and colleagues (10). Visual improvement by two or more lines was obtained in 25% of treated eyes. Blankenship (3) first reported a randomized clinical trial of macular photocoagulation that included eyes treated with grid photocoagulation for diffuse macular edema. Although he found that the rate of visual improvement was 17% in treated eyes compared with 5% in untreated eyes after 2 years, these results were not statistically significant. Olk (4) reported the results of a randomized clinical trial of modified grid photocoagulation for diffuse macular edema. His study included a large number of patients (160 eyes of 92 patients). A surprisingly higher rate of visual improvement (45%) in treated eyes compared with the control group (8%) was observed. McDonald and Schatz (11), however, reported that 67% of eyes with diffuse macular edema that were treated with grid photocoagulation had decreased edema posttreatment, but only 17% of treated eyes showed improved visual acuity.

Thus, visual improvement following grid treatment for diffuse macular edema may not be sufficiently great, and

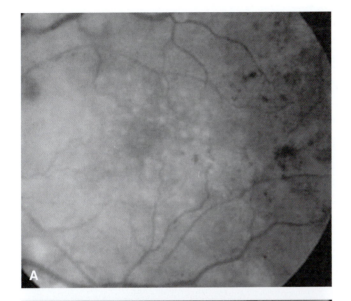

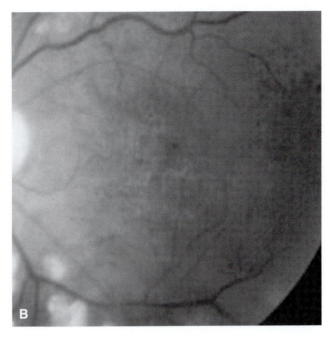

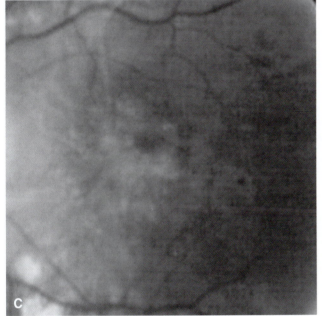

**Figure 21-7.** Progressive enlargement of laser scars following grid photocoagulation. **A:** Left eye. immediately after grid photocoagulation, small white dots indicate photocoagulation burns. **B:** Left macula 6 months after grid photocoagulation. Note the finely pigmented, small discrete laser scars in the macular area. **C:** Four years after grid photocoagulation. Note the area of atrophy in the central macula caused by enlargement and coalescence of laser scars.

progressive enlargement of laser scars following grid photocoagulation may occur (12) (Fig. 21-7). For these reasons, alternative methods for treating macular edema have been developed.

## ALTERNATIVE LASER TREATMENTS FOR MACULAR EDEMA

Conventional grid photocoagulation causes visible laser scars that can enlarge postoperatively (12), as well as complications including choroidal neovascularization, subretinal fibrosis

and visual field loss (13–15). Intrinsic damage from visible end point laser photocoagulation has prompted interest in developing alternative methods for treating macular edema such as vitrectomy (16), subthreshold micropulse diode laser photocoagulation (17–18), and intravitreal or subtenon injection of triamcinolone acetonide (TA) (19).

Management of macular edema using vitrectomy is discussed in another chapter.

Shortening a laser pulse limits the spread of photocoagulation damage caused by heat conduction during laser exposure (17). Subthreshold micropulse diode laser photocoagulation does not create ophthalmoscopically or angiographically detectable lesions. Laursen et al. studied the visual and morphological outcomes of subthreshold micropulse diode laser photocoagulation and conventional argon laser photocoagulation in eyes with diabetic macular edema (18). Changes in macular edema were measured by optical coherence tomography. Subthreshold micropulse diode laser and conventional argon laser treatment produced equally good effects on visual acuity. Subthreshold micropulse diode laser treatment stabilized or even improved macular edema.

Intravitreal injection of TA reportedly improves visual acuity and reduces macular thickness in eyes with diffuse diabetic macular edema (19). However, these beneficial effects do not persist in the long term. Several reports have shown that beneficial effects on visual acuity and macular thickness last less than 24 weeks after treatment because of the macular edema recurrence (20–22). Such recurrence can be treated with repeat intravitreal injections. However, subsequent TA injections might not be as effective as the initial treatment, and may increase the risk of complications such as raised intraocular pressure, cataract development and endophthalmitis. Kang and associates reported the clinical outcomes of modified macular grid laser coagulation performed 3 weeks after an intravitreal injection of TA for diffuse diabetic macular edema (23). This combination therapy seemed to improve visual acuity and reduce macular edema at 3 and 6 months after treatment, as compared with an intravitreal injection only. They concluded that macular laser coagulation reduces macular edema recurrence after intravitreal TA injection.

Posterior subtenon injection of TA has also been reported to effectively reduce macular edema (24). However, its efficacy is likely to be temporary. Shimura and coworkers hypothesized that subtenon injection of TA prior to grid photocoagulation would reduce macular edema, allowing the grid photocoagulation to be performed with minimal laser power, thereby improving prognosis for visual acuity, macular thickness, and visual field sensitivity (25). The effectiveness of this combination therapy against diffuse diabetic macular edema was evaluated in a prospective controlled study comparing it to grid laser treatment alone. Patients previously treated with TA were found to require less laser power and have fewer adverse side effects from grid laser photocoagulation than those treated with the laser alone. TA-assisted grid photocoagulation maintained the improvements in visual acuity and macular thickness for up to 24 weeks without macular edema recurrence.

## References

1. Patz A, Schatz H, Berkow TW, et al. Macular edema—an overlooked complication of diabetic retinopathy. *Trans. Am Academy of Ophthalmol and Otolaryngol* 1973;77:34–42.
2. British Multicenter Study Group. Photocoagulation for diabetic maculopathy: a randomized controlled clinical trial using xenon arc. *Diabetes* 1983;32:1010–1016.
3. Blankenship GW. Diabetic macular edema and argon laser photocoagulation: a prospective randomized study. *Ophthalmology* 1979;86:69–78.
4. Olk RJ. Modified grid argon (blue-green) laser photocoagulation for diffuse macular edema. *Ophthalmology* 1986;93:938–950.
5. Early Treatment Diabetic Retinopathy Study Research Group. Photocoagulation for diabetic macular edema: Early Treatment Diabetic Retinopathy Study report number 1. *Arch Ophthalmol* 1985;103:1796–1806.
6. Early Treatment Diabetic Retinopathy Study Research Group. Early photocoagulation for diabetic retinopathy: Early Treatment Diabetic Retinopathy Study report number 9. *Ophthalmology* 1991;98:766–785.
7. Bresnick GH. Diabetic maculopathy: a critical review highlighting diffuse macular edema. *Ophthalmology* 1983;90:1301–1317.
8. Bresnick GH. Diabetic macular edema: a review. *Ophthalmology* 1986;93:989–997.
9. Diabetic Retinopathy Study Research Group. Four risk factors for severe visual loss in diabetic retinopathy: Diabetic Retinopathy Study report number 3. *Arch Ophthalmol* 1979;97:654–655.
10. Whitelocke RAF, Kearns M, Blach RK, et al. The diabetic maculopathies. *Trans Ophthal Soc UK* 1979;99:314–320.
11. McDonald HR, Schatz H. Grid photocoagulation for diffuse macular edema. *Retina* 1985;5:65–72.
12. Schatz H, Madeira D, McDonald HR, et al. Progressive enlargement of laser scars following grid laser photocoagulation for diffuse diabetic macular edema. *Arch Ophthalmol* 1991;109:1549–1551.
13. Lewis H, Schachat AP, Haimann MH, et al. Choroidal neovascularization after laser photocoagulation for diabetic macular edema. *Ophthalmology* 1990;97:503–510.
14. Rutledge BK, Wallow IHL, Poulsen GL. Sub-pigment epithelial membranes after photocoagulation for diabetic macular edema. *Arch Ophthalmol* 1993;111:608–613.
15. Striph GG, Hart WM Jr, Olk RJ. Modified grid laser photocoagulation for diabetic macular edema. The effect on the central visual field. *Ophthalmology* 1988;95:1673–1679.
16. Tachi N, Ogino N. Vitrectomy for diffuse macular edema in cases of diabetic retinopathy. *Am J Ophthalmol* 1996;122:258–260.
17. Luttrull JK, Musch DC, Mainster MA. Subthreshold diode micropulse photocoagulation for the treatment of clinically significant diabetic macular oedema. *Br J Ophthalmol* 2005;89:74–80.
18. Laursen ML, Moeller F, Sander B, et al. Subthreshold micropulse diode laser treatment in diabetic macular oedema. *Br J Ophthalmol* 2004;88:1173–1179.
19. Jonas JB, Sofker A. Intraocular injection of crystalline cortisone as adjunctive treatment of diabetic macular edema. *Am J Ophthalmol* 2001;132:425–427.
20. Martidis A, Duker JS, Greenberg PB, et al. Intravitreal triamcinolone for refractory diabetic macular edema. *Ophthalmology* 2002;109:920–957.
21. Jonas JB, Kreissig I, Sofker A, et al. Intravitreal injection of triamcinolone for diffuse diabetic macular edema. *Arch Ophthalmol* 2003;121:57–61.
22. Massin P, Audren F, Haouchine B, et al. Intravitreal triamcinolone acetonide for diabetic diffuse macular edema. Preliminary results of a prospective controlled trial. *Ophthalmology* 2004;111:218–225.
23. Kang SW, Sa H, Cho HY, et al. Macular grid photocoagulation after intravitreal triamcinolone acetonide for diffuse diabetic macular edema. *Arch Ophthalmol* 2006;124:653–658.
24. Ohguro N, Okada AA, Tano Y. Trans-Tenon's retrobulbar triamcinolone infusion for diffuse diabetic macular edema. *Grafe's Arch Clin Exp Ophthalmol* 2004;242:444–445.
25. Shimura M, Nakazawa T, Yasuda K, et al. Pretreatment of posterior subtenon injection of triamcinolone acetonide has beneficial effects for grid pattern photocoagulation against diffuse diabetic macular edema. *Br J Ophthalmol* 2007;91:449–454.

# Vitreous Surgery for Diabetic Retinopathy

Monica Rodriguez-Fontal ■ John B. Kerrison

# INTRODUCTION

Laser therapy and tight metabolic control of blood glucose are indispensable strategies in full-scope management of diabetic retinopathy. A number of eyes, however, will progress toward candidacy for surgical treatment despite aggressive implementation of these valuable interventions. According to the Early Treatment Diabetic Retinopathy Study, 5.3% of eyes receiving optimal medical treatment will still have progressive retinopathy that requires laser treatment and *pars plana* vitrectomy (PPV) (1).

Several complications of advanced diabetic retinopathy can be treated surgically. Vitrectomy can clear media opacities, relieve traction on the retina, make adequate laser treatment of the retina possible, and stabilize the proliferation process. Removal of premacular vitreous may also improve diabetic macular edema (DME).

Machemer and colleagues developed the PPV technique in 1971. The objective for Machemer vitrectomy was treating nonclearing vitreous hemorrhage from proliferative diabetic retinopathy. There have been many changes in the indications and in the timing for vitrectomy in diabetic retinopathy. New instrumentation, better understanding of the pathophysiology of the disease, development of surgical skills, and supplementary pharmacotherapy have improved surgical results (2–5).

The Diabetic Retinopathy Vitrectomy Study (6–8) was designed to evaluate the risks and benefits of performing early PPV in eyes with advanced proliferative diabetic retinopathy. The results from this study provide a better-defined role and timing of vitrectomy surgery for these conditions. The results of the study were obtained before the development of endolaser photocoagulation. Endophotocoagulation may be considered one of the most important reasons for performing a vitrectomy (9–12).

This book chapter will review the indications, techniques, results and complications of performing PPV for diabetic retinopathy.

# INDICATIONS

Vitreous hemorrhage, traction retinal detachment involving the macula, and combined traction/rhegmatogenous retinal detachment are the classic indications (13,14). The major indications for vitrectomy in diabetic retinopathy are summarized in Table 22-1. In 1987, Aaberg et al. (14) published a review that found that 15% of cases were performed exclusively for vitreous hemorrhage, 40% for traction macular detachment, and 35% for combined traction/rhegmatogenous retinal detachment. The remaining indications were severe fibrovascular proliferation, dense preretinal (premacular) hemorrhage, and other less common conditions (massive postvitrectomy fibrin response, progressive fibrolental proliferation). DME associated or not with posterior hyaloidal traction has been recognized as an indication for vitrectomy (15–17). Vitreopapillary traction may be an additional indication for vitrectomy (18).

## TABLE 22-1 INDICATIONS FOR VITRECTOMY

**Media opacities**
A. Nonclearing hemorrhage
  1. Vitreous
  2. Subhyaloid, premacular hemorrhage
  3. Anterior segment neovascularization with posterior segment opacity
B. Cataract preventing treatment of severe proliferative diabetic retinopathy (lensectomy)

**Traction defects**
A. Progressive fibrovascular proliferation
B. Traction retinal detachment involving the macula
C. Combined traction and rhegmatogenous retinal detachment
D. Macular edema associated with taut, persistently attached posterior hyaloids
E. Vitreopapillary traction

**Other indications**
A. Ghost cell glaucoma
B. Anterior hyaloidal fibrovascular proliferation
C. Fibrinoid syndrome
D. Epiretinal membrane (nonvascularized)

# VITREOUS HEMORRHAGE

Historically, the first indication for PPV was severe diabetic vitreous hemorrhage. As a result of the development of new techniques, the distribution of cases undergoing vitrectomy for vitreous hemorrhage decreased from about 70% in 1977 to about 20% in 1987 (14). Despite the extensive use of the panretinal photocoagulation, severe vitreous hemorrhages remain a very common reason for vitreous surgery. The surgical objectives include removal of vitreous hemorrhage to provide a clear medium, excision of the posterior hyaloid and epiretinal fibrovascular membranes to relieve vitreoretinal traction, and endolaser photocoagulation to achieve regression of proliferative tissue. The Diabetic Retinopathy Vitrectomy Study (7) demonstrated that diabetic type 1 patients had a more favorable visual outcome if the vitrectomy was performed in the first 6 months than with deferral for 1 year. For type 2 diabetic patients, the study did not show a significant difference in the 2 groups.

In general the recommended timing of vitrectomy for severe vitreous hemorrhage is before 3 months for type 1 patients and before 6 months for type 2 patients (19). Since type 2 diabetics more commonly have spontaneous resolution of hemorrhage and slower progression of fibrovascular proliferation, the usual approach for patients with type 2 diabetes is to defer surgical intervention longer than for patients with type 1 diabetes.

Several clinical features influence the recommended timing of vitrectomy for diabetic vitreous hemorrhage. Earlier surgical intervention is generally recommended when no previous laser treatment has been performed, when the fibrovascular proliferation complexes are more extensive and more vascular, when the fellow eye has rapidly progressive visual loss, or when the fellow eye is blind.

## TRACTION AND COMBINED RETINAL DETACHMENT

The tractional defects constitute the majority of patients undergoing vitrectomy for complications of diabetic retinopathy. The spectrum of tractional involvement includes macular heterotopia, traction retinal detachment, and rhegmatogenous retinal detachment with a retinal break caused by progressive traction.

The most common indication for vitrectomy in diabetic patients is a traction detachment involving the macula. The main goal with the vitrectomy in these eyes is to relieve vitreoretinal traction by excision of the posterior hyaloid and epiretinal fibrovascular membranes (14,20–23). The prognosis is better in cases with a short duration of the detachment, limited extension of the detachment, the presence of previous photocoagulation, and the absence of vitreous hemorrhage or severe neovascularization (21,23,24).

It is hard to predict when an extramacular detachment is going to progress and involve the macula. Because peripheral or midperipheral traction retinal detachments progress to involve the macula in only about 15% of cases per year, (25) caution is advised in recommending vitrectomy. Studies have demonstrated that early vitrectomy may benefits patients with progressive traction detachment that threatens the macula. (26). Macular detachment for a period greater than 6 months precludes the return of useful vision, and surgery may not be indicated.

Combined traction and rhegmatogenous detachment is an indication of vitrectomy regardless of the macular status. Combined detachment cases account for 17% to 35% of the diabetic eyes undergoing vitrectomy (14,27). Progressive fibrosis and traction may lead to a retinal break resulting in a combined detachment. The break is usually small, posterior to the equator, and adjacent to the fibrovascular proliferation. Combined retinal detachment in proliferative diabetic retinopathy may occur in the setting of active fibrovascular proliferation or as a late complication. It is frequently associated with tightly adherent preretinal tissue and extensive detachment. Preoperative visual acuity best predicts visual prognosis (28).

## SEVERE FIBROVASCULAR PROLIFERATION

Vitrectomy is indicated for patients with an attached hyaloid with active neovascular and fibrovascular proliferation despite extensive photocoagulation. If the vitreous and hyaloid is not removed, the fibrovascular tissue can undergo contraction, resulting in vitreous hemorrhage and retinal detachment. The vitrectomy study demonstrated more favorable visual and anatomic outcome with early vitrectomy than with conventional management (29,30).

## DIABETIC MACULAR EDEMA

DME accounts for 72% of blind patients with diabetes mellitus (31). Of the diabetic population, 9% develop macular edema, and 40% of these individuals have central macular involvement. (32). A small percentage of these patients have thickened posterior hyaloid associated with macular traction and diffuse macular edema. The patients with macular traction and diffuse macular edema have usually failed to respond to one or more prior macular photocoagulation sessions, and visual acuity is moderately reduced.

The vitreous is may contribute to the pathogenesis of DME. In the presence of vitreomacular separation, the macula edema is more likely to resolve (33). Lewis et al. (34) were first to describe a positive effect of PPV on diabetic patients who had a thickened posterior hyaloid membrane with traction on the macula. Tangential vitreomacular tractional forces combined with the local presence of a number of cytokines and growth factors (35) are thought to contribute to the development of DME.

From the pathophysiological point of view, vitrectomy could relieve the retina from the traction forces. Optical coherence tomography (OCT) facilitates the visualization of the vitreoretinal interface and the identification of eyes with diffuse macula edema that should benefit from surgery. Vitrectomy may also improve the oxygen and nutrients supply from the vitreous cavity to the macula. The condensed posterior premacular hyaloid may prevent diffusion caused by the accumulation of cytokines (produced by the ischemic retina) which may lead to a diffuse breakdown of the inner blood-retinal barrier, thus generating diffuse edema. After vitrectomy, these cytokines may escape easier into the vitreous cavity.

Several studies have reported favorable outcomes of PPV for diabetic eyes with or without visible taut and thickened posterior hyaloid (36,37). The surgical goals in these cases include opening, elevating, and removing the posterior hyaloid with or without peeling of the internal limiting membrane (ILM).

Combinations of the mechanical surgical approach with pharmacological adjuncts (intravitreal bevacizumab or intravitreal triamcinolone) may further improve success rates for the treatment of diffuse DME.

## OTHER INDICATIONS: PREMACULAR HEMORRHAGE

This is characterized by blood that is tightly confined between the macula and the posterior vitreous face of an incomplete vitreous detachment without a fully separated posterior hyaloid. 6% to 10% of vitrectomies are performed for this indication (38,39).

Usually, the hemorrhage is oval and obscures the fundus detail. Some of these hemorrhages clear spontaneously; in spite of that, surgical intervention should be considered relatively early in course to prompt recovery of visual acuity and to prevent severe macular traction or wrinkling of the fovea. The presence of hemorrhage in contact with the hyaloid face and ILM stimulates the growth of fibrous tissue. The fibrovascular tissue may contract and result in macular traction detachment.

## OTHER INDICATIONS: ANTERIOR SEGMENT NEOVASCULARIZATION

When iris or angle neovascularization is present in eyes with vitreous hemorrhage, panretinal photocoagulation cannot be performed; so, vitrectomy surgery with endolaser photocoagulation is indicated. The goal of the vitrectomy in these cases is preventing the neovascular glaucoma (40,41).

In eyes with established neovascular glaucoma, vitrectomy surgery in conjunction with a glaucoma procedure (tube implantation) is sometimes indicated (42,43).

## OTHER INDICATIONS: GHOST-CELL/HEMOLYTIC GLAUCOMA

After vitreous hemorrhage, glaucoma can develop. The reason for elevation of intraocular pressure (IOP) may result from impedance of outflow in the trabecular meshwork. Erythroclastic cells (ghost cells) are large in size and cannot pass through the trabecular meshwork. Blood-induced open-angle glaucoma may also result from erythrocytic debris and/or macrophages containing erythrocytic debris (hemolytic cells). The indication for vitrectomy surgery is uncontrolled IOP despite maximal medical therapy (44,45).

## SURGICAL TECHNIQUE

The surgical objectives of vitrectomy are to address the complications of proliferative diabetic retinopathy that result in visual loss. The goals of vitrectomy are to remove axial opacities, relieve anterior-posterior and tangential traction, control hemostasis, deliver laser treatment, and treat retinal breaks.

A variety of equipment and instruments may be used to achieve these objectives. Instruments like intraocular infusion fluids, contact lenses and wide-angle viewing systems, vitreous cutting instruments, ultrasonic phacofragmentation devices, fiberoptic illuminators, diathermy instruments, photocoagulation devices, cryoprobes, as well as a variety of intraocular blades, cannulas, scissors, forceps, and picks. Long-acting gases and silicone oil are additional agents that remain in the eye for an extended period of time. The typical vitreous cutter is 20-gauge; however, 23-gauge and 25-gauge instruments are available.

## VITRECTOMY AND MEMBRANECTOMY FOR VITREORETINAL TRACTION

The degree of posterior vitreous separation and pathoanatomy determine the approach to vitrectomy. In most cases, the selected surgical approach is customized as a hybrid of all techniques.

## Complete Posterior Vitreous Detachment

The usual indication for surgery in this case is nonclearing vitreous hemorrhage. A core vitrectomy is performed to remove the central vitreous. After one opening is created in the hyaloid, it should be enlarged circumferentially; hemorrhage over the posterior pole is aspirated with a soft tipped cannula. Peripheral vitreous should be excised in order to allow more complete laser treatment and improved postoperative fundus examination. In phakic eyes, extensive peripheral vitrectomy is not usually done because of the risk of damage to the lens and peripheral retina.

## Incomplete Posterior Vitreous Detachment and No Posterior Vitreous Detachment

The surgery is directed at separating the posterior hyaloid. Several surgical techniques for membrane removal have been developed, including segmentation, delamination, and en bloc segmentation. In an incomplete posterior vitreous detachment, the outer cortical vitreous can usually be identified as the central formed vitreous is removed. In areas with wide separation between the cortical vitreous and retina, the vitreous cutter may be used to incise the posterior hyaloid to gain access to the subhyaloid space. In the presence of a small separation, care must be taken to avoid damage to the retina while entering the subhyaloid space. When minimal vitreous separation is present, an opening may be made with a myringo-vitreal-retinal (MVR) blade. In eyes with no posterior vitreous separation, the subhyaloid space cannot be entered in the mid periphery with the cutter; usually the separations are easily founded adjacent to fibrovascular epicenter of proliferation or areas of clotted blood. The peripapillary area is typically a good place to start dissection with an MVR blade used to enter the subhyaloid space adjacent to the optic nerve head. In some cases, a condensed vitreous strand inserts at a vascular epicenter and forms a bridge between the membrane and the vitreous base, creating the illusion of a partially separated posterior hyaloid (vitreoschisis). The extent of the split is variable and may range from only a partial division surrounding a single vascular epicenter to a total division where there is no separation of the entire posterior hyaloid. The presence of posterior vitreoschisis should be recognized. If this phenomenon is unrecognized when extirpating a vitreoretinal adhesion, only the inner wall of the vitreoschisis cavity will be excised and the traction may be unrelieved.

Several surgical techniques have been developed for a membranectomy: the segmentation technique, the delamination technique, and the en bloc technique.

## Segmentation

In the segmentation technique, the traction is sequentially dissected and isolated in independent segments. The vertical scissors are the preferable instrument for this step. The bottom blade of the scissors is used as a pick to define and as a blunt dissector. The direction of the dissection should be from posterior to anterior to avoid excess of unrecognized traction on thinner peripheral retina. The cleavage plane can be developed at the edge of the optic disc, directly over a region of subhyaloid hemorrhage, or in some cases, the posterior hyaloid may be seen to be shallowly elevated from some portion of the retina.

## Delamination

This technique involves cutting the connections between the posterior hyaloid and fibrovascular tissue and the ILM. The anterior to posterior traction is commonly removed first. Horizontal scissors are used to remove preretinal tissue at the retinal plane as one or more pieces.

## En Bloc Technique

The surface of the traction is removed with scissors as a confluent piece, with the anteroposterior vitreous traction used for counter-traction. The counter-traction retracts tissue from the retinal surface to facilitate the dissection. The en bloc technique clearly makes the dissection with vitreoretinal scissors easier by maintaining fixation of the epicenter during cutting. Removal of the anteroposterior traction and vitreous is the last step.

## Adjunctive Maneuvers

Several adjunctive maneuvers have been described to facilitate the membranectomy.

Viscodissection involves the use of viscoelastic material in the space between the sheet of fibrovascular membrane and the retina (46,47). Viscodissection, first described by Stenkula and Tornquist (46), is a surgical dissection technique that facilitates removal of epiretinal membranes. The idea is to use less force and distribute the forces more evenly in order to avoid retinal breaks. This technique also better defines the fibrovascular tissue and isolates possible hemorrhage. This step is also an especially useful technique in the presence of atrophic, thin retina.

Tissue plasminogen activator (tPA) injection 15 minutes before the surgery has been proposed to help with the membrane dissection (48).

Perfluorocarbon liquids were introduced in retina surgery in 1987 by Chang (49). The main use is retina stabilization in case of large retinal detachments. The heavy liquids help to keep the posterior retina attached while the anterior dissection is completed, and also contain the intraoperative bleeding. Recently it has been proposed that perfluorocarbon liquids facilitate the dissection of epiretinal membranes and the posterior hyaloid. The perfluorodissection requires the injection of the perfluorocarbon in between the retina and the posterior hyaloid to separate the epiretinal tissue from the adjacent retina (50).

## PHOTOCOAGULATION AND HEMORRHAGE CONTROL

An important surgical objective is endolaser panretinal photocoagulation. Laser endophotocoagulation is performed during diabetic vitrectomy in order to achieve regression of neovascular proliferation and to create chorioretinal adhesions around retinal breaks.

Intraoperative hemostasis can be achieved by using intravitreal diathermy, increasing the intraocular infusion pressure, or by using intraocular thrombin.

## TAMPONADE

After fluid-air exchange, air, long-acting gas ($SF_6$ or $C_3F_8$) or silicon oil can be used as tamponade. Liquid silicone provides a permanent tamponade which, can be used in eyes with recurrent hemorrhage, in patients that require early visual recovery especially after failed vitrectomy, in eyes with multiple and large retinal defects, and in cases of progressive anterior segment neovascularization. It is important to remove all the traction tissue before tamponade with silicone. Growth factors can reach a high concentration in the fluid in between the retina and the silicone bubble which may increase the tendency for fibrovascular reproliferation. In the presence of anterior segment neovascularization, silicon oil prevents the diffusion of the growth factors from the retina to the anterior segment.

## ADDITIONAL PROCEDURES

Scleral buckling and relaxing retinectomies are procedures used in cases of severe proliferation and adhesions. A buckle can relieve peripheral traction in cases where the vitrectomy and the membranectomy were insufficient or in case of combined retinal detachment with a peripheral break. Relaxing retinectomy should be performed when other methods have failed or have a poor chance of success. Classic indications of retinectomy during reoperation are redetachment with anterior fibrovascular proliferation and redetachment with fibrous proliferation and contraction at prior sclerotomy sites. Diabetic eyes requiring relaxing retinectomy have a poorer prognosis than those not requiring retinectomy (51).

## COMPLICATIONS

Postoperative complications are common after vitrectomy for diabetic retinopathy. Elevated IOP, corneal defects, and lens opacification are common to the surgery and not unique in diabetic retinopathy. The principal complications of PPV in diabetic retinopathy are: vitreous hemorrhage, retinal detachment and rubeosis iridis with neovascular glaucoma.

## VITREOUS HEMORRHAGE

Some degree of vitreous hemorrhage after vitrectomy surgery can be observed in all the cases (52). The published incidence is as high as 75% of the cases. It is considered severe in around 30% of the cases (52). Postoperative vitreous hemorrhage is more common and resolves more slowly in phakic eyes than in aphakic eyes (53,54). The majority of recurrent hemorrhages occur in the first 6 months after surgery, and 80% occur within the first year.

Early postoperative vitreous cavity hemorrhage may occur from residual fibrovascular tissue or from dispersion of residual blood remaining on the retinal surface or within the peripheral vitreous skirt. Usually these hemorrhages clear spontaneously within days to weeks of their onset.

Some hemorrhages do not clear spontaneously. These hemorrhages are associated to fibrovascular proliferation of the sclerotomy site or with recalcitrant retinal fibrovascular proliferation. Fluid-gas exchange (procedure performed at the doctor's office), or repeat vitrectomy (performed in the operating room) are some of the treatment options for these cases.

## NEOVASCULAR GLAUCOMA

The incidence of iris neovascularization after diabetic vitrectomy was 8% to 26% in phakic eyes and 31% to 55% in aphakic eyes in early studies (55,56). More recently, with current vitreoretinal instrumentation and techniques, the incidence of postoperative rubeosis and neovascular glaucoma is lower, around 8.5% (57).

The mechanism involved in the development of iris neovascularization is related to the degree of retinal ischemia and growth factors. In eyes with active preretinal neovascularization these new vessels contribute to the supply of oxygen and nutrients to the inner retina. Surgical removal of these vessels will, in theory, aggravate retinal ischemia and stimulate production of growth factors. The vitreous removal also provides an easier diffusion of these growth factors to the anterior segment. The surgical removal of the lens makes the diffusion of these factors easier.

An extensive laser photocoagulation can help to prevent this complication. Silicone oil is a good tamponade option in cases of iris neovascularization. Regression of neovascularization after silicone oil infusion has been reported in 36 -43% of the cases (58,59). In patients with poorly controlled neovascular glaucoma, procedures such as Molteno or Baerveldt tube placement may be considered.

## RETINAL DETACHMENT

Vitrectomy surgery in diabetic patients may lead to breakdown of the blood-retinal barrier that can subsequently results in intraocular fibrin deposition. In some patients, fibrin forms in the anterior chamber and may lead to pupillary block; in others, massive fibrin formation (fibrinoid syndrome) occurs in the vitreous cavity and may lead traction retinal detachment, ciliary body detachment with resultant hypotony, or rubeosis with neovascular glaucoma. Risk factors for fibrin formation after diabetic vitrectomy include lensectomy, extensive membrane dissection, scleral buckle placement, and extensive panretinal photocoagulation.

Steroid injection at the end of surgery and frequent topical corticosteroid treatment are given as prophylaxis against postoperative inflammation and fibrin. When a significant fibrin response occurs, select patients should be treated with recombinant tPA. Indications for tPA are pupillary block with elevation of the IOP or fibrin that obstructs the pupil and interferes with postoperative management.

## ANTERIOR HYALOIDAL FIBROVASCULAR PROLIFERATION

Anterior hyaloidal fibrovascular proliferation (AHFVP) typically occurs in young patients with long standing diabetes and extensive retinal ischemia with a progressive neovascularization despite aggressive laser treatment. This condition is seen in up to 13% of cases (60) and becomes apparent with hemorrhage into the vitreous cavity 3 to 12 weeks after vitrectomy. The hemorrhage is the result of fibrovascular proliferation from the peripheral retina extending toward the equator of the lens and on to the posterior lens capsule. In early stages, extensive photocoagulation can help, otherwise another vitrectomy is indicated.

In general, eyes undergoing several vitrectomies for complications of previous surgeries have a poor visual prognosis. Brown et al. (61) published in 1992 their results for reoperations in 41 eyes. The primary causes for reoperation included rhegmatogenous retinal detachment in 44% of the eyes, recurrent vitreous hemorrhage in 51%, and glaucoma in 5%. Among the total group of 41 eyes that required subsequent surgery, the retina eventually remained detached in 18 eyes (44%), and phthisis bulbi occurred in 13 eyes (32%). Rubeosis iridis developed in 17 (94%) of 18 eyes in which the retina remained detached.

Intravitreal Avastin (bevacizumab) is being used as an adjunct therapy before the vitrectomy to prevent complications during surgery and as treatment for some of the complications after the surgery. Intravitreal Avastin 5 to 7 days before surgery has been proposed in order to reduce potential intraoperative bleeding and surgical timing (62). It is worth noting that Maya and Flynn found the incidence of tractional retinal detachment after the injection to be of 4.7%. The authors thought the detachment was related to the fast neovascular involution with fibrosis contraction (Maya M, Flynn HW et al., 2007 ARVO poster abstract 1430).

## SURGICAL RESULTS

### Vitreous Hemorrhage and Severe Fibrovascular Proliferation

The results of vitrectomy for nonclearing vitreous hemorrhage have been reported and reviewed extensively. Vision improves in 59% to 83% of patients, and final visual acuity of 20/200 or better is achieved in 40% to 62% of the cases.

The Diabetic Retinopathy Vitrectomy Study (DRVS) enrolled and managed patients between 1976 and 1980, during the early days of vitrectomy surgery. The first report was published in 1985 (6). Three groups were part of the vitrectomy trial: 2 groups involving vitrectomy (groups H and NR) and 1 a natural history group (N).

Group H involved eyes with severe vitreous hemorrhage for 1 to 6 months and visual acuity of 5/200 or less; the eyes of this group were randomized to early vitrectomy group versus deferral group. After 2 years, 25% of the eyes in the early vitrectomy group had visual acuity of 10/20 or better versus 15% of the eyes in the deferral group. There was an advantage of performing early vitrectomy in patients with type 1 diabetes. Of the patients with type 1 diabetes, 36% of eyes in the early vitrectomy group had 10/20 or better visual acuity versus 12% of eyes in the deferral group. There did not appear to be a significant advantage of early vitrectomy in patients with Type 2 diabetes; 18% of eyes in the early vitrectomy group had 10/20 or better visual acuity versus 16% of eyes in the deferral group (7). The advantage for early vitrectomy remained after 4 years of follow up.

The DRVS also demonstrated that progression to no light perception was similar for the early and the deferral groups at 2 years (25% versus 19%).

Group NR involved eyes with active proliferative diabetic retinopathy or fibrovascular proliferation and vision better than 10/200. After 4 years, 44% of eyes in the early vitrectomy group had 20/40 or better versus 28% in the conventional group (observation, photocoagulation, or vitrectomy only after traction macular detachment or 6 months of nonclearing vitreous hemorrhage). The advantage of early vitrectomy was most evident in eyes with severe proliferation. The final recommendations were to perform early vitrectomy in cases of severe extensive neovascularization (30).

These results were obtained before the development of endolaser photocoagulation, and the surgeries were performed without the benefit of using glucose-fortified solutions to reduce intraoperative lens opacity. These advances have contributed to more favorable results.

## RETINAL DETACHMENT

Vitrectomy for retinal detachment in diabetic patients has a 49% to 75% rate of visual improvement (20,21,23). Macular reattachment was achieved in 66% to 88% of the eyes. 59% to 71% of the eyes had a final visual acuity of 5/200 or better (23,63). The visual results remain limited by preoperative alterations in retinal function; macular ischemia and macular edema, often present, are the main reason for the visual acuity results.

Eyes with combined retinal detachment have slightly worse results. Forty-eight percent to 70% improved visual acuity after surgery; 45% to 56% had a final visual acuity better than 5/200 (28,63–65). The preoperative visual acuity is the factor most associated with postoperative visual outcome.

## DIABETIC MACULAR EDEMA

Several uncontrolled studies have shown the beneficial effects of the vitrectomy on eyes with macular edema associated with thickened and persistent attached posterior hyaloid. The anatomical results after vitrectomy with or without peeling of the ILM are very promising, even though the visual acuity recovery does not always shows the same promising results (Table 22-2) (66–70).

| TABLE 22-2 | VISUAL ACUITY RESULTS AFTER PARS PLANA VITRECTOMY FOR DME | | | |
|---|---|---|---|---|
| Author | Eyes | Technique | Improved VA | Reduction on OCT |
| Jahn 2004 (66) | 30 | PPV/ILM removal | 56% | – |
| Rosenblatt 2005 (67) | 26 | PPV/ILM removal | 50% | – |
| Dillinger 2004 (68) | 60 | PPV/ILM removal | 43% | 93% |
| Yanyali 2007 (69) | 27 | PPV/ILM removal | 37% | 81% |
| Hartley 2008 (70) | 24 | PPV/ILM removal | 25% | – |

PPV, pars plana vitrectomy; ILM, internal limiting membrane; OCT, optical coherence tomography.

## CONCLUSION

Many complications of advanced diabetic retinopathy can be treated surgically. Vitrectomy can clear media opacities, relieve traction on the retina, make adequate laser treatment of the retina possible, and stabilize the proliferation process. Removal of premacular vitreous may also improve DME. Despite new surgical techniques, advanced diabetic retinopathy is a severe disease with a guarded prognosis. The 5 year survival rate for patients who undergo vitrectomy is 75%. Factors associated with a lower survival rate include age, duration of the diabetes, and complications of diabetes.

### References

1. Flynn HW, Chew EY, Simons BD, et al. Pars plana vitrectomy in the Early Treatment Diabetic Retinopathy Study. ETDRS report number 17. The Early Treatment Diabetic Retinopathy Study Research Group. *Ophthalmology* 1992;99:1351–1357.
2. Helbig H, Sutter FK. Surgical treatment of diabetic retinopathy. *Graefes Arch Clin Exp Ophthalmol* 2004;242:704–709.
3. Mason JO III, Colagross CT, Haleman T, et al. Visual outcome and risk factors for light perception vision after vitrectomy for diabetic retinopathy. *Am J Ophthalmol* 2005;140:231–235.
4. Blankenship GW. Preoperative prognostic factors in diabetic pars plana vitrectomy. *Ophthalmology* 1982;89:1246–1249.
5. Machemer R, Hickingbotham D. The three-port microcannular system for closed vitrectomy. *Am J Ophthalmol* 1985;100:590–592.
6. Diabetic Retinopathy Study Research Group. Preliminary report on effects of photocoagulation therapy. *Am J Ophthalmol* 1976;81:383–3967.
7. Diabetic Retinopathy Vitrectomy Study Research Group. Early vitrectomy for severe vitreous hemorrhage in diabetic retinopathy: two-year results of a randomized trial, Diabetic Retinopathy Vitrectomy Study report 2. *Arch Ophthalmol* 1985;103:1644–1652.
8. Diabetic Retinopathy Vitrectomy Study Research Group. Early vitrectomy for severe vitreous hemorrhage in diabetic retinopathy: four-year results of a randomized trial, Diabetic Retinopathy Vitrectomy Study report 5. *Arch Ophthalmol* 1990;108:958–964.
9. Charles S. Endophotocoagulation. *Retina* 1981;1:117–120.
10. Fleischman JA, Swartz M, Dixon JA. Argon laser endophotocoagulation: an intraoperative trans-pars plana technique. *Arch Ophthalmol* 1981;99:1610–1612.
11. Landers MB, Trese MT, Stefansson E, et al. Argon laser intraocular photocoagulation. *Ophthalmology* 1982;89:785–788.

12. Parke DW III, Aaberg TM. Intraocular argon laser photocoagulation in the management of severe proliferative vitreoretinopathy. *Am J Ophthalmol* 1984;97:434–443.

13. Aaberg TM. Vitrectomy for diabetic retinopathy. In: Freeman HM, Hirose T, Schepens CL (eds). *Vitreous surgery and advances in fundus diagnosis and treatment*. New York: Appleton-Century-Crofts, 1977;297–313.

14. Aaberg TM, Abrams GW. Changing indications and techniques for vitrectomy in management of complications of diabetic retinopathy. *Ophthalmology* 1987;94:775–779.

15. Harbour JW, Smiddy WE, Flynn HW Jr, et al. Vitrectomy for diabetic macular edema associated with a thickened and taut posterior hyaloid membrane. *Am J Ophthalmol* 1996;121:405–413.

16. Lewis H, Abrams GW, Blumenkranz MS, et al. Vitrectomy for diabetic macular traction and edema associated with posterior hyaloidal traction. *Ophthalmology* 1992;99:753–759.

17. Rosenblatt BJ, Shah GK, Sharma S, et al. Pars plana vitrectomy with internal limiting membranectomy for refractory diabetic macular edema without a taut posterior hyaloid. *Graefes Arch Clin Exp Ophthalmol* 2005; 243:20–25.

18. Kroll P, Wiegand W, Schmidt J. Vitreopapillary traction in proliferative diabetic vitreoretinopathy. *Br J Ophthalmol* 1999;83:261–264.

19. Ho T, Smiddy WE, Flynn HW. Vitrectomy in the management of diabetic eye disease. *Surv Ophthalmol* 1992;37:190–202.

20. Aaberg TM. Clinical results in vitrectomy for diabetic traction retinal detachment. *Am J Ophthalmol* 1979;88:246–253.

21. Aaberg TM. Pars plana vitrectomy for diabetic traction retinal detachment. *Ophthalmology* 1981;88:639–642.

22. Hutton WL, Bernstein I, Fuller D. Diabetic traction retinal detachment. *Ophthalmology* 1980;87:1071–1077.

23. Thompson JT, de Bustros S, Michels RG, et al. Results and prognostic factors in vitrectomy for diabetic traction retinal detachment of the macula. *Arch Ophthalmol* 1987;105:497–502.

24. Peyman GA, Huamonte FU, Goldberg MF, et al. Four hundred consecutive pars plana vitrectomies with the vitreophage. *Arch Ophthalmol* 1978;96: 45–50.

25. Charles S, Flinn CE. The natural history of diabetic extramacular traction retinal detachment. *Arch Ophthalmol* 1981;99:66–68.

26. Ratner CM, Michels RG, Auer C, et al. Pars plana vitrectomy for complicated retinal detachments. *Ophthalmology* 1983;90:1323–1327.

27. Thompson JT, Bustros S, Michels RG, et al. Results and prognostic factors in vitrectomy for diabetic traction-rhegmatogenous retinal detachment. *Arch Ophthalmol* 1987;105:503–507.

28. Yang CM, Su PY, Yeh PT, et al. Combined rhegmatogenous and traction retinal detachment in proliferative diabetic retinopathy: clinical manifestations and surgical outcome. *Can J Ophthalmol* 2008;43:192–198.

29. Diabetic Retinopathy Vitrectomy Study Research Group. Early vitrectomy for severe proliferative diabetic retinopathy in eyes with useful vision: results of a randomized trial, Diabetic Retinopathy Vitrectomy Study report 3. *Ophthalmology* 1988;95:1307–1320.

30. Diabetic Retinopathy Vitrectomy Study Research Group. Early vitrectomy for severe proliferative diabetic retinopathy in eyes with useful vision: clinical application of results of a randomized trial, Diabetic Retinopathy Vitrectomy Study report 4. *Ophthalmology* 1988;95:1321–1334.

31. Clark J, Grey R, Lim K, et al. Loss of vision before ophthalmic referral in blind and partially sighted diabetics in Bristol. *Br J Ophthalmol* 1994;78: 741–744.

32. Klein R, Klein B, Moss S, et al. The Wisconsin Epidemiologic Study Of Diabetic Retinopathy. IV. Diabetic macular edema. *Ophthalmology* 1984;91: 464–474.

33. Hikichi T, Fujio N, Akiba J, et al. Association between the short-term natural history of diabetic macular edema and the vitreomacular relationship in type II diabetes mellitus. *Ophthalmology* 1997;104:473–478.

34. Lewis H, Abrams G, Blumenkranz M, et al. Vitrectomy for diabetic macular traction edema associated with posterior hyaloidal traction. *Ophthalmology* 1992;99:753–759.

35. Kent D, Vinores S, Campochiaro P. Macular oedema: the role of soluble mediators. *Br J Ophthalmol* 2000;84:542–545.

36. Ikeda TSK, Katano T, Hayashi Y. Vitrectomy for cystoid macular oedema with attached posterior hyaloid membrane in patients with diabetes. *Br J Ophthalmol* 1999;83:12–14.

37. Tachi N, Ogino N. Vitrectomy for diffuse macular oedema in cases of diabetic retinopathy. *Am J Ophthalmol* 1996;122:258–260.

38. O'Hanley GP, Canny CLB. Diabetic dense premacular hemorrhage: a possible indication for prompt vitrectomy. *Ophthalmology* 1985;92:507–511.

39. Ramsay RC, Knobloch WH, Cantrill HL. Timing of vitrectomy for active proliferative diabetic retinopathy. *Ophthalmology* 1986;93:283.

40. Blankenship G. Preoperative iris rubeosis and diabetic vitrectomy results. *Ophthalmology* 1980;87:176–182.

41. Wand M, Dueker DK, Aiello LM, et al. Effects of panretinal photocoagulation of rubeosis iridis, angle neovascularization, and neovascular glaucoma. *Am J Ophthalmol* 1978;86:332–339.

42. Lloyd MA, Heuer DK, Baerveldt G, et al. Combined Molteno implantation and pars plana vitrectomy for neovascular glaucomas. *Ophthalmology* 1991;98:1401–1405.

43. Luttrell JK, Avery RL. Pars plana implant and vitrectomy for treatment of neovascular glaucoma. *Retina* 1995;15:379–387.

44. Ghartey KN, Tolentino FL, Freeman HM. Closed vitreous surgery. XVII. Results and complications of pars plana vitrectomy. *Arch Ophthalmol* 1980;98:1248–1252.

45. Singh H, Grand MG. Treatment of blood-induced glaucoma by trans pars plana vitrectomy. *Retina* 1981;1:255–257.

46. Stenkula S, Tornquist R. Healon: a guide to its use in ophthalmic surgery. In: Miller D, Stegman R (eds). *Use of healon in vitrectomy and difficult retinal detachments*. New York: Wiley, 1983:207–221.

47. Grigorian RA, Castellarin A, Bhagat N, et al. Use of viscodissection and silicone oil in vitrectomy for severe diabetic retinopathy. *Semin Ophthalmol* 2003;18:121–126.

48. Hesse L, Chofflet J, Kroll P. Tissue plasminogen activator as a biochemical adjuvant in vitrectomy for proliferative diabetic vitreoretinopathy. *Ger J Ophthalmol* 1995;4:323–327.

49. Chang S, Zimmerman NJ, Iwamoto T, et al. Experimental vitreous replacement with perfluorotributylamine. *Am J Ophthalmol* 1987;103:29–37.

50. Arevalo JF. En bloc perfluorodissection in vitreoretinal surgery: a new surgical technique. *Retina* 2008;28:653–656.

51. Eliott D, Lewis JM, Townsend-Pico W. Relaxing retinotomy performed during vitrectomy for proliferative diabetic retinopathy. *Invest Ophthalmol Vis Sci* 1997;38:483.

52. Schachat AP, Oyakawa RT, Michels RG, et al. Complications of vitreous surgery for diabetic retinopathy. II. Postoperative complications. *Ophthalmology* 1983;90:522–530.

53. Mieler WF, Wolf MD. Management of postvitrectomy diabetic vitreous hemorrhage. In: Lewis H, Ryan SJ (eds). *Medical and surgical retina: advances, controversies, and management*. St. Louis: Mosby, 1994:330–340.

54. Novak MA, Rice TA, Michels RG, et al. Vitreous hemorrhage after vitrectomy for diabetic retinopathy. *Ophthalmology* 1984;91:1485–1489.

55. Rice TA, Michels RG, Maguire MG, et al. The effect of lensectomy on the incidence of iris neovascularization and neovascular glaucoma after vitrectomy for diabetic retinopathy. *Am J Ophthalmol* 1983;95:1–11.

56. Blankenship G, Cortez R, Machemer R. The lens and pars plana vitrectomy for diabetic retinopathy complications. *Arch Ophthalmol* 1979;97: 1263–1267.

57. Helbig H, Kellner U, Bornfeld N, et al. Rubeosis iridis after vitrectomy for diabetic retinopathy. *Graefes Arch Clin Exp Ophthalmol* 1998;236: 730–733.

58. Brourman ND, Blumenkranz MS, Cox MS, et al. Silicone oil for the treatment of severe proliferative diabetic retinopathy. *Ophthalmology* 1989;96: 759–764.

59. Castellarin A, Grigorian R, Bhagat N, et al. Vitrectomy with silicone oil infusion in severe diabetic retinopathy. *Br J Ophthalmol* 2003;87:318–321.

60. Lewis H, Abrams GW, Williams GA. Anterior hyaloidal fibrovascular proliferation after diabetic vitrectomy. *Am J Ophthalmol* 1987;104:607–613.

61. Brown GC, Tasman WS, Benson WE, et al. Reoperation following diabetic vitrectomy. *Arch Ophthalmol* 1992;110:506–510.

62. Rizzo S, Genovesi-Ebert F, Di Bartolo E, et al. Injection of intravitreal bevacizumab (Avastin) as a preoperative adjunct before vitrectomy surgery in the treatment of severe proliferative diabetic retinopathy (PDR). *Graefes Arch Clin Exp Ophthalmol* 2008;246:837–842.

63. Tolentino FI, Freeman HM, Tolentino FL. Closed vitrectomy in the management of diabetic traction retinal detachment. *Ophthalmology* 1980;87: 1078–1089.

64. Rice TA, Michels RG, Rice EF. Vitrectomy for diabetic rhegmatogenous retinal detachment. *Am J Ophthalmol* 1983;95:34–44.

65. Thompson JT, de Bustros S, Michels RG, et al. Results and prognostic factors in vitrectomy for diabetic traction-rhegmatogenous retinal detachment. *Arch Ophthalmol* 1987;105:503–507.

66. Jahn CE, Töpfner von Schutz K, Richter J, et al. Improvement of visual acuity in eyes with diabetic macular edema after treatment with pars plana vitrectomy. *Ophthalmologica* 2004;218:378–384.

67. Rosenblatt BJ, Shah GK, Sharma S, et al. Pars plana vitrectomy with internal limiting membranectomy for refractory diabetic macular edema without a taut posterior hyaloid. *Graefes Arch Clin Exp Ophthalmol* 2005;243: 20–25.

68. Dillinger P, Mester U. Vitrectomy with removal of the internal limiting membrane in chronic diabetic macular oedema. *Graefes Arch Clin Exp Ophthalmol* 2004;242:630–637.

69. Yanyali A, Horozoglu F, Celik E, et al. Long-term outcomes of pars plana vitrectomy with internal limiting membrane removal in diabetic macular edema. *Retina* 2007;27:557–566.

70. Hartley KL, Smiddy WE, Flynn HW Jr, et al. Pars plana vitrectomy with internal limiting membrane peeling for diabetic macular edema. *Retina* 2008;28:410–419.

# Macular Edema

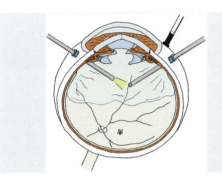

C H A P T E R

# 23

# Macular Edema Associated with Aphakia and Pseudophakia

Hiroko Terasaki

193

## INTRODUCTION

Cystoid macular edema (CME) is characterized by cystoid spaces in the macular area with perifoveal fluorescein leakage, increased thickness of the retina, and visual impairment. This form of CME is referred to as clinically significant CME. CME can also be present without the increased macular thickness and is referred to as angiographic CME (1–5). CME is not a frequent complication of recent, modern, and successful cataract extraction and posterior intraocular lens (IOL) implantation (1). There are some factors that predispose eyes to CME after uneventful cataract surgery, including uveitis, retinal vein occlusion, and diabetes mellitus, and also after complicated cataract surgery (2,3). CME tends to resolve spontaneously or with pharmacological treatment (6–11); however, if it remains chronic, a permanent loss of central vision can occur. Clinical improvement can occur in eyes with no apparent vitreous traction.

Vitrectomy has been reported to be effective in treating CME, and some pseudophakic eyes with chronic CME that is unresponsive to medical treatment will recover good vision after vitrectomy (12–18). In this chapter, we discuss the rationales for vitrectomy to treat aphakic/pseudophakic CME and report the indications and effectiveness of recent surgical techniques in treating CME.

## PATHOGENESIS OF APHAKIC/ PSEUDOPHAKIC CYSTOID MACULAR EDEMA

Inflammatory responses are activated to different degrees in eyes that have undergone intraocular surgery. Prostaglandins (PGs) are released postoperatively by a disruption of the blood–retinal barrier caused by inflammation, hypotony, vitreous traction, and other complications. The PGs are metabolic breakdown products of arachidonic acid, and they have been postulated to be causative of CME (19). The products of the arachidonic acid cascade are not only chemical transmitters but also consist of complement, platelet-activation factor, lysosomal enzymes, and interleukin 6. In addition to these chemical mediators, vascular endothelial growth factor (VEGF) also acts with PGs as key mediators in the breakdown of the blood-aqueous-barrier (BAB) or blood-retinal-barrier (BRB). In fact, the efficacy of intravitreal injection of anti-VEGF has been reported to treat eyes with CME (11), which would indicate that there was an upregulation of VEGF in eyes with CME. This upregulation is not limited to the macular area but is present diffusely in the eye, which suggests that soluble chemical mediators are released by the primary lesion (20). In addition to the inflammation, vitreous traction on the retina in the macular area has been postulated to be the cause of CME in a small number of patients.

## ROLE OF VITRECTOMY

Releasing the vitreous traction on the iris or the ciliary body is expected to inactivate the inflammatory response and enhance the passive transport of chemical mediators through the non-pigmented epithelium of the ciliary body. Removing the entire vitreous as a reservoir for cytokines may contribute to a faster clearance of chemical mediators.

Eyes in which the posterior hyaloid remains attached to the retina may benefit from separation of the vitreous from the retina and release of traction. Peeling the internal limiting membrane (ILM) has not been proven to alleviate the CME in a cohort study, although there are some case reports that found an improvement of CME after ILM peeling (21).

## EVALUATION OF CYSTOID MACULAR EDEMA

The basic ophthalmological examinations required to examine eyes with suspected CME are visual acuity, ophthalmoscopy, biomicroscopy, and fluorescein angiography. The recent development of high-resolution optical coherence tomography (OCT) instruments has allowed clinicians to detect different degrees of increased macular thickness, cystoid spaces in the middle layers of the retina, and the presence or absence of the IS/OS line, a high-reflective line in OCT images present at the border of photoreceptor inner and outer segments. Vitreous traction on the macular area can also be documented by high-resolution OCT techniques (Figs. 23-1 to 23-4).

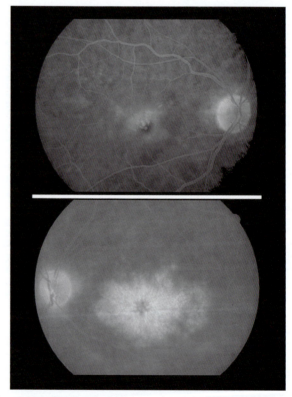

**Figure 23-1.** Fluorescein angiogram of pseudophakic eye with cystoid macular edema. Grade II° with circumferential leakage of fluorescein (**top**). Grade III° with typical honeycomb appearance of fluorescein pooling in the cystic spaces (**bottom**) (From Miyake K, Ota I, Maekubo K, et al. Latanoprost accelerates disruption of the blood-aqueous barrier and the incidence of angiographic cystoid macular edema in early postoperative pseudophakias. *Arch Ophthalmol* 1999;117:34).

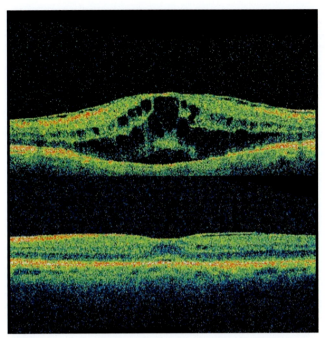

**Figure 23-2.** Typical optical coherence tomography (OCT) findings in eye with cystoid macular edema (before treatment). There is an increase in the thickness of the macula with cystic space in the middle and outer layer of the retina. After vitreous injection of bevasizmub, the macular thickness is markedly decreased. A thin epiretinal membrane can be seen in the OCT sections.

The fluorescein angiographic images have been classified (22): Grade 0° = no sign of fluorescein leakage; grade I° = slight fluorescein leakage into the cystic space but not sufficient enough to cover the entire fovea centralis; grade II° = complete circular accumulation of fluorescein in the cystic space but its diameter is <2 mm; and grade III° = circular accumulation of fluorescein whose diameter is >2 mm. The resolution of the newer OCT instruments is high enough to demonstrate the very small cystic spaces; however, fluorescein angiography is still necessary to determine whether a breakdown of the BAB and BRB is present.

## TREATMENT OPTIONS

Early after development of CME, topical steroids, topical nonsteroidal anti-inflammatory drops, and cessation of latanoprost (if being used) are recommended. In cases of recalcitrant CME, a subtenon or intravitreal injection of triamcinolone is recommended. Bevacizumab, 1.25 mg/0.05 mL, has been reported to be efficacious; however, recurrences are common. Such pharmacological treatments can lead to increased intraocular pressure and/or frequent recurrences. Vitrectomy is indicated in chronic cases with no special vitreous involvement or with vitreous-related complications.

## VITRECTOMY PROCEDURES

Eyes without retinal complications such as lattice degeneration, proliferative diabetic retinopathy, and other retinal diseases are good candidates for transconjunctival, small gauge vitrectomy. Adequate vitreous gel should be removed with the creation of a posterior vitreous detachment (PVD) if the eye does not have a PVD. Triamcinolone acetonide may be useful in making the vitreous gel on the surface of the posterior retina (23,24) or anterior vitreous strand incarcerated in corneoscleral wounds (25) more visible. ILM peeling may be used to remove all of the vitreous fibers over the macula area in order to prevent epiretinal proliferation.

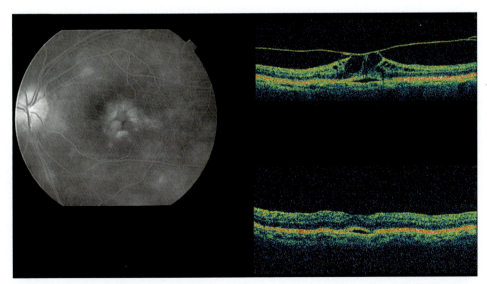

**Figure 23-3.** Fluorescein angiogram of a pseudophakic eye in a patient with sarcoidosis (**left**). Cystoid macular edema with fluorescein leakage can be seen. Optical coherence tomography shows vitreomacular traction, which is an indication for vitrectomy (**top right**). The shape of the macula after surgery is markedly improved; however, serous retinal detachment can still be seen at the fovea (**bottom right**).

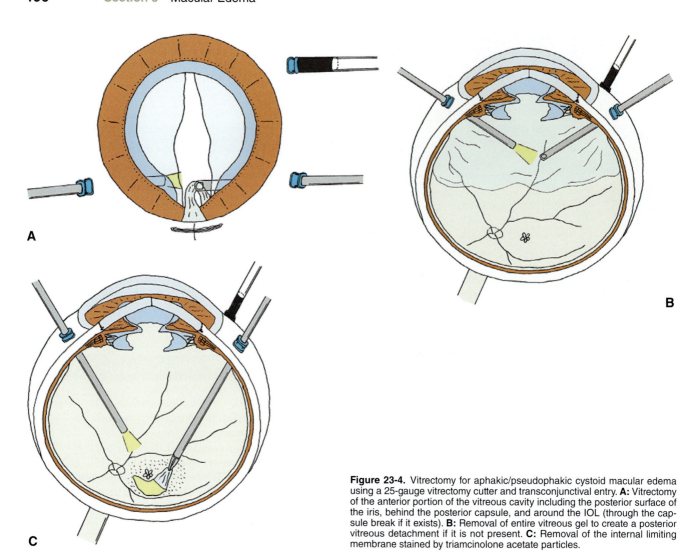

**Figure 23-4.** Vitrectomy for aphakic/pseudophakic cystoid macular edema using a 25-gauge vitrectomy cutter and transconjunctival entry. **A:** Vitrectomy of the anterior portion of the vitreous cavity including the posterior surface of the iris, behind the posterior capsule, and around the IOL (through the capsule break if it exists). **B:** Removal of entire vitreous gel to create a posterior vitreous detachment if it is not present. **C:** Removal of the internal limiting membrane stained by triamcinolone acetate particles.

## CONCLUSIONS

Acute CME that develops after cataract surgery can be treated with topical corticosteroids and/or cyclooxygenase inhibitors; subtenon or intravitreal injections of triamcinolone; or intravitreal injection of bevacizmab. In chronic cases or cases with vitreous-related complications, vitrectomy should be considered. The best surgical approach may be vitrectomy through the pars plana with the use of small gauge instruments if other retinal complications are not present.

### References

1. Wolf EJ, Braunstein A, Shih C, et al. Incidence of visually significant pseudophakic macular edema after uneventful phacoemulsification in patients treated with nepafenac. *J Cataract Refract Surg* 2007;33:1546.
2. Henderson BA, Kim JY, Ament CS, et al. Clinical pseudophakic cystoid macular edema: risk factors for development and duration after treatment. *J Cataract Refract Surg* 2007;33:1550.
3. Arcieri ES, Santana A, Rocha FN, et al. Blood-aqueous barrier changes after the use of prostaglandin analogues in patients with pseudophakia and aphakia: a 6-month randomized trial. *Arch Ophthalmol* 2005;123:186.
4. Irvine AR, Bresky R, Crowder BM, et al. Macular edema after cataract extraction. *Ann Ophthalmol* 1971;3:1234.
5. Gass JDM. Cystoid macular edema after cataract extraction. In: Gass JDM (ed). *Stereoscopic atlas of macular diseases: diagnosis and treatment*, 3rd ed, St. Louis: CV Mosby, 1987:368.
6. Koutsandrea C, Moschos MM, Brouzas D, et al. Intraocular triamcinolone acetonide for pseudophakic cystoid macular edema: optical coherence tomography and multifocal electroretinography study. *Retina* 2007;27:159.
7. Sørensen TL, Haamann P, Villumsen J, et al. Intravitreal triamcinolone for macular oedema: efficacy in relation to aetiology. *Acta Ophthalmol Scand* 2005;83:67.
8. Benhamou N, Massin P, Haouchine B, et al. Intravitreal triamcinolone for refractory pseudophakic macular edema. *Am J Ophthalmol* 2003;135:246.
9. Conway MD, Canakis C, Livir-Rallatos C, et al. Intravitreal triamcinolone acetonide for refractory chronic pseudophakic cystoid macular edema. *J Cataract Refract Surg* 2003;29:27.
10. Rho DS. Treatment of acute pseudophakic cystoid macular edema: diclofenac versus ketorolac. *J Cataract Refract Surg* 2003;29:2378.
11. Mason JO III, Albert MA Jr, Vail R. Intravitreal bevacizumab (Avastin) for refractory pseudophakic cystoid macular edema. *Retina* 2006;26:356.
12. Wilkinson CP. Vitrectomy for chronic pseudophakic cystoid macular edema. *Am J Ophthalmol* 2000;129:310.
13. Pendergast SD, Margherio RR, Williams GA, et al. Vitrectomy for chronic pseudophakic cystoid macular edema. *Am J Ophthalmol* 1999;128:317.
14. Aaberg TM. Pars plana vitrectomy for persistent aphakic cystoid macular edema secondary to vitreous incarceration in the cataract wound. In:

McPherson A (ed). *New and controversial aspects of vitrectomy surgery*, vol 3. St. Louis: Mosby, 1977:230.

15. Federman JL, Annesley WH Jr, Sarin LK, et al. Vitrectomy and cystoid macular edema. *Ophthalmology* 1980;87:622.
16. Fung WE. Anterior vitrectomy for chronic aphakic cystoid macular edema. *Ophthalmology* 1980;87:189.
17. Young PW, Shea M. Pars plasma vitrectomy in the management of the Irvine-Gass syndrome. *Can J Ophthalmol* 1980;15:172.
18. Fung WE. Vitrectomy –ACME Study Group: vitrectomy for chronic aphakic cystoid macular edema: results of a national, collaborative, prospective, randomized investigation. *Ophthalmology* 1985;92:1102.
19. Miyake K, Ibaraki N. Prostaglandins and cystoid macular edema. *Surv Ophthalmol* 2002;47:S203.
20. Terasaki H, Miyake K, Miyake Y. Reduced oscillatory potentials of the full-field electroretinogram of eyes with aphakic or pseudophakic cystoid macular edema. *Am J Ophthalmol* 2003;135:477.
21. Peyman GA, Canakis C, Livir-Rallatos C. The effect of internal limiting membrane peeling on chronic recalcitrant pseudophakic cystoid macular edema: a report of two cases. *Am J Ophthalmol* 2002;133:571.
22. Miyake K, Ota Ì, Maekubo K, et al. Latanoprost accelerates disruption of the blood-aqueous barrier and the incidence of angiographic cystoid macular edema in early postoperative pseudophakias. *Arch Ophthalmol* 1999; 117:34.
23. Tognetto D, Zenoni S, Sanguinetti G, et al. Staining of the internal limiting membrane with intravitreal triamcinolone acetonide. *Retina* 2005; 25:462.
24. Kimura H, Kuroda S, Nagata M. Triamcinolone acetonide-assisted peeling of the internal limiting membrane. *Am J Ophthalmol* 2004;137:172.
25. Yamakiri K, Uchino E, Kimura K, et al. Intracameral triamcinolone helps to visualize and remove the vitreous body in anterior chamber in cataract surgery. *Am J Ophthalmol* 2004;138:650.

# 24

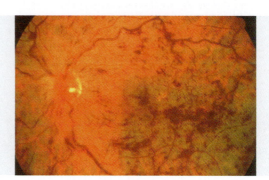

# Macular Edema Associated with Vascular Occlusion

Jawad Ahmad Qureshi ■ Sharon Fekrat ■ Daniel Finkelstein

Occlusion within retinal veins may occur in the central retinal vein, producing a central retinal vein occlusion (CRVO), or in a branch retinal vein, producing a branch retinal vein occlusion (BRVO) or a hemiretinal vein occlusion (HRVO). Approximately 2 in 1,000 persons aged 40 years or older developed a retinal vein occlusion over a 4-year period in a population-based study performed in Israel (1). In persons aged 65 years or older, this increased to 5 per 1,000 individuals.

The likelihood of some of the ocular consequences of venous occlusive disease, such as decreased visual acuity from perfused macular edema in eyes with BRVO, vitreous hemorrhage, and neovascular glaucoma, may be decreased by early diagnosis and laser treatment (2–5).

## BRANCH RETINAL VEIN OCCLUSION

Occlusion of a retinal venous branch typically occurs in the seventh decade of life (6) and develops because the blood flow in the affected retinal venous branch is slowed or interrupted. It usually occurs where a retinal artery crosses a retinal vein, the retinal arteriovenous intersection (7–9). Rarely, a BRVO may occur at a site other than an arteriovenous crossing in eyes with ocular inflammatory disease.

An increased risk of developing a BRVO was noted in persons with histories of cardiovascular disease, systemic hypertension, glaucoma, increased body mass index at 20 years of age, or higher serum levels of $a_2$-globulin in the Eye Disease Case-Control Study (10). In this study, those persons with higher serum high-density lipoprotein cholesterol levels and greater levels of alcohol consumption had a decreased risk of BRVO; diabetes mellitus was not a strong independent risk factor for BRVO (10). Other studies have suggested an increased risk of BRVO in eyes with shorter axial lengths (11–14).

### Clinical Features

An *acute* BRVO is one that has been present for less than 6 months and displays characteristic ophthalmoscopic findings. In the affected distribution, variable amounts of superficial and deep retinal hemorrhage, retinal edema, venous tortuosity and dilation, and cotton-wool spots may coexist in a segmental pattern (Fig. 24-1). The presence of cotton-wool spots in the involved area, however, does not necessarily imply that the vein occlusion is ischemic. In the acute phase, the diagnosis of a BRVO is usually straightforward, unless the affected segment is either small or well perfused, with complete recovery of function. If another retinal vascular disease, such as diabetic retinopathy, coexists, or if there are several BRVOs in one eye, the diagnosis may not be so obvious.

A BRVO may lead to compromise of visual acuity or may be asymptomatic, depending on the location of the occluded segment. If the visual acuity is affected, it may be attributed to involvement of the macula with hemorrhage, edema, or ischemia. If the venous blockage is peripheral to those veins draining the macula, the macula may not be involved, and

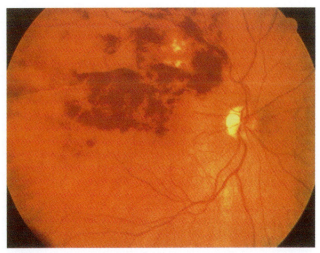

**Figure 24-1.** An acute branch retinal vein occlusion is characterized ophthalmoscopically by a segmental distribution of varying amounts of intraretinal hemorrhage and segmental venous dilatation and tortuosity.

visual acuity may be unaffected. Nasal BRVOs seem less common, but this may be a result, in part, of the asymptomatic location of these occlusions (15). The superotemporal venous branch is involved more frequently (63%); the inferotemporal branch is affected in almost all other cases (15). The apex of the segmentally distributed intraretinal hemorrhage usually marks the approximate location of the arteriovenous intersection at which the occlusion occurred (Fig. 24-1). With some exceptions, the closer the BRVO occurs to the optic disc, the greater the distribution of affected retina and the more serious the sequelae (15,16). If the BRVO occurs at the optic disc, two quadrants of the retina may be involved, whereas if the occlusion is peripheral to the disc, one quadrant or less may be affected.

A BRVO may be categorized as chronic 6 months or more after its onset. The diagnosis may be more challenging ophthalmoscopically in these eyes, because the intraretinal hemorrhage may have been mostly reabsorbed. Ophthalmoscopically, retinal capillary abnormalities, such as capillary dilation, capillary nonperfusion, microaneurysms, and collateral vessel formation, may be noted in the involved distribution. In these cases, fluorescein angiography may facilitate the diagnosis by better delineating the segmental retinal capillary abnormalities. If the occlusion is deemed ischemic, sclerosis and sheathing of the retinal vasculature in the distribution of the occlusion may also be identified.

### Perfusion Status

If the ophthalmoscopic diagnosis of BRVO has been determined, it is useful to determine whether the BRVO is perfused (nonischemic) or nonperfused (ischemic), using high-quality fluorescein angiography (2). If less than five disc areas in diameter of retinal capillary nonperfusion is present in the affected distribution on fluorescein angiography, the occlusion is classified as perfused or nonischemic. If five or more disc areas in diameter of nonperfusion are present on angiography, the occlusion is classified as nonperfused or ischemic. Of eyes with a BRVO affecting one quadrant of the retina or more, about half are ischemic.

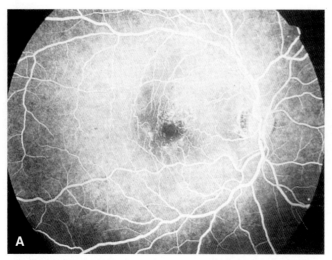
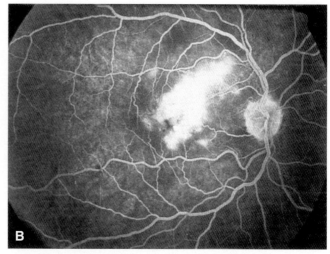

**Figure 24-2.** Perfused macular edema in an eye with branch retinal vein occlusion. **A:** The transit phase of the fluorescein angiogram shows an intact parafoveal retinal capillary network. **B:** Late accumulation of fluorescein dye parafoveally and in the foveal center is present.

Identification of retinal capillary nonperfusion may not be feasible on fluorescein angiography in those eyes with moderate to marked amounts of intraretinal hemorrhage, because the hemorrhage may block the fluorescein outline of the parafoveal vascular network as well as patches of retinal capillary nonperfusion. As a result, fluorescein angiography cannot be utilized diagnostically until the hemorrhage resorbs sufficiently to allow the observation of underlying capillary architecture. The hemorrhage may take up to 1 year to clear in some eyes.

## Macular Edema

Macular edema may be categorized angiographically in eyes with a BRVO as perfused (nonischemic), nonperfused (ischemic), or mixed (perfused and nonperfused) (5,17). Rarely, the macular edema may not be characterizable into one of these three classes, because it may have developed in association with a distant BRVO. After sufficient resorption of the intraretinal hemorrhage, careful evaluation of the parafoveal vascular architecture with ophthalmoscopy and high-quality fluorescein angiography is necessary to identify the type of macular edema (17). Optical coherence tomography has also become increasingly useful in evaluating, characterizing, and following macular edema.

If fluorescein angiography demonstrates an intact parafoveal retinal capillary network during the transit phase of the angiogram (Fig. 24-2A) followed by the late accumulation of fluorescein dye both parafoveally and in the foveal center (Fig. 24-2B), the macular edema is classified as perfused.

If fluorescein angiography demonstrates an irregular parafoveal vascular network with para- and perifoveal areas of retinal capillary nonperfusion (Fig. 24-3) followed by the absence of any late accumulation of fluorescein dye in the foveal center, the macular edema is classified as nonperfused.

If fluorescein angiography demonstrates parafoveal retinal capillary dilation and leakage admixed with areas of capillary nonperfusion, the macular edema is classified as

mixed (17). In the late phase of the angiogram in these eyes, fluorescein dye accumulates in the foveal center. In eyes with mixed edema, however, it is not possible to discern how much of the foveal cystoid edema may be attributed to perfused edema and how much may be attributed to nonperfused edema. Spontaneous resolution of the nonperfused portion of the macular edema within 6 to 12 months may permit reassessment.

Distant macular edema may develop in an eye with a peripheral BRVO, in which the occluded venous branch is peripheral to the macular area. Fluorescein angiography may demonstrate leakage. The pathophysiology of the macular edema in these eyes has not been elucidated.

## Optic-disc and Retinal Neovascularization

Approximately 40% of eyes with an ischemic BRVO develop retinal or disc neovascularization. If laser photocoagulation is not performed, approximately 60% of those that have

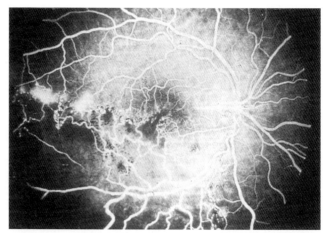

**Figure 24-3.** Nonperfused macular edema is present if fluorescein angiography demonstrates an irregular parafoveal vascular network with para- and perifoveal areas of retinal capillary nonperfusion and no late accumulation of fluorescein dye in the foveal center.

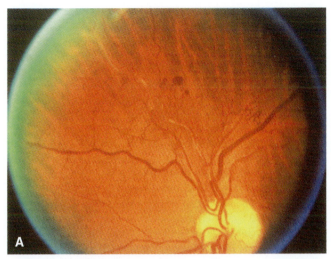
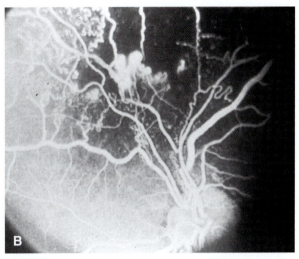

**Figure 24-4.** **A:** Retinal neovascularization may be difficult to differentiate from collateral channels in eyes with vein occlusion. **B:** Fluorescein angiography may help distinguish whether the abnormal vessels are true neovascularization or collateral vessels, because fluorescein leakage is more prominent from the neovascularization than from collateral vessels.

neovascularization develop vitreous hemorrhages (2). Neovascularization of the optic disc and retina (Fig. 24-4A) may develop in eyes with an ischemic BRVO, usually within the first 6 to 12 months after onset but possible at any time within the first 3 years. Retinal neovascularization almost always occurs within the involved segment; however, rarely, it may develop outside the affected area, usually at an arteriovenous crossing.

Ophthalmoscopically, disc and retinal neovascularization may be mistaken for collateral vessels. Collateral vessels may develop on the disc or within the retina along the horizontal raphe or around the site of occlusion (Fig. 24-4B). These venule-to-venule channels bypass the occluded vein and appear as dilated, and occasionally tortuous, vessels. Fluorescein angiography may help to distinguish whether these vessels are collateral or represent true neovascularization, because the fluorescein leakage is much greater from neovascularization than from collateral vessels.

## Iris Neovascularization

Iris neovascularization and neovascular glaucoma are infrequent sequelae in eyes with BRVO. The coexistence of diabetes mellitus, with or without retinopathy, may increase the likelihood of developing iris neovascularization.

## Pathogenesis and Histopathology

Although branch venous occlusive disease has been attributed primarily to arterial insufficiency (18), in animal studies, common manifestations of BRVO, including retinal capillary nonperfusion and secondary retinal arteriolar changes, can be duplicated by the experimental occlusion of a retinal vein alone (19,20). In human eyes, the blocked venous branch is almost always localized to a nearby arteriovenous crossing (8). Histopathologic examination of the involved branch retinal vein has demonstrated a thrombus as the cause of the venous occlusion at the arteriovenous intersection (21); despite this, the pathogenesis of thrombus formation remains unclear. In a histopathologic study, a fresh or recanalized thrombus was

present at the site of venous occlusion in each of nine eyes with BRVO (21); thus the primary event was thought to be intravenous thrombosis with secondary arterial and capillary manifestations and ultimately neovascular proliferation. Thrombus formation was not observed in any of the corresponding retinal arterioles, even though all but one of the corresponding arterioles had moderate to severe sclerosis.

Because branch venous occlusive disease almost always occurs at arteriovenous intersections (7–9,22,23), associated arterial disease may be in part a cause of the occlusion. Retinal arterioles cross anterior to retinal veins at approximately 55% to 70% of all arteriovenous crossings in normal eyes (7–9). The artery was located anterior to the vein at the obstructed site in 99% of 106 eyes with BRVO (8). Histopathologically, the retinal artery and vein share a common adventitial sheath at the crossing site, and the lumen of the vein may be compressed up to 33% at the site in some cases (21,22). Atherosclerosis may contribute to increased rigidity of the crossing artery and contraction of the common adventitia, resulting in turbulent venous blood flow, endothelial cell injury, and thrombotic venous occlusion.

In an animal model, certain histopathologic sequelae develop after the complete occlusion of a branch retinal vein (19,20,24). Within 1 to 6 hours following the occlusion, there is a suspected elevation in intravascular pressure, resulting in capillary leakage and retinal edema. Within 6 hours to 1 week following the obstruction, necrosis of the vascular endothelium leads to exposure of the basement membrane with thrombus development. Complete microvascular stasis results, followed by the development of retinal hemorrhages. Within 1 to 5 weeks following the occlusion, irreversible capillary closure has developed, with the invasion of proliferating glial cells into the ghost vessels.

## Treatment and Clinical Course
### Medical Intervention

Systemic anticoagulation has not been demonstrated to prevent or alter the clinical outcome of the venous occlusion.

Because the administration of anticoagulants may result in systemic bleeding complications, and because anticoagulants may promote the development of intraretinal hemorrhage acutely, anticoagulant therapy currently is not recommended. Other agents, such as troxerutin, and ticlopidine, have been suggested as potential treatments by reducing blood viscosity and improving retinal microcirculation. Studies on the use of troxerutin and ticlopidine have shown a trend toward improving visual acuity in eyes with BRVO, but the evidence to support these treatments is limited at this time (25,26).

## Laser Photocoagulation

Some basic knowledge of laser treatment techniques is essential in treating these eyes; a meticulous approach helps decrease the likelihood of developing complications. Laser photocoagulation should not be done over substantial intraretinal hemorrhage, because the energy of the laser is absorbed by the hemorrhage and may damage the nerve fiber layer, producing preretinal fibrosis. If intraretinal edema is present, higher laser powers may be necessary for adequate uptake.

The Collaborative Branch Vein Occlusion Study (BVOS) (2,5), supported by the National Eye Institute, was a multicenter, randomized clinical trial constructed to answer three questions about the management of complications of BRVO:

1. Does grid argon laser photocoagulation improve visual acuity in eyes with visual acuity of 20/40 because of perfused macular edema (5)?
2. Does peripheral scatter argon laser photocoagulation prevent the development of neovascularization (2)?
3. Does segmental peripheral scatter argon laser photocoagulation prevent vitreous hemorrhage in eyes with neovascularization (2)?

## Macular Edema

The BVOS was designed to determine if grid argon laser photocoagulation can improve the visual acuity in eyes with an acuity of 20/40 or worse resulting from macular edema from BRVO of 3 to 18 months' duration (5). The BVOS data demonstrate that grid photocoagulation may improve the visual acuity in treated eyes. The timing of laser treatment of perfused macular edema, after the onset of a BRVO, did not affect the visual acuity. Early photocoagulation did not appear to be more beneficial. In a different nonrandomized study of 161 treated eyes with macular edema, those eyes treated 12 months or longer after the onset of the BRVO improved less than those treated within the first year (27).

Clinical information must be collected prior to treating macular edema with laser (5,17). First, the visual acuity in the eye with the BRVO should be documented. In the BVOS, treated eyes had a corrected visual acuity better than 20/40. Second, high-quality fluorescein angiography must be feasible to demonstrate foveal dye accumulation and an absence of moderate to marked para- and perifoveal capillary nonperfusion. Hemorrhage may interfere with determination of visual acuity, angiographic interpretation, and subsequent laser treatment. Third, fluorescein-proven perfused macular edema

involving the foveal center must be documented to be the cause of visual loss. Blood should not be in the foveal center, because subsequent clearing of this blood may lead to some spontaneous improvement in visual acuity. Fourth, one must be confident that the macular edema is not resorbing spontaneously. Untreated foveal macular edema of less than 12 months' duration can improve during the first 6 to 12 months after the onset of a BRVO; approximately one third of patients may improve two or more Snellen lines of visual acuity without treatment (5). Individuals who are hypertensive or have had decreased visual acuity for greater than 1 year from macular edema, however, are less likely to regain vision spontaneously. For the nonperfused and mixed forms of macular edema, a small study suggested that the spontaneous rate of improvement was much greater, approximately 90% (17). If some capillary nonperfusion is present along the edge of the foveal avascular zone, the acuity may be more likely to improve; if larger areas of capillary nonperfusion exist at the border of the foveal avascular zone, the acuity often does not improve.

Argon laser photocoagulation was placed in a "grid" pattern within the area of vascular leakage on fluorescein angiography (Fig. 24-5) in the BVOS (5). The treatment could extend from the edge of the foveal avascular zone to the major vascular arcade. Suggested treatment parameters include a spot size of 50 to 100 mm in diameter, a 0.1-second duration, and a power setting sufficient to produce a light to medium white burn. Grid laser photocoagulation is not performed to directly and immediately close the leaking and dilated capillary vasculature; instead, laser absorption occurs at the level of the retinal pigment epithelium. Although it is not understood how the laser treatment may act in lessening edema if laser absorption occurs at this level, experimental studies in normal primates have shown a decrease in capillary diameter if this form of therapy is used (28). Grid treatment may produce retinal thinning that permits the choroidal vasculature to provide for the inner retina; this may lead to autoregulatory constriction of the retinal vasculature in the leaking area and ultimately result in decreased macular edema (28).

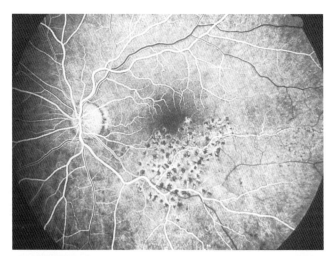

**Figure 24-5.** In the Branch Vein Occlusion Study (5), argon laser photocoagulation was placed in a "grid" pattern within the region of leakage on fluorescein angiography. Treatment extended no closer to the fovea than the margin of the capillary free zone and no farther peripherally than the major vascular arcade.

Identifying distinct landmarks may help avoid accidental laser photocoagulation of the fovea (5,17,29). If sufficient landmarks cannot be identified, then the treatment may be started far away from the foveal avascular zone. At the 3-month follow-up visit, fluorescein angiography outlines the previous area of grid laser photocoagulation and defines the amount of additional treatment needed. If macular edema with foveal involvement is still present, another treatment session may bring the grid treatment pattern closer to the edge of the foveal avascular zone. This staged method may be less risky and as effective as a single treatment in some cases (29).

A follow-up evaluation is recommended approximately 3 months following treatment (5). If macular edema persists ophthalmoscopically and the acuity has not improved, fluorescein angiography is suggested. If residual fluorescein leakage is observed, another session of laser photocoagulation may be necessary. In the BVOS at 3 years, treated eyes were more likely to have visual improvement, a final visual acuity of 20/40 or better, and an average visual acuity better than that of untreated eyes (5). Sixty-three percent of treated eyes improved two or more lines compared with 36% of untreated eyes at 3 years. The mean visual acuity improvement in treated eyes, however, was only one more Snellen line than in untreated eyes. Because approximately 10% of individuals with BRVO have a second venous occlusion in the same or fellow eye, the acuity gain from treatable macular edema may be important (5,29).

## Neovascularization

The BVOS sought to determine if segmental peripheral scatter argon laser photocoagulation could prevent the development of neovascularization in eyes with ischemic BRVO (2), and whether, if neovascularization develops in untreated eyes with nonperfused branch vein occlusion, segmental peripheral scatter laser photocoagulation could prevent a vitreous hemorrhage (2).

Data from the BVOS demonstrated that prophylactic scatter laser photocoagulation can decrease the likelihood of subsequent neovascularization, and, if neovascularization is already present, scatter laser photocoagulation can lessen subsequent vitreous hemorrhage (2). Treatment should cover the entire area of ischemic retina, except within two disc diameters of the fovea, and consist of medium-intensity 200- to 500-mm argon laser burns spaced one burn width apart.

Neovascularization develops in approximately 40% of untreated eyes with ischemic BRVO (2). Disc or retinal neovascularization may develop any time within the initial 3 years following a BRVO but usually appears during the first 6 to 12 months. The incidence of neovascularization may be decreased to approximately 20% if peripheral scatter laser photocoagulation is administered (2). If routine photocoagulation were applied to all eyes with nonperfused BRVO before the development of neovascular proliferation, however, the 60% that would never develop neovascularization would receive unnecessary scatter laser photocoagulation. As a result, prophylactic laser treatment in these eyes has not been advocated.

Of the 40% of untreated eyes with nonperfused BRVO that do develop neovascularization, approximately 60% develop a vitreous hemorrhage (2). If neovascularization is definitely present, as documented by fluorescein angiography in the BVOS, peripheral scatter laser photocoagulation can decrease the likelihood of vitreous hemorrhage to 30% (2).

The BVOS did not determine whether ischemic eyes should receive prophylactic photocoagulation or be observed and photocoagulated only if neovascularization should develop. Analysis of the available data suggests that there may be no benefit to treating prior to the development of neovascularization (2). If fluorescein angiography demonstrates that the BRVO is ischemic, then an examination every 4 months to look for neovascularization is suggested. If neovascularization is noted, then scatter photocoagulation is recommended to the ischemic region. Data from the BVOS suggest that laser photocoagulation following the development of neovascularization is just as effective in preventing vitreous hemorrhage as is photocoagulation prior to the development of neovascularization (2).

## Vitreous Hemorrhage

A vitreous hemorrhage in eyes with BRVO usually develops either from disc or retinal neovascularization, with or without prior scatter laser photocoagulation, or from the breakthrough of retinal hemorrhage through the internal limiting membrane into the vitreous cavity. B-scan ultrasonography may be useful to rule out a traction retinal detachment and other intraocular causes of bleeding. The long-term sequelae of visual loss from vitreous hemorrhage in BRVO have not been investigated, but in some individuals, vitreous hemorrhage from neovascularization results in prolonged visual loss. In other eyes, however, the hemorrhage resolves spontaneously without resulting in permanent visual impairment.

Retinal or disc neovascularization should be excluded if a vitreous hemorrhage is present in eyes with BRVO, whether or not previous scatter laser photocoagulation has been administered. If ophthalmoscopy is not feasible because of a dense hemorrhage, fluorescein angiography or angioscopy may permit visualization of neovascularization. If a neovascular source cannot be identified, it is possible that the hemorrhage resulted from the breakthrough of retinal hemorrhage; however, this is less likely. If the vitreous hemorrhage does not clear spontaneously over time, a *pars plana* vitrectomy with endolaser photocoagulation is recommended, especially in eyes that have not had previous scatter laser photocoagulation.

## Vitrectomy (with and without Sheathotomy)

Evidence exists suggesting that vitreomacular attachment alone may contribute to the development of macular edema in BRVO (30). Kurimoto and coworkers found that vitrectomy with separation of the posterior hyaloid resulted in decreased macular edema. Six of the seven eyes had improved visual acuity at 3 months follow up (31). Saika and coworkers reported similar results (32). Increased oxygenation of the macula, removal of vitreous traction, and tamponade of the macula by intraocular gas are possible explanations for the clinical improvements seen in these studies.

As discussed previously, the blocked venous branch in a BRVO is almost always localized to nearby arteriovenous crossing (8). It has been suggested that removal of the compressive factors affecting the vein by sectioning the adventitial sheath (sheathotomy) may be an effective treatment for BRVO (33). Osterloh and Charles reported significant visual improvement in the first report of sheathotomy (20/200 to 20/25+ over 8 months) (34). Opermcak and Bruce reported equal or improved visual acuity in 12 of 15 patients undergoing sheathotomy. All of the patients in this study had marked resolution of edema and intraretinal hemorrhages (35). Mason and coworkers compared sheathotomy to control groups in which patients were treated with laser or no treatment. Of the 20 eyes that underwent surgical intervention, 75% percent achieved a halving of their visual angle compared with only 40% of control patients (36). In contrast, Cahill and colleagues reported 27 cases of BRVO treated with sheathotomy without a statistically significant improvement in postoperative median visual acuity (37). No randomized, controlled study evaluating the benefits of sheathotomy has been published. This procedure has been largely abandoned.

## Intraocular Corticosteroids

Recently, intraocular injection of steroids has been added as an option for the treatment of macular edema. Although the exact mechanism of macular edema development from BRVO has not been elucidated, breakdown of the blood-retinal barrier is thought to play a role. A corticosteroid suspension, triamcinolone acetonide, has been shown experimentally to reduce breakdown of the blood-retinal barrier when injected intravitreally (38). A human pharmacokinetics study of non-vitrectomized eyes found a single 4 mg injection of triamcinolone to have a mean elimination half-life of 18.6 days with measurable concentrations expected to last approximately 3 months (39). The administration of intravitreal corticosteroids to treat macular edema has gained popularity due to the potential of minimizing side effects while allowing higher drug concentrations to the eye. A number of studies have reported improvements in visual acuity and macular edema by optical coherence tomography and clinically (40–48). The results appear to be transitory, requiring reinjection to maintain improvement (41–45,48). Side effects of intravitreal corticosteroids include increased intraocular pressure, cataract formation in phakic patients, vitreous hemorrhage, sterile and infectious endophthalmitis, and retinal detachment (40,44–47,49–50).

The Standard Care vs. Corticosteroid for Retinal Vein Occlusion (SCORE) Study is a multicenter, randomized, Phase III trial sponsored by the National Eye Institute currently underway to assess the efficacy and safety of standard of care versus intravitreal triamcinolone injection for treatment of macular edema associated with CRVO and BRVO. The study has recruited 1260 patients randomized to standard care, laser treatment, intravitreal triamcinolone (IVTA) 4 mg, or IVTA 1 mg. (51). Two multicenter phase III trials evaluating the safety and efficacy of an intravitreal implant of dexamethasone (Posurdex, Allergan Inc.) for the treatment of macular edema from retinal vein occlusion are also currently recruiting patients.

## ANTI-VEGF Intravitreal Therapy

Anti-VEGF (vascular endothelial) therapies such as pegaptanib sodium (Macugen; Eyetech Pharmaceuticals and Pfizer), ranibizumab and bevacizumab (Lucentis and Avastin, respectively; Genentech) may play a role in treating macular edema related to RVO and preventing neovascular complications. Further study is underway with these agents in BRVO.

## CENTRAL RETINAL VEIN OCCLUSION

CRVO is a common cause of visual loss in individuals 50 years of age and older (52). In young individuals, CRVO has been termed as *"papillophlebitis"* and considered a different disease entity, with an assumed inflammatory cause (53). There is little basis, however, on which to differentiate these eyes from those in older individuals with CRVO, except for the younger age of these patients.

In the Eye Disease Case-Control Study (54), relationships between certain risk factors, including glaucoma, systemic hypertension, and diabetes mellitus, and the development of CRVO were suggested. Others report that increased plasma viscosity and increased hematocrit also may contribute to the development of venous occlusive disease (55).

## Clinical Features

A collection of ophthalmoscopic manifestations characterizes eyes with CRVO, rarely creating a diagnostic dilemma, and includes varying quantities of superficial and deep intraretinal hemorrhage emanating from the optic disc into the peripheral fundus in all four quadrants, optic nerve-head congestion, and a tortuous and dilated retinal venous tree. A mild or chronic CRVO, however, may create diagnostic confusion. In eyes with scattered, blot-shaped, intraretinal hemorrhage, predominantly in the peripheral retina, atherosclerotic carotid artery disease should be sought as the underlying cause. In an eye with carotid insufficiency and decreased arterial perfusion, gentle digital pressure on the globe may produce pulsations of the central retinal artery. If simultaneous bilateral intraretinal hemorrhage is observed, even if asymmetric, an underlying systemic hyperviscosity disorder must be considered.

In eyes with CRVO, the clinical course varies (3,4,56,57). In eyes with mild disease, the ophthalmoscopic characteristics may resolve within several months, with subtle or no sequelae. In moderate cases, some hemorrhage may persist, with retinal vascular abnormalities and macular edema. In eyes with ischemic CRVO, however, complications may develop, such as iris or angle neovascularization with neovascular glaucoma, vitreous hemorrhage, and optic-disc or retinal neovascularization, among others.

The Central Vein Occlusion Study (CVOS) collected and tabulated data to determine the visual prognosis of eyes with CRVO (4). The best corrected visual acuity, on presentation, may be a predictor of the final visual outcome. For example, if the initial visual acuity is 20/40 or better, the acuity in the affected eye is likely to remain good. If the visual acuity is

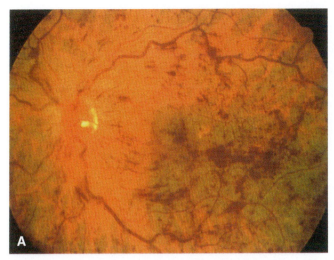
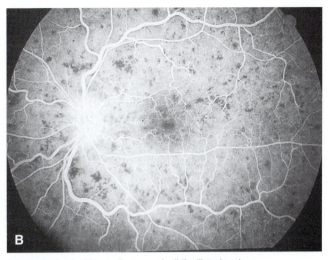

**Figure 24-6. A:** In eyes with perfused central retinal vein occlusion, a few small, scattered retinal hemorrhages and mildly dilated and tortuous retinal veins may be present. **B:** Fluorescein angiography in an eye with a perfused central retinal vein occlusion demonstrates less than 10 disc areas of capillary nonperfusion. Blocked fluorescence from the scattered hemorrhage and, in some cases, a prolonged venous transit time may be present.

20/50 to 20/200, however, the visual prognosis varies; the acuity may improve (20%), may not change (approximately 50%), or may worsen. If the initial visual acuity is worse than 20/200, the visual prognosis is poor (80% remain the same or deteriorate), and the CRVO is usually ischemic.

## Perfusion Status

Both the extent and number of retinal hemorrhages offer clues regarding the perfusion status of the vein occlusion. Based on fluorescein angiographic findings, a CRVO may be categorized as perfused (nonischemic), nonperfused (ischemic), or indeterminate (3,57). The fluorescein angiogram should be performed with a wide-angle fundus camera; sweep views of the midperiphery 30 seconds following fluorescein administration should be obtained (57).

A perfused or nonischemic CRVO is a milder disease in symptomatology, ophthalmoscopic appearance, and course

than a nonperfused or ischemic CRVO (3,4,56,57). In an eye with a nonischemic vein occlusion, mildly tortuous and dilated retinal veins and some small, scattered retinal hemorrhages may be noted (57) (Fig. 24-6A). In an eye with an ischemic vein occlusion, many superficial and deep retinal hemorrhages, almost confluent, and obviously tortuous and dilated retinal veins may be noted (3) (Fig. 24-7A). Even though the ophthalmoscopic manifestations of a central vein occlusion may suggest its perfusion status, high-quality fluorescein angiography is needed for definitive determination.

## Perfused Central Retinal Vein Occlusion

A perfused (nonischemic) CRVO is characterized by less than 10 disc diameters of retinal capillary nonperfusion on fluorescein angiography (57). Many synonyms for this type of CRVO exist, including nonischemic, partial, mild, imminent, incomplete, incipient, threatened, impending, and edematous.

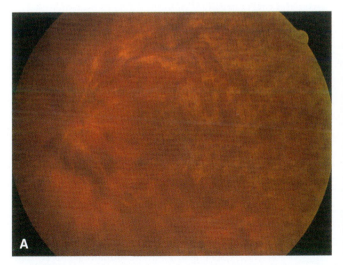
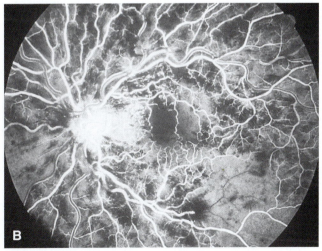

**Figure 24-7. A:** In eyes with ischemic central retinal vein occlusion, many almost confluent retinal hemorrhages, both superficial and deep, and markedly dilated, tortuous retinal veins may be present. **B:** Fluorescein angiography in an eye with an ischemic central retinal vein occlusion demonstrates 10 or more disc areas of retinal capillary nonperfusion. Other manifestations include delayed venous filling and capillary and venous dilation.

Eyes with an acute, perfused CRVO (Fig. 24-6A) may demonstrate disc hyperemia with or without edema, variable amounts of retinal hemorrhage, minimal or no retinal capillary nonperfusion, and mild venous tortuosity and dilation. Rarely, cottonwool spots are present.

Fluorescein angiographic findings include blocked fluorescence from the scattered hemorrhage and, in some eyes, a prolonged venous transit time. Variable amounts of disc and parafoveal dye leakage, dilation of the retinal venous circulation, and mild staining of the venous walls may be present. Less than 10 disc diameters of capillary nonperfusion is present (57) (Fig. 24-6B).

The perfusion status may change during follow-up, and the CRVO may be classified as ischemic (4,57). A significant proportion of those eyes in the CVOS with perfused CRVO were recognized as nonperfused during follow-up. About one third of eyes with an initially perfused CRVO were nonperfused at 3 years (4). Progression to an ischemic status was most likely in the first 4 months (4,57). If the vein occlusion remains perfused, most hemorrhages slowly resolve over many months. The associated macular edema may improve, worsen, or remain unchanged.

## Nonperfused Central Retinal Vein Occlusion

A nonperfused (ischemic) CRVO demonstrates 10 or more disc diameters of retinal capillary nonperfusion on fluorescein angiography (3,57). Synonyms for nonperfused CRVO include ischemic, hemorrhagic, and complete. Eyes with an acute, nonperfused central vein occlusion (Fig. 24-7A) may demonstrate nearly confluent hemorrhages; scattered cotton-wool spots; retinal, macular, and disc edema; and extensive nonperfusion (if vascular detail can be appreciated on fluorescein angiography in the presence of overlying hemorrhage). The disc margins are indistinct, with an absence of the physiologic cup because of disc edema and overlying splinter hemorrhages. The retinal hemorrhage is usually more extensive posterior to the equator; however, the configuration varies. Some intraretinal hemorrhage may break through into the vitreous cavity. The retinal venous tree is congested, with dilated and tortuous vessels. Spontaneous venous pulsations are not present and usually cannot be induced prior to arterial pulsation. Cotton-wool spots may be present.

Fluorescein angiography demonstrates 10 or more disc areas of retinal capillary nonperfusion (3,57) (Fig. 24-7B). In the acute phase of the CRVO, extensive overlying intraretinal hemorrhage may obscure the underlying architecture of the retinal capillary vasculature. Other findings include delayed venous filling, capillary and venous dilation, and in some cases microaneurysms. Late-phase frames of the angiogram demonstrate varying amounts of fluorescein leakage into the retinal tissue and staining of the venous walls. Parafoveal fluorescein leakage from the retinal capillary network is rarely present in eyes with ischemic CRVO, because patent macular vessels are usually absent.

In eyes with chronic CRVO, the majority of retinal hemorrhages slowly resorb over many months (Fig. 24-8); however, scattered dot- and flame-shaped hemorrhages may be

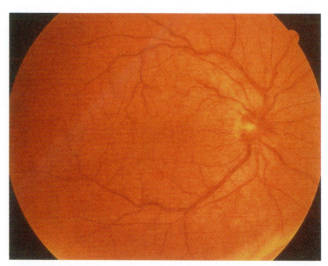

**Figure 24-8.** In eyes with chronic central vein occlusion, most hemorrhages disappear slowly over subsequent months; however, scattered dot- and flame-shaped hemorrhages may be found for much longer. Microaneurysms and cotton-wool spots may disappear after several months; microaneurysms may remain in some eyes. Over time, the retinal veins become less dilated and tortuous, whereas the disc remains congested.

observed for years, especially in the periphery. Microaneurysms and cotton-wool spots also tend to resolve after several months; however, microaneurysms may remain in some eyes. The veins become less dilated and tortuous over time, and collateral vessels may develop (described here subsequently).

## Indeterminate Central Retinal Vein Occlusion

If a significant amount of intraretinal hemorrhage prevents the angiographic interpretation of the perfusion status of the vein occlusion, it is categorized as indeterminate (57). Following sufficient resorption of hemorrhage, evaluation of retinal vascular detail on fluorescein angiography is possible; in these eyes, the CRVO usually is determined to be ischemic (4,57). Within 6 months of enrollment into the CVOS, 38 (83%) of 46 eyes that had extensive retinal hemorrhage, preventing the determination of perfusion status on the baseline angiogram, were determined to be nonperfused. Eight eyes (17%) were determined to be perfused.

## Macular Edema

Macular edema may be categorized angiographically as perfused (nonischemic), nonperfused (ischemic), or mixed (perfused and nonperfused) (56). Characterizing the perfusion status of macular edema angiographically is not as significant therapeutically in eyes with CRVO as it is in eyes with BRVO. Laser photocoagulation has not been determined to be significantly beneficial for eyes with any angiographic category of macular edema from CRVO (56). A clinical trend, however, suggesting that visual acuity in individuals younger than 65 years old may be more likely to improve following grid laser photocoagulation, was demonstrated.

## Intraocular Neovascularization

In eyes with ischemic CRVO, the development of iris or angle neovascularization is more likely than the development of disc or retinal neovascularization.

### Iris and Angle Neovascularization

Iris or angle neovascularization may form in eyes with ischemic CRVO. Close examination of the undilated pupillary margin using high slit-lamp magnification is necessary every month for the first several months to detect early neovascularization in all eyes with ischemic CRVO. Gonioscopy also is recommended.

In the entire CVOS population of 714 eyes (nonischemic and ischemic), 117 eyes (16%) developed at least two clock hours of iris or any angle neovascularization during the follow-up period (4). In 10 (five treated with panretinal photocoagulation [PRP] prophylactically, five treated with PRP after early iris neovascularization) of the 117 eyes, the iris or angle neovascularization did not regress following laser treatment but instead progressed to neovascular glaucoma, defined as an intraocular pressure greater than 30 mm Hg with two clock hours of iris or angle neovascularization. Of these 10 eyes, four had poor outcomes, with progressive neovascular glaucoma (3,4).

Normal vessel variants observed on the pupillary margin may be identified inadvertently as early iris neovascularization. Specific clinical findings, however, may help differentiate these iris vessels from true iris neovascularization. For example, if the vessels on the pupillary margin also are noted in a contralateral eye that does not have a vein occlusion, then the vessels may represent a congenital variant or an aging change and not neovascularization. Moreover, if prominent vessels in the angle of the affected eye are also present in the fellow eye or if peripheral anterior synechiae are not present in the affected eye, then the vessels in the angle may not represent true angle neovascularization. Angiography of iris vasculature is not currently helpful in distinguishing true iris neovascularization from normal iris-vessel variants. As a result, it may not be feasible to differentiate true iris or angle neovascularization from normal vessel variants in some cases. Close follow-up of the vessels, with comparison with baseline iris photographs, may facilitate clinical decision making in these cases, because vessel growth would imply true neovascular proliferation.

### Disc and Retinal Neovascularization

In the CVOS, neovascularization of the disc, elsewhere on the retina or in both places, developed in 11 of the 90 eyes that underwent prophylactic PRP and in 16 of the 91 eyes that were not treated ($p < .3$) (3). In these eyes, posterior-segment neovascularization developed later during follow-up than anterior-segment neovascularization. Approximately half of the eyes with retinal neovascular proliferation also had anterior segment neovascularization at some point during the follow-up period (3).

Neovascularization on the disc should be distinguished from collateral vessels on the disc. Collateral vessels may form

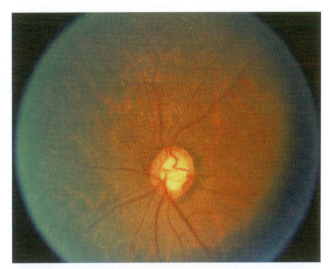

**Figure 24-9.** Collateral vessels, between the obstructed disc capillaries and unobstructed choroidal or pial capillaries, may form on the surface of the optic disc from preexisting retinal vessels (arrow). Collateral channels are tortuous vascular loops on or adjacent to the disc.

on the surface of the optic nerve from preexisting retinal vessels and connect obstructed disc capillaries to unobstructed choroidal or pial capillaries (Fig. 24-9). Collateral channels appear as tortuous vascular loops adjacent to or on the optic disc. It has been suggested that these channels may be associated with improved visual acuity (58,59); this finding, however, has not been substantiated widely (60).

## Pathogenesis and Histopathology

The pathophysiology of CRVO is not understood completely. The suggested cause is intravascular thrombus formation within the central retinal vein in the region of the lamina cribrosa (61,62). Histopathologic examination of eyes with CRVO has demonstrated occlusions at or just behind the level of the lamina cribrosa (61). There are certain anatomic factors at this location that may predispose the central retinal vein to thrombus formation. First, the central retinal artery and vein are bound by a common adventitial sheath and their lumina narrow as they pass through the lamina cribrosa. In addition, the close anatomic position of these vessels in the region of the lamina cribrosa also may lead to turbulent flow and the formation of a thrombus. Second, the lamina cribrosa is a sieve-like structure of connective tissue that may limit the expansion and displacement of the optic nerve and these vessels within it. A perioperative intraocular pressure change with an associated shift in the position of the lamina cribrosa may contribute to the blockage of venous outflow in susceptible eyes (63). A posterior shift in the cribrosa from an elevation in intraocular pressure or an anterior shift in the lamina cribrosa from a sudden decrease in intraocular pressure may result in turbulent flow and thrombus formation within the central retinal vein.

Activated protein C resistance and factor V Leiden recently have been identified as the most common genetic predisposition to venous thrombosis (64–67). Investigators have attempted to implicate activated protein C resistance and factor V Leiden as the cause of retinal vein occlusion; however, the literature has contradictory findings, and further investigation is necessary (68,69).

Few eyes have been studied histopathologically soon after a CRVO. Many cases in the literature involve eyes that have been enucleated because of chronic neovascular glaucoma; secondary changes that did not result in the original occlusion may interfere with the microscopic interpretation in these eyes. In evaluating the histopathology, Green and colleagues (61) suggested that the time interval between the venous occlusion and histopathologic examination must be considered. Twenty-nine eyes, enucleated 6 hours to 10 years following the occlusion, were studied. Thrombosis within the central retinal vein in the region of the lamina cribrosa was a consistent histopathologic observation. Green and coworkers (61) hypothesized that as the vein progressively narrows at the lamina cribrosa, where it may be impinged on further by arteriosclerosis of the adjacent central retinal artery, blood flow through the central retinal vein may become increasingly turbulent. The intravascular turbulence may damage the endothelium in the retrolaminar vein, stimulate platelet aggregation, and lead to thrombus formation. Endothelial cell proliferation and recanalization of the vein often occur as reparative events. Inflammation, appearing as periphlebitis, phlebitis, or obliterating endophlebitis, may be a late consequence. A thickened vein with one channel may form many years later.

Koizumi and colleagues recently suggested that complete thrombotic vein occlusion may not be as important in CRVO formation as once thought (70). Additional investigation into the pathophysiology of venous occlusion with histopathologic examination of eyes with recent CRVO is necessary to better understand and possibly prevent the occlusion.

## Management and Course

All eyes with ischemic, or potentially ischemic, CRVO should be evaluated each month to identify early anterior segment neovascularization and, if detected, to begin PRP promptly to promote vessel regression and prevent progression to neovascular glaucoma (3,4). Slit-lamp examination of the undilated pupillary margin using high magnification is necessary to detect early neovascular proliferation; angle neovascularization rarely may develop before iris neovascularization and requires gonioscopy for detection (3,4,57). Normal iris or angle vessels may resemble iris or angle neovascularization, and in these cases, photographs may be useful for comparison during subsequent examinations.

Approximately one third of initially nonischemic eyes later are determined to be ischemic (4,57). If visual acuity is 20/40 or better, the patient should be reexamined every 2 months for the first 6 months, decreasing to once per year as the clinical condition stabilizes. If the acuity is between 20/50 and 20/200, a CRVO is more likely to become nonperfused; monthly follow-up is recommended for 6 months after the onset, decreasing to once per year as the clinical condition stabilizes. If the acuity is worse than 20/200, the patient is examined once per month for the initial 6-month period. If the acuity should decrease to less than 20/200 during follow-up, the vein occlusion may have progressed to an ischemic perfusion status, requiring immediate examination. The follow-up schedule then should be modified to monthly visits, as would be recommended for a new patient presenting with a similar acuity (4).

## Medical Management

In the CVOS, the medical evaluation and management of patients with central vein occlusion were not addressed (3,4,56,57). Systemic pharmacologic substances, such as aspirin, heparin, warfarin, or other anticoagulants, have not been shown to prevent the development of vein occlusion. Intravenous pentoxifylline, a synthetic xanthine derivative, has been demonstrated to increase pulsatile ocular blood flow in eyes without vein occlusion, possibly by decreasing blood viscosity and promoting vasodilation (71). Its ability to prevent CRVO has not been investigated.

## Laser Photocoagulation

The CVOS was a multicenter, randomized, clinical trial that addressed three issues concerning the management of the common ocular sequelae of CRVO, macular edema and neovascularization (3,4,56,57). First, would macular grid pattern laser photocoagulation improve visual acuity in CRVO eyes with perfused macular edema (56)? Second, would early PRP prevent iris neovascularization in eyes with nonperfused CRVO (3,4)? Third, is early PRP more effective than PRP at the first identification of iris neovascularization in preventing neovascular glaucoma in eyes with nonperfused CRVO (3,4)?

### Macular Edema

The CVOS sought to determine whether macular grid pattern laser photocoagulation would improve visual acuity in eyes with CRVO with perfused macular edema on fluorescein angiography and visual acuity worse than 20/50 (56).

The CVOS data did not support a recommendation of grid pattern laser photocoagulation for perfused macular edema (56). Although laser treatment significantly decreased macular edema angiographically, it did not result in visual acuity improvement. No quantifiable macular edema was observed angiographically in 21 (31%) of 68 treated eyes at the 1-year visit; however, some macular edema was present in 72 untreated eyes ($p < .0001$) (56). This observation was similar for eyes with duration of CRVO of less than 12 months or of 12 months or longer, and in both younger and older persons. The visual outcome was comparable in both untreated and treated eyes. Initial median visual acuity was 20/125 in untreated eyes and 20/160 in treated eyes. The final median visual acuity was 20/160 in untreated eyes and 20/200 in treated eyes. The acuity improved by two or more lines in 17 treated eyes, 11 of which were in persons younger than 65 years of age. The number of eyes was too small for a significant conclusion; however, if the affected person is younger than 65 years of age, grid pattern laser photocoagulation for perfused macular edema may be considered (56). Additional study is warranted to better guide the management of patients younger than 65 years old with perfused macular edema from CRVO.

## Intraocular Neovascularization

The CVOS was designed to determine whether early PRP would prevent iris neovascularization in eyes with ischemic CRVO and whether early PRP would be more effective than PRP at the first detection of iris neovascularization in preventing progression to neovascular glaucoma (3,4).

The data from the CVOS does not support a recommendation for prophylactic PRP (3), because PRP does not always prevent the development of anterior-segment neovascularization. Neovascularization developed less often in eyes treated prophylactically than in untreated eyes; however, the difference was not statistically significant. PRP prior to the development of any iris or angle neovascularization may be considered only for nonperfused eyes if monthly examinations are not possible. Even with prophylactic PRP, frequent follow-up visits are needed to ensure that iris or angle neovascularization does not develop, requiring supplementation of the PRP (3,4).

PRP should be initiated only after the detection of neovascular proliferation, to save many eyes from receiving unnecessary photocoagulation, because many eyes with ischemic vein occlusion never develop iris or angle neovascularization (3,4). Because PRP results in prompt regression of neovascular proliferation in eyes that have not received prophylactic photocoagulation, it should be begun promptly at the first detection of early definite neovascularization. Following PRP, examination every 2 to 4 weeks is recommended to be certain that the neovascularization is not increasing; if it is progressing, supplemental photocoagulation is needed. The two clock hours of iris or angle neovascularization did not regress immediately after PRP in 11% of eyes in both groups in the CVOS study; instead, the neovascularization gradually regressed over a 2- to 30-month period (median, 9 months) (3,4). Except for 5 (5%) of the 90 treated eyes that received prophylactic PRP and 5 (5%) of the 91 initially untreated eyes, all eyes eventually stabilized and did not develop neovascular glaucoma. PRP similarly should be administered to eyes that develop disc or retinal neovascularization.

Various consequences of CRVO may hamper the sufficient placement of PRP. Iris neovascularization and associated posterior synechiae may interfere with pupillary dilation and the adequate delivery of PRP. Laser photocoagulation may disrupt the synechiae in early cases, allow pupillary dilation, and facilitate PRP. Moreover, corneal edema from elevated intraocular pressure may interfere with photocoagulation. The pharmacologic lowering of the intraocular pressure, the use of atropine and intensive topical corticosteroids, and the topical placement of glycerin may lessen the corneal edema and permit the delivery of PRP. Nonclearing vitreous hemorrhage and extensive retinal hemorrhage also may interfere with photocoagulation. If sufficient PRP is not possible, circumferential cryotherapy (72) or vitrectomy combined with endolaser photocoagulation may be considered.

## Vitreous Hemorrhage

In eyes with CRVO, a vitreous hemorrhage usually results from disc or retinal neovascularization, with or without previous PRP, or from the breakthrough of retinal hemorrhage through the internal limiting membrane into the vitreous cavity. If retinal detail cannot be evaluated in an eye with a vitreous hemorrhage, B-scan ultrasonography should be performed to exclude a traction retinal detachment and possibly other unrelated, intraocular causes of the bleeding.

In an eye with a CRVO and a vitreous hemorrhage, the presence or absence of disc or retinal neovascularization would direct the clinical decision of whether to initiate or supplement scatter laser photocoagulation. If the density of the hemorrhage precludes ophthalmoscopy, fluorescein angiography or angioscopy may facilitate visualization of any neovascularization. If a neovascular cause cannot be found, the hemorrhage may have resulted from the breakthrough of retinal hemorrhage. Identification of a neovascular source may be feasible as the hemorrhage spontaneously clears. If iris or angle neovascularization develops and the vitreous hemorrhage prevents adequate ophthalmoscopy, a pars plana vitrectomy with endolaser photocoagulation is recommended.

## Investigational Treatment Options

Conventionally, management has been directed at the treatment of sequelae of a CRVO, including macular edema and neovascularization, with laser photocoagulation (3,56) and has not been aimed toward reestablishing retinal venous outflow and possibly altering the natural history of the occlusive process. Prevention of the occlusion itself would be desirable; however, if a CRVO does occur, avoiding the ocular sequelae altogether, instead of treating them, is preferable. Consequently, treatment modalities recently have been directed toward restoring venous outflow (73–81) but are slowly shifting back to treating the ocular sequelae again.

### Bypass of the Retinal Vein: Chorioretinal Anastomosis Formation

Creation of a chorioretinal anastomosis (Fig. 24-10) between the choroid and a retinal vein may bypass the occluded vein and potentially relieve the venous congestion (73–75). The rationale for attempting to reestablish venous outflow with chorioretinal anastomosis formation has been to alter the natural history of eyes with perfused CRVO by improving visual acuity, through lessening of associated macular edema, and by decreasing the conversion rate to nonperfusion.

In eyes with a nonperfused vein occlusion, bypassing the occluded retinal vein has not been advocated, because reestablishing venous outflow in these eyes would not likely result in improved visual acuity or reperfusion of the regions of retinal capillary nonperfusion.

Creation of a chorioretinal venous anastomosis using laser photocoagulation has been successful in some eyes (73,75). Of 24 treated eyes with a perfused CRVO in one study, 8 (33%) developed an anastomosis within 7 weeks after treatment with some visual improvement, whereas only 12% of the 24 treated eyes had marked visual improvement of at least six lines (73). None of these eight eyes progressed to a nonperfused status. Of 30 eyes with a perfused vein occlusion in another study, 12 (40%) developed an anastomosis with some visual improvement; however, only two (8%) had marked visual improvement of at least 6 lines (75). Leonard and colleagues successfully created chorioretinal anastomoses by applying laser energy to

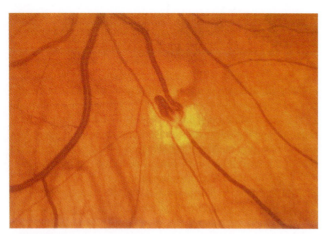

**Figure 24-10.** The formation of a chorioretinal anastomosis (arrow) between a retinal vein and the choroid may bypass the occluded venous segment and subsequently relieve the venous congestion.

rupture Bruch's membrane directly adjacent to the candidate branch vein site, avoiding laser-associated trauma to the retinal vein (82). Chang and Finkelstein reported a case of perfused CRVO of 22-month duration treated by the procedure of Leonard and colleagues (83). After successful CRA creation, visual acuity improved from 20/100 to 20/30 over a 9-month period. Successful CRA creation is reported in 10-54% of perfused CRVO with subsequent conversion to ischemic CRVO in 0-8% of eyes (84–87).

Major complications after this technique may occur (88–92). Possible treatment complications include longstanding, vision-limiting hemorrhage (88,91), preretinal fibrosis with or without traction retinal detachment (75,91), choroidal neovascularization (89,91), and choriovitreal neovascularization (90,91). Laser anastomosis is no longer commonly performed but with increased success rates, it may be re-visited.

Vitreoretinal surgical techniques are being explored to create a chorioretinal anastomosis (76). A few authors have attempted to create chorioretinal anastomoses surgically through a variety of techniques including transretinal venipuncture with variable results (93,94). The intraoperative removal of the posterior hyaloid in these eyes may lessen the likelihood of developing choriovitreal neovascularization (95).

## Reperfusion of the Retinal Vein

Modalities to reperfuse the blocked central retinal vein have included the use of recombinant tissue plasminogen activator (rt-PA) (77,78,96), transvitreal cannulation of the retinal vein (79), and radial optic neurotomy (RON) (97–103).

rt-PA is a synthetic, fibrinolytic, clot-selective agent that converts plasminogen to plasmin in the presence of fibrin. Tissue plasminogen activator has been utilized to lyse the thrombus within the central retinal vein (77). In 28 rabbit eyes, the thrombolytic effect of intravenous rt-PA to disrupt the clot in the retinal vein was examined (96). In 16 treated eyes (100%), the retinal vein became patent, whereas only 1 (8%) of 16 eyes treated with placebo was patent.

The administration of intravenous rt-PA may result in unwanted systemic hemorrhage causing injury and, in some cases, death. In individuals with CRVO, the local administra-

tion of rt-PA may be safer. A small pilot trial evaluated the effect of 75 mg of intravitreal rt-PA in eyes with acute (less than 1 week), perfused CRVO and suggested that rt-PA may be effective in treating these eyes (77). Three of nine treated eyes had return of visual acuity and resolution of the ophthalmoscopic manifestations of CRVO. This small study did not have a control group; therefore, it is not known if the presumed effect resulted from the use of intravitreal rt-PA or would have been the clinical course of the vein occlusion without treatment in these three eyes. Transvitreal retinal vein cannulation may provide direct access to an intravenous thrombus. In rabbit and cat eyes, cannulation of the retinal vasculature has been accomplished with glass micropipettes prepared from standard capillary tubing (79). Published case reports have used intravitreal tissue plasminogen activator (tPA) (104–107) and, more recently, vitrectomy followed by cannulation of a branch retinal vein and direct injection of tPA (108–111). Overall, the data available represent small uncontrolled case series. An increase in visual acuity (VA) of ≥3 lines has been reported in 50% to 59% (111,112) of patients with recent-onset CRVO and VA of 20/50 or worse. Unwanted side effects have included cataract, anterior segment and retinal neovascularization, vitreous hemorrhage, and rhegmatogenous and tractional retinal detachments (111–113).

Opremcak and colleagues proposed combining vitrectomy with transvitreal incision of the nasal scleral ring to release pressure on the central retinal vein at the level of the scleral outlet (97). RON is performed by vitrectomy followed by the use of a 20-gauge microvitreoretinal (MVR) blade to incise the lamina cribrosa and adjacent retina, usually nasally. The initial report by Opremcak and colleagues was a retrospective review of 11 eyes. Successful RON was performed with no complications, and clinical improvement in retinal hemorrhages and venous congestions was seen. In a prospective interventional trial, Garcia-Arumi and colleagues reported successful RON surgery in 14 eyes (98). In this study, 57% percent gained one line of visual acuity, and visual recovery was found to be related to reduction in macular edema. Six (43%) developed a postoperative chorioretinal anastomosis (CRA) at the RON site; those with CRA trended toward better final visual acuity compared to those without anastomosis formation (20/60 vs. 20/110). Seventy-three percent of patients had improved Snellen acuity. A retrospective case series of 5 patients and another nonrandomized prospective case series of 10 patients reported less impressive or no improvement (99,100). Complications associated with the RON procedure include severe immediate hemorrhage, visual field (VF) defects (101), postoperative neovascularization of the anterior segment and neurotomy site (100,102), and RD originating at the incision site (103).

## Intraocular Corticosteroids

Corticosteroids have been explored as a treatment of CRVO-related macular edema. Although the exact mechanism of action of corticosteroids in decreasing macular edema is not known, it is believed that a combination of stabilization of the blood-retinal barrier and anti-inflammatory effects may be involved.

Intravitreal delivery of corticosteroids allows for localized delivery of the drug to the macular region while limiting potential systemic side effects. Intravitreal injection of triamcinolone acetonide (Kenalog, TA) has gained in popularity due to reported improvements in visual acuity, low complication rates, a favorable safety profile, and ease of single or repeated administration with TA (45,114–120). Park and colleagues retrospectively reported ophthalmoscopic reduction in macular edema which corresponded to significant improvement in visual acuity and macular thickness by volumetric optical coherence tomography in 10 eyes with chronic perfused CRVO (121). Although no complications from the procedure were noted, 40% of patients had elevated intraocular pressure requiring topical aqueous suppressants. Potential complications include cataract progression, elevated intraocular pressure, retinal detachment, vitreous hemorrhage, and sterile and infectious endophthalmitis.

As a potential alternative, an intravitreal sustained release fluocinolone acetonide device (Retisert, Bausch and Lomb) is being implanted via *pars plana* incision. Currently, clinical trials are ongoing.

With respect to intravitreal corticosteroid treatment, controversies remain regarding the optimal dosing, long term effectiveness, adverse effects, and timing and need for retreatment. The SCORE study (discussed in the previous BRVO section), a multicenter phase III trial, has the potential to answer many of these questions (51).

## ANTI-VEGF Intravitreal Therapy

As discussed previously, anti-VEGF therapies such as pegaptanib sodium (Macugen; Eyetech Pharmaceuticals and Pfizer), ranibizumab and bevacizumab (Lucentis and Avastin, respectively; Genentech) may play a role in treating macular edema related to RVO and preventing neovascular complications (122–127). We are currently awaiting the results from a phase II randomized, double-blind, multicenter trial evaluating the efficacy, safety, and pharmacokinetics of intravitreal injections of pegaptanib sodium (Macugen) versus sham injections in patients with recent vision loss due to CRVO-related macular edema (128). Also, the RAVE (Rubeosis Anti-VEGF) Trial is evaluating the role of complete VEGF blockade with intravitreal ranibizumab (Lucentis, Genentech) in preventing neovascular glaucoma in ischemic CRVO (129).

## HEMIRETINAL VEIN OCCLUSION

The terms hemiretinal, hemispheric, and hemicentral retinal vein occlusion describe those eyes in which the superior or inferior retinal venous vasculature has been occluded. An HRVO may be diagnosed ophthalmoscopically if the intraretinal hemorrhage and venous tortuosity and dilation, characteristic of eyes with vein occlusion, involve either the superior or inferior half of the fundus. Systemic hypertension and a history of diabetes mellitus have been associated with an increased risk for HRVO (130). A consensus as to whether HRVO is a variant of CRVO or BRVO has not been reached (131–133); we categorize and manage eyes with HRVO as we do eyes with BRVO. Major differences in the natural history of HRVO compared with BRVO have not been identified.

Different configurations of the branches of the central retinal vein are found within the population (131). In approximately 20% of eyes, the branch retinal veins draining the superior and inferior halves of the retina enter the lamina cribrosa separately before joining to form a single central retinal vein (133). The occlusion of one of these dual trunks of the central retinal vein within the nerve produces a hemicentral retinal vein occlusion (131,133). In some eyes, the nasal retina is drained by a branch of either the superior or inferior temporal vein, instead of a separate vein. The obstruction of one of the veins draining both the nasal retina and the superior or inferior retina near the optic nerve head results in HRVO (134).

### References

1. David R, Zangwill L, Badarna M, et al. Epidemiology of retinal vein occlusion and its association with glaucoma and increased intraocular pressure. *Ophthalmologica* 1988;197:69.
2. Branch Vein Occlusion Study Group. Argon laser scatter photocoagulation for prevention of neovascularization and vitreous hemorrhage in branch vein occlusion: a randomized clinical trial. *Arch Ophthalmol* 1986;104:34.
3. The Central Vein Occlusion Study Group. A randomized clinical trial of early panretinal photocoagulation for ischemic central vein occlusion: the central vein occlusion study group N report. *Ophthalmology* 1995;102:1434.
4. The Central Vein Occlusion Study Group. Natural history and clinical management of central retinal vein occlusion. *Arch Ophthalmol* 1997;115:486.
5. Branch Vein Occlusion Study Group. Argon laser photocoagulation for macular edema in branch vein occlusion. *Am J Ophthalmol* 1984;98:271.
6. Johnston RL, Brucker AJ, Steinmann W, et al. Risk factors of branch retinal vein occlusion. *Arch Ophthalmol* 1985;103:1831.
7. Weinberg D, Dodwell DG, Fern SA. Anatomy of arteriovenous crossings in branch retinal vein occlusion. *Am J Ophthalmol* 1990;109:298.
8. Duker JS, Brown GC. Anterior location of the crossing artery in branch retinal vein occlusion. *Arch Ophthalmol* 1989;107:998.
9. Zhao J, Sastry SM, Sperduto RD, et al. Arteriovenous crossing patterns in branch retinal vein occlusion: The Eye Disease Case-Control Study Group. *Ophthalmology* 1993;100:423.
10. The Eye Disease Case-Control Study Group. Risk factors for branch retinal vein occlusion. *Am J Ophthalmol* 1993;116:286.
11. Ariturk N, Oge Y, Erkan D, et al. Relation between retinal vein occlusions and axial length. *Br J Ophthalmol* 1996;80:633.
12. Majji AB, Janarthanan M, Naduvilath TJ. Significance of refractive status in branch retinal vein occlusion: a case-control study. *Retina* 1997;17:200.
13. Timmerman EA, de Lavalette VW, van den Bron HJ. Axial length as a risk factor to branch retinal vein occlusion. *Retina* 1997;17:196.
14. Simons BD, Brucker AJ. Branch retinal vein occlusion: axial length and other risk factors. *Retina* 1997;17:191.
15. Gutman FA, Zegarra H. The natural course of temporal retinal branch vein occlusion. *Trans Am Acad Ophthalmol Otolaryngol* 1974;78:178.
16. Blankenship GW, Okun E. Retinal tributary vein occlusion. *Arch Ophthalmol* 1973;89:363.
17. Finkelstein D. Ischemic macular edema: recognition and favorable natural history in branch vein occlusion. *Arch Ophthalmol* 1992;119:1427.
18. Paton A, Rubenstein K, Smith VH. Arterial insufficiency in retinal venous occlusion. *Trans Ophthalmol Soc UK* 1964;84:559.
19. Hamilton AM, Kohner EM, Rosen D, et al. Experimental retinal branch vein occlusion in rhesus monkeys: I. Clinical appearances. *Br J Ophthalmol* 1979;63:377.
20. Rosen DA, Marshall J, Kohner EM, et al. Experimental retinal branch vein occlusion in rhesus monkeys: II. Retinal blood flow studies. *Br J Ophthalmol* 1979;63:388.
21. Frangieh GT, Green WR, Barraquer-Somers E, et al. Histopathologic study of nine branch retinal vein occlusions. *Arch Ophthalmol* 1982;100:1132.
22. Leber T. Die krankheiten der netzhaut und des schnerven. In: Graefe A, Saemisch T (eds). *Handbuch der gesammten augenheilkunde*, vol 5. Leipsig: Verlag von Wilhelm Engelmann, 1877:521.
23. Seitz R (Blodi FC, trans). The crossing phenomenon. In: Blodi FC (ed). *The retinal vessels.* St Louis: Mosby, 1964:20.
24. Hockley DJ, Tripathi RC, Ashton N. Experimental retinal branch vein occlusion in rhesus monkeys: III. Histopathological and electron microscopic studies. *Br J Ophthalmol* 1979;63:393.
25. Glacet-Bernard A, Coscas G, Chabanel A, et al. A randomized, double-masked study on the treatment of retinal vein occlusion with troxerutin. *Am J Ophthalmol* 1994;118:421–429.

26. Houtsmuller AJ, Vermeulen JA, Klompe M, et al. The influence of ticlopidine on the natural course of retinal vein occlusion. *Agents Actions Suppl* 1984;15:219–229.

27. Magargal LE, Kimmel AS, Sanborn GE, et al. Temporal branch retinal vein obstruction: a review. *Ophthalmic Surg* 1986;17:240.

28. Wilson DJ, Finkelstein D, Quigley HA, et al. Macular grid photocoagulation: an experimental study on the primate retina. *Arch Ophthalmol* 1988;106:100.

29. Finkelstein D. Laser treatment of macular edema resulting from branch vein occlusion. *Semin Ophthalmol* 1994;9:23.

30. Takahashi M, Hikichi T, Akiba J, et al. Role of the vitreous and macular edema in branch retinal vein occlusion. *Ophthalmic Surg Lasers* 1997;28:294–299.

31. Kurimoto M, Takagi H, Suzuma K, et al. Vitrectomy for macular edema secondary to retinal vein occlusion: evaluation by retinal thickness analyzer. *Jpn J Clin Ophthalmol* 1999;53:717–720.

32. Saika S, Tanaka T, Miyamoto T, et al. Surgical posterior vitreous detachment combined with gas/air tamponade for treating macular edema associated with branch retinal vein occlusion: retinal tomography and visual outcome. *Graefes Arch Clin Exp Ophthalmol* 2001;239:729–732.

33. Kumar B, Yu DY, Morgan WH, et al. The distribution of angioarchitectural changes within the vicinity of the arteriovenous crossing in branch retinal vein occlusion. *Ophthalmology* 1998;105:424–427.

34. Osterloh MD, Charles S. Surgical decompression of branch retinal vein occlusions. *Arch Ophthalmol* 1988;106:1469–1471.

35. Opremcak EM, Bruce RA. Surgical decompression of branch retinal vein occlusion via arteriovenous crossing sheathotomy: a prospective review of 15 cases. *Retina* 1999;19:1–5.

36. Mason J III, Feist R, White M Jr, et al. Sheathotomy to decompress branch retinal vein occlusion. A matched control study. *Ophthalmology* 2004;111:540–545.

37. Cahill MT, Kaiser PK, Sears JE, et al. The effect of arteriovenous sheathotomy on cystoid macular oedema secondary to branch retinal vein occlusion. *Br J Ophthalmol* 2003;87:1329–1332.

38. Wilson CA, Berkowitz BA, Sato Y, et al. Treatment with intravitreal steroid reduces blood-retinal barrier breakdown due to retinal photocoagulation. *Arch Ophthalmol* 1992;110:1155–1159.

39. Beer PM, Bakri SJ, Singh RJ, et al. Intraocular concentration and pharmacokinetics of triamcinolone^Rx^ acetonide^Rx^ after a single intravitreal injection. Ophthalmology 2003;110:681–686.

40. Jonas JB, Akkoyun I, Kamppeter B, et al. Branch retinal vein occlusion treated by intravitreal triamcinolone acetonide. *Eye* 2005;19:65–71.

41. Krepler K, Ergun E, Sacu S, et al. Intravitreal triamcinolone acetonide in patients with macular oedema due to branch retinal vein occlusion: a pilot study. *Acta Ophthalmol Scand* 2005;83:600–604.

42. Salinas-Alaman A, Garcia-Layana A, Sadaba-Echarri LM, et al. Branch retinal vein occlusion treated by intravitreal triamcinolone [in Spanish]. *Arch Soc Esp Oftalmol* 2005;80:463–465.

43. Karacorlu M, Ozdemir H, Karacorlu SA. Resolution of serous macular detachment after intravitreal triamcinolone acetonide treatment of patients with branch retinal vein occlusion. *Retina* 2005;25:856–860.

44. Cekic O, Chang S, Tseng JJ, et al. Intravitreal triamcinolone injection for treatment of macular edema secondary to branch retinal vein occlusion. *Retina* 2005;25:851–855.

45. Tewari HK, Sony P, Chawla R, et al. Prospective evaluation of intravitreal triamcinolone acetonide injection in macular edema associated with retinal vascular disorders. *Eur J Ophthalmol* 2005;15:619–626.

46. Bakri SJ, Shah A, Falk NS, et al. Intravitreal preservative-free triamcinolone acetonide for the treatment of macular oedema. *Eye* 2005;19:686–688.

47. Ozkiris A, Evereklioglu C, Erkilic K, et al. The efficacy of intravitreal triamcinolone acetonide on macular edema in branch retinal vein occlusion. *Eur J Ophthalmol* 2005;15:96–101.

48. Yepremyan M, Wertz FD, Tivnan T, et al. Early treatment of cystoid macular edema secondary to branch retinal vein occlusion with intravitreal triamcinolone acetonide. *Ophthalmic Surg Lasers Imaging* 2005;36:30–36.

49. Kaushik S, Gupta V, Gupta A, et al. Intractable glaucoma following intravitreal triamcinolone in central retinal vein occlusion. *Am J Ophthalmol* 2004;137:758–760.

50. Jonas JB, Degenring RF, Kreissig I, et al. Intraocular pressure elevation after intravitreal triamcinolone acetonide injection. *Ophthalmology* 2005;112:593–598.

51. U.S. National Institutes of Health. Clinicaltrials.gov. The standard care versus corticosteroid for retinal vein occlusion(SCORE) study. http://www.clinicaltrials.gov/ct/gui/show/NCT00105027. Accessed December 10, 2007.

52. Gutman FA. Evaluation of a patient with central retinal vein occlusion. *Ophthalmology* 1983;90:481.

53. Fong AC, Schatz H, McDonald HR, et al. Central retinal vein occlusion in young adults (papillophlebitis). *Retina* 1992;12:3.

54. The Eye Disease Case-Control Study Group. Risk factors for central retinal vein occlusion. *Arch Ophthalmol* 1996;114:545.

55. Arend O, Remky A, Jung F, et al. Role of rheologic factors in patients with acute central retinal vein occlusion. *Ophthalmology* 1996;103:80.

56. The Central Vein Occlusion Study Group. Evaluation of grid pattern photocoagulation for macular edema in central vein occlusion: the central vein occlusion study group M report. *Ophthalmology* 1995;102:1425.

57. Central Vein Occlusion Study Group. Baseline and early natural history report: the Central Vein Occlusion Study. *Arch Ophthalmol* 1993;111:1087.

58. Priluck IA, Robertson DM, Hollenhorst RW. Long-term follow-up of occlusion of the central retinal vein in young adults. *Am J Ophthalmol* 1980;90:190.

59. Blinder KJ, Khan JA, Giangiacomo J, et al. Optociliary veins and visual prognosis after central retinal vein occlusion. *Ann Ophthalmol* 1989;21:192.

60. Quinlan PM, Elman MJ, Bhatt AK, et al. The natural course of central retinal vein occlusion. *Am J Ophthalmol* 1990;110:118.

61. Green WR, Chan CC, Hutchins GM, et al. Central retinal vein occlusion: a prospective histopathologic study of 29 eyes in 28 cases. *Retina* 1981;1:27.

62. Green WR. Retina. In: Spencer WH (ed). *Ophthalmic pathology, an atlas and textbook*, 3rd ed. Philadelphia, PA: WB Saunders, 1985:589.

63. Dev S, Herndon L, Shields MB. Retinal vein occlusion after trabeculectomy with mitomycin C. *Am J Ophthalmol* 1996;122:574.

64. Dahlback B, Carlsson M, Svensson PJ. Familial thrombophilia due to a previously unrecognized mechanism characterized by poor response to activated protein C: prediction of a cofactor to activated protein C. *Proc Natl Acad Sci USA* 1993;90:1004.

65. Bertina RM, Koeleman BPC, Koster T, et al. Mutation in blood coagulation factor V associated with resistance to activated protein C. *Nature* 1994;369:64.

66. Greengard JS, Sun X, Xu X, et al. Activated protein C resistance caused by Arg506Gln mutation in factor V. *Lancet* 1994;343:1361.

67. Zoller B, Svensson PJ, He X, et al. Identification of the same factor V gene mutation in 47 out of 50 thrombosis-prone families with inherited resistance to activated protein C. *J Clin Invest* 1994;94:2521.

68. Williamson TH, Rumley A, Lowe GDO. Blood viscosity, coagulation, and activated protein C resistance in central retinal vein occlusion: a population controlled study. *Br J Ophthalmol* 1996;80:203.

69. Ciardella AP, Yannuzzi LA, Freund KB, et al. Factor V Leiden, activated protein C resistance, and retinal vein occlusion. *Retina* 1998;18:308.

70. Koizumi H, Ferrara DC, Brue C, et al. Central retina vein occlusion case control study. *Am J Ophthalmol* 2007;144(6):858–863.

71. Schmetterer L, Kemmler D, Breiteneder H, et al. A randomized, placebo-controlled, double-blind crossover study of the effect of pentoxifylline on ocular fundus pulsations. *Am J Ophthalmol* 1996;121:169.

72. Stefaniotou M, Paschides CA, Psilas K. Panretinal cryopexy for the management of neovascularization of the iris. *Ophthalmologica* 1995;209:141.

73. McAllister IL, Constable IJ. Laser-induced chorioretinal venous anastomosis for treatment of nonischemic central retinal vein occlusion. *Arch Ophthalmol* 1995;113:456.

74. Finkelstein D, Clarkson JG. Retinal vessel bypass: a promising new clinical investigative procedure. *Arch Ophthalmol* 1995;113:421.

75. Fekrat S, Goldberg MF, Finkelstein D. Laser-induced chorioretinal venous anastomosis for nonischemic central or branch retinal vein occlusion. *Arch Ophthalmol* 1998;116:43.

76. Fekrat S, de Juan E Jr. Chorioretinal anastomosis for vein occlusion: transvitreal venipuncture. *Ophthalmic Surg Lasers* 1999;30: 52–55.

77. Lahey JM, Kearney JJ. A pilot study for the treatment of acute central retinal vein occlusion with intravitreal tissue plasminogen activator [abstract]. *Ophthalmology* 1996;103(S):185.

78. Elman MJ. Thrombolytic therapy for central retinal vein occlusion: results of a pilot study. *Trans Am Ophthalmol Soc* 1996;94:471.

79. Allf BE, de Juan E Jr. In vivo cannulation of retinal vessels. *Graefes Arch Clin Exp Ophthalmol* 1987;225:221.

80. Vasco-Posada J. Modification of the circulation in the posterior pole of the eye. *Ann Ophthalmol* 1972;4:48.

81. Rodriquez J, Rodriquez FJ, Betancourt F. Presumed occlusion of posterior ciliary arteries following central retinal vein decompression surgery. *Arch Ophthalmol* 1994;112:54.

82. Leonard BC, Coupland SG, Kertes PJ, et al. Long-term follow-up of a modified technique for laser-induced chorioretinal venous anastomosis in nonischemic central retinal vein occlusion. *Ophthalmology* 2003;110(5):948–954.

83. Chang MA, Finkelstein D. Modified laser-induced chorioretinal anastomosis for treatment of longstanding perfused central retinal vein occlusion. *Retina* 2006;26(7):824–825.

84. Fekrat S, de Juan E Jr. Chorioretinal venous anastomosis for central retinal vein occlusion: transvitreal venipuncture. *Ophthal Surg Lasers* 1999;30:52–55.

85. Browning DJ, Antoszyk AN. Laser chorioretinal venous anastomosis for nonischemic central retinal vein occlusion. *Ophthalmology* 1998;105:670–677; discussion 7–9.

86. McAllister IL, Constable IJ. Laser-induced chorioretinal venous anastomosis for treatment of nonischemic central retinal vein occlusion [comment]. *Arch Ophthalmol* 1995;113:456–462.

87. McAllister IL, Douglas JP, Constable IJ, et al. Laser-induced chorioretinal venous anastomosis for nonischemic central retinal vein occlusion: evaluation of the complications and their risk factors. *Am J Ophthalmol* 1998;126:219–229.

88. Browning DJ, Rotberg MH. Vitreous hemorrhage complicating laser-induced chorioretinal anastomosis for central retinal vein occlusion. *Am J Ophthalmol* 1996;122:588.

89. Eccarius SG, Moran MJ, Slingsby JG. Choroidal neovascular membrane after laser-induced chorioretinal anastomosis. *Am J Ophthalmol* 1996;122:590.

90. Yarng S-S, Hsieh C-L. Choriovitreal neovascularization following laser-induced chorioretinal venous anastomosis [abstract]. *Ophthalmology* 1996;103(S):136.

91. McAllister IL, Douglas JP, Constable IJ, et al. Laser-induced chorioretinal venous anastomosis for nonischemic central retinal vein occlusion: evaluation of the complications and their risk factors. *Am J Ophthalmol* 1998;126:219.

92. Browning DJ, Antoszyk AN. Laser chorioretinal venous anastomosis for nonischemic central retinal vein occlusion. *Ophthalmology* 1998;105:670.

93. Peyman GA, Kishore K, Conway MD. Surgical chorioretinal venous anastomosis for ischemic central retinal vein occlusion. *Ophthalmic Surg Lasers* 1999;30:605–614.

94. Mirshahi A, Roohipoor R, Lashay A, et al. Surgical induction of chorioretinal venous anastomosis in ischaemic central retinal vein occlusion: a non-randomised controlled clinical trial. *Br J Ophthalmol* 2005;89:64–69.

95. Hikichi T, Konno S, Trempe CL. Role of the vitreous in central retinal vein occlusion. *Retina* 1995;15:29.

96. Oncel M, Peyman GA, Khoobehi B. Tissue plasminogen activator in the treatment of experimental retinal vein occlusion. *Retina* 1989;9:1.

97. Opremcak EM, Bruce RA, Lomeo MD, et al. Radial optic neurotomy for central retinal vein occlusion: A retrospective pilot study of 11 consecutive cases. *Retina* 2001;21:408–415.

98. Garcia-Arumi J, Boixadera A, Martinez-Castillo V, et al. Chorioretinal anastomosis after radial optic neurotomy for central retinal vein occlusion. *Arch Ophthalmol* 2003;121:1385–1391.

99. Martínez-Jardón CS, Meza-de Regil A, Dalma-Weiszhausz J, et al. Radial optic neurotomy for ischaemic central vein occlusion. *Br J Ophthalmol* 2005;89:558–561.

100. Weizer JS, Stinnett SS, Fekrat S. Radial optic neurotomy as treatment for central retinal vein occlusion. *Am J Ophthalmol* 2003;136:814–819.

101. Schneider U, Inhoffen W, Grisanti S, et al. Characteristics of visual field defects by scanning laser ophthalmoscope microperimetry after radial optic neurotomy for central retinal vein occlusion. *Retina* 2005;25:704–712.

102. Schneider U, Inhoffen W, Grisanti S, et al. Chorioretinal neovascularization after radial optic neurotomy for central retinal vein occlusion. *Ophthalmic Surg Lasers Imaging* 2005;36:508–511.

103. Samuel MA, Desai UR, Gandolfo CB. Peripapillary retinal detachment after radial optic neurotomy for central retinal vein occlusion. *Retina* 2003;23:580–583.

104. Lahey JM, Fong DS, Kearney J. Intravitreal tissue plasminogen activator for acute central retinal vein occlusion. *Ophthalmic Surg Lasers* 1999;30:427–434.

105. Glacet-Bernard A, Kuhn D, Vine AK, et al. Treatment of recent onset central retinal vein occlusion with intravitreal tissue plasminogen activator: a pilot study. *Br J Ophthalmol* 2000;84:609–613.

106. Ghazi NG, Noureddine B, Haddad RS, et al. Intravitreal tissue plasminogen activator in the management of central retinal vein occlusion. *Retina* 2003;23:780–784.

107. Elman MJ, Raden RZ, Carrigan A. Intravitreal injection of tissue plasminogen activator for central retinal vein occlusion. *Trans Am Ophthalmol Soc* 2001;99:219–221; discussion 222–223.

108. Weiss JN. Retinal surgery for treatment of central retinal vein occlusion. *Ophthalmic Surg Lasers* 2000;31:162–165.

109. Weiss JN. Treatment of central retinal vein occlusion by injection of tissue plasminogen activator into a retinal vein. *Am J Ophthalmol* 1998;126:142–144.

110. Bynoe LA, Weiss JN. Retinal endovascular surgery and intravitreal triamcinolone acetonide for central vein occlusion in young adults. *Am J Ophthalmol* 2003;135:382–384.

111. Bynoe LA, Hutchins RK, Lazarus HS, et al. Retinal endovascular surgery for central retinal vein occlusion: initial experience of four surgeons. *Retina* 2005;25:625–632.

112. U.S. National Institutes of Health. Clinicaltrials.gov. The standard care versus corticosteroid for retinal vein occlusion (SCORE) study. http://www.clinicaltrials.gov/ct/gui/show/NCT00105027. Accessed December 15, 2007.

113. Weiss JN, Bynoe LA. Injection of tissue plasminogen activator into a branch retinal vein in eyes with central retinal vein occlusion. *Ophthalmology* 2001;108:2249–2257.

114. Jonas JB, Kreissig I, Degenring RF. Intravitreal triamcinolone[Rx] acetonide[Rx] as treatment of macular edema in central retinal vein occlusion. *Graef Arch Clin Exp Ophthalmol* 2002;240:782–783.

115. Ip MS, Kumar KS. Intravitreous triamcinolone[Rx] acetonide[Rx] as treatment for macular edema from central retinal vein occlusion. *Arch Ophthalmol* 2002;120:1217–1219.

116. Greenberg PB, Martidis A, Rogers AH, et al. Intravitreal triamcinolone[Rx] acetonide[Rx] for macular oedema due to central retinal vein occlusion. *Br J Ophthalmol* 2002;86:247–248.

117. Jonas JB, Akkoyun I, Kamppeter B, et al. Intravitreal triamcinolone acetonide for treatment of central retinal vein occlusion. *Eur J Ophthalmol* 2005;15:751–758.

118. Ip MS, Gottlieb JL, Kahana A, et al. Intravitreal triamcinolone for the treatment of macular edema associated with central retinal vein occlusion. *Arch Ophthalmol* 2004;122:1131–1136.

119. Cekiç O, Chang S, Tseng JJ, et al. Intravitreal triamcinolone treatment for macular edema associated with central retinal vein occlusion and hemiretinal vein occlusion. *Retina* 2005;25:846–850.

120. Bashshur ZF, Maíluf RN, Allam S, et al. Intravitreal triamcinolone for the management of macular edema due to nonischemic central retinal vein occlusion. *Arch Ophthalmol* 2004;122:1137–1140.

121. Park CH, Jaffe GJ, Fekrat S. Intravitreal triamcinolone[Rx] acetonide[Rx] in eyes with cystoid macular edema associated with central retinal vein occlusion. *Am J Ophthalmol* 2003;136:419–425.

122. Hsu J, Kaiser RS, Sivalingam A, et al. Intravitreal bevacizumab (Avastin) in central retinal vein occlusion. *Retina* 2007;27(8):1013–1019.

123. Priglinger SG, Wolf AH, Kreutzer TC, et al. Intravitreal bevacizumab injections for treatment of central retinal vein occlusion: six-month results of a prospective trial. *Retina* 2007;27(8):1004–1012.

124. Ferrara DC, Koizumi H, Spaide RF. Early bevacizumab treatment of central retinal vein occlusion. *Am J Ophthalmol* 2007;144(6):864–871.

125. Stahl A, Agostini H, Hansen LL, et al. Bevacizumab in retinal vein occlusion-results of a prospective case series. *Graefes Arch Clin Exp Ophthalmol* 2007;245(10):1429–1436.

126. Pai SA, Shetty R, Vijayan PB, et al. Clinical, anatomic, and electrophysiologic evaluation following intravitreal bevacizumab for macular edema in retinal vein occlusion. *Am J Ophthalmol* 2007;143(4):601–606.

127. Iturralde D, Spaide RF, Meyerle CB, et al. Intravitreal bevacizumab (Avastin) treatment of macular edema in central retinal vein occlusion: a short-term study. *Retina* 2006;26(3):279–284.

128. U.S. National Institutes of Health. Clinicaltrials.gov. Pegaptanib sodium compared to sham injection in patients with recent vision loss due to macular edema secondary to central retinal vein occlusion (CRVO). http://www.clinicaltrials.gov/show/NCT00088283. Accessed December 15, 2007.

129. The RAVE (Rubeosis Anti-VEGF Trial). http://www.houstonretina.com/research.html. Accessed December 15, 2007.

130. Sperduto RD, Hiller R, Chew E, et al. Risk factors for hemiretinal vein occlusion: comparison with risk factors for central and branch retinal vein occlusion: the Eye Disease Case-Control Study. *Ophthalmology* 1998;105:765.

131. Hayreh SS, Hayreh MS. Hemi-central retinal vein occlusion: pathogenesis, clinical features, and natural history. *Arch Ophthalmol* 1980;98:1600.

132. Appiah AP, Trempe CL. Differences in contributory factors among hemicentral, central, and branch retinal vein occlusions. *Ophthalmology* 1989;96:364.

133. Chopdar A. Dual trunk central retinal vein incidence in clinical practice. *Arch Ophthalmol* 1984;102:85.

134. Sanborn GE, Magargal LE. Characteristics of the hemispheric retinal vein occlusion. *Ophthalmology* 1984;91:1616.

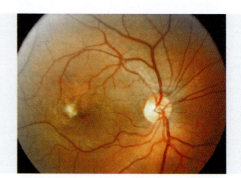

# Macular Edema Associated with Idiopathic Telangiectasias and Macroaneurysm

Peter Liggett ■ Nauman Chaudry

# PARAFOVEAL TELANGIECTASIS

"Retinal telangiectasis" is a term first proposed by Reese in 1956 (1) to describe a retinal vascular disorder associated with ectasia and irregular dilation of capillaries in the macula or peripheral retina. Fundoscopic and fluorescein angiographic findings of eyes with loss of macular function associated with retinal telangiectasis have been well described by Gass (2) in 1968. The term "parafoveal telangiectasis" (PT), however, first was used in 1978 by Hutton and colleagues (3), describing the presence of dilated capillaries in the juxtafoveal area. The cause of this condition is unknown; Gass & Oyakama (4) termed this condition "idiopathic juxtafoveal retinal telangiectasis" and divided the disease into several groups based on clinical findings and the purported underlying cause. Gass (2) proposed that in some patients, the telangiectatic capillaries were of congenital or developmental origin (a variant of Coat's disease), whereas in others, they were an acquired anomaly. Gass and Blodi (5) later modified the original classification system and sub-divided the group into three categories (Table 25-1).

# EPIDEMIOLOGY

PT is a relatively rare condition, and precise incidence and prevalence figures have not been established. Patients typically first present in adulthood with decreased vision or scotoma in one or both eyes. Patient characteristics differ for each of these subgroups proposed by Gass and Blodi (Table 25-1). Group 1 patients are usually male and typically have only one eye involved. Patients with group 2 or 3 disease are older and typically have bilateral disease. Both males and females are affected with equal frequency with group 2 disease. Group 3A patients are typically women, whereas group 3B patients are usually men.

A familial tendency may be present in some subtypes (2B, 3A, 3B) (5), and one case of father-to-son transmission of PT has been reported (6).

# CONGENITAL PARAFOVEAL TELANGIECTASIS

The common finding on fluorescein angiography in all three groups is the presence of retinal capillary telangiectasis localized to the parafoveal region. Other features are typical (Table 25-1) of a particular group.

## Group 1A: Unilateral Congenital Parafoveal Telangiectasis

Group 1A consists typically of men whose mean age at onset of the disease is 40 years. Only one eye is involved in these patients. The telangiectatic vessels are confined to the temporal parafoveal region, and the zone of involvement typically straddles the horizontal raphe (Fig. 25-1A-B). In patients with subtype 1A, the zone of involvement is usually one to two disc diameters in size. The telangiectatic vessels appear as microaneurysmal or saccular dilation of retinal capillaries and are visible biomicroscopically. Retinal capillary leakage is believed to be the principal abnormality in these eyes, and thus exudation is a prominent feature. Lipid exudates are often present at the margin of the zone of telangiectasis. Macular edema and exudation are the major causes of visual loss in these eyes. Visual acuity at presentation usually ranges from 20/25 to 20/40, although 20/200 may occur.

# ACQUIRED PARAFOVEAL TELANGIECTASIS

## Group 1B: Unilateral Idiopathic Parafoveal Telangiectasis

According to Gass (2), idiopathic PT (IPT) is found in middle-aged men who have more localized disease, with less than two clock hours of telangiectasis. The foveal avascular zone (FAZ)

## TABLE 25-1   PARAFOVEAL TELANGIECTASIS CLASSIFICATION (4)

|  | Group 1A unilateral congenital parafoveal telangiectasis | Group 1B unilateral idiopathic parafoveal telangiectasis | Group 2 bilateral acquired parafoveal telangiectasis | Group 3 bilateral idiopathic parafoveal telangiectasis and capillary obliteration |
|---|---|---|---|---|
| Mean age (years) | 40 | 40 | 50–60 | 50 |
| Gender | Males | Males | Males and Females | – |
| Parafoveal area involved | Temporal 1–2 disc diameters | One clock-hour area only | Temporal or the entire parafoveal network | Progressive obliteration of the entire parafoveal network |
| Other retinal features |  |  | Eventual retinal pigment epithelial hyperplasia, right-angle venule, yellow lesion at the center of the fovea avascular zone, subretinal neovascularization | Optic disc pallor |

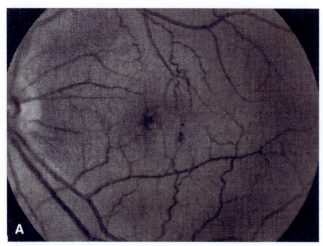
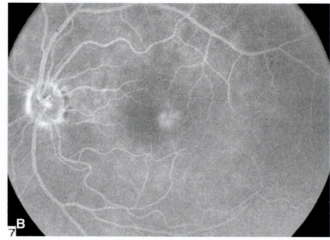

**Figure 25-1.** Group 1A unilateral congenital parafoveal telangiectasis and macular edema. **A:** Left eye. **B:** Late phase fluorescein angiography.

may be significantly smaller in these patients. Mansour and Schachat (7) found that the FAZ was almost completely vascularized in 65% of eyes with IPT studied by fluorescein angiography. The median FAZ in eyes with Group 1 PT was 0.0 mm$^2$ compared with 0.405 mm$^2$ in control eyes. Rarely does this area of telangiectasis have much leakage on fluorescein angiography. Visual acuity is usually better than 20/25.

## Group 2: Bilateral Acquired Parafoveal Telangiectasis

This is the most common form of IPT. Men and woman are affected equally, and the disease is nearly always bilateral. The telangiectatic capillaries are difficult to see biomicroscopically and often require fluorescein angiography for detection. The telangiectasis always involves the entire parafoveal retina. Multiple refractile, glistening deposits may be seen in the superficial retina overlying the zone of telangiectasis (8). A round yellow spot, 100–300 microns in size, may be present in the foveal center in some eyes.

Gass has described five stages in eyes with Group 2 IPT (5). In the first stage, there is minimal or no evidence of retinal telangiectasis, with only mild staining at the level of the outer parafoveal retina in the late phase of the fluorescein angiography. Stage 3 is characterized by the appearance of dilated venules that extend at right angles from the inner to the outer retina. The right angle venules may appear to drain the outer telangiectatic retinal capillary bed. In stage 4, retinal pigment epithelial hyperplasia develops. The hyperplastic retinal pigment epithelium may form intraretinal pigment plaques and may surround the right angle venules. In stage 5, subretinal neovascularization (SRNV) and fibrosis (Fig. 25-2) develop, typically in the region of intraretinal pigment epithelial migration. SRNV occurs in approximately 14% of eyes with Group 2 IPT. Optical coherence tomography (OCT) has provided further insight into the retinal thickness at the different stages of the natural course of the disease. It appears that, in the presence of retinal staining with fluorescein angiography, there may be no associated retinal thickening. Albani et al. (9) reported the presence of foveal cysts revealed by OCT in

stage 3 IPT, but no correlation with fluorescein angiogram was found. Paunescu et al. (10) reported the following OCT features of IPT: a lack of correlation between retinal thickening on OCT and leakage on fluorescein angiography; loss of disruption of the photoreceptor layer; cystlike structures in the fovea and within the internal layers; a unique internal limiting membrane draping across the fovea related to underlying loss of tissue; intraretinal neovascularization near the fovea; and, central intraretinal deposits and plaques.

Gass and Blodi (5) identified a separated subtype of patients, Group 2B, that showed a familial pattern. Group 2B was distinguished from the more common nonfamilial Group 2A by the lack of right-angle venules, superficial retina refractile deposits, and hyperplastic retinal pigment plaques. Acute central visual loss occurs in some patients with the development of neovascularization, which may begin as intraretinal neovascularization. Later follow-up of such cases shows the presence of retinochoroidal anastomosis, which often involves the foveal avascular zone (11).

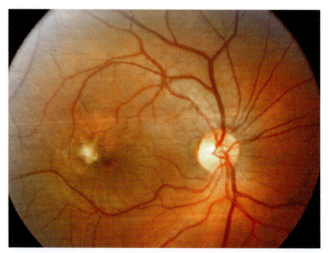

**Figure 25-2.** Group 2 bilateral acquired parafoveal telangiectasis. Subretinal neovascularization (SRNV) and fibrosis associated with parafoveal telangiectasis.

## Group 3: Occlusive Idiopathic Parafoveal Telangiectasis

The occlusive form is the rarest form of IPT and is characterized by extensive occlusion and loss of parafoveal capillary network, associated with telangiectasis of the remaining parafoveal capillaries. The disease is typically bilateral. Parafoveal fluorescein leakage is virtually absent in these patients. In contrast to Group 1 IPT, in which the FAZ may be small or absent, the FAZ in eyes with Group 3 IPT is enlarged markedly. Despite this marked capillary loss, visual acuity may remain good (20/25 or better in 67%) (5). An atypical case of Group 3 IPT associated with peripheral retinal ischemia and anterior and posterior segment neovascularization has been reported (12).

Gass distinguished patients with subtype 3A from those with subtype 3B, by the presence of an associated central nervous system vasculopathy in patients with 3B. Manifestations of central nervous system disease include optic disc pallor, exaggerated deep tendon reflexes, gait abnormalities, and multiple brain infarcts on magnetic resonance imaging (5).

## HISTOPATHOLOGY

Green and colleagues (13) reported on the histopathologic and ultrastructural features of an eye with IPT. The patient was a 58-year-old woman who underwent orbital exenteration for squamous cell carcinoma. Prior to removal of the globe, fluorescein angiography was obtained and revealed bilateral telangiectatic capillaries temporal to the fovea and a clinical picture consistent with Group 2A IPT. On histological examination, however, no telangiectatic capillaries were observed. Rather, there was marked thickening of the capillary wall and narrowing of the lumen. Electron microscopy revealed that the capillary wall thickening resulted from marked proliferation and reduplication of basement membrane in a multilayer arrangement. There was marked degeneration of pericytes and, in some areas, degeneration of endothelial cells. The histopathologic changes observed in this eye are strikingly similar to the retinal vascular abnormalities in patients with diabetes. The patient studied by Green and colleagues had no history of diabetes. Given the lack of true telangiectatic vessels histopathologically, Green and colleagues questioned the use of term "telangiectasis" to describe this condition. They hypothesized that the appearance of telangiectasis of fluorescein angiogram was a result of the diffusion of fluorescein dye through endothelial defects and into the thickened capillary wall.

Gass has suggested that this capillary-wall abnormality was a physical substrate for the "diffusion defect" in patient with group 2 IPT. The histopathology of patients with Group 1 or Group 2 IPT has not been studied.

## ASSOCIATION WITH DIABETES MELLITUS

An association between diabetes mellitus and Group 2 IPT has been suggested (13). The histopathologic similarity between the two diseases provides further support for the existence of a relationship. Some investigators have speculated that abnormal glucose metabolism may lead to parafoveal telangiectasis based on findings that 35% of patients with IPT have abnormal glucose tolerance test results (14). Gass and Blodi (5), however, who reported on the largest number of patients, found that only 6.5% of patients with Group 2 IPT developed diabetes. They suggested that diabetes may predispose some patients to develop Group 2 IPT, but that its relative importance is small. Another systemic disease that has been reported to be associated with cases of PT is celiac sprue (15).

A histopathologic study by Eiliassi-Rad and Green (16) showed dilation and proliferation of retinal capillaries into the other retinal and subretinal space. There was a migration of the retinal pigment epithelium within the retina along the telangiectasic vessels. Preretinal neovascularization was also found. Interestingly, there was a sharp demarcation between the edematous and nonedematous retina. With the staining of the retina with fluorescein in eyes with minimal edema, Gas has postulated that it possible that the primary abnormality may be found in the parafoveal retina neural of Muller cells (17).

## DIFFERENTIAL DIAGNOSIS

The diagnosis of PT may be made by careful biomicroscopy and fluorescein angiography. PT is a clinical entity that is distinctly different from secondary telangiectasis, which can result from various other diseases. The most common causes of secondary telangiectasis include diabetic retinopathy, venous occlusive disease, radiation retinopathy, hypertensive retinopathy, and ocular ischemic syndrome (5,18). Most of these secondary causes of telangiectasis tend to produce a diffuse vasculopathy, unlike IPT, which is localized to the parafoveal region (predominantly temporally). Moreover, the presence of associated retinal abnormalities such intraretinal hemorrhage, cotton-wool spots, and retinal neovascularization can help distinguish secondary telangiectasis from IPT.

Venous occlusive disease (particularly small retinal vein occlusions) can produce localized vascular abnormalities, including telangiectasias. The telangiectatic vessels, however, are confined to the distribution of the involved vein, distal to the point of blockage. Thus, the telangiectatic vessels usually do not cross the horizontal raphe. In contrast, in IPT, the telangiectatic vessels typically straddle the horizontal raphe.

Age-related macular degeneration is another entity for which PT may be mistaken. In this disease, the choroidal neovascularization is accompanied by drusen and retinal pigment epithelium (RPE) abnormalities with no evidence of retina capillary disease.

## MANAGEMENT

The treatment of macular edema in patients with PT is controversial. There have been no controlled clinical trials. Grid laser photocoagulation to the area of angiographic leakage has been advocated by some investigators (3,19) who have observed a reduction in macular edema and improvement of visual acuity in treated patients. Others have reported favorable results in a case series in which a number of cases of classic choroidal neovascularization, including PT, received photodynamic therapy (20).

Recently, there has been an increase in the use of intraocular antivascular endothelial growth factor (anti-VEGF). Mandal et al. (21) reported 6 patients treated with intravitreal bevacizumab (Avastin) for subretinal neovascularization secondary to type 2A idiopathic juxtafoveal telangiectasia. After a follow-up of 4.2 months, the visual acuity improved two or three lines as did the mean central foveal thickness. This is a small series and longer follow-up is required. Moon et al. (22) reported one case with complete resolution of macular edema after intravitreal bevacizumab injection in short term follow-up. Intravitreal triamcinolone injection is been also reported for the treatment of macular edema secondary to idiopathic juxtafoveal telangiectasis in one patient (23).

## RETINAL ARTERY MACROANEURYSMS

Retinal arterial macroaneurysms are an acquired retinal vascular abnormality. These isolated dilations of the major retinal arterial branches are found within the posterior pole and are associated with systemic hypertension, arteriosclerosis, retinal emboli and cardiovascular disease. Robertson, in 1973 (24), coined the term "macroaneurysm" for a retinal arterial lesion with the following characteristics: saccular or fusiform arterial swelling, located within the first three orders of the retinal arteriole tree, and usually situated at the arterial bifurcation. Most commonly, retinal macroaneurysm affects patients in the sixth and seventh decades of life. Numerous studies have found 70% to 80% of the patients to be women. A large collaborative series by Schatz et al. described the findings in 130 eyes of 120 patients; they found two-thirds of these patients to be hypertensive (25,26). It presents unilaterally in more than 90% of patients.

## CLINICAL SYMPTOMS AND FINDINGS

The majority of patients are asymptomatic if the macula is not involved, but the most common clinical symptom is acute decrease in central visual acuity due to retinal edema, exudation, or hemorrhage (27). Patients may have also other visual changes such as shadows of "floaters."

Macroaneurysms typically present as round or fusiform dilation of the retinal arteriole that may be several times the caliber of the arteriole (Fig. 25-3A). Variable degrees of arterial wall hyalinization and surrounding intraretinal lipid and hemorrhage are frequently present. They occur mostly in the superotemporal retinal vasculature (52%), followed by inferotemporal (38%), inferotemporal (5%), and superonasal vessels (5%) (28). If pulsatile macroaneurysm is present, some investigators speculate that a greater risk of vitreous hemorrhage exists (29). Schatz et al. (26) coined the term *hourglass hemorrhage* to describe the simultaneous presence of both a subretinal and preretinal hemorrhage secondary to the macroaneurysm. Secondary vitreous hemorrhage occurs in approximately 10% of eyes but is rarely recurrent. Hemorrhage in the space beneath the retinal pigment epithelium may produce a dark lesion simulating an ocular melanoma (30) or a lesion associated with age-related macular degeneration. Table 25-2 shows the most common retinal disorders to be considered in the differential diagnosis of retinal artery macroaneurysms.

## ANGIOGRAPHIC FEATURES

Fluorescein angiography in an eye with retinal macroaneurysm may disclose early uniform filling (Fig. 25-3B). The hemorrhage may also partially or completely obscure the aneurysm. In those cases, indocyanine green angiography could be helpful in establishing the diagnosis and influencing the management of these patients who present with submacular or premacular hemorrhage (31). The appearance of the late

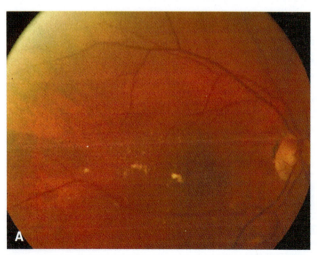
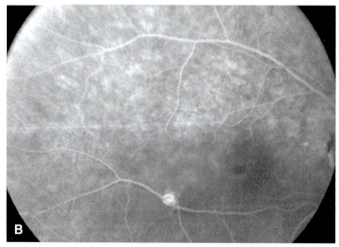

**Figure 25-3. A:** Retinal arterial macroaneurysm with surrounding lipid exudate. **B:** Early phase fluorescein angiography showing complete filling of retinal artery macroaneurysm.

**TABLE 25-2 RETINAL DISORDERS TO BE CONSIDERED IN THE DIFFERENTIAL DIAGNOSIS OR RETINAL ARTERY MACROANEURYSMS**

Leber's miliary aneurysm

Coat's syndrome

Idiopathic parafoveal telangiectasis

Angiomatosis retinae

Hemorrhagic pigment epithelium

Detachment

Diabetic retinopathy

Cavernous hemangioma

Malignant choroidal melanoma

Disciform scar secondary to ARMD.

ARMD, age-related macular degeneration.

phase of the fluorescein angiography varies, ranging from little staining of the vessel wall to marked leakage. The lipid often present in the macular area fails to block fluorescein unless the amount of exudation is massive.

## HISTOPATHOLOGY

Fichte and associates (32) described aneurysmal sites showing thickening of the blood vessel wall secondary to a fibrin-laminated clot, with accompanying hypertrophy of the muscularis. Hyaline, hemorrhage, and foamy macrophages may be seen in the vessel wall.

## MANAGEMENT

All patients with retinal macroaneurysm should undergo complete medical evaluation due to the high association with systemic hypertension and retinal emboli. Some investigators believe the visual prognosis is excellent in most patients who have macroaneurysms and do not undergo treatment, because the lesions can thrombose and spontaneously regress with clearing of the macular exudate (33). However, the exudative process could progress and cause structural damage to the macula with loss of vision. Although formal indications for photocoagulation treatment remain uncertain, most investigators agree that laser photocoagulation should be performed if lipid exudate threatens or involve the fovea. Laser photocoagulation may be performed either directly or indirectly. Direct photocoagulation of the macroaneurysm, with or without treatment of the surrounding retina has been successful in closing macroaneurysms (34,35). Potential complications of direct laser treatment include rupture of the macroaneurysm with subsequent hemorrhage and branch retina artery occlusion involving the feeding arteriole.

## References

1. Reese AB. Telangiectasis of the retina and Coat's disease. *Am J Ophthalmol* 1956;42:1.
2. Gass JDM. A fluorescein angiogram study of macular dysfunction secondary to retinal vascular disease. Part V: retinal telangiectasis. *Arch Ophthalmol* 1968;80:592.
3. Hutton WL, Snyder WB, Fuller D, et al. Focal parafoveal telangiectasis. *Arch Ophthalmol* 1978;96;1362.
4. Gass JD, Oyakama RT. Idiopathic juxtafoveolar retinal telangiectasis. *Arch Ophthalmol* 1982;100:769–780.
5. Gass JDM, Blodi BA. Idiopathic juxtafoveal retinal telangiectasis: update on classification and follow-up study. *Ophthalmology* 1993;100:1536–1546.
6. Devenyi RG, Castillejos-Rios D. Familial parafoveal telangiectasis. *Can J Ophthalmol* 1993;28:76.
7. Manssur AM, Schachat AP. Foveal avascular zone in idiopathic juxtafoveal telangiectasis. *Ophthalmologica* 1993;207:9.
8. Moisseiev J, Lewis H, Bartov E, et al. Superficial retinal refractile deposits in juxtafoveal telangiectasis. *Am J Ophthalmol* 1990;109:604.
9. Albini TA, Benz MS, Coffee RE, et al. Optical coherence tomography of idiopathic juxtafoveolar telangiectasia. *Ophthalmic Surg Lasers Imaging* 2006;37(2):120–128.
10. Paunescu LA, Ko TH, Duker JS, et al. Idiopathic juxtafoveal retinal telangiectasis: new findings by ultrahigh-resolution optical coherence tomography. *Ophthalmology* 2006;113(1):48–57.
11. Gass JDM. Histological study of presumed parafoveal telangiectasia. *Retina* 2000;20:226–227.
12. Lim JI, Bressler NM. Atypical parafoveal telangiectasis with subsequent anterior and posterior segment neovascularization. *Retina* 1992;12:351.
13. Chew EY, Murphy RP, Newsome DA, et al. Parafoveal telangiectasis and diabetic retinopathy. *Arch Ophthalmol* 1986;104:71.
14. Millary R, Klein M, Handelman I, et al. Abnormal glucose metabolism and parafoveal telangiectasis. *Arch Ophthalmol* 1986;102:363.
15. Lee HC, Liu M, Ho AC. Idiopathic juxtafoveal telangiectasis in association with celiac sprue. *Arch Ophthalmol* 2004;122:411–413.
16. Eliassi-Rad B, Green WR. Histopathologic study of presumed parafoveal telangiectasis. *Retina* 1999;19:332–335.
17. Green WR, Quigley HA, de la Cruz Z, et al. Parafoveal retinal telangiectasis: Light and electrón microscopy studies. *Trans Ophthalmol Soc UK* 1980;100:162–170.
18. Terasvirta M, Touvinen E. Idiopathic uniocular juxtafoveal retinal telangiectasis in a female patient. *Arch Ophthalmol* 1985;63:60.
19. Chopdar A. Retinal telangiectasis in adults: fluorescein angiographic findings and treatment by argon laser. *Br J Ophthalmol* 1978;62:243.
20. Muller-Velten R, Michels S, Schimdt-Erfurth U, et al. Photodynamic therapy: extended indication. *Ophthalmologe* 2003;100:384–390.
21. Mandal S, Venkatesh P, Abbas Z, et al. Intravitreal bevacizumab (Avastin) for subretinal neovascularization secondary to type 2A idiopathic juxtafoveal telangiectasia. *Graefes Arch Clin Exp Ophthalmol* 2007;245(12):1895–1899.
22. Moon SJ, Berger AS, Tolentino MJ, et al. Intravitreal bevacizumab for macular edema from idiopathic juxtafoveal retinal telangiectasis. *Ophthalmic Surg Lasers Imaging* 2007;38:164–166.
23. Maia Junior OO, Takahashi WY, Bonanomi MT, et al. Intravitreal triamcinolone injection in the treatment of idiopathic juxtafoveal telangiectasis. *Arq Bras Oftalmol* 2006;69:941–944.
24. Robertson D. Macroaneurysms of the retinal arteries. *Trans Am Acad Ophthalmol Otolaryngol* 1973;77:OP55–OP67.
25. Palestine AG, Robertson DM, Goldstein BG. Macroaneurysm of the retinal arteries. *Am J Ophthalmol* 1982;93:164–171.
26. Schatz H, Gitter K, Yanuzzi J, et al. Retinal arterial macroaneurysm: a large collaborative study. Presented at the American Academy of Ophthalmology Annual Meeting; November 1990; Chicago.
27. Lavin MJ, Marsh RJ, Peart S, et al. Retinal arterial macroaneurysms: a retrospective study for 40 patients. *Br J Ophthalmol* 1987;71:817–825.
28. Tezel T, Gunalp I, Tezel G. Morphometrical analysis of retinal arterial macroaneurysms. *Doc Ophthalmol* 1994;88:113–125.
29. Shults WT, Swan KC. Pulsatile aneurysm of the retinal tree. *Am J Ophthalmol* 1974;77:304–309.
30. Perry HD, Zimmerman LE, Benson WE. Hemorrhage from isolated aneurysm of a retinal artery; report of two cases simulating malignant melanoma. *Arch Ophthalmol* 1977;95:281.
31. Townsend-Pico WA, Meyers SM, Lewis H. Indocyanine green angiography in the diagnosis of retinal arterial macroaneurysms associated with submacular and preretinal hemorrhages: a case series. *Am J Ophthalmol* 2000;129:33–37.
32. Fichte C, Streeten BW, Friedman AH. A histopathologic *study of retinal arterial aneurysms. Am J Ophthalmol* 1978;85:509–518.
33. Asdourian GK, Goldberg MJ, Jampol L, et al. Retinal macroaneurysms. *Arch Opthalmol* 1977;95:624–628.
34. Lewis Ra, Norton EWD, Gass JDM. Acquired arterial macroaneurysm of the retina. *Br J Ophthalmol* 1976;60:21–30.
35. Abdel-Khalek MN, Richardson J. Retinal macroaneurysm: natural history and guidelines for treatment. *Br J Ophthalmol* 1986;70:2–11.

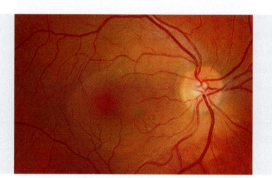

# Macular Edema Associated with Ocular Inflammatory Diseases

J. Peter Campbell ■ Diana V. Do ■ Quan Dong Nguyen

Cystoid macular edema (CME) is one of the most common causes of visual loss in patients with ocular inflammatory disease or uveitis (1–5). Due to the chronic nature of uveitic inflammation, CME can be especially difficult to treat, and uncontrolled CME can lead to macular scarring, irreversible visual loss, and blindness. The primary treatment for uveitis-associated CME is therapy of the underlying disease, which varies by uveitis syndrome, though adjunctive therapy targeting CME is often needed. Oral and periocular corticosteroids have represented the mainstay of treatment for years, though the introduction of intravitreal triamcinolone acetate and the development of modern nonsteroidal immunomodulatory and biologic therapies may change the way that this sight-threatening complication is managed in the years to come.

The incidence of CME depends on the anatomic location of the uveitis syndrome (2,6,7). The rate of CME is highest in panuveitis (66%), intermediate uveitis (60%), and posterior uveitis (34%). Uveitis entities commonly associated with CME are: pars planitis, Adamantiades-Behçet's disease, sarcoidosis, juvenile rheumatoid arthritis (JRA), birdshot chorioretinopathy, and HLA-B27 associated uveitis. Approximately one in three uveitis patients will develop serious visual impairment or legal blindness in at least one eye (2,3,7). In the majority of cases, CME is responsive to therapy, though it often becomes resistant to treatment (8,9). Table 26-1 lists the frequency of CME and visual loss by anatomic location and etiology. CME can complicate the course of uveitis at any stage of disease, including when the uveitic inflammation has been controlled. Treating physicians must be aware of this complication and aggressively pursue the etiology of decreased vision in patients with uveitis as CME may develop even in the absence of overt inflammation (6,9).

## PATHOGENESIS

The pathogenesis of uveitis-associated CME remains unclear but probably implicates a number of inflammatory mediators leading to a transient breakdown of the inner or outer blood retinal barrier (BRB) and vascular leakage. The involvement of multiple mediators and cascades has been proposed, including: free radicals, serotonin, prostaglandins, histamine, bradykinin substance P, leukotrienes, TNFα, multiple interleukins (IL-1, IL-6, IL-8), multiple cell adhesion molecules (sICAM, sVCAM), interferons and IP-10, vascular endothelial growth factor (VEGF) and other factors (10–13). Several cytokines have been implicated in the disruption of the blood-ocular barrier, which is the likely mechanism of uveitic CME; however, the lack of good experimental models has made elucidation of the exact mechanism difficult (10,11).

The vitreous may also contribute to uveitic CME through several possible mechanisms. Vitreomacular traction may contribute to mechanical dysfunction of the inner BRB as vitreous fibers connect to the Muller cells in the macular areas, which are responsible for maintaining fluid balance in the retina, and are known to be swollen and damaged in CME (14–16). Supporting this concept, it has been demonstrated that in patients with uveitis, eyes with posterior vitreous detachments are significantly less likely to experience macular damage (10,17). The vitreous may also act as a depot for inflammatory mediators, allowing longer lasting physiological effects. In certain uveitic syndromes, e.g. Vogt-Koyanagi-Harada disease and sympathetic ophthalmia, choroidal inflammation may also contribute to retinal and macular edema (10).

## MANAGEMENT

The management of uveitic CME is primarily targeted at the control of the underlying inflammation. Therapy has historically consisted of anti-inflammatory medications (corticosteroids, nonsteroidal immunomodulators, targeted biologic agents), carbonic anhydrase inhibitors, and vitrectomy. Specific therapy is based on ocular involvement (unilateral or bilateral), degree of visual symptoms, associated systemic disease, previous response to medications, and a patient's history and preference. Recent advances in management have been in the delivery methods of conventional therapies such as intravitreal injection and implantation of corticosteroids. Given the high side effect profile of corticosteroids over the long term, corticosteroid-sparing immunomodulators have received much interest. New biologic agents targeting specific mediators in the inflammatory cascade have been developed and have shown early promise. As our understanding of the pathogenesis of uveitis grows, new potential therapeutic targets, such as intercellular adhesion molecule (ICAM) inhibitors, are frequently identified and much recent work has been focused on finding less toxic, more convenient, and more effective treatments.

| TABLE 26-1 | UVEITIS ASSOCIATED WITH CYSTOID MACULAR EDEMA (CME)[a] | |
|---|---|---|
| | Proportion with CME (%) | Proportion with CME and visual acuity <20/60 |
| **Location** | | |
| Anterior | 23/213 (11%) | 7/23 (30%) |
| Intermediate | 43/72 (60%) | 17/43 (40%) |
| Posterior | 41/122 (34%) | 13/41 (32%) |
| Pan | 65/99 (66%) | 34/65 (52%) |
| Scleritis | 3/23 (13%) | 3/3 (100%) |
| **Cause of uveitis** | | |
| HLA-B27 associated | 7/58 (12%) | 2/7 (29%) |
| Sarcoidosis | 17/29 (59%) | 6/17 (35%) |
| Fuch's heterochromic iridocyclitis | 3/22 (14%) | 2/3 (67%) |
| JRA | 6/10 (60%) | 2/6 (33%) |
| Behcet's | 5/8 (63%) | 2/5 (40%) |
| Birdshot chorioretinopathy | 6/6 (100%) | 5/6 (83%) |

[a]Adapted from Lardenoye CW, van Kooij B, Rothova A, et al. Impact of macular edema on visual acuity in uveitis. *Ophthalmology* 2006;(7):1446–1449.

## Nonsteroidal Anti-Inflammatory Drugs

Although prostaglandins have been implicated in the pathogenesis of macular edema, the role of prostaglandin inhibitors in uveitis is unclear. It has been conventional wisdom that nonsteroidal anti-inflammatory drugs (NSAIDS) such as topical ketorolac, are of benefit in pseudophakic and aphakic macular edema, but less so in uveitis; however, a recent systematic review failed to find convincing evidence for the use of topical NSAIDS in either acute or chronic CME of any etiology (6,18).

## Acetazolamide

Carbonic anhydrase enzymes attached to the pigment epithelium facilitate fluid removal from the retina. Carbonic anhydrase inhibitors can accelerate this process and have played a role in the management of CME in a variety of conditions (19,20). Acetazolamide has been shown to benefit patients with aphakic CME but has often failed to control uveitic CME in trials (6,20–22). A recent long-term study demonstrated a benefit to low dose acetazolamide in uveitic CME but mostly limited to the subgroup of patients with no active inflammation (19). Given its recognizable but often tolerable side effect profile, acetazolamide probably represents an appropriate treatment option in cases of uveitic CME with controlled inflammatory activity, approximately half of whom can be completely weaned off all medications (19). Its benefit in more severe cases, or as adjunctive therapy with immunomodulators, is not well established.

## Corticosteroids

Corticosteroids have represented the mainstay of treatment for sight-threatening uveitis (9,10,23–26). They can be administered orally, topically, periocularly, intravitreally, or via steroid implant. The advantage to corticosteroids is their broad anti-inflammatory effect and rapid onset of action. Corticosteroids act on several pathways involved in intraocular inflammation and decrease both the cellular inflammatory response as well as the degree of vascular leakage (27,28). The effect of corticosteroids on the retinal vasculature is dose-related, favoring the trend towards local therapy with the highest intraocular concentrations. Local therapy, whether periocular injection, intravitreal injection, or intraocular implant, has the further advantage of minimizing the systemic side effects of corticosteroids. Unfortunately, high intraocular concentration of steroids raises the incidence of ocular side effects, predominantly elevated intraocular pressure (AOP) and cataract (24).

### Oral Corticosteroids

Oral corticosteroids are utilized in the management of many uveitic syndromes and associated disease states. In the management of CME, oral prednisone is preferred in patients with bilateral uveitis or severe unilateral inflammation resistant to local or regional steroids. A recent trial comparing sub-Tenon's corticosteroid injection (for unilateral CME) versus a short course of oral corticosteroids (for bilateral CME) found that the short course of oral corticosteroids results in significantly faster visual recovery, suggesting a possible role for oral corticosteroid in conjunction with sub-Tenon's injection in unilateral cases (29,30). Patients who require high doses of systemic steroids for longer periods of time are often considered for immunosuppressive therapy with a nonsteroidal immunomodulator to decrease the risk of developing the myriad complications of systemic steroids.

### Topical Corticosteroids

Topical corticosteroids are used most often in the treatment of anterior uveitis, less commonly in intermediate uveitis, and rarely for isolated uveitic CME (31). Effectiveness is limited by suboptimal posterior segment penetration and complicated dosing regimen. The combination of topical corticosteroids and topical NSAIDs can provide synergistic effects in managing CME and can yield better efficacy than either class alone. Given the high ocular morbidity of persistent macular edema, there should be a low threshold for use of periocular, intravitreal, or systemic therapy in patients with complicated or recurrent CME associated with anterior uveitis (7).

### Periocular Corticosteroids

Periocular steroid injections have played a key role in the management of intermediate and posterior uveitis (32). The periocular approach provides a large bolus of steroid at the site of inflammation with extended duration of efficacy and minimal systemic toxicity. The sub-Tenon's approach has been favored over the orbital floor approach due to its proximity to the macula (10,33). The majority of patients respond well to periocular corticosteroid injection; however patients may become resistant to therapy (26,32,34–36). Complications of periocular injection include globe penetration, cataract, and increased intraocular pressure. A study of 53 patients by Dafflon et al. found that 23/64 eyes (36%) experienced an increase in IOP >8 mm Hg compared to baseline, with 6 (9%) requiring surgery (32). Though intravitreal injection has been gaining popularity in recent years, there is a paucity of randomized controlled data and risk-benefit analysis to confirm its superiority over periocular administration; the periocular approach will most likely remain a part of the management algorithm of macular edema (37).

### Intravitreal Corticosteroids

Efficacy of intravitreal injection of steroids has been demonstrated in treating numerous intraocular complications, including choroidal neovascularization (CNV), often in conjunction with other therapies such as VEGF antagonists or photodynamic therapy, proliferative vitreoretinopathy (PVR), and CME from multiple etiologies (38–43). Although triamcinolone acetonide (TA) is most commonly used, other types of steroids, such as dexamethasone, can also be injected intravitreally. The clinical effect is usually seen for 8 to 12 weeks (for TA), though repeat injections are almost always necessary, which raises the risk of adverse events (26,44,45). On the other hand, intravitreal

TA (IVTA) often succeeds in controlling CME in patients who have failed other therapies and may justify the increased risk of intravitreal injection in these patients (26). The majority of patients with treatment-resistant uveitic CME respond rapidly to IVTA, though many will eventually relapse (26,40, 45–48). Patients who require chronic therapy for control of the underlying inflammation can often be weaned off (or to lower doses of) systemic corticosteroids and immunomodulators (49).

The main adverse effects include elevated IOP, cataract, and a small risk of endophthalmitis. Increased intraocular pressure is common following IVTA injection (44,45,50,51). IOP elevations >21 mm Hg (absolute) are seen in 30% to 50% of patients, and can occur months after initial therapy (26,52). In most cases, the IOP elevation can be treated with topical medication, though some (<10%) may require filtering surgery (45,51,52). The incidence and degree of cataract progression appears to be related to the duration of follow-up and the number of injections (26). It is important to note that these numbers are consistent with the rate of cataract progression with sub-Tenon's injections of TA (26). In a randomized, controlled trial, Gillies et al. found that cataract surgery was performed in 29% of the eyes treated with IVTA compared with 5% in placebo (51). A recent review put the overall risk of endophthalmitis at 0.3% per injection, or 0.9% per eye, but noted that the risk varied based on technique. A distinction was also made between true bacterial endophthalmitis and "pseudo-endophthalmitis," thought to be an inflammatory reaction to the preservative (26,53).

## Implantable Corticosteroids

Intraocular sustained released fluocinolone acetonide delivery devices have demonstrated great promise at controlling intraocular inflammation, providing high local concentration with minimal systemic toxicity, and a duration of action of more than two years (31). In recent phase III trial results, the 34-week recurrence rate decreased from 51.4% preimplantation to 6.1% postimplantation, with 87% of eyes experiencing an improvement in visual acuity (VA) and decreased fluorescein angiography (FA) hyperfluorescence (54). Of patients with evidence of CME at baseline, 25% demonstrated a ≥3-line increase in VA at 34 weeks. Overall, the adverse event profile is similar to IVTA and other routes of corticosteroid administration, with 51.1% of eyes requiring ocular hypertensive therapy, 5.8% of patients requiring glaucoma surgery, and 9.9% requiring cataract surgery (54). Currently, the major prohibition to the FA implant is the cost, which can exceed US$20,000 (31). However, one must take into consideration the cost of systemic medications employed in the management of uveitis, which often is significantly higher over the duration of the implant. In addition, one needs to consider the adverse events associated with systemic therapy compared to those associated with the implants. Longer term clinical trials are underway to evaluate the costs and benefits of this effective and longer acting, but expensive, therapy.

The dexamethasone delivery system (DDS) represents another promising therapeutic option. It consists of a biodegradable copolymer of lactic acid and glycolic acid that safely biodegrades in the eye over time, releasing a steady concentration of dexamethasone. A recent trial reported the results of a single 700 ug application of dexamethasone with promising results in patients with CME secondary to various causes, including uveitis (30,55).

## Traditional Nonsteroidal Immunomodulatory Therapy

Though corticosteroids are often the initial treatment in patients with intermediate and posterior uveitis and related CME, their long term use is seriously limited by their systemic side-effects (56–58). Nonsteroidal immunomodulators are often introduced in order to decrease the daily corticosteroid dose to acceptable systemic levels (less than 10 mg per day of prednisone or equivalent) (23,56). These alternatives to corticosteroids can be classified into traditional immunosuppressive agents and the newer biological agents. The traditional agents are the antimetabolites, alkylating agents, and T-cell inhibitors. These agents are the most common second-line agents due to their long history and safety record, though they all have the potential for serious side effects, including bone marrow toxicity and neoplasm. The use of these medications is directed at the control of the underlying disease state. They would rarely, if ever, be used for the treatment of isolated CME in the absence of inflammation. This review will focus on those with proven benefit in the treatment of CME.

## Antimetabolites

Methotrexate, azathioprine, and mycophenolate mofetil are the three main antimetabolites used in the treatment of uveitis (23,56–59). Methotrexate is often used in the treatment of anterior uveitis associated with juvenile idiopathic arthritis and the seronegative spondyloarthropathies (60,61). Its use in posterior and intermediate uveitis is institution-specific, but some believe that it should be the first line corticosteroid-sparing agent (23,56,62). Mycophenolate mofetil has largely replaced use of azathioprine due to its similar mechanism and efficacy and better side effect profile. There are several reports of its efficacy and safety in uveitis; however, there is insufficient evidence to support the role of antimetabolites in managing uveitic CME (63–65).

## Alkylating Agents

Cyclophosphamide is rarely used except in severe cases of treatment-resistant uveitis, scleritis, ocular cicatricial pemphigoid, and ocular inflammation due to Wegener granulomatosis (23,56,57). Chlorambucil may also be useful in severe, treatment resistant ocular inflammation, especially in patients with Behcet's-related uveitis (56,57). Both agents suffer from severe systemic side effects including bone marrow suppression, teratogenicity, and risks of malignancy (23,57).

## T-Cell Inhibitors

Cyclosporine and tacrolimus have received much attention for the treatment of noninfectious posterior uveitis due to their inhibition of IL-2 in the inflammatory cascade. There are multiple reports of their efficacy in intermediate and posterior uveitis (23,56). Low-dose cyclosporine is often considered as a first-line therapy, occasionally in conjunction with low-dose corticosteroids, in patients with ocular inflammation, such as birdshot chorioretinopathy (57). The advantage to tacrolimus is that it can be titrated to clinical effect, minimizing the side serious side effects of renal impairment, hypertension, and metabolic abnormalities that plague these therapies; however there are not as many reports of its use in uveitis (23,57). Recent work has investigated the possibility of local delivery of T-cell inhibitors in these patients, whether by intravitreal injection or deep scleral implant (23). Sirolimus is a noncalcineurin T-cell inhibitor recently developed. It has shown early benefit in the treatment of uveitis, though the data are early and more validating work is needed (66).

Voclosporin is a newer generation of calcineurin inhibitor that is currently being investigated in three phase-3 randomized clinical trials as a potential therapeutic agent for controlling active posterior uveitis, intermediate uveitis, panuveitis, or anterior uveitis, or as an agent that can maintain the uveitis in remission after it has been controlled by corticosteroids or another immunomodulatory agent. Resolution of macular edema associated with the uveitis will be evaluated in the studies as one of the parameters of bioactivity of voclosporin.

## Biologic Agents

There has been much recent interest in the role of biological agents in the management of uveitis (56–58,61,62,67–76). These agents are promising due to their selective inhibition of target mediators in the inflammatory cascade. The majority of the research has been in tumor necrosis factor (TNF) antagonists and the role of interferon, and in patients with therapy-resistant CME (23).

## Biologic Agents: TNF-α Antagonists

There is good rationale for the use of TNF-α inhibitors in uveitis, based on their success in multiple rheumatologic diseases (23,61,67,76). The efficacy of infliximab has been demonstrated in several recent reports on the treatment of anterior and posterior uveitis, with anatomic and functional improvement in eyes with chronic, refractory CME (56,67,71,76). There is also growing interest in adalimumab due to the fact that it can be administered subcutaneously, every one to two weeks (23). It has demonstrated promise in JRA and ocular Behcet's disease, though its role in treatment of CME in the absence of inflammation is unknown (77–79).

## Biologic Agents: Interferon-α

IFN therapy has demonstrated similar efficacy to TNF-α antagonists in intermediate and posterior uveitis, especially in patients with ocular involvement due to Behcet's disease, though the lack of head-to-head trials makes comparison difficult (23,56,57,80–82). The main differences are in the route of administration and side-effect profile (23,70). IFN-α-2 a is

the most common formulation, and is given by subcutaneous injection. Side effects, including a flu-like syndrome, are severe enough to discontinue therapy in approximately 5% of patients (23).

## Vascular Endothelial Growth Factor Antagonists

There is good reason to believe that VEGF antagonists may play a role in the treatment of uveitic CME. VEGF concentrations are higher in the aqueous of patients with uveitic CME than in that of patients with uveitis but no CME (12). Further, bevacizumab has already demonstrated efficacy in treating CME secondary to central retinal vein occlusion (CRVO) and diabetes. (83,84) Cordero Coma et al. recently published the first report of intravitreal bevacizumab for treatment of uveitic CME, which demonstrated anatomic but not functional improvement (85). A second small case series reported similarly disappointing results (86). While these short-term safety and efficacy studies provide less than compelling clinical results, given the experience with bevacizumab and other VEGF antagonists in the treatment of diabetic macular edema (DME) and age-related macular degeneration (AMD), this therapy merits further evaluation in larger, randomized controlled trials (84).

## Biologic Agents: Other

Rituximab is an anti-CD20 (B-cell antigen) monoclonal antibody that was developed for the treatment of B cell lymphomas, but has emerged as a promising therapy for a number of T cell-mediated autoimmune diseases, including rheumatoid arthritis, lupus, and Wegener granulomatosis; however, thus far its use in uveitis is limited to case reports (87,88).

Several interleukin family mediators have received interest as potential therapeutic targets. Daclizumab is a monoclonal antibody against IL-2, which has shown mixed results in the treatment of resistant noninfectious intermediate and posterior uveitis (23,56,72,89,90). Its role in the primary treatment of uveitic CME has not been studied. Both anakinra (an IL-1 antagonist) and tocilizumab (an IL-6 receptor antagonist) have shown early promise in the treatment of rheumatologic disease, but neither has been evaluated in uveitis.

Abatacept is a CTLA-4 blocker that has been evaluated in patients with rheumatoid arthritis, but not in uveitis (87). There have also been a few published reports on the use of octreotide in uveitis and uveitic CME with promising results, in small studies (68,74,91). The authors emphasized the need for further study.

Following a report that trace microalbuminuria was associated with patients with uveitis and patients with CME, but not those without, van Kooij et al. investigated the potential efficacy of lisinopril in the treatment of uveitic CME (92,93). In one of the few decent sized ($n = 40$) randomized, double-blind, placebo-controlled trials in the field, they concluded that lisinopril had no effect on inflammatory CME or visual acuity, though it did lower blood pressure and decrease morning urinary albumin excretion (93).

## Surgical Management

The literature on the use of vitrectomy for the treatment of uveitic CME has spanned more than twenty years (15,94). Becker et al. recently reviewed the subject and found 44 articles published through early 2005; however the lack of standardization of inclusion/exclusion criteria, outcome measures, and follow-up limited the analysis, and there were no randomized controlled trials at the time (95). Nevertheless, the authors were able to draw some conclusions from the study. First, they concluded that pars plana vitrectomy (PPV) is indicated for the treatment of structural complications of uveitis, including cataract, retinal detachment, and epiretinal membrane. They found insufficient evidence to conclude that vitrectomy had an independent visual benefit in CME apart from the removal of debris in the vitreous. Second, as most of the literature focused on intermediate uveitic syndromes, the positive outcomes reported overall seem to generalize to these entities, but conclusions on specific syndromes were more difficult to make. They also noted that pediatric patients may respond especially well, an outcome confirmed in a recent retrospective study (96). Third, they noted that PPV was usually associated with visual improvement, though it was difficult to separate the effect of PPV from frequent concomitant surgical procedures such as cataract extraction. Fourth, no firm conclusions could be drawn regarding the disease modifying effect of the PPV, though there was some evidence that PPV decreased inflammation in some patients through removal of stimulants. Finally, the authors suggested that when the evidence for PPV from other etiologies of CME is included, it affirms the suggestive trend in the data that PPV may benefit some patients with uveitic CME. Without further comparative studies between PPV and medical therapy, however, it is impossible to work out the appropriate role of PPV in the management of uveitic CME.

Since that publication, Tranos et al. published the first prospective, interventional, randomized, controlled study on the effect of PPV on chronic CME associated with uveitis (97). They reported the results in 23 eyes of 23 patients with CME secondary to chronic intermediate or posterior uveitis unresponsive to medical treatment. 12 were randomized into a surgical group who underwent PPV, and 11 had standard medical therapy. Vision improved by two or more lines in 50% of the surgery group as opposed to 18% of the medical group, which was statistically significant despite the small sample size. There was also a trend for angiographic improvement in the vitrectomized eyes, though this was not statistically significant. It is important to note, however, that 66% demonstrated no angiographic improvement after 6 months of follow-up, again raising the question of the confounding effect of the vitreous clearing effect of PPV. The authors did not find a significant difference in the need for systemic medications between the two groups in the six months following randomization. This pilot study demonstrated the potential efficacy of PPV in chronic uveitic CME in a prospective, randomized controlled trial, and confirms the need for larger prospective trials in the future.

The current indications for vitrectomy are decreased visual acuity in chronic CME, visual obstruction from vitreous debris, macular pucker, retinal detachment, and proliferative tractional retinopathy (22,98). PPV has demonstrated benefit for patients with these ocular complications of chronic uveitis (95). It may have further benefit as primary treatment of both uveitis and uveitic CME due to its role as a depot of inflammatory mediators, though this effect has yet to be convincingly demonstrated. Longer term, larger studies are needed to confirm this effect and comparative studies are needed to determine the appropriate role of vitrectomy in the management of these patients.

## CONCLUSION

The management of uveitis associated macular edema can be frustrating and challenging for the patient and provider, but much work is currently being performed to provide superior treatment alternatives for this complex condition. Table 26-2 lists the currently ongoing clinical trials for the management of uveitis and/or uveitic CME demonstrating the diversity of therapeutic strategies being explored. There are two research questions that will impact the future management of uveitis associated CME. First, how can we better control the underlying uveitis syndromes? Many of the trials in Table 26-2 are targeting uveitis, rather than CME, as primary outcome measures. As new therapies are developed to better treat the various forms of ocular inflammatory disease, the incidence of associated CME may decrease. However, even with controlled uveitis we know that CME can occur and lead to visual loss and blindness. Thus, the second question is: in the patient with isolated CME, among all of the new biological molecules, delivery vehicles, and surgical options being explored, what is the optimal strategy to control a given patient's CME, balancing efficacy, tolerability, convenience, and cost?

This review attempted to provide a broad consensus on the current answers to this second question. Figure 26-1 displays a typical management algorithm for a patient with uveitis-associated CME. For unilateral CME, local or regional therapy is preferred, with corticosteroids often as first-line, though biologics and VEGF antagonists may demonstrate utility as first-line agents. In cases of bilateral (or severe) CME, either local or systemic therapy (or a combination) may be used, depending on disease characteristics. In many cases, there are a plethora of treatment options with few demonstrating clear superiority (most often due to lack of adequate trials). As new therapies are developed, head to head trials are necessary to definitively guide therapeutic decision making. Until then, uveitis specialists will need to balance the hope in newer therapies with demonstrated efficacy of the better established options. With the many ongoing clinical trials, participation in a trial ought to be an option discussed with patients, especially for those who are poorly controlled and at high risk for vision loss.

## TABLE 26-2 ONGOING CLINICAL TRIALS FOR UVEITIS AND/OR UVEITIC CME[a]

| Intervention | Phase | Single or multicenter | Primary outcome | Sponsor |
|---|---|---|---|---|
| To compare therapeutic effect of intravitreal bevacizumab and triamcinolone in resistant uveitic cystoid macular edema | I | Single | CME resorption on OCT and exam | Shaheed Beheshti Medical University |
| Lucentis (ranibizumab) for inflammatory macular edema (LIME) | I/II | Single | Change in visual acuity at 3 months | UCSF Genentech |
| Adalimumab (Humira) in the treatment of refractory Noninfectious uveitis | II | Multiple | (1) Snellen Visual acuity improvement greater than 2 lines (2) Reduction in systemic steroid dose (3) Two-step improvement in control of ocular inflammation (4) Reduction of CME on angiography | Oregon Health and Science University |
| Evaluation of birdshot retinochoroidopathy treatment by either steroid or interferon alpha2a (BIRDFERON) | II | Single | Decrease in OCT-measured macular thickness at 4 months | Assistance Publique - Hôpitaux de Paris |
| Randomized, controlled trial to test the efficacy of interferon beta in the treatment of intermediate uveitis | III | Single | Change in visual acuity (3 lines ETDRS) at months 1, 3, 6, and 12 | University of Heidelberg Serono GmbH |
| Adalimumab in uveitis refractory to conventional therapy (ADUR trial) | II/III | Single | Improvement of visual acuity (3 lines EDTRS) at weeks 0, 2, 6, 12, and 24 | University of Heidelberg Abbott |
| A study of LX211 in clinically quiescent noninfectious intermediate, anterior and intermediate, posterior or Pan-uveitis (LUMINATE) | III | Multiple | Recurrence of ocular inflammation | Lux Biosciences |
| Safety, tolerability, and efficacy of AEB071 in the treatment of uveitis | II | Multiple | Change in macular edema from baseline to week 8 | Novartis |
| Multicenter uveitis steroid treatment (MUST) trial | IV | Multiple | Visual acuity | National Eye Institute |
| Human anti-tac (daclizumab) to treat JIA-associated uveitis | II | Single | Collect preliminary information on the utility of acute daclizumab theraphy on active ocular inflammation in a pediatric population. | National Eye Institute |
| Efalizumab to treat uveitis | II | Single | Reduction of macular edema | National Eye Institute |
| Phase 2 study of MM-093 to treat patients with uveitis | II | Single | Safety and tolerability | Merrimack Pharmaceuticals |
| Daclizumab and sirolimus to treat uveitis | I | Single | Ability to taper off drug while disease remains quiet at week 108 while receiving no concomitant systemic immunosuppressive medications | National Eye Institute |
| Reimplantation of a fluocinolone acetonide implant for noninfectious uveitis affecting the posterior segment | IV | Single | Inflammatory recurrence | Bosch & Lomb Duke University |
| Multicenter prospective registry of infliximab use for childhood uveitis | IV | Single | Effects on disease activity | Duke University Childhood Arthritis & Rheumatology Research Alliance |
| Interferon-alpha2a versus cyclosporin A for severe ocular Behcet's disease (INCYTOB) | III | Single | Time to improvement and remission | University Hospital Tuebingen |
| The safety and efficacy of a tumor necrosis factor receptor fusion protein on uveitis associated with juvenile rheumatoid arthritis | III | Single | Safety and tolerability | National Eye Institute |
| Intravitreal ranibizumab treatment of central serous chorioretinopathy | I | Single | Safety and tolerability | Genentech Vitreous Retina-Macula Consultants of New York |

[a]Adapted from the Web site at www.clinicaltrials.gov database for uveitis. If there was only one location listed, the trial is being considered as single center in this table. CME, Cystoid macular edema; EDTRS, Early Treatment Diabetic Retinopathy Study; OCT, optical coherence tomography;

Management Algorithm for Uveitic CME

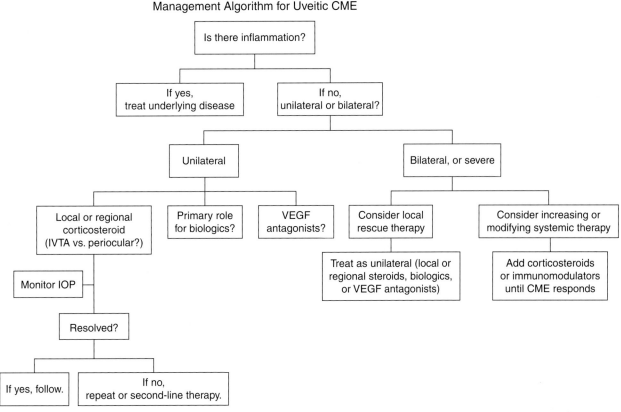

**Figure 26-1.** Management of uveitic cystoid macular edema. IOP, intraocular pressure; IVTA, intravitreal triamcinolone acetonide; VEGF, vascular endothelial growth factor.

## References

1. Bonfioli AA, Damico FM, Curi AL, et al. Intermediate uveitis. *Semin Ophthalmol* 2005;20(3):147–154.
2. Rothova A, Suttorp-van Schulten MS, Frits Treffers W, et al. Causes and frequency of blindness in patients with intraocular inflammatory disease. *Br J Ophthalmol* 1996;80(4):332–336.
3. Durrani OM, Tehrani NN, Marr JE, et al. Degree, duration, and causes of visual loss in uveitis. *Br J Ophthalmol* 2004;88(9):1159–1162.
4. Durrani OM, Meads CA, Murray PI. Uveitis: A potentially blinding disease. *Ophthalmologica* 2004;218(4):223–236.
5. Bodaghi B, Cassoux N, Wechsler B, et al. Chronic severe uveitis: Etiology and visual outcome in 927 patients from a single center. *Medicine (Baltimore)* 2001;80(4):263–270.
6. Okhravi N, Lightman S. Cystoid macular edema in uveitis. *Ocul Immunol Inflamm* 2003;11(1):29–38.
7. Lardenoye CW, van Kooij B, Rothova A. Impact of macular edema on visual acuity in uveitis. *Ophthalmology* 2006;113(8):1446–1449.
8. Markomichelakis NN, Halkiadakis I, Pantelia E, et al. Course of macular edema in uveitis under medical treatment. *Ocul Immunol Inflamm* 2007;15(2):71–79.
9. Rojas B, Zafirakis P, Christen W, et al. Medical treatment of macular edema in patients with uveitis. *Doc Ophthalmol* 1999;97(3–4):399–407.
10. Freeman G, Matos K, Pavesio CE. Cystoid macular oedema in uveitis: An unsolved problem. *Eye* 2001;15(Pt 1):12–17.
11. Guex-Crosier Y. The pathogenesis and clinical presentation of macular edema in inflammatory diseases. *Doc Ophthalmol* 1999;97(3–4):297–309.
12. Fine HF, Baffi J, Reed GF, et al. Aqueous humor and plasma vascular endothelial growth factor in uveitis-associated cystoid macular edema. *Am J Ophthalmol* 2001;132(5):794–796.
13. van Kooij B, Rothova A, Rijkers GT, et al. Distinct cytokine and chemokine profiles in the aqueous of patients with uveitis and cystoid macular edema. *Am J Ophthalmol* 2006;142(1):192–194.
14. Schepens CL, Avila MP, Jalkh AE, et al. Role of the vitreous in cystoid macular edema. *Surv Ophthalmol* 1984;28(Suppl):499–504.
15. Schubert HD. Cystoid macular edema: The apparent role of mechanical factors. *Prog Clin Biol Res* 1989;312:277–291.

16. Fine BS, Brucker AJ. Macular edema and cystoid macular edema. *Am J Ophthalmol* 1981;92(4):466–481.
17. Hirokawa H, Takahashi M, Trempe CL. Vitreous changes in peripheral uveitis. *Arch Ophthalmol* 1985;103(11):1704–1707.
18. Sivaprasad S, Bunce C, Wormald R. Non-steroidal anti-inflammatory agents for cystoid macular oedema following cataract surgery: A systematic review. *Br J Ophthalmol* 2005;89(11):1420–1422.
19. Schilling H, Heiligenhaus A, Laube T, et al. Long-term effect of acetazolamide treatment of patients with uveitic chronic cystoid macular edema is limited by persisting inflammation. *Retina* 2005;25(2):182–188.
20. Whitcup SM, Csaky KG, Podgor MJ, et al. A randomized, masked, cross-over trial of acetazolamide for cystoid macular edema in patients with uveitis. *Ophthalmology* 1996;103(7):1054–1062; discussion 1062–1063.
21. Wolfensberger TJ. The role of carbonic anhydrase inhibitors in the management of macular edema. *Doc Ophthalmol* 1999;97(3–4):387–397.
22. Gutfleisch M, Spital G, Mingels A, et al. Pars plana vitrectomy with intravitreal triamcinolone: Effect on uveitic cystoid macular oedema and treatment limitations. *Br J Ophthalmol* 2007;91(3):345–348.
23. Imrie FR, Dick AD. Nonsteroidal drugs for the treatment of noninfectious posterior and intermediate uveitis. *Curr Opin Ophthalmol* 2007;18(3):212–219.
24. Becker MD, Smith JR, Max R, et al. Management of sight-threatening uveitis: New therapeutic options. *Drugs* 2005;65(4):497–519.
25. Rothova A. Medical treatment of cystoid macular edema. *Ocul Immunol Inflamm* 2002;10(4):239–246.
26. van Kooij B, Rothova A, de Vries P. The pros and cons of intravitreal triamcinolone injections for uveitis and inflammatory cystoid macular edema. *Ocul Immunol Inflamm* 2006;14(2):73–85.
27. Choi JY, Buzney SM, Weiter JJ. Cystoid macular edema: Current modes of therapy. *Int Ophthalmol Clin* 2005;45(4):143–151.
28. Wilson CA, Berkowitz BA, Sato Y, et al. Treatment with intravitreal steroid reduces blood-retinal barrier breakdown due to retinal photocoagulation. *Arch Ophthalmol* 1992;110(8):1155–1159.
29. Venkatesh P, Abhas Z, Garg S, et al. Prospective optical coherence tomographic evaluation of the efficacy of oral and posterior subtenon corticosteroids in patients with intermediate uveitis. *Graefes Arch Clin Exp Ophthalmol* 2007;245(1):59–67.

30. Rothova A. Inflammatory cystoid macular edema. *Curr Opin Ophthalmol* 2007;18(6):487–492.

31. Mohammad DA, Sweet BV, Elner SG. Retisert: Is the new advance in treatment of uveitis a good one? *Ann Pharmacother* 2007;41(3): 449–454.

32. Lafranco Dafflon M, Tran VT, Guex-Crosier Y, et al. Posterior sub-tenon's steroid injections for the treatment of posterior ocular inflammation: Indications, efficacy and side effects. *Graefes Arch Clin Exp Ophthalmol* 1999;237(4):289–295.

33. Tranos PG, Wickremasinghe SS, Stangos NT, et al. Macular edema. *Surv Ophthalmol* 2004;49(5):470–490.

34. Sivaprasad S, McCluskey P, Lightman S. Intravitreal steroids in the management of macular oedema. *Acta Ophthalmol Scand* 2006;84(6): 722–733.

35. Helm CJ, Holland GN. The effects of posterior subtenon injection of triamcinolone acetonide in patients with intermediate uveitis. *Am J Ophthalmol* 1995;120(1):55–64.

36. Yoshikawa K, Kotake S, Ichiishi A, et al. Posterior sub-tenon injections of repository corticosteroids in uveitis patients with cystoid macular edema. *Jpn J Ophthalmol* 1995;39(1):71–76.

37. Ryan SJ, (ed). *Retina*. 4th ed, vol. 3. Philadelphia, PA: Elsevier Mosby, 2006.

38. Atmaca LS, Yalcindag FN, Ozdemir O. Intravitreal triamcinolone acetonide in the management of cystoid macular edema in Behcet's disease. *Graefes Arch Clin Exp Ophthalmol* 2007;245(3):451–456.

39. Dhir L, Prasad SD. Psoriatic uveitis-associated cystoid macular oedema treated with intravitreal triamcinolone acetonide. *Acta Ophthalmol Scand* 2006;84(3):436–437.

40. Karacorlu M, Arf Karacorlu S, Ozdemir H. Intravitreal triamcinolone acetonide in Vogt-Koyanagi-Harada syndrome. *Eur J Ophthalmol* 2006;16(3):481–483.

41. Martidis A, Duker JS, Puliafito CA. Intravitreal triamcinolone for refractory cystoid macular edema secondary to birdshot retinochoroidopathy. *Arch Ophthalmol* 2001;119(9):1380–1383.

42. Morrison VL, Kozak I, LaBree LD, et al. Intravitreal triamcinolone acetonide for the treatment of immune recovery uveitis macular edema. *Ophthalmology* 2007;114(2):334–339.

43. Sirimaharaj M, Robinson MR, Zhu M, et al. Intravitreal injection of triamcinolone acetonide for immune recovery uveitis. *Retina* 2006;26(5):578–580.

44. Androudi S, Letko E, Meniconi M, et al. Safety and efficacy of intravitreal triamcinolone acetonide for uveitic macular edema. *Ocul Immunol Inflamm* 2005;13(2–3):205–212.

45. Angunawela RI, Heatley CJ, Williamson TH, et al. Intravitreal triamcinalone acetonide for refractory uveitic cystoid macular oedema: Long term management and outcome. *Acta Ophthalmol Scand* 2005;83(5):595–599.

46. Sorensen TL, Haamann P, Villumsen J, et al. Intravitreal triamcinolone for macular oedema: Efficacy in relation to aetiology. *Acta Ophthalmol Scand* 2005;83(1):67–70.

47. Young S, Larkin G, Branley M, et al. Safety and efficacy of intravitreal triamcinolone for cystoid macular oedema in uveitis. *Clin Experiment Ophthalmol* 2001;29(1):2–6.

48. Karacorlu M, Mudun B, Ozdemir H, et al. Intravitreal triamcinolone acetonide for the treatment of cystoid macular edema secondary to Behcet disease. *Am J Ophthalmol* 2004;138(2):289–291.

49. Kok H, Lau C, Maycock N, et al. Outcome of intravitreal triamcinolone in uveitis. *Ophthalmology* 2005;112(11):1916.

50. Jonas JB, Schlichtenbrede F. Visual acuity and intraocular pressure after high-dose intravitreal triamcinolone acetonide in selected ocular diseases. *Eye* 2008;22(7):869–873.

51. Gillies MC, Simpson JM, Billson FA, et al. Safety of an intravitreal injection of triamcinolone: Results from a randomized clinical trial. *Arch Ophthalmol* 2004;122(3):336–340.

52. Jonas JB, Degenring RF, Kreissig I, et al. Intraocular pressure elevation after intravitreal triamcinolone acetonide injection. *Ophthalmology* 2005;112(4):593–598.

53. Jager RD, Aiello LP, Patel SC, et al. Risks of intravitreous injection: A comprehensive review. *Retina* 2004;24(5):676–698.

54. Jaffe GJ, Martin D, Callanan D, et al. Fluocinolone acetonide implant (Retisert) for noninfectious posterior uveitis: Thirty-four-week results of a multicenter randomized clinical study. *Ophthalmology* 2006;113(6): 1020–1027.

55. Kuppermann BD, Blumenkranz MS, Haller JA, et al. Randomized controlled study of an intravitreous dexamethasone drug delivery system in patients with persistent macular edema. *Arch Ophthalmol* 2007;125(3): 309–317.

56. Kim EC, Foster CS. Immunomodulatory therapy for the treatment of ocular inflammatory disease: Evidence-based medicine recommendations for use. *Int Ophthalmol Clin* 2006;46(2):141–164.

57. Okada AA. Immunomodulatory therapy for ocular inflammatory disease: A basic manual and review of the literature. *Ocul Immunol Inflamm* 2005;13(5):335–351.

58. Hemady RK, Chan AS, Nguyen AT. Immunosuppressive agents and nonsteroidal anti-inflammatory drugs for ocular immune and inflammatory disorders. *Ophthalmol Clin North Am* 2005;18(4):511–528.

59. Malik AR, Pavesio C. The use of low dose methotrexate in children with chronic anterior and intermediate uveitis. *Br J Ophthalmol* 2005;89(7): 806–808.

60. Dev S, McCallum RM, Jaffe GJ. Methotrexate treatment for sarcoid-associated panuveitis. *Ophthalmology* 1999;106(1):111–118.

61. Dunn JP. Review of immunosuppressive drug therapy in uveitis. *Curr Opin Ophthalmol* 2004;15(4):293–298.

62. Baker KB, Spurrier NJ, Watkins AS, et al. Retention time for corticosteroid-sparing systemic immunosuppressive agents in patients with inflammatory eye disease. *Br J Ophthalmol* 2006;90(12):1481–1485.

63. Baltatzis S, Tufail F, Yu EN, et al. Mycophenolate mofetil as an immunomodulatory agent in the treatment of chronic ocular inflammatory disorders. *Ophthalmology* 2003;110(5):1061–1065.

64. Choudhary A, Harding SP, Bucknall RC, et al. Mycophenolate mofetil as an immunosuppressive agent in refractory inflammatory eye disease. *J Ocul Pharmacol Ther* 2006;22(3):168–175.

65. Thorne JE, Jabs DA, Qazi FA, et al. Mycophenolate mofetil therapy for inflammatory eye disease. *Ophthalmology* 2005;112(8):1472–1477.

66. Shanmuganathan VA, Casely EM, Raj D, et al. The efficacy of sirolimus in the treatment of patients with refractory uveitis. *Br J Ophthalmol* 2005;89(6):666–669.

67. Hale S, Lightman S. Anti-TNF therapies in the management of acute and chronic uveitis. *Cytokine* 2006;33(4):231–237.

68. Kafkala C, Choi JY, Choopong P, et al. Octreotide as a treatment for uveitic cystoid macular edema. *Arch Ophthalmol* 2006;124(9):1353–1355.

69. Kiss S, Ahmed M, Letko E, et al. Long-term follow-up of patients with birdshot retinochoroidopathy treated with corticosteroid-sparing systemic immunomodulatory therapy. *Ophthalmology* 2005;112(6):1066–1071.

70. Mackensen F, Max R, Becker MD. Interferon therapy for ocular disease. *Curr Opin Ophthalmol* 2006;17(6):567–573.

71. Markomichelakis NN, Theodossiadis PG, Pantelia E, et al. Infliximab for chronic cystoid macular edema associated with uveitis. *Am J Ophthalmol* 2004;138(4):648–650.

72. Nussenblatt RB, Peterson JS, Foster CS, et al. Initial evaluation of subcutaneous daclizumab treatments for noninfectious uveitis: A multicenter noncomparative interventional case series. *Ophthalmology* 2005;112(5): 764–770.

73. Onal S, Foster CS, Ahmed AR. Efficacy of intravenous immunoglobulin treatment in refractory uveitis. *Ocul Immunol Inflamm* 2006;14(6): 367–374.

74. Papadaki T, Zacharopoulos I, Iaccheri B, et al. Somatostatin for uveitic cystoid macular edema (CME). *Ocul Immunol Inflamm* 2005;13(6): 469–470.

75. Sobaci G, Bayraktar Z, Bayer A. Interferon alpha-2 a treatment for serpiginous choroiditis. *Ocul Immunol Inflamm* 2005;13(1):59–66.

76. Theodossiadis PG, Markomichelakis NN, Sfikakis PP. Tumor necrosis factor antagonists: Preliminary evidence for an emerging approach in the treatment of ocular inflammation. *Retina* 2007;27(4):399–413.

77. Mushtaq B, Saeed T, Situnayake RD, et al. Adalimumab for sight-threatening uveitis in Behcet's disease. *Eye* 2007;21(6):824–825.

78. Biester S, Deuter C, Michels H, et al. Adalimumab in the therapy of uveitis in childhood. *Br J Ophthalmol* 2007;91(3):319–324.

79. Mansour AM. Adalimumab in the therapy of uveitis in childhood. *Br J Ophthalmol* 2007;91(3):274–276.

80. Bodaghi B, Gendron G, Wechsler B, et al. Efficacy of interferon alpha in the treatment of refractory and sight threatening uveitis: A retrospective monocentric study of 45 patients. *Br J Ophthalmol* 2007;91(3):335–339.

81. Deuter CM, Koetter I, Guenaydin I, et al. Interferon alfa-2 a: A new treatment option for long lasting refractory cystoid macular edema in uveitis? A pilot study. *Retina* 2006;26(7):786–791.

82. Becker MD, Heiligenhaus A, Hudde T, et al. Interferon as a treatment for uveitis associated with multiple sclerosis. *Br J Ophthalmol* 2005;89(10): 1254–1257.

83. Rosenfeld PJ, Fung AE, Puliafito CA. Optical coherence tomography findings after an intravitreal injection of bevacizumab (avastin) for macular edema from central retinal vein occlusion. *Ophthalmic Surg Lasers Imaging* 2005;36(4):336–339.

84. Arevalo JF, Fromow-Guerra J, Quiroz-Mercado H, et al. Primary intravitreal bevacizumab (Avastin) for diabetic macular edema: Results from the Pan-American Collaborative Retina Study Group at 6-month follow-up. *Ophthalmology* 2007;114(4):743–750.

85. Cordero Coma M, Sobrin L, Onal S, et al. Intravitreal bevacizumab for treatment of uveitic macular edema. *Ophthalmology* 2007;114(8):1574–1579.

86. Ziemssen F, Deuter CM, Stuebiger N, et al. Weak transient response of chronic uveitic macular edema to intravitreal bevacizumab (avastin). *Graefes Arch Clin Exp Ophthalmol* 2007;245(6):917–918.

87. Lim L, Suhler EB, Smith JR. Biologic therapies for inflammatory eye disease. *Clin Experiment Ophthalmol* 2006;34(4):365–374.

88. Tappeiner C, Heinz C, Specker C, et al. Rituximab as a treatment option for refractory endogenous anterior uveitis. *Ophthalmic Res* 2007;39(3):184–186.

89. Gallagher MJ, Quinones K, Cervantes-Castaneda RA, et al. Biologic response modifier therapy for refractory childhood uveitis. *Br J Ophthalmol* 2007;91(10):1341–1344.

90. Buggage RR, Levy-Clarke G, Sen HN, et al. A double-masked, randomized study to investigate the safety and efficacy of daclizumab to treat the ocular complications related to Behcet's disease. *Ocul Immunol Inflamm* 2007;15(2):63–70.

91. Kuijpers RW, Baarsma S, van Hagen PM. Treatment of cystoid macular edema with octreotide. *N Engl J Med* 1998;338(9):624–626.

92. van Kooij B, Fijnheer R, Roest M, et al. Trace microalbuminuria in inflammatory cystoid macular edema. *Am J Ophthalmol* 2004;138(6):1010–1015.

93. van Kooij B, Fijnheer R, de Boer J, et al. A randomized, masked, cross-over trial of lisinopril for inflammatory macular edema. *Am J Ophthalmol* 2006;141(4):646–651.

94. Algvere P, Alanko H, Dickhoff K, et al. Pars plana vitrectomy in the management of intraocular inflammation. *Acta Ophthalmol (Copenh)* 1981;59(5):727–736.

95. Becker M, Davis J. Vitrectomy in the treatment of uveitis. *Am J Ophthalmol* 2005;140(6):1096–1105.

96. Trittibach P, Koerner F, Sarra GM, et al. Vitrectomy for juvenile uveitis: Prognostic factors for the long-term functional outcome. *Eye* 2006;20(2):184–190.

97. Tranos P, Scott R, Zambarajki H, et al. The effect of pars plana vitrectomy on cystoid macular oedema associated with chronic uveitis: A randomized, controlled pilot study. *Br J Ophthalmol* 2006;90(9):1107–1110.

98. Accorinti M, Pirraglia MP, Paroli MP, et al. Infliximab treatment for ocular and extraocular manifestations of Behçet's disease. *Jpn J Ophthalmol* 2007;51(3):191–196.

# six

# Vitreous Traction Maculopathies

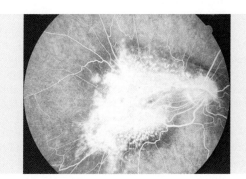

# 27

# Epiretinal Membrane

Richard C. Lin ■ William F. Mieler ■ William J. Wirostko

Epiretinal membranes (ERMs) are proliferations of fibrous tissue along the inner retinal surface. Since their initial description by Iwanoff in 1865 (1), ERMs have been referred to by many names, including surface wrinkling retinopathy (2), macular pucker (3–5), cellophane maculopathy (6,7), and wrinkling of the internal limiting membrane (ILM) (8). Other names are preretinal macular fibrosis (8,9), macular ERM, primary retinal folds (10), idiopathic preretinal macular gliosis (11–13), and vitreoretinal interface changes (14). ERMs can be primary (or idiopathic) versus secondary; underlying conditions for secondary ERMs include retinal breaks with or without retinal detachment, blunt or penetrating ocular trauma, inflammation, vitreous hemorrhage, retinal vascular disorders, and ocular surgery (15).

When located within the macula, ERMs can produce visual symptoms, namely decreased visual acuity (VA), metamorphopsia, micropsia, or monocular diplopia (16). If symptomatic enough to bother patients, ERMs can be treated by pars plana vitrectomy (PPV) with membrane peeling. In this chapter, we will discuss the clinical features of ERMs, their pathogenesis, and operative considerations including preoperative evaluation and surgical approaches, along with results and complications of surgery.

## CLINICAL FEATURES

Most ERMs are peripheral to the macula and produce no visual symptoms (17). However, visual changes may develop if the ERM occurs in the macula. Symptoms include decreased VA, micropsia, metamorphopsia, and monocular diplopia. These may develop either slowly or rapidly (8,15–19). Absolute scotomas are rare (8,20). Mechanisms for visual changes involve ERM opacities overlying the fovea, macular traction and distortion, macular edema, or traction-induced ischemic changes (15–18). Severity of symptoms relates to ERM type, with a thin ERM producing the mildest symptoms. Eyes with thin idiopathic ERMs retain 20/200 vision or better in 95% of cases, and commonly maintain 20/50 VA (8,19–21). Thin idiopathic ERMs are generally stable, produce no further decrease in VA after diagnosis in 87% of cases, and undergo no change in clinical appearance after 38 months in 83% of cases (11,19). ERMs associated with proliferative vitreoretinopathy (PVR) are typically thicker and possess an avascular, fibrocellular appearance (Fig. 27-1) (22). Diabetic ERMs are commonly fibrovascular (23). Visual prognosis with these membranes may be limited by associated macular disease. Occasionally, visual symptoms from an ERM may spontaneously resolve after a PVD separates the ERM from the retina (24,25).

Biomicroscopically, ERMs demonstrate a spectrum of clinical signs. In the mildest cases, the ERM may be just a glinting, shifting light reflex on the retinal surface seen only with red-free light (Fig. 27-2) (14,16). In more severe cases, the ERM may be opaque and produce additional fundus changes. Superficial retinal striae may form adjacent to the ERM (Fig. 27-3)

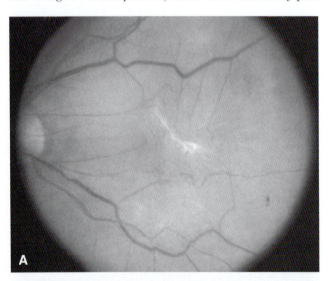

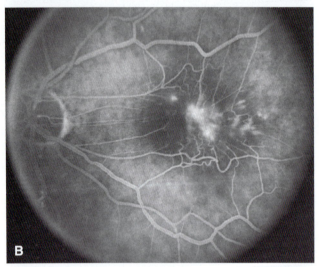

**Figure 27-1. A:** Color fundus photograph OS of a dense opaque epiretinal membrane (ERM) following a rhegmatogenous retinal detachment. **B:** Fluorescein angiogram (FA) demonstrating late leakage of dye along the temporal border of the macular region from breakdown of the retinal vasculature under the ERM.

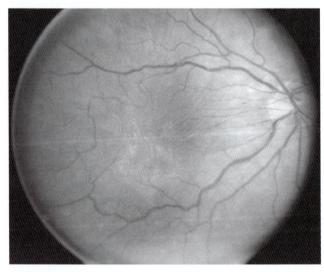

**Figure 27-2.** Color retinal photograph OD demonstrating mild glistening and retinal sheen from a thin epiretinal membrane.

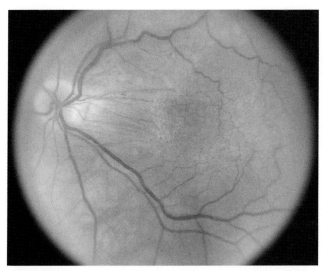

**Figure 27-3.** Color retinal photograph OS showing tortuous, dragged retinal vessels and retinal striae from an epiretinal membrane.

(12,14). Retinal capillaries may become dark, dilated, and tortuous from ERM retinal traction. Major retinal vessels may appear straightened and drawn together (6,14). Typically, retinal dragging, macular heterotopia, and tractional retinal detachment only occur when ERM contraction is severe (Fig. 27-4) (7,12,16). Pseudoholes may form (Fig. 27-5) (16,26), and these represent contractions of perimacular ERM that do not extend over the fovea. Pseudoholes must be distinguished from lamellar and full-thickness holes since treatment for each is different. Pseudoholes contain retinal tissue and vessels in their base, have no retinal edge, display no cuff of subretinal fluid, and show no central hyperfluorescence on fluorescein angiography (FA) (12,14). It should be remembered that ERMs can occur in eyes with full thickness macular holes (14). Microaneurysms, blot hemorrhages, and yellow hard exudates may develop, with or without retinal edema (8,12,16,20). In cases of severe retinal thickening, one sees shadows of the superficial retinal vessels on the retinal pigment epithelium (RPE) (20). Frequently, FA demonstrates irregular leakage of dye in this region (14). Typical cystoid leakage may not be apparent because of retinal distortion. Retinal cystoid spaces may form as the retinal edema coalesces. One should always consider choroidal neovascularization (CNV) as an etiology for retinal edema and hard exudates in older patients. Cotton wool spots and fluffy white retinal opacities may form. These are felt to be from blockage of axoplasmic flow from retinal traction (27). They usually resolve within several days after ERM removal. Retinal pigmentary changes may occur, namely RPE hypertrophy and atrophy. These are poor prognostic signs and can be from ERM-induced retinal traction or the original event that induced ERM formation (trauma or inflammation). Occasionally, pigment may be seen within the ERM itself (14). This represents ingestion of melanin or hemosiderin by macrophages within the ERM, or the proliferation of RPE cells in the ERM. Intraocular inflammatory cells are usually not seen with the ERM. Their presence suggests an underlying inflammatory etiology (14). A thorough funduscopic examination with peripheral retinal assessment is recommended in all patients with ERM to rule

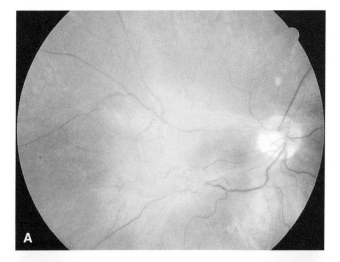

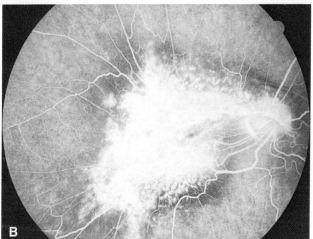

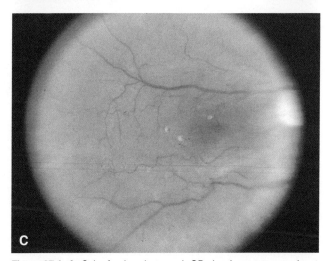

**Figure 27-4. A:** Color fundus photograph OD showing a very prominent epiretinal membrane (ERM) with mild pigmentation (possibly consistent with a combined hamartoma of the retina/retinal pigment epithelium). **B:** Fluorescein angiogram reveals marked dragging of the retinal vessels along with extensive leakage of dye from the retinal vasculature. **C:** Postoperative fundus photograph of the same eye after pars plana vitrectomy and ERM removal.

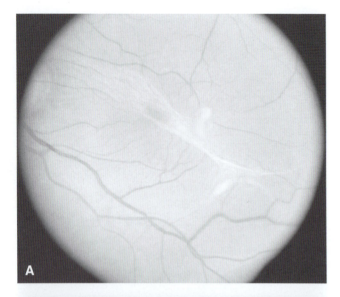

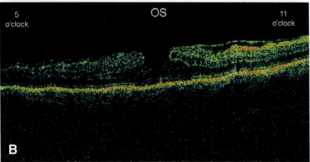

**Figure 27-5. (A)** Color retinal photograph OS displaying a pseudohole from an epiretinal membrane, with **(B)** accompanying optical coherence tomography (OCT). At the time of pars plana vitrectomy, no full thickness macular hole was detected.

out retinal vascular disease or the presence of a retinal break. FA may be obtained prior to surgery to document retinal changes, to rule out the presence of CNV, and to exclude the possibility of macular ischemia from retinal vascular occlusive disease. Optical coherence tomography (OCT) is also routinely obtained to document the appearance of the ERM, and it is also employed in the decision-making process of deciding whether or not to perform surgical removal of the ERM. The use of OCT will be discussed in greater detail later in this chapter.

## TERMINOLOGY

No standard nomenclature is currently used to describe ERMs, although several systems have been proposed. Gass (14) offered the following classification of ERMs based on clinical appearance:

*Grade 0*: Translucent membranes unassociated with retinal distortion (*cellophane maculopathy*)

*Grade 1*: Membranes causing irregular wrinkling of the inner retina (*crinkled cellophane maculopathy*)

*Grade 2*: Opaque membranes obscuring the underlying vessels with prominent retinal distortion (*macular pucker*)

Joondeph (28) stratified ERMs into four grades depending on their appearance and anatomic severity:

*Grade 1*: Transparent ERMs characterized by changes in the light reflex without any appreciable distortion of the retinal tissue; the membrane is completely transparent and is in its earliest stage

*Grade 2*: Translucent ERMs obscuring some of the underlying retinal landmarks with mild distortion of the retinal architecture but no distinct striae

*Grade 3*: Translucent to opaque ERMs showing marked distortion of the underlying retina, frequently with retinal striae

*Grade 4*: ERMs exhibiting severe retinal distortion with complications such as tractional elevation or macular holes

## PATHOGENESIS

Depending on the age range and race examined, ERMs occur in about 4% to 18% of the adult population and are bilateral in up to 20% of patients (17,29–35). The stimulus for ERM formation remains poorly understood. In a recent study, no etiology for ERM formation was found in 68% of cases. In the remaining 32%, factors associated with ERM formation included retinal surgery (scleral buckling, laser photocoagulation, cryotherapy, or vitrectomy) (28%), ocular inflammation (2%), ocular trauma (<1%), or retinal vascular disease (<1%) (36). Additional risk factors for ERM are proliferative diabetic retinopathy (PDR), vitreous hemorrhage, and nonretinal ocular surgery such as cataract extraction (2,4–6,8,12,15–17,30,37,38).

Numerous cytokines, receptors, and extracellular matrix proteins have been implicated in ERM formation. In ERMs in diabetic eyes, for example, immunohistochemistry has identified insulinlike growth factor receptor/binding proteins, erythropoietin receptors, hypoxia inducible factor, angiopoietin, and vascular endothelial growth factor (39–42). These factors are likely to play a role in the proliferation of endothelial cells and the development of vascular ERMs. PVR membranes have been shown to express inflammatory mediators and growth factors such as interleukins, tumor necrosis factor alpha, urokinase, tissue plasminogen activator, endothelin 1, and platelet-derived growth factor (PDGF) (43–46). Interestingly, PDGF induces migration of RPE cells across the retina *in vitro* and *in vivo* (47–51). Finally, in addition to endothelial cells and RPE cells, glial cells are also likely to play a role in ERM formation through the expression of trophic factors, transcription factors, and cell cycle molecules such as NF-kappaB and cyclin D1 (52,53).

Mechanical stimuli may also play a role in the formation of ERMs. In particular, the process of posterior vitreous detachment (PVD) has been proposed to cause ERM formation by introducing a small amount of trauma or causing discontinuities in the ILM. Several lines of evidence point to an association between PVD and ERM formation. First, the incidence of idiopathic membranes and PVD both increase with age. One study noted a 10-fold increase in ERMs, from 2% to 20%, when two groups of patients, aged 50 and 75 years, respectively, were compared (2). Second, PVDs have been estimated to be present in 80% to 95% of eyes with ERMs (2,6,11,20–22,29,54–56).

Third, Wiznia (19) described 9% of eyes developing an ERM within 7 days of a PVD, and 41% within 18 months, which suggests that a PVD may directly cause ERM formation. Finally, in PVDs associated with retinal breaks, dispersion of RPE cells through the break can contribute to ERM formation.

On the other hand, a PVD is certainly not required for ERM formation. If PVDs are present in 80% to 95% of eyes with ERMs, this leaves 5% to 20% of eyes with ERMs but no PVDs. Moreover, an ERM can develop on the surface of an attached hyaloid membrane (57). These findings, in combination with the low incidence of ERMs superior to the macula (the site where PVDs often first occur), argue against the requirement of PVD for ERM formation (2). Foos (58) suggested that an ERM may actually induce a PVD by disturbing the vitreolaminar interface, and thus PVDs may be both a cause and an effect of ERMs.

Hirokawa et al. (56) studied 250 eyes with idiopathic ERMs and classified them into four categories based on relationship with the vitreous:

*Group 1*: No PVD

*Group 2*: Partial PVD but no vitreoretinal adhesion or traction to the area of preretinal macular fibrosis

*Group 3*: Partial PVD with vitreous traction to the area of preretinal fibrosis

*Group 4*: Complete PVD

Interestingly, the worst VA was found in eyes in Group 3 as opposed to patients with a complete PVD or no PVD whatsoever. This configuration of vitreous traction to the area of an ERM is now called vitreomacular traction (VMT) syndrome (18). It is readily diagnosed using OCT (as is discussed later in the chapter).

In short, the exact pathogenesis underlying ERM formation is not precisely understood and depends on a combination of chemical and mechanical factors. The stimulus for ERM formation differs in different clinical settings such as PDR or PVR. Whatever the initiating stimulus, ERM formation is likely an immune process of ocular wound healing and extracellular matrix protein remodeling (59,60).

## HISTOPATHOLOGY

ERMs are fibrocellular sheets of collagen with interspersed cells. Their composition most commonly involves collagen, glial cells, RPE cells, and macrophages (6,37,47,61–63). They may vary in thickness and display a spectrum of histologic composition. In one study of 168 ERMs, one of six predominant matrices was present: glial cells (36%), fibrovascular tissue (17%), cortical vitreous (13%), RPE cells (10%), fibroinflammatory tissue (10%), or a combination (14%) (54). All ERMs contain collagen (63). Specific cells commonly found in ERMs include fibrous astrocytes, RPE cells, fibrocytes, and macrophages. Myofibroblasts, hyalocytes, and inflammatory cells occur less frequently (6,37,47,61,62). ERM histopathology varies with clinical scenario. Idiopathic ERMs frequently contain glial cells (15,22,37,61–69), diabetic ERMs are commonly fibrovascular, and postretinal detachment ERMs typically contain RPE cells (54).

The cellular origin of ERMs remains debated. Previously, it was believed that glial cells proliferated through defects in the ILM and that RPE cells originated from breaks in the retina (22,70). While this theory explained the frequency of glial cells in idiopathic ERMs and the presence of RPE cells in postretinal detachment ERM, it failed to explain the presence of RPE cells or macrophages within idiopathic ERMs (15,22). Now, it is suspected that RPE cells can also originate from non-RPE cells that have undergone transformation into RPE cells, from transretinal migration of RPE cells or from developmental rests of epithelial cells on the surface of the retina, which have undergone activation (18,68). The contribution from each source is unknown. Macrophages are felt to arise from either local tissue or blood. The latter is more likely, as macrophages are uncommon in normal retina (71). Furthermore, macrophages have been induced in ERMs by autologous intravitreal blood injection in an animal model (72). Recently, it has been demonstrated using electron microscopy that the cellular components of ERMs can lie strictly underneath the ILM (i.e., on the retinal side rather than the vitreous side); thus, breaks in the ILM are not required for ERM formation (73).

## EVALUATION BY OPTICAL COHERENCE TOMOGRAPHY

OCT provides noninvasive, high-resolution cross-sectional imaging of the macula and is useful in the preoperative evaluation (Fig. 27-6) and postoperative follow-up of patients with ERMs (Fig. 27-7). OCT imaging is very helpful in identifying associated macular edema (Figs. 27-6 and 27-7) or VMT (Fig. 27-8), which can be difficult to detect by clinical examination or via FA. VMT refers to a configuration in which adhesion between the posterior hyaloid face and the retinal surface leads to traction in an anteroposterior direction, in contrast to the tangential traction exerted on the retinal surface by a contracting ERM. Do et al. (74) specifically examined the impact of OCT imaging on surgical decision making for ERMs. This study discovered that OCT imaging was more sensitive than clinical examination in detecting macular edema and VMT associated with ERMs. Of the 84 eyes in this study, 19 eyes were recommended for surgery based on clinical examination alone, while 33 eyes were recommended for surgery when the OCT findings were used in conjunction with clinical examination. Gallemore et al. (75) also found OCT to be much more sensitive than clinical examination in detecting VMT in eyes with a variety of conditions including ERMs.

ERMs have also been examined using spectral domain OCT, which provides faster and higher resolution imaging than time domain OCT. Again, spectral domain OCT imaging is useful in identifying macular edema, VMT, and photoreceptor defects that are not apparent on clinical examination (76). In short, OCT imaging is useful in determining the amount of adherence between an ERM and the retina, the amount of associated retinal edema, and the configuration of the ERM (77). This information is extremely helpful to the retinal surgeon both in making the decision as to whether or not to perform surgery, and once a decision is made, in guiding the surgery itself.

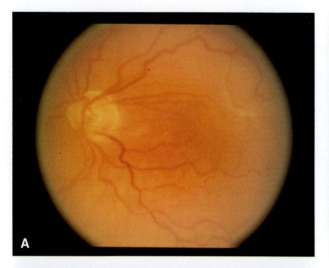

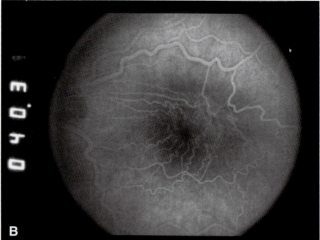

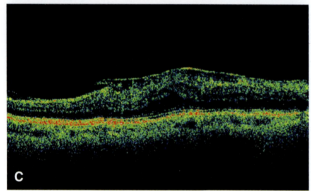

**Figure 27-6.** **(A)** Color photograph OS showing prominent epiretinal membrane (ERM), **(B)** fluorescein angiogram reveals moderate leakage, and **(C)** optical coherence tomography documents the ERM with a distinct edge, along with underlying macular edema.

## TREATMENT

No treatment is indicated for asymptomatic or minimally symptomatic ERMs (11,14). The majority of ERMs can be observed and are expected to remain stable; for instance, in the Blue Mountains Eye Study, only 29% of ERMs showed significant progression over a 5-year period (32). Treatment for symptomatic ERMs involves PPV with membrane peeling. This is most appropriate when symptoms are significant and VA is decreased. Some wait an additional 6 to 8 weeks after the development of symptoms to allow further ERM maturation. Mature ERMs are often easier to visualize, engage, and remove than immature ERMs (78). PPV with ERM peeling improves vision in up to 75% of cases (16,36,55,79,80). Laser photocoagulation of ERMs is not recommended, even when leaking capillaries are seen on FA. This modality is ineffective and aggravates ERM contraction (12,14). Similarly, corticosteroids appear ineffective for treating ERMs and retinal edema.

PPV with ERM peeling is achieved with a three port approach, and any gauge system (20 vs. 23 vs. 25 gauge) can be effectively utilized. First, a core vitrectomy is performed with particular attention to the posterior vitreous. The postlenticular anterior vitreous and peripheral vitreous may also be vitrectomized, although care must be taken not to touch the lens or cause a peripheral retinal tear. Next, an edge of the ERM is visualized, engaged on a barbed instrument, and separated from the retina with an elevating and a side-to-side

motion. Visualization is best if the barb faces the light source. With a 20-gauge vitrectomy system, a barbed MVR blade can be used for this step (the barb is created by pressing the blade tip against a metallic surface). Some surgeons employ a 1.5 inch 23-gauge needle with its tip bent toward its lumen by 80 degrees. Filling the hub and shaft of the needle with a balanced salt solution prevents air from entering the eye (16). If no edge to the ERM is seen, oblique illumination from the light pipe may identify an area of the ERM that is elevated above the retina and can be safely incised to create an edge (20). Other options for engaging an edgeless ERM involve scraping a diamond-dusted silicone-tipped cannula or barbed instrument tangentially from the periphery toward the center of the membrane (78,81), or engaging the ERM with a 20-gauge blunt flute catheter (82). Once an edge is elevated, it is grasped with the vitreous cutter or intraocular forceps and the instrument is used to remove the remaining ERM (62). Margherio (16,26) advocates removing the ERM with a tangential rather than anteroposterior motion to decrease the incidence of retinal tears. ERM removal beyond the arcades may best limit recurrent symptoms (79); however, if this is not possible, residual fragments of epiretinal tissue can usually be left behind with no undesirable effect as long as the perifoveal area has been relieved of epimacular tissue. Frequently, the ERM is larger than originally observed on clinical exam. The presence of abnormal underlying retinal sheen or wrinkling after ERM removal suggests that residual layers of ERM are present and additional peeling may be required. However, a second layer of

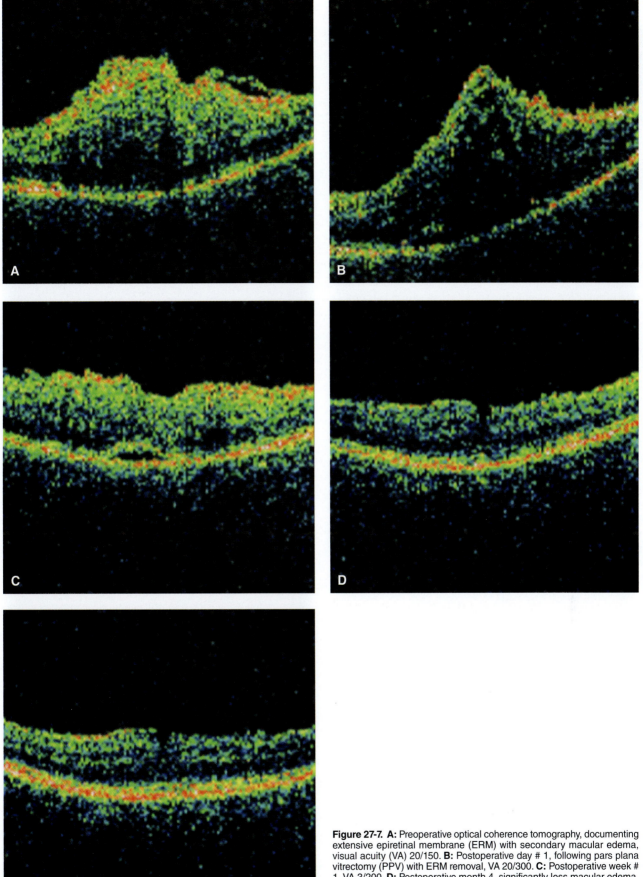

**Figure 27-7. A:** Preoperative optical coherence tomography, documenting extensive epiretinal membrane (ERM) with secondary macular edema, visual acuity (VA) 20/150. **B:** Postoperative day # 1, following pars plana vitrectomy (PPV) with ERM removal, VA 20/300. **C:** Postoperative week # 1, VA 3/200. **D:** Postoperative month 4, significantly less macular edema, VA 20/150. **E:** Postoperative year 2, following cataract surgery 6 months earlier, VA 20/30.

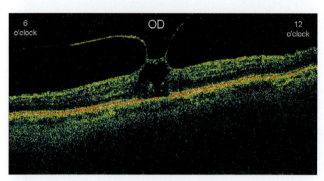

**Figure 27-8.** Optical coherence tomography of vitreomacular traction (VMT) syndrome documenting the anteroposterior traction commonly seen in this condition.

ERM is quite rare. These changes must not be confused with the fluffy white retinal opacities and axoplasmic stasis that develop from ERM. Attempting to peel these areas can produce nerve fiber layer (NFL) damage and retinal breaks. The development of petechial hemorrhages on the retinal surface after ERM removal suggests that separation has properly occurred at the level of the ILM. Removal of the ILM itself is generally not necessary, though on occasion some surgeons will remove it as well. Once the ERM is removed, the peripheral retina is inspected for breaks and the eye is surgically closed (15,16,78,80,83).

Over the past several years, small-gauge sutureless transconjunctival vitrectomy has become increasingly popular for ERM surgery because of its ease of opening and closing. A 25-gauge sutureless system was first introduced in 2002 (84). The surgical approach is the same as that for 20-gauge surgery and still involves removal of the vitreous prior to peeling of the membrane. An MVR blade cannot be used to start an edge because it does not fit through the trochar, but a 25-gauge diamond-dusted silicone tip can be used to start the edge. Alternatively, the membrane can be grasped with forceps without starting an edge first. Studies comparing 20-gauge to 25-gauge surgery for ERM peels have shown similar long-term visual outcomes, although patients may experience less initial discomfort and faster visual recovery after 25-gauge surgery (85,86). More recently, 23-gauge sutureless vitrectomy has been introduced and probably produces similar results to 25- and 20-gauge surgery (87). Finally, 27-gauge surgery has been described to peel ERMs, and in some cases, this is done without removing any vitreous (nonvitrectomizing vitreous surgery) (88). However, this technique is still controversial and has not been widely adopted.

Various dyes and agents have been used to stain ERMs during surgery to improve visualization (89–91). These agents include indocyanine green (ICG) (92–97), trypan blue (98–103), and triamcinolone acetonide (104). Sequential use of more than one agent during surgery has also been described (105). Triamcinolone acetonide crystal can be used to dust the posterior hyaloid face, ERM, or ILM. It is relatively inexpensive and does not have any known retinal toxicity, although it does have the potential to cause ocular hypertension and cataract formation. Trypan blue stains cellular membranes such as ERMs more strongly than the acellular ILM, so it can be useful in cases where the ERM edge is difficult to visualize directly.

ICG stains the ILM more strongly than the ERM, so it is useful in cases in which ILM peeling is desired. However, ICG may cause toxicity to RPE cells (95). Furthermore, as noted previously, there is no consensus whether ILM peeling is beneficial in straightforward ERM surgery. While some authors suggest that ILM removal may lead to better visual outcomes and less recurrence of ERMs (106,107), others have found that removal of large segments of ILM is associated with worse postoperative VA (108).

In brief, the principles of surgery include removing the vitreous, elevating an edge of the ERM, removing the ERM, inspecting the peripheral retina for breaks, and closing the eye. No large prospective randomized studies have established definite, long-term benefits based on gauge of instrumentation, use of staining agent, or removal of ILM.

## TREATMENT OUTCOME

PPV with ERM stripping improves VA two lines or more in up to 90% of eyes, although incomplete recovery of VA is the rule (16,78,109,110). In one study, median VA improved from 20/200 preoperatively to 20/70 by 10 months after surgery (18). Final VA is achieved within 8 weeks postoperatively in 82% of eyes, and persists for 3 to 5 years in 58% of eyes (36,111). Decreased metamorphopsia occurs in 85% of patients (80), and this can result in improved quality of life even in the absence of improved VA (112). Additional benefits from ERM removal include less micropsia, resolution of diplopia, and a more normal fundus appearance with less vascular tortuosity, fewer retinal striae, and decreased retinal exudate (Fig. 27-5) (15,16,20). Postoperative OCT imaging usually shows a decrease in retinal thickness compared to preoperative measurements, although the macular topography often does not completely return to normal (113).

Final outcomes appear to be dependent on several variables, most of which are beyond the surgeon's control. Multiple authors have attempted to define prognostic indicators for outcomes following ERM removal; commonly examined indicators have been preoperative VA, duration of symptoms prior to surgery, presence of preoperative continuing medical education (CME), patient age, thickness of epiretinal tissue, cause of the membrane, presence of RPE window defects on FA, and presence of ILM in the specimen obtained during surgery.

Preoperative VA is probably the most reliable prognostic indicator for ERM surgery. As a rule of thumb, postoperative VA tends to stabilize about halfway between preoperative acuity and normal acuity (26). Thus, eyes with better preoperative VA tend to gain less lines of vision but end up with better acuity compared to eyes with worse preoperative acuity (36,114). For example, an eye with preoperative acuity of 20/50 would tend to gain about two lines and end up around 20/30, while an eye with preoperative acuity of 20/200 would tend to gain about four lines and end up around 20/60.

Several other factors may also play a role in outcomes following ERM surgery. A shorter duration of symptoms is associated with good visual outcome (15,36,114). Pesin et al. (36), for instance, determined that eyes with duration of symptoms less than 6 months recover 2.9 more Snellen lines of VA than eyes with greater than 6 months of visual changes. Phakic status also influences visual outcome after ERM surgery, most likely because vitrectomy causes cataract formation (36). Thompson (115) reviewed a series of 40 patients undergoing ERM surgery with preoperative vision of 20/50 or better; patients who were phakic by the end of follow-up had a mean postoperative acuity of 20/50, while patients who were pseudophakic at the end of follow-up had a mean postoperative acuity of 20/30. The presence or absence of other macular disease, patient age, and the occurrence of intraoperative complications also play a significant role in postoperative VA (15,36).

The importance of the cause of the membrane as a prognostic indicator is unclear. Margherio et al. (26) treated 328 patients with membranes with various causes and concluded that those with the idiopathic variety had significantly better outcomes than those with membranes secondary to retinal tears or detachment. On the other hand, Rice et al. (114) discovered that eyes with antecedent retinal detachments had significantly better outcomes versus eyes with membranes in the idiopathic category. Pesin et al. (36) found no statistically significant difference in visual outcomes between the idiopathic and postretinal reattachment groups.

Other factors with unclear prognostic value are the presence of preoperative CME on FA and the thickness of the ERM. In some studies, these factors are associated with a worse prognosis (63,78,110,114), while in others they are not (15,36). The source of the conflicting results remains unclear, but the reason could be uncontrolled factors such as associated macular pathology.

Patients should be counseled accordingly regarding the decision to undergo surgery for ERMs. The most important decision is whether to defer surgery awaiting further visual loss or proceed with surgery at better levels of acuity. It is evident that the prospects to achieve best postoperative acuity lie in pursuing surgery at relatively better levels of acuity preoperatively and before symptoms have been present for more than 6 months. Still, the eyes that have the most to gain from surgery are commonly those with lower levels of preoperative acuity. Patients should also be counseled that symptoms and quality of life may improve even if VA does not. The type of ERM itself is probably not important in counseling patients, although their expectations should be lowered if they have concomitant macular pathology besides the ERM.

Phakic patients should be advised that they may need staged PPV, followed by eventual cataract surgery. Often, a surgeon will perform combined surgery to remove the ERM and perform cataract surgery at the same time, especially in the setting of mild to moderate cataract formation. However, there is no comparative study indicating better or worse surgical outcomes in the setting of combination surgery. At least in this situation, a second surgery is avoided.

## TREATMENT COMPLICATIONS

As in any surgery, complications can occur in PPV with ERM removal. Fortunately, sight-threatening complications following ERM surgery are relatively rare. Iris rubeosis and endophthalmitis, for example, develop in less than 0.5% of cases (15,79). Retinal breaks have been reported to occur between 4% and 9% during or after membrane peeling (55,114). Eyes at greatest risk include those with severe myopia, an edgeless ERM, or an ERM that is evenly adherent to the retina (78). Eyes with a high scleral buckle are also at risk. These eyes have limited access to the posterior pole, and membrane removal is often more difficult (15,78). Retinal breaks are usually confined to the retinal periphery and easily treated with laser or cryoretinopexy (16).

Retinal detachment has been reported to occur following vitrectomy for ERM in 3% to 6% of cases, with the highest frequency among eyes that have had previous retinal detachment repair (114,116). Retinal detachment may occur in the postoperative period because of iatrogenic breaks occurring in the region of the sclerotomies, or it may occur later as the result of ongoing vitreous traction exerted by residual peripheral vitreous gel. The risk of detachment should be lowered with appropriate vigilance in the search for iatrogenic tears at the time of surgery, in conjunction with meticulous effort to remove as much cortical vitreous as possible. This should reduce convection forces that may be imparted to the retinal periphery in the later postoperative period. Retinal detachments are successfully managed in the majority of cases with scleral buckle procedure or PPV (36).

Macular hole formation has been reported after ERM surgery (117). The risk for macular breaks is greatest in eyes with dense epimacular proliferation occurring in conjunction with advanced thinning or cyst formation at the fovea. In such cases, it may be necessary to generate peeling forces centripetally with respect to the macular center, often with amputation of the epicenter of tissue over the foveola in lieu of complete excision.

Surface hemorrhages are usually limited and of little visual significance. On occasion, rupture of a retinal vessel results in more sizable accumulation of hemorrhage. Often, this is easily treated by raising the intraocular pressure or with diathermy if necessary (16,36).

Choroidal neovascular membrane (CNVM) formation has been reported very rarely following ERM surgery, with six cases described in the literature (118). It is conceivable that surgical trauma to the macula caused small breaks in Bruch's membrane and subsequent CNVM formation. However, given the high incidence of ERMs and CNVMs particularly in the elderly population, these CNVMs may have developed purely coincidentally following surgery and not as a direct result of this.

Among phakic eyes, the most important complication encountered is progression of nuclear sclerosis cataract. Accelerated nuclear sclerosis develops after ERM removal in 12% to 60% of eyes and, not surprisingly, is more common with longer follow-up (15,16,36,78–80,111,119). The precise cause of this phenomenon following vitrectomy is still not known, though it is probably a combination of physical, chemical, and oxidative damage to the lens both during and after surgery. As mentioned above, the prospect of cataract progression and surgery must be a central component of preoperative counseling for phakic patients.

The rate of ERM recurrence after surgical removal varies according to ERM etiology. Recurrence is low in cases with idiopathic ERM (5% to 7%), but higher in eyes with an ERM due to retinal vascular disease (31%), inflammation (20%), and trauma (17%) (15,79). Most recurrences are mild and require no surgical intervention. ERM recurrence appears unrelated to the thickness of the ERM or to incomplete removal of ERM during PPV. ERM recurrence conveys no worse prognosis for visual outcome as compared to eyes without ERM recurrence (120). The surgical approach for visually significant recurrent membranes is identical to the methods employed for primary membranes. A possible role for local or systemic immunosuppressive agents in reducing the incidence of recurrent membranes has not been established.

## SUMMARY

ERMs are proliferations of fibrous tissue along the inner retinal surface. Their composition involves glial cells, fibrocytes, RPE cells, and macrophages. Although they are frequently asymptomatic, they can produce significant visual changes when they occur in the macula. Visual symptoms include decreased VA, metamorphopsia, micropsia, and monocular diplopia. In most cases, symptoms are stable or only slowly progressive. Risk factors for ERM formation include retinal breaks or detachments, ocular trauma, retinal vascular disease, uveitis, ocular surgery, or vitreous hemorrhage. Treatment involves surgical removal through PPV and ERM peeling. An improvement in visual symptoms and anatomic changes can be expected in the majority of cases. Final acuity following ERM removal tends to stabilize approximately halfway between preoperative acuity and normal acuity. As with any surgical procedure, case selection and preoperative counseling are paramount in achieving optimal results. Refinements in preoperative OCT imaging, surgical techniques and instrumentation, and stains for intraoperative visualization may continue to minimize surgical trauma, with reduction in complication rates and improved visual outcomes.

### References

1. Iwanoff A. Beitrage zur normalen und pathologischen anatomie des auges. *Graefes Arch Clin Exp Ophthalmol* 1865;11:135–170.
2. Roth, AM, Foos RY. Surface wrinkling retinopathy in eyes enucleated at autopsy. *Trans Am Acad Ophthalmol Otolaryngol* 1971;75:1047–1059.
3. Francois J, Verbraeken H. Relationship between the drainage of the subretinal fluid in retinal detachment surgery and the appearance of macular pucker. *Ophthalmologica* 1979;179:111–114.
4. Tanenbaum HL, Schepens CL, Elzeneiny I, et al. Macular pucker following retinal detachment surgery. *Arch Ophthalmol* 1970;83:286–293.
5. Tanenbaum HL, Schepens CL, Elzeneiny I, et al. Macular pucker following retinal surgery: a biomicroscopic study. *Can J Ophthalmol* 1969;4:20–23.
6. Jaffe NS. Macular retinopathy after separation of vitreoretinal adherence. *Arch Ophthalmol* 1967;78:585–591.
7. Maumenee AE. Further advances in the study of the macula. *Arch Ophthalmol* 1967;78:151–165.
8. Wise GN. Preretinal macular fibrosis (an analysis of 90 cases). *Trans Ophthalmol Soc UK* 1972;92:131–140.
9. Mills PV. Preretinal macular fibrosis. *Trans Ophthalmol Soc UK* 1979;99: 50–53.
10. Kleinert H. Primare netzhaufaltelung im maculabereich. *Graefes Arch Clin Exp Ophthalmol* 1954;155:350–358.
11. Sidd RJ, Fine SL, Owens SL, et al. Idiopathic preretinal gliosis. *Am J Ophthalmol* 1982;94:44–48.
12. Noble KG, Carr RE. Idiopathic preretinal gliosis. *Ophthalmology* 1982;89:521–523.
13. Yagoda AD, Walsh JB, Henkind P. Idiopathic preretinal macular gliosis. *Int Ophthalmol Clin* 1981;21:107–118.
14. Gass JDM. *Stereoscopic atlas of macular diseases: diagnosis and treatment.* 4th ed, St. Louis, MO: Mosby; 1997:938–950.
15. Michels RG. A clinical and histopathologic study of epiretinal membranes affecting the macula and removed by vitreous surgery. *Trans Am Ophthalmol Soc* 1982;80:580–656.
16. Margherio RR. Epiretinal macular membranes. In: Albert DM, Jakobiec FA (eds). *Principles and practice of ophthalmology*, vol 2. Philadelphia, Pa: WB Saunders; 1994:919–924.
17. Klein R, Klein BE, Wang Q, et al. The epidemiology of epiretinal membranes. *Trans Am Ophthalmol Soc* 1994;92:403–430.
18. Smiddy WE, Michels RG, Green WR. Morphology, pathology, and surgery of idiopathic vitreoretinal macular disorders. *Retina* 1990;10:288–296.
19. Wiznia RA. Natural history of idiopathic preretinal macular fibrosis. *Ann Ophthalmol* 1982;14:876–878.
20. Wise GN. Clinical features of idiopathic preretinal macular fibrosis. *Am J Ophthalmol* 1975;79:349–357.
21. Scudder MJ, Eifrig DE. Spontaneous surface wrinkling retinopathy. *Ann Ophthalmol* 1975;7:333–336,339–341.
22. Vinores SA, Campochiaro PA, Conway BP. Ultrastructural and electron-immunocytochemical characterization of cells in epiretinal membranes. *Invest Ophthal Vis Sci* 1990;31:14–28.
23. Hiscott P. Macrophages in the pathobiology of epiretinal membranes: multifunctional cells for a multistage process. *Br J of Ophthalmol* 1993;77(11):686–687.
24. Sumers KD, Jampol LM, Goldberg MF, et al. Spontaneous separation of epiretinal membranes. *Arch Ophthalmol* 1980;98:318–320.
25. Messner KH. Spontaneous separation of preretinal macular fibrosis. *Am J Ophthalmol* 1977;83:9–11.
26. Margherio RR, Cox MS Jr., Trese MT, et al. Removal of epimacular membranes. *Ophthalmology* 1985;92:1075–1083.
27. Arroyo JG, Irvine AR. Retinal distortion and cotton-wool spots associated with epiretinal membrane contraction. *Ophthalmology* 1995;102:662–668.
28. Joondeph HC. The incidence of epiretinal membrane with retinal breaks and detachments. In: Fine SL, Owens SL (eds). *Management of retinal vascular and macular disorders.* Baltimore, MD: WSW Publishers; 1983.
29. Pearlstone AD. The incidence of idiopathic preretinal macular gliosis. *Ann Ophthalmol* 1985;17:378–380.
30. Mitchell P, Smith W, Chey T, et al. Prevalence and association of epiretinal membranes. The Blue Mountains Eye Study. *Ophthalmology* 1997;104:1033–1040.
31. Hikichi T, Trempe CL. Risk of bilateral idiopathic preretinal macular fibrosis. *Eye* 1995;9:64–66.
32. Fraser-Bell S, Guzowski M, Rochtchina E, et al. Five-year cumulative incidence and progression of epiretinal membranes: the Blue Mountains Eye Study. *Ophthalmology* 2003;110:34–40.
33. Miyazaki M, Nakamura H, Kubo M, et al. Prevalence and risk factors for epiretinal membranes in a Japanese population: the Hisayama study. *Graefes Arch Clin Exp Ophthalmol* 2003;241:642–646.
34. Fraser-Bell S, Ying-Lai M, Klein R, et al. Prevalence and associations of epiretinal membranes in Latinos: the Los Angeles Latino Eye Study. *Invest Ophthalmol Vis Sci* 2004;45:1732–1736.
35. McCarty DJ, Mukesh BN, Chikani V, et al. Prevalence and associations of epiretinal membranes in the visual impairment project. *Am J Ophthalmol* 2005;140:288–294.
36. Pesin SR, Olk RJ, Grand MG, et al. Vitrectomy for premacular fibroplasia: prognostic factors, long-term follow-up, and time course of visual improvement. *Ophthalmology* 1991;98:1109–1114.
37. Kampik A, Kenyon KR, Michels RG, et al. Epiretinal and vitreous membranes: comparative study of 56 cases. *Arch Ophthalmol* 1981;99:1445–1454.
38. Constable IJ. Pathology of vitreous membranes and the effect of haemorrhage and new vessels on the vitreous. *Trans Ophthalmol Soc UK* 1975;95:382–386.
39. Augustin AJ, Spitznas M, Koch F, et al. Indicators of oxidative tissue damage and inflammatory activity in epiretinal membranes of proliferative diabetic retinopathy, proliferative vitreoretinopathy, and macular pucker. *Ger J Ophthalmol* 1995;4:47–51.
40. Ulbig MW, Wolfensberger TJ, Hiscott P, et al. Insulin-like growth factor I (IGF-I) receptor/binding protein in human diabetic epiretinal membranes. *Ger J Ophthalmol* 1995;4:264–268.
41. Kase S, Saito W, Yokoi M, et al. Expression of glutamine synthetase and cell proliferation in human idiopathic epiretinal membrane. *Br J Ophthalmol* 2006;90:96–98.
42. Abu El-Asrar AM, Missotten L, Geboes K. Expression of hypoxia-inducible factor-1alpha and the protein products of its target genes in diabetic fibrovascular epiretinal membranes. *Br J Ophthalmol* 2007;91:822–826.
43. Limb GA, Earley O, Jones SE, et al. Expression of mRNA coding for TNF alpha, IL-1 beta and IL-6 by cells infiltrating retinal membranes. *Graefes Arch Clin Exp Ophthalmol* 1994;232:646–651.

44. Vinores SA, Henderer JD, Mahlow J, et al. Isoforms of platelet-derived growth factor and its receptors in epiretinal membranes: immunolocalization to retinal pigmented epithelial cells. *Exp Eye Res* 1995;60: 607–619.

45. Immonen I, Vaheri A, Tommila P, et al. Plasminogen activation in epiretinal membranes. *Graefes Arch Clin Exp Ophthalmol* 1996;234:664–669.

46. Roldán-Pallarés M, Rollín R, Mediero A, et al. Immunoreactive ET-1 in the vitreous humor and epiretinal membranes of patients with proliferative vitreoretinopathy. *Mol Vis* 2005;11:461–471.

47. Machemer R, van Horn D, Aaberg TM. Pigment epithelial proliferation in human retinal detachment with massive periretinal proliferation. *Am J Ophthalmol* 1978;85:181–191.

48. Campochiaro PA, Jerdan JA, Glaser BM. Serum contains chemoattractants for human retinal pigment epithelial cells. *Arch Ophthalmol* 1984;102:1830–1833.

49. Campochiaro PA, Glaser BM. Platelet-derived growth factor is chemotactic for human retinal pigment epithelial cells. *Arch Ophthalmol* 1985;103: 576–579.

50. Campochiaro PA, Glaser BM. Endothelial cells release a chemoattractant for retinal pigment epithelial cells in vitro. *Arch Ophthalmol* 1985;103:1876–1880.

51. Machemer R, Laqua H. Pigment epithelium proliferation in retinal detachment (massive periretinal proliferation). *Am J Ophthalmol* 1975;80:1–23.

52. Harada C, Mitamura Y, Harada T. The role of cytokines and trophic factors in epiretinal membranes: involvement of signal transduction in glial cells. *Prog Retin Eye Res* 2005;25:149–164.

53. Kase S, Saito W, Ohgami K, et al. Expression of erythropoietin receptor in human epiretinal membrane of proliferative diabetic retinopathy. *Br J Ophthalmol* 2007;91:1376–1378.

54. Clarkson JG, Green WR, Massof D. A histopathologic review of 168 cases of preretinal membrane. *Am J Ophthalmol* 1977;84:1–17.

55. de Bustros S, Thompson JT, Michels RG, et al. Vitrectomy for idiopathic epiretinal membranes causing macular pucker. *Br J Ophthalmol* 1988;72:692–695.

56. Hirokawa H, Jalkh AE, Takahashi M, et al. Role of the vitreous in idiopathic preretinal macular fibrosis. *Am J Ophthalmol* 1986;101:166–169.

57. Heilskov TW, Massicotte SJ, Folk JC. Epiretinal macular membranes in eyes with attached posterior cortical vitreous. *Retina* 1996;16:279–284.

58. Foos RY. Vitreoretinal juncture; epiretinal membranes and vitreous. *Invest Ophthalmol Vis Sci* 1977;16:416–422.

59. Kmera-Muszynska M, Pratnicki A. Current views on the etiopathogenesis of proliferative vitreoretinopathy. *Klinika Oczna* 1995;97:44–47.

60. Ioachim E, Stefaniotou M, Gorezis S, et al. Immunohistochemical study of extracellular matrix components in epiretinal membranes of vitreoproliferative retinopathy and proliferative diabetic retinopathy. *Eur J Ophthalmol* 2005;15:384–391.

61. Green WR, Kenyon KR, Michels RG, et al. Ultrastructure of epiretinal membranes causing macular pucker after retinal reattachment surgery. *Trans Ophthalmol Soc UK* 1979;99:63–77.

62. Kenyon KR, Michels RG. Ultrastructure of epiretinal membrane removed by pars plana vitreoretinal surgery. *Am J Ophthalmol* 1977;83:815–823.

63. Trese MT, Chandler DB, Machemer R. Macular pucker. *Graefes Arch Clin Exp Ophthalmol* 1983;221:16–26.

64. Robertson DM, Buettner H. Pigmented preretinal membranes. *Am J Ophthalmol* 1977;83:824–829.

65. Kampik A, Green WR, Michels RG, et al. Ultrastructural features of progressive idiopathic epiretinal membrane removed by vitreous surgery. *Am J Ophthalmol* 1980;90:797–809.

66. McDonald HR, Abrams GW, Burke JM, et al. Clinicopathologic results of vitreous surgery for epiretinal membranes in patients with combined retinal and retinal pigment epithelial hamartomas. *Am J Ophthalmol* 1985;100:806–813.

67. Rentsch FJ. The ultrastructure of preretinal macular fibrosis. *Graefes Arch Clin Exp Ophthalmol* 1977;203:321–337.

68. Smiddy WE, Maguire AM, Green R, et al. Idiopathic epiretinal membranes. Ultrastructural characteristics and clinicopathologic correlation. *Ophthalmology* 1989;96:811–821.

69. Van Horn DL, Aaberg TM, Machemer R, et al. Glial cell proliferation in human retinal detachment with massive periretinal proliferation. *Am J Ophthalmol* 1977;84:383–393.

70. Bellhorn MB, Friedman AH, Wise GN, et al. Ultrastructure and clinicopathologic correlation of idiopathic preretinal macular fibrosis. *Am J Ophthalmol* 1975;79:366–373.

71. Nicolai U, Eckardt C. The occurrence of macrophages in the retina and periretinal tissues in ocular diseases. *Ger J Ophthalmol* 1993;2: 195–201.

72. Kono T, Kohno T, Inomata H. Epiretinal membrane formation. Light and electron microscopic study in an experimental rabbit model. *Arch Ophthalmol* 1995;113:359–363.

73. Haritoglou C, Schumann RG, Kampik A, et al. Glial cell proliferation under the internal limiting membrane in a patient with cellophane maculopathy. *Arch Ophthalmol* 2007;125:1301–1302.

74. Do DV, Cho M, Nguyen QD, et al. Impact of optical coherence tomography on surgical decision making for epiretinal membranes and vitreomacular traction. *Retina* 2007;27:552–556.

75. Gallemore RP, Jumper JM, McCuen BW II, et al. Diagnosis of vitreoretinal adhesions in macular disease with optical coherence tomography. *Retina* 2000;20:115–120.

76. Michalewski J, Michalewska Z, Cisiecki S, et al. Morphologically functional correlations of macular pathology connected with epiretinal membrane formation in spectral optical coherence tomography (SOCT). *Graefes Arch Clin Exp Ophthalmol* 2007;245:1623–1631.

77. Mori K, Gehlbach PL, Sano A, et al. Comparison of epiretinal membranes of differing pathogenesis using optical coherence tomography. *Retina* 2004;24:57–62.

78. Michels RG. Vitreous surgery for macular pucker. *Am J Ophthalmol* 1981;92:628–639.

79. Dellaporta A. Macular pucker and peripheral retinal lesions. *Trans Am Ophthalmol Soc* 1973;71:329–340.

80. Poliner LS, Olk RJ, Grand MG, et al. The surgical management of premacular fibroplasia. *Arch Ophthalmol* 1988;106:761–764.

81. Lewis JM, Park I, Ohji M, et al. Diamond-dusted silicone cannula for epiretinal membrane separation during vitreous surgery. *Am J Ophthalmol* 1997;124(4):552–554.

82. Kanawati C, Wono D, Hiscott P, et al. "En bloc" dissection of epimacular membranes using aspiration delamination. *Eye* 1996;10:47–52.

83. Michels RG, Rice TA, Ober RR. Vitreoretinal dissection instruments. *Am J Ophthalmol* 1979;87:836–837.

84. Fujii GY, De Juan E Jr., Humayun MS, et al. A new 25-gauge instrument system for transconjunctival sutureless vitrectomy surgery. *Ophthalmology* 2002;102:1807–1812.

85. Kadonosono K, Yamakawa T, Uchio E, et al. Comparison of visual function after epiretinal membrane removal by 20-gauge and 25-gauge vitrectomy. *Am J Ophthalmol* 2006;142:513–515.

86. Rizzo S, Genovesi-Ebert F, Murri S, et al. 25-gauge, sutureless vitrectomy and standard 20-gauge pars plana vitrectomy in idiopathic epiretinal membrane surgery: a comparative pilot study. *Graefes Arch Clin Exp Ophthalmol* 2006;244:472–479.

87. Fine HF, Iranmanesh R, Iturralde D, et al. Outcomes of 77 consecutive cases of 23-gauge transconjunctival vitrectomy surgery for posterior segment disease. *Ophthalmology* 2007;114:1197–1200.

88. Sawa M, Ohji M, Kusaka S, et al. Nonvitrectomizing vitreous surgery for epiretinal membrane long-term follow-up. *Ophthalmology* 2005;112:1402–1408.

89. Collaer N, Stalmans P. Which colour suits the vitreoretinal surgeon? *Br J Ophthalmol* 2007;91:1101–1102.

90. Kampik A, Haritoglou C, Gandorfer A. What are vitreoretinal surgeons dyeing for? *Retina* 2006;26:599–601.

91. Bhisitkul RB. Second generation vital stains in retinal surgery. *Br J Ophthalmol* 2003;87:664–665.

92. Hillenkamp J, Saikia P, Herrmann WA, et al. Surgical removal of idiopathic epiretinal membrane with or without the assistance of indocyanine green: a randomised controlled clinical trial. *Graefes Arch Clin Exp Ophthalmol* 2007;245:973–979.

93. Mavrofrides E, Smiddy WE, Kitchens JW, et al. Indocyanine green-assisted internal limiting membrane peeling for macular holes: toxicity? *Retina* 2006;26:637–644.

94. Lai TY, Kwok AK, Au AW, et al. Assessment of macular function by multifocal electroretinography following epiretinal membrane surgery with indocyanine green-assisted internal limiting membrane peeling. *Graefes Arch Clin Exp Ophthalmol* 2007;245:148–154.

95. Maia M, Haller JA, Pieramici DJ, et al. Retinal pigment epithelial abnormalities after internal limiting membrane peeling guided by indocyanine green staining. *Retina* 2004;24:157–160.

96. Kwok AK, Lai TY, Yew DT, et al. Internal limiting membrane staining with various concentrations of indocyanine green dye under air in macular surgeries. *Am J Ophthalmol* 2003;136:223–230.

97. Haritoglou C, Gandorfer A, Gass CA, et al. The effect of indocyanine-green on functional outcome of macular pucker surgery. *Am J Ophthalmol* 2003;135:328–337.

98. Lesnik Oberstein SY, Mura M, Tan SH, et al. Heavy trypan blue staining of epiretinal membranes: an alternative to infracyanine green. *Br J Ophthalmol* 2007;91:955–957.

99. Vote BJ, Russell MK, Joondeph BC. Trypan blue-assisted vitrectomy. *Retina* 2004;24:736–738.

100. Haritoglou C, Gandorfer A, Schaumberger M, et al. Trypan blue in macular pucker surgery: an evaluation of histology and functional outcome. *Retina* 2004;24:582–590.

101. Teba FA, Mohr A, Eckardt C, et al. Trypan blue staining in vitreoretinal surgery. *Ophthalmology* 2003;110:2409–2412.

102. Haritoglou C, Eibl K, Schaumberger M, et al. Functional outcome after trypan blue-assisted vitrectomy for macular pucker: a prospective, randomized, comparative trial. *Am J Ophthalmol* 2004;138: 1–5.

103. Perrier M, Sébag M. Epiretinal membrane surgery assisted by trypan blue. *Am J Ophthalmol* 2003;135:909–911.

104. Shah GK, Rosenblatt BJ, Blinder KJ, et al. Triamcinolone-assisted internal limiting membrane peeling. *Retina* 2005;25:972–975.

105. Kwok AK, Lai TY, Li WW, et al. Trypan blue- and indocyanine green-assisted epiretinal membrane surgery: clinical and histopathological studies. *Eye* 2004;18:882–888.

106. Kwok AKH, Lai TY, Yuen KS. Epiretinal membrane surgery with or without internal limiting membrane peeling. *Clin Experiment Ophthalmol* 2005;33:379–385.

107. Bovey EH, Uffer S, Achache F. Surgery for epimacular membrane: impact of retinal internal limiting membrane removal on functional outcome. *Retina* 2004;24:728–735.

108. Sivalingam A, Eagle RC Jr., Duker JS, et al. Visual prognosis correlated with the presence of internal-limiting membrane in histopathologic specimens obtained from epiretinal membrane surgery. *Ophthalmology* 1990;97:1549–1552.

109. Michels RG. Vitrectomy for macular pucker. *Ophthalmology* 1984;91:1384–1387.

110. Charles S. Epimacular proliferation. In: Schachet WS (ed). *Vitreous microsurgery*. Baltimore, MD: Williams & Wilkins; 1981:131–133.

111. McDonald HR, Verre WP, Aaberg TM. Surgical management of idiopathic epiretinal membranes. *Ophthalmology* 1986;93:978–983.

112. Ghazi-Nouri SM, Tranos PG, Rubin GS, et al. Visual function and quality of life following vitrectomy and epiretinal membrane peel surgery. *Br J Ophthalmol* 2006;90:559–562.

113. Massin P, Allouch C, Haouchine B, et al. Optical coherence tomography of idiopathic macular epiretinal membranes before and after surgery. *Am J Ophthalmol* 2000;130:732–739.

114. Rice TA, de Bustros S, Michels RG, et al. Prognostic factors in vitrectomy for epiretinal membranes of the macula. *Ophthalmology* 1986;93:602–610.

115. Thompson JT. Vitrectomy for epiretinal membranes with good visual acuity. *Trans Am Ophthalmol Soc* 2004;102:97–103.

116. de Bustros S, Thompson JT, Michels RG, et al. Nuclear sclerosis after vitrectomy for idiopathic epiretinal membranes. *Am J Ophthalmol* 1988;105:160–164.

117. Mason JO III, Feist RM, Albert MA Jr. Eccentric macular holes after vitrectomy with peeling of epimacular proliferation. *Retina* 2007;27:45–48.

118. Warden SM, Pachydaki SI, Christoforidis JB, et al. Choroidal neovascularization after epiretinal membrane removal. *Arch Ophthalmol* 2006;124:1652–1654.

119. de Bustros S, Rice TA, Michels RG, et al. Vitrectomy for macular pucker: use after treatment of retinal tears or retinal detachment. *Arch Ophthalmol* 1988;106:758–760.

120. Grewing R, Mester U. Results of surgery for epiretinal membranes and their recurrences. *Br J of Ophthalmol* 1996;80:323–326.

# seven

# Macular Holes

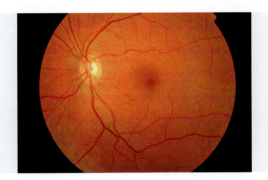

# Macular Hole

Borja Corcostegui ■ Lorena Patricia Pimentel

## INTRODUCTION

A macular hole is a full thickness defect of retinal tissue involving the anatomic fovea and the foveola of the eye. Macular holes were first described in 1869 by Knapp and later by Noyes in young patients mainly in relation to trauma (1,2). Recent studies have shown that the vast majority occur as an age-related primary idiopathic condition with a female predominance in the seventh decade of life.

They may also occur in association with cystoid macular edema in the setting of inflammation, retinal vascular disease (diabetic retinopathy, vascular occlusion, hypertensive retinopathy) highly myopic eyes, macular pucker, retinal detachment, and in less frequency with lightning strike (3,4).

## PATHOGENESIS

There are three basic historical theories regarding the etiology of macular holes:

Traumatic Theory: In the first reported cases, trauma was estimated to account for as many as 50% of cases.

Cystoid Degeneration Theory: In the first histopathologic descriptions of macular holes, Coats in 1907 noted cystic retinal changes adjacent to the macular hole and thought that these changes could be caused by trauma as well as other mechanisms. In cases where there was not an immediate hole formation, trauma was believed to cause reactive vasoconstriction followed by vasodilatation, thus leading to cystic degeneration of the central macula and full thickness macular hole formation by coalescence of the cysts (5). Cystoid degeneration of the macula with secondary macular hole formation has been uncommonly described in association with a variety of conditions that include Coat's disease, retinal vascular occlusions, severe hypertension, syphilis, solar maculopathy, arc welding maculopathy, electrocution, and vitreous traction (6).

Vascular Theory: Coats and Kuhnt believed that aging-related changes of the retinal vasculature (also characterized as ocular angiospasm) led to cystoid degeneration and subsequent macular hole formation.

Other theories:

Vitreous Theory: In 1912, Zeeman described the histopathology of the premacular vitreous condensation adjacent to foveal cystoid degeneration. Later on, as noted by Aaberg, Lister described anteroposterior fibrous vitreous traction bands, which were believed to cause macular distortion that led to tractional macular detachment, cystoid macular degeneration, and subsequently, macular hole formation (7). Based on these observations, the vitreous theory proposed that both forms of vitreous actions—preretinal condensation and contracting vitreous bands—were involved in the pathogenesis of macular holes. Around 1960, different studies began to highlight the relationship of the vitreous and the macula in eyes with macular holes. Worst described the premacular vitreous bursa as a vitreous pocket anterior to the macula and attached to it. This bursa, despite the fluid in the prefoveal interface, could exert anteroposterior traction from the margins. However, the problem with all these observations was that although the presence of a firm vitreofoveal adhesion was known, an obvious anteroposterior vitreous traction band was rarely observed.

Other investigators emphasized that the process of vitreous separation from the macula was the critical event in the pathogenesis of a macular hole. For example, Reese et al. proposed that vitreous separation from the fovea could cause avulsion of the fovea, resulting in a lamellar or full thickness macular hole (8). Because of the preponderance of women with macular hole, McDonnell et al. speculated that systemic estrogen fluctuations might promote destabilization and liquefaction of the vitreous, resulting eventually in vitreous separation with formation of a macular hole (9,10).

Involutional Macular Thinning: Morgan and Schatz incorporated vitreous, vascular, and cystic degeneration theories and proposed that initially, choroidal vascular changes would take place and then lead to altered submacular choroidal vascular perfusion and cystic degeneration of the retina. This would cause a progressive involutional macular thinning that, in addition to vitreous traction generated from attached posterior vitreous, would cause macular hole formation (11).

Muller Cell "Cone": In 1999, Gass emphasized the importance of the foveal Muller cell "cone," originally described by Yamada and Hogan et al. in histological studies of the normal human foveola. These studies showed that the foveola is composed of an inverted cone of Muller glia with a truncated apex up to the external limiting membrane (ELM). Radially oriented inner cone segments that radiate toward the beginning of the outer nuclear layer of cone nuclei are located between the apex and the ELM. The base of the cone formed the umbo and extended into the clivus in the perifoveolar region (12). Gass suggested that the Muller cell cone has three important roles in the formation of a macular hole:

- Glia contain concentrated superficial xanthophyll, which migrates centrifugally during the formation of a full thickness macular hole and may be seen as a yellow spot or a yellow ring. This hypothesis is supported by the presence of xantophyll in the operculum.
- The Muller cone provides structural support for the radiating inner cone segments at the foveola and its disruption may lead to damage and atrophy of the cone cells located in this area.
- Muller cells within the cone invade the prefoveolar vitreous cortex and initiate cellular remodeling and contraction. This, results in tangential traction on the foveola, centrifugal migration of photoreceptors and xantophyll, causing further disruption of the Muller cone and eventually umbo dehiscence (12).

Hydration Theory: Tornambe in 2003, on the basis of optical coherence tomography (OCT) 3 images and a simple model, proposed the Hydration theory. In this theory, susceptible eyes have a firm point of adherence between the posterior hyaloid face and the central macula. Stages 1A and 1B holes are explained by this foveal traction that lifts the fovea, distorting the foveal depression and displacing deeper yellow pigment. If the posterior hyaloid traction tears the inner foveal retina,

OCT 3 suggests that vitreous fluid soaks into the layers of the macula initially creating a cavity in the inner retina, and then dissecting deeper, laterally accumulating in the outer plexiform layer. As the swelling increases, the hole enlarges. Because the internal limiting membrane (ILM) at its junction with the inner retina is a more rigid structure than the deeper retinal tissue, this complex (ILM/inner retina) retracts and elevates as the swelling increases. If the posterior hyaloid separates from the macula (stage 4), it may pull a tag of inner retinal tissue (ILM/nerve fiber layer/Muller cell/inner nuclear cells) (13).

## CLINICAL STAGING

In 1988, Gass and then Johnson and Gass (14,15) developed a classification scheme for idiopathic macular holes and their precursor lesions (Fig. 28-1).

Stage 1 (Foveolar Detachment). It is also known as "impending hole." Patients usually note metamorphopsia and blurred vision, although visual acuity at this stage is reasonably good (20/20–20/60) (14–16). These symptoms may be unnoticed in the first eye involved but are the rule not the exception if the fellow eye becomes affected. There is a progressive loss of foveal depression in the absence of posterior vitreous detachment or vitreofoveal separation, associated with the appearance of an enhanced lipofucsin-colored yellow spot of approximately 100 to 150 μm at the fovea (stage 1A). The foveal retina then elevates to the level of the surrounding perifoveal retina, elongating the foveal retina around the umbo and creating a small yellow ring of 200 to 300 μm in diameter (stage 1B). Fine radiating striae surrounding the central area can be demonstrated and are best observed with retroillumination (17). Fluorescein angiography may be normal or may show fluorescence in the normally dark fovea that fades in later phases and is consistent with a window defect. The OCT scan may show a perifoveal separation of the posterior hyaloid with focal vitreous attachment to the fovea, a foveal detachment or an intraretinal space termed as pseudocyst. There is no evidence of a full thickness retinal defect. Johnson and Gass (14,15) and Kokame (16) observed that 66% of stage 1 macular holes progressed to stage 2, while Akiba et al. and Guyer et al. reported that 37% and 10.5% of stage 1 holes progressed to stage 2, respectively (18,19).

Stage 2 (Early Full Thickness Macular Hole). Further traction results in the formation of a small, full thickness macular hole that can be seen centrally within the yellow ring or eccentrically at the margin of the ring. The eccentric location is typical in the majority of cases (80%–90%) and it extends in a "can opener" fashion to form a crescentic hole that progresses to a horseshoe shaped hole, and eventually, to a round hole with a fully detached operculum. The visual symptoms become more severe as metamorphopsia increases and visual acuity deteriorates to a level of 20/40 to 20/100 (5,6). The vitreous has the same appearance as that in stage 1. As the hole enlarges, the yellow ring often turns gray as the retina surrounding the hole begins to detach from the underlying retinal pigment epithelium (RPE), creating an annular neurosensory

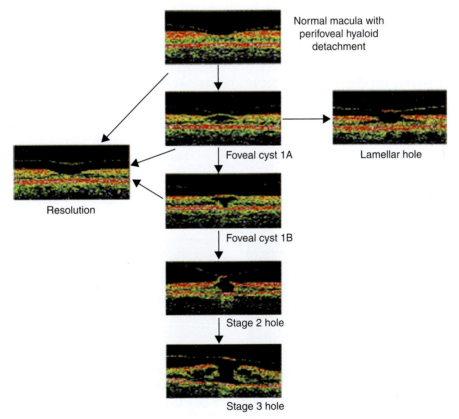

Normal macula with perifoveal hyaloid detachment

Foveal cyst 1A

Lamellar hole

Resolution

Foveal cyst 1B

Stage 2 hole

Stage 3 hole

**Figure 28-1.** Staging of macular hole.

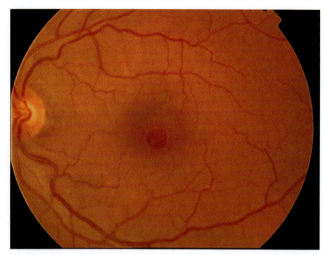

**Figure 28-2.** Left eye of a 64-year-old female patient with an initial visual acuity of 20/200 and a stage 3 macular hole with yellowish deposits at the level of retinal pigment epithelium.

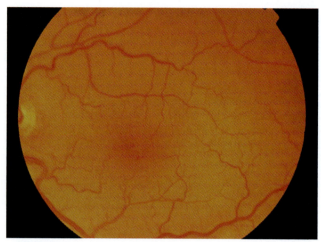

**Figure 28-4.** Fundus color photograph shows closure of the macular hole and some retinal pigment epithelium disturbances at the foveal area with two pinpoint hemorrhages at inferotemporal margin of the fovea. Final visual acuity improved to 20/60.

retinal detachment. Fluorescein angiography may have a more intense central fluorescence, but it is not reliable in differentiating the two stages. The OCT scan shows a small full thickness retinal defect or a rupture of the roof of the pseudocyst. Approximately, 67% of stage 2 holes progress to stage 3 as noted by Hikichi et al. (20). Kim et al. reported a 55% progression rate to stage 3 for centric stage 2 holes, and 100% for eccentric (can opener) holes, with an overall 74% progression rate of all stage 2 holes to either stage 3 or 4 (21). There are some eyes with "stage 2-like" holes that appear to have small retinal defects that remain stable for years without progression. These eyes probably do not have a true full thickness defect but rather, a lamellar macular hole that can be demonstrated with an OCT scan (14). Clinical differentiation between these two entities is not easy but it is important to decide if surgical intervention is needed. For this reason, surgery for very small or questionable full thickness macular holes should be deferred until progression can be demonstrated clinically.

Stage 3 (Fully Developed Full Thickness Macular Hole without Posterior Vitreous Detachment).

Stage 4 (Fully Developed Full Thickness Macular Hole with Posterior Vitreous Detachment).

The visual acuity drops between 20/80 and 20/200. In stage 3, vitreofoveal separation occurs at the macula and is usually only detected because of the presence of the operculum

suspended on it, lying a short distance anterior to retinal plane. In stage 4, 20% to 40% of patients present evidence of posterior vitreous separation, such as partial or complete remnants of Weiss' ring and 50% to 70% of patients present a retinal operculum that can be seen freely floating on the posterior hyaloid face (Figs. 28-2 to 28-5). In these two stages, a full thickness retinal defect of 300 to 1500 µm in diameter associated with a surrounding neurosensory retinal detachment can be easily detected clinically, although the full extent of the detachment might be underestimated, since there is often a much larger area of shallow detachment surrounding the retina around the retinal hole. Discrete white deposits, which represent nodular proliferations of RPE cells, may appear on the surface of the RPE at the base of the hole or under the surrounding retinal detachment in approximately 50% of the patients (7). In long standing cases, a pigmented demarcation line at the level of RPE may be seen surrounding the cuff of fluid along with cystic changes. Fluorescein angiography demonstrates a window defect with early fluorescence in the area of neurosensory retinal defect followed by gradual fading of the fluorescence. OCT scan shows a full thickness retinal defect with a sharp edge that changes over time to become a rounded edge and that is associated with an adjacent neurosensory retinal detachment. Intraretinal edema and epiretinal membranes may also be observed.

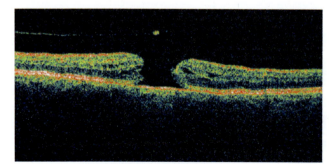

**Figure 28-3.** Optical coherence tomography scan shows retinal edema at the margins of the macular hole and the operculum lying in the posterior hyaloid face, which is detached.

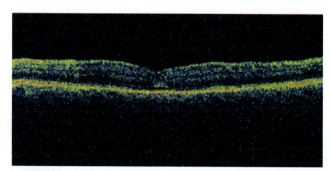

**Figure 28-5.** Optical coherence tomography scan 1-month postoperative shows complete closure of the hole with a partial recovery of the foveal depression, and there is a tiny pocket of subfoveal fluid.

In 1995, Gass reappraised his theory of macular hole formation and introduced the concept of "occult macular hole" in the revised classification. This revised theory is characterized by a dehiscence at the umbo with lateral displacement of photoreceptors; the operculum represents the overlying prefoveal tissue and not necessarily neurosensory retina (19). The hole may become evident in two ways—as a centric or as an eccentric hole caused by separation of the prefoveolar vitreous cortex from the edge or the center of the round, previously occult macular hole. Spontaneous vitreofoveal separation then occurs, creating a pseudo-operculum (semitranslucent prefoveal opacity) that is often larger than the underlying occult foveolar hole. Biomicroscopically, a full thickness defect can be detected at stage 2 holes and may be obscured by the overlying pseudo-operculum (22). Also Gass described that most macular operculum probably are not composed of retinal receptors;– instead, they are composed of vitreous condensations and reactive glial proliferation.

OCT scans have recently shown that foveal pseudocysts are the first step of full thickness macular hole formation, but they also may evolve into a lamellar hole, may persist unchanged for months, or may resolve completely. Foveal pseudocyst formation may be the result of the incomplete separation of the vitreous cortex at the foveal center and the particular structure of the foveal Müller cells (23).

## EXAMINATION AND DIAGNOSIS

As many lesions can simulate macular holes or macular hole precursor lesions, careful slit lamp biomicroscopy with a fundus contact lens (90–78D) should be performed in all cases where doubt exists. The Watzke-Allen test entails placing a narrow vertical slit beam through the fovea and asking the patient to describe the line. A positive test results when the patient detects a break in the line. Those with small holes or other lesions associated with metamorphopsia may report "thinning" of the line and that can be interpreted as a negative Watzke sign. The laser aiming beam test is probably more sensitive and specific for full thickness macular holes. It is performed by placing the 50 μm laser photocoagulator such that the beam is aimed onto the center of the suspected macular hole; a positive test is observed when the patient cannot detect the aiming beam in the center but is able to detect it in the surrounding intact retinal tissue (24). Amsler Grid abnormalities are sensitive to macular lesions but not specific to macular holes. Bowing of the lines and micropsia can be appreciated perhaps because of the edema of the surrounding retinal tissue. The early central hyperfluorescence observed in fluorescein angiography is not helpful for differentiating because it appears in 79% of true and 63% of pseudomacular holes. B-scan ultrasonography is not sensitive enough to distinguish macular holes from masquerade lesions but may be helpful in macular hole staging and surgical planning because it allows to evaluate vitreomacular relationship (25). Macular microperimetry using a scanning laser ophthalmoscope can evaluate the absolute and relative scotoma associated with a macular hole. This technique has demonstrated that visual loss in eyes with macular holes is due to the absence of retinal function (neurosensory defect) in the area of the hole as well as reduction in retinal function in the area of the surrounding neurosensory retinal detachment (26). Confocal laser tomography, laser biomicroscopy, and OCT have the advantage of improving the resolution of the vitreomacular interface.

## DIFFERENTIAL DIAGNOSIS

The most common lesions simulating a full thickness macular hole are lamellar macular holes (LMH) and macular pseudoholes (MPH). The pathogenesis is different. MPH are the result of epiretinal membrane (ERM) contraction, which results in the verticalization of the foveal slopes, whereas LMH result from an aborted process of macular hole formation and there is avulsion of part of the macular tissue (23,27). MPH associated with epiretinal membranes can be differentiated because of the presence of retinal vascular tortuosity and compression, a median visual acuity of 20/30, and the absence of a rim with subretinal fluid (28). LMH are characterized by a flat, reddish hue-type lesion with intact outer retinal tissue that can be observed with a careful contact lens biomicroscopic evaluation. Patients usually report a negative Watzke sign and are also able to see the laser-aiming beam within the lesion.

Differentiating between MPH and LMH may still be difficult at biomicroscopy in some cases, especially when the LMH is surrounded by an ERM or when the ERM causing the MPH is thin, transparent, and not associated with obvious retinal folds. For these cases, Haochine B, Massin P, Gaudric A reported two different OCT profiles. In LMH, the foveal center is thinner than normal and its profile is irregular. This thinning fits well with the mechanism of LMH formation, which involves avulsion of the roof of a foveal cyst without the opening of the outer retinal layer. In MPH, the mean thickness of the macular center is nearly normal or slightly increased (24). The thickening of the macular area and verticalization of the foveal slope causes the foveal pit to acquire a cylindrical appearance, as suggested by Allen and Gass (25).

Premacular hole lesions are also simulated by other macular lesions and the most important diagnostic tool is careful slit lamp biomicroscopic evaluation. For example, yellow macular lesions are observed in pseudo-opercula; vitreomacular traction; vitelliform and pattern dystrophies; cystoid macular edema; acute solar maculopathy; macular neurosensory elevations such as central serous chorioretinopathy; post-traumatic maculopathy; and less commonly, inflammatory or infectious chorioretinopathies (29). It is important to remember that in true premacular hole lesions, there is not a significant elevation of the fovea above the surrounding tissue, and at this stage no vitreofoveal separation has occurred. Nowadays, OCT is a very useful tool to evaluate and diagnose all the types of macular holes as is demonstrated by many articles in the literature (23,28).

## TREATMENT

Initially, macular holes were considered untreatable and surgery was only indicated if an extensive retinal detachment occurred. Later, the attention was focused on preventing macular hole formation in patients believed to be at risk. A clinical trial in which patients with stages 1A and 1B lesions in one eye and a full thickness macular hole in their fellow eyes were randomized to vitrectomy or observation showed that vitrectomy does not provide a benefit in the prevention of macular holes (30). Due to the refinement of surgical techniques, the attention was then diverted to treat full thickness macular holes. Initially, the attempts were centered on creation of a strong chorioretinal adhesion along the margin of the hole to allow for flattening of the surrounding neurosensory retinal detachment. This was achieved by applying laser photocoagulation to the rim of the macular hole, but poor visual outcomes were reported because laser photocoagulation caused damage to the neurosensory retina and RPE (31).

Nowadays, the indication and timing for surgery mostly depends on the extent of progression of the macular hole and its resultant symptoms. Coexisting conditions such as severe traumatic maculopathy, choroidal rupture, diabetic retinopathy, retinal vascular abnormalities, macular degeneration, severe glaucoma, and optic nerve disorders should be taken into consideration because the prognosis for postoperative visual improvement may be worse when they are present. Surgery is indicated in most eyes with moderate to large stage 3 or 4 holes that cause symptoms and reduce visual acuity in the range of 20/60 to 20/400, and also in eyes with small full thickness stage 2 or 3 holes, causing symptoms and reducing visual acuity to a range between 20/40 and 20/60. Macular hole surgery in eyes with visual acuity better than 20/40 is rarely indicated. It is now well known that preoperative visual acuity is a prognostic factor for visual outcome and that it is inversely correlated with the absolute amount of visual improvement. Therefore, eyes with worse preoperative acuity experience the greatest amount of improvement after surgery, gaining two or more lines approximately. Moreover, eyes with better preoperative visual acuity end up with better postoperative visual acuity, even though they will not experience as many lines of improvement after surgery. Other predictors of visual outcome include the size of the macular hole and preoperative lens opacification. Smaller holes and less lens opacification are associated with better postoperative acuity (32,33). If the patient is more than 55 years old and presents with lens opacification, a phacoemulsification can precede the retinal surgery.

Currently, the surgical technique consists of a conventional pars plana vitrectomy with a three-port system. Historically, a 20-gauge system has been employed; however, over the past years, 23-gauge and 25-gauge systems have been introduced and adopted by some retinal surgeons. After removal of the central vitreous, the posterior cortical vitreous must be identified and separated from the retinal surface. Cortical vitreous can be easily identified with the tip of the vitrectome or using a soft-tipped silicon cannula. With the tip of the vitrectome and after elevating intraocular pressure and vacuum pressure, aspiration over the temporal vascular arcades while exerting a soft tangential traction toward the periphery of the retina makes the cortical vitreous easy to catch and exposes the subhyaloid space. With the silicon cannula, after suction is applied, the orifice of the cannula becomes occluded by the cortical vitreous and the cannula flexes. This is called the "fish-strike" sign or the "divining-rod" sign (34,35). Cortical vitreous

can also be visualized by staining it with trypan blue and indocyanine green (ICG), although some concerns over the potential toxicity of ICG have been expressed. Triamcinolone may also be used for this purpose and appears to be well tolerated but any remains of it inside the vitreous cavity may be associated with complications such as cataract, ocular hypertension, and sterile uveitis. After creation of posterior vitreous detachment, a floating Weiss' ring can be usually visualized and vitrectomy must then be completed. At this point, ERM and ILM may be stained with ICG, trypan blue, or triamcinolone and removed if the surgeon desires. Here it is important to remember that in small full thickness macular holes, ILM peeling can be avoided but in stages 3 and 4 macular holes, ILM peeling seems to be highly recommended to improve anatomical success. Then, careful peripheral examination for retinal iatrogenic breaks should be performed, followed by fluid-air exchange and aspiration of the accumulated intravitreal fluid from the preretinal space before closure of the sclerotomies and air-gas exchange. Nonexpansile concentrations of C3F8 (14%–15%) and SF6 (20%–25%) are used as long standing tamponades to improve surgical success. In recent onset or very small full thickness macular holes, the use of air as a tamponade can also be considered. SF6 can be used for stages 1 and 2 macular holes and C3F8 for stages 3 and 4. Silicon oil can also be used in long standing cases, in high myopes, in previously operated eyes with recurrence of the macular hole and in children or elder people who are not able to maintain face-down positioning. Face-down positioning in the postoperative period is required to provide tamponade, reduce intraocular fluid currents, and promote closure of the macular hole. During the surgery, it is important to remember the potential toxicity of light to the photoreceptors, and the surgeon should try to reduce to a minimum the time of focusing the light directly to the macula.

In Kelly and Wendell's original description of macular hole surgery, 58% of cases achieved anatomical success performing a pars plana vitrectomy and posterior hyaloid detachment (34). Later, the addition of ERM peeling and sulfur hexafluoride as a tamponade to the technique led to 60% to 70% of anatomic success (36). With ILM peeling, some authors have reported anatomic success of 90% (37).

Anatomic surgical success is indicated by complete resolution of the neurosensory retinal detachment and absence of visible edges of the prior hole. Closure of the hole can be demonstrated as early as 24 hours postoperatively by OCT scan (38). Two patterns of OCT macular hole closure have been described: in the first and the most frequent one, the macula takes on a normal appearance with an absence of retinal defect and with a normal foveal depression (Figs. 28-6 to 28-9), while in the second one, there is a persistent outer retinal space simulating a foveal neurosensory retinal detachment (39). This latter pattern may be associated with poorer visual acuity, may progress into the first pattern of closure, or may lead to an early recurrence of macular hole. With anatomic success, retinal function usually improves; patients usually report an improvement in symptoms of metamorphopsia and gain resolution or improvement of preoperative symptomatic central scotoma. Most importantly, visual acuity improves subjectively and objectively in most eyes. After surgery, foveolar lucencies can be observed by OCT in approximately 26% of cases. They

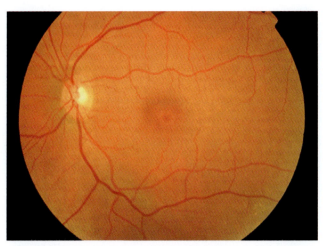

**Figure 28-6.** Left eye of a 57-year-old female patient showing a stage 2 macular hole with an initial visual acuity of 20/200.

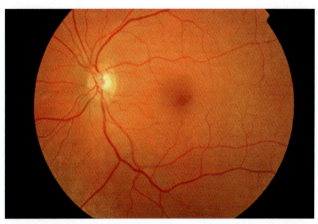

**Figure 28-8.** Fundus color photograph 1-month postoperative showing complete closure of the macular hole. Final visual acuity improved to 20/50.

occur with and without ICG-assisted peeling of the ILM and gradually decrease and resolve with time without the need for additional surgical intervention and with further improvement of visual acuity (40).

Actually, some controversies exist about the necessity, efficacy, preferred technique, and complications of epiretinal and ILM peeling. For example, some authors report that ICG-assisted ILM peeling improves anatomic success in surgery but it may potentially lead to unfavorable visual outcome and peripheral visual field loss due to posterior RPE atrophy, while others report equivalent anatomic and visual outcomes with and without the use of ICG (41,42).

Moreover, some authors advocate ILM peeling in all cases, based on the observation that macular hole reopening takes place due to tangential contraction of ERM formed postoperatively and that ILM peeling would prevent the reopening by inhibiting recurrence of the epiretinal membrane (43). Others describe that ILM peeling does not significantly improve visual acuity in case of larger holes, and therefore, is not necessary in all cases (44).

As face-down positioning is inconvenient, and may be impossible to attain in patients with physical and mental limitations, the choice of intravitreal gas tamponade and duration of postoperative face-down positioning remains controversial. In the early descriptions of macular hole surgery, the authors

used a nonexpansile concentration of sulfur hexafluoride and face-down positioning for at least a week. There have been some reports about macular hole surgery without face-down positioning combined with cataract surgery in the case of phakic patients. Tornambe PE and Madgula IM have reported success rates between 79% and 96% using a complete 15% C3F8 vitreous cavity fill, combined with cataract extraction and intraocular lens insertion in phakic cases without postoperative posturing (45,46). Moreover, Rubinstein and Wickens have reported that pars plana vitrectomy, ILM peeling, and C3F8 gas tamponade with a shortened period of face-down position or without positioning provides anatomical and functional results comparable to those cases with posturing, and that this technique is not associated with significant adverse outcomes (47,48). Unfortunately, there are few well-designed studies comparing the efficacy of different gases, gas concentrations, and durations of face-down positioning on anatomic and visual outcomes. Silicone oil may be used to reduce dependence of surgical outcome on face-down positioning, and usually is removed 6 to 12 weeks postoperatively.

Nowadays, most surgeons indicate face-down positioning and strongly recommend a 100% compliance for at least a week. Longer face-down positioning may be beneficial in maximizing surgical success, but the ideal duration of face-down position still unclear.

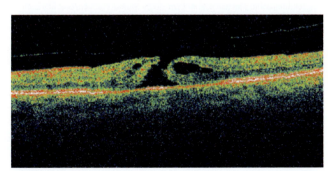

**Figure 28-7.** Optical coherence tomography scan of the same patient shows a full thickness retinal defect with retinal edema at the margins and an incomplete posterior vitreous detachment.

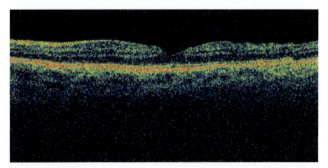

**Figure 28-9.** Optical coherence tomography scan 1-month postoperative showing complete closure of the macular hole with recovery of the foveal contour and a slight defect at the level of the external photoreceptor layer at the central fovea.

In an effort to increase anatomic and visual success rates, several surgical adjunctive agents have been used. Intravitreal transforming growth factor-B2 (TGF-B2) derived from bovine bone was reported to have a dose dependent efficacy and a higher anatomic success rate than placebo (49). Autologous concentrated platelets have been seen to have a high success rate in age-related idiopathic and pediatric macular hole. Futures studies may further elucidate any benefit of adjunctive agents (50).

Late reopening of previously repaired macular holes can occur due to any process that modifies the foveolar anatomy, such as progressive ERM formation, macular cystoid edema after cataract surgery or inflammation, or intraretinal and preretinal cellular remodeling and resultant traction. Spontaneous closure of a macular hole after previous vitrectomy can occur due to ERM contracture and bridging glial cell proliferation (51).

## References

1. Knapp H. Uber isolirte Z erreissungen der Aderhaut in Folge von Traumen auf dem Augapfel. *Arch Augenheilkd* 1869;1:6–29.
2. Noyes HD. Detachment of the retina with laceration at the macular lutea. *Trans Am Ophthalmol Soc* 1871;1:128–129.
3. Campo RV, Lewis RS. Lightning-induced macular hole. *Am J Ophthalmol* 1984;97:792–794.
4. Cohen SM, Gass JD. Macular hole following severe hypertensive retinopathy [letter]. *Arch Ophthalmol* 1994;112:878–879.
5. Frangieh GT, Green WR, Engel HM. A histopathologic study of macular cysts and holes. *Retina* 1981;1:311–336.
6. Cohen SM, Gass JDM. Macular hole following severe hypertensive retinopathy. *Arch Ophthalmol* 1994;112:878–879.
7. Aaberg TM. Macular holes: a review. *Surv Ophthalmol* 1970;15:139–162.
8. Reese AB, Jones IS, Cooper W. Macular changes secondary to vitreous traction. *Am J Ophthalmol* 1967;64:544–549.
9. Kornzweig AL, Feldstein M. Studies of the eye in old age. Hole in the macula: a clinico-pathologic study. *Am J Ophthalmol* 1950;33:243–247.
10. McDonnell PJ, Fine SL, Hillis AI. Clinical features of idiopathic macular cysts and holes. *Am J Ophthalmol* 1982;93:777–786.
11. Morgan CM, Schatz H. Involutional macular thinning: a premacular hole condition. *Ophthalmology* 1986;93:153–161.
12. Gass JDM. Muller cell cone, an overlooked part of the anatomy of the fovea centralis. Hypotheses concerning its role in the pathogenesis of macular hole and foveomacular retinoschisis. *Arch Ophthalmol* 1999;117:821–823.
13. Tornambe P. Macular Hole Genesis: the hydration theory (hypothesis). *Retina* 2003;23:421–424.
14. Gass JDM. Idiopathic senile macular holes its early stages and development. *Arch Ophthalmol* 1988;106:629–639.
15. Johnson RN, Gass JDM. Idiopathic macular holes. Observations, stages of formation, and implications for surgical intervention. *Ophthalmology* 1988;95:917–934.
16. Kokame GT, de Bustros S. The Vitrectomy for Prevention of Macular Hole Study Group: Visual acuity as a prognostic indicator in stage 1 macular holes. *Am J Ophthalmol* 1995;119:112–114.
17. Ho A, Guyer D, Fine S. Macular Hole. *Surv of Ophthalmol* 1998;42:393–416.
18. Akiba J, Kakehashi A, Arzabe CW, et al. Risk of developing a macular hole. *Arch Ophthalmol* 1990;108: 1088–1090.
19. Guyer Dr, de Bustros S, Diener-West M, et al. The natural history of idiopathic macular holes and cysts. *Arch Ophthalmol* 1992;110:1264–1268.
20. Hikichi T, Yoshida A, Akiba J, et al. Prognosis of stage 2 macular holes. *Am J Ophthalmol* 1995;119:571–575.
21. Kim JW, Freeman WR, El-Haig W, et al. Baseline characteristics, natural history, and risk factors to progression in eyes with stage 2 macular holes. Results from a prospective randomized clinical trial. *Ophthalmology* 1995;102:1818–1829.
22. Gass JDM. Reappraisal of biomicroscopic classification of the stages of development of a macular hole. *Am J Ophthalmol* 1995;119:752–759.
23. Haochine B, Massin P, Gaudric A. Foveal pseudocyst as the first step in macular hole formation: a prospective study by optical coherence tomography. *Ophthalmology* 2001;108:15–22.
24. Martinez J, Smiddy WE, Kim J, et al. Differentiating macular holes from macular pseudoholes. *Am J Ophthalmol* 1994;117:762–767.
25. Dugel PU, Smiddy WE, Byrne SF, et al. Macular hole syndromes. Echographic findings with clinical correlation. *Ophthalmology* 1994;101:815–821.
26. Sjaarda RN, Frank DA, Glaser BM, et al. Assessment of vision in idiopathic macular holes with macular microperimetry using the scanner laser ophthalmoscope. *Ophthalmology* 1993;100:1513–1518.
27. Allen AW, Gass JD. Contraction of a perifoveal epiretinal membrane simulating a macular hole. *Am J Ophthalmol* 1976;82:684–691.
28. Fish RH, Arnand R, Izbrand DJ. Macular pseudoholes: clinical features and accuracy of diagnosis. *Ophthalmology* 1992;99:1665–1670.
29. Gass JD, VanNewkirk M. Xanthic scotoma and yellow foveolar shadow caused by a pseudo-operculum after vitreofoveal separation. *Retina* 1992;12: 242–244.
30. de Bustros S. Vitrectomy for prevention of macular holes: results of a randomized multicenter clinical trial. Vitrectomy for Prevention of Macular Hole Study Group. *Ophthalmology* 1994;101:1055–1059.
31. Cox MS, Lakhanpal V, Xiaoping M, et al. Laser treatment of macular holes. *Ophthalmology* 1988;95:581–582.
32. Ullrich S, Haritoglou C, Gass C, et al. Macular hole size as a prognostic factor in macular hole surgery. *Br J Ophthalmol* 2002;86:390–393.
33. Sjaarda RN, Glaser BM, Thompson JT, et al. Effect of preoperative visual acuity in the treatment of macular holes with vitrectomy and TGF- beta. *Ophthalmology* 1991;100(suppl):73.
34. Kelly NE, Wendell RT. Vitreous surgery for idiopathic macular holes: results of a pilot study. *Arch Ophthalmol* 1991;109:654–659.
35. Mein CE, Flynn HW Jr. Recognition and removal of the posterior cortical vitreous during vitreoretinal surgery for impending macular hole. *Am J Ophthalmol* 1991;111:611–613.
36. Wendell RT, Patel AC, Kelly NE. Vitreous surgery for macular holes. *Ophthalmology* 1993;100:1671–1676.
37. Park DW, Sipperley JO, Sneed SR. Macular hole surgery with internal limiting membrane peeling and intravitreous air. *Ophthalmology* 1999;106: 1392–1398.
38. Kasuga Y, Arai J, Akimoto M, et al. Optical coherence tomography to confirm early closure of macular holes. *Am J Ophthalmol* 2000;130:675–676.
39. Takahashi H, Hishi S. Tomographic features of early macular hole closure after vitreous surgery. *Am J Ophthalmol* 2000;130:192–196.
40. Mahmoud TH, McCuen BW II. Natural history of foveolar lucencies observed by optical coherence tomography after macular holes surgery. *Retina* 2007;27(1):95–100.
41. Ando F, Sasano K, Ohba N. Anatomic and visual outcomes after indocyanine green-assisted peeling of the retinal internal limiting membrane in idiopathic macular hole surgery. *Am J Ophthalmol* 2004;13(4): 609–614.
42. Kumagai K, Furukawa M, Ogino N. Long-term outcomes of internal limiting membrane peeling with or without indocyanine green in macular hole surgery. *Retina* 2006;26(6):613–617.
43. Yoshida M, Kishi S. Pathogenesis of macular hole recurrence and its prevention by internal limiting membrane peeling. *Retina* 2007;27(2): 169–173.
44. Kumagai K, Furukawa M, Ogino N. Vitreous surgery with and without internal limiting membrane peeling for macular hole repair. *Retina* 2004;24(5):721–727.
45. Tornambe PE, Poliner LS, Grote K. Macular hole surgery without face-down positioning. A pilot study. *Retina* 1997;17(3):179–185.
46. Madgula IM, Costen M. Functional outcome and patient preferences following combined phaco-vitrectomy for macular hole without prone posturing [published online ahead of print April 13, 2007]. *Eye* 2007. doi:10.1038/sj. eye.6702835.
47. Rubinstein A, Ang A, Patel CK. Vitrectomy without postoperative posturing for idiopathic macular holes. *Clin Experiment Ophthalmol* 2007;35(5): 458–461.
48. Wickens JC, Shah GK. Outcomes of macular hole surgery and shortened face-down positioning. *Retina* 2006;26(8):902–904.
49. Glaser BM, Michels RG, Kuppermann BD, et al. Transforming growth factor-B for the treatment of full-thickness macular holes: a prospective randomized study. *Ophthalmology* 1992;99:1162–1173.
50. Sjaarda R, Thompson J. Macular hole. In: Ryan S (ed). *Retina*, 4th ed. Philadelphia, PA: Elsevier Inc, 2006:2527–2544.
51. Gross J. Late reopening and spontaneous closure of previously repaired macular holes. *Am J Ophthalmol* 2005;140(3):556–558.

# 29

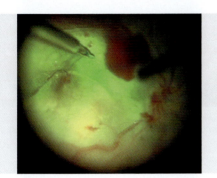

# Intraocular Dyes for Vitreoretinal Surgery

Michel E. Farah ■ Eduardo B. Rodrigues ■ Mauricio Maia ■ Lihteh Wu ■ J. Fernando Arevalo

255

## INTRODUCTION

The intraocular application of dyes to assist visualization of preretinal tissues during vitreoretinal surgery, "chromovitrectomy," has become a very popular technique in the past few years (1). Chromovitrectomy was motivated by the difficulty in visualizing the several thin and transparent tissues in the vitreoretinal interface (2,3). Staining the internal limiting membrane (ILM), the epiretinal membrane (ERM), and the vitreous with a vital dye may assist the visualization of those fine transparent tissues, thereby leading to improvement in the postoperative visual acuity. The first vital dye used in chromovitrectomy, indocyanine green (ICG), facilitated the identification of the fine and transparent ILM (2). Following ICG, trypan blue (TB) has been introduced as an appropriate agent to identify the several ERMs, and triamcinolone acetonide (TA) has been found to stain the vitreous well. Recently, additional vital dyes such as infracyanine green (IfCG) and patent blue (PB) have been proposed for intraocular application during vitrectomy (4,5). In this chapter the current knowledge involving the use of dyes in chromovitrectomy will be discussed. In order to minimize the risk of toxic effects of dyes in chromovitrectomy, surgical recommendations are presented.

## INDOCYANINE GREEN

The application of intravitreal ICG was first reported in cadaver eyes to improve the visualization of the ILM. Since then, many articles have been released regarding the use of ICG as a surgical adjuvant to facilitate the identification and removal of the ILM in macular surgery (Figs. 29-1 and 29-2). ICG-assisted macular hole surgery demonstrated closure rates above 75% as well as visual improvements varying from 18% to 94% (3). However, soon after the introduction of ICG for the treatment of macular holes, caution among vitreoretinal surgeons took

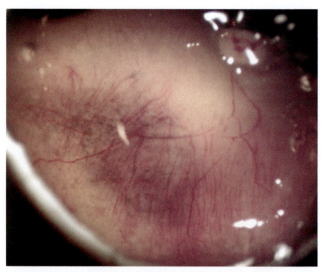

**Figure 29-2.** Internal limiting membrane peeling guided by indocyanine green staining in macular hole surgery using diamond dusted scraper (DDS).

over the previous enthusiasm, as Gandorfer et al. in 2001 (6) postulated that intravitreous ICG-assisted ILM-peeling promoted worse visual outcomes in macular surgery. Histopathological analysis of tissue harvested during ICG-assisted vitreomacular surgery revealed various retinal elements adherent to the ILM. On electron microscopy, these retinal structures on the inner surface of the ILM were identified mainly as the plasma membrane of Müller cells (7,8). They are thought to originate from an altered cleavage plane induced by the ICG application. Most toxicity studies in animals have shown dose-dependent toxicity of ICG to various types of retinal cells. Interestingly, recent clinical reports have shown better surgical outcomes of ICG-guided chromovitrectomy, which may be explained by a more selective and controlled ICG application (9,10).

## INFRACYANINE GREEN

IfCG is the modified iodine-free version of ICG that does not contain 5% sodium iodide used for the lyophilized form necessary for dye-solubility. The dilution of IfCG in glucose 5% generates an iso-osmotic solution, thereby reducing the risks of hypo-osmotic-induced toxicity previously reported with ICG. Similar to ICG, IfCG has been demonstrated to avidly stain the ILM. In contrast to ICG, most animal studies demonstrated a safe profile of IfCG for chromovitrectomy. ILM-specimens excised after IfCG-staining have not shown any neural retinal disruption (11).

## TRYPAN BLUE

The anionic hydrophilic azo-dye TB has a molecular weight of 960 Daltons. The vital stain traverses cell membranes only in dead cells and therefore colors only dead tissues or cells blue. In the late 1990s, TB was shown to have a great affinity to the

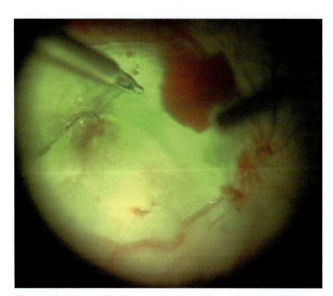

**Figure 29-1.** Internal limiting membrane peeling guided by indocyanine green staining in macular hole surgery using the intraocular forceps.

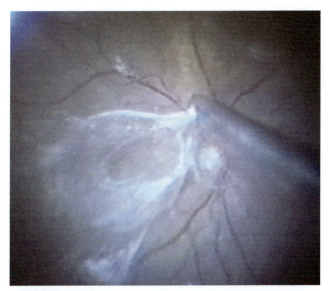

**Figure 29-3.** Epiretinal membranes are stained prominently with 1.5 mg/ml of trypan blue dye. The dye is mixed with 5% glucose (1 ml of trypan blue and 0.5 ml of glucose) to keep the blue dye heavier than BSS. This results in easy epiretinal membrane identification.

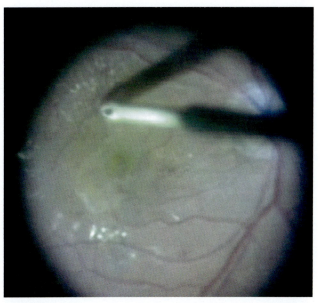

**Figure 29-4.** Internal limiting membrane peeling guided by triamcinolone acetonide deposition in macular hole surgery using the intraocular forceps.

anterior capsule of the lens which facilitated capsulorrhexis in cataract surgery. Soon thereafter, TB was tried as a stain for preretinal tissues such as the ILM and ERM in chromovitrectomy (Fig. 29-3) (4). However, ILM staining with TB is more subtle than ICG stained ILM. If TB is used for ILM staining, the dye should be kept in contact with the ILM for a longer period of time than ICG. Consecutive clinical studies reveal that TB exerted only mild toxic effects on the retina, while some experimental data disclosed mild irreversible retinal damage after retinal exposure to TB.

## PATENT BLUE

PB is a hydrophilic triarylmethane dye with a molecular weight of 582 Daltons. The biostain has been certified for capsule staining during cataract surgery at a concentration of 0.24%. Animal studies and preliminary clinical data demonstrated a moderate affinity of PB to ERM and vitreous, with a poor affinity to the ILM. Our clinical evaluation revealed PB to be a great vital dye useful for coloring the glial ERM in a similar manner to TB. Toxicology studies revealed safety data regarding retinal toxicity of PB. PB has been found to induce only mild and reversible retinal toxicity in *in vitro* and *in vivo* experimental studies (12,13). Our rabbit subretinal toxicity model demonstrated that subretinal injection of PB resulted only in mild ultrastructural retinal damage during follow-up; the histological damage induced by TB was more severe than that by PB.

## TRIAMCINOLONE ACETONIDE

TA is a corticosteroid with a molecular weight of 434 Daltons. The introduction of TA for chromovitrectomy was facilitated by the familiarity in previous clinical ophthalmic situations.

The white-steroid has been applied intravitreally in the treatment of proliferative, angiogenic, and edematous disorders (14). TA has great affinity for the acellular vitreous gel and enables complete posterior vitreous and anterior vitreous base removal. Although some proposed that TA may stain the thin ILM, the steroid crystals only deposit on the ILM by gravity and therefore facilitate the contrast between the ILM and the underlying retina (15). Therefore, the vitreous is the best target for TA application in macular surgery (Fig. 29-4). Most experimental data revealed that intravitreal 4 mg TA induced little or no retinal toxicity (16).

## RELEVANCE OF THE SURGICAL TECHNIQUE ON INTRAVITREAL DYE TOXICITY

Several different surgical approaches have been used to inject vital dyes into the vitreous cavity. Various concentrations (between 0.025% and 0.5%) and volumes (ranging from 3 drops to 2 ml) of ICG have been proposed. Variations in the technique for intravitreal dye application include the air-filled against the fluid-filled technique. The contact time of the dye on the retinal surface is another important issue in dye application. Immediate wash out from the vitreous cavity has been reported, whereas others reported contact times of up to 5 minutes before dye aspiration. Studies report a higher rate of complications, such as frequent change in retinal pigmented epithelium (RPE), when a long ICG-retina contact time is used. Of further concern is the reinjection of ICG on the bare retina after ILM peeling. This may induce a harmful direct contact of vital dye to the neuroretinal cells. Lastly, intravitreal dye solutions should be within the iso-osmolar range since hypo- or hyper-osmolar solutions may yield severe retinal damage. A new instrument similar to a painting brush has been recently developed to prevent uncontrolled staining of the entire retina. The Vitreoretinal Internal limiting membrane Color Enhancer (VINCE) (Dutch Ophthalmic, Netherlands) enables a selective painting of preretinal membranes. The device allows the dye to paint in a minimal ILM area.

## CONCLUSIONS

The current rationale of ILM-peeling in macular holes was validated by an earlier meta-analysis that demonstrated better functional and anatomical results after vitrectomy with additional ILM-peeling. Intraoperative visualization of the ILM and ERM is difficult. Furthermore, there is a high risk of retinal damage by light exposure plus surgical trauma. All this should encourage dye application during macular surgery.

When vital dyes including ICG are used, some important surgical recommendations should be followed:

– The dye should be injected in concentrations as low as possible, just enough to distinguish the preretinal membranes from the underlying reddish retina
– Avoid repeat injections onto bare retina, i.e., areas where ILM has already been removed
– Avoid injecting dye directly through the macular hole by any method to control the ILM staining including slow injection, VINCE, and perfluorocarbons on the macular hole
– Shorten the time that the vital dye is in the vitreous cavity to diminish the concentration in contact with the retinal tissue
– Keep the light pipe far from the retina throughout the whole surgical procedure in order to minimize dye-induced photosensitizer effects

– Adjust the osmolarity of the dye solution so that it remains in the iso-osmolar range

## References

1. Rodrigues EB, Meyer CH, Kroll P. Chromovitrectomy: a new field in vitreo-retinal surgery. *Graefes Arch Clin Exp Ophthalmol* 2005;243:291–293.
2. Burk SE, Da Mata AP, Snyder ME, et al. Indocyanine green-assisted peeling of the retinal internal limiting membrane. *Ophthalmology* 2000;107:2010–2014.
3. Rodrigues EB, Meyer CH, Farah ME, et al. Intravitreal staining of the internal limiting membrane using indocyanine green in the treatment of macular holes. *Ophthalmologica* 2005;219:251–262.
4. Wong KL, Hiscott P, Stanga P, et al. Trypan blue staining of the internal limiting membrane and epiretinal membrane during vitrectomy: visual results and histopathological findings. *Br J Ophthalmol* 2003;87:216–219.
5. Hiebl W, Gunther B, Meinert H. Substances for staining biological tissues: use of dyes in ophthalmology. *Klin Monatsbl Augenheilkd* 2005;222:309–311.
6. Gandorfer A, Haritoglou C, Gass CA, Ulbig MW, Kampik A. Indocyanine green-assisted peeling of the internal limiting membrane may cause retinal damage. *Am J Ophthalmol*. 2001;132(3):431–433.
7. Maia M, Haller JA, Pieramici DJ, et al. Retinal pigment epithelium abnormalities after internal limiting membrane peeling guided by indocyanine green staining. *Retina* 2004;24:157–160.
8. Nakamura T, Murata T, Hisatomi T, et al. Ultrastructure of the vitreoretinal interface following the removal of the internal limiting membrane using indocyanine green. *Curr Eye Research* 2004;27:395–399.
9. Sheidow TG, Blinder KJ, Holekamp N, et al. Outcome results in macular hole surgery: an evaluation of internal limiting membrane peeling with and without indocyanine green. *Ophthalmology* 2003;110:1697–1701.
10. Lochhead J, Jones E, Chui D, et al. Outcome of ICG-assisted ILM peel in macular hole surgery. *Eye* 2004;18:804–808.
11. La Heij EC, Dieudonne SC, Mooy CM, et al. Immunohistochemical analysis of the internal limiting membrane peeled with infracyanine green. *Am J Ophthalmol* 2005;140:1123–1125.
12. Veckeneer M, van Overdam K, Monzer J, et al. Ocular toxicity study of trypan blue injected into the vitreous cavity of rabbit eyes. *Graefes Arch Clin Exp Ophthalmol* 2001;239:698–704.
13. Narayanan R, Kenney MC, Kamjoo S, et al. Trypan blue: effect on retinal pigment epithelial and neurosensory retinal cells. *Invest Ophthalmol Vis Sci* 2005;46:304–309.
14. Jonas JB, Kreissig I, Degenring R. Intravitreal triamcinolone acetonide for treatment of intraocular proliferative, exudative, and neovascular diseases. *Prog Retin Eye Res* 2005;24:587–611.
15. Burk SE, Da Mata AP, Snyder ME, et al. Visualizing vitreous using Kenalog suspension. *J Cataract Refract Surg* 2003;29:645–651.
16. Yu SY, Damico FM, Viola F, et al. Retinal toxicity of intravitreal triamcinolone acetonide: a morphological study. *Retina* 2006;26:531–536.

# Choroidal Neovascularization and Age-Related Macular Degeneration

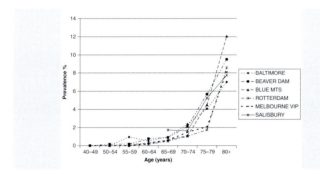

# Age-Related Macular Degeneration

Jie Jin Wang ■ Ronald Klein

Age-related macular degeneration (AMD), also termed age-related maculopathy (ARM), is the leading cause of irreversible blindness and visual impairment in older persons, and will remain a major threat to vision in coming decades (1). Research on AMD has progressed rapidly in recent decades (2–9). In particular, the identification of genetic variants responsible for AMD susceptibility (6,7,10–12) and environmental risk or protective factors for AMD, has pointed to likely pathogenetic mechanisms for this condition (7,9,13–15).

## PREVALENCE AND INCIDENCE OF AGE-RELATED MACULAR DEGENERATION

In the last two decades there has been a growing number of large population-based studies conducted in different countries, providing estimates of AMD prevalence (16–33) and incidence (34–48).

## AGE-RELATED MACULAR DEGENERATION PREVALENCE IN WHITES

The meta-analysis conducted by the Eye Disease Prevalence Research Group (49), using data collected from multiple populations, including the Baltimore Eye Survey (20), the Beaver Dam Eye Study (BDES) (16) and the Salisbury Eye Evaluation (SEE) project (50) in the USA, the Rotterdam Study (RS) (17) in the Netherlands, and the Blue Mountains Eye Study (BMES) (18) and Visual Impairment Project (VIP) (22) in Australia, showed high consistency in the age-specific prevalence of late

AMD (Fig. 30-1) and large soft drusen (≥125 μm in diameter) (Fig. 30-2) in whites. The prevalence of late AMD (geographic atrophy and neovascular AMD) increased exponentially with increasing age, rising from less than 0.5% at age 60 years to around 10% at age 80+ years (49) (Fig. 30-1). The prevalence of large drusen showed a similar age-related increasing trend but the association with age is more linear than exponential (49) (Fig. 30-2). The natural course of AMD (involving the disappearance of large drusen associated with the progression to a more advanced AMD stage with aging (36) could explain the observed age-related linear (rather than exponential) pattern in the prevalence of large drusen.

## AGE-RELATED MACULAR DEGENERATION PREVALENCE IN OTHER RACES AND ETHNICITIES

Ethnic variation in the prevalence of AMD and AMD lesions was observed in studies with multiracial groups such as the Baltimore Eye Survey (20), National Health and Nutrition Examination Survey (NHANES III) (51) and the Multi-Ethnic Study of Atherosclerosis (MESA) (33), and was previously summarized from studies conducted prior to this century (52).

### Blacks

Findings from the Baltimore Eye Survey (20), and the Barbados Eye Study (53) which examined a sample of blacks, have suggested that the prevalence of some AMD lesions, particularly late AMD, is lower in blacks than in whites. The same observation has been consistently reported by a number of studies conducted in populations in the USA (21,23,33,50). Possible selection bias may have occurred in some studies due to either low participation rate (21), a high proportion with ungradable

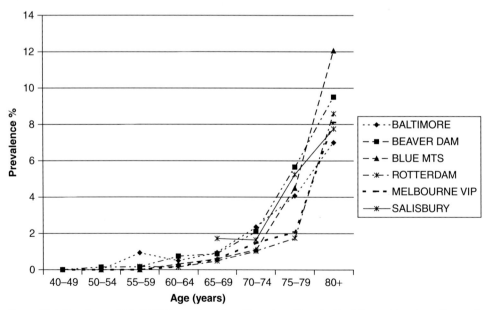

**Figure 30-1.** Prevalence of late ARMD by age in whites. (Reproduced from the Eye Disease Prevalence Research Group report, Friedman DS, O'Colmain BJ, Munoz B, et al. Prevalence of age-related macular degeneration in the United States. *Arch Ophthalmol* 2004;122:564–572.)

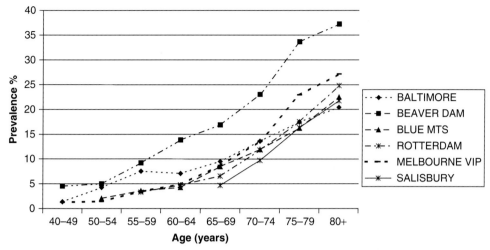

**Figure 30-2.** Prevalence of large drusen (≥125 µm in diameter) by age in whites. (Reproduced from the Eye Disease Prevalence Research Group report, Friedman DS, O'Colmain BJ, Munoz B, et al. Prevalence of age-related macular degeneration in the United States. *Arch Ophthalmol* 2004;122:564–572.)

retinal photographs (20,21,23), or poor survival in the eldest among black participants (20). Other factors may also be responsible for the racial variations in AMD frequency, including choroidal melanin density (23) and gene polymorphisms that may predispose whites to a more severe AMD than blacks (19,20).

## Mexican Americans

Mexican Americans (Hispanic whites) have been found to have a relatively low prevalence of late AMD but a similar prevalence of signs of early AMD compared to non-Hispanic whites (19,51). This observation was confirmed by data from the Los Angeles Latino Eye Study (LALES) (25) and the Proyecto Vision Evaluation and Research (VER) (32), both with large population-based samples of Hispanic whites, and the MESA Study (33), which used the same study methods, grading protocol and graders to assess AMD lesions in participants of four racial/ethnic groups (blacks, Hispanic, Chinese and whites).

## Asians

Relatively well-conducted population-based studies of AMD prevalence in Asian populations have emerged in recent years, including studies conducted in Japan (28) (Funagata Study, unpublished data), India (29,31), and China (30).

The prevalence of early and late AMD in Japanese and Indian populations does not appear to be substantially different from that in whites of the Western world, according to the two studies that used retinal photographic grading to diagnose AMD and AMD lesions (28,31). However, the prevalence of soft drusen and retinal pigmentary abnormalities varies across studies (28,31) and differs from the corresponding prevalence reported in white populations of similar age (soft distinct drusen 10–16%, soft indistinct drusen 5–8%, and pigmentary abnormalities 7–13%)(16,18). While soft indistinct drusen were relatively infrequent in both Japanese (0.5%) (28) and Indians (2.2%) (31), the predominant early AMD lesion in the Japanese population was soft distinct drusen (8.4%) and not retinal pigmentary abnormalities (3.2%) (28), whereas in the

Indian population, both soft distinct drusen (34.0%) and retinal pigmentary abnormalities (10.8%) were frequent (31). In a Chinese population aged 40+ years, the Beijing Eye Study team reported a very low prevalence of both early (1.4%) and late AMD (0.2%) (30).

Comparability of study findings from Asian populations to those of Western countries is still limited, due to different methods used across studies. Although the Wisconsin Age-Related Maculopathy Grading System has been used in these recent studies in Asia, the AMD grading used has not been validated either internally or externally (28,30,31). Standardized methodology in retinal photography and AMD grading, together with the use of uniform AMD definitions, are critical for new studies in Asia to confirm whether the differences in AMD frequency between Asian and Western populations are real.

There are other possible reasons that could explain the observed differences in AMD prevalence across studies and racial groups. It is worth noting that two Japanese studies both reported high prevalence rates of neovascular AMD in Japanese men, similar to those observed in whites but sharply contrasting with the much lower prevalence in Japanese women (28) (Funagata Study, unpublished data). Possible explanations for this gender difference may include a high prevalence of smoking among Japanese men and a higher frequency of polypoidal choroidal vasculopathy (PCV) among Japanese men compared to Japanese women (54). The complement factor H (CFH) polymorphism (the Y402H) has consistently been documented as a major AMD genetic marker in white patient samples. However, in Japanese and Chinese with late AMD, the frequency of the variant high risk genotypes (CC) or the risk allele (C) of CFH was much lower than that reported in whites with late AMD (55–57). This may partly explain the low prevalence of late AMD observed in the Japanese and the Chinese. Different AMD-related gene variants may be manifest in Asian with AMD. The lack of an association of CFH Y402H polymorphism with late AMD in two independent case studies of Japanese patients suggest that different gene polymorphisms may play a role in the pathogenesis of AMD in Asians compared to non-Asian cohorts (55,56).

## AGE-RELATED MACULAR DEGENERATION INCIDENCE IN WHITES

After the turn of the century a number of population-based studies, following the BDES (34,37), have provided AMD incidence in older white populations (36,38–43,46,47).

The cumulative 5-year, person-specific incidence of early AMD has been reported to range from 7.9% to 8.7%, and the corresponding incidence of late AMD ranges from 0.9% to 1.1% in the three predominantly white populations across three continents, the BDES (34), RS (38) and the BMES (36), all of which used similar study protocols in AMD phenotype ascertainment. Similar to AMD prevalence, incidence of this condition is strongly age-related (34,36,38,39), showing an exponential increase with age (see Fig. 30-2 of the report by the RS (38)).

The long-term (10 or more years) cumulative incidence and progression of AMD has been reported by the BDES (37,48), BMES (47), and the Copenhagen City Eye Study (42). Estimates from the two studies with reasonable follow-up rates (37,47) indicate that the person-specific 10-year incidence of early AMD ranged from 10.8% to 12.1%, and the corresponding incidence of late AMD ranged from 2.1% to 2.8%, after age-standardization of the BMES to the BDES population (47). The 15-year cumulative incidence of late AMD was 3.1% and of early AMD was 14.3% in the BDES (48). In addition to age, incidence of late AMD was also strongly related to the severity of early AMD lesions at baseline (37,47,48).

A substantially higher incidence of neovascular AMD has been observed in the second eye of clinic patients presenting unilateral neovascular AMD, observed not only in whites (58–61) but also in Japanese (62). In the BMES population, 29% of second eyes developed end-stage AMD (neovascular AMD or geographic atrophy involving the fovea) in subjects with unilateral end-stage AMD (36).

## PROGRESSION

Progression of AMD from soft (distinct or indistinct) drusen, reticular drusen, or retinal pigmentary abnormalities to geographic atrophy or neovascular AMD has been well documented in clinical case series (60,63,64). In the BDES and BMES, early ARM lesion characteristics have been studied in detail in terms of distribution, location, size, lesion type, and area involved in relation to the risk of subsequent development of late AMD (37,65,66). Large soft drusen (≥125 μm in diameter), soft drusen with indistinct margins (indistinct soft or reticular drusen), or pigmentary changes involving large macular areas plus close proximity to the fovea indicate a much higher risk of subsequent late AMD development (37,65).

The Age-Related Eye Disease Study (AREDS) developed an ordinal AMD severity for risk prediction from pre-existing early AMD lesions defined from baseline retinal photographs (67,68). The BMES 10-year AMD incidence data validated this AREDS AMD Simplified Severity Scale and provided further evidence supporting that incidence of late AMD strongly relates to the severity of early AMD lesions at baseline (47).

## AGE-RELATED MACULAR DEGENERATION INCIDENCE IN OTHER ETHNICITIES

### Blacks

The Barbados Eye Study reported 4-year (40) and 9-year incidence (46) of AMD in a black population aged 40–84 years at baseline. At the 4-year visit (40), incident neovascular AMD was observed in one of the 2362 persons at risk (0.04%) and incident geographic atrophy in none of the 2419 at risk (0%). The incidence of early AMD lesions, including intermediate-sized drusen, was also low (5.2%, 60/1160). However, at the 9-year visit, the long-term incidence of early AMD was 12.6% and of late AMD 0.7% (46). This 9-year incidence of early AMD is similar to that reported from the BDES and BMES (37,47), but the 9-year incidence of late AMD is lower than that observed in whites (37,47). In the AREDS participants who had early or intermediate AMD at baseline, the risk of progression to neovascular AMD over a median follow-up period of 6.3 years was nearly 7-fold in whites than in blacks (odds ratio 6.8, 95% confidence interval 1.2-36.9) (69).

### Other Ethnicities

To date, there are no Hispanic white population-based data available on AMD incidence, and only one report from a Japanese population on the 5-year incidence of AMD (44). Early AMD incidence was 8.5% and late AMD incidence was 0.8% in Japanese aged 50+ years at baseline, with 1.9% in men but only 0.2% in women. The nearly 10-fold difference in incidence rates between Japanese men and women is consistent with findings of AMD prevalence among Japanese, possibly due to high frequency of smoking and high incident PCV cases in Japanese men (54).

## EMERGING AMD RISK AND PROTECTIVE FACTORS

### Smoking

Smoking is a major modifiable risk factor for AMD, consistently found not only in cross-sectional population-based studies (70–73) (Fig. 30-3A), but also in longitudinal studies (69,74–80) (Fig. 30-3B). Pooled data estimated that risk for 5-year incidence of late AMD was more than double (odds ratio [OR] 2.35, 95% confidence interval [CI] 1.30–4.27) in current smokers compared to persons who never smoked (77) (Fig. 30-3B). Overall, the magnitude of risk for late AMD in current versus noncurrent smokers, or in past versus nonsmokers, ranges between 2- and 5-fold (80). In the BMES population (76), current smokers developed late AMD at a mean age of 67 years,

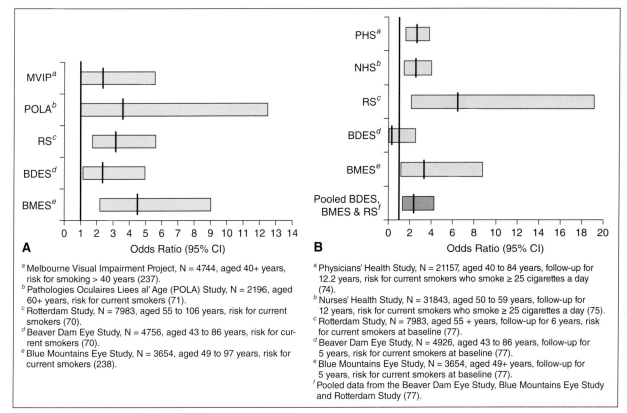

**Figure 30-3. A:** Smoking and prevalence of late age-related macular degeneration. **B:** Smoking and incidence of late age-related macular degeneration.

while past smokers developed late AMD at a mean age of 73 years and nonsmokers at a mean age of 77 years. This 10-year average difference in the mean age of developing late AMD in smokers versus nonsmokers implies a substantial increase in the burden on affected individuals, their families, and aged disability care. Evidence supporting a causal role for smoking in AMD includes its dose-response relationship with pack-years of smoking (81,82), reduced risk after smoking cessation (the earlier smoking cessation occurs, the lower the risk of developing AMD later in life (71,81–84), and evidence from animal models (85). Passive smoking exposure has also been documented to be associated with AMD in a case control study (81), but not in a population-based study (86). Smoking as a major AMD risk factor has also been documented in Mexican American (87), Indian (88), and Japanese (44) populations.

Evidence of synergistic effects of history of smoking with other factors contributing to high AMD risk has been emerging recently (82,89–94). Carriers of the APOE ε2 allele had a much higher risk of neovascular AMD if they smoked, compared to APOE ε4 or APOE ε3 carriers who also smoked (89). For the two confirmed AMD-related gene loci (CFH and LOC387715), smoking exerts a much greater effect on AMD risk in persons homozygous for the risk alleles of either of these two gene polymorphisms (Y402H in CFH and rs10490924 in LOC387715), compared to subjects homozygous for the nonrisk alleles (90–95) (Figs. 30-4 and 30-5). The odds ratio (OR) for AMD among individuals homozygous for the risk alleles who also smoked was two- or three-fold compared to subjects with either factor alone (nonsmoking, or absence of the risk alleles)

(91,92,94,96). In the BMES 10-year follow-up data, biological synergism of smoking with the lowest level of serum high-density lipoprotein (HDL) cholesterol, the highest total to HDL cholesterol ratio, or history of low fish consumption with AMD risk was suggested (82).

Based on currently available evidence, cigarette smoking is considered an important trigger or promoter in the course of the development of late AMD (80,85). Emerging evidence indicates that combined effects of smoking with other AMD-related

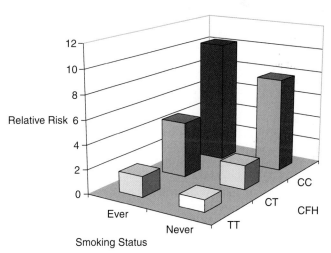

**Figure 30-4.** Joint effect of *CFH-Y402H* gene and smoking on risk of age-related macular degeneration (93). CFH, complement factor H; CC; CT; TT.

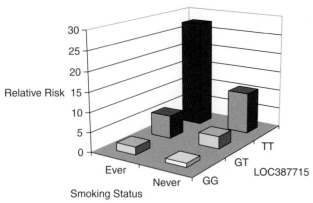

**Figure 30-5.** Joint effect of the *Loc387715-A69S* gene and smoking on risk of age-related macular degeneration (95). GG; GT; TT.

factors most likely contribute to the high risk of AMD among smokers (82,94,96). No statistically significant interaction on multiplicative scales has been established (96–98), but biological interaction on an additive scale (82,92,94,96) is not uncommon (99).

## ANTIOXIDANT NUTRIENTS

The hypothesis that oxidative damage may be involved in the pathogenesis of AMD (100) is supported by a number of factors: (a) the high concentration of polyunsaturated fatty acids present in the outer segments of photoreceptors of the retina; (b) high photo-oxidative stress and relatively high oxygen tension in this region, and; (c) the well-known susceptibility of polyunsaturated fatty acids to undergo oxidation in the presence of oxygen or oxygen-derived radical species (100). However, evidence of a protective effect of antioxidant nutrients against AMD has been inconsistent (101–109), as has the association between AMD and serum carotenoids (110–113).

Currently, evidence as to the effectiveness of intervention with antioxidant vitamin and mineral supplementation on slowing AMD progression is dominated by findings from one large randomized clinical trial, the AREDS (114,115). In this study, a modest beneficial effect (25% reduction) from antioxidant and zinc supplementation on progression to late AMD was observed in persons with moderate to relatively advanced early AMD (114). While the majority of intervention trials conducted so far were underpowered to detect small differences (115), there is limited evidence at present suggesting that people with less advanced early AMD lesions should take supplements (115,116), and the AREDS findings should only be applied to appropriate at-risk patients with caution (117). The UK Drug and Therapeutics Bulletin (118) published a very thorough evaluation of the use of nutritional supplements for AMD: subgroup analysis of AREDS data suggested that in patients with unilateral advanced AMD, the AREDS formula (a specific combination of high doses of zinc and antioxidant vitamins) may assist in preventing advanced disease and deterioration of visual acuity in the fellow eye, though there is no convincing evidence to support the use of nutritional supplements in other groups (118). The Food and Drug Administration

(FDA) of the USA also concluded that no credible evidence exists for a health claim about the intake of lutein or zeaxanthin (or both) and the risk of AMD (119). The AREDS-2 is currently investigating this relationship.

## DIETARY FATTY ACIDS, FISH CONSUMPTION, AND LIPIDS

The underlying hypothesis for associations between serum cholesterol and dietary fat intake and AMD arose from the speculation that AMD and cardiovascular disease may share common risk factors (120,121) or similar pathogenesis (such as atherosclerosis and arterioscleroses) (121,122). Another consistently documented factor associated with low AMD risk is regular fish consumption (72,121–124) or dietary omega 3 fatty acid intake (125) (Fig. 30-6A, 30-6B). In the BMES cohort, joint exposure to low frequency of a history of fish consumption and current smoking was found to be associated with a much higher long-term risk of late AMD than the effect of either exposure alone (82). In comparison with nonsmoking individuals who consumed fish at least once per month, the relative risk of late AMD from current smoking increased from 2.7 (95% confidence interval, [CI], 0.9-7.7) in persons who regularly consumed fish at least once per month to 7.3 (95% CI 2.4-22.4) in those who consumed fish less than once a month, with an estimated synergy index of 4.2 (82) for biological interaction (99). In addition, BMES 10-year AMD incidence data showed that the protective effect from weekly fish consumption is only evident among subjects homozygous for the CHF Y402H C allele, with a statistically significant interaction (unpublished).

In three separate studies of largely different study samples, the Eye Disease Case-Control Study (125), the Age-related Macular Degeneration Study (121) and the US Twin Study of Age-related Macular Degeneration (72), Seddon et al. reported a possible joint effect of linoleic acid (a major component of omega-6 fatty acid) and omega-3 fatty acids or fish consumption on the risk of AMD. A trend of reduced AMD risk associated with increasing intake of omega-3 fatty acids (72,125), or a reduced risk of AMD progression associated with fish consumption at least twice a week (121), was only evident in persons who consumed a diet low in linoleic acid. Similarly, in the BMES population, weekly consumption of fish was protective against early AMD incidence over 10 years only in subjects with low intake (below median) of linoleic acid (unpublished data).

No consistent evidence has been found for associations of AMD with other dietary fats (23,121–129) or serum lipids (120,129,130–133). Use of cholesterol-lowering medications (statins) has also shown inconsistent findings of a protective effect on AMD prevalence (134–136) and incidence (137–141). Conflicting findings on these associations between intake of other mono- and poly-unsaturated fats, or serum lipids, and AMD suggest that these associations, if they exist, are unlikely to be major AMD risk factors.

Interpretation of findings regarding dietary data should be made with caution because these findings may be due, in part,

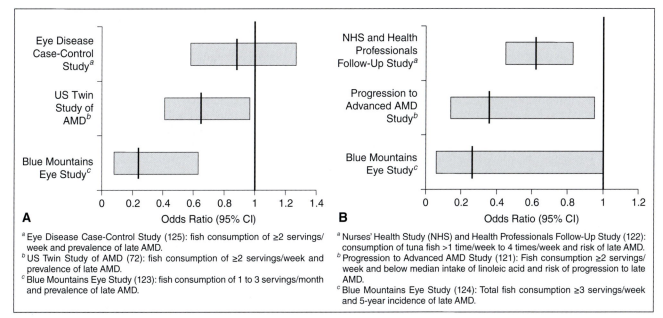

**Figure 30-6. A:** Regular fish intake and prevalence of late age-related macular degeneration. **B:** Regular fish consumption and incidence of late age-related macular degeneration.

to uncontrolled confounding. It is possible that participants with a previous diagnosis of early AMD subsequently changed to a healthier diet, or that persons with a better diet were more likely to have a better overall lifestyle and receive better medical care, accounting for the lower frequency of AMD. Such biases have been used to explain why data from longitudinal observational studies showed a benefit of hormone replacement therapy while a large randomized control trial, the Women's Health Initiative, did not (142).

## INFLAMMATORY MARKERS

Inflammation may play a role in the pathogenesis of AMD. Supporting this hypothesis is the fact that leucocytes have been observed in choroidal neovascularization (CNV) tissues from post-mortem eyes with neovascular AMD (14,143). In laser-induced CNV mice models, macrophages have been shown to have a role in the extent of CNV (144). This hypothesis has received further support from findings on some AMD-related genetic markers located on complement-related genes: CFH (complement regulatory gene) (11), C2/BF (complement pathway-associated genes) (13,14,145,146) and C3 (the most abundant complement component) (147). CFH is known to modulate the complement cascade by inactivating components of the cascade and by binding initiation factors such as C-reactive protein (CRP) (14,146,148,149). Age has been shown to be associated with increasing, and smoking associated with reducing, plasma levels of CFH (150). However, the CFH Y402H polymorphism was not found to be associated with CRP level (151,152), nor did the genetic variation in CRP appear to be associated with risk of AMD (153).

A recent finding that the CFH Y402H polymorphism affects binding affinity to CRP has led to the hypothesis that reduced binding of CFH Y402H to CRP leads to impaired targeting of CFH to cellular debris, accumulation of which increases inflammation at the retinal pigment epithelium–choroid interface in subjects with AMD (154). This hypothesis is in keeping with one proposed by Anderson et al. (13) and Hageman et al. (155), namely, that local, immune-mediated, inflammation plays a role in drusen biogenesis (9,13,155), possibly analogous to processes observed in other age-related conditions such as Alzheimer's disease and atherosclerosis (14,156).

Some inflammatory markers, such as high leukocyte count, have been documented to be associated with long-term AMD incidence in two well-conducted population-based studies (157,158). Other large studies have provided inconsistent evidence on the association between CRP and AMD incidence (159–163). A joint effect of AMD genetic susceptibility, indicated by the CFH Y402H CC genotype, with high CRP level or leukocyte count on AMD progression has been suggested in a population-based sample (92). Associations between AMD and factors related to hemostasis or endothelial dysfunction have also been reported inconsistently (164,165).

It is has been speculated that certain microbial infections could be environmental triggers for AMD pathogenesis. Chlamydia pneumoniae infection has been thought to be a trigger, but its association with AMD has not been consistently documented (166–170). Use of systemic anti-inflammatory medications has not been found to have an effect on AMD prevalence or incidence (137,171–173).

Despite the plausible hypothesis that AMD pathogenesis involves inflammatory processes, the associations of systemic inflammatory markers with AMD have been inconsistent. This could be explained by possible discordance between local and systemic inflammation, and that AMD pathogenesis involves other joint factors in addition to local inflammation or low-level systemic inflammation (92).

## SUNLIGHT EXPOSURE

Although biologically plausible, the hypothesis of an association between sunlight or short wavelength blue light (174) exposure and AMD has proven difficult to investigate, due to lack of precise, quantitative measures on life-time exposure and confounding by sun-avoidance behavior in subjects with very fair skin susceptible to sun-related skin damage (175). Surrogate factors (questionnaires, sun-related skin damage or presence of pterygium) have been used in epidemiological studies (175–181), with inconsistent associations found to date (180).

In the BDES population some consistency is revealed across baseline cross-sectional data (178), 5-year (182) and 10-year (183) longitudinal data. Time spent outdoors in summer, particularly earlier in life (teens to thirties), was associated with an increased risk of early AMD later in life (182,183), while the use of hats or sunglasses appeared to provide some protection against development of early AMD lesions later in life (182,183).

In the BMES (181) persons presenting with pterygium or reporting a past history of pterygium surgery at baseline had an increased risk of 5-year incident late (adjusted OR 3.3, 95% CI 1.1-10.3) and early AMD (adjusted OR 1.8, 95% CI 1.1-2.9). A recent report from a UK case-control study found no association between late AMD and sunlight exposure-related factors, except for the suggestion of an association between skin type prone to sunburn and geographic atrophy (184), a finding consistent with observations from a previous population-based case-control study (175). Although accumulated data suggest the possibility of a sunlight exposure–AMD link, inconsistent evidence does not support the association to be strong (5).

## POST CATARACT SURGERY

Light exposure to eyes may increase after cataract surgery (including eyes with intraocular lens implantation). Whether the risk of late AMD is increased in eyes following cataract surgery is a longstanding but unresolved clinical question. Conflicting findings exist between clinical and population-based studies (174). A higher risk of developing late-stage AMD in eyes following cataract surgery has previously been documented in both clinic (185,186) and population-based cross-sectional (50,88), case-control (187) and longitudinal studies (188–190) (Fig. 30-7A, 30-7B). A report from postmortem eyes also suggested that neovascular AMD was more frequent in pseudophakic than phakic eyes (191). In contrast, the AREDS (192) and some clinical studies could not confirm a definite link (193,194).

Potential confounding factors could be operative in this observed association. Cataract surgery could be recommended for some patients with early AMD signs, to enable a better view of the fundus to facilitate diagnosis and therapy. Cataract in the fellow eye of persons with unilateral late AMD may cause substantial disability and a greater need for surgical intervention. As AMD tends to be bilateral, the risk of AMD developing in the second eye of such cases would be much higher than the risk of AMD occurring in the first eye (58–61), irrespective of cataract surgery. Analogous to recently documented synergisms between smoking and genetic variants (90–95), cataract surgery or the nonphakic ocular status alone may not accelerate AMD progression but could act as a trigger to modify the risk of late AMD development and accelerate AMD progression if in combination with other genetic and systemic AMD risk factors. Longitudinal cohort studies on cataract surgical patients are needed to answer this important clinical question. It is important for patients who already have AMD risk signs or

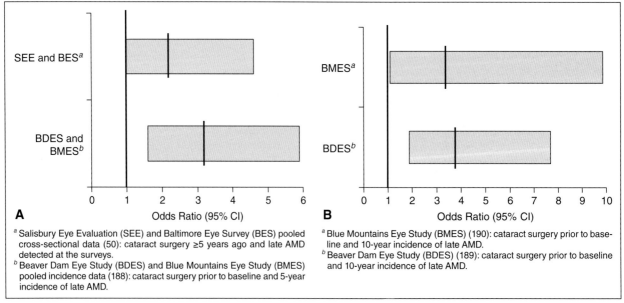

<sup>a</sup> Salisbury Eye Evaluation (SEE) and Baltimore Eye Survey (BES) pooled cross-sectional data (50): cataract surgery ≥5 years ago and late AMD detected at the surveys.
<sup>b</sup> Beaver Dam Eye Study (BDES) and Blue Mountains Eye Study (BMES) pooled incidence data (188): cataract surgery prior to baseline and 5-year incidence of late AMD.

<sup>a</sup> Blue Mountains Eye Study (BMES) (190): cataract surgery prior to baseline and 10-year incidence of late AMD.
<sup>b</sup> Beaver Dam Eye Study (BDES) (189): cataract surgery prior to baseline and 10-year incidence of late AMD.

**Figure 30-7. A:** Prior cataract surgery and 5-year risk of late age-related macular degeneration. **B:** Cataract surgery prior to baseline and 10-year incidence of late age-related macular degeneration in the Blue Mountains and Beaver Dam Eye Studies.

AMD genetic susceptibility to be informed about findings of cataract surgery and higher risk in some studies and to discuss this with their doctors before undergoing cataract surgery.

## LESS CONSISTENTLY DOCUMENTED RISK FACTORS

### Female Gender and Hormones

Gender differences have been observed in the prevalence of AMD lesions in white populations (16,18,22), but the differences are not consistent across different populations (2,17,21,23–26,53,70). No statistically significant gender difference has been found for AMD incidence (34,37–39), though in the BMES population, women were nonsignificantly more likely to develop both early and late AMD (36) while in the BDES population a similar trend was observed in persons aged >75 years (34).

An association between exogenous estrogen exposure and AMD was postulated by investigators of the Eye Disease Case-Control Study Group based on findings from a hospital-based clinic sample (126). This hypothesis has been investigated in basic research (195,196) and supported by some, but not all, observational studies (197–204). No evidence from longitudinal population-based cohort studies supports the estrogen–AMD hypothesis (77,205). However, in a randomized clinical trial (206), treatment with conjugated equine estrogens with or without progestin was associated with a reduced risk of soft drusen (OR, 0.83; 95% CI, 0.68-1.00) and a reduced risk of neovascular AMD (OR, 0.29; 95% CI, 0.09-0.92), after adjustment for covariables. Estrogen receptor α gene polymorphisms were found to be associated with an increased risk of late AMD in the RS population (207).

### Other Cardiovascular Disease Risk Factors

AMD and cardiovascular disease have been speculated to share common antecedents or etiologic pathways (2,120,126,208). Apart from age and smoking, other cardiovascular risk factors that have been evaluated for their associations with AMD include atherosclerosis (209), blood pressure (131,177,210), serum total cholesterol (126) or serum high-density lipoprotein (HDL) levels (129,131–133,211), plasma homocysteine level (208,212), body mass index (130,177,213,214) or waist circumference (215), alcohol consumption (79,216,217) and physical activity (218).

Inconsistent findings on the association between serum HDL cholesterol and AMD have been reported, with a positive association observed in some studies (129,131,132,211) but an inverse association observed in the BMES (133). The longitudinal associations between high levels of HDL and an increased AMD risk (129,211), and an inverse association between total serum cholesterol and incident neovascular AMD (77) run counter to the cardiovascular disease associations with these lipids. These observed lipid–AMD associations could also be influenced by genetic susceptibility (129) or other environmental/systemic factors (82).

In the BDES, no positive cross-sectional associations were found between blood pressure or history of cardiovascular disease and late AMD at baseline (219). In the 5- and 10-year follow-up examinations of the same study population, positive associations between pulse pressure or blood pressure and incident late AMD or retinal pigment epithelial abnormalities emerged (211,220). These findings gained support from the RS (221) but not from the BMES (no association) (133) or the cross-sectional Women's Health Initiative Study (association in the opposite direction) (141).

Measures of atherosclerosis (221) and hypertensive retinal vessel wall signs (222,223) have been reported to be to be associated with incident AMD. Associations between AMD and subsequent cardiovascular disease events and mortality have also been reported in some but not all studies (224–229). An active lifestyle such as regular walking exercise at baseline was found to be associated with a reduced risk of neovascular AMD over the next 15 years in the BDES population (218).

The use of antihypertensive medications or low-dose aspirin has not been found to have a significant protective effect on AMD prevalence (230) or incidence (137,171,173) in large population-based samples.

## ALCOHOL CONSUMPTION

In a sub-sample of the NHANES I study population (216) persons who reported moderate wine consumption were significantly less likely to have AMD than nondrinkers. This association has not been confirmed in either cross-sectional (231,232) or longitudinal population-based studies (217,233–235). The BDES 5-year follow-up data showed that beer drinking in men was associated with an increased risk of soft indistinct drusen (217). In the 10-year follow-up, heavy drinking at baseline was found to be associated with a higher risk of late AMD (79), while in the 15-year follow-up, heavy drinking at baseline predicted a higher incidence of geographic atrophy in men (235). The longitudinal association between alcohol consumption and incident AMD was not observed in the BMES (unpublished data). The inconsistency in these findings suggests that alcohol consumption is unlikely to play a major role in the development of AMD (5,236).

## SUMMARY

Investigation of AMD risk factors has led to the identification of a few consistent, modifiable deleterious (smoking) and protective risk factors (fish consumption and intake of antioxidants). Risk of AMD from smoking has a magnitude of impact larger than the 20-30% reduction in AMD progression from intake of antioxidant supplements.

Joint contribution from multiple factors, including gene variants, environmental triggers and systemic conditions, is likely to explain a high proportion of AMD development. There are likely to be diverse biological processes involved in the etiology of AMD (9,155). Mechanisms by which genes and environmental factors interact to promote AMD development are still not understood. AMD pathogenesis is likely to prove analogous to that of other complex systemic conditions (13,14).

Measures to promote smoking cessation are important to reducing the burden of AMD. While there are no clinical trial data to demonstrate that regular consumption of fish and a healthy diet will contribute to reduction of risk of incident AMD, the mounting evidence epidemiological data suggest possible benefit. Cost-effective approaches to prevent or delay the onset of AMD may include lifestyle adjustments and new preventive treatments targeting at high genetically at-risk individuals who are susceptible to AMD at early stages of the disease (9).

## References

1. Fine SL. Age-related macular degeneration 1969–2004: A 35-year personal perspective. *Am J Ophthalmol* 2005;139:405–420.
2. Evans JR. Risk factors for age-related macular degeneration. *Prog Retin Eye Res* 2001;20:227–253.
3. Ambati J, Ambati BK, Yoo SH, et al. Age-related macular degeneration: etiology, pathogenesis, and therapeutic strategies. *Surv Ophthalmol* 2003;48:257–293.
4. Klein R, Peto T, Bird A, et al. The epidemiology of age-related macular degeneration. *Am J Ophthalmol* 2004;137:486–495.
5. Seddon JM, Chen CA. The epidemiology of age-related macular degeneration. *Int Ophthalmol Clin* 2004;44:17–39.
6. Tuo J, Bojanowski CM, Chan CC. Genetic factors of age-related macular degeneration. *Prog Retin Eye Res* 2004;23:229–249.
7. Haddad S, Chen CA, Santangelo SL, et al. The genetics of age-related macular degeneration: a review of progress to date. *Surv Ophthalmol* 2006;51:316–363.
8. Klein R. Overview of progress in the epidemiology of age-related macular degeneration. *Ophthalmic Epidemiol* 2007;14:184–187.
9. Gehrs KM, Anderson DH, Johnson LV, et al. Age-related macular degeneration—emerging pathogenetic and therapeutic concepts. *Ann Med* 2006;38:450–471.
10. Fisher SA, Abecasis GR, Yashar BM, et al. Meta-analysis of genome scans of age-related macular degeneration. *Hum Mol Genet* 2005;14:2257–2264.
11. Thakkinstian A, Han P, McEvoy M, et al. Systematic review and meta-analysis of the association between complement factor H Y402H polymorphisms and age-related macular degeneration. *Hum Mol Genet* 2006;15:2784–2790.
12. Chamberlain M, Baird P, Dirani M, et al. Unraveling a complex genetic disease: age-related macular degeneration. *Surv Ophthalmol* 2006;51:576–586.
13. Anderson DH, Mullins RF, Hageman GS, et al. A role for local inflammation in the formation of drusen in the aging eye. *Am J Ophthalmol* 2002;134:411–431.
14. Donoso LA, Kim D, Frost A, et al. The Role of Inflammation in the Pathogenesis of Age-related Macular Degeneration. *Surv Ophthalmol* 2006;51:137–152.
15. Espinosa-Heidmann DG, Sall J, Hernandez EP, et al. Basal laminar deposit formation in APO B100 transgenic mice: complex interactions between dietary fat, blue light, and vitamin E. *Invest Ophthalmol Vis Sci* 2004;45:260–266.
16. Klein R, Klein BE, Linton KL. Prevalence of age-related maculopathy. The Beaver Dam Eye Study. *Ophthalmology* 1992;99:933–943.
17. Vingerling JR, Dielemans I, Hofman A, et al. The prevalence of age-related maculopathy in the Rotterdam Study. *Ophthalmology* 1995;102:205–210.
18. Mitchell P, Smith W, Attebo K, et al. Prevalence of age-related maculopathy in Australia. The Blue Mountains Eye Study. *Ophthalmology* 1995;102:1450–1460.
19. Cruickshanks KJ, Hamman RF, Klein R, et al. The prevalence of age-related maculopathy by geographic region and ethnicity. The Colorado-Wisconsin Study of Age-Related Maculopathy. *Arch Ophthalmol* 1997;115:242–250.
20. Friedman DS, Katz J, Bressler NM, et al. Racial differences in the prevalence of age-related macular degeneration: the Baltimore Eye Survey. *Ophthalmology* 1999;106:1049–1055.
21. Klein R, Clegg L, Cooper LS, et al. Prevalence of age-related maculopathy in the Atherosclerosis Risk in Communities Study. *Arch Ophthalmol* 1999;117:1203–1210.
22. VanNewkirk MR, Nanjan MB, Wang JJ, et al. The prevalence of age-related maculopathy: the visual impairment project. *Ophthalmology* 2000;107:1593–1600.
23. Klein R, Klein BE, Marino EK, et al. Early age-related maculopathy in the cardiovascular health study. *Ophthalmology* 2003;110:25–33.
24. Jonasson F, Arnarsson A, Sasaki H, et al. The prevalence of age-related maculopathy in Iceland: Reykjavik eye study. *Arch Ophthalmol* 2003;121:379–385.
25. Varma R, Fraser-Bell S, Tan S, et al. Prevalence of age-related macular degeneration in Latinos: the Los Angeles Latino eye study. *Ophthalmology* 2004;111:1288–1297.
26. Augood CA, Vingerling JR, De Jong PT, et al. Prevalence of age-related maculopathy in older Europeans: the European Eye Study (EUREYE). *Arch Ophthalmol* 2006;124:529–535.
27. Topouzis F, Coleman AL, Harris A, et al. Prevalence of age-related macular degeneration in Greece: the Thessaloniki Eye Study. *Am J Ophthalmol* 2006;142:1076–1079.
28. Oshima Y, Ishibashi T, Murata T, et al. Prevalence of age related maculopathy in a representative Japanese population: the Hisayama study. *Br J Ophthalmol* 2001;85:1153–1157.
29. Nirmalan PK, Katz J, Robin AL, et al. Prevalence of vitreoretinal disorders in a rural population of southern India: the Aravind Comprehensive Eye Study. *Arch Ophthalmol* 2004;122:581–586.
30. Li Y, Xu L, Jonas JB, et al. Prevalence of age-related maculopathy in the adult population in China: the Beijing eye study. *Am J Ophthalmol* 2006;142:788–793.
31. Gupta SK, Murthy GV, Morrison N, et al. Prevalence of early and late age-related macular degeneration in a rural population in northern India: the INDEYE feasibility study. *Invest Ophthalmol Vis Sci* 2007;48:1007–1011.
32. Munoz B, Klein R, Rodriguez J, et al. Prevalence of age-related macular degeneration in a population-based sample of Hispanic people in Arizona: Proyecto VER. *Arch Ophthalmol* 2005;123:1575–1580.
33. Klein R, Klein BE, Knudtson MD, et al. Prevalence of age-related macular degeneration in 4 racial/ethnic groups in the multi-ethnic study of atherosclerosis. *Ophthalmology* 2006;113:373–380.
34. Klein R, Klein BE, Jensen SC, et al. The five-year incidence and progression of age-related maculopathy: the Beaver Dam Eye Study. *Ophthalmology* 1997;104:7–21.
35. Klaver CC, Assink JJ, van Leeuwen R, et al. Incidence and progression rates of age-related maculopathy: the Rotterdam Study. *Invest Ophthalmol Vis Sci* 2001;42:2237–2241.
36. Mitchell P, Wang JJ, Foran S, et al. Five-year incidence of age-related maculopathy lesions: The blue mountains eye study. *Ophthalmology* 2002;109:1092–1097.
37. Klein R, Klein BE, Tomany SC, et al. Ten-year incidence and progression of age-related maculopathy: The Beaver Dam eye study. *Ophthalmology* 2002;109:1767–1779.
38. van Leeuwen R, Klaver CC, Vingerling JR, et al. The risk and natural course of age-related maculopathy: follow-up at 6 1/2 years in the Rotterdam study. *Arch Ophthalmol* 2003;121:519–526.
39. Mukesh BN, Dimitrov PN, Leikin S, et al. Five-year incidence of age-related maculopathy: the Visual Impairment Project. *Ophthalmology* 2004;111:1176–1182.
40. Leske MC, Wu SY, Hyman L, et al. Four-year incidence of macular changes in the Barbados Eye Studies. *Ophthalmology* 2004;111:706–711.
41. Jonasson F, Arnarsson A, Peto T, et al. 5-year incidence of age-related maculopathy in the Reykjavik Eye Study. *Ophthalmology* 2005;112:132–138.
42. Buch H, Nielsen NV, Vinding T, et al. 14-year incidence, progression, and visual morbidity of age-related maculopathy: the Copenhagen City Eye Study. *Ophthalmology* 2005;112:787–798.
43. Delcourt C, Lacroux A, Carriere I. The three-year incidence of age-related macular degeneration: the "Pathologies Oculaires Liees a l'Age" (POLA) prospective study. *Am J Ophthalmol* 2005;140:924–926.
44. Miyazaki M, Kiyohara Y, Yoshida A, et al. The 5-year incidence and risk factors for age-related maculopathy in a general Japanese population: the Hisayama study. *Invest Ophthalmol Vis Sci* 2005;46:1907–1910.
45. Arnarsson A, Sverrisson T, Stefansson E, et al. Risk factors for five-year incident age-related macular degeneration: the Reykjavik Eye Study. *Am J Ophthalmol* 2006;142:419–428.
46. Leske MC, Wu SY, Hennis A, et al. Nine-year incidence of age-related macular degeneration in the Barbados Eye Studies. *Ophthalmology* 2006;113:29–35.
47. Wang JJ, Rochtchina E, Lee AJ, et al. 10-year incidence and progression of age-related maculopathy: the Blue Mountains Eye Study. *Ophthalmology* 2007;114:92–98.
48. Klein R, Klein BE, Knudtson MD, et al. Fifteen-year cumulative incidence of age-related macular degeneration: the Beaver Dam Eye Study. *Ophthalmology* 2007;114:253–262.
49. Friedman DS, O'Colmain BJ, Munoz B, et al. Prevalence of age-related macular degeneration in the United States. *Arch Ophthalmol* 2004;122:564–572.
50. Freeman EE, Munoz B, West SK, et al. Is there an association between cataract surgery and age-related macular degeneration? Data from three population-based studies. *Am J Ophthalmol* 2003;135:849–856.
51. Klein R, Klein BE, Jensen SC, et al. Age-related maculopathy in a multiracial United States population: the National Health and Nutrition Examination Survey III. *Ophthalmology* 1999;106:1056–1065.

52. Klein R, Klein BE, Cruickshanks KJ. The prevalence of age-related maculopathy by geographic region and ethnicity. *Prog Retin Eye Res* 1999;18:371–389.

53. Schachat AP, Hyman L, Leske MC, et al. Features of age-related macular degeneration in a black population. The Barbados Eye Study Group. *Arch Ophthalmol* 1995;113:728–735.

54. Maruko I, Iida T, Saito M, et al. Clinical characteristics of exudative age-related macular degeneration in Japanese patients. *Am J Ophthalmol* 2007;144:15–22.

55. Fuse N, Miyazawa A, Mengkegale M, et al. Polymorphisms in Complement Factor H and Hemicentin-1 genes in a Japanese population with dry-type age-related macular degeneration. *Am J Ophthalmol* 2006;142:1074–1076.

56. Uka J, Tamura H, Kobayashi T, et al. No association of complement factor H gene polymorphism and age-related macular degeneration in the Japanese population. *Retina* 2006;26:985–987.

57. Lau LI, Chen SJ, Cheng CY, et al. Association of the Y402H polymorphism in complement factor H gene and neovascular age-related macular degeneration in Chinese patients. *Invest Ophthalmol Vis Sci* 2006;47:3242–3246.

58. Macular Photocoagulation Study Group. Five-year follow-up of fellow eyes of patients with age-related macular degeneration and unilateral extrafoveal choroidal neovascularization. Macular Photocoagulation Study Group. *Arch Ophthalmol* 1993;111:1189–1199.

59. Chang B, Yannuzzi LA, Ladas ID, et al. Choroidal neovascularization in second eyes of patients with unilateral exudative age-related macular degeneration. *Ophthalmology* 1995;102:1380–1386.

60. Pieramici DJ, Bressler SB. Age-related macular degeneration and risk factors for the development of choroidal neovascularization in the fellow eye. *Curr Opin Ophthalmol* 1998;9:38–46.

61. Sandberg MA, Weiner A, Miller S, et al. High-risk characteristics of fellow eyes of patients with unilateral neovascular age-related macular degeneration. *Ophthalmology* 1998;105:441–447.

62. Uyama M, Takahashi K, Ida N, et al. The second eye of Japanese patients with unilateral exudative age related macular degeneration. *Br J Ophthalmol* 2000;84:1018–1023.

63. Holz FG, Wolfensberger TJ, Piguet B, et al. Bilateral macular drusen in age-related macular degeneration. Prognosis and risk factors. *Ophthalmology* 1994;101:1522–1528.

64. Arnold JJ, Sarks SH, Killingsworth MC, et al. Reticular pseudodrusen. A risk factor in age-related maculopathy. *Retina* 1995;15:183–191.

65. Wang JJ, Foran S, Smith W, et al. Risk of age-related macular degeneration in eyes with macular drusen or hyperpigmentation: the Blue Mountains Eye Study cohort. *Arch Ophthalmol* 2003;121:658–663.

66. Knudtson MD, Klein R, Klein BE, et al. Location of lesions associated with age-related maculopathy over a 10-year period: the Beaver Dam Eye Study. *Invest Ophthalmol Vis Sci* 2004;45:2135–2142.

67. Age-Related Eye Disease Research Study Group. A simplified severity scale for Age-Related Macular Degeneration: AREDS report number 18. *Arch Ophthalmol* 2005;123:1570–1574.

68. Age-Related Eye Disease Research Study Group. The Age-Related Eye Disease Study severity scale for Age-Related Macular Degeneration: AREDS report number 17. *Arch Ophthalmol* 2005;123:1484–1498.

69. Clemons TE, Milton RC, Klein R, et al. Risk factors for the incidence of Advanced Age-Related Macular Degeneration in the Age-Related Eye Disease Study (AREDS) AREDS report no. 19. *Ophthalmology* 2005;112:533–539.

70. Smith W, Assink J, Klein R, et al. Risk factors for age-related macular degeneration: Pooled findings from three continents. *Ophthalmology* 2001;108:697–704.

71. Delcourt C, Diaz JL, Ponton Sanchez A, et al. Smoking and age-related macular degeneration. The POLA Study. Pathologies Oculaires Liees a l'Age. *Arch Ophthalmol* 1998;116:1031–1035.

72. Seddon JM, George S, Rosner B. Cigarette smoking, fish consumption, omega-3 fatty acid intake, and associations with age-related macular degeneration: the US Twin Study of Age-Related Macular Degeneration. *Arch Ophthalmol* 2006;124:995–1001.

73. Chakravarthy U, Augood C, Bentham GC, et al. Cigarette smoking and age-related macular degeneration in the EUREYE Study. *Ophthalmology* 2007;114:1157–1163.

74. Christen WG, Glynn RJ, Manson JE, et al. A prospective study of cigarette smoking and risk of age-related macular degeneration in men. *JAMA* 1996;276:1147–1151.

75. Seddon JM, Willett WC, Speizer FE, et al. A prospective study of cigarette smoking and age-related macular degeneration in women. *JAMA* 1996;276:1141–1146.

76. Mitchell P, Wang JJ, Smith W, et al. Smoking and the 5-year incidence of age-related maculopathy: the Blue Mountains Eye Study. *Arch Ophthalmol* 2002;120:1357–1363.

77. Tomany SC, Wang JJ, van Leeuwen R, et al. Risk factors for incident age-related macular degeneration: pooled findings from 3 continents. *Ophthalmology* 2004;111:1280–1287.

78. Klein R, Klein BE, Moss SE. Relation of smoking to the incidence of age-related maculopathy. The Beaver Dam Eye Study. *Am J Epidemiol* 1998;147:103–110.

79. Klein R, Klein BE, Tomany SC, et al. Ten-year incidence of age-related maculopathy and smoking and drinking: the Beaver Dam Eye Study. *Am J Epidemiol* 2002;156:589–598.

80. Thornton J, Edwards R, Mitchell P, et al. Smoking and age-related macular degeneration: a review of association. *Eye* 2005;19:935–944.

81. Khan JC, Thurlby DA, Shahid H, et al. Smoking and age related macular degeneration: the number of pack years of cigarette smoking is a major determinant of risk for both geographic atrophy and choroidal neovascularisation. *Br J Ophthalmol* 2006;90:75–80.

82. Tan JS, Mitchell P, Kifley A, et al. Smoking and the long-term incidence of age-related macular degeneration: the Blue Mountains Eye Study. *Arch Ophthalmol* 2007;125:1089–1095.

83. Vingerling JR, Hofman A, Grobbee DE, et al. Age-related macular degeneration and smoking. The Rotterdam Study. *Arch Ophthalmol* 1996;114:1193–1196.

84. Evans JR, Fletcher AE, Wormald RP. 28,000 Cases of age related macular degeneration causing visual loss in people aged 75 years and above in the United Kingdom may be attributable to smoking. *Br J Ophthalmol* 2005;89:550–553.

85. Suner IJ, Espinosa-Heidmann DG, Marin-Castano ME, et al. Nicotine increases size and severity of experimental choroidal neovascularization. *Invest Ophthalmol Vis Sci* 2004;45:311–317.

86. Klein R, Knudtson MD, Cruickshanks KJ, et al. Further observations on the association between smoking and the long term incidence and progression of age-related macular degeneration. *Arch Ophthalmol* 2008;126(1):115–121.

87. Fraser-Bell S, Wu J, Klein R, et al. Smoking, alcohol intake, estrogen use, and age-related macular degeneration in Latinos: the Los Angeles Latino Eye Study. *Am J Ophthalmol* 2006;141:79–87.

88. Krishnaiah S, Das T, Nirmalan PK, et al. Risk factors for age-related macular degeneration: findings from the Andhra Pradesh eye disease study in South India. *Invest Ophthalmol Vis Sci* 2005;46:4442–4449.

89. Schmidt S, Haines JL, Postel EA, et al. Joint effects of smoking history and APOE genotypes in age-related macular degeneration. *Mol Vis* 2005;11:941–949.

90. Sepp T, Khan JC, Thurlby DA, et al. Complement factor H variant Y402H is a major risk determinant for geographic atrophy and choroidal neovascularization in smokers and nonsmokers. *Invest Ophthalmol Vis Sci* 2006;47:536–540.

91. Schmidt S, Hauser MA, Scott WK, et al. Cigarette smoking strongly modifies the association of LOC387715 and age-related macular degeneration. *Am J Hum Genet* 2006;78:852–864.

92. Despriet DD, Klaver CC, Witteman JC, et al. Complement factor H polymorphism, complement activators, and risk of age-related macular degeneration. *JAMA* 2006;296:301–309.

93. Seddon JM, George S, Rosner B, et al. CFH Gene Variant, Y402H, and Smoking, Body Mass Index, Environmental Associations with Advanced Age-Related Macular Degeneration. *Hum Hered* 2006;61:157–165.

94. Schaumberg DA, Hankinson SE, Guo Q, et al. A prospective study of 2 major age-related macular degeneration susceptibility alleles and interactions with modifiable risk factors. *Arch Ophthalmol* 2007;125:55–62.

95. Francis PJ, George S, Schultz DW, et al. The LOC387715 Gene, Smoking, Body Mass Index, Environmental Associations with Advanced Age-Related Macular Degeneration. *Hum Hered* 2007;63:212–218.

96. Seddon JM, Francis PJ, George S, et al. Association of CFH Y402H and LOC387715 A69S with progression of age-related macular degeneration. *JAMA* 2007;297:1793–1800.

97. DeAngelis MM, Ji F, Kim IK, et al. Cigarette Smoking, CFH, APOE, ELOVL4, and Risk of Neovascular Age-Related Macular Degeneration. *Arch Ophthalmol* 2007;125:49–54.

98. Scott WK, Schmidt S, Hauser MA, et al. Independent effects of complement factor H Y402H polymorphism and cigarette smoking on risk of age-related macular degeneration. *Ophthalmology* 2007;114:1151–1156.

99. Greenland S, Rothman KJ. Concepts of interaction. In: Rothman KJ, Greenland S (eds). *Modern epidemiology.* Philadelphia, PA: Lippincott-Raven, 1998:329–342.

100. Winkler BS, Boulton ME, Gottsch JD, et al. Oxidative damage and age-related macular degeneration. *Mol Vis* 1999;5:32.

101. Cooper DA, Eldridge AL, Peters JC. Dietary carotenoids and certain cancers, heart disease, and age-related macular degeneration: a review of recent research. *Nutr Rev* 1999;57:201–214.

102. Seddon JM, Ajani UA, Sperduto RD, et al. Dietary carotenoids, vitamins A, C, and E, and advanced age-related macular degeneration. Eye Disease Case-Control Study Group. *Journal of the American Medical Association* 1994;272:1413–1420.

103. VandenLangenberg GM, Mares Perlman JA, Klein R, et al. Associations between antioxidant and zinc intake and the 5-year incidence of early age-related maculopathy in the Beaver Dam Eye Study. *Am J Epidemiol* 1998;148:204–214.

104. Christen WG, Ajani UA, Glynn RJ, et al. Prospective cohort study of anti-oxidant vitamin supplement use and the risk of age-related maculopathy. *Am J Epidemiol* 1999;149:476–484.

105. Flood V, Smith W, Wang JJ, et al. Dietary antioxidant intake and incidence of early age-related maculopathy: the Blue Mountains Eye Study. *Ophthalmology* 2002;109:2272–2278.

106. Cho E, Seddon JM, Rosner B, et al. Prospective study of intake of fruits, vegetables, vitamins, and carotenoids and risk of age-related maculopathy. *Arch Ophthalmol* 2004;122:883–892.

107. van Leeuwen R, Boekhoorn S, Vingerling JR, et al. Dietary intake of anti-oxidants and risk of age-related macular degeneration. *JAMA* 2005;294:3101–3107.

108. Delcourt C, Carriere I, Delage M, et al. Plasma lutein and zeaxanthin and other carotenoids as modifiable risk factors for age-related maculopathy and cataract: the POLA Study. *Invest Ophthalmol Vis Sci* 2006;47:2329–2335.

109. Age-Related Eye Disease Study Research Group. The Relationship of Dietary Carotenoid and Vitamin A, E, and C Intake With Age-Related Macular Degeneration in a Case-Control Study: AREDS Report No. 22. *Arch Ophthalmol* 2007;125:1225–1232.

110. West S, Vitale S, Hallfrisch J, et al. Are antioxidants or supplements protective for age-related macular degeneration? *Arch Ophthalmol* 1994;112:222–227.

111. Mares-Perlman JA, Brady WE, Klein R, et al. Serum antioxidants and age-related macular degeneration in a population-based case-control study. *Arch Ophthalmol* 1995;113:1518–1523.

112. Smith W, Mitchell P, Rochester C. Serum beta carotene, alpha tocopherol, and age-related maculopathy: the Blue Mountains Eye Study. *Am J Ophthalmol* 1997;124:838–840.

113. Mares-Perlman JA, Fisher AI, Klein R, et al. Lutein and Zeaxanthin in the Diet and Serum and Their Relation to Age-Related Maculopathy in the Third National Health and Nutrition Examination Survey. *Am J Epidemiol* 2001;153:424–432.

114. Age-Related Eye Disease Study Research Group. A Randomized, Placebo-Controlled, Clinical Trial of High-Dose Supplementation With Vitamins C and E, Beta Carotene, and Zinc for Age-Related Macular Degeneration and Vision Loss: AREDS Report No. 9. *Arch Ophthalmol* 2001;119:1417–1436.

115. Evans JR. Antioxidant vitamin and mineral supplements for age-related macular degeneration. *Cochrane Database Syst Rev* 2002;1–24.

116. Chong EW, Wong TY, Kreis AJ, et al. Dietary antioxidants and primary pre-vention of age related macular degeneration: systematic review and meta-analysis. *BMJ* 2007;335:755, doi:10.1136/bmj.39350.500428.47.

117. Constable IJ. Age-related macular degeneration and its possible prevention. Despite well publicised claims of the therapeutic value of dietary supple-ments and other new treatments, the evidence for their effectiveness is modest. *Med J Aust* 2004;181:471–472.

118. Nutritional supplements for macular degeneration. *Drug Ther Bull* 2006;44:9–11.

119. Trumbo PR, Ellwood KC. Lutein and zeaxanthin intakes and risk of age-related macular degeneration and cataracts: an evaluation using the Food and Drug Administration's evidence-based review system for health claims. *Am J Clin Nutr* 2006;84:971–974.

120. Snow KK, Seddon JM. Do age-related macular degeneration and cardiovas-cular disease share common antecedents? *Ophthalmic Epidemiol* 1999;6:125–143.

121. Seddon JM, Cote J, Rosner B. Progression of age-related macular degenera-tion: association with dietary fat, transunsaturated fat, nuts, and fish intake. *Arch Ophthalmol* 2003;121:1728–1737.

122. Cho E, Hung S, Willett WC, et al. Prospective study of dietary fat and the risk of age-related macular degeneration. *Am J Clin Nutr* 2001;73:209–218.

123. Smith W, Mitchell P, Leeder SR. Dietary fat and fish intake and age-related maculopathy. *Arch Ophthalmol* 2000;118:401–404.

124. Chua B, Flood V, Rochtchina E, et al. Dietary fatty acids and the 5-year incidence of age related maculopathy. *Arch Ophthalmol* 2006;124:981–986.

125. Seddon JM, Rosner B, Sperduto RD, et al. Dietary fat and risk for advanced age-related macular degeneration. *Arch Ophthalmol* 2001;119:1191–1199.

126. Eye Disease Case-Control Study Group. Risk factors for neovascular age-related macular degeneration. *Arch Ophthalmol* 1992;110:1701–1708.

127. Mares-Perlman JA, Brady WE, Klein R, et al. Dietary fat and age-related maculopathy. *Arch Ophthalmol* 1995;113:743–748.

128. Heuberger RA, Mares-Perlman JA, Klein R, et al. Relationship of dietary fat to age-related maculopathy in the Third National Health and Nutrition Examination Survey. *Arch Ophthalmol* 2001;119:1833–1838.

129. van Leeuwen R, Klaver CC, Vingerling JR, et al. Cholesterol and age-related macular degeneration: is there a link? *Am J Ophthalmol* 2004;137:750–752.

130. Delcourt C, Michel F, Colvez A, et al. Associations of cardiovascular disease and its risk factors with age-related macular degeneration: the POLA study. *Ophthalmic Epidemiol* 2001;8:237–249.

131. Hyman L, Schachat AP, He Q, et al. Hypertension, cardiovascular disease, and age-related macular degeneration. Age-Related Macular Degeneration Risk Factors Study Group. *Arch Ophthalmol* 2000;118:351–358.

132. Klein R, Klein BE, Knudtson MD, et al. Subclinical atherosclerotic cardio-vascular disease and early age-related macular degeneration in a multiracial cohort: the Multiethnic Study of Atherosclerosis. *Arch Ophthalmol* 2007;125:534–543.

133. Tan JS, Mitchell P, Smith W, et al. Cardiovascular Risk Factors and the Long-term Incidence of Age-Related Macular Degeneration The Blue Mountains Eye Study. *Ophthalmology* 2007;114:1143–1150.

134. McGwin G Jr, Owsley C, Curcio CA, et al. The association between statin use and age related maculopathy. *Br J Ophthalmol* 2003;87:1121–1125.

135. McGwin G Jr, Modjarrad K, Hall TA, et al. 3-hydroxy-3-methylglutaryl coen-zyme a reductase inhibitors and the presence of age-related macular degen-eration in the Cardiovascular Health Study. *Arch Ophthalmol* 2006;124:33–37.

136. Guymer RH, Chiu AW, Lim L, et al. HMG CoA reductase inhibitors (statins): do they have a role in age-related macular degeneration? *Surv Ophthalmol* 2005;50:194–206.

137. van Leeuwen R, Tomany SC, Wang JJ, et al. Is medication use associated with the incidence of early age-related maculopathy? Pooled findings from 3 continents. *Ophthalmology* 2004;111:1169–1175.

138. van Leeuwen R, Vingerling JR, Hofman A, et al. Cholesterol lowering drugs and risk of age related maculopathy: prospective cohort study with cumula-tive exposure measurement. *BMJ* 2003;326:255–256.

139. Klein R, Knudtson MD, Klein BE. Statin use and the five-year incidence and progression of age-related macular degeneration. *Am J Ophthalmol* 2007;144:1–6.

140. Tan JS, Mitchell P, Rochtchina E, et al. Statins and the Long-term Risk of Incident Age-related Macular Degeneration: The Blue Mountains Eye Study. *Am J Ophthalmol* 2007;143:685–687.

141. Klein R, Deng Y, Klein BE, et al. Cardiovascular disease, its risk factors and treatment, and age-related macular degeneration: Women's Health Initiative Sight Exam ancillary study. *Am J Ophthalmol* 2007;143:473–483.

142. Enserink M. Women's health. The vanishing promises of hormone replace-ment. *Science* 2002;297:325–326.

143. Penfold PL, Madigan MC, Gillies MC, et al. Immunological and aetiological aspects of macular degeneration. *Prog Retin Eye Res* 2001;20:385–414.

144. Espinosa-Heidmann DG, Suner IJ, Hernandez EP, et al. Macrophage deple-tion diminishes lesion size and severity in experimental choroidal neovas-cularization. *Invest Ophthalmol Vis Sci* 2003;44:3586–3592.

145. Gold B, Merriam JE, Zernant J, et al. Variation in factor B (BF) and comple-ment component 2 (C2) genes is associated with age-related macular degeneration. *Nat Genet* 2006;38:458–462.

146. Bok D. Evidence for an inflammatory process in age-related macular degen-eration gains new support. *Proc Natl Acad Sci U S A* 2005;102:7053–7054.

147. Yates JR, Sepp T, Matharu BK, et al. Complement C3 Variant and the Risk of Age-Related Macular Degeneration. *N Engl J Med* 2007;357:553–561.

148. Daiger SP. Was the Human Genome Project Worth the Effort? *Science* 2005;308:362–364.

149. Sivaprasad S, Chong NV. The complement system and age-related macular degeneration. *Eye* 2006;20:867–872.

150. Esparza-Gordillo J, Soria JM, Buil A, et al. Genetic and environmental fac-tors influencing the human factor H plasma levels. *Immunogenetics* 2004;56:77–82.

151. Zee RY, Diehl KA, Ridker PM. Complement factor H Y402H gene polymor-phism, C-reactive protein, and risk of incident myocardial infarction, ischae-mic stroke, and venous thromboembolism: A nested case-control study. *Atherosclerosis* 2006;187:332–335.

152. Kardys I, Klaver CC, Despriet DD, et al. A common polymorphism in the complement factor H gene is associated with increased risk of myocardial infarction: the Rotterdam Study. *J Am Coll Cardiol* 2006;47:1568–1575.

153. Schaumberg DA, Christen WG, Kozlowski P, et al. A prospective assessment of the Y402H variant in complement factor H, genetic variants in C-reactive protein, and risk of age-related macular degeneration. *Invest Ophthalmol Vis Sci* 2006;47:2336–2340.

154. Laine M, Jarva H, Seitsonen S, et al. Y402H polymorphism of complement factor H affects binding affinity to C-reactive protein. *J Immunol* 2007;178:3831–3836.

155. Hageman GS, Luthert PJ, Victor Chong NH, et al. An integrated hypothesis that considers drusen as biomarkers of immune-mediated processes at the RPE-Bruch's membrane interface in aging and age-related macular degen-eration. *Prog Retin Eye Res* 2001;20:705–732.

156. Barouch FC, Miller JW. The role of inflammation and infection in age-related macular degeneration. *Int Ophthalmol Clin* 2007;47:185–197.

157. Klein R, Klein BE, Tomany SC, et al. Association of emphysema, gout, and inflammatory markers with long-term incidence of age-related maculopathy. *Arch Ophthalmol* 2003;121:674–678.

158. Shankar A, Mitchell P, Rochtchina E, et al. Association between circulating white blood cell count and long-term incidence of age-related macular degeneration: the Blue Mountains Eye Study. *Am J Epidemiol* 2007;165:375–382.

159. Seddon JM, Gensler G, Milton RC, et al. Association between C-reactive protein and age-related macular degeneration. *JAMA* 2004;291:704–710.

160. Klein R, Klein BE, Knudtson MD, et al. Systemic markers of inflammation, endothelial dysfunction, and age-related maculopathy. *Am J Ophthalmol* 2005;140:35–44.

161. McGwin G, Hall TA, Xie A, et al. The relation between C reactive protein and age related macular degeneration in the Cardiovascular Health Study. *Br J Ophthalmol* 2005;89:1166–1170.

162. Seddon JM, George S, Rosner B, et al. Progression of age-related macular degeneration: prospective assessment of C-reactive protein, interleukin 6, and other cardiovascular biomarkers. *Arch Ophthalmol* 2005;123:774–782.

163. Schaumberg DA, Christen WG, Buring JE, et al. High-sensitivity C-reactive protein, other markers of inflammation, and the incidence of macular degeneration in women. *Arch Ophthalmol* 2007;125:300–305.

164. Lip PL, Blann AD, Hope-Ross M, et al. Age-related macular degeneration is associated with increased vascular endothelial growth factor, hemorheology and endothelial dysfunction. *Ophthalmology* 2001;108:705–710.

165. Wu KH, Tan AG, Rochtchina E, et al. Circulating inflammatory markers and hemostatic factors in age-related maculopathy: a population-based case-control study. *Invest Ophthalmol Vis Sci* 2007;48:1983–1988.

166. Kalayoglu MV, Galvan C, Mahdi OS, et al. Serological association between Chlamydia pneumoniae infection and age-related macular degeneration. *Arch Ophthalmol* 2003;121:478–482.

167. Miller DM, Espinosa-Heidmann DG, Legra J, et al. The association of prior cytomegalovirus infection with neovascular age-related macular degeneration. *Am J Ophthalmol* 2004;138:323–328.

168. Robman L, Mahdi O, McCarty C, et al. Exposure to Chlamydia pneumoniae infection and progression of age-related macular degeneration. *Am J Epidemiol* 2005;161:1013–1019.

169. Kessler W, Jantos CA, Dreier J, et al. Chlamydia pneumoniae is not detectable in subretinal neovascular membranes in the exudative stage of age-related macular degeneration. *Acta Ophthalmol Scand* 2006;84:333–337.

170. Robman L, Mahdi OS, Wang JJ, et al. Exposure to Chlamydia pneumoniae Infection and Age-Related Macular Degeneration: The Blue Mountains Eye Study. *Invest Ophthalmol Vis Sci* 2007;48:4007–4011.

171. Klein R, Klein BE, Jensen SC, et al. Medication use and the 5-year incidence of early age-related maculopathy: the Beaver Dam Eye Study. *Arch Ophthalmol* 2001;119:1354–1359.

172. Wang JJ, Mitchell P, Smith W, et al. Systemic use of anti-inflammatory medications and age-related maculopathy: the Blue Mountains Eye Study. *Ophthalmic Epidemiol* 2003;10:37–48.

173. Christen WG, Glynn RJ, Ajani UA, et al. Age-related maculopathy in a randomized trial of low-dose aspirin among US physicians. *Arch Ophthalmol* 2001;119:1143–1149.

174. Glazer-Hockstein C, Dunaief JL. Could blue light-blocking lenses decrease the risk of age-related macular degeneration? *Retina* 2006;26:1–4.

175. Darzins P, Mitchell P, Heller RF. Sun exposure and age-related macular degeneration. An Australian case-control study. *Ophthalmology* 1997;104:770–776.

176. Taylor HR, Munoz B, West S, et al. Visible light and risk of age-related macular degeneration. *Trans Am Ophthalmol Soc* 1990;88:163–173.

177. Age-Related Eye Disease Study Research Group. Risk factors associated with age-related macular degeneration. A case-control study in the age-related eye disease study: AREDS Report No. 3. *Ophthalmology* 2000;107:2224–2232.

178. Cruickshanks KJ, Klein R, Klein BE. Sunlight and age-related macular degeneration. The Beaver Dam Eye Study. *Arch Ophthalmol* 1993;111:514–518.

179. Mitchell P, Smith W, Wang JJ. Iris color, skin sun sensitivity, and age-related maculopathy. The Blue Mountains Eye Study. *Ophthalmology* 1998;105:1359–1363.

180. Delcourt C, Carriere I, Ponton-Sanchez A, et al. Light exposure and the risk of age-related macular degeneration: the Pathologies Oculaires Liees a l'Age (POLA) study. *Arch Ophthalmol* 2001;119:1463–1468.

181. Pham TQ, Wang JJ, Rochtchina E, et al. Pterygium/pinguecula and the five-year incidence of age-related maculopathy. *Am J Ophthalmol* 2005;139:536–537.

182. Cruickshanks KJ, Klein R, Klein BE, et al. Sunlight and the 5-year incidence of early age-related maculopathy: the beaver dam eye study. *Arch Ophthalmol* 2001;119:246–250.

183. Tomany SC, Cruickshanks KJ, Klein R, et al. Sunlight and the 10-year incidence of age-related maculopathy: the Beaver Dam Eye Study. *Arch Ophthalmol* 2004;122:750–757.

184. Khan JC, Shahid H, Thurlby DA, et al. Age related macular degeneration and sun exposure, iris colour, and skin sensitivity to sunlight. *Br J Ophthalmol* 2006;90:29–32.

185. Pollack A, Marcovich A, Bukelman A, et al. Age-related macular degeneration after extracapsular cataract extraction with intraocular lens implantation. *Ophthalmology* 1996;103:1546–1554.

186. Pollack A, Marcovich A, Bukelman A, et al. Development of exudative age-related macular degeneration after cataract surgery. *Eye* 1997;11:523–530.

187. Kaiserman I, Kaiserman N, Elhayany A, et al. Cataract surgery is associated with a higher rate of photodynamic therapy for age-related macular degeneration. *Ophthalmology* 2007;114:278–282.

188. Wang JJ, Klein R, Smith W, et al. Cataract surgery and the 5-year incidence of late-stage age-related maculopathy: pooled findings from the Beaver Dam and Blue Mountains eye studies. *Ophthalmology* 2003;110:1960–1967.

189. Klein R, Klein BE, Wong TY, et al. The association of cataract and cataract surgery with the long-term incidence of age-related maculopathy: the Beaver Dam eye study. *Arch Ophthalmol* 2002;120:1551–1558.

190. Cugati S, Mitchell P, Rochtchina E, et al. Cataract surgery and the 10-year incidence of age-related maculopathy: the Blue Mountains Eye Study. *Ophthalmology* 2006;113:2020–2025.

191. van der Schaft TL, Mooy CM, de Bruijn WC, et al. Increased prevalence of disciform macular degeneration after cataract extraction with implantation of an intraocular lens. *Br J Ophthalmol* 1994;78:441–445.

192. Martin DF, Gensler G, Klein BEK, et al. The effect of cataract surgery on progression to advanced AMD. *Invest Ophthalmol Vis Sci* 2002;43, E-Abstract 1907.

193. Armbrecht AM, Findlay C, Aspinall PA, et al. Cataract surgery in patients with age-related macular degeneration: one-year outcomes. *J Cataract Refract Surg* 2003;29:686–693.

194. Sutter FK, Menghini M, Barthelmes D, et al. Is pseudophakia a risk factor for neovascular age-related macular degeneration? *Invest Ophthalmol Vis Sci* 2007;48:1472–1475.

195. Marin-Castano ME, Elliot SJ, Potier M, et al. Regulation of estrogen receptors and MMP-2 expression by estrogens in human retinal pigment epithelium. *Invest Ophthalmol Vis Sci* 2003;44:50–59.

196. Espinosa-Heidmann DG, Marin-Castano ME, Pereira-Simon S, et al. Gender and estrogen supplementation increases severity of experimental choroidal neovascularization. *Exp Eye Res* 2005;80:413–423.

197. Klein BE, Klein R, Jensen SC, et al. Are sex hormones associated with age-related maculopathy in women? The Beaver Dam Eye Study. *Trans Am Ophthalmol Soc* 1994;92:289–295.

198. Vingerling JR, Dielemans I, Witteman JC, et al. Macular degeneration and early menopause: a case-control study. *BMJ* 1995;310:1570–1571.

199. Smith W, Mitchell P, Wang JJ. Gender, oestrogen, hormone replacement and age-related macular degeneration: results from the Blue Mountains Eye Study. *Aust N Z J Ophthalmol* 1997;25(Suppl 1):S13–S15.

200. Snow KK, Cote J, Yang W, et al. Association between reproductive and hormonal factors and age-related maculopathy in postmenopausal women. *Am J Ophthalmol* 2002;134:842–848.

201. Abramov Y, Borik S, Yahalom C, et al. The effect of hormone therapy on the risk for age-related maculopathy in postmenopausal women. *Menopause* 2004;11:62–68.

202. Defay R, Pinchinat S, Lumbroso S, et al. Sex steroids and age-related macular degeneration in older French women: the POLA study. *Ann Epidemiol* 2004;14:202–208.

203. Nirmalan PK, Katz J, Robin AL, et al. Female reproductive factors and eye disease in a rural South Indian population: the Aravind Comprehensive Eye Survey. *Invest Ophthalmol Vis Sci* 2004;45:4273–4276.

204. Freeman EE, Munoz B, Bressler SB, et al. Hormone replacement therapy, reproductive factors, and age-related macular degeneration: the Salisbury Eye Evaluation Project. *Ophthalmic Epidemiology* 2005;12:37–45.

205. Klein BE, Klein R, Lee KE. Reproductive exposures, incident age-related cataracts, and age-related maculopathy in women: the beaver dam eye study. *Am J Ophthalmol* 2000;130:322–326.

206. Haan MN, Klein R, Klein BE, et al. Hormone therapy and age-related macular degeneration: the Women's Health Initiative Sight Exam Study. *Arch Ophthalmol* 2006;124:988–992.

207. Boekhoorn SS, Vingerling JR, Uitterlinden AG, et al. Estrogen receptor alpha gene polymorphisms associated with incident aging macula disorder. *Invest Ophthalmol Vis Sci* 2007;48:1012–1017.

208. Seddon JM, Gensler G, Klein ML, et al. Evaluation of plasma homocysteine and risk of age-related macular degeneration. *Am J Ophthalmol* 2006;141:201–203.

209. Vingerling JR, Dielemans I, Bots ML, et al. Age-related macular degeneration is associated with atherosclerosis. The Rotterdam Study. *Am J Epidemiol* 1995;142:404–409.

210. Miyazaki M, Nakamura H, Kubo M, et al. Risk factors for age related maculopathy in a Japanese population: the Hisayama study. *Br J Ophthalmol* 2003;87:469–472.

211. Klein R, Klein BEK, Tomany SC, et al. The Association of Cardiovascular Disease with the Long-term Incidence of Age-related Maculopathy. The Beaver Dam Eye Study. *Ophthalmology* 2003;110:1273–1280.

212. Rochtchina E, Wang JJ, Flood VM, et al. Elevated serum homocysteine, low serum vitamin B12, folate, and age-related macular degeneration: the Blue Mountains Eye Study. *Am J Ophthalmol* 2007;143:344–346.

213. Smith W, Mitchell P, Leeder SR, et al. Plasma fibrinogen levels, other cardiovascular risk factors, and age-related maculopathy: the Blue Mountains Eye Study. *Arch Ophthalmol* 1998;116:583–587.

214. Schaumberg DA, Christen WG, Hankinson SE, et al. Body mass index and the incidence of visually significant age-related maculopathy in men. *Arch Ophthalmol* 2001;119:1259–1265.

215. Dawn AG, Santiago-Turla C, Lee PP. Patient expectations regarding eye care: focus group results. *Arch Ophthalmol* 2003;121:762–768.

216. Obisesan TO, Hirsch R, Kosoko O, et al. Moderate wine consumption is associated with decreased odds of developing age-related macular degeneration in NHANES-1. *J Am Geriatr Soc* 1998;46:1–7.

217. Moss SE, Klein R, Klein BE, et al. Alcohol consumption and the 5-year incidence of age-related maculopathy: the Beaver Dam eye study. *Ophthalmology* 1998;105:789–794.

218. Knudtson MD, Klein R, Klein BE. Physical activity and the 15-year cumulative incidence of age-related macular degeneration: the Beaver Dam Eye Study. *Br J Ophthalmol* 2006;90:1461–1463.

219. Klein R, Klein BE, Franke T. The relationship of cardiovascular disease and its risk factors to age-related maculopathy. The Beaver Dam Eye Study. *Ophthalmology* 1993;100:406–414.

220. Klein R, Klein BE, Jensen SC. The relation of cardiovascular disease and its risk factors to the 5-year incidence of age-related maculopathy: the Beaver Dam Eye Study. *Ophthalmology* 1997;104:1804–1812.

221. van Leeuwen R, Ikram MK, Vingerling JR, et al. Blood pressure, atherosclerosis, and the incidence of age-related maculopathy: the Rotterdam Study. *Invest Ophthalmol Vis Sci* 2003;44:3771–3777.

222. Wang JJ, Mitchell P, Rochtchina E, et al. Retinal vessel wall signs and the 5 year incidence of age related maculopathy: the Blue Mountains Eye Study. *Br J Ophthalmol* 2004;88:104–109.

223. Liew G, Kaushik S, Rochtchina E, et al. Retinal Vessel Signs and 10-Year Incident Age-Related Maculopathy The Blue Mountains Eye Study. *Ophthalmology* 2006;113:1481–1487.

224. Voutilainen-Kaunisto RM, Terasvirta ME, Uusitupa MI, et al. Age-related macular degeneration in newly diagnosed type 2 diabetic patients and control subjects: a 10-year follow-up on evolution, risk factors, and prognostic significance. *Diabetes Care* 2000;23:1672–1678.

225. Clemons TE, Kurinij N, Sperduto RD. Associations of mortality with ocular disorders and an intervention of high-dose antioxidants and zinc in the Age-Related Eye Disease Study: AREDS Report No. 13. *Arch Ophthalmol* 2004;122:716–726.

226. Wong TY, Klein R, Sun C, et al. Age-related macular degeneration and risk for stroke. *Ann Intern Med* 2006;145:98–106.

227. Wong TY, Tikellis G, Sun C, et al. Age-related macular degeneration and risk of coronary heart disease: the Atherosclerosis Risk in Communities Study. *Ophthalmology* 2007;114:86–91.

228. Duan Y, Mo J, Klein R, et al. Age-related macular degeneration is associated with incident myocardial infarction among elderly Americans. *Ophthalmology* 2007;114:732–737.

229. Cugati S, Cumming RG, Smith W, et al. Visual impairment, age-related macular degeneration, cataract, and long-term mortality: the Blue Mountains Eye Study. *Arch Ophthalmol* 2007;125:917–924.

230. Wu KH, Wang JJ, Rochtchina E, et al. Angiotensin-converting enzyme inhibitors (ACEIs) and age-related maculopathy (ARM): cross-sectional findings from the Blue Mountains Eye Study. *Acta Ophthalmol Scand* 2004;82:298–303.

231. Ritter LL, Klein R, Klein BE, et al. Alcohol use and age-related maculopathy in the Beaver Dam Eye Study. *Am J Ophthalmol* 1995;120:190–196.

232. Smith W, Mitchell P. Alcohol intake and age-related maculopathy. *Am J Ophthalmol* 1996;122:743–745.

233. Ajani UA, Christen WG, Manson JE, et al. A prospective study of alcohol consumption and the risk of age-related macular degeneration. *Ann Epidemiol* 1999;9:172–177.

234. Cho E, Hankinson SE, Willett WC, et al. Prospective study of alcohol consumption and the risk of age-related macular degeneration. *Arch Ophthalmol* 2000;118:681–688.

235. Knudtson MD, Klein R, Klein BE. Alcohol consumption and the 15-year cumulative incidence of age-related macular degeneration. *Am J Ophthalmol* 2007;143:1026–1029.

236. Hyman L, Neborsky R. Risk factors for age-related macular degeneration: an update. *Curr Opin Ophthalmol* 2002;13:171–175.

237. McCarty CA, Mukesh BN, Fu CL, et al. Risk factors for age-related maculopathy: the Visual Impairment Project. *Arch Ophthalmol* 2001;119:1455–1462.

238. Smith W, Mitchell P, Leeder SR. Smoking and age-related maculopathy. The Blue Mountains Eye Study. *Arch Ophthalmol* 1996;114:1518–1523.

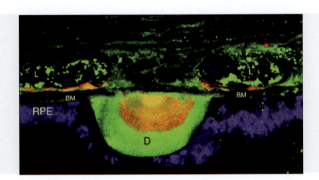

# Genetics of Age-Related Macular Degeneration

Mike Grassi ■ Josephine Hoh

Ophthalmology has a rich tradition of providing major contributions to the field of genetics. For instance, the first inherited disease to be linked to a human autosome was the pulverulent cataract, which was linked to the Duffy blood group antigen by Renwick and Lawler in 1963 (1). The first tumor suppressor gene to be discovered, which was also one of the first positionally cloned genes, was the retinoblastoma gene (2). More recently, the implication of the complement factor H (CFH) gene in age-related macular degeneration (AMD) resulted from the first successful genome-wide association (GWA) study for a complex trait (3,4,5).

Support for a genetic component to AMD has grown slowly and was initially based on conjecture and anecdotal observation. AMD was initially referred to as "senile macular degeneration" because of the mistaken belief that all elderly individuals would eventually develop this condition and that there was no underlying genetic component. In 1973, Gass et al. published a retrospective case series reporting a 20% prevalence of central vision loss in family members of patients with AMD (6). A more sophisticated epidemiologic approach, the familial aggregation study, was later employed to compare the frequency of AMD in siblings and children of affected individuals to the frequency of AMD in family members of controls. Several studies of this nature have suggested that a first-degree relative of an individual with AMD is five times more likely to develop AMD than a family member of a control (7,8,9,10). Twin studies not only confirm this genetic association but also demonstrate striking phenotypic similarities between monozygotic twins, which intuitively demonstrate the major role genes play in this condition (Fig. 31-1) (11).

## INITIAL GENETIC STUDIES OF AGE-RELATED MACULAR DEGENERATION

Candidate gene studies (12) have been successful for complex diseases but rely on having the correct identity of the gene or pathway as a biologic basis for that condition predicted in advance. For the study of AMD, candidate gene studies were initially performed on genes implicated in Mendelian maculopathies, such as Best disease (13), Pattern dystrophy (14), Sorsby fundus dystrophy (14), Malattia Leventinese (15), and Stargardt disease (16–19). These diseases were chosen because they recapitulate many features of AMD, such as the deposition of drusenoid-like material, atrophy or choroidal neovascularization (CNV) (Fig. 31-2). To date, these genes have been associated with only a small fraction of the total cases of AMD (2%-3% or less) or have been inconclusive (16,20).

Linkage mapping studies have the advantage of being hypothesis free and have enjoyed great success in the study of Mendelian conditions but have suffered when applied to complex disorders like AMD due to a lack of statistical power to detect mild effects and lack of resolution produced by low marker density. As an example, the PPAR gene association with diabetes (21) would never have been identified with a linkage approach as it would have required the sample population to include over one million affected sibling pairs to generate this association. Linkage studies for AMD have found only

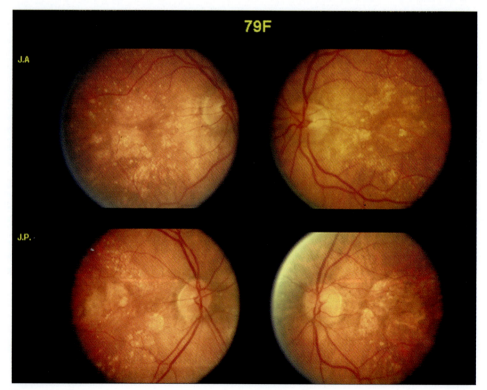

**Figure 31-1.** Fundus photographs from monozygotic twins with age-related macular degeneration. (From Klein ML, Mauldin WM, Stoumbos VD. Heredity and age-related macular degeneration. Observations in monozygotic twins. *Arch Ophthalmol* 1994;112:932–937.)

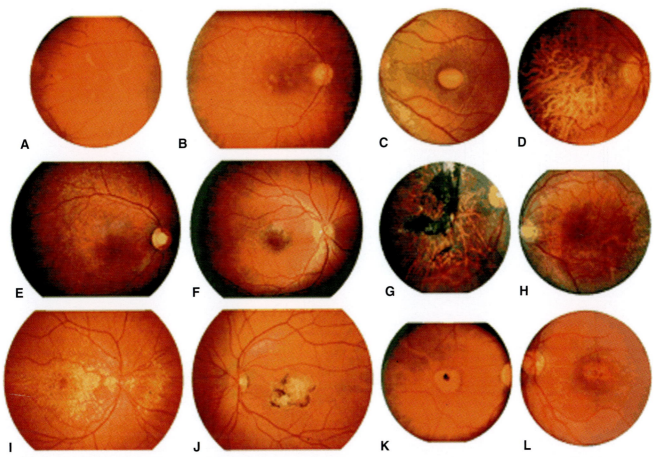

**Figure 31-2.** Ophthalmoscopic phenotypes of patients affected with molecularly confirmed early-onset heritable macular dystrophies. The left panel of each pair shows the more typical clinical appearance of each disease while the right panel depicts a variant appearance that could be confused with AMD or one of the other heritable dystrophies. **A** and **B:** *RDS*-associated pattern dystrophy (*RDS* Gly167Asp); **C** and **D:** Best disease (*VMD2* Ala243Thr); **E:** Stargardt disease (*ABCA4* Phe608Ile/Leu2027Phe); **F:** Stargardt disease (*ABCA4* Cys1488Phe/Cys2150Tyr); **G:** Sorsby fundus dystrophy (*TIMP3* Gly167Cys; photograph courtesy of Dr Samuel Jacobson); **H:** Sorsby fundus dystrophy (*TIMP3* Ser181Cys; photograph courtesy of Dr Michael Klein); **I** and **J:** ML (*EFEMP1* Arg345Trp); **K** and **L:** Stargardt-like dominant macular dystrophy (*ELOVL4* common 5 bp deletion). (From Stone EM, Sheffield VC, Hageman GS. Molecular genetics of age-related macular degeneration. *Hum Mol Genet* 2001;10:2285–2292.)

suggestive areas of linkage by standard statistical criteria (22,23). However, both the CFH gene and LOC387715/HTRA1 locus were found within previously mapped linkage loci (1q31 and 10q26, respectively).

## GENOME-WIDE ASSOCIATION STUDIES

Such challenges have spurred recent interest in the application of GWA studies using single nucleotide polymorphisms (SNPs) as an approach that has a better capability to localize disease susceptibility genes harboring smaller effects. Two GWA studies for AMD using drusen and neovascularization as the primary phenotypes have implicated two major genes in this disease. The first GWA study discovered variants in the CFH gene (3), and the second GWA study discovered variants in the LOC387715/HTRA1 locus (4). Fig. 31-3 shows results from the GWA study indicating association with the CFH gene. Subsequent resequencing based on the principle of linkage

disequilibrium (LD) showed that the causal mutation in CFH may be a missense variant in amino acid residue 402 where a tyrosine is replaced by a histidine.

When one looks at the successful design of GWA studies, one immediately appreciates that cases and controls were ascertained from clusters of subjects at the two extremes (Fig. 31-4). In the Klein study (11), cases were comprised of subjects with end-stage AMD as defined by the presence of geographic atrophy or CNV with controls having little to no drusen, which at a mean age of 80 turns out to be typically more difficult to ascertain than AMD patients. The DeWan study (4) was designed to ascertain only Asian individuals given their higher incidence of polypoidal CNV in the absence of drusen. These individuals were compared to age matched controls with no ophthalmoscopic findings of AMD. This thoughtful design enabled the identification of a novel association in the LOC387715/HTRA1 locus, which was not discerned in prior analyses due to greater "noise."

In summary, to achieve success in GWA studies, study power needs to be increased. There are two ways to do this. The first is by increasing the subject number, as in the WTCC

**A**

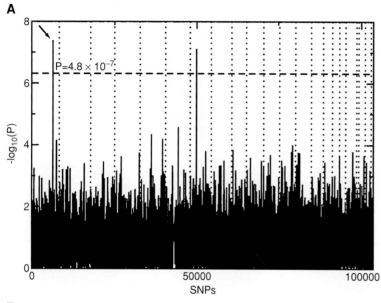

**B**

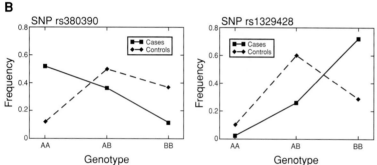

**Figure 31-3. A:** *P* values of genome-wide association scan for genes that affect the risk of developing AMD. -log$_{10}$(*p*) is plotted for each SNP in chromosomal order. The spacing between SNPs on the plot is uniform and does not reflect distances between SNPs on the chromosomes. The dotted horizontal line shows the cutoff for *p* = .05 after Bonferroni correction. The vertical dotted lines show chromosomal boundaries. The arrow indicates the peak for SNP rs380390, the most significant association, which was studied further. **B:** Variation in genotype frequencies between cases and controls. (From Klein RJ, Zeiss C, Chew EY, et al. Complement Factor H Polymorphism in Age-Related Macular Degeneration. *Science* 2005;308:385–389.)

study (24), and future genetic studies of AMD will likely involve tens of thousands of subjects. Secondly, and *possibly more importantly*, clinical insight plays a critical role in the study design because well characterized, homogeneous cohorts at polar ends of the disease spectrum also increase statistical power. The bottom line with genetic association studies is that, from a phenotypic standpoint, if you put "garbage in" you will get "garbage out." An example is the lack of associations to date for heterogeneous phenotypic conditions such as primary open-angle glaucoma, for which this approach has not yet been successful. In contradistinction, GWA studies have successfully identified multiple SNPs in the 15q24.1

region as an important risk factor for pseudoexfoliation glaucoma (25), which is a much cleaner, more homogenous phenotype.

## THE COMPLEMENT FACTOR H GENE, DRUSEN, AND AGE-RELATED MACULAR DEGENERATION

Genotype–phenotype correlations have been made between variations in the CFH gene and the cuticular drusen phenotype. In retrospect, this is not surprising. In 1985 Kenyon and Maumenee (26) described a peculiar fundus pattern characterized biomicroscopically by diffuse, 25-75 μm, yellow, circular drusen. These drusen often cluster in groups of 15-20 resembling streptococci seen on Gram stain (Fig. 31-5A). Commonly appearing in early adulthood, this phenotype is best appreciated on fluorescein angiography, which reveals a "starry-sky" appearance (Fig. 31-5B)(27). Russell and coworkers have demonstrated that histopathologically, these drusen are indistinguishable from those found in typical AMD (28). It has been a long standing clinical observation that individuals

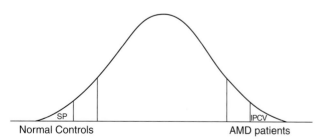

**Figure 31-4.** Normal curve indicating distribution of phenotypes. AMD, age-related macular degeneration; IPCV, idiopathic polypoidal choroidal vasculopathy; SP, super controls (no drusen at age 80 years).

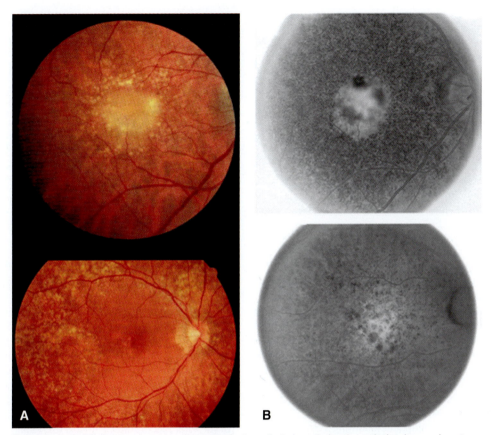

**Figure 31-5.** Ophthalmoscopic and angiographic features that characterize the cuticular drusen phenotype. **A:** Thirty-degree color fundus photograph centered on the macula demonstrating classic features of cuticular drusen, including a vitelliform macular detachment. **B:** Negative fluorescein angiogram of the same patient taken at 55.2 seconds revealing multiple pinpoint areas of hyperfluorescence corresponding to drusen in a "starry sky" distribution. Note the fluorescein blockage and associated early leakage due to a drusenoid pigment epithelial detachment. **C:** Sixty-degree fundus photograph centered on the macula of a patient with membranoproliferative glomerulonephritis type II demonstrating diffuse cuticular drusen. **D:** Threshold photograph used for grading the cuticular drusen phenotype. Classification required the presence of cuticular drusen on fluorescein angiography of equal or greater number and extent than that visualized in this frame. (From Grassi MA, Folk JC, Scheetz TE, et al. Complement Factor H Polymorphism p.Tyr402His and Cuticular Drusen. *Arch Ophthalmol* 2007;125: 93–97.)

with membranoproliferative glomerulonephritis type II (MPGN2) develop cuticular drusen (27,29–37).

Animal models for the study of MPGN2 have been generated through the targeted deletion of the CFH gene. These CFH knockout models recapitulate many of the systemic features of MPGN2 including the ocular manifestations. Moreover, a histopathologic study of drusen substructure identified many terminal complement components (38). Such observations, taken together, led Hageman and coworkers to pursue the CFH gene as plausible candidate gene in AMD (12). It was found that 70% of individuals with MGPN2 harbored the CFH histidine risk variant at amino acid position 402.

Subsequent work by Grassi and coworkers revealed that individuals with the cuticular drusen phenotype had a similarly increased prevalence of the CFH risk allele, firmly establishing this genotype-phenotype correlation (39). Confirmation and extension was provided by Boone et al. who demonstrated that the monogenic inheritance of rare variants in the CFH gene, together with the histidine risk allele, results in familial cuticular drusen (40). Heterozygous, nonsense, missense, and splice-site variants in the CFH gene segregated with the cuticular phenotype in five of the ascertained families.

## COMPLEMENT, INFLAMMATION, AND AGE-RELATED MACULAR DEGENERATION

The association of polymorphisms in the CFH gene firmly implicates alterations in innate immunity as being important in the pathobiology of AMD. Subsequent studies have identified polymorphisms in the C2/CFB gene (41) and C3 gene (42) as well. Factor B is a positive activator of the alternative complement pathway and competes with CFH for binding C3b. CFH is the primary inhibitor of the alternate cascade of the complement pathway. CFH binds to activated C3 and promotes its proteolytic inactivation by complement factor I (Fig. 31-6). It is conjectured that the tyrosine to histidine polymorphism at position 402 decreases CFH activity, thereby allowing an

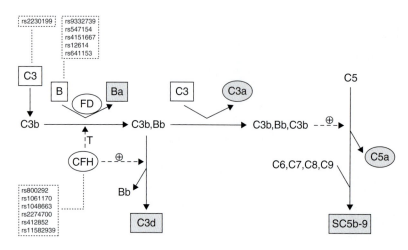

**Figure 31-6.** The Alternative Pathway of Complement: Polymorphic Variants and Complement Proteins under Study. Complement gene SNPs (boxed with dotted lines) and protein plasma concentrations (boxed with solid lines) were determined in all AMD patients and controls. C3, C4 and factor B are substrates (open rectangles), factor H and factor D are regulators (open ellipses), Ba, C3d and SC5b-9 are markers of chronic activation (filled rectangles), and C3a and C5a are markers of acute activation (filled ellipses) of the alternative complement pathway. doi:10.1371/journal.pone.0002593. g001. (From Scholl HPN, Issa PC, Walier M, et al. Systemic complement activation in age-related macular degeneration. *PlosOne* 3(7):e2593.doi:10.1371, 2008.). CFH, complement factor H.

upregulated immune response. Recent work by Ormsby (43) suggests that the mechanism by which this might occur is to decrease interaction between CFH and C reactive protein (CRP) (44).

Histopathologic studies clearly implicate the role of the alternative complement pathway in drusen substructure (Fig. 31-7). Cellular remnants and debris derived from degenerate RPE cells constitute a chronic inflammatory stimulus. This entrapped cellular debris then becomes the target of encapsulation by a variety of inflammatory mediators, which results in drusen biogenesis.

From an evolutionary standpoint, mounting a more robust immune response to infection was advantageous and provided a survival benefit. When the lifespan was 40 years, this did not have a deleterious effect. However, during present times we see the manifestations of this low-grade persistent inflammatory activity. Given the firm genetic associations with biologic correlates, current work is exploring mechanisms by which the alternate complement cascade can be modulated to prevent or alleviate AMD.

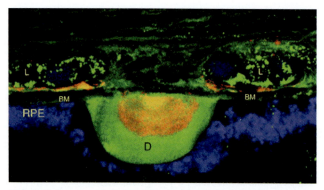

**Figure 31-7.** Immunocytochemistry of a druse (D) from the eye of an 85-year-old donor. The entire druse is stained with antibodies against complement factor H (green). In the center of the druse, factor H colocalizes with the C5b-9 membrane attack complex of complement (orange). The retinal pigment epithelium (RPE), which is distorted by the druse, contains autofluorescent lipofuscin granules (blue). Factor H staining is also visible in the lumen (L) of the capillaries, which are separated from the RPE by Brüch's membrane (BM). Colocalization of factor H and C5b-9 is also observed in the capillary wall (orange). Image is courtesy of Patrick Johnson and Kellen Betts (University of California, Santa Barbara). (From Bok D. Evidence for an inflammatory process in age-related macular degeneration gains new support. *Proc Natl Acad Sci* 2005;102:7227–7232.)

## CLINICAL IMPLICATIONS

Recent headlines stating that current genetic variants explain 74% of AMD are misleading. What these statistics are referring to is an individual's attributable risk in the presence of these genetic variants. Hence, the interpretation is not that 74% of AMD heritability is known, but rather, in a given individual, 74% of the reason why they developed the disease can be attributed to those genetic variations if they harbor them (45,41). For instance, in patients with the CFH risk allele, 50% of the total risk of AMD is due to this exposure.

Both epistasis, which is gene to gene interaction, and gene environmental interactions have been invoked to explain the incomplete penetrance and variable expressivity of these risk alleles in the complex phenotype of AMD. Schmidt et al. elegantly demonstrated how the LOC387715 and CFH risk variants interact with the environmental exposure of smoking to predispose to AMD in their cohort (46). Similar studies (45) are of critical importance to better understand the nature of these interactions. However, it is clear that these reports are consistent with the early epidemiologic studies implicating the three major risk factors for AMD: age, heredity, and smoking.

The question that patients ask in the clinic is: If I have the risk allele what is my chance of developing AMD? While genetic based treatments for AMD have not yet arrived, many clinicians wonder if genetic testing is possible for this condition. A major limitation of the current era of GWA studies is that they have been performed on case-control cohorts. As such there is no natural history or prognostic information present in these studies, which from a clinical perspective is critical. Seddon and coworkers (45) addressed this question by looking at progression from early or intermediate AMD to advanced stages in the Age-Related Eye Disease Study (AREDS) cohort over a six year period and found that individuals homozygous for the CFH risk allele were almost 3 times as likely to develop geographic atrophy or CNV. When they looked at both known genetic and environmental risk factors combined, the risk increased 19-fold.

The association of CFH with AMD is a major scientific breakthrough. Genetic studies have definitively linked variations in the CFH gene to AMD predisposition. Inflammation and dysregulation of the alternative complement pathway are now implicated in the pathogenesis of this condition. Insights from these early genetic studies will require future translational studies focused on resequencing of implicated genes in large cohorts, functional characterization of associated variants, extension to cell based assays, study of animal models, genotype-phenotype correlations, and studies of therapeutic proof of concept over the coming years, all of which should allow the medical community to move rapidly towards improved treatments for AMD.

## References

1. Renwick JH, Lawler SD. Probable linkage between a congenital cataract locus and the Duffy blood group locus. *Ann Hum Genet* 1963;27:67–76.
2. Friend SH, Bernards R, Rogelj S, et al. A human DNA segment with properties of the gene that predisposes to retinoblastoma and osteosarcoma. *Nature* 1986;323:642–646.
3. Klein RJ, Zeiss C, Chew EY, et al. Complement factor H polymorphism in age-related macular degeneration. *Science* 2005;308:385–389.
4. DeWan A, Liu M, Hartman S, et al. HTRA1 promoter polymorphism in wet age-related macular degeneration. *Science* 2006;314(5801):989–992.
5. Fritsche LG, Loenhardt T, Janssen A, et al. Age-related macular degeneration is associated with an unstable ARMS2 (LOC387715) mRNA. *Nat Genet* 2008;40:892–896.
6. Gass JD. Drusen and disciform macular detachment and degeneration. *Arch Ophthalmol* 1973;90(3):206–217.
7. Meyers SM. A twin study on age-related macular degeneration. *Trans Am Ophthalmol Soc* 1994;92:775–843.
8. Seddon JM, Ajani UA, Mitchell BD. Familial aggregation of age-related maculopathy. *Am J Ophthalmol* 1997;123:199–206.
9. Klein BEK, Klein R, Lee EL, et al. Risk of incident age-related diseases in people with an affected sibling: the Beaver Dam Eye Study. *Am J Epidemiol* 2001;154:207–211.
10. Hammond CJ, Webster AR, Sneider H, et al. Genetic influence on early age-related maculopathy: a twin study. *Ophthalmology* 2002;109:730–736.
11. Klein ML, Mauldin WM, Stoumbos VD. Heredity and age-related macular degeneration. Observations in monozygotic twins. *Arch Ophthalmol* 1994;112:932–937.
12. Hageman GS, Anderson DH, Johnson LV, et al. A common haplotype in the complement regulatory gene factor H (HF1/CFH) predisposes individuals to age-related macular degeneration. *PNAS* 2005;102:7227–7232.
13. Lotery AJ, Munier FL, Fishman GA, et al. Allelic variation in the VMD2 gene in best disease and age-related macular degeneration. *Invest Ophthalmol Vis Sci* 2000;42:1291–1296.
14. Stone EM, Sheffield VC, Hageman GS. Molecular genetics of age-related macular degeneration. *Hum Mol Genet* 2001;10:2285–2292.
15. Stone EM, Lotery AJ, Munier FL, et al. A single EFEMP1 mutation associated with both Malattia Leventinese and Doyne honeycomb retinal dystrophy. *Nat Genet* 1999;22:199.
16. Allikmets R, Shroyer NF, Singh N, et al. Mutation of the Stargardt disease gene (ABDR) in age-related macular degeneration. *Science and Culture* 1997;277:1805–1807.
17. Allikmets R. Further evidence for an association of ABDR alleles with age-related macular degeneration. The International ABCR Screening Consortium. *Am J Hum Genet* 2000;67:487–491.
18. Stone EM, Webster AR, Vandenburgh K, et al. Allelic variation in ABCR associated with Stargardt disease but not age-related macular degeneration. *Nat Genet* 1998;20:328.
19. Guymer RH, Heon E, Lotery AJ, et al. Variation of Codons 1961 and 2177 of the Stargardt Disease Gene Is Not Associated With Age-Related Macular Degeneration. *Arch Ophthalmol* 2001;119:745–751.
20. Allikmets R. Further evidence for an association of ABCR alleles with age-related macular degeneration. The International ABCR Screening Consortium. *Am J Hum Genet* 2000;67:487–491.
21. Altshuler D, Pollara VJ, Cowles CR, et al. An SNP map of the human genome generated by reduced representation shotgun sequencing. *Nature* 2000;407:513–516.
22. Majewski J, Schultz D, Weleber RG, et al. Age-related Macular Degeneration – a Genome Scan in Extended Families. *Am J Hum Genet* 2003;73:540–550.
23. Weeks D. Age-related maculopathy: an expanded genome-wide scan with evidence of susceptibility loci within the 1q31 and 17q25 regions. *Am J Ophthalmol* 2001;132:682–692.
24. Bowcock AM. Guilt by association. *Nature* 2007;445:646–647.
25. Thorleifsson G, Magnusson KP, Sulem P, et al. Common sequence variants in the LOXL1 gene confer susceptibility to exfoliation glaucoma. *Am J Ophthalmol* 2007;144:974–975.
26. Kenyon KR, Maumenee AE, Ryan SJ, et al. Diffuse drusen and associated complications. *Am J Ophthalmol* 1985;100:119–128.
27. Gass JDM. *Stereoscopic atlas of macular diseases diagnosis and treatment*, 4th ed. St. Louis: Mosby; 1997:599.
28. Russell SR, Mullins RF, Schneider BL, et al. Location, substructure, and composition of basal laminar drusen compared with drusen associated with aging and age-related macular degeneration. *Am J Ophthalmol* 2000;129:205–214.
29. Leys A, Proesmans W, Van Damme-Lombaerts R, et al. Specific eye fundus lesions in type II membranoproliferative glomerulonephritis [erratum appears in Pediatr Nephrol 1991 May;5(3):364]. *Pediatr Nephrol* 1991;5:189–192.
30. Leys A, Vanrenterghem Y, Van Damme B, et al. Fundus changes in membranoproliferative glomerulonephritis type II. A fluorescein angiographic study of 23 patients. *Graefes Arch Clin Exp Ophthalmol* 1991;229:406–410.
31. Leys A, Van Damme B, Verberckmoes R. Ocular complications of type 2 membranoproliferative glomerulonephritis. *Nephrol Dial Transplant* 1996;11:211–214.
32. Leys A, Vanrenterghem Y, Van Damme B, et al. Sequential observation of fundus changes in patients with long standing membranoproliferative glomerulonephritis type II (MPGN type II). *Eur J Ophthalmol* 1991;1:17–22.
33. Michielsen B, Leys A, Van Damme B, et al. Fundus changes in chronic membranoproliferative glomerulonephritis type II. *Doc Ophthalmol* 1990;76:219–229.
34. Leys A, Michielsen B, Leys M, et al. Subretinal neovascular membranes associated with chronic membranoproliferative glomerulonephritis type II. *Graefes Arch Clin Exp Ophthalmol* 1990;228:499–504.
35. O'Brien C, Duvall-Young J, Brown M, et al. Electrophysiology of type II mesangiocapillary glomerulonephritis with associated fundus abnormalities. *Br J Ophthalmol* 1993;77:778–780.
36. McAvoy CE, Silvestri G. Retinal changes associated with type 2 glomerulonephritis. *Eye* 2005;19:985–989.
37. Mullins RF, Aptsiauri N, Hageman GS. Structure and composition of drusen associated with glomerulonephritis: implications for the role of complement activation in drusen biogenesis. *Eye* 2001;15:390–395.
38. Hageman GS, Luthert PJ, Victor Chong NH, et al. An integrated hypothesis that considers drusen as biomarkers of immune-mediated processes at the RPE-Bruch's membrane interface in aging and age-related macular degeneration. *Prog Retin Eye Res* 2001;20:705–732.
39. Grassi MA, Folk JC, Scheetz TE, et al. Complement factor H polymorphism p.Tyr402His and cuticular drusen. *Arch Ophthalmol* 2007;125:93–97.
40. Boone CJF, Klevering BJ, Hoyng CB, et al. Basal laminar drusen caused by compound heterozygous variants in the CFH gene. *Am J Hum Genet* 2008;82:516–523.
41. Gold B, Merriam JE, Zernant J, et al. Variation in factor B (BF) and complement component 2 (C2) genes is associated with age-related macular degeneration. *Nat Genet* 2006;38:458–462.
42. Yates JR, Sepp T, Matharu G, et al. Complement C3 variant and the risk of age-related macular degeneration. *N Engl J Med* 2007;357:553–561.
43. Ormsby RJ, Ranganathan S, Tong JC, et al. Functional and structural implications of the complement factor HY402H polymorphism associated with age-related macular degeneration. *Invest Ophthalmol Vis Sci* 2008;49:1763–1770.
44. Johnson PT, Betts KE, Radeke MJ, et al. Individuals homozygous for the age-related macular degeneration risk-conferring variant of complement factor H have elevated levels of CRP in the choroid. *PNAS* 2006;103:17456–17461.
45. Seddon JM, Francis PJ, George S, et al. Association of CFH Y402H and LOC387715 A69S with progression of age-related macular degeneration. *JAMA* 2007;297:1793–1800.
46. Schmidt S, Hauser Michael A, Scott WK, et al. Cigarette Smoking Strongly Modifies the Association of LOC387715 and Age-Related Macular Degeneration. *Am J Hum Genet* 2006;78:852–864.

32

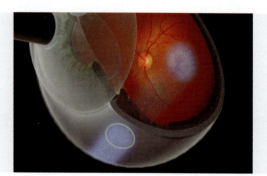

# Radiotherapy Treatment for Age-Related Macular Degeneration

Raul Velez-Montoya ■ Virgilio Morales-Canton ■ Hugo Quiroz-Mercado

## INTRODUCTION

Age-related macular degeneration (AMD) is a complex disease and difficult to define. Since its first description by Holloway and Verhoeff in 1929 as a condition characterized by the loss of vision in older patients due to degenerative changes in the retina pigment epithelium (RPE) (1), the amount of knowledge about this disease, as well as the interest in finding an adequate therapy, has been increasing exponentially. Eighty years later, despite all the resources and efforts put forth to better understand the etiology and pathophysiology of AMD, many of its mechanisms remain elusive.

As life expectancy in developed countries and around the world has increased, AMD incidence has also risen to become the leading cause of vision loss among individuals aged 50 years or older (2–4). It is believed that the annual incidence of some degree of AMD among patients 60 years or older reaches 40% to 50%. AMD-related disability and poor quality of life have become heavy socioeconomic burdens in industrialized countries (5–7).

Although most AMD patients suffer the atrophic or "dry" form, the neovascular or "wet" form will be found in more than 10% of the cases. Wet AMD is characterized by deep choroidal neovascularization (CNV), subretinal fluid (SRF), subretinal hemorrhage (SRH), exudates, scarring, and severe visual loss (8–11). The natural history of the disease dictates that approximately 75% of the patients with subfoveal exudative lesions will become legally blind after 2 years (12,13). Population studies such as the Beaver Dam Eye Study demonstrated that approximately 10% to 20% of patients with the dry form of AMD will progress to the exudative form (especially if the patient's retina exhibits large drusen [≥125 μm], soft indistinct drusen, retinal pigment epithelium abnormalities, or exudative and geographic lesions). This phenomenon of dry to wet progression was likely responsible for most of the estimated 1.2 million cases of visual loss due to AMD (14–16) which occurred in the 1990s in the United States and may lead to 7 million by the year 2025, given that 4% of the wet AMD cases are classified as severe (17) (Fig. 32-1).

Although the etiology of the AMD is still largely unknown, there has been an improvement in understanding the pathophysiology of the disease. In a normal eye, the byproducts of photoreceptor metabolism are usually removed by the RPE cells (18). It is believed that the aging process slows down RPE metabolism, diminishing its phagocytosis and lysosomal capacity, and resulting in accumulation of cell debris, clinically seen as drusen (5,18,19). Over time, these changes gradually thicken Bruch's membrane and make it more hydrophobic, impairing oxygen delivery to photoreceptors (19–21). It is not clear why this aging process ends in cell loss and atrophy in dry AMD, while in the wet form it stimulates a choroidal neovascular response. What we do know is that the hypoxia induces a low-grade inflammatory cascade which ends in the production of several growth factors, including vascular endothelial growth factor (VEGF), found to have a key role in CNV pathogenesis (2,22). VEGF is a dimeric lipoprotein whose principal biological activity is to produce an increase in the vascularization of hypoxic

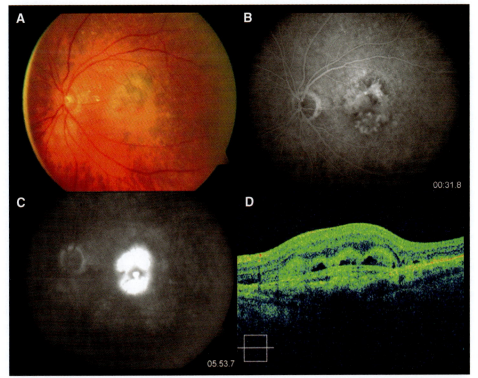

**Figure 32-1.** Color picture **(A)**, fluorescein angiography **(B and C)**, and spectral domain optical coherence tomography **(D)** of a 65-year-old female with clinical diagnosis of wet age-related macular degeneration. The color picture shows the presence of subretinal fibrosis and subretinal hemorrhage. **B** and **C** show middle and late fluorescein leakage, which indicates an active lesion. **D** shows the presence of a subretinal hyperreflective lesion (fibrosis) and hyperreflective spaces, which may indicate the presence of blood or subretinal fluid.

tissues (23,24). This is accomplished through several mechanisms: increase in the mitotic activity of vascular endothelial cells; increase in vascular permeability via leukocyte-mediated endothelial cell injury, formation of fenestrae and dissolution of tight junctions; and induction of activated endothelial cells to produce enzymes and metalloproteinases which digest the capillaries' basement membrane, the surrounding ground substance, and Bruch's membrane, thus forming spaces and breaks through which newly formed vessels pass into the subretinal space (2,18,23–26).

It has also been demonstrated by histological studies that a granulomatous inflammatory response to the degenerated Bruch's membrane is additionally responsible for the formation of breaks (23–30). This is supported by the observation of lymphocyte and macrophage infiltration of Bruch's membrane and accumulation of macrophages at the site of neovascularization in some animal models of laser-induced CNV (23–30). However, it is still unknown whether this inflammatory response is part of the aging process of the eye or if the macrophage and lymphocyte activation is necessary for the CNV process (23).

Once the CNV reaches the subretinal space, the visual impairment will be closely related to the lesion size, the amount of exudates, and thickness of the disciform fibrosis. Any therapeutic approach that helps to control or reduce the three pathways of VEGF action described earlier may result in the stabilization or improvement of visual acuity in patients with wet AMD (31,32).

## Basics About Radiation Therapy for AMD

The application of radiation to treat AMD is based on the concept that CNV formation is analogous to a wound-healing process, where the high rate of proliferating endothelial cells makes them more sensitive to the effects of radiation (33–35). Reinhold described that a single dose of 8.7 Gy on normal capillaries leads within hours to swelling and vacuolation of the endothelium cells' cytoplasm and local vasodilation (8,36). Reinhold also describes that the radiation effects continue through time, until the loss of endothelial nuclei occurs and a reduction is seen in the number and length of the capillaries and occlusive changes (8,36,37). The clinical effect of radiation on the eye vessels was first described in plaque-irradiated choroidal melanoma patients where, following plaque removal, a ring of choroidal atrophy with decreased or absent blood flow by fluorescein angiography (FA) was observed around the tumor's base (18,38). A similar response has also been seen in choroidal hemangiomas and intracerebral arteriovenous malformations, where radiation is used to induce regression, and in ocular and cutaneous wounds, where radiation stunts the growth of newly formed vessels without thermal injury associated with lasers and cautery (8,18,34,39–41).

Although the biological justification to use radiation to treat CNV seems clear, there is controversy regarding the exact mechanism that drives the radio effect (42). The use of ionizing radiation induces the formation of free radicals (mainly from water molecules), which in turn cause irreparable damage to the DNA backbone and disrupt protein synthesis. The irradiated cell loses its ability to replicate and migrate but does not lose its cellular integrity nor undergoes necrosis (33–35). On the other hand, there is evidence that radiation induces

programmed cell death *in vivo* (33–35,43,44). Miyamoto *et al.* studied the histologic appearance of rabbit eyes with experimental CNV, 4 weeks after a single fraction exposure to 20 Gy of focal X-ray irradiation (45,46). The degree of vascular formation and the number of endothelial cells in the CNV of irradiated eyes were less than in those of control eyes. And although the pathogenesis of experimental CNV and CNV due to AMD are not identical (45,46), the selective toxicity of radiation on rapidly dividing endothelial cells seems clear.

The use of sublethal radiation doses, low enough to spare cell life but high enough to induce DNA damage, can produce growth arrest by altering the genes of endothelial-growth–regulating cytokines and genes of inflammatory cytokines interactively affecting different cell populations (8,47,48). *In vitro* investigations of radiated endothelial cells showed an upregulation of basal intracellular adhesion molecule-1, which participates in the radiation-induced inflammatory reaction of the endothelium, facilitating inflammatory cells adhesion (49). All these actions decrease the CNV growth profile and the inflammatory response, which is thought by many to play a role in the formation of CNV (18,50,51).

Although radiation effects on endothelial cells are important in its ability to impact CNV, the power of radiation to affect inflammatory cells and fibroblasts is also a key factor, as it alters the formation and deposition of collagen, ultimately inhibiting scarring and fibrosis, which are important components of end-stage AMD (32,39,40,52). The results of the Belfast Study Group, showing that deterioration of visual acuity is less marked and scars are smaller in irradiated eyes than in untreated eyes at 6 to 24 months of follow-up, and that there is a positive correlation between scar size and better visual acuity, seem to support this assertion (53,54). Radiation reduces the expression of basic fibroblast growth factor and transforming growth factor β1, as well as the synthesis of prostacyclin (32,55), which decreases fibroblast proliferation and collagen deposition *in vitro*, and may play a role in reshaping the disciform scars in radiated eyes (32).

Despite the fact that radiation is potentially damaging to the retina, optic nerve, and the lacrimal system, the most frequently described adverse effects of clinical radiation in the eye are epiphora and transient conjunctival irritation (14). The rod photoreceptors are the most radiosensitive cells in the retina; cell death, however, is not seen at doses less than 10 Gy and RPE cell loss does not occur at less than 20 Gy (14). Radiation retinopathy is unlikely to occur at doses of 25 Gy or less, especially if delivered in fractions and/or over small volumes of the retina (8,56–58). But even though the retina and REP are the most radiosensitive tissue of the eye (59), it is the lens that is the most sensitive to long-term exposure. Radiation damage to the lens occurs on two levels: acute radical reactions involving lens crystallins or enzymes of the carbohydrate metabolism and the oxidative defense system, leading to transient or definitive transparency changes, and radiation-induced damage to DNA of lens epithelial cells (14,59–62).

We can therefore speculate that there is a therapeutic window where radiation can spare normal tissue but yet have a selective toxicity over the endothelium, fibroblasts, and inflammatory cascade, targeting specific pathways that pharmacologic anti-VEGF therapy does not presently reach by itself (18).

## EARLY EXPERIENCE WITH RADIATION THERAPY FOR AMD

For over 30 years, studies investigating the use of radiotherapy in the treatment of AMD have shown mixed results. To recount every single published paper on the subject would be impractical, if not tedious. Since many of these publications addressed case series, uncontrolled small studies, and other less reliable data, only the most relevant (in the authors' opinion) will be mentioned here. The general treatment options consisted of two broad strategies: (a) teletherapy (delivering a beam of radiation over a distance to the patient) using external beam, proton beam, charged particles, or gamma-knife and (b) plaque brachytherapy using radioactive isotopes (I-125, Palladium-103 [Pd-103], Strontium-90 [Sr-90], ruthenium [Rhu]) (Fig. 32-2). Broadly speaking, plaque brachytherapy was superior to teletherapy with respect to targeting and complications. This is primarily because the brachytherapy plaque was sewn onto the sclera directly over the macula. The treatment volume was constrained to a limited region, and the optic nerve and nonmacular retina received much less energy than with teletherapy, unless, of course, the plaque became dislodged over the course of the several-day–long treatment. The obvious drawback to plaque brachytherapy was that, due to its position immediately over the macula, the plaque (and the radiation) was directly aimed at the lens. For all intents and purposes, this meant that every phakic patient developed a cataract shortly after therapy. The second drawback was that it required two surgeries—one to place the radioactive plaque and the second to remove it. These surgeries often necessitated disinsertion of one or more muscles, and double vision was not an uncommon complication. Of course, the development of a cataract often required yet another operation to replace the lens.

### Experience with Plaque Brachytherapy

The first isotope employed in a pilot study for the treatment of wet AMD using plaque brachytherapy was Pd-103 (63). In this first study, Finger *et al.* treated six patients with 12-15 Gy, resulting in a decrease in hemorrhage, exudates, and leakage on FA, while sparing the neurosensory retina, with no evidence of radiation retinopathy or optic neuropathy (63). Based on the positive result of this preliminary study, a pilot open label, uncontrolled, nonrandomized phase I study was designed, where 23 patients received Pd-103 plaque brachytherapy for the treatment of wet AMD, with a dose ranging from 12.5 to 23.62 Gy (64). The mean follow-up was 19 ± 10.7 months. In this second study, a moderate visual acuity loss (≤3 ETDRS lines) was seen in 16% of subjects at 6 months, 31% at 12 months, and 22% at 24 months of follow-up (64). For data analysis, the funduscopic and angiographic findings were grouped in the following categories: (a) improved lesions—decreased or resolved hemorrhage, exudates, and/or fluid; (b) stable lesions—relatively unchanged or minimal enlargement; and (c) progressive—increased lesion size (64). For all lesions at last follow-up, there was an 87% rate of stable or improved funduscopic and angiographic findings, but approximately 30% of the cases developed recurrent lesions (64). The rate of progression at 19 months was 9%, and 61% were stable or improved (64). There were no reported cases of radiation retinopathy, optic nerve injury, or complications related to the surgical technique. The same authors, in a separate report (2003), described the outcomes of a 7-year follow-up of 31 eyes treated with Pd-103 brachytherapy (65). The mean radiation dose was 17.25 Gy (range 12.5 to 24 Gy) in a single fraction. The visual acuity results at last follow-up (mean 33.3 months, range 3 to 84 months) included loss of >3 ETDRS lines at 55%; improvement of >3 ETDRS lines at 16%; and within 2 ETDRS lines from baseline at 29% (65). The most common anatomic outcome (69%) was regression or stabilization of the exudative process. The authors reported a rate of severe visual loss (>6 ETDRS lines) at 6 months in 4% of the subjects, which progressed to 5% at 12 months and 25% at 48 months. At last follow-up, no patient had developed radiation retinopathy, optic neuropathy, or cataract (65).

Another isotope which has also been extensively explored as plaque brachytherapy is Sr-90 (66). In a study carried out by Jaakkola *et al.* in 1998, 20 patients received a 54-minute

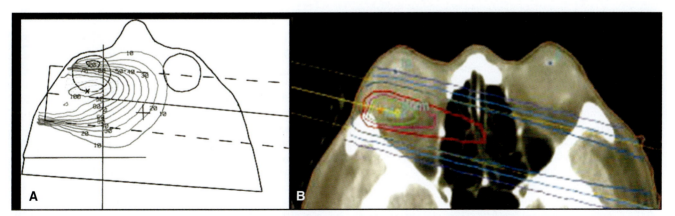

**Figure 32-2.** Treatment plan and schematization of teletherapy for AMD. **A:** Dose distribution and treatment plan of a 16-MV electron beam of 4 × 4 cm². The macula is enclosed by the 100% isodose, while the rest of the orbit also receives radiation. **B:** Computer tomography with superimposed treatment plan showing the isodose distribution for 6-MV photon beam. The green circle shows the 95% isodose, focused on the fovea. (Part A from Lambooij AC, Kuijpers RW, Mooy CM, et al. Radiotherapy of exudative age-related macular degeneration; a clinical and pathologic study. *Graefes Arch Clin Exp Ophthalmol* 2001;239:539–543. Part B from Eter N, Wegener A, Schüller H, et al. Radiotherapy for age related macular degeneration causes transient lens transparency changes. *Br J Ophthalmol* 2000;84:757–760.)

application of Sr-90 to achieve a dose of 15 Gy. The visual acuity was within 5 letters of baseline or improved in 55% of patients, and 74% of patients demonstrated either a decrease in CNV size or a decrease in the amount of late leakage on FA (66). At 12 months of follow-up, 74% of patients demonstrated partial or total occlusion of the CNV (66). Two years later, the same authors published a larger randomized controlled clinical study which appeared to include the previous 20 patients (67). On this occasion, 86 patients divided into a study (43) and a control (43) group were included. The study group was again divided into two subgroups. The first one (18 patients) received a 54-minute therapy consisting of 15 Gy, and the second one (25 patients) received an 11-minute therapy consisting of 12.6 Gy (67). During the first 12 months of the study, the treated group had a significantly lesser risk of moderate visual loss (>15 ETDRS letters), but that advantage diminished by 24 and 36 months of follow-up. The 15-Gy dose seemed to be superior to the 12.6 Gy in terms of moderate visual acuity loss (67). The FA outcomes demonstrated statistically significantly less lesion activity with respect to baseline at the 6-month follow-up in 37.5% of the patients and 56.4% at the 12-month follow-up, favoring the study group (67).

Other isotopes have additionally been investigated for plaque brachytherapy treatment of wet AMD, including ruthenium-106 (Rhu-106), without reported adverse effects to the retina (68,69).

## Experience with Teletherapy

In this treatment modality, the most broadly explored techniques were the use of proton beam, external beam megavoltage X-ray (EBRT), and the gamma-knife. The theoretical advantage of proton beam over EBRT to treat AMD is based on the superior distribution of radiation dose due to the physical properties of the protons, which allow low-dose delivery at entry, a focused delivery at the target, and a minimal exit dose (70,71). Therefore, proton beams, unlike EBRT photons, can be designed to yield a uniform dose across the target, allowing the treatment of relatively small areas with critical structures nearby (71).

The clinical effect, however, was essentially the same, as each tissue has a threshold below which radiation exposure results in damage that is repaired contemporaneously and above which radiation exposure results in pathologic changes and complications (72). The volume of tissue exposed to the radiation plays a significant role in potential development of undesirable effects. This volume is not readily apparent in most teletherapy experience with wet AMD treatment, as it depends on multiple and dynamic factors. For proton beam and EBRT, the beam size ranges from 1 to 1.2 cm. The patient is seated in a restrained position, with a thermoplastic mask and bite block to hold the head, and a fixation target to guide the eye (70–72). The beam is transmitted from a source located across the room; the radiation technician is monitoring the patient's eye with a video camera and is instructed to cut off the radiation if the eye strays from a predetermined coordinate. There is also a temporal component; the radiation is delivered in multiple fractions over 10 to 20 days. Thus, for the targeting to be as prescribed, the patient has to be positioned so that the head does not move or rotate in any axis, that the eye likewise does not move or rotate, and such that the head and eye are located in the same coordinate for 10 to 20 consecutive treatments, often with different operators on various treatment days. As one might imagine, under such circumstances, targeting is not constrained to the macula; hence, the need for bigger spot size to ensure that the macula is being treated (57,72–74).

Therefore, due to the reasons outlined earlier, the historical evidence about the results of traditional teletherapy in treating wet AMD is somewhat contradictory. Some studies report success in stabilizing visual acuity and reducing the size of lesion and scarring; however, most of these studies also report high rates of recurrence and short-term effect. Other studies simply cannot find a difference in disease progression between the control groups and treated groups (8,12, 18,45,53,75–79). The Cochrane review of radiotherapy for AMD evaluated 11 studies with 1078 patients who received external beam radiotherapy ranging in doses from 7.5 to 24 Gy in 1 to 10 fractions and made the following conclusions: (a) most trials demonstrated beneficial effects, although there was considerable heterogeneity in patients, dose, and lesion composition (79); (b) uncontrolled reports demonstrated a trend toward greater efficacy, supported by lesion composition on FA, particularly with respect to classic CNV (79); (c) not all studies specifically looked at FA as an outcome, and of the five that did, one demonstrated a beneficial effect of therapy (change in lesion size), while four showed no difference compared with controls (79). The most common adverse effect was cataract (59–62,79) and there were no reported cases of radiation retinopathy, optic neuropathy, or malignancy in the 1078 patients (79).

A Harvard group evaluated 166 patients over 24 months in a randomized, open-label, uncontrolled, single-center study using two doses: 16 and 24 cobalt gray equivalent (CGE) in two fractions over 2 to 3 days (70). The treatment plan included the entire CNV lesion plus a 2-mm surrounding margin (70). The group found no dose-dependent differences in the rates of moderate visual acuity loss, with 42% versus 35% and 62% versus 53% at the 16 versus 24 CGE doses at 12 and 24 months of follow-up, respectively ($p = .40$) (70).

## CURRENT RESEARCH ON RADIOTHERAPY FOR WET AMD

The high variability of results that has, up to now, been demonstrated in the use of radiotherapy for wet AMD has prevented this treatment modality from becoming a mainstay in the management of the disease. This variability, coupled with the relatively good results (in terms of visual acuity and safety) seen with other treatment modalities such as intravitreal administration of antiangiogenic drugs, has relegated radiotherapy to only a secondary or supportive role (26,80,81). Nevertheless, currently accepted therapeutics for wet AMD (antiangiogenic compounds, photodynamic therapy, and intravitreal steroids) exhibit some significant drawbacks (81,82). The lack of effect durability and the need for frequent retreatments (often monthly) are two of the most important.

Consequently, there has been an evolution in the way in which radiation has been historically delivered to the eye for the treatment of wet AMD, and newer technologies are presently under investigation. These allow more precise localization of energy on the CNV target, with less exposure to the surrounding retina and other eye structures. The newer technologies are being clinically tested in conjunction with antiangiogenic therapy, and preliminary results appear to show considerable promise, both in terms of safety and efficacy improvements upon the prior radiotherapy experience described earlier. The current approaches to radiation treatment of wet AMD include both improved brachytherapy and a novel low-voltage stereotactic external beam system.

## Intraocular Brachytherapy Approach

This interesting research is based on the previous success of plaque brachytherapy and the notion that radiation delivery from outside the eye leads to a "supertherapeutic" dose which potentially adversely affects the choroid and sclera. A device has been built which allows focal delivery of beta radiation intraocularly, directly over the CNV (35,83). This device consists of a hollow stainless steel handpiece with a Sr-90 seed in equilibrium with yttrium-90 on the tip, the latter being the daughter product of Sr-90 after beta decay (Fig. 32-3). Yttrium-90 is a stronger beta emitter than Sr-90 and is the main component of the therapeutic effect. The position of the radioactive source is controlled by a hand-activated slide mechanism. When the mechanism is in the storage (retracted) position, the radioactive seed is shielded inside an aluminum and tungsten alloy shaft. When activated into the treatment position, the radioactive seed is deployed to the tip of the shaft, which has minimum shielding (0.1 mm stainless steel), allowing the radiation to treat the CNV. The shaft is completely sealed, preventing direct contact of the radioactive seed with the intraocular tissue. A mark on the tip of the probe aids in the positioning of the device (35,83). The instrument is calibrated to deliver doses of 15 and 24 Gy in as little as 3 to 5 minutes. The treatment procedure consists of a conventional pars plana core vitrectomy, followed by the introduction of the probe containing the radioactive seed. The surgeon holds the tip of the probe over the CNV and activates the device.

The safety of the surgical procedure, as well as the safety of the radiation procedure, was validated in two separate animal studies. In the first, 10 rabbits went through the entire treatment as designed, but using a dummy device (no radiation). None of the rabbits showed any complication during the procedure or after 1 month of follow-up (35,83). In the second study, 120 rabbits were irradiated with the device, using escalated doses up to 246 Gy. The authors did not observe any retinal or subretinal tissue damage in doses below 103 Gy (data on file, not published; NeoVista, Inc.) (35,83).

There are two published clinical reports about the use of this technique in humans (35,83). In the first one, Avila et al. describe the safety and visual acuity results at 12-month follow-up in a nonrandomized, multicenter study (83). The study included 34 patients with either predominantly or minimally classic or occult CNV due to AMD, with baseline best-corrected visual acuity (BCVA) between 20/70 and 20/400. The population was divided into two subgroups for later analysis: the first one included all the patients, regardless of the existence of deviations from protocol ($N = 34$), and the second included only those patients who did not have major protocol deviations ($N = 23$). In the first group, 8 patients received treatment at 15 Gy and 26 patients received treatment at the 24-Gy dose. In the second group, 5 patients received treatment at 15 Gy and 18 patients received treatment at 24 Gy. The follow-up appointments were scheduled to be every 3 months during the first year and every 6 months during the rest of the follow-up. This study mentions only the results of the first 12 months' follow-up (83). In the safety analysis, the reported adverse effects were attributed to the surgical technique and not to the radiation procedure (two retinal tears and 11 patients developed cataract). During the first year of follow-up, 9 of the 11 patients who developed cataract had it removed, with intraocular lens implantation. The study report did not mention if the

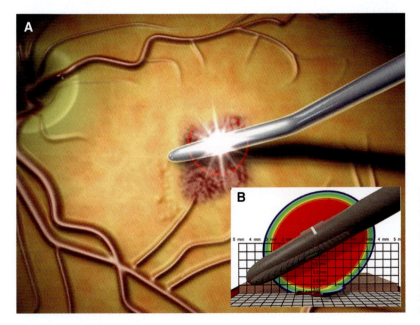

**Figure 32-3.** Graphic representation of the epiretinal radiation device. **A:** Shows how the device is placed over the macular after a core vitrectomy for the local treatment of AMD. **B:** Shows the critical relationship between the actual position of the handpiece and the dose of radiation delivered to the tissue, since any variation in distance of the probe tip from the retina could result in a significant variation in the actual dose. (From Avila MP, Farah ME, Santos A, et al. Twelve-month safety and visual acuity results from a feasibility study of intraocular, epiretinal radiation therapy for the treatment of subfoveal CNV secondary to AMD. *Retina* 2009;29:157–169.)

phacoemulsification was part of the original protocol; however, the visual acuity results could be altered due to this procedure, and the study outcomes must therefore be considered accordingly. All patients in the second group lost fewer than 15 letters (3 lines) at 12 months. Forty percent of the patients treated with 15 Gy had no loss or improved vision at 12 months. Among patients treated with 24 Gy, 72% had no loss or improved vision at 12 months and 28% experienced gains more than 15 letters (83).

In the second report, again Avila *et al.* described the safety and visual acuity results of a 12-month prospective multicenter study, where a combined therapy of intraocular bevacizumab and 24 Gy epiretinal radiation was applied (35). Patients with all types of CNV lesions were included. Thirty-four treatment-naïve patients were enrolled in this study, but only 24 met all the inclusion/exclusion criteria. The adverse events reported were related to the device or to the procedure, and no radiation-related events were noted (35). There were one case of SRH, one retinal tear, two cases of subretinal fibrosis, one case of epiretinal membrane, and six patients developed cataract (25% of the phakic study eyes) during follow-up. Eight patients showed evidence of CNV activity by optical coherence tomography (OCT) during follow-up and were retreated with intravitreal bevacizumab. Only one patient needed more than one retreatment (35).

At 12 months, 91% of patients treated with 24 Gy and intravitreal bevacizumab lost fewer than 15 letters and 68% had stable or improved vision. Nearly 40% (13/34) of patients gained 15 or more letters at the end of follow-up. There was also a 71.8-µm reduction on central retinal thickness measured by OCT at the last observation (35).

Recruitment for a multicenter randomized, controlled trial of epiretinal brachytherapy was completed in 2009, although results of the study have not yet become available at the time of this writing (for more information, visit www.clinicaltrials.gov, CABERNET study).

In summary, epiretinal brachytherapy is a new approach to radiotherapy for wet AMD. The results of the early investigations are promising but there are some drawbacks. First, there is a relatively high rate of adverse events, some of which are potentially sight threatening (although attributed to the surgical procedure and not radiation). Second, the high incidence of cataract formation and the need of surgery to correct this problem can discourage the patients from trying this new treatment. And finally, but perhaps most importantly, the low tissue penetration of the Sr-90 beta radiation requires the surgeon to keep the tip of the device in close, steady contact with the retina throughout the entire exposure time, since any deviation in probe tip position, no matter how small, could significantly reduce the dose to the CNV and spread the radiation to unintended regions of the retina, or to other eye structures, like the optic nerve (35,83).

## Low-Voltage Stereotactic Radiosurgery Approach

Another approach currently being investigated to improve the delivery of radiation to the CNV lesion involves a system specifically designed to stereotactically place low-voltage X-rays directly onto the macula, avoiding surrounding critical structures of the eye and irradiating only a very small volume of the retina. The device consists of a robotically positioned low-energy X-ray tube, an eye stabilization, alignment and tracking component, and automated safety features. The system delivers up to 24 Gy to the macular target, using three highly collimated sequential beams, which project through the pars plana via distinct sclera entry positions and overlap at the retina. The individual beams are approximately 4 mm wide at the target, comprising a 6-mm treatment diameter at the 80% to 90% isodose line. Energy fall-off is extremely sharp, such that exposure to the optic nerve and other nontargeted structures is minimized. The device has built-in shielding, providing radiation safety for the clinical staff and obviating the need for extrinsic radiation protection, as required for linear accelerators and other radiotherapeutic devices (Fig. 32-4).

Safety of this radiation system was confirmed in an animal study using Yucatan mini-swine, in which data to 9 months' follow-up indicate a dose-dependent progressive radiological effect in the retina of the investigational animals, consistent with the design parameters of the device (data not published, personal communication). In this study, 12 eyes were randomized to 6 treatment groups. Ten eyes were doused with radiation and two eyes served as untreated controls. The device was used to deliver X-rays stereotactically to the retina of each eye, in doses of 0, 16, 24, 42, 60, and 90 Gy. Animals were evaluated on days 7, 30, 90, 150, 210, and 270 with a full ocular examination, intraocular pressure measurements, fundus photography/FA, OCT, and routine veterinary assessments. An additional assessment involving indocyanine green angiograms was added during the study to provide further imaging of the choroidal vasculature. Examinations were performed at approximately day 110 and were repeated at the end of the study. Computer tomography (CT) and magnetic resonance imaging (MRI) were also performed at the conclusion of the study to further evaluate orbital bone and cranial neurological tissues for any possible radiation effects. Histopathology was obtained at the conclusion of the investigation. Ophthalmic examinations revealed progressively more pronounced retinal hypopigmented lesions as early as the first month of follow-up in both 90 Gy eyes, one 60 Gy eye and the other 42 Gy eye. A small focal lesion was also observed at month 7 in a second 42 Gy eye. These lesions were anatomically located in the area expected to have been targeted by the X-ray beams. Fundus photographs and angiography provided clear evidence of dose-dependent progressive changes in the retina beyond those observed on ophthalmoscopy. The higher dose eyes (42 Gy and above) showed well-demarcated circular lesions approximately equal to beam diameter, thus confirming the accuracy of the convergent beams. OCT was consistent with the fundus photography findings. A clear transition zone was seen, indicating injury within the area targeted by radiation. This effect was progressive over time, but confined to the irradiated zone, with no propagation in area. Postmortem histopathology confirmed the dose–response seen via imaging and demonstrated no radiation effects outside of the zone targeted on the retina. No adverse radiation effects were observed on histopathology at the clinically relevant doses of 16 and 24 Gy.

At the time of this writing, no data have yet been published about human clinical trials involving this stereotactic device, though there have been numerous presentations and

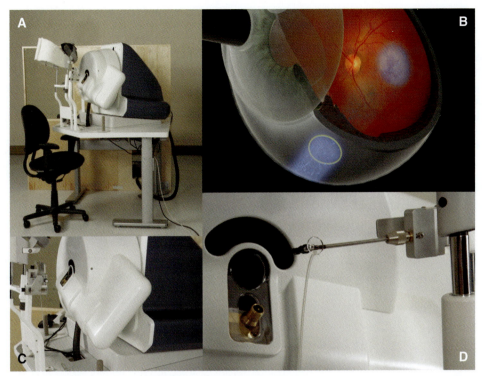

**Figure 32-4.** Investigational stereotactic low-voltage X-ray device. **A** and **C:** The system and a close-up of the robotically positioned X-ray tube. **B:** A graphic representation of how the highly collimated beams pass through the sclera at the pars plana, sparing the lens and optic disk and targeting the macula. **D:** The eye stabilization and tracking device.

posters at various ophthalmology conferences worldwide (ARVO meeting 2009; Poster 5007/A608, SOE 2009, E-Poster, ARVO meeting 2010; Poster 85/A132, ASRS New York 2009, ASRS Vancouver 2010). In an ongoing clinical pilot study, the device was used to deliver an 11, 16, or 24 Gy dose of radiation to the macula, in conjunction with intravitreal injection of ranibizumab. The radiotherapy was delivered in a single session utilizing three sequential beams, each depositing up to 3.6, 5.3, or 8 Gy (for the 11, 16, and 24 Gy doses, respectively) at the macula through calculated scleral entry points and crossing the pars plana region of the eye. Ranibizumab 0.5 mg was administered by intravitreal injection at days 0 and 30 and subsequently as required according to specified rescue criteria. Radiation was administered at day 14. Subjects were evaluated monthly with a full ocular examination, visual acuity measurement (ETDRS chart at a distance of 4 m), FA, and spectral domain OCT.

A total of 62 subjects were enrolled, representing both anti-VEGF treatment-naïve and previously treated cohorts of wet AMD patients. The study shows a favorable safety profile and demonstrates that treatment with this system may be effective in the management of wet AMD, as indicated by the outcomes on visual acuity, OCT, and FA. Overall, there have been few adverse events in the study population, and, other than mild, transient superficial keratopathy postprocedure, only one other event (mild headache), was considered to be related to the study intervention because of its temporal relationship to the treatment. There were five serious adverse events, all nonocular and unrelated to radiotherapy.

Stabilization or improvement in BCVA has been demonstrated for the majority of patients in this study. On average, subjects gained 8 to 10 letters of BCVA, and this has generally been maintained through the available subject follow-up. In addition, stability and improvement in BCVA is associated with the majority of subjects not requiring further concomitant treatment with anti-VEGF. In fact, 52% of subjects in the 16 Gy cohort (14/27) did not require further injections after month 1 through month 12; during this time period, the other 48% required a total of 26 injections. For those subjects who did require further injections, the average number was 2; for the group as a whole, the average number of injections per patient was 0.9 during the first year. This finding suggests that radiotherapy might be able to decrease a patient's dependency on continued, frequent anti-VEGF treatment.

In addition, visual acuity findings in this study correlate with anatomic data, which show that, on average, OCT images exhibit a consistent trend toward decreased retinal thickness, and FAs demonstrate mean decreased total lesion and CNV sizes.

At the time of this writing, a double-masked, sham-controlled, dose-ranging multicenter clinical study evaluating this stereotactic system has also been initiated, with more than 75 patients treated to date (data not published yet, personal communication). This study will involve 150 to 300 subjects with CNV secondary to neovascular AMD at multiple sites across Europe. The objective is to confirm the safety of low-voltage external beam radiosurgery using at two dose levels (16 and 24 Gy) and to determine if the system is effective in sparing the number of anti-VEGF injections during the first 12 months. Patients will be randomized (2:1:1:1) to 16 Gy radiation + PRN ranibizumab:sham 16 Gy radiation + PRN ranibizumab:24 Gy radiation + PRN ranibizumab:sham 24 Gy radiation + PRN ranibizumab and will be followed for 2 years.

In summary, low-voltage stereotactic radiation is another new approach to radiotherapy for wet AMD. The results of the early investigations are promising, and further data from randomized, sham-controlled trials are expected to shed additional light upon this emerging treatment modality.

## ACKNOWLEDGMENTS

The authors thank E. Mark Shusterman, M.D., and Darius Moshfeghi, M.D., for their help in completing this manuscript and Oraya, Inc. and NeoVista, Inc. for contributing information regarding their respective technologies and research data. The authors do not have any economic, proprietary, or financial interest to disclose, in the publication of this chapter.

## References

1. Holloway TB, Verhoeff FH. Disklike degeneration of the macula: with microscopic report of a tumor-like mass in the macular region. *Arch Opthal* 1929;1:219–230.
2. Do DV. Antiangiogenic approaches to age-related macular degeneration in the future. *Ophthalmology* 2009;116(10, Suppl):S24–S26.
3. Friedman DS, O'Colmain BJ, Munoz B, et al. Prevalence of age-related macular degeneration in the United States. *Arch Ophthalmol* 2004;122:564–572.
4. Kellner U, Kellner S, Weinitz S. Fundus autofluorescence (488 NM) and near-infrared autofluorescence (787 NM) visualize different retinal pigment epithelium alterations in patients with age-related macular degeneration. *Retina* 2010;30:6–15.
5. Ivandic BT, Ivandic T. Low-level laser therapy improves vision in patients with age-related macular degeneration. *Photomed Laser Surg* 2008;26:241–245.
6. Apte RS, Scheufele TA, Blomquist PH. Etiology of blindness in an urban community hospital setting. *Ophthalmology* 2001;108:693–696.
7. Evans J, Wormald R. Is the incidence of registrable age-related macular degeneration increasing? *Br J Ophthalmol* 1996;80:9–14.
8. Krott R, Staar S, Müller RP, et al. External beam radiation in patients suffering from exudative age-related macular degeneration. A matched-pairs study and 1-year clinical follow-up. *Graefes Arch Clin Exp Ophthalmol* 1998;236:916–921.
9. Bird AC. Bruch's membrane change with age. *Br J Ophthalmol* 1992;76:166–168.
10. Hyman LG, Lilienfeld AM, Ferris FL III, et al. Senile macular degeneration: a case-control study. *Am J Epidemiol* 1983;118:213–227.
11. Klein BE, Klein R. Cataracts and macular degeneration in older Americans. *Arch Ophthalmol* 1982;100:571–573.
12. Haas A, Papaefthymiou G, Langmann G, et al. Gamma knife treatment of subfoveal, classic neovascularization in age-related macular degeneration: a pilot study. *J Neurosurg* 2000;93:172–176.
13. Bressler NM, Frost LA, Bressler SB, et al. Natural course of poorly defined choroidal neovascularization associated with macular degeneration. *Arch Ophthalmol* 1988;106:1537–1542.
14. Ciulla TA, Danis RP, Harris A. Age-related macular degeneration: a review of experimental treatments. *Surv Ophthalmol* 1998;43:134–146.
15. Tielsch JM, Javitt JC, Coleman A, et al. The prevalence of blindness and visual impairment among nursing home residents in Baltimore. *N Eng J Med* 1995;332:1205–1209.
16. Klein R, Klein BE, Lee KE. Changes in visual acuity in a population. The Beaver Dam Eye Study. *Ophthalmology* 1996;103:1169–1178.
17. Klein R, Klein BE, Lee KE, et al. Changes in visual acuity in a population over 15-year period: The Beaver Dam Eye Study. *Am J Ophthalmol* 2006;142:539–549.
18. Flaxel CJ. Use of radiation in the treatment of age-related macular degeneration. *Ophthalmol Clin North Am* 2002;15:437–444.
19. Moore DJ, Clover GM. The effect of age on the macromolecular permeability of human Bruch's membrane. *Invest Ophthalmol Vis Sci* 2001;42:2970–2975.
20. Liang FQ, Godley BF. Oxidative stress-induced mitochondrial DNA damage in human retinal pigment epithelial cells: a possible mechanism for RPE aging and age-related macular degeneration. *Exp Eye Res* 2003;76:397–403.
21. Ambati J, Ambati BK, Yoo SH, et al. Age-related macular degeneration: etiology, pathogenesis, and therapeutic strategies. *Surv Ophthalmol* 2003;48:257–293.
22. Barouch FC, Miller JW. Anti-vascular endothelial growth factor strategies for the treatment of choroidal neovascularization from age-related macular degeneration. *Int Ophthalmol Clin* 2004;44:23–32.
23. Kulkarni AD, Kuppermann BD. Wet age-related macular degeneration. *Adv Drug Deli Rev* 2005;57:1994–2009.
24. Leung DW, Cachianes G, Kuang WJ, et al. Vascular endothelial growth factor is a secreted angiogenic mitogen. *Science* 1989;46:1306–1309.
25. Ishida S, Usui T, Yamashiro K, et al. VEGF164-mediated inflammation is required for pathological, but not physiological, ischemia-induced retinal neovascularization. *J Exp Med* 2003;198:483–489.
26. Velez-Montoya R, Fromow-Guerra J, Burgos O, et al. The effect of unilateral intravitreal bevacizumab (Avastin), in the treatment of diffuse bilateral diabetic macular edema: a pilot study. *Retina* 2009;29:20–26.
27. Penfold PL, Killingsworth MC, Sarks SH. Senile macular degeneration: the involvement of immunocompetent cells. *Graefes Arch Clin Exp Ophthalmol* 1985;233:69–76.
28. Löffler HU, Lee WR. Basal lineal deposit in the human macula. *Graefes Arch Clin Exp Ophthalmol* 1986;224:493–501.
29. Penfold PL, Provis JM, Billson FA. Age-related macular degeneration: ultrastructural studies of the relationship of leucocytes to angiogenesis. *Graefes Arch Clin Exp Ophthalmol* 1987;225:70–76.
30. Ryan SJ. Subretinal neovascularization. Natural history of an experimental model. *Arch Ophthalmol* 1982;100:1804–1809.
31. Weiter JJ, Wing GL, Trempe CL, et al. Visual acuity related to retinal distance from the fovea in macular disease. *Ann Ophthalmol* 1984;16:174–176.
32. Haas A, Prettenhofer U, Stur M, et al. Morphologic characteristics of disciform scarring after radiation treatment for age-related macular degeneration. *Ophthalmology* 2000;107:1358–1363.
33. Kirwan JF, Constable PH, Murdoch IE, et al. Beta irradiation: new uses for an old treatment: a review. *Eye* 2003;17:207–215.
34. De Gowin RL, Lewis LJ, Hoak JC, et al. Radiosensitivity of human endothelial cells in culture. *J Lab Clin Med* 1974;84:42–48.
35. Avila MP, Farah ME, Santos A, et al. Twelve-month short-term safety and visual-acuity results from a multicentre prospective study of epiretinal strontium-90 brachytherapy with bevacizumab for the treatment of subfoveal choroidal neovascularisation secondary to age-related macular degeneration. *Br J Ophthalmol* 2009;93:305–309.
36. Reinhold HS. Vasculoconnective tissue. In: Scherer E, Streffer C, Trott KR (eds). *Radiopathology of organs and tissues.* Berlin, Heidelberg/New York: Springer, 1988:263–268.
37. Chakravarthy U, Houston FR, Archer DB. Treatment of age-related subfoveal neovascular membranes by teletherapy: a pilot study. *Br J Ophthalmol* 1993;77:265–273.
38. Finger PT. Radiation therapy for choroidal melanoma. *Surv Ophthalmol* 1997;42:215–232.
39. Chakravarthy U, Biggart JH, Gardiner TA, et al. Focal irradiation of perforating eye injuries. *Curr Eye Res* 1989;8:1241–1250.
40. Chakravarthy U, Gardiner TA, Archer DB, et al. A light microscopic and autoradiographic study of non-irradiated and irradiated ocular wounds. *Curr Eye Res* 1989;8:337–348.
41. Engenhart R, Wowra B, Debus J, et al. The role of high-dose, single-fraction irradiation in small and large intracranial arteriovenous malformations. *Int J Radiat Oncol Biol Phys* 1994;30:521–529.
42. Zhan Q, Carrier F, Fornace AJ Jr. Induction of cellular p53 activity by DNA-damaging agents and growth arrest. *Mol Cell Biol* 1993;13:4242–4250.
43. Verin V, Popowski Y, de Bruyne B, et al. Endoluminal beta-radiation therapy for the prevention of coronary restenosis after balloon angioplasty. The Dose-Finding Study Group. *N Engl J Med* 2001;344:243–249.
44. Wallace SS. Enzymatic processing of radiation-induced free radical damage in DNA. *Radiat Res* 1998;150:S60–S79.
45. Lambooij AC, Kuijpers RW, Mooy CM, et al. Radiotherapy of exudative age-related macular degeneration; a clinical and pathologic study. *Graefes Arch Clin Exp Ophthalmol* 2001;239:539–543.
46. Miyamoto H, Kimura H, Yasukawa T, et al. Effect of focal X-ray irradiation on experimental choroidal neovascularization. *Invest Ophthalmol Vis Sci* 1999;40:1496–1502.
47. Haimovitz-Friedman A, Vlodavsky I, Chaudhuri A, et al. Autocrine effects of fibroblast growth factor in repair of radiation damage in endothelial cells. *Cancer Res* 1991;51:2552–2558.
48. Hallahan DE, Virudachalam S, Schwartz JL, et al. Inhibition of protein kinases sensitizes human tumor cells to ionizing radiation. *Radiat Res* 1992;129:345–350.
49. Gaugler MH, Squiban C, van der Meeren A, et al. Late and persistent up-regulation of intercellular adhesion molecule-1 (ICAM-1) expression by ion-

izing radiation in human endothelial cells in vitro. *Int J Radiat Biol* 1997;72:201–209.

50. Finger PT, Chakravarthy U, Augsburger JJ. Radiotherapy and the treatment of age-related macular degeneration. External beam radiation therapy is effective in the treatment of age-related macular degeneration. *Arch Ophthalmol* 1998;116:1507–1511.

51. Krishnan L, Krishnan EC, Jewell WR. Immediate effect of irradiation on microvasculature. *Int J Radiat Oncol Biol Phys* 1988;15:147–150.

52. Velikay M, Stolba U, Wedrich A, et al. The antiproliferative effect of fractionalized radiation therapy: optimization of dosage. *Doc Ophthalmol* 1994;87:265–269.

53. Berginik GJ, Hoyng CB, van der Maazen RW, et al. A randomized controlled clinical trial on the efficacy of radiation therapy in the control of subfoveal choroidal neovascularization in age-related macular degeneration: radiation versus observation. *Graefes Arch Clin Exp Ophthalmol* 1998;236:321–325.

54. Hart PM, Chakravarthy U, MacKenzie G, et al. Teletherapy for subfoveal choroidal neovascularisation of age-related macular degeneration: results of follow up in a non-randomised study. *Br J Ophthalmol* 1996;80:1046–1050.

55. Noel F, Ijichi A, Chen JJ, et al. X-ray-mediated reduction in basic fibroblast growth factor expression in primary rat astrocyte cultures. *Radiat Res* 1997;147:484–489.

56. Chan RC, Shukovsky LJ. Effects of irradiation on the eye. *Radiology* 1976;120:673–675.

57. Parsons JT, Fitzgerald CR, Hood CI, et al. The effects of irradiation on the eye and optic nerve. *Int J Radiat Oncol Biol Phys* 1983;9:609–622.

58. Plowman PN, Harnett AN. Radiotherapy in benign orbital disease. I: Complicated ocular angiomas. *Br J Ophthalmol* 1988;72:286–288.

59. Amoaku WM, Frew L, Mahon GJ, et al. Early ultrastructural changes after low-dose X-irradiation in the retina of the rat. *Eye* 1989;3:638–646.

60. Eter N, Wegener A, Schüller H, et al. Radiotherapy for age related macular degeneration causes transient lens transparency changes. *Br J Ophthalmol* 2000;84:757–760.

61. MacFaul PA, Bedford MA. Ocular complications after therapeutic irradiation. *Br J Ophthalmol* 1970;54:237–247.

62. Gordon KB, Char DH, Segerman RH. Late effects of radiation on the eye and ocular adnexa. *Int Radiat Oncol Biol Phys* 1995;30:1123–1139.

63. Finger PT, Berson A, Sherr D, et al. Radiation therapy for subretinal neovascularization. *Ophthalmology* 1996;103:878–889.

64. Finger PT, Berson A, Ng T, et al. Ophthalmic plaque radiotherapy for age-related macular degeneration associated with subretinal neovascularization. *Am J Ophthalmol* 1999;127:170–177.

65. Finger PT, Gelman YP, Berson AM, et al. Palladium-103 plaque radiation therapy for macular degeneration: results of a 7 year study. *Br J Ophthalmol* 2003;87:1497–1503.

66. Jaakkola A, Heikkonen J, Tommila P, et al. Strontium plaque irradiation of subfoveal neovascular membranes in age-related macular degeneration. *Graefes Arch Clin Exp Ophthalmol* 1998;263:24–30.

67. Jaakkola A, Heikkonen J, Tommila P, et al. Strontium plaque brachytherapy for exudative age-related macular degeneration: three-year results of a randomized study. *Ophthalmology* 2005;112:567–573.

68. Furdová A, Strmen P. Brachytherapy in the treatment of age-related macular degeneration. *Bratisl Lek Listy* 2000;101:234–236.

69. Sari B, Siki J, Katusi D, et al. Brachytherapy—optional treatment for choroidal neovascularization secondary to age-related macular degeneration. *Coll Antropol* 2001;25(Suppl):89–96.

70. Zambarakji HJ, Lane AM, Ezra E, et al. Proton beam irradiation for neovascular age-related macular degeneration. *Ophthalmology* 2006;113:2012–2019.

71. Hahn SM, Maity A. General principles of radiation and chemoradiation. *Retina* 2009;29:S30–S31.

72. Adams JA, Paiva KL, Munzenrider JE, et al. Proton beam therapy for age-related macular degeneration: development of a standard plan. *Med Dosim* 1999;24:233–238.

73. Ciulla TA, Danis RP, Klein SB, et al. Proton therapy for exudative age-related macular degeneration: a randomized, sham-controlled clinical trial. *Am J Ophthalmol* 2002;134:905–906.

74. Parsons JT, Bova FJ, Fitzgerald CR, et al. Radiation optic neuropathy after megavoltage external-beam irradiation: analysis of time-dose factors. *Int J Radiat Oncol Biol Phys* 1994;30:755–763.

75. Eter N, Schüller H, Spitznas M. Radiotherapy for age-related macular degeneration: is there a benefit for classic CNV? *Int Ophthalmol* 2001;24:13–19.

76. Prettenhofer U, Haas A, Mayer R, et al. Long-term results after external radiotherapy in age-related macular degeneration. A prospective study. *Strahlenther Onkol* 2004;180:91–92.

77. Hayashi M, Chernov M, Usukura M, et al. Gamma knife surgery for choroidal neovascularization in age-related macular degeneration. Technical note. *J Neurosurg* 2205;102:S200–S203.

78. Hanlon J, Lee C, Chell E, et al. Kilovoltage stereotactic radiosurgery for age-related macular degeneration: assessment of optic nerve dose and patient effective dose. *Med Phys* 2009;36:2671–3681.

79. Evans JR, Sivagnanavel V, Chong V. Radiotherapy for neovascular age-related macular degeneration. *Cochrane Database Syst Rev* 2010;5:CD004004.

80. Quiroz-Mercado H, Velez-Montoya R, Fromow-Guerra J, et al. Mexican clinical experience in ocular anti-angiogenic therapy. *Gac Med Mex* 2008;144:245–253.

81. Wu L, Arevalo FJ, Maia M, et al. Comparing outcomes in patients with subfoveal choroidal neovascularization secondary to age-related macular degeneration treated with two different doses of primary intravitreal bevacizumab: results of the Pan-American Collaborative Retina Study Group (PACORES) at the 12-month follow-up. *Jpn J Ophthalmol* 2009;53:125–130.

82. Gordon-Angelozzi M, Velez-Montoya R, Fromow-Guerra J, et al. Bevacizumab local complications. *Ophthalmology* 2009;116:2264.e1–2264.e3.

83. Avila MP, Farah ME, Santos A, et al. Twelve-month safety and visual acuity results from a feasibility study of intraocular, epiretinal radiation therapy for the treatment of subfoveal CNV secondary to AMD. *Retina* 2009;29:157–169.

# 33

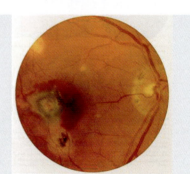

# Ocular Histoplasmosis and Non-AMD Disorders Associated with Choroidal Neovascularization

Odette M. Houghton ■ Travis A. Meredith

Choroidal neovascularization (CNV) can occur in presumed ocular histoplasmosis syndrome (POHS) as well as in other non–age-related macular degeneration (AMD) related disorders including pathologic myopia, angioid streaks, punctate inner choroidopathy (PIC), and multifocal choroiditis (MFC) (1–5). Since CNV can lead to severe loss of central vision in these disorders, several treatment approaches have been explored.

Various surgical techniques have been proposed as a treatment for CNV attributable to POHS and other non-AMD related disorders. The earliest reports on the surgical intervention of CNV were in patients with end-stage AMD. De Juan and Machemer were the first to describe the surgical excision of CNV (6). They gained direct exposure of the membrane by the creation of a large flap retinotomy. Blinder et al. subsequently described a surgical technique which similarly permitted direct access to the membrane (7). Unlike De Juan and Machemer, who describe the creation of a 180-degree peripheral retinotomy, Blinder et al. created a flap retinotomy, which encompassed the macula. Although the membranes were successfully removed using these methods, the postoperative result was complicated by poor visual acuity.

An alternative surgical approach, in which the subretinal space was accessed via a small retinotomy, was described in two patients with POHS by Thomas and Kaplan in 1991 (8). Subretinal manipulation of the membrane was aided by the creation of an overlying neurosensory retinal detachment via a subretinal infusion of fluid. This enabled the passage of instruments to dislodge and grasp the membrane. Both patients in this report experienced a dramatic improvement in visual acuity. Modifications of this technique have been used extensively in studies regarding the surgical removal of CNV (9–13).

Macular translocation has recently emerged as a strategy for the management of subfoveal CNV. The objective of this technique is to create a retinal detachment to relocate the fovea to a bed of healthier retinal pigment epithelium (RPE) (14). The first presentation of macular translocation in humans was in patients with submacular hemorrhage from AMD (14). Relocation of the fovea was accomplished by the creation of a total retinal detachment and a 360 degrees retinotomy, followed by rotation then reattachment of the retina. A different technique of limited translocation with scleral imbrication was used by de Juan et al. (15). Their approach involved creating a subtotal retinal detachment via a subretinal infusion, scleral shortening by suturing crescent shaped partial thickness scleral resections and retinal reattachment. Preliminary results were encouraging. This technique plus modifications of this technique, with scleral shortening achieved via scleral sutures without scleral resection, appear to be the most predominant method used in more recent studies (16–20).

In entertaining a decision of surgery for CNV, the intraoperative and postoperative risks of the procedure must be taken into consideration. In addition to the specific complications associated with excising the CNV or relocating the macula, risks inherent to pars plana vitrectomy are also associated with these surgeries. Some of the reported intraoperative and postoperative complications are listed in Table 33-1.

The outcomes of CNV excision are varied and depend on the etiology of the CNV. The visual outcome of non–AMD-related CNV are listed in Table 33-2. The best candidates for this

| TABLE 33-1 | COMPLICATIONS OF SURGERY FOR CHOROIDAL NEOVASCULARIZATION IN NON–AMD-RELATED DISORDERS |
|---|---|
| **Intraoperative complications** | |
| Submacular surgery | Subretinal hemorrhage (9,11) |
| | Macular dehiscence (9,10,12) |
| | Neurosensory retinal damage (21) |
| | Retinal tears |
| Macular translocation | Subretinal hemorrhage |
| | Retinal tears |
| **Postoperative complications** | |
| Submacular surgery | Identified peripheral breaks |
| | Retina detachment (9–13) |
| | Epimacular proliferation (8) |
| Macular translocation | Identified peripheral breaks (20) |
| | Retinal Detachment (19) |
| | Epimacular proliferation |
| | Macular hole (16,20) |
| | Macular folds (16,20) |
| | Transient diplopia or cyclotorsion (16,19,20) |

approach are considered to be those with POHS (10). Early studies investigating submacular surgery for CNV attributable to POHS were retrospective, noncontrolled and had limited follow-up (9–12). Together these studies showed that 74% to 83% of eyes experienced stable or improved visual acuity after the surgical removal of subfoveal CNV.

The Submacular Surgery Trial (SST) group H directly compared surgical intervention versus observation for the management of subfoveal CNV secondary to POHS and idiopathic membranes in a randomized manner (13). The findings of this study indicate that surgical removal of CNV did not offer an advantage over observation. The results did suggest that surgical removal of subfoveal CNV may be beneficial in patients with a best-corrected visual acuity <20/100. However, in light of the complications observed no strong recommendations can be made from these data.

Based on short term and retrospective results, encouraging submacular surgical outcomes have been obtained for patients with peripapillary CNV secondary to POHS extending to the subfoveal region (21–31). It appears that there may be a more favorable prognosis in younger patients with peripapillary CNV (32).

There have been studies indicating that the surgical intervention of CNV associated with high myopia may offer better restoration and preservation of visual function compared to observation in these eyes (13,16,17,19,20,29). A retrospective

**TABLE 33-2   VISUAL OUTCOME OF CHOROIDAL NEOVASCULARIZATION IN NON–AMD-RELATED DISORDERS**

| Intervention | Study | Etiology | n | Average follow-up (months) | Improved | Unchanged | Worse | Recurrence |
|---|---|---|---|---|---|---|---|---|
| Submacular surgery | Holekamp et al. (12) | POHS | 117 | 13 | 40% | 41% | 19% | 44% |
| | Berger et al. (11) | POHS | 63 | 24 | 35% | 44% | 21% | 38% |
| | Thomas et al. (10) | POHS | 67 | 11 | 34% | 49% | 17% | 37% |
| | SST (13) | POHS/idiopathic | 103 | 24 | 28% | 26% | 48% | 58% |
| | Atebara et al. (22) | Peripapillary CNV/POHS | 14 | 33 | 71% | 22% | 7% | 33% |
| | Uemura et al. (23) | Myopia | 48 | 24 | 39% | 26% | 35% | 57% |
| | Hamelin et al. (18) | Myopia | 18 | 14 | 33% | 11% | 56% | 39% |
| | Essex et al. (24) | Mixed | 57 | 24 | 63% | 24% | 12% | 33% |
| | Adelberg et al. (25) | Mixed | 17 | 16 | 35% | 59% | 6% | 24% |
| | Joseph et al. (26) | Juxtafoveal | 46 | 20 | 56% | 22% | 22% | 56.5% |
| Macular translocation | Ichibe et al. (17) | Myopia | 10 | 16 | 90% | 10% | 0% | 30% |
| | Glacet-Bernard et al. (19) | Myopia | 9 | 10 | 89% | 11% | 0% | 11% |
| | Glacet-Bernard et al. (20) | Myopia | 34 | 28 | 55% | 40% | 5% | 41% |
| | Hamelin et al. (18) | Myopia | 14 | 11 | 50% | 43% | 7% | 14% |
| | Fujii et al. (16) | Mixed | 23 | 11 | 48% | 30% | 2% | |
| PDT | Rosenfeld et al. (37) | POHS | 22 | 24 | 45% | 36% | 18% | |
| Natural History | SST (13) | POHS/idiopathic | 97 | 24 | 21% | 37% | 40% | |
| | Ho et al. (28) | Idiopathic | 19 | | 32% | 63% | 5% | |
| | VIP (29) | Myopia | 39 | 24 | 13% | 31% | 57% | |

POHS, Presumed ocular histoplasmosis syndrome; SST, Submacular Surgery Trial Group; CNV, choroidal neovascularization; VIP, verteporfin in photodynamic therapy.

case series compared limited macular translocation versus surgical removal in patients with subfoveal CNV in myopia. Visual acuity improved by three lines in 50% of patients undergoing macular translocation versus 33% of patients undergoing surgical removal of the CNV (18).

There have been a few noncontrolled studies on submacular surgery for CNV in PIC and MFC (3,24). Although outcomes appear promising, recurrences were common and often led to loss of vision (3). The surgical outcomes for CNV secondary to angioid streaks are disappointing (25).

Case selection appears to be very important in the successful surgical removal of choroidal neovascularization. The presence of RPE and prevention of choriocapillaris atrophy appears to be essential to good visual recovery (33). Thus type 2 CNV, such as those associated with POHS, where new vessels extend through focal abnormalities of the RPE and the membrane is anterior to the RPE are likely to have better outcomes than type 1 membranes, where the CNV is intertwined with the RPE (30). Better outcomes have also been associated with CNV that have extrafoveal ingrowth sites rather than subfoveal ingrowth sites (34). Clinical findings suggestive of type 2 CNV

were described by Gass in 1994. Angiographic features may aid the identification of type 2 CNV and ingrowth site. The SST confirmed that those with classic lesions had a subretinal component in POHS (13). The newer generations of optical coherence tomography could also potentially aid this distinction (35).

Nonsurgical therapies have been used in the treatment of CNV. In randomized trials, the Macular Photocoagulation Study (MPS) demonstrated that laser photocoagulation is effective in reducing the risk of vision loss in patients with well-defined, classic extrafoveal, juxtafoveal, and peripapillary CNV lesions secondary to POHS (36–37). Since spontaneous improvement was expected without therapy in some cases, and since laser photocoagulation is not a recommended treatment for subfoveal CNV in patients with POHS, subfoveal CNV was not studied in the POHS arm of the MPS (38). Laser photocoagulation of juxtafoveal CNV in pathologic myopia is also not recommended, partly due to the extensive enlargement of the laser scar over time.

The Verteporfin in Photodynamic Therapy (VIP) Study showed no benefit for patients with subfoveal CNV secondary to pathologic myopia assigned to photodynamic therapy compared to observation at two years (29). To date there have been no randomized, controlled clinical trials suggesting photodynamic therapy (PDT) treatment to be beneficial for patients with subfoveal CNV associated with POHS. However, the two year results of an uncontrolled, prospective study of patients with subfoveal CNV secondary to POHS receiving PDT demonstrate improvement from baseline without serious adverse events (27).

Recently, there has been a breakthrough in the successful treatment of CNV in AMD with antiangiogenesis agents (39). Lack of well defined, effective treatment strategies for non–AMD-related CNV has encouraged the investigation into the use of such agents for these disorders. Although current evidence is limited, regarding this approach, early studies are encouraging.

Management options for non–AMD-related CNV are currently evolving. Current options include observation, laser photocoagulation, PDT, surgical excision, and macular translocation. This may change in the new era of antiangiogenesis agents. These agents hold hope for the successful treatment of these disorders, either alone or in combination with more established treatment options.

## References

1. Gunby P. Ocular histoplasmosis syndrome. *J Am Med Assoc* 1980;243:626–627.
2. Watzke RC, Packer AJ, Folk JC, et al. Punctate inner choroidopathy. *Am J Ophthalmol* 1984;98:572–584.
3. Olsen TW, Capone A Jr, Sternberg P Jr, et al. Subfoveal choroidal neovascularization in punctate inner choroidopathy. *Ophthalmology* 1996;103:2061–2069.
4. Shields JA, Federman JL, Tomer TL, et al. Ophthalmoscopic variations and diagnostic problems. *Br J Ophthalmol* 1975;59:257–266.
5. Brown J Jr, Folk JC, Reddy CV, et al. Visual prognosis of multifocal choroiditis, punctate inner choroidopathy, and the diffuse subretinal fibrosis syndrome. *Ophthalmology* 1996;103:1100–1105.
6. De Juan E, Machemer R. Vitreous surgery for hemorrhagic fibrous complications of age-related macular degeneration. *Am J Ophthalmol* 1988;105:25–29.
7. Blinder KJ, Peyman GA, Paris CL, et al. Submacular scar excision in age-related macular degeneration. *Int Ophthalmol* 1991;15:215–222.
8. Thomas MA, Kaplan HJ. Surgical removal of subfoveal neovascularization in the presumed ocular histoplasmosis syndrome. *Am J Ophthalmol* 1991;111:1–7.
9. Thomas MA, Grand MD, Williams DF, et al. Surgical management of subfoveal choroidal neovascularization. *Ophthalmology* 1992;99:952–976.
10. Thomas MA, Dickinson JD, Melberg NS, et al. Visual results following the surgical removal of subfoveal choroidal neovascularization. *Ophthalmology* 1994;101:1384–1396.
11. Berger AS, Conway M, Del Priore LV, et al. Submacular surgery for subfoveal choroidal neovascular membranes in patients with presumed ocular histoplasmosis. *Arch Ophthalmol* 1997;115:991–996.
12. Holekamp NM, Thomas MA, Dickinson JD, et al. Surgical removal of subfoveal choroidal neovascularization in presumed ocular histoplasmosis. Stability of early visual results. *Ophthalmology* 1997;104:22–26.
13. Submacular Surgery Trials Research Group. Surgical removal versus observation for subfoveal choroidal neovascularization, either associated with the ocular histoplasmosis syndrome or idiopathic. I. Ophthalmic findings from a randomized clinical trial: submacular surgery trials (SST) group H trial: SST Report No. 9. *Arch Ophthalmol* 2004;122:1597–1611.
14. Machemer R, Steinhorst UH. Retinal separation, retinotomy and macular relocation: II. A surgical approach for age related macular degeneration. *Graefes Arch Clin Exp Ophthalmol* 1993;231:635–641.
15. De Juan E Jr, Loewenstein A, Bressler NM, et al. Translocation of the retina for management of subfoveal choroidal neovascularization, II: A preliminary report in humans. *Am J Ophthalmol* 1998;125:635–646.
16. Fujii GY, Au Eong K-G, Humayun MS, et al. Initial experience of inferior limited macular translocation for subfoveal choroidal neovascularization resulting from causes other than age-related macular degeneration. *Am J Ophthalmol* 2001;131:90–100.
17. Ichibe M, Imai K, Ohta M, et al. Foveal translocation with scleral imbrication in patients with myopic neovascular maculopathy. *Am J Ophthalmol* 2001;132:164–171.
18. Hamelin N, Glacet-Bernard A, Brindeau C, et al. Surgical treatment of subfoveal neovascularization in myopia: macular translocation versus surgical removal. *Am J Ophthalmol* 2002;133:530–536.
19. Glacet-Brenard A, Benyelles N, Dumas S, et al. Photodynamic therapy versus limited macular translocation in the management of subfoveal choroidal neovascularization in pathologic myopia: a two-year study. *Am J Ophthalmol* 2007;143:68–76.
20. Glacet-Bernard A, Simon P, Hamelin N, et al. Translocation of the macular for management of subfoveal choroidal neovascularization comparison of results in age-related macular degeneration and degenerative myopia. *Am J Ophthalmol* 2001;131:78–89.
21. Hsu JK, Thomas MA, Ibanez H, et al. Clinicopathologic studies of an eye after submacular membranectomy for choroidal neovascularization. *Retina* 1995;15:43–52.
22. Atebara NH, Thomas MA, Holekamp NM, et al. Surgical removal of extensive peripapillary choroidal neovascularization associated with presumed ocular histoplasmosis syndrome. *Ophthalmology* 1998;105:1598–1605.
23. Uemura A, Thomas A. Subretinal surgery for subfoveal choroidal neovascularization. *Ophthalmology* 1992;99:952–968.
24. Essex RW, Tufail A, Bunce C, et al. Two-year results of surgical removal of choroidal neovascular membranes related to non-age-related macular degeneration. *Br J Ophthalmol* 2007;91:649–654.
25. Adelberg DA, Del Priore L, Kaplan HJ. Surgery for subfoveal membranes in myopia, angioid streaks, and other disorders. *Retina* 1995;15:198–205.
26. Joseph DP, Uemura A, Thomas MA. Subretinal surgery for juxtafoveal choroidal neovascularization. *Retina* 2003;23:463–468.
27. Rosenfeld PJ, Saperstein DA, Bressler NM, et al. Photodynamic therapy with verteporfin in ocular histoplasmosis: uncontrolled, open-label 2-year study. *Ophthalmology* 2004;111:1725–1733.
28. Ho AC, Yanuzzi LA, Pisicano K, et al. The natural history of idiopathic subfoveal choroidal neovascularization. *Ophthalmology* 1995;102:782–789.
29. Blinder KJ, Blumenkranz MS, Bressler NM, et al. Verteporfin therapy of subfoveal choroidal neovascularization in pathologic myopia: 2-year results of a randomized clinical trial–VIP Report No. 3. *Ophthalmology* 2003;110(4):667–673.
30. Gass DJ. Biomicroscopic and histopathologic considerations regarding the feasibility of surgical excision of subfoveal neovascular membranes. *Am J Ophthalmol* 1994;118:285–298.
31. Kertes PJ. Massive peripapillary subretinal neovascularization. An indication for submacular surgery. *Retina* 2004;24:219–225.
32. Bains HS, Patel MR, Singh H, et al. Surgical treatment of extensive peripapillary choroidal neovascularization in elderly patients. *Retina* 2003;23:469–474.
33. Akduman L, Del Priore LV, Desai VN, et al. Perfusion of the subfoveal choriocapillaris affects visual recovery after submacular surgery in presumed ocular histoplasmosis syndrome. *Am J Ophthalmol* 1997;123:90–96.
34. Melberg NS, Thomas MA, Burgess D. The surgical removal of subfoveal choroidal neovascularization. Ingrowth site as a predictor of visual outcome. *Retina* 1996;16:190–195.
35. Alam S, Zawadzki RJ, Chou S, et al. Clinical application of rapid serial Fourier-domain optical coherence tomography for macular imaging. *Ophthalmology* 2006;113:1425–1431.
36. Macular Photocoagulation Study Group. Argon laser photocoagulation for idiopathic neovascularization: results of a randomized clinical Trial. *Arch Ophthalmol* 1983;101:1358–1361.
37. Macular Photocoagulation Study Group. Laser photocoagulation for neovascular lesions nasal to fovea: results from clinical trials for lesions secondary to ocular histoplasmosis or idiopathic causes. *Arch Ophthalmol* 1995;113:56–61.
38. Fine SL, Wood WJ, Isernhagen RD. Laser treatment for subfoveal neovascular membranes in ocular histoplasmosis syndrome: results of a pilot randomized clinical trial. *Arch Ophthalmol* 1993;111:19–20.
39. Rosenfeld PJ, Rich RM, Lalwani GA. Ranibizumab: Phase III clinical trial results. *Ophthalmol Clin North Am* 2006;19(3):361–372.

# 34

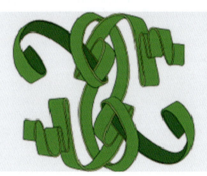

# Pharmacotherapy of Choroidal Neovascularization

Wayne W. Wu ■ Franco M. Recchia ■ Paul Sternberg Jr.

# MECHANISM OF CHOROIDAL NEOVASCULARIZATION

Angiogenesis is the formation of new blood vessels by the sprouting and splitting of existing vessels, a process that is implicated in both normal physiological processes such as the female reproductive cycle, hair growth, and wound healing, and in diseases such as cancer, psoriasis, rheumatoid arthritis, and various ocular conditions (1). Retinal angiogenesis is central to such conditions as proliferative diabetic retinopathy, advanced retinopathy of prematurity, neovascular glaucoma, and proliferative sickle cell retinopathy (2). Neovascular (exudative or "wet") age-related macular degeneration (AMD) arises most often from choroidal neovascularization (CNV) or choroidal angiogenesis. While the most common cause for visual impairment from retinal neovascularization is vitreous hemorrhage, CNV most commonly leads to subretinal hemorrhage and only rarely leads to vitreous hemorrhage. Similarly, while retinal neovascularization can lead to preretinal fibrous proliferation and traction retinal detachment, CNV frequently leads to subretinal fibrous proliferation with disciform scar formation.

However, the molecular mechanism underlying retinal neovascularization and CNV share similarities, and much of our knowledge of the pathophysiology and therapeutics of CNV arises from experimental models of retinal angiogenesis. Normally, endothelial cells lining the blood vessels are "silent" as a result of an intricate balance of pro-angiogenic and anti-angiogenic (angiostatic) factors. Pathological conditions such as hypoxia and ischemia perturb this balance and lead to an increased expression of pro-angiogenic factors and/or a down-regulation of angiostatic factors (3–5). The resulting angiogenic drive "activates" endothelial cells and precipitates a complex cascade of cellular events: proliferation of endothelial cells, migration of endothelial cells, tube formation, and ultimately formation of blood vessel loops from endothelial cell tubes (Fig. 34-1). Many stimulatory and inhibitory molecules are thought to be involved in this complex cascade: growth factors, adhesion molecules, extracellular matrix components, proteinase enzymes, upstream and downstream regulators, and others (4). Therapies can be targeted at one or more steps of the angiogenic process.

Angiostatic factors include thrombospondin, angiostatin, endostatin, and pigment epithelium-derived factor (PEDF) (3,4). Identified pro-angiogenic factors include vascular endothelial growth factor (VEGF), fibroblast growth factor (FGF) families, transforming growth factors-alpha and -beta (TGF-alpha and TGF-beta), angiopoietin-1 and -2 (3,4). Members of the VEGF gene family include VEGF-A, VEGF-B, VEGF-C, VEGF-D, VEGF-E, and placental growth factor (PIGF) (6). VEGF-A has been shown to play a key role in normal vasculogenesis and in angiogenesis in animals and humans, while the role of other members of the VEGF family appears more limited (6,7). VEGF-A was first described in 1983 as a "tumor vascular permeability factor" (VPF) that induced vascular leakage in skin (8). VPF was subsequently found to be identical to an endothelial cell mitogen named VEGF (9). Therefore, VEGF-A has two important functions: stimulation of angiogenesis and enhancement of vascular permeability. Both these properties are important in the pathogenesis of CNV in neovascular AMD.

As a result of alternative splicing and cleavage of signal sequences, multiple isoforms and cleavage products of VEGF-A exist. There are six major isoforms consisting of 121, 145, 165, 183, 189, and 206 amino acids (10,11). VEGF121 is the highly diffusible isoform, while VEGF165 is the most abundantly expressed in humans with only a portion of it being diffusible (12). Both VEGF189 and VEGF206 are almost completely sequestered in the extracellular matrix (12). While all isoforms are important in angiogenesis, VEGF165 has been purported to be the isoform most allied with neovascularization (10,13). All isoforms can be mobilized through extracellular cleavage by plasmin to generate the diffusible VEGF110 (14).

The biological effects of VEGF-A are mediated through the VEGF-specific tyrosine-kinase receptors VEGFR-1 (Flt-1), VEGFR-2 (Flk-1), and VEGFR-3 (Flt-4), and the neuropilins

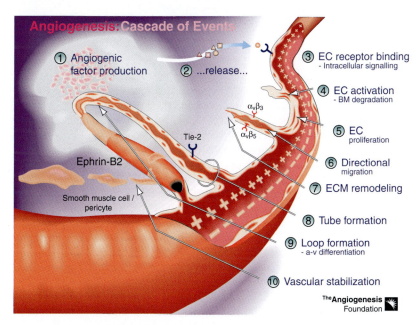

Angiogenesis: Cascade of Events

① Angiogenic factor production

② ...release...

③ EC receptor binding
- Intracellular signalling

④ EC activation
- BM degradation

⑤ EC proliferation

⑥ Directional migration

⑦ ECM remodeling

⑧ Tube formation

⑨ Loop formation
- a-v differentiation

⑩ Vascular stabilization

$\alpha_v\beta_3$

$\alpha_v\beta_5$

Tie-2

Ephrin-B2

Smooth muscle cell / pericyte

The Angiogenesis Foundation

**Figure 34-1.** The resulting angiogenic drive "activates" endothelial cells and precipitates a complex cascade of cellular events: proliferation of endothelial cells; migration of endothelial cells; tube formation; and ultimately formation of blood vessel loops from endothelial cell tubes. (From http://angio.org/understanding/understanding.html. © 2000 The Angiogenesis Foundation, Inc. All rights reserved.).

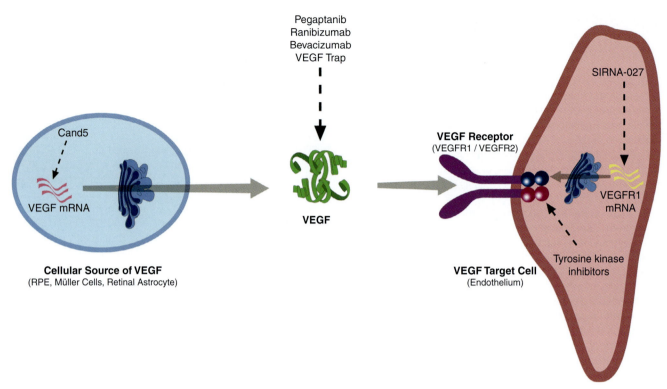

**Figure 34-2.** The biological effects of vascular endothelial growth factor (VEGF)-A are mediated through the VEGF-specific tyrosine-kinase receptors VEGFR-1 (Flt-1), VEGFR-2 (Flk-1), and VEGFR-3 (Flt-4), and the neuropilins (NP1, NP2).

(NP1, NP2) (Fig. 34-2) (6,15). VEGFR-2 appears to be the main receptor responsible for the angiogenic effects of VEGF-A. NP1 may enhance the effectiveness of VEGFR-2-mediated signaling by presenting isoform VEGF165 to VEGFR-2 (16). In humans, VEGFR-3 is thought to play a role in lymphangiogenesis (17).

Laboratory and clinical findings implicate VEGF-A in the pathogenesis of neovascular AMD. VEGF-A expression can be induced in cultured retinal pigment epithelial (RPE) cells under hypoxic conditions (18,19). Increased VEGF-A concentrations are found in surgically excised CNV membranes (20), in vitreous samples from patients with submacular hemorrhage and AMD (21), and in RPE cells in the early stages of AMD (22).

There is increasing evidence supporting the role of inflammation in both nonneovascular and neovascular stages of AMD (23,24). The complement system is part of the innate immune system. Polymorphisms in the gene encoding complement factor H, one component of the native immune system, are strongly associated with subtypes of neovascular AMD (25). An illustration of current understanding of the pathogenesis of neovascular AMD is depicted in Figure 34-3.

## TREATMENTS DIRECTED AGAINST VASCULAR ENDOTHELIAL GROWTH FACTOR AND ITS RECEPTORS

The primary target for pharmacologic treatment of CNV in AMD has been VEGF, and strategies have been devised to interrupt different steps along the VEGF signaling pathway

(Fig. 34-2). Blockage of VEGF effect may be achieved by extracellular inactivation of VEGF-A by direct binding or "trapping," by intracellular inhibition of VEGF gene transcription, or by inhibition of VEGF tyrosine receptor kinases.

## INACTIVATION OF EXTRACELLULAR VASCULAR ENDOTHELIAL GROWTH FACTOR

### Pegaptanib

Pegaptanib sodium (Macugen, OSI/Eyetech Pharmaceuticals, New York, NY, USA) was the first anti-VEGF agent approved by the United States Food and Drug and Administration (FDA) for the treatment of neovascular AMD. Pegaptanib is a ribonucleic acid (RNA) aptamer, a sequence of 28 ribonucleotides generated through a systemic evolution of ligands by exponential enrichment (SELEX) to achieve high specific affinity for VEGF165 (26). The attachment of a polyethylene glycol (PEG) moiety increases the half-life of the compound to provide a desired intraocular concentration in excess of minimal inhibitory concentration for VEGF165 for approximately 6 weeks (27,28). Unlike peptides and monoclonal antibodies, an important feature of aptamers such as pegaptanib is that they are essentially nonimmunogenic even when administered in excess of therapeutic doses.

The VEGF Inhibition Study in Ocular Neovascularization (VISION) involved two concurrent, prospective, randomized, double-masked, sham-controlled, dose-ranging Phase III clinical

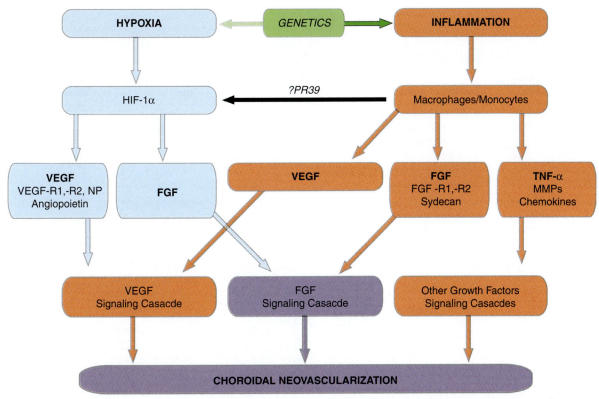

**Figure 34-3.** The current understanding of the pathogenesis of neovascular age-related macular degeneration (AMD). FGF, fibroblast growth factor; HIF, hypoxia inducible factor; MMP, matrix metalloproteinases; TNF, tumor necrosis factor; VEGF, vascular endothelial growth factor.

trials of intravitreal pegaptanib for the treatment of neovascular AMD (Table 34.1) (29). A total of 1,186 patients were randomized 1:1:1:1 to receive pegaptanib (0.3 mg, 1.0 mg, or 3.0 mg) or sham injection every 6 weeks for 48 weeks. The primary endpoint was the proportion of patients losing fewer than 15 letters of visual acuity at 54 weeks. Compared with those receiving sham injection, patients treated with 0.3 mg pegaptanib were significantly more likely to lose fewer than 15 letters of visual acuity (70% vs. 55%), more likely to maintain or improve visual acuity (33% vs. 23%), and less likely to lose 30 or more letters of visual acuity (10% vs. 22%). However, only 6% of treated patients gained 15 letters or more in visual acuity. Serious adverse events were primarily those associated with intravitreal injection: endophthalmitis, in 1.3% of patients; lens trauma, in 0.7%; and retinal detachment, in 0.6%. These events were associated with a severe loss of visual acuity in 0.1% of patients. Two-year results of the VISION study confirmed the benefit of 0.3 mg pegaptanib in reducing moderate visual acuity loss and progression to legal blindness. Advantages of pegaptanib over the prevailing standard of care, photodynamic therapy (PDT) with verteporfin, included its equal efficacy for all angiographic types of CNV and the relative ease and portability of the treatment (30). However, the treatment only demonstrated moderate improvement in visual outcome for patients and requirement of treatment at 6-week intervals versus 3-month intervals for PDT.

## Ranibizumab

Approximately 18 months following the release of pegaptanib, the FDA approved ranibizumab (Lucentis, Genentech, Inc., South San Francisco, California, USA), for the intravit-

real treatment of neovascular AMD on June 30, 2006. Ranibizumab is the active portion (antibody fragment, or Fab) of a full-length humanized murine monoclonal antibody directed against all isoforms and degradation products of human VEGF-A (31). A closely related molecule, bevacizumab (Avastin, Genentech, Inc., South San Francisco, California, USA), had previously been approved for the treatment of metastatic colorectal cancer (32). Ranibizumab was developed because it was thought that its smaller size would afford better retinal penetration and more precise targeting of subretinal CNV (33,34). Additionally, its lack of a fragment crystallizable (Fc) region should eliminate binding of ranibizumab to Fc gamma receptors and avoid a complement-mediated immune response.

Ranibizumab was studied in two Phase III, multicenter, double-masked, randomized, sham-controlled clinical trials of patients with subfoveal CNV from AMD (Table 34-1) (35,36). In the Anti-VEGF Antibody for the Treatment of Predominantly Classic Choroidal Neovascularization in AMD (ANCHOR) study (36), 423 patients were randomly assigned patients in a 1:1:1 ratio to receive monthly intravitreal injections of ranibizumab (0.3 mg or 0.5 mg) plus sham PDT with verteporfin or monthly sham injections plus active PDT. At 12 months, 94.3% of those in the 0.3 mg group and 96.4% of those in the 0.5 mg group lost fewer than 15 letters, as compared with 64.3% of those in the verteporfin group. Mean visual acuity increased by 8.5 letters in the 0.3 mg group and 11.3 letters in the 0.5 mg group, as compared with a decrease of 9.5 letters in the verteporfin group. Perhaps the most exciting result was that visual acuity improved by 15 letters or more in 35.7% of the 0.3 mg group and 40.3% of the 0.5 mg group, in contrast to 5.6% of

**TABLE 34-1   PUBLISHED PHASE III CLINICAL TRIALS OF PHARMACOLOGICAL TREATMENT OF CHOROIDAL NEOVASCULARIZATION SECONDARY TO AGE-RELATED MACULAR DEGENERATION**

| Phase III clinical trial | Inclusion criteria[a] | Treatment arms | <15 Letter vision loss | >3 Line vision gain | Serious ocular adverse events |
|---|---|---|---|---|---|
| VISION (1 year) | Subfoveal CNV of all types | A. 0.3 mg pegaptanib<br>B. 1.0 mg pegaptanib<br>C. 3.0 mg pegaptanib<br>D. Sham<br><br>(Randomized 1:1:1:1 to Q6 weeks intravitreal injection) | 0.3 mg group: 70%<br>Sham group: 55% | 0.3 mg group: 6%<br>Sham group: 2% | Endophthalmitis (1.3%)<br>Retinal detachment (0.6%)<br>Traumatic lens injury (0.7%) |
| ANCHOR (1 year) | Predominantly classic subfoveal CNV | A. 0.3 mg ranibizumab/sham PDT<br>B. 0.5 mg ranibizumab/sham PDT<br>C. sham/active PDT<br><br>(monthly intravitreal injection) | 0.3 mg group: 94.3%<br>0.5 mg group: 96.4%<br>Sham/PDT: 64.3% | 0.3 mg group: 35.7%<br>0.5 mg group: 40.3%<br>PDT/sham: 5.6% | Endophthalmitis (1.4%)<br>Serious uveitis (0.7%) |
| MARINA (2 years) | Minimally classic or occult without classic subfoveal CNV | A. 0.3 mg ranibizumab<br>B. 0.5 mg ranibizumab<br>C. Sham<br><br>(monthly intravitreal injection) | 1 year<br>0.3 mg group: 94.5%<br>0.5 mg group: 94.6%<br>Sham group: 62.2%<br>1 year<br>0.3 mg group: 92%<br>0.5 mg group: 92%<br>Sham group: 52.9% | 1 year<br>0.3 mg group: 24.8%<br>0.5 mg group: 33.8%<br>Sham group: 5.0%<br>2 years<br>0.3 mg group: 26.1%<br>0.5 mg group: 33.1%<br>Sham group: 3.8% | Endophthalmitis (1%)<br>Serious uveitis (1.3%) |
| C-01-99 Comparison trial (1 year) | Predominantly classic subfoveal CNV | A. 15 mg (anecortate acetate or AA) juxtascleral injection (at month 1, 6)<br>B. PDT | AA group: 45%<br><br>PDT group: 49% | N/A<br><br>N/A | None |

[a]All lesions are subfoveal CNV<5400 μm in the greatest linear dimension.
VISION, VEGF Inhibition Study in Ocular Neovascularization; CNV, choroidal neovascularization; ANCHOR, Anti-VEGF Antibody for the Treatment of Predominantly Classic Choroidal Neovascularization in AMD; PDT, photodynamic therapy; MARINA, Minimally Classic/Occult Trial of the Anti-VEGF Antibody Ranibizumab in the Treatment of Neovascular AMD.

the verteporfin group. A subgroup analysis of 12-month data from the ANCHOR study showed ranibizumab to be superior to PDT in all evaluated subgroups (37).

Similar results emerged from the Minimally Classic/Occult Trial of the Anti-VEGF Antibody Ranibizumab in the Treatment of Neovascular AMD (MARINA) study (35), in which 716 patients were randomly assigned to receive 24 monthly intravitreal injections of ranibizumab (either 0.3 mg or 0.5 mg) or sham injections. At 12 months, 94.5% of the patients in the 0.3 mg group and 94.6% of those in the 0.5 mg group lost fewer than 15 letters, as compared with 62.2% of patients in the sham injection group. It is noteworthy that 24.8% of the 0.3 mg group and 33.8% of the 0.5 mg group experienced visual acuity improvement by 15 or more letters, as compared with 5.0% of the sham injection group. Mean increases in visual acuity were 6.5 letters in the 0.3 mg group and 7.2 letters in the 0.5 mg group, as compared with a decrease of 10.4 letters in the sham injection group. The benefit in visual acuity was maintained at 24 months. Retrospective, subgroup analyses of 24-month data from the MARINA study and 12-month data from the ANCHOR study demonstrated that the most important predictors of improved visual acuity outcome were, in decreasing order of importance, worse baseline visual acuity score, smaller CNV lesion size, and younger age (37,38).

The primary ocular adverse events associated with intravitreal ranibizumab were presumed to be endophthalmitis and

uveitis, each occurring with a frequency of roughly 1%. The incidence of systemic thromboembolic events (0.7% to 2.2%) was approximately equal among all groups, but the studies were not sufficiently powered to detect significant differences in uncommon events.

Ranibizumab is the first treatment for neovascular AMD to improve visual acuity in a significant number of patients regardless of lesion size or angiographic subtype. What remains unclear is the optimal frequency and duration of treatments. The pivotal MARINA and ANCHOR studies employed monthly injections over 2 years. On the basis of collective clinical experience, however, there is wide variability in patient response to treatment, as some patients require monthly injections to maintain their level of visual acuity, while others may require only bimonthly or quarterly injections. It is hoped that this ambiguity may be clarified by ongoing studies of variable dosing regimens (39).

## Bevacizumab

Encouraged by the results of the ranibizumab treatment and awaiting its FDA approval, Rosenfeld and other researchers (40–42) explored the off-label use of bevacizumab. The higher molecular weight and presence of two antigen-binding domains as well as the longer systemic half-life of bevacizumab suggested that its intravitreal half-life may be longer than that of ranibizumab. An open-label, uncontrolled clinical study showed short-term efficacy of systemic bevacizumab, with elevated blood pressure as the primary adverse effect (40). Subsequently, a few small, uncontrolled trials and retrospective studies suggested that an intravitreal injection of bevacizumab (typically 1.25 mg) was well tolerated and associated with improvement in visual acuity, reduction in macular thickening, and reduction in angiographic leakage in most patients (41,42). The primary advantage of bevacizumab over ranibizumab is its significantly lower cost, since approximately 40 intravitreal doses can be obtained from a single vial of bevacizumab. However, questions regarding the efficacy and long-term safety of bevacizumab remain and will only be answered definitively by controlled clinical trials. The first of the Comparison of AMD Treatment Trials (CATT), a pivotal clinical trial involving comparison of both fixed and interval dosing regimens of bevacizumab versus ranibizumab, is presently underway.

## Vascular Endothelial Growth Factor Trap

VEGF-trap R1R2 (Regeneron, Tarrytown, New York, USA) is a recombinant soluble receptor protein in which the immunoglobulin (Ig) domain 2 of the VEGF receptor VEGFR-1 and Ig domain 3 are combined with the Fc portion of human IgG1 (43). The receptor-binding domains confer high specific affinity (Kd < 1 pm) for all isoforms of VEGF-A, all other forms of VEGF (B, C, D), and PIGF (placental growth factors 1 and 2). Therefore, VEGF-trap differs from ranibizumab because of its high potency to neutralize all VEGF family members. The Fc portion slows the clearance of the drug by conferring a long circulating half-life of an Ig molecule to the fusion protein. Subcutaneous injection of VEGF-trap R1R2 (25 mg/kg) has been shown to effectively neutralize VEGF in mice with VEGF-secreting tumors (44). Intravenous or intravitreal administration of VEGF-trap into mice has also shown that VEGF-trap suppresses CNV and VEGF-induced breakdown of the blood-retinal barrier (45). The Clinical Evaluation of Antiangiogenesis in the Retina (CLEAR) AMD-1 study was a randomized, multicenter, dose-ranging placebo-controlled Phase 1 clinical trial of intravenous VEGF-trap (46). Despite reduction of macular thickening, a dose-dependent increase in blood pressure among treated patients led to the discontinuation of this trial and to the development and clinical study of an intravitreal formulation. Phase 2 and 3 studies of intravitreal VEGF-trap are ongoing.

## INHIBITION OF GENE TRANSCRIPTION OF VASCULAR ENDOTHELIAL GROWTH FACTOR AND ITS RECEPTORS

### Small Interfering RNA-Based Therapies

Small interfering RNA (siRNAs) are double-stranded sequences of 21 to 23 ribonucleotides that assemble intracellularly into a multiprotein complex, termed RNA-induced silencing complex

(RISC), to induce RNA degradation through a natural gene-silencing pathway called RNA interference (RNAi) (Fig. 34-4) (47). siRNAs have rapidly become the most widely used approach for gene knockdown because of their high potency. Chemically modified short siRNAs targeting VEGF-A or VEGFR-1 were shown to inhibit neovascularization in several preclinical models (48–50). Encouraging results from Phase I trials have been observed with siRNAs targeting VEGF-A (Cand5 [Acuity Pharmaceuticals, Philadelphia, Pennsylvania, USA] and ALN-VEG01 [Alnylam, Cambridge, Massachusetts, USA]) and with siRNA targeting VEGFR-1 (SiRNA-027, Sirna Therapeutics, Boulder, Colorado, USA).

## INHIBITION OF VASCULAR ENDOTHELIAL GROWTH FACTOR RECEPTOR TYROSINE KINASES

VEGF signals through two major tyrosine receptor kinases: VEGFR-1 (flt-1) and VEGFR-2 (Flk-1 or KDR) (6). Some evidence suggests that flt-1 serves as a "decoy receptor," regulating the amount of free VEGF available in the extracellular space, while VEGF binding to KDR causes receptor dimerization and autophosphorylation, and activation of downstream pathways essential for endothelial cell proliferation and angiogenesis (51,52). Although VEGF clearly plays a central role in the development of neovascular diseases, other growth factor pathways acting through additional tyrosine kinases, such as platelet-derived growth factor receptor (PDGFR), fibroblast growth factor receptors (FGFRs), and Flt-4, have all been implicated in neovascularization and ocular disease (53,54). Studies, which demonstrate that inhibition of these receptor kinases leads to more potent decreases in angiogenesis, suggest that inhibition of multiple tyrosine kinase receptors may be a desirable approach in treating ocular neovascularization (55).

Such compounds that have progressed to Phase I and I/II clinical trials include vatalanib (PTK787; Norvartis, East Hanover, New Jersey, USA), a potent inhibitor of all known VEGF receptor tyrosine kinases; AG-013958 (Pfizer, San Diego, California, USA), a selective inhibitor of VEGFR and PDGFR and; a series of novel indolyl quinolinones (Merck Inc., Whitehouse Station, New Jersey, USA) with activity against KDR and several other closely related tyrosine kinases.

## TREATMENTS DIRECTED AGAINST PIGMENT EPITHELIUM-DERIVED FACTOR

PEDF is one of several naturally occurring endogenous antiangiogenic factors, others being angiostatin, thrombospondin-1, and endostatin. A member of the serine protease inhibitor (serpin) superfamily, PEDF is secreted into the surrounding interphotoreceptor matrix by human RPE cells and has higher angiostatic potency than other endogenous factors (56). In the vitreous of neovascular AMD patients, an increased expression

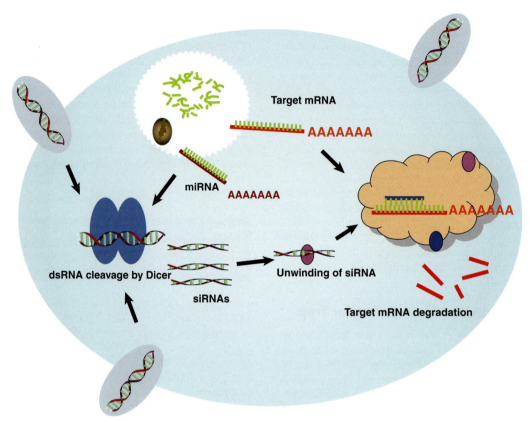

**Figure 34-4.** Small interfering ribonucleic acids (SiRNAs) are double-stranded sequences of 21 to 23 ribonucleotides that assemble intracellularly into a multiprotein complex, termed RNA-induced silencing complex (RISC), to induce RNA degradation through a natural gene-silencing pathway called RNA interference (RNAi).

of VEGF was accompanied by decreased expression of PEDF (57). Preclinical studies have shown regression of experimental CNV following intraocular delivery of the PEDF gene via an adenoviral vector (58–60) and led to human trials of AdGVPEDF.11D (AdPEDF, GenVec, Gaithersburg, Maryland, USA).

## TREATMENTS DIRECTED AGAINST INFLAMMATION AND HYPERPERMEABILITY

Folkman et al. (61,62) demonstrated the angiostatic effects of certain steroids, although their mechanism of action is not clearly understood. Triamincinolone acetonide (TA) has been widely used as an intravitreal treatment of a number of ocular conditions, including diabetic macular edema and neovascular AMD. Periocular anecortave acetate has been investigated as pharmacotherapy for neovascular AMD.

## TRIAMCINOLONE ACETONIDE

The angiostatic and antiedematous properties of TA have been known for some time (63). Penfold et al. (64) were the first to inject TA intravitreally to treat neovascular AMD. Although early nonrandomized studies showed promising results in patients with neovascular AMD (64–66), the results of a double-masked, placebo-controlled, randomized clinical study by Gillies et al. (67) were disappointing. The study was designed to determine whether a single intravitreal injection of 4 mg of TA in patients with classic CNV associated with AMD could safely reduce the risk of severe visual loss. In both treated and control groups, the 12-month risk of severe visual loss was 35%. The change in size of the CNV at 3 months, however, was significantly less in eyes receiving TA.

Although monotherapy with intravitreal TA is not recommended for neovascular AMD, the combination of intravitreal TA and PDT with verteporfin (Visudyne) has shown promising results. Spaide et al. (68) first reported a pilot study of 26 eyes in 26 patients with CNV secondary to AMD; 13 eyes were treatment-naïve and 13 eyes had experienced visual loss during treatment with PDT alone. Of the 13 patients with no prior PDT therapy, the mean visual acuity change at 3 months was an improvement of 1.9 lines, and four (30.8%) had an improvement of at least three lines. The treatment effect was less notable in the remaining 13 patients who had prior PDT therapy. Subsequent studies have demonstrated an improvement in visual acuity and a reduction in the number of PDT sessions required (69,70), although these investigations were not multicenter, randomized controlled trials.

Intravitreal triamcinolone for neovascular AMD remains an off-label use. The most common complications are cataract and elevated intraocular pressure, which occurs in up to 50% of patients (68–71) and may require glaucoma filtering surgery. Other adverse effects associated with intravitreal injection include infectious endophthalmitis, sterile endophthalmitis, vitreous hemorrhage, and rhegmatogenous retinal detachment.

## ANECORTAVE ACETATE

Anecortave acetate (Retaane, Alcon Research Ltd., Fort Worth, Texas, USA) is a structural analog of cortisol that is modified specifically to achieve angiostatic activity, but without glucocorticoid receptor-mediated side effects such as cataract and glaucoma and without anti-inflammatory effects (72). Posterior juxtascleral depot administration of anecortave acetate was found to be a safe and effective method for delivering therapeutic concentrations of drug to the macular region of the choroid and retina for up to 6 months (73).

Anecortave acetate was evaluated in three safety and efficacy studies of patients with subfoveal CNV secondary to AMD (Monotherapy Trial C-98-03, Combination Trial C-00-07, and Comparison C-01-99) (74). These demonstrated that 15 mg of anecortave acetate was superior to the vehicle and comparable to PDT with verteporfin, for preventing loss of 15 letters of visual acuity.

## SQUALAMINE

Squalamine lactate (Evizon, Genaera, Inc., Plymouth Meeting, Pennsylvania, USA) is one of a class of naturally occurring, pharmacologically active, small molecules known as aminosterols. Squalamine blocks the action of a number of angiogenic growth factors, including VEGF, cytoskeleton, and integrin expression (75). When taken up by activated endothelial cells, the drug inhibits membrane Na+/H+ exchange pump and leads to suppression of endothelial cell proliferation. In a Phase II multicenter, prospective, randomized, dose-ranging clinical trial of squalamine administered weekly for 4 weeks, 83% of treated patients lost fewer than 15 letters of visual acuity at 4 months, compared with 60% of untreated controls and 71% of those treated with PDT.

## OTHER POTENTIAL TARGETS FOR PHARMACOTHERAPY OF CHOROIDAL NEOVASCULARIZATION

Basic FGF-2 has been detected in RPE cells of surgically removed CNV membranes (76), and its level is elevated in laser-induced CNV lesions in rats (77). However, targeted inhibition of FGF-2 gene in mice did not inhibit CNV formation in laser-induced CNV model of mice, suggesting that it is not required for CNV development (78).

Angiopoietins are involved in regulating vascular integrity and neovascularization (79). Angiopoietin-1 protects adult vasculature against plasma leakage (80). Angiopoietin-2 enhances the effect of VEGF in ischemia-induced angiogenesis (81). Hypoxia and VEGF up-regulate the expression of angiopoietin-2 but not angiopoietin-1 (82). Both angiopoietin-1 and -2 were identified in CNV membranes in AMD patients (83). It is therefore possible that the inhibition of both VEGF and angiopoietin-2 may have additive inhibition of ischemia-induced retinal and choroidal disorders (84). Systemically expressed soluble Tie2 receptor (receptor to angiopoietin-2) with adenoviral-mediated gene delivery markedly inhibits the laser-induced CNV formation in mice (85), via a mechanism analogous to VEGF trap. Angiopoietin-1 may also have therapeutic potential because it suppresses VEGF-induced leukostasis and inflammation and preserves vascular integrity (86).

Another important group of molecules in angiogenesis are extracellular matrix molecules. Matrix metalloproteinases and their inhibitors play a role in the penetration of blood vessels into the extracellular matrix. Preclinical studies in inhibiting CNV by suppressing integrin function or by overexpression of tissue inhibitors of metalloproteinase-3 have been promising (87,88).

Other angiostatic agents in preclinical or clinical development include cyclooxygenase inhibitors, thalidomide, prolactin, octreotide, thrombospondin-2, angiostatin, endostatin, plasminogen kringle 5, and TNP-470 (10,89). Intravitreal administration of indomethacin, a cyclooxygenase inhibitor, inhibits the development of laser-induced CNV in monkeys (90). Angiostatin is an internal proteolytic fragment of plasminogen, inhibiting endothelial cell proliferation *in vitro* and angiogenesis *in vivo* (91). Overexpression of angiostatin with adenovirus-associated vectors causes regression of CNV in a murine model (92). Endostatin, a proteolytic fragment of the C-terminal fragment of collagen XVIII, also inhibits endothelial cell proliferation *in vitro* and angiogenesis *in vivo* (93–95).

## COMBINATION THERAPY

Like anticancer or antiviral (e.g., HIV) therapy, combination therapy for CNV may have synergistic effects, extending duration of effect and reducing doses or frequency of treatment. Combination therapy using intravitreal dexamethasone with verteporfin PDT and bevacizumab with verteporfin PDT has yielded encouraging results (96).

The RhuFab V2 Ocular Treatment Combining the Use of Visudyne to Evaluate Safety (FOCUS) study was a 2-year, phase I/II, multicenter, randomized, single-masked, controlled study to investigate the safety and efficacy of intravitreal ranibizumab treatment combined with verteporfin PDT in patients with predominantly classic CNV (97). Patients received monthly ranibizumab ($n = 106$) or sham ($n = 56$) injections. The PDT was performed 7 days before initial ranibizumab or sham treatment and then quarterly as needed. At 12 months, 90.5% of the ranibizumab/PDT-treated patients, as compared with 67.9% of the control patients (PDT monotherapy), had lost less than 15 letters. However, when comparing the ANCHOR results with the FOCUS results, it appears that the combination of ranibizumab with PDT does not necessarily result in better visual acuity outcomes, and the use of PDT may even reduce the visual acuity benefits achieved with ranibizumab alone. It seems unlikely that combination therapy provides any significant advantage over ranibizumab alone unless the combination of PDT and ranibizumab can decrease the need for frequent retreatment.

Two large trials of a combination of PDT and pegaptanib are also ongoing. Combination of various anti-VEGF agents (such as monoclonal antibodies and siRNAs) or combination of anti-VEGF agents with steroid and analogs may provide a more complete blockade of CNV by targeting different stages of the angiogenic process.

## DELIVERY SYSTEMS OF PHARMACOTHERAPY

The mode of drug delivery is largely dependent on the drug being delivered. Most current studies are focused on delivery systems for anti-VEGF drugs. There are two general modes of drug delivery: local or systemic. Local delivery to the eye has presumably fewer side effects than systemic administration but raises the concerns of infection, intraocular damage, and long-term safety from repeated VEGF inhibition. Modalities for local delivery include intravitreal injection, extraocular depot injection, gene therapy, and intraocular/extraocular slow-release implant devices (98).

Gene therapy for delivery of anti-angiogenic factors has been an intense area of research and is promising because the RPE cell is an easy target of viral transfection. A major concern, however, is the safety profile of viral vectors. Intravitreal polymer implants/pellets with release of first-order kinetics have been developed to deliver the anti-VEGF receptor (KDR) antibody over an extended duration to inhibit retinal neovascularization in an animal model (99). Transscleral delivery may be an innovative way of delivering drugs to the posterior segment (100). Transscleral delivery was shown to be possible by the loading of aptamer EYE001-containing polyacid microsphere into a device and placing it onto the scleral surface (101). Iontophoresis (use of electricity) and sonophoresis (ultrasound) have been used to facilitate the transscleral delivery of drugs in animal models (102). Recently, a sub-Tenon's posterior juxtascleral depot (PJD) approach has been shown to be safe and effective in delivering anecortave acetate to the posterior segment in patients with neovascular AMD (73).

## IMPLICATIONS OF CURRENT PHARMACOTHERAPY ON PATIENT CARE

### Approach to the Patient with Age-Related Macular Degeneration

Clinical trials of thermal laser and PDT with verteporfin provided clinicians with important knowledge of the clinical course of AMD and established unique parameters for the evaluation, treatment, and counseling of patients with AMD. For example, a treatment benefit was defined not as visual improvement but as prevention of moderate vision loss (less than three lines). Both the MARINA and ANCHOR studies demonstrated a prevention of moderate vision loss in 95% of patients at 12 months. More promisingly, an improvement in visual acuity of at least three lines was observed in roughly one-third of the patients. Dissemination of these results in the medical, business, and popular media raised patients' hopes for a treatment that might restore vision. With ranibizumab currently in use and other promising anti-angiogenic treatments on the horizon, physicians now hope to share in their patient's euphoria rather than commiserate with their frustration.

The clinical trials of PDT with verteporfin (Verteporfin In Photodynamic Therapy [VIP] and Treatment of Age-Related Macular Degeneration in Photodynamic Therapy [TAP]) established a clear endpoint for treatment: angiographic closure of the CNV (103,104). They also established the number and duration of treatments required to achieve this endpoint; most patients required between five and six PDT sessions over 2 years, and virtually no patient required treatment beyond 4 years (105). By contrast, in the MARINA and ANCHOR trials, patients were assigned *a priori* to receive monthly intravitreal injections of ranibizumab. Since no treatment endpoint was specified, the duration of treatment with ranibizumab remains indeterminate.

Fluorescein angiography (FA) has historically been integral to the evaluation and management of exudative AMD. A subgroup analysis of patients in the TAP study suggested a greater benefit from verteporfin in eyes with predominantly classic CNV, and exploratory analyses of data from the VIP and TAP studies further indicated lesion size (less than four disc areas) as the primary determinant of response to PDT. Therefore, FA was valuable for providing anatomic data that determined the choice and duration of treatment. The use of anti-VEGF therapies such as ranibizumab, by contrast, does not rely so heavily on FA findings, since the MARINA and ANCHOR trials showed treatment benefits irrespective of lesion size or angiographic characteristics. It is conceivable that physicians will use FA for the initial confirmation of exudative AMD, while using OCT during the course of treatment to evaluate therapeutic response. Such a paradigm is a significant change from the predictable, trimonthly "FA with possible retreatment" approach that was common with PDT.

## IMPACT ON PRACTICE DYNAMICS AND ECONOMICS

The efficacy of ranibizumab raised patients' and doctors' expectations and suggested that the vast majority of patients with exudative AMD be offered treatment of some kind. A greater number of patients being treated, coupled with an increasing frequency of treatments, translates into a dramatic increase in the number of patient visits for a practice. For example, if a physician initiates a 1 year course of monthly ranibizumab in two new patients each week, then he/she should expect to perform 624 injections in the first year, including 96 in the twelfth month alone. With the duration of treatment unknown, the total number of injections and total number of patient visits (and hence scheduling and staffing needs) cannot be accurately predicted.

Intravitreal injections carry with them infrequent but significant complications, most notably infectious endophthalmitis. The MARINA and ANCHOR study protocols provided for a safety visit 1 week following injection. While this practice may not be routinely performed by all physicians because of logistical constraints or inconvenience to the patient, potential side effects must still be considered. One approach is to document each injection performed, to discuss warning signs of infection with the patient, and to call the patient shortly after the injection. Such an approach may require organizational changes within a practice.

The overhead expenses associated with PDT (an infusionist, a dedicated laser, and the medication) were considerable and limited the number of offices at which treatments could be administered. The primary expenditure associated with ranibizumab is the medication. In order to avoid the time and expense associated with drug procurement and billing, physicians are more likely to participate in a competitive acquisition program (CAP), in which the medication can be obtained directly from a third-party vendor. Administration of ranibizumab in multiple offices is more feasible than with PDT but still requires an exam or treatment room, assistant, sterile equipment, and provisions for appropriate storage.

Given the significant cost of ranibizumab and concerns over complete and timely reimbursement for their capital outlay, many physicians have adopted the use of bevacizumab exclusively for the treatment of neovascular AMD. This practice raises medicolegal and ethical concerns regarding off-label applications as well as concerns over the supply and procurement of bevacizumab for intravitreal use.

## IMPACT ON FUTURE CLINICAL TRIALS AND NEWER TREATMENTS

Traditionally, a primary outcome measure in clinical trials of AMD has been the prevention of moderate vision loss (loss of fewer than three lines). Given the substantial number of patients in the ANCHOR and MARINA trials who maintained or improved their visual acuity, a reappraisal of this outcome measure is likely. Moreover, since ranibizumab has demonstrated superiority over prevailing standard-of-care treatments for many patients with exudative AMD, the appropriate incorporation of ranibizumab as a treatment arm (with its attendant costs) in new phase III trials will have to be addressed.

In summary, advances in our understanding of the pathophysiology of angiogenesis, ocular pharmacokinetics, and modes of drug delivery translate into the rapid development and investigation of new therapies for neovascular AMD. It is hoped that results from ongoing clinical trials will elucidate novel and better treatment paradigms and offer greater hope to patients with neovascular AMD.

## References

1. Folkman J, Klagsbrun M. Angiogenic factors. *Science* 1987;235:442–447.
2. Adamis AP, Shima DT. The role of vascular endothelial growth factor in ocular health and disease. *Retina* 2005;25:111–118.
3. Eugene WMN, Adamis AP. Targeting angiogenesis, the underlying disorder in neovascular age-related macular degeneration. *Can J Ophthalmol* 2005;40:352–368.
4. Ming L, Adamis AP. Molecular biology of choroidal neovascularization. *Ophthalmol Clin N Am* 2006;19:323–334.
5. Tong JP, Yao YF. Contribution of VEGF and PEDF to choroidal angiogenesis: a need for balanced expressions. *Clin Biochem* 2006;39(3):267–276.
6. Otrock ZK, Makarem JA, Shamseddine AI. Vascular endothelial growth factor family of ligands and receptors: Review. *Blood Cells Mol Dis* 2007;38(3):258–268.
7. Ferrara N, Carver-Moore K, Chen H, et al. Heterozygous embryonic lethality induced by targeted inactivation of the VEGF gene. *Nature* 1996;380(6573):439–442.
8. Senger DR, Galli SJ, Dvorak AM, et al. Tumor cells secret a vascular permeability factor that promotes accumulation of ascites fluid. *Science* 1983;219:983–985.
9. Ferrara N, Henzel WJ. Pituitary follicular cells secrete a novel heparin-binding growth factor specific for vascular endothelial cells. *Biochem Biophys Res Commun* 1989;161:851–858.
10. Ferrara N. Vascular endothelial growth factor: basic sciences and clinical progress. *Endocr Rev* 2004;25:581–611.
11. Houck KA, Ferrara N, Winer J, et al. The vascular endothelial growth factor family: identification of a fourth molecular species and characterization of alternative splicing of RNA. *Mol Endocrinol* 1991;5:1801–1814.
12. Park JE, Keller GA, Ferrara N. The vascular endothelial growth factor (VEGF) isoforms: differential deposition into the subepithelial extracellular matrix and bioactivity of extracellular matrix-bound VEGF. *Mol Biol Cell* 1993;4:317–1326.
13. Ishida S, Usui T, Yamashira K, et al. VEGF-165-mediated inflammation is required for pathological, but not physiological, ischemia-induced retinal neovascularization. *J Exp Med* 2003;198:483–489.
14. Keyt BA, Berleau LT, Nguyen HV, et al. The carboxyl-terminal domain (111-165) of vascular endothelial growth factor is critical for its mitogenic potency. *J Biol Chem* 1996;271:7788–7795.
15. Ferrara N, Gerber HP, LeCouter J. The biology of VEGF and its receptors. *Nat Med* 2003;9:669–676.
16. Klagsbrun M, Folkman J. Angiogenesis. In: Sporn MB, Roberts AB (eds). *Peptide growth factors and their receptors*. New York, NY: Springer-Verlag New York; 1991:549–586.
17. Paavonen K, Puolakkainen P, Jussila J, et al. Vascular endothelial growth factor receptor-3 in lymphangiogenesis in wound healing. *Am J Pathol* 2000;156:1499–1504.
18. Aiello LP, Norrhrup JM, Keyt BA, et al. Hypoxic regulation of vascular endothelial growth factor in retinal cells. *Arch Ophthalmol* 1995;113:1538–1544.
19. Blaauwgeers HG, Holtkamp GM, Rutten H, et al. Polarized vascular endothelial growth factor secretion by human retinal pigment epithelium and localization of vascular endothelial growth factor receptors on the inner choriocapillaris. Evidence for a trophic paracrine relation. *Am J Pathol* 1999;155:421–428 (As cited in Scopus).
20. Kvanta A, Algvere PV, Berglin L, et al. Subfoveal fibrovascular membranes in age-related macular degeneration express vascular endothelial growth factor. *Invest Ophthalmol Vis Sci* 1996;37:1929–1934.
21. Wells JA, Murthy R, Chibber R, et al. Levels of vascular endothelial growth factor are elevated in the vitreous of patients with subretinal neovascularisation. *Br J Ophthalmol* 1996;80:363–366.
22. Kliffen M, Sharma HS, Mooy CM, et al. Increased expression of angiogenic growth factors in age-related maculopathy. *Br J Ophthalmol* 1997;81:154–162.
23. Donoso LA, Kim D, Frost A, et al. The role of inflammation in the pathogenesis of age-related macular degeneration. *Surv Ophthalmol* 2006;51:137(2):137–152.
24. Moshfeqhi DM, Blumenkranz MS. Role of genetic factors and inflammation in age-related macular degeneration. *Retina* 2007;27(3):269–275.
25. Thakkinstian A, Han P, McEvoy M, et al. Systematic review and meta-analysis of the association between complementary factor H Y402H polymorphisms and age-related macular degeneration. *Hum Mol Genet* 2006;15(18):2784–2790.
26. Ruckman J, Green LS, Beeson J, et al. 2'-Fluoropyrimidine RNA-based aptamers to the 165-amino acid form of vascular endothelial growth factor (VEGF$_{165}$). Inhibition of receptor binding and VEGF-induced vascular permeability through interactions requiring the exon 7-encoded domain. *J Biol Chem* 1998;273:20556–20567.
27. Puliafito CA, Duker JS, Blumenkranz MS, et al. Targeting VEGF in vascular diseases. *Dulaney Foundation Webcast* 2004.
28. Eugene WM Ng, Shima DT, Calias P, et al. Pegaptanib, a targeted anti-VEGF aptamer for ocular vascular disease. *Nat Rev Drug Discov* 2006;5:123–132.

29. Gragoudas ES, Adamis AP, Cunningham ET Jr., et al. Pegaptanib for neovascular age-related macular degeneration. *N Engl J Med* 2004;351:2805–2816.

30. Charkravarthy U, Adamis AP, Cunningham ET, et al. VEGF Inhibition Study in Ocular Neovascularization (V.I.S.I.O.N) clinical trial group: Year 2 efficacy results of 2 randomized controlled clinical trials of pegaptanib for neovascular age-related macular degeneration. *Ophthalmology* 2006;113(9): e1–e25.

31. Kim KJ, Li B, Houck K, et al. The vascular endothelial growth factor proteins: identification of biologically relevant regions by neutralizing monoclonal antibodies. *Growth Factors* 1992;7:53–64.

32. Marshall J. The role of bevacizumab as first-line therapy for colon cancer. *Semin Oncol* 2005;32(6 suppl 9):S43–S47.

33. Mordenti J, Cuthbertson RA, Ferrara N, et al. Comparisons of the intraocular tissue distribution, pharmacokinetics, and safety of 125I-labeled full-length and Fab antibodies in rhesus monkeys following intravitreal administration. *Toxicol Pathol* 1999;27:536–544.

34. Gaudreault J, Fei D, Rusit J, et al. Preclinical pharmacokinetics of ranibizumab (rhuFabV2) after a single intravitreal administration. *Invest Ophthalmol Vis Sci* 2005;46:726–733.

35. Brown DM, Kaiser PK, Michels M, et al. The ANCHOR Study Group (2006). Ranibizumab versus verteporfin for neovascular age-related macular degeneration. *New Eng J Med* 2006;355:1432–1444.

36. Rosenfeld PJ, Brown DM, Heier JS, et al. The MARINA Study Group, (2006). Ranibizumab for neovascular age-related macular degeneration. *New Eng J Med* 2006;355: 1419–1431.

37. Kaiser PK, Brown DM, Zhang K, et al. Ranibizumab for predominantly classic neovascular age-related macular degeneration: subgroup analysis of first-year ANCHOR results. *Am J Ophthalmol* 2007;144(6):850–857.

38. Boyer DS, Antoszyk AN, Awh CC, et al. Subgroup analysis of the MARINA study of ranibizumab in neovascular age-related macular degeneration. *Ophthalmology* 2007;114(2):246–252.

39. Rosenfeld PJ, Rich RM, Lalwani GA. Ranibizumab: Phase III clinical trial results. *Ophthalmol Clin North Am* 2006;19(3):361–372.

40. Moshfeghi AA, Rosenfeld PJ, Puliofito CA, et al. Systemic bevacizumab (Avastin) therapy for neovascular age-related macular degeneration: twenty-four-week results of an uncontrolled open-label clinical study. *Ophthalmology* 2006;113(11):2002.e1–2002.e12 (Epub Oct 5, 2006).

41. Emerson MV, Lauer AK, Flaxel CJ, et al. Intravitreal bevacizumab (avastin) treatment of neovascular age-related macular degeneration. *Retina* 2007;27(4):439–444.

42. Golf MJ, Johnson RN, McDonald HR, et al. Intravitreal bevacizumab for previously treated choroidal neovascularization from age-related macular degeneration. *Retina* 2007;27(4):432–438.

43. Wulff C, Wilson H, Wiegand SJ, et al. Prevention of thecal angiogenesis, antral follicular growth, and ovulation in the primate with vascular endothelial growth factor trapR1R2. *Endocrinology* 2002;143:2797–2807.

44. Wong AK, Alfert M, Castrillon DH, et al. Excessive tumor-elaborated VEGF and its neutralization define a lethal paraneoplastic syndrome. *Proc Natl Acad Sci USA* 2001;98:7481–7486.

45. Saishin Y, Saishin Y, Takahashi K, et al. VEGF-TRAP(R1R2) suppresses choroidal neovascularization and VEGF-induced breakdown of the blood-retinal barrier. *J Cell Physiol* 2003;195(2):241–248.

46. Ngyen QD, Shah SM, Hafiz G, et al. A phase I trial of an IV-administered vascular endothelial growth factor trap for treatment in patients with choroidal neovascularization due to age-related macular degeneration. *Ophthalmology* 2006;113(9):1522.e1–1522.e14 (Epub Jul 28, 2006).

47. Pushparai PN, Melendez AJ. Short interfering RNA(SiRNA) as a novel therapeutic. *Clin Exp Pharmacol Physiol* 2006;33(5-6):504–510.

48. Reich SJ, Fosnot J, Kuroki A, et al. Small interfering RNA (siRNA) targeting VEGF effectively inhibits ocular neovascularization in a mouse model. *Mol Vis* 2003;9:210–216.

49. Cashman SM, Bowman L, Christofferson J, et al. Inhibition of choroidal neovascularization by adenovirus-mediated delivery of short hairpin RNAs targeting VEGF as a potential therapy for AMD. *Invest Ophthalmol Vis Sci* 2006;47(8):3496–3504 (As cited in Scopus).

50. Shen J, Samul R, Silva RL, et al. Suppression of ocular neovascularization with siRNA targeting VEGF receptor 1. *Gene Therapy* 2006;13(3):225–234.

51. Takahashi T, Ueno H, Shibuya M. VEGF activates protein kinase C-dependent, but Ras-independent Raf-MEK-MAP kinase pathway for DNA synthesis in primary endothelial cells. *Oncogene* 1999;18:2221–2230.

52. Gerber HP, McMurtrey A, Kowalski J, et al. Vascular endothelial growth factor regulates endothelial cell survival through the phosphatidylinositol 3′-kinase/Akt signal transduction pathway. Requirement for Flk-1/KDR activation. *J Biol Chem* 1998;273:30336–30343.

53. Jain RK. Molecular regulation of vessel maturation. *Nat Med* 2003;9:685–693.

54. Bikfalvi A, Bicknell R. Recent advances in angiogenesis, anti-angiogenesis and vascular targeting. *Trends Pharmacol Sci* 2002;23:576–582.

55. Bergers G, Song S, Meyer-Morse N, et al. Benefits of targeting both pericytes and endothelial cells in the tumor vasculature with kinase inhibitors. *J Clin Invest* 2003;111:1287–1295.

56. Tombran-Tink J, Barnstable CJ. PEDF: a multifaceted neurotrophic factor. *Nat Rev Neurosci* 2003;4(8):628–636.

57. Tong JP, Chan WM, Liu DT, et al. Aqueous humor levels of vascular endothelial growth factor and pigment epithelium-derived factor in polypoidal choroidal vasculopathy and choroidal neovascularization. *Am J Ophthalmol* 2006;141(3):456–462.

58. Mori K, Gehlbach P, Yamamoto S, et al. AAV-mediated gene transfer of pigment epithelium-derived factor inhibits choroidal neovascularization. *Invest Ophthalmol Vis Sci* 2002;43:1994–2000.

59. Mori K, Gehlbach P, Ando A, et al. Regression of ocular neovascularization in response to increased expression of pigment epithelium-derived factor. *Invest Ophthalmol Vis Sci* 2002;43:2428–2434.

60. Rassmussen H, Chu KW, Campochiaro P, et al. Clinical protocol: an open-label, phase I, single administration, dose-escalation study of ADGVPEDF.11D (ADPEDF) in neovascular age-related macular degeneration (AMD). *Hum Gene Therapy* 2001;12:2029–2032.

61. Folkman J, Ingber DE. Angiostatic steroids. Method of discovery and mechanism of action. *Ann Surg* 1987;206:374–383.

62. Folkman J, Weisz BV, Joullie MM, et al. Control of angiogenesis with synthetic heparin substitutes. *Science* 1989;243:1490–1493.

63. Jonas JB. Intravitreal triamcinolone acetonide: a change in a paradigm. *Ophthamic Res* 2006;38:218–245.

64. Penfold PL, Gyory JF, Hunyor AB, et al. Exudative macular degeneration and intravitreal triamcinolone. A pilot study. *Aust N Z J Ophthalmol* 1995; 23(4):293–298.

65. Jonas JB, Degenring RF, Kreissig I, et al. Exudative age-related macular degeneration treated by intravitreal triamcinolone acetonide: a prospective comparative non-randomized study. *Eye* 2005;19:163–170.

66. Nicolo M, Ghiglione D, Lai S, et al. Intravitreal triamcinolone in the treatment of serous pigment epithelial detachment and occult choroidal neovascularization secondary to age-related macular degeneration. *Eur J Ophthalmol* 2005;15:415–419.

67. Gillies MC, Simpson JM, Luo W, et al. A randomized clinical trial of a single dose of intravitreal triamcinolone acetonide for neovascular age-related macular degeneration: one-year results. *Arch Ophthalmol* 2003;121:667–673.

68. Spaide RF, Sorenson J, Maranan L. Combined photodynamic therapy with verteporfin and intravitreal triamcinolone acetonide for choroidal neovascularization. *Ophthalmology* 2003;110:1517–1525.

69. Arias L, Garcin-Arami J, Ramon JM, et al. Photodynamic therapy with intravitreal triamcinolone in predominantly classic choroidal neovascularization: one-year results of a randomized study. *Ophthalmology* 2006;113(2):2243–2250.

70. Augustin AJ, Schmidt-erfurth U. Verteporfin therapy combined with intravitreal triamcinolone in all types of choroidal neovascularization due to age-related macular degeneration. *Ophthalmology* 2006;113(1): 14–22.

71. Ozkiris A, Erkilic K. Complications of intravitreal injection of triamcinolone acetonide. *Can J Ophthalmol* 2005;40:63–68.

72. Clark AF. AL-3789: a novel ophthalmic angiostatic steroid. *Expert Opin Investig Drugs* 1997;6:1867–1877.

73. Kaiser PK, Goldberg MF, Davis AA; Anecortave Acetate Clinical Study Group. Posterior juxtascleral depot administration of anecortave acetate. *Surv Ophthalmol* 2007;52(Suppl 1):S62–S69.

74. Russell SR, Hudson HL, Jerdan JA; Anecortave Acetate Clinical Study Group. Anecortave acetate for the treatment of exudative age-related macular degeneration–a review of clinical outcomes. *Surv Ophthalmol* 2007;52(Suppl 1):S79–S90.

75. Connolly B, Desai A, Garcia CA, et al. Squalamine lactate for exudative age-related macular degeneration. *Ophthalmol Clin North Am* 2006;19(3):381–389.

76. Frank RN, Amin RH, Eliott D, et al. Basic fibroblast growth factor and vascular endothelial growth factor and vascular endothelial growth factor are present in epiretinal and choroidal neovascular membranes. *Am J ophthalmol* 1996;122:393–403.

77. Yi X, Ogata N, Komada M, et al. Vascular endothelial growth factor expression in choroidal neovascularization in rats. *Graefe Arch Clin Exp Ophthalmol* 1997;235:313–319.

78. Tobe T, Ortega S, Luna JD, et al. Targeted disruption of the FGF2 gene does not prevent choroidal neovascularization in a murine model. *Am J Pathol* 1998;153:1641–1646.

79. Yancopoulos GD, Davis S, Gale NW, et al. Vascular-specific growth factors and blood vessel formation. *Nature* 2000;407:242–248.

80. Thurston G, Rudge JS, Joffe E, et al. Angiopoietin-1 protects the adult vasculature against plasma leakage. *Nat Med* 2000;6:460–463.

81. Oh H, Takagi H, Suzuma K, et al. Hypoxia and vascular endothelial growth factor selectively up-regulate angiopoietin/tie 2 system in ischemia-induced retinal neovascularization. *Invest ophthalmol Vis Sci* 2003;44: 393–402.

82. Oh H, Takagi H, Suzuma K, et al. Hypoxia and vascular endothelial growth factor selectively up-regulate angiopoietin-2 in bovine microvascular endothelial cells. *J Biol Chem* 1999;274:15732–15739.

83. Otani A, Takagi H, Oh H, et al. Expressions of angiopoietins and Tie2 in human choroidal neovascular membranes. *Invest Ophthalmol Vis Sci* 1999;40:1912–1920.

84. Takagi H, Koyama S, Seike H, et al. Potential role of the angiopoietins/Tie2 system in ischemia-induced retinal neovascularization. *Invest Ophthalmol Vis Sci* 2003;44:393–402.

85. Hangai M, Moon YS, Kitaya N, et al. Systemically expressed soluble tie2 inhibits intraocular neovascularization. *Hum Gen Ther* 2001;12:1311–1321.

86. Kim I, Moon SO, Park SK, et al. Angiopoietin-1 reduces VEGF-stimulated leukocyte adhesion to endothelial cells by reducing ICAM-1, VCAM-1, and E-selectin expression. *Circ Res* 2001;89:477–479.

87. Hammes HP, Brownlee M, Jonczyk A, et al. Subcutaneous injection of a cyclic peptide antagonist of vitronectin receptor-type integrins inhibits retinal neovascularization. *Nat Med* 1996;2:529–533.

88. Takahashi T, Nakamura T, Hayashi A, et al. Inhibition of experimental choroidal neovascularization by overexpression of tissue inhibitor of metalloproteinases-3 in retinal pigment epithelium cells. *Am J Ophthalmol* 2000;130(6):774–781.

89. Witmer AN, Vrensen GF, Van Noorden CJ, et al. Vascular endothelial growth factors and angiogenesis in eye disease. *Pro Retin Eye Res* 2003;22:1–29.

90. Sakamoto T, Soriano D, Nassaralla J, et al. Effect of intravitreal administration of indomethacin on experimental subretinal neovascularization in subhuman primate. *Arch Ophthalmol* 1995;113:222–226.

91. Wahl ML, Kenan DJ, Gonzalez-Gronow M, et al. Angiostatin's molecular mechanism: aspects of specificity and regulation elucidated. *J. Cell Biochem* 2005;96:242–261.

92. Balaggan KS, Binkley K, Esapa M, et al. EIAV vector-mediated delivery of endostatin or angiostatin inhibits angiogenesis and vascular hyperpermeability in experimental CNV. *Gene Therapy* 2006;13(15):1153–1165 (Epub Jun 13, 2006).

93. Digtyar AV, Pozdnyakova NV, Feldman NB, et al. Endostatin: current concepts about its biological role and mechanisms of action. *Biochemistry (Mosc)* 2007;72(3):235–246.

94. Yamagucchi N, Anand-Apte N, Lee M, et al. Endostatin inhibits VEGF-induced endothelial cell migration and tumor growth independently of zinc binding. *EMBO J* 1999;18(16):4414–4423.

95. Tatar O, Shinoda K, Adam A, et al. Expression of endostatin in human choroidal neovascular membranes secondary to age-related macular degeneration. *Exp Eye Res* 2006;83(2):329–338 (Epub Apr 11, 2006).

96. Augustin AJ, Puls S, Offermann I. Triple therapy for choroidal neovascularization due to age-related macular degeneration: verteporfin PDT, bevacizumab, and dexamethasone. *Retina* 2007;27(2):133–140.

97. Heier JS, Boyer DS, Ciulla TA, et al. Ranibizumab in combination with verteporfin photodynamic therapy in neovascular age-related macular degeneration (FOCUS): year 1 results. *Arch Ophthalmol* 2006;124(11):1532–1542.

98. Lu M, Adamis AP. Ocular delivery of angiostatic agents. *Int Ophthalmol Clin* 2004;44:41–51.

99. Mcleod DS, Taomoto M, Cao J, et al. Localization of VEGF receptor-2 (KDR/Flk-1) and effects of blocking it in oxygen-induced retinopathy. *Invest Ophthalmol Vis Sci* 2002;43:474–482.

100. Ambati J, Adamis AP. Transscleral drug delivery to the retina and choroid. *Prog Retin Eye Res* 2002;21:145–151.

101. Carrasquillo KG, Ricker JA, Rigas IK, et al. Controlled delivery of the anti-VEGF aptamer EYE001 with poly(lactic-co-glycolic) acid microspheres. *Invest Ophthalmol Vis Sci* 2003;44:290–299.

102. Myles ME, Neumann DM, Hill JM. Recent progress in ocular drug delivery for posterior segment disease: emphasis on transscleral iontophoresis. *Adv Drug Deliv Rev* 2005;57(14):2063–2079.

103. Bressler NM; Treatment of Age-Related Macular Degeneration with Photodynamic Therapy (TAP) Study Group. Photodynamic therapy of subfoveal choroidal neovascularization in age-related macular degeneration with verteporfin: two-year results of 2 randomized clinical trials – TAP report 2. *Arch Ophthalmol* 2001;119(2):198–207.

104. Verteporfin in Photodynamic Therapy Study Group. Verteporfin therapy of subfoveal choroidal neovascularization in age-related macular degeneration: two-year results of a randomized clinical trial including lesions with occult with no classic choroidal neovascularization–verteporfin in photodynamic therapy report 2. *Am J Ophthalmol* 2001;131(5):541–560.

105. Bressler NM, Bressler SB, Haynes LA, et al. Verteporfin therapy for subfoveal choroidal neovascularization in age-related macular degeneration: four-year results of an open-label extension of 2 randomized clinical trials: TAP Report No. 7. *Arch Ophthalmol* 2005;123(9):1283–1285.

# 35

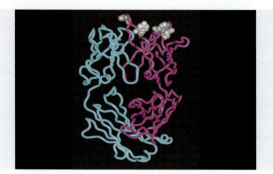

# Ranibizumab (Ranibizumab™) in the Treatment of Wet Macular Degeneration

Monica Rodriguez-Fontal ■ D. Virgil Alfaro III ■ John B. Kerrison

## INTRODUCTION

Pathologic angiogenesis and vascular leakage have been recognized as major causes of visual loss in the wet form of age-related macular degeneration (AMD) (1). Although a combination of molecular regulators is involved in this complex process (2), multiple studies evidence the role of the vascular endothelial growth factor (VEGF) as the main signal in the ocular neovascularization (3,4,5).

The VEGF, also known as VEGF-A, is a heparin-binding glycoprotein that belongs to a gene family that includes VEGF-C, VEGF-D, VEGF-B, and placenta growth factor (PIGF) (1). The human VEGF-A has 4 different isoforms as a result of the alternative exon splicing, $VEGF_{121}$, $VEGF_{165}$, $VEGF_{189}$, $VEGF_{206}$; the numbers show how many amino acids the VEGF molecule has after each cleavage. Other less frequent variants that have been reported are $VEGF_{145}$ and $VEGF_{183}$ (1). The $VEGF_{165}$ is the major isoform (6) (Fig. 35-1). Inhibiting the action of the VEGF (the isoform$_{165}$ or all the isoforms) has been postulated as a possible treatment in several diseases including solid tumors and ocular diseases that involved visual loss as a result of vascular leakage or pathologic angiogenesis.

The use of VEGF inhibition as a treatment for human disease has been studied for many years, and different therapeutic agents targeting the VEGF have been developed. A humanized monoclonal anti-VEGF antibody, Bevacizumab (Avastin®; Genentech, CA) was approved by the FDA in 2004 for intravenous therapy of metastatic colorectal cancer; in early 2004, Rosenfeld et al, initiated the use of bevacizumab in the treatment of wet AMD. In their first study SANA (Systemic Avastin for Neovascular AMD) the investigators used the drug intravenously and subsequent studies have used it, off-label, with intravitreal injections (7,8,9,10).

Macugen® (pegaptanib sodium; Eyetech Pharmaceuticals, NY), an anti-VEGF aptamer, was the first anti-VEGF agent proved to be efficacious in patients with wet AMD (11); its complex structure allows it to specifically bind the $VEGF_{165}$ isoform.

In June 2006, the U. S. Food and Drug Administration (FDA) approved ranibizumab for the treatment of neovascular wet AMD. Ranibizumab (Lucentis™; Genentech, CA) is a recombinant, humanized, monoclonal anti-VEGF antibody fragment, with the ability to bind to all the isoforms of the VEGF (12) (Fig. 35-2).

This chapter reviews the science and clinical trials of Lucentis™ (ranibizumab) and the role of this drug in the treatment of subfoveal choroidal neovascularization (CNV) secondary to AMD.

## BACKGROUND

The observation that solid tumor growth can be accompanied by increase vascularity was made one century ago (1). Ide et al. (13) postulated in 1939 the existence of a tumor-derived blood vessel growth-stimulating factor that may be responsible for inducing the neovascularization in the growing tumor. In 1948, Isaac Michaelson (14) proposed that a diffusible angiogenic "factor X" produced by the retina may be responsible for the retinal and iris neovascularization that occurs in proliferative diabetic retinopathy and other retinal disorders, such a central vein occlusion. In 1971, Folkman et al. (15) proposed that anti-angiogenesis might be an effective treatment for human cancer and initiated the efforts to isolate a "tumor angiogenesis factor." In 1983, Senger et al. (16) described the partial purification of a tumor protein able to induce vascular leakage, named "tumor vascular permeability factor." Because it was not isolated and sequenced, it remained molecularly unknown at that time. In 1989, Ferrera et al. (17) reported the isolation of a diffusible endothelial cell-specific mitogen, named VEGF; that was demonstrated later to be the same molecule that Senger found. After these initials steps, numerous papers have been published supporting the theory that VEFG is an endothelial cell mitogen and vascular permeability factor.

Aiello et al. (5) and Malecaze et al. (18) reported elevations of the VEGF in the aqueous humor and vitreous humor of the human eyes with proliferative retinopathy secondary to diabetes and other retinal disorders, demonstrating a temporal correlation between the VEGF elevations and the active proliferative retinopathy.

Studies by Kvanta et al. (19) and Lopez et al. (20) suggest a role for VEGF in the progression of the CNV in AMD; the authors

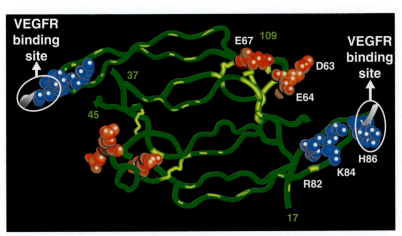

**Figure 35-1.** Vascular endothelial growth factor (VEGF), a homodimeric glycoprotein that is secreted in response to hypoxia and ischemia. VEGF induces angiogenesis and vascular permeability. Arrows show the binding site VEGF receptor.

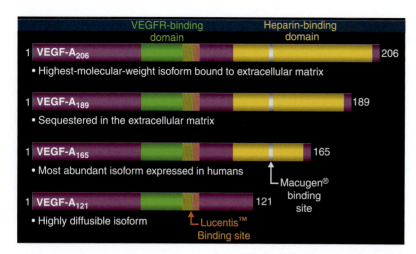

**Figure 35-2.** Ranibizumab (Ranibizumab™ Genentech, CA) is a recombinant, humanized, monoclonal anti–vascular endothelial growth factor (VEGF) antibody fragment, with ability to bind to all the isoforms of the VEGF. (From Ferrara et al. *Nat Med* 2003;9:669; Robinson and Stringer. *J Cell Sci* 2001;114:853, with permission; Macugen® (pegaptanib) PI 2005. Genetech, data on file.).

demonstrated the immunohistochemical localization of the VEGF in surgically resected CNV membranes from AMD patients.

Significant experimental evidence began to support the theory that VEGF inhibition could lead to suppression of ocular angiogenesis. Aiello et al. (21) evaluated *in vitro* and *in vivo* the inhibition of the VEGF and subsequent CNV using VEGF-neutralizing chimaeric proteins in a murine model of ischemic retinopathy. With this study Aiello clearly demonstrated that stimulation of the bovine retinal endothelial cell growth by both exogenous VEGF and hypoxia-induced VEGF was effectively suppressed with *in vitro* use of VEGF-receptor chimaeric proteins. Furthermore, he demonstrated, using a highly reproducible murine model of ischemia-induced retinal neovascularization, that inhibition of the VEGF reduces retinal neovascularization *in vivo*. Aiello (21) also highlighted another interesting theory, when he realized that the VEGF-neutralizing chimaeric proteins incompletely inhibited retinal neovascularization. The author theorized that penetration of the VEGF-neutralizing chimaeric proteins (human Flt-IgG and murine Flt-1-IgG both consist of entire VEGF receptors bound to IgG heavy chain) into the retinal tissue was unlikely, because of the size of the bulky chimaeric proteins, limiting the protein actions to the capillaries on the inner retinal surface.

Adamis et al. (4) also demonstrated that the VEGF was necessary for the retinal ischemia-associated iris neovascularization in a monkey model. The authors prevented iris neovascularization in monkey eyes with injections of an anti-VEGF monoclonal antibody.

## Synthesis of Ranibizumab: Humanization, Affinity-Maturation, and Fragmentation

Murine antibodies (muMAb VEGF) are effective in the primate model (4), but their use as a human therapy was limited by the anti-globulin secondary immune reaction (22,23). Chimaeric molecules, where human constant regions are fused with variable rodent domains, are still capable of eliciting an immune response (24). Humanization of the murine monoclonal antibodies was an effective solution to overcome this clinical limitation. Presta et al. (25) described how the transfer of six complimentary-determining regions (CDR) from muMAB VEGF A 4.6.1 to a human framework by site direct mutagenesis and subsequently reduce its binding to VEGF over 1000 fold, humanizing the murine antibody (Fig. 35-3). To achieve binding equivalent to the original muMab, seven framework residues in the humanized variable light domain were changed from human to murine. Comparison of the humanized and the chimaeric antibodies revealed the same activity.

It remained to be investigated whether such recombinant proteins would reach their target following intravitreal administration. Mordenti et al. (26) suggested that rhuMAb VEGF Fab (fragment of the entire antibody with affinity for the

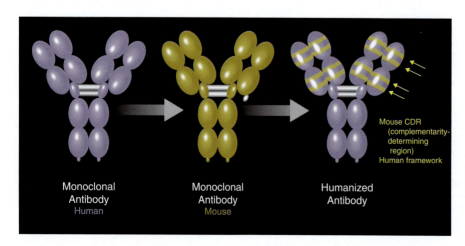

**Figure 35-3.** The humanization of muMAb VEGF A.4.6.1 involved the transfer of six complimentary-determining regions (CDR) from muMAb VEGF A.4.6.1 to a human framework by site-directed mutagenesis. The final antibody is a rhuMAb (recombinant, humanized, monoclonal antibody).

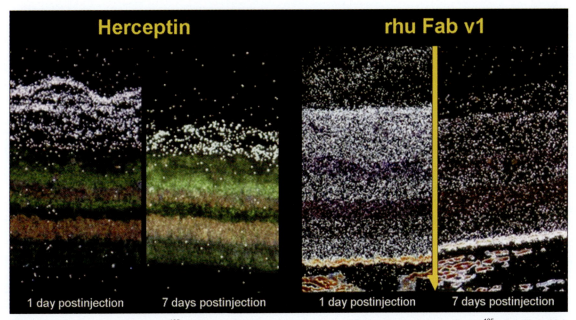

**Figure 35-4.** Histoautoradiograph of [125]I-rhuMab VEGF Fab V1, the humanized Fab antibody (Column B) and [125]Iodine (I)-rhuMab HER2, the full-length humanized antibody (Column A) following bilateral intravitreal injections in Rhesus monkeys. The Fab fragment penetrated all of the layers of the retina evenly extending as far back as the retinal pigment epithelium while the full-length antibody failed to penetrate farther than the ILM at any point during the study.

VEGF) might be a more effective therapy for AMD than full-length rhuMAb antibody because of its ability to diffuse into the retinal-choroidal boundary. Mordenti et al. (26) studied the safety, the pharmacokinetics, and the retinal distribution of rhuMab HER2 (the full-length humanized antibody, 148 kD) and rhuMab VEGF Fab (the humanized Fab antibody 48.3 kD), following bilateral intravitreal injections in Rhesus monkeys. Retinal tissue distribution of [125]I-labeled rhuMab HER2 and rhuMAb VEGF Fab was evaluated with microautoradiography. One hour post-injection, rhuMab VEGF Fab was detected throughout the retinal layers while rhuMab HER2 was found only in the vitreous cavity. RhuMab HER2 failed to penetrate the inner limiting membrane (ILM) (Fig. 35-4). RhuMab VEGF Fab was detected throughout the retinal layers as far as the retinal pigment epithelium (RPE) in the medial and lateral portions. By day 1, rhuMab VEGF Fab was evenly distributed throughout all of the retinal layers and remained so through day 4. Signals peaked to a maximum at day 1 and did not

persist past day 7. Analysis of vitreous fluids revealed a half-life of 5.6 days of the full-length rhuMAb HER2 antibody and 3.2 days for the rhuMAb VEGF Fab, supporting the conclusion that the rate of vitreous clearing is directly affected by the molecular size of the molecules. Plasma levels of rhuMAb VEGF Fab remained constant below the assay limit of detection (7.8 ng/ml) throughout the study. Plasma levels of rhuMAb HER2 ranged from <4% to 30%. The authors suggested that Bruch's membrane may act as a barrier for rhuMAb VEGF fab, preventing further diffusion into the choroid and resulting in an accumulation of fragmented antibody in the RPE. The ILM may also act as a physical barrier to the full-length antibody. Based on this assay, rhuMAb was fragmented to obtain Fab fragment with the same affinity as the whole antibody but with greater ability for penetration in the tissue (Fig. 35-5).

Following humanization, the Fab portion of the antibody (known as rhuMAb VEGF or recombinant humanized Monoclonal Antibody VEGF) was affinity-matured through CDR

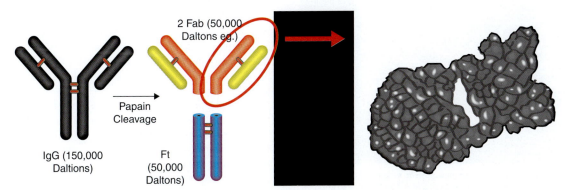

**Figure 35-5.** Papain cleavage of IgG antibody into two Fab fragments and the Fc fragment. The Fab portion is approximately a third of the original IgG.

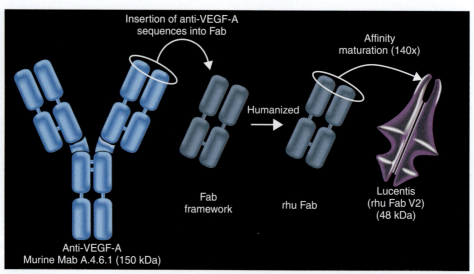

**Figure 35-6.** RhuMAb vascular endothelial growth factor (VEGF) was fragmented and affinity matured through complementarity-determining region (CDR) mutation and affinity selection by monovalent phage display.

mutation and affinity selected by monovalent phage display (27). It was possible to improved contacts between antibody and antigen. Two mutations resulted in increased van der Waals contact and improved hydrogen bonding (Figs. 35-6 and 35-7). The final antibody (affinity-matured rhuMAb) has improved affinity for several VEGF variants as compared with the parental antibody.

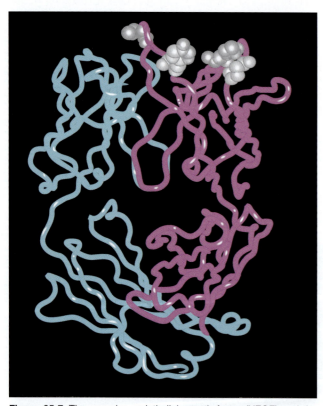

**Figure 35-7.** The vascular endothelial growth factor (VEGF) and the affinity-matured Fab fragment complex. Locally, it was possible to improve the contact between the antibody and the antigen through two mutations that improved the hydrogen bonding and van der Waals contact.

# PHARMACOKINETICS AND MECHANISM OF ACTION OF RANIBIZUMAB

## Pharmacokinetics

Graudreault et al. (28) studied the ranibizumab (rhuFabV2, the rhuFab with affinity-matured) pharmacokinetic (PK) profile in cynomolgus monkeys. The selection of these monkeys was based on the idea of using the same animal model that was used to characterize the ranibizumab profile. The authors found that ranibizumab clears equivalently from all ocular compartments, with a half life of 3 days; 50% of the drug reached the circulation after 2 days, consistent with the half life and also suggesting that intraocular metabolism does not play a significant role in the elimination of ranibizumab from the vitreous. The authors observed the ability of the drug to penetrate the retina in cynomolgus monkeys, a finding consistent with the previous study in Rhesus monkeys using the first generation of rhuFab (rhuFabV1 without maturation) (26).

The same results were obtained after intravitreal administration of ranibizumab in rabbits. Ranibizumab clears from rabbits' vitreous cavity in 2.9 days (29). The distribution of $^{125}$I-labeled ranibizumab determined by microautoradiography was consistent with specific sites of VEGF production and binding (ganglion cell and photoreceptor layer) (29). Avery et al. have shown that ranibizumab penetrates the full thickness retina at 1 to 3 days (30). In patients with neovascular AMD the pharmacokinetic profile was investigated following monthly intravitreal administration of ranibizumab; the maximum ranibizumab serum concentrations were low (0.3 ng/ml to 2.36 ng/ml). These levels were below the concentration of ranibizumab (11 ng/ml to 27 ng/ml) thought to be necessary to inhibit the biological activity of VEGF-A by 50%, as measured in an *in vitro* cellular proliferation assay. The maximum observed serum concentration was dose proportional over the dose range of 0.05 to 1.0 mg/eye. Based on a population pharmacokinetic

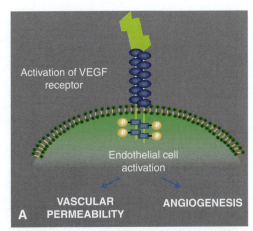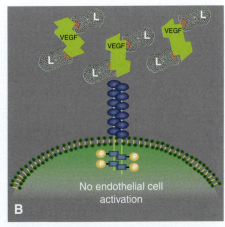

**Figure 35-8. A:** Activation of the vascular endothelial growth factor (VEGF) receptor (VEGFR1 and VEGFR2) of the endothelial cell by the VEGF generates an endothelial cell activation that increases the vascular permeability and induces angiogenesis. (From Ferrara et al. *Nat Med* 2003;9:669.) **B:** Ranibizumab binds to the receptor binding site of active forms of VEGF-A, avoid the interaction of VEGF-A with its receptors, on the surface of endothelial cells, reducing endothelial cell proliferation, vascular leakage, and new blood vessel formation.

analysis, maximum serum concentrations of 1.5 ng/ml are predicted to be reached at approximately 1 day after monthly intravitreal administration of ranibizumab 0.5 mg/eye. Based on the disappearance of ranibizumab from serum, the estimated average vitreous elimination half-life was approximately 9 days. Steady-state minimum concentration is predicted to be 0.22 ng/ml with a monthly dosing regimen. In humans, serum ranibizumab concentrations are predicted to be approximately 90,000-fold lower than vitreal concentrations.

## Mechanism of Action

Ranibizumab binds to the receptor binding site of active forms of VEGF-A, including the biologically active, cleaved form of this molecule, $VEGF_{110}$. With binding of ranibizumab to VEGF-A, the interaction of VEGF-A with its endothelial cell surface receptors, VEGFR1 and VEGFR2, is impaired leading to a reduction in endothelial cell proliferation, vascular leakage, and new blood vessel formation (Fig. 35-8A and B).

## Assays in Animal Models

Krystolik et al. (31) designed a two phase study to evaluate the safety and efficacy of intravitreal rhuFab (monoclonal, recombinant, humanized, Fab fragment antibody) injection in a monkey model (cynomolgus monkeys) of CNV. The assay had 2 phases: phase 1 or prevention phase and phase 2 or treatment phase.

During phase 1, the possibility of preventing the formation of significant CNV with intravitreal rhuFab VEGF injections was investigated. In this phase each monkey was randomly assigned a prevention eye and a control eye, and nine CNV lesions were induced in the macula of each eye with argon green laser burns. The prevention eyes were treated with intravitreal injections of 500 μg of reconstituted rhuFab per eye, pre and post the induction of the lesions while the control eyes received a vehicle with the same components as the reconstituted rhuFab minus the rhuFab VEGF protein. Analysis of the

CNV lesions using color photographs and fluorescein angiography revealed that the rhuFab injected eyes had less chance of reaching grade 4 leakage than the vehicle treated eyes, indicating that the formation of significant CNV can be prevented with intravitreal rhuFab VEGF injections.

During phase 2, the effect of intravitreal rhuFab therapy on existing CNV lesions was assessed. This phase began 3 weeks after the laser treatments at approximately the time when CNV lesions in the control eyes began to form, the control eyes were switched over into a treatment group and received injections of 500 μg per eye of rhuFab VEGF, and the injections were repeated 14 days later. Analysis showed a significant decrease in amount of leakage from already formed CNV membranes after rhuFab treatment. The results from phase 2 suggest that rhuFab therapy is a beneficial treatment for established CNV lesions (Fig. 35-9).

The blood and vitreous samples collected to test antibodies to rhuFab VEGF show that one of the ten monkeys developed antibodies to rhuFab VEGF in the vitreous following the first injection and accumulating with subsequent treatments as well as slightly elevated serum levels of rhuFab VEGF. The antibodies were generated toward the humanized rhuFab VEGF backbone (not the mouse-derived binding epitope) and are thereby not neutralizing (31).

Over the course of the study, researchers had the opportunity to evaluate the safety of intravitreal rhuFab VEGF through clinical examination and fundus photographs. No choroidal or retinal hemorrhages were found as a result of the intravitreal injections in either the rhuFab treated eyes or the vehicle receiving eyes. No perivascular lesions associated with higher rhuFab levels in some animals were noted. Consistent throughout phase 1 and phase 2 was the development of acute inflammation in each rhuFab-treated eye following the first injection with intravitreal rhuFab VEGF, and subsequent treatments resulted in less inflammation. Vehicle-treated eyes had little or no inflammation throughout the study (31).

Gaudreault et al. (32) characterized the effect of rhuFab V2 (Ranibizumab) inhibition on VEGF-induced permeability in

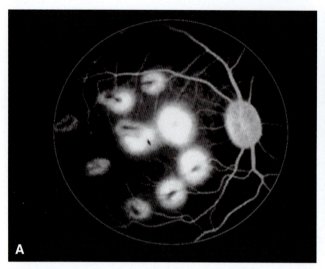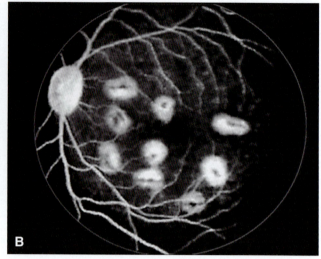

**Figure 35-9.** Krystolik assay. Cynomolgus monkeys, model of choroidal neovascularization. **A:** Pre-rhuFab injection. **B:** After rhuFab injection.

guinea pigs (Miles assay). Following intracardiac injection of Evans Blue, hairless guinea pigs received intradermal dorsum injections of rhuFab V2 (0–6000 ng/ml) concomitantly with rhVEGF$_{165}$ (100 ng/ml). One hour following intradermal injection, the animals were euthanized; pelts were harvested and photographed for quantification of dye leakage into the injection sites. The relationship between rhuFab V2 concentration and dye leakage was characterized using an E$_{max}$ model. RhuFab V2 inhibition of VEGF-induced permeability occurred in a concentration-dependent manner and this inhibition of VEGF-induced permeability was demonstrated in a Miles Assay (Fig. 35-10).

## CLINICAL TRIALS

### Ranibizumab for Age-Related Macular Degeneration: Phase I/II Studies

Three studies (phase I and I/II) were designed to investigate the doses of ranibizumab that would be appropriate for the treatment of neovascular AMD in large, multicenter, randomized phase III clinical trials. The first, FVF 1770 g, a

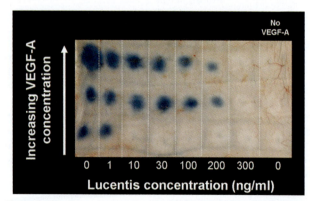

**Figure 35-10.** Characterizing the effect of rhuFab V2 (Ranibizumab) inhibition on vascular endothelial growth factor (VEGF)-induced permeability in guinea pigs (Miles assay). (From Gaudreault J, Reich M, Arata A, et al. Ocular pharmacokinetics and antipermeability effect of rhuFab V2 in animals. ARVO 2003. Poster B645).

phase I dose-escalating study with patients with neovascular AMD (33); the second, a larger, phase I/II clinical study, investigated the tolerability and efficacy of multiple monthly intravitreal injections of ranibizumab at doses of 0.3 mg or 0.5 mg in patients with neovascular AMD (34); and the third trial, a phase I clinical study, investigated doses of ranibizumab above 0.5 mg to determine if doses higher than the maximum tolerated single dose could be well accepted when injected in an escalating stepwise fashion every 2 or 4 weeks (35).

A Phase IA (FVF 1770 g) open-label, 5-center, uncontrolled, prospective, dose-ranging, interventional case series enrolled 27 patients (33). A single intravitreal injection of ranibizumab (ranging from 50 µg to 1000 µg) was given to 27 patients with occult or mix CNV to determine ocular and systemic safety. Visual acuity was measured 3 months post injection. While 11% of patients experienced a transient decline of 3 or more lines maximized by day 3, all 27 patients ended the study 3 months later with visual acuity similar to or improved from baseline. Dose-limiting toxicity resulting in ocular inflammation was reached at 1000 µg/eye. A dose of 500 µg/eye was determined to be the maximum tolerated dose. Furthermore there was initial concern that the humanized protein containing the residual mouse sequences might elicit a human anti-mouse immunoresponse that might decrease ranibizumab's efficacy. At the end of the 3 month trial, no serum antibodies against ranibizumab were observed.

A Phase IB/II (FVF 2128 g) multicenter, randomized, controlled trial evaluating the safety and tolerability of repeated intravitreal ranibizumab injections in treating neovascular AMD was designed (34). Sixty-four patients with subfoveal predominantly or minimally classic AMD-related CNV were included. Patients were randomized to 300 µg/eye or 500 µg/eye regimes of ranibizumab, or to standard therapy (observation or photodynamic therapy [PDT]). In part 1, subjects were randomized to monthly intravitreal ranibizumab for 3 months (4 injections of 0.3 mg or 1 injection of 0.3 mg followed by 3 injections of 0.5 mg; n = 53 patients) or usual care (11 patients). In part 2, subjects could continue their regimen for 3 additional months or cross over to the alternative treatment. The results were very enthusiastic. The visual acuity improved from baseline 15 letters or more in 45% (at day 210) of subjects on ranibizumab while none of the "standard care" patients had 15 letters or more (at day 98). These results showed that intravitreal injections of ranibizumab had a good safety profile and were associated with improved visual acuity (VA) and decreased leakage from CNV in subjects with neovascular AMD.

The third FVF 2425 g study was a phase I open-label, 2-center, uncontrolled, randomized study designed to investigate whether multiple intravitreal doses of up to 2 mg of ranibizumab can be tolerated and are biologically active when injected using a dose-escalating strategy in eyes of patients with neovascular AMD (35). The study enrolled 32 patients with wet AMD; the treatment regimens consisted of 5, 7, or 9 intravitreal injections of ranibizumab at 2 or 4-week intervals for 16 weeks, with escalating doses ranging from 0.3 mg to 2.0 mg; 27 patients completed the study through day 140. Results were similar across the 3 treatment groups. The ocular adverse events were mild, and the most common were iridocyclitis (83%) although the inflammation did not increase with repeated injections, despite the increasing ranibizumab doses. No serum anti-ranibizumab antibodies were detected. The team concluded that multiple intravitreal injections of ranibizumab at escalating doses ranging from 0.3 mg to 2.0 mg were well tolerated, but these results did not seem to add any benefit beyond that seen with repeated injections at lower doses in the larger phase I/II study.

## FOCUS Study (RhuFab V2 Ocular Treatment Combining the Use of Visudyne to Evaluate Safety)

Based on these results, Genentech initiated another phase I/II study: the *FOCUS* Study. This trial was a single-masked, multicenter study evaluating the safety, tolerability and efficacy of multiple-dose intravitreal injections of ranibizumab used in combinations with PDT in patients with predominantly classic AMD. One hundred and sixty-two patients were randomized 2:1 to receive PDT in combination with monthly intravitreal injection of 0.5 mg of ranibizumab (106 patients) and PDT with sham injection (56 patients). All patients received initial treatment with PDT but were only retreated at the judgment of the treating physician.

At month 12, the patients in the ranibizumab group gained an average of 5 letters in visual acuity compared to study entry, while those in the control group lost an average of 8 letters (Fig. 35-11) (36). Twenty-four percent of patients treated with ranibizumab in combination with PDT versus 5% of patients treated with PDT alone improved vision by 15 letters or more compared to study entry (36). At month 24, 88% of the patients in the ranibizumab group lost fewer than 15 letters compared with 75% of the patients of the PDT group. The visual acuity benefit of adding ranibizumab to PDT in year 1 persisted through year 2. On average, ranibizumab + PDT patients exhibited less lesion growth and greater reduction of CNV leakage and subretinal fluid accumulation, and required fewer PDT retreatments, than PDT-alone patients (mean = 0.4 vs 3.0 PDT retreatments) (37). An analysis of the 1 year data showed there was an increased risk of the serious ocular adverse events: uveitis in patients treated with ranibizumab in combination with PDT compared to patients treated with PDT alone. An amendment to the study protocol was made after data safety monitoring identified this imbalance. Endophthalmitis was the second most common ocular serious adverse event occurring in patients treated with ranibizumab; endophthalmitis and serious intraocular inflammation occurred, respectively, in 2.9% and 12.4% of ranibizumab + PDT patients and 0% of PDT-alone patients (37). Among non-ocular serious adverse events, the frequency of cerebral vascular events was higher in those treated with ranibizumab, while the frequency of myocardial infarctions was higher in the PDT-alone arm. In both cases, the difference between groups was not statistically significant.

## Ranibizumab for Age-Related Macular Degeneration: Phase III Studies

### MARINA (Minimally Classic/Occult Trial of the Anti-VEGF Antibody Ranibizumab in the Treatment of Neovascular AMD)

MARINA, the first phase III clinical trial, was a prospective, multicenter, randomized, double-masked, placebo-controlled study of the safety, tolerability, and efficacy of repeated injections of ranibizumab in patients with minimally classic or occult subfoveal CNV secondary to AMD.

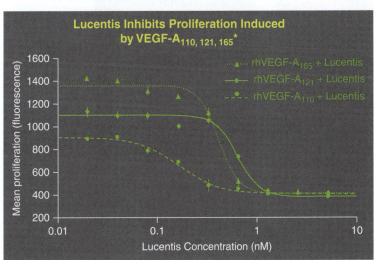

**Figure 35-11.** Human umbilical vein endothelial cell (HUVEC) proliferation assay. rhuFab V2 Ranibizumab is capable of binding all three VEGF isoforms and thereby inhibiting vascular endothelial growth factor (VEGF)-isoforms-induced endothelial cell proliferation.

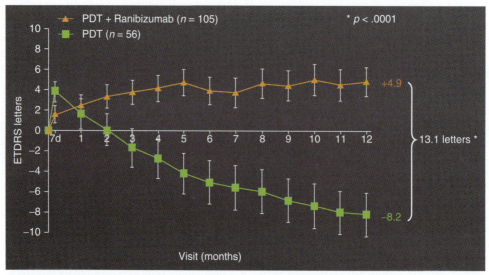

**Figure 35-12.** Mean change in visual acuity in FOCUS Study. PDT, photodynamic therapy.

Between March 2003 and December 2003, 716 patients were enrolled and randomly assigned to study treatment. Groups were balanced for demographic and baseline ocular characteristics. More than 90% of patients in each treatment group remained in the study at 12 months, and approximately 80% to 90% remained at 24 months. The patients were enrolled and randomized to receive ranibizumab 0.3 mg, ranibizumab 0.5 mg or sham injections. Subjects received monthly intravitreal injections for 2 years (38).

In this clinical trial, 90% to 92% of the patients in the ranibizumab arm (0.3 mg and 0.5 mg) lost fewer than 15 letters compared with 53% of the patients of control group. Patients treated with ranibizumab gained an average of 5.4 and 6.6 letters (ranibizumab 0.3 mg and 0.5 mg) in visual acuity compared to study entry, while those in the control group lost

an average of 14 letters (Fig. 35-12). Twenty-six percent to 33% of patients treated with ranibizumab (0.3 mg and 0.5 mg) versus 4% of the control group improved vision by 15 letters or more compared to study entry; 34% to 42% ended the second year with a visual acuity of 20/40 or better compared with 6% of the control arm.

Visual acuity benefits observed with ranibizumab were accompanied by corresponding benefits on fluorescein angiography and optical coherence tomography (OCT) (39). The lesions in ranibizumab-treated patients did not recede or disappear, but did demonstrate less fibrosis and exudation, as measured by a decrease in the area of leakage from the CNV, subretinal fluid area, and center point retinal thickness on OCT (Fig. 35-13) (39). The most influential predictor of visual acuity outcomes were the visual acuity score at baseline, lesion

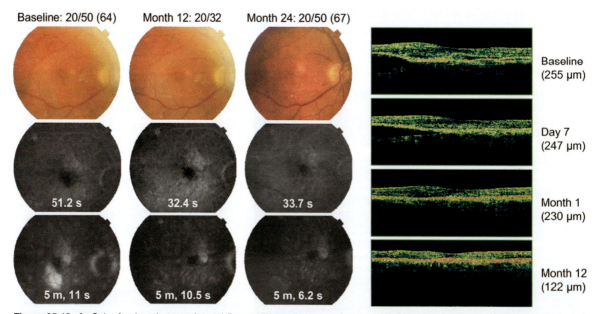

**Figure 35-13. A:** Color fundus photographs and fluorescein angiography of patient number 1. At month 12 and 24 no leakage was observed. **B:** Optical coherence tomography shows normal foveal contour by month 12 (Kaiser PK, Blodi BA, Shapiro H et al. Angiographic and optical coherence tomographic results of the MARINA study of ranibizumab in neovascular age-related macular degeneration. *Ophthalmology* 2007;114:1868–1875).

size, and patient age; better visual acuity score, smaller lesion and younger patients ended at 2 years with better visual results (40). Side effects reported occurred more frequently in the ranibizumab groups than in the control group and were mild to moderate. Side effects included conjunctival hemorrhage, increased intraocular pressure, and vitreous floaters. Serious ocular adverse events reported were more frequently in the ranibizumab-treated arms; endophthalmitis (cumulative 1.3% or less over 2 years) and intraocular inflammation (cumulative 1.7% or less over 2 years). Among nonocular serious adverse events, the combined cumulative rate of cerebral vascular events and myocardial infarctions at 2 years was 3% (7/236) in the sham injection group, 4.6% (11/238) in the 0.3 mg ranibizumab group and 4.2% (10/239) in the 0.5 mg group.

## ANCHOR (Anti-VEGF Antibody for the Treatment of Predominantly Classic CNV in AMD)

ANCHOR, a second phase III clinical trial, was multicenter, randomized, double-masked, head-to-head comparison of ranibizumab to verteporfin (Visudyne®) photodynamic therapy (PDT) for patients with predominantly classic subfoveal CNV secondary to AMD.

Between June 2003 and September 2004, 423 patients were enrolled and randomly assigned to a study treatment. One hundred and forty-three patients were assigned to the verteporfin group and 140 patients to each of the ranibizumab groups (0.3 mg or 0.5 mg dose). More than 90% of patients in each group (91.5% overall) were receiving treatment at 12 months. During the first year of this 2 year study the patients receive monthly intravitreal injections of ranibizumab plus sham verteporfin therapy or monthly sham injections plus active verteporfin therapy (41).

Ninety-four percent of patients treated with 0.3 mg of ranibizumab and 96% of those treated with 0.5 mg of ranibizumab lost fewer than 15 letters compared to baseline, compared with 64% of those treated with PDT. Almost 36% of patients treated with 0.3 mg of ranibizumab and 40% of patients treated with 0.5 mg of ranibizumab gained 15 letters or more compared with approximately 6% of patients treated with PDT. Thirty-one percent of patients treated with 0.3 mg of ranibizumab and practically 39% of patients treated with 0.5 mg of ranibizumab achieved visual acuity of 20/40 or better at 12 months compared with approximately 3% of those treated with PDT. Finally, the patients treated with ranibizumab gained an average of 8.5 and 11.3 letters (ranibizumab 0.3 mg and 0.5 mg) in visual acuity compared to study entry, while those in the PDT group lost an average of 9.5 letters (Fig. 35-14). Subgroup analysis of 12-month data from the ANCHOR study showed ranibizumab to be superior to PDT in all subgroups evaluated and was consistent with the subgroup analysis of 24 month from MARINA. The analysis showed that the most important predictors of visual acuity outcomes were, in decreasing order of impact, the patient's baseline visual acuity score, CNV lesion size, and age of the patient (42). An analysis of the 1 year data showed that adverse events were similar to those seen in MARINA and the other early clinical trials of ranibizumab.

## PIER Study

PIER was a study designed to determine the safety and efficacy of quarterly dosing regimen for ranibizumab in patients with AMD: Phase IIIb, Multicenter, Randomized, Double-Masked, Sham Injection-Controlled Study of the Efficacy and Safety of Ranibizumab in Subjects with Subfoveal CNV with or without Classic CNV Secondary to AMD. PIER study enrolls 184 patients in the United States.

In this study patients receive ranibizumab (0.3 mg or 0.5 mg respectively) or sham injections once per month for the first 3 months followed thereafter by doses once every 3 months for a total of 24 months.

Patients treated with ranibizumab demonstrated an initial increase in mean visual acuity compared to baseline after 3 monthly injections; at month 3, patients treated with ranibizumab gained 2.9 letters and 4.3 letters (0.3 mg and 0.5 mg dose groups, respectively) compared to a loss of 8.7 letters among patients in the sham group (Fig. 35-15). Following month 3, patients treated with ranibizumab received additional

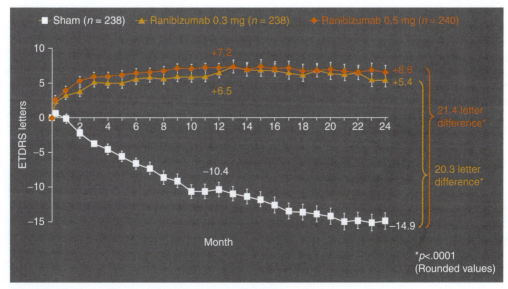

**Figure 35-14.** Mean change in visual acuity in MARINA Study.

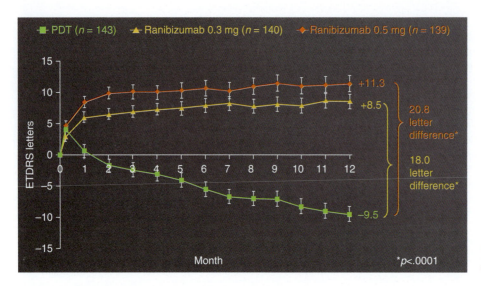

**Figure 35-15.** Mean change in visual acuity in ANCHOR Study. PDT, photodynamic therapy.

doses at months 6, 9, and 12. On average, patients treated with ranibizumab returned to baseline visual acuity by month 12, while patients in the sham group experienced significant vision loss. At month 12, patients treated with ranibizumab lost 1.6 letters and 0.2 letters (0.3 mg and 0.5 mg) compared to a loss of 16.3 letters in the sham group. Patients treated with ranibizumab, 83% (0.3 mg) and 90% (0.5 mg) lost fewer than 15 letters in visual acuity compared to baseline, compared with 49% in the control group; 12% (0.3 mg) and 13% (0.5 mg) of those treated with ranibizumab improved vision by a gain of 15 letters or more versus approximately 10% of those in the control group; 30% (0.3 mg) and 28% (0.5 mg) of those treated with ranibizumab achieved 20/40 vision at 12 months compared to 11% in the sham group. Consistent with earlier trials, common side effects occurred more frequently in the ranibizumab groups than in the control group. After 1 year the side effects were mild to moderate and included conjunctival hemorrhage, eye pain, and increased intraocular pressure. There were no reported cases of endophthalmitis, serious intraocular inflammation, or other key ocular serious adverse events. There were no deaths, myocardial infarctions, or cerebral vascular events in the first year of the study (43).

The PIER study met its primary efficacy endpoint by preventing vision loss, and demonstrated an initial increase in mean visual acuity compared to baseline after 3 monthly injections. Although quarterly ranibizumab therapy maintained baseline visual acuity, this regimen was associated with a 4.5 letter loss in the maximal visual acuity benefit achieved with monthly induction therapy during months 1 to 3. This loss was accompanied, with an increase in vascular leakage and increases in mean retinal thickness. This observation suggested that monthly or individualize retreatment schedule is probably more accurate in achieving sustainable improvement in visual acuity than quarterly doses.

## PrONTO Study (Prospective OCT Imaging of Patients with Neovascular AMD Treated with Intraocular Lucentis)

An investigator-sponsored study, PrONTO, was a 2 year, 40 patient study initiated in 2004 with the goal of determining,

through OCT, how quickly visual acuity improves and central retinal thickness (CRT) decreases following ranibizumab therapy in all types of AMD lesions. In the 1 year results, patients received an average of 5 to 6 intravitreal injections, after all patients had received a monthly injection for the 3 first months. The OCT was used to follow patients and determine when the retreatment was necessary. Overall, average vision improved in the treated eye almost 2 lines. Eighty-two percent of patients had the same visual acuity or better at the end of 1 year, and 35% of patients experienced a 3 line improvement in visual acuity. Also, PrONTO shows an improvement in the macular anatomy (by OCT) within 1 day following the injection. After 1 year of follow up, 17.5% of the patients did not need another injection and 20% needed 1 additional injection. These results indicated a highly variable individual response to treatment (44).

## SAILOR Study (Safety Assessment of Intravitreal Ranibizumab for AMD)

In November 2005, Genentech began enrollment in a Phase IIIb study, SAILOR, to make ranibizumab available to eligible patients before FDA approval. This clinical trial enrolled patients with all subtypes of new or recurrent active subfoveal wet AMD. One-year study designed to evaluate the safety of two different doses (0.3 mg and 0.5 mg) of ranibizumab administered once a month for 3 months and thereafter as needed based on retreatment criteria. The study was conducted at more than 100 sites in the United States and enrolled around 5,000 patients. Results are not available for the time that this chapter was printed.

## CONCLUSION

Ranibizumab (Lucentis™) is the first recombinant, humanized, monoclonal anti-VEGF antibody fragment, approved by the FDA for the treatment of neovascular AMD; the ability of this molecule to bind all the isoforms of the VEGF-A makes it a powerful drug for VEGF inhibition. Several clinical trials were

**TABLE 35-1   RESULTS FOR THE THREE PHASE III STUDIES**

| Study findings | Anchor study (N:423) Classic CNV | | | Marina study (N:716) Occult CNV | | | Pier study (N:184) Quarterly dosing | | |
|---|---|---|---|---|---|---|---|---|---|
| | 0.3 mg | 0.5 mg | PDT arm | 0.3 mg | 0.5 mg | Sham arm | 0.3 mg | 0.5 mg | Sham arm |
| Main change VA | (+)8.5 | (+)11.3 | (−)9.5 | (+)5.4 | (+)6.6 | (−)14 | (−)1.6 | (−)0.2 | (−)16.3 |
| >15 Letters gain | 36% | 40% | 6% | 26% | 33% | 4% | 12% | 13% | 10% |
| Lost <15 Letters | 94% | 96% | 64% | 90% | 92% | 53% | 83% | 90% | 49% |
| 20/40 or better | 31% | 39% | 3% | 34% | 42% | 6% | 30% | 28% | 11% |

conducted and are still being conducted to prove the efficacy of ranibizumab in the management of one of the leading causes of blindness in the United States, the wet form of AMD.

Ranibizumab therapy is the first treatment for neovascular AMD to improve vision for most patients. Nearly all patients (95%) treated with ranibizumab maintained their vision in the Phase III clinical trials. The vision improved by at least 3 lines (or 15 letters) on the study eye in more than 40% of these patients at 1 year (Table 35-1). The benefits apply to all angiographic subtypes of neovascular AMD and across all lesion sizes. The combination therapy does not provide any significant advantage over ranibizumab alone. Comparing ANCHOR results with FOCUS results, it becomes apparent that the combination of ranibizumab with PDT does not necessarily result in better visual acuity outcomes.

The main studies also proved that ranibizumab-treated patients were more likely than sham-treated patients to report visual function improvements (45). The most common adverse reactions among patients treated with ranibizumab included: conjunctival hemorrhage, eye pain, vitreous floaters, increased intraocular pressure, and intraocular inflammation. Although there was a low rate (less than 4%) of arterial thromboembolic events (ATEs) observed in the ranibizumab clinical trials, that was not statistically different for the treatment group and the control. The combined rate of myocardial infarction and stroke during the first year of ANCHOR and MARINA was similar

**TABLE 35-2   MAIN ADVERSE EVENTS REPORT FOR THE THREE PHASE III STUDIES**

| Main adverse event | Lucents arm | Control arm |
|---|---|---|
| Conjuctival hemorrhage | 77%–43% | 66%–29% |
| Vitreous floaters | 32%–3% | 10%–3% |
| Retinal hemorrhage | 26%–15% | 56%–37% |
| Intraocular pressure increased | 24%–8% | 7%–3% |
| Intraocular inflammation | 18%–5% | 11%–3% |
| Eye irritation | 19%–4% | 20%–6% |
| Cataract | 16%–5% | 16%–6% |
| Foreign body sensation in eyes | 19%–6% | 14%–6% |

in the control and the 0.3 mg ranibizumab arms (1.3% and 1.6% respectively); these adverse events were higher in the 0.5 mg ranibizumab arm (2.9%). These differences were not statistically significant. Serious adverse events related to the injection procedure occurred in less than 0.1% of intravitreal injections, including endophthalmitis, retinal detachments, and traumatic cataracts. Other serious ocular adverse events observed, occurred in less than 2% of patients, included intraocular inflammation and increased intraocular pressure (Table 35-2).

After monthly dosing with ranibizumab for 12 to 24 months, low titers of antibodies to ranibizumab were detected in approximately 1% to 6% of patients. The immunogenicity data reflect the percentage of patients whose test results were considered positive, in an electro-luminescence assay and are highly dependent on the sensitivity and specificity of the assay. The clinical significance of immunoreactivity to ranibizumab is unclear at this time, although some patients with the highest levels of immunoreactivity were noted to have iritis or vitritis.

Six cases of RPE tears have been reported to occur after intravitreal injection of ranibizumab in patients with neovascular AMD, 4 of them with AMD associated with pigment epithelial detachments (PED). Further study is needed to determine whether CNV membranes associated with PED are more likely to develop RPE tears after treatment with anti-VEGF agents (46,47,48).

Ranibizumab 0.5 mg is recommended for intravitreal injection once a month. Patients should be evaluated regularly; we recommend ophthalmoscopy evaluation, fluorescein angiography, the use of OCT, and visual acuity as the main criteria to decided retreatment in the patients.

### References

1. Ferrara N. Vascular endothelial growth factor: basic science and clinical progress. *Endocr Rev* 2004;25:581–611.
2. Folkman J, Klagsbrun M. Angiogenic factors. *Science* 1987;235:442–447.
3. Adamis AP, Miller JW, Bernal MT, et al. Increased vascular endothelial growth factor levels in the vitreous of eyes with proliferative diabetic retinopathy. *Am J Ophthalmol* 1994;118:445–450.
4. Adamis AP, Shima DT, Tolentino MJ, et al. Inhibition of vascular endothelial growth factor prevents retinal ischemia-associated iris neovascularization in a nonhuman primate. *Arch Ophthalmol* 1996;114:66–71.
5. Aiello LP, Avery RL, Arrigg PG, et al. Vascular endothelial growth factor in ocular fluid of patients with diabetic retinopathy and other retinal disorders. *N Engl J Med* 1994;331:1480–1487.
6. Houck KA, Leung DW, Rowland AM, et al. Dual regulation of vascular endothelial growth factor bioavailability by genetic and proteolytic mechanisms. *J Biol Chem* 1992;267:26031–26037.
7. Rosenfeld PJ, Moshfeghi AA, Puliafito CA. Optical coherence tomography findings after an intravitreal injection of bevacizumab (avastin) for neovascular age-related macular degeneration. *Ophthalmic Surg Lasers Imaging* 2005;36:331–335.

8. Avery RL, Pieramici DJ, Rabena MD, et al. Intravitreal Bevacizumab (Avastin) for neovascular age-related macular degeneration. *Ophthalmol* 2006;113:363–372.

9. Spaide RF, Laud K, Fine HF, et al. Intravitreal bevacizumab treatment of choroidal neovascularization secondary to age-related macular degeneration. *Retina* 2006;26:383–390.

10. Bashshur ZF, Bazarbachi A, Schakal A, et al. Intravitreal bevacizumab for the management of choroidal neovascularization in age-related macular degeneration. *Am J Ophthalmol* 2006;142:1–9.

11. Gragoudas ES, Adamis AP, Cunningham ET Jr, et al for the VEGF Inhibition Study in Ocular Neovascularization Clinical Trial Group. Pegaptanib for neovascular age-related macular degeneration. *N Engl J Med* 2004;351:2805–2816.

12. Lowe J, Araujo J, Palma M, et al. RhuFab V2 inhibits VEGF-Isoforms-Stimulated HUVEC proliferation. ARVO 2003, B724.

13. Ide AG, Baker NH, Warren SL. Vascularization of the Brown Pearce rabbit epithelioma transplant as seen in the transparent ear chamber. *Am J Roentgenol* 1939;42:891–899.

14. Michaelson IC. The mode of development of the vascular system of the retina with some observations on its significance for certain retinal disorders. *Trans Ophthalmo Soc UK* 1948;68:137–180.

15. Folkman J. Tumor angiogenesis: therapeutic implications. *N Engl J Med* 1971;285:1182–1186.

16. Senger DR, Galli SJ, Dvorak AM, et al. Tumor cells secrete a vascular permeability factor that promotes accumulation of ascites fluid. *Science* 1983;219:983–985.

17. Ferrara N, Henzel WJ. Pituitary follicular cells secrete a novel heparin-binding growth factor specific for vascular endothelial cells. *Biochem Biophys Res Commun* 1989;161:851–858.

18. Malecaze F, Clamens S, Simorre-Pinatel V, et al. Detection of vascular endothelial growth factor messenger RNA and vascular endothelial growth factor-like activity in proliferative diabetic retinopathy. *Arch Ophthalmol* 1994;112:1476–1482.

19. Kvanta A, Algvere PV, Berglin L, et al. Subfoveal fibrovascular membranes in age-related macular degeneration express vascular endothelial growth factor. *Invest Ophthalmol Vis Sci* 1996;37:1929–1934.

20. Lopez PF, Sippy BD, Lambert HM, et al. Transdifferentiated retinal pigment epithelial cells are immunoreactive for vascular endothelial growth factor in surgically excised age-related macular degeneration-related choroidal neovascular membranes. *Invest Ophthalmol Vis Sci* 1996;37: 855–868.

21. Aiello LP, Pierce EA, Foley ED, et al. Suppression of retinal neovascularization in vivo by inhibition of vascular endothelial growth factor (VEGF) using soluble VEGF-receptor chimeric proteins. *Proc Natl Acad Sci USA* 1995;92:10457–10461.

22. Miller RA, Oseroff AR, Stratte PT, et al. Monoclonal antibody therapeutic trials in seven patients with T-cell lymphoma. *Blood* 1983;62:988–995.

23. Schroff RW, Foon KA, Beatty SM, et al. Human anti-murine immunoglobulin responses in patients receiving monoclonal antibody therapy. *Cancer Res* 1985;45:879–885.

24. Neuberger MS, Williams GT, Mitchell EB, et al. A hapten-specific chimaeric IgE antibody with human physiological effector function. *Nature* 1985;314: 268–270.

25. Presta LG, Chen H, O'Connor SJ, et al. Humanization of an anti-vascular endothelial growth factor monoclonal antibody for the therapy of solid tumors and other disorders. *Cancer Res* 1997;57:4593–4599.

26. Mordenti J, Cuthbertson RA, Ferrara N, et al. Comparisons of the intraocular tissue distribution, pharmacokinetics, and safety of 125I-labeled full-length and Fab antibodies in rhesus monkeys following intravitreal administration. *Toxicol Pathol* 1999;27:536–544.

27. Chen Y, Wiesmann C, Fuh G, et al. Selection and analysis of an optimized anti-VEGF antibody: crystal structure of an affinity-matured Fab in complex with antigen. *J Mol Biol* 1999;293:865–881.

28. Gaudreault J, Fei D, Rusit J, et al. Preclinical pharmacokinetics of Ranibizumab (rhuFabV2) after a single intravitreal administration. *Invest Ophthalmol Vis Sci* 2005;46:726–733.

29. Gaudreault J, Fei D, Beyer JC, et al. Pharmacokinetics and retinal distribution of ranibizumab, a humanized antibody fragment directed against VEGF-A, following intravitreal administration in rabbits. *Retina* 2007; 27:1260–1266.

30. Bakri JS, Snyder MR, Reid JM, et al. Pharmacokinetics of intravitreal Ranibizumab (Lucentis). *Ophthalmology* 2007;114:2179–2182.

31. Krzystolik MG, Afshari MA, Adamis AP, et al. Prevention of experimental choroidal neovascularization with intravitreal anti-vascular endothelial growth factor antibody fragment. *Arch Ophthalmol* 2002;120:338–346.

32. Gaudreault J, Reich M, Arata A, et al. Ocular pharmacokinetics and antipermeability effect of rhuFab V2 in animals. ARVO 2003. Poster B645. *Invest Ophthalmol Vis Sci* 2003;44: E-Abstract 3942.

33. Rosenfeld PJ, Schwartz SD, Blumenkranz MS, et al. Maximum tolerated dose of a humanized anti-vascular endothelial growth factor antibody fragment for treating neovascular age-related macular degeneration. *Ophthalmology* 2005;112:1048–1053.

34. Heier JS, Antoszyk AN, Pavan PR, et al. Ranibizumab for treatment of neovascular age-related macular degeneration: a phase I/II multicenter, controlled, multidose study. *Ophthalmology* 2006;113:642.

35. Rosenfeld PJ, Heier JS, Hantsbarger G, et al. Tolerability and efficacy of multiple escalating doses of Ranibizumab (Ranibizumab) for neovascular age-related macular degeneration. *Ophthamol* 2006;113:632–642.

36. Heier JS, Boyer DS, Ciulla TA, et al; FOCUS Study Group. Ranibizumab combined with verteporfin photodynamic therapy in neovascular age-related macular degeneration. Year 1 results of the FOCUS Study. *Arch Ophthalmol* 2006;124:1532–1542.

37. Antoszyk AN, Tuomi L, Chung CY, et al; FOCUS STUDY GROUP. Ranibizumab combined with verteporfin photodynamic therapy in neovascular age-related macular degeneration (FOCUS): Year 2 results. *Am J Ophthalmol* 2008;145(5):862–874.

38. Rosenfeld PJ, Brown DM, Heier JS, et al; MARINA Study Group. Ranibizumab for neovascular age-related macular degeneration. *N Engl J Med* 2006;355:1419–1431.

39. Kaiser PK, Blodi BA, Shapiro H, et al; MARINA Study Group. Angiographic and optical coherence tomographic results of the MARINA study of ranibizumab in neovascular age-related macular degeneration. *Ophthalmology* 2007;114:1868–1875.

40. Boyer DS, Antoszyk AN, Awh CC, et al; MARINA Study Group. Subgroup analysis of the MARINA study of ranibizumab in neovascular age-related macular degeneration. *Ophthalmology* 2007;114:246–252.

41. Brown DM, Kaiser PK, Michels M, et al; ANCHOR Study Group. Ranibizumab versus Verteporfin for Neovascular Age-Related Macular Degeneration. *N Engl J Med* 2006;355:1432–1444.

42. Kaiser PK, Brown DM, Zhang K, et al. Ranibizumab for predominantly classic neovascular age-related macular degeneration: subgroup analysis of first-year ANCHOR results. *Am J Ophthalmol* 2007;144:850–857.

43. Regillo CD, Brown DM, Abraham P, et al. Randomized, double-masked, sham-controlled trial of ranibizumab for neovascular age-related macular degeneration: PIER Study year 1. *Am J Ophthalmol* 2008;145:239–248.

44. Rosenfeld PJ, Fung AE, Lalwani GA, et al. Presented at ARVO Annual Meeting, Ft. Lauderdale, FL, 2006.

45. Chang TS, Bressler NM, Fine JT, et al; MARINA Study Group. Improved vision-related function after ranibizumab treatment of neovascular age-related macular degeneration: results of a randomized clinical trial. *Arch Ophthalmol* 2007;125:1460–1469.

46. Kiss C, Michels S, Prager F, et al. Retinal pigment epithelium tears following intravitreal ranibizumab therapy. *Acta Ophthalmol Scand* 2007;85:902–903.

47. Bakri SJ, Kitzmann AS. Retinal pigment epithelial tear after intravitreal ranibizumab. *Am J Ophthalmol* 2007;143:505–507.

48. Carvounis PE, Kopel AC, Benz MS. Retinal pigment epithelium tears following ranibizumab for exudative age-related macular degeneration. *Am J Ophthalmol* 2007;143:504–505.

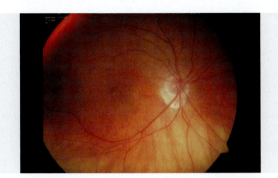

# Bevacizumab (Avastin™)

Monica Rodriguez-Fontal ■ Craig M. Greven

## INTRODUCTION

Bevacizumab is a monoclonal antibody to vascular endothelial growth factor developed for the treatment of cancer. Over the past years, it has been used in the management of complicated retinal and choroidal vascular conditions like diabetic retinopathy, retinal venous occlusive disease, retinopathy of prematurity, neovascular glaucoma, and exudative age-related macular degeneration (AMD). The following chapter will address the pharmacology and pharmacokinetics of Bevacizumab and its utility in the management of ophthalmic diseases.

## BACKGROUND

The idea of using antibodies that target malignant tumor cells was originally suggested by Ehrlich at the beginning of the 20th century (1). Creation of somatic hybridization to generate "hybridoma" cell lines brought this idea closer to reality in 1976. Initially the monoclonal antibodies (mAbs) failed to show efficacy in clinical trials mainly due to intrinsic immunogenicity (rodent-derived mAbs). These issues were quickly overcome by newly developed molecular antibody engineering methods that allowed humanization of antibodies. The advance in technology led investigators to develop monoclonal antibodies for specific targets. Antibodies are currently engineered to customize their size, binding specificity, affinity, effectors function, and ability to be produced on a large scale suitable for clinical use.

Bevacizumab is a humanized antibody (IgG1) designed to recognize all isoforms of a diffusible endothelial cell-specific mitogen, the vascular endothelial growth factor (VEGF) with high affinity (Kd, 0.8 nM). Bevacizumab inhibits VEGF-induced proliferation of endothelial cells and VEGF-induced vascular leakage. Angiogenesis is an essential process required for tumor growth, as well as for new vessel formation. The VEGF pathway is well established as one of the key regulators of the angiogenesis process. Elevation of VEGF was found in aqueous humor and vitreous humor in human eyes with proliferative diabetic retinopathy and other retinal disorders. VEGF was also found to be elevated in surgically extracted choroidal neovascular membranes from AMD patients (2,3).

Bevacizumab was Food and Drug Administration (FDA) approved in 2004 for first-line therapy in combination with irinotecan, 5-fluorouracil (5-FU), and leucovorin in metastatic colorectal cancer. This approval was based in the results of a phase III trial (4), where over 800 previously untreated metastatic colon cancer patients were given bolus irinotecan, 5-FU, and leucovorin plus placebo or bevacizumab. The overall response rate was 44.8% in the bevacizumab group and 34.8% in the placebo group, with duration of response of 10.4 and 7.1 months, respectively. The median progression-free survival (PFS) was 10.55 versus 6.24 months, and median survival was 20.34 versus 15.61 months. The main toxicities in the bevacizumab group were grade 3 hypertension (11% versus 2.3%), proteinuria, and arterial thromboembolic events (4.4% vs 1.9%). In 2006, bevacizumab was approved by the FDA for second-line treatment for metastatic colon cancer in combination with intravenous 5-FU-based chemotherapy, and first-line

treatment for nonsmall cell lung cancer. In February 2008, the FDA granted accelerated approval of bevacizumab in combination with paclitaxel for first-line treatment of metastatic HER2-negative breast cancer.

Bevacizumab has structural and functional similarities to another anti VEGF agent, ranibizumab. When initial clinical trial data suggested a significant benefit with ranibizumab in AMD, and with ranibizumab unavailable for use because it was awaiting licensing approval by the FDA, ophthalmologists began treating AMD and subsequently diabetic retinopathy and macular edema with bevacizumab, When ranibizumab was eventually licensed for use in America, bevacizumab was already well established in the retina community as a potentially effective and apparently safe therapy. The use of the drug for intravitreous injection increased exponentially without the evidence base that usually guides the rational and safe use of new medicines, namely large randomized controlled clinical trials. The current Comparisons of Age-Related Macular Degeneration Treatments Trials (CATT) is a randomized controlled clinical trial designed to compare the efficacy and safety of two dosing strategies of bevacizumab and ranibizumab.

## BEVACIZUMAB SYNTHESIS

Bevacizumab (rhuMAb VEGF) is a recombinant humanized IgG1 antibody derived from the murine VEGF monoclonal antibody A4.6.1 (5). It is a full-length antibody of 149 kilodaltons, bigger than ranibizumab (antibody fragment of 48 kilodaltons). Bevacizumab has 93% human and 7% murine protein sequences. The humanization process of bevacizumab was performed by site-directed mutagenesis of a human framework. Several framework residues and the six complementary-determining regions were changed from human to murine. The final result was a humanized anti-VEGF F(ab), rhuMAb VEGF, agent with the same biochemical and pharmacologic properties as the parental antibody, but with reduced immunogenicity, and a longer biological half-life (5).

Bevacizumab binds and inhibits all biologically active forms of VEGF, much like ranibizumab (6). It is a full-length, humanized monoclonal antibody, whereas ranibizumab is a humanized antigen-binding fragment. Both proteins were genetically engineered from the same murine monoclonal antibody against VEGF (5). Although bevacizumab has two binding sites for VEGF, ranibizumab has only a single binding site, which has been affinity matured to have an increased binding affinity for VEGF compared with the antigen-binding fragment derived from the original murine antibody (7).

## BEVACIZUMAB CHARACTERISTICS: PHARMACOKINETICS, MECHANISM OF ACTION

### Intravenous Pharmacokinetics

The pharmacokinetic profile of bevacizumab administered intravenously in patients with tumors was collected in phase I to phase III trials (8). Pharmacokinetics were assessed after analyzing 491 patients (a total of 4,629 bevacizumab concentrations) who received 1 to 20 mg/kg of bevacizumab weekly, every 2 weeks, or every 3 weeks (9). The estimated half-life of bevacizumab was approximately 20 days (range 11 to 50 days). The predicted time to reach a steady state was 100 days. The accumulation ratio following a dose of 10 mg/kg of bevacizumab every 2 weeks was 2.8. The clearance of bevacizumab varied by body weight, by gender, and by tumor burden. After correcting for body weight, males had a higher bevacizumab clearance (0.262 L/day vs. 0.207 L/day) and a larger Vc (3.25 L vs. 2.66 L) than females. Clearance was 26% faster in men than in women. Patients with higher tumor burden had a higher clearance (0.249 L/day vs. 0.199 L/day) than patients with tumor burdens below the median.

## Intravitreal Pharmacokinetics: Animal Models

Bakri et al. (10) published the first intravitreal pharmacokinetic study. They used a rabbit model to analyze the pharmacokinetics of 1.25 mg of intravitreal bevacizumab. They found that vitreous concentrations of bevacizumab reach a peak concentration of 400μg/mL 1 day after intravitreal injection and declined in a monoexponential fashion with a half-life of 4.32 days. Concentrations of >10μg/mL bevacizumab were maintained in the vitreous humor for 30 days. Bevacizumab concentrations in the aqueous humor of the injected eye reached a peak concentration of 37.7μg/mL 3 days after drug administration. Serum concentrations were low; a maximum serum concentration of 3.3μg/mL was achieved 8 days after intravitreal injection and the concentration fell 29 days after injection. Elimination of bevacizumab from aqueous humor and serum paralleled elimination found in vitreous humor, with half-life values of 4.88 days and 6.86 days, respectively.

Bakri also detected very low concentrations of bevacizumab in the fellow uninjected eye (0.35 ng/mL at 1 day to 11.17 ng/mL at 4 weeks). Concentrations of bevacizumab in aqueous humor of the fellow eye reached their peak at 1 week and declined to 4.56 ng/ml at 4 weeks.

Ranibizumab pharmacokinetics were analyzed using the same rabbit model (11). After injecting 0.5 mg of intravitreal ranibizumab into rabbit eye, the half-life in vitreous was 2.88 days (compared 4.32 days of bevacizumab). No ranibizumab concentration was detected in the serum or in the fellow eye.

## Intravitreal Pharmacokinetics: Human Eyes

Csaky and associates (12) report a half-life of 10 days in vitreous samples of 18 patients after injection of 1.25 mg of bevacizumab. In accordance with these results Krohne et al. (13) found a half-life of 9.82 days after analyzing aqueous humor sample of 30 eyes that received 1.5 mg bevacizumab. In the Csaky study, bevacizumab concentrations in vitreous are reported to reach peak values of 80 to 170μg/mL. Krohne showed that concentration of the drug in aqueous humor peaked on the first day after injection with a mean concentration of 33.3μg/mL and declined in monoexponential fashion. The higher concentrations in vitreous compared with aqueous

humor measurements are to be expected considering the intravitreal delivery of the drug.

Zhu et al. (14) found a relatively lower half-life (6.7 days) after analyzing vitreous samples of 11 patients with choroidal neovascularization injected with 1.25 mg of bevacizumab. The investigators showed a peak concentration of the drug 2 days after injection, and a minimum concentration to completely block the VEGF-A-induced endothelial cell proliferation (>500 ng/mL) for 48 days. They also investigated the relationship between intravitreal bevacizumab and vitreous VEGF-A. Free VEGF-A levels in the vitreous ranged from 0.2 to 33.9 pg/mL and showed a negative correlation with the bevacizumab concentration, confirming in vivo binding affinity of bevacizumab to VEGF-A.

## PENETRATION THOUGH THE RETINAL LAYERS

Assays in cynomolgus monkeys (15) and albino rabbits (16) showed that bevacizumab penetrated inner layers of the retina on the first day of injection and reached the choroid during the following days. An active transport mechanism is probably involved in the process.

### Retina Toxicity

Safety of intravitreal bevacizumab was evaluated in several animal assays and in vitro studies. Electroretinograms performed after various doses of bevacizumab injections in rabbits show no retinal toxicity, with no alterations in scotopic and photopic a-wave and b-wave amplitude. No histopathology changes or toxicity to the cells were noted (16–20).

### Mechanism of Action

Bevacizumab binds to the receptor-binding site of active forms of VEGF-A, including the biologically active (cleaved form of this molecule) VEGF$_{110}$. With the binding of bevacizumab to VEGF-A, the interaction of this molecule with its receptors (Flt-1 [VEGFR-1] and KDR [VEGFR-2]) on the surface of endothelial cells reduces endothelial cell proliferation, vascular leakage, and new blood vessel formation (21).

VEGF inhibition generates ultrastructural changes in blood vessels. Some of these alterations explain the efficacy of bevacizumab in the treatment of macular edema and choroidal neovascularization.

Structural changes, like reduction in number of open fenestrations in blood vessels, and close-tight junctions between adjacent endothelial cells, lead to a reduction in vascular leakage and new vessel formation (22). Electron microscopic quantification demonstrated a highly significant reduction of endothelial cell fenestrations at choriocapillaris level after intravitreal injection of bevacizumab. In an animal model, blockage of the VEGF causes secondary atrophy of the choriocapillaris and results in a loss of endothelial cell fenestrations. The loss of fenestrations starts within 24 hours of bevacizumab injection into the vitreous, and regeneration of fenestrated capillaries is detected within two weeks after VEGF inhibition.

Electron microscopic evaluation after intravitreal bevacizumab also demonstrated some degree of capillary blockage. Regionally altered arrangement of leukocytes, thrombocytes, and erythrocytes were found closing the capillaries lumen (22).

Moreover, in vitro studies with human umbilical vein endothelial cells incubated with bevacizumab demonstrated reduction of the number of proliferating cells, prevention of cell growth, induction of apoptosis, and, significantly, reduction of migration capacity of the cells (23). These results demonstrate that clinical doses of bevacizumab are able to prevent several steps of the angiogenic process.

## CLINICAL INDICATIONS OF BEVACIZUMAB

Following FDA approval of Bevacizumab for treatment of metastatic colorectal cancer, ophthalmologists from around the world extended treatment indications. Currently, bevacizumab is being used for a variety of eye diseases that involve new vessel formation and macular edema.

The first outcomes of bevacizumab in ophthalmology were published in 2006. The encouraging results observed with intravitreal ranibizumab in the earlier phase I/II studies gave the initial impulse to investigate the systemic effect of bevacizumab in neovascular age-related macular degeneration (ARMD) patients.

SANA (Systemic Avastin for Neovascular AMD) was designed to look at the safety, efficacy, and durability of systemic bevacizumab for the treatment of neovascular ARMD. Two cohorts of 9 patients were followed for 24 consecutive weeks following intravenous administration of Bevacizumab at doses of 5 mg/Kg. Improved visual acuity with resolution of leakage from neovascular lesions was observed after 2 or 3 doses of bevacizumab (24). Mild elevation in blood pressure was the only adverse event identified. In spite of the lack of severe adverse events in this first trial, some investigators were concerned with the potential risk for uncontrolled hypertension and thromboembolic events, as had been observed in cancer patients (25,26). With that concern in mind, and because of the pharmacologic similarity with the ranibizumab, intravitreal delivery was tested. It was assumed that, theoretically, a 400-fold lower dose of bevacizumab injected into the eye was safer for the patient than a higher dose given systemically.

Since that first publication in 2006, several studies have been done using bevacizumab for multiple retinal pathologies. New vessel formation, macular edema, choroidal neovascularization, and as an adjuvant in vitreous and glaucoma surgery have been some of the indications for bevacizumab in ophthalmology.

## BEVACIZUMAB IN MACULAR EDEMA

The pathogenesis of macular edema is multifactorial and not completely understood. Disruption in the blood-retinal barrier secondary to inflammatory mediators like VEGF, prostaglandins, cytokines, and other vasopermeability factors, have been involved in the increased permeability of the perifoveal capillaries and the resulting macular edema.

Recent studies show the efficacy of an intravitreal injection of bevacizumab in reduction of pseudophakic cystoid macular edema (27), macular edema secondary to retinal venous occlusions, diabetes (28,29), and other eye diseases like retinitis pigmentosa (30).

## DIABETIC MACULAR EDEMA

The Early Treatment Diabetic Retinopathy Study (ETDRS) (31) established that focal laser photocoagulation for diabetic macular edema (DME) reduced moderate visual loss by 50%. Based on these results, laser treatment for DME has been the only well demonstrated treatment that reduces the risk of vision loss in these patients. However, in the ETDRS, 12% of treated eyes lost $\geq$15 ETDRS letters at a 3-year follow-up interval. Furthermore, only 3% of the laser-treated eyes gained $\geq$3 lines of vision. Given that most of the eyes laser-treated for DME do not experience an improvement in visual acuity, alternative management strategies like intravitreal steroids and anti-VEGF are being considered.

Bevacizumab has been used as a treatment for DME since 2006. Several studies have been published showing good results with this new approach (Table 36-1). It has been proposed that the use of intravitreal bevacizumab may reduce the risk of vision loss in eyes with DME by 96% (29). This risk reduction is lower when the investigators include eyes with advanced stages of DME and macular ischemia (32–34). The benefit appears evident during the first month of treatment and may continue improving for the next 6 months. Re-injections are often necessary, however, to reach maximum improvement. The optimal treatment schedule is yet to be determined but probably variable, depending on multiple factors. There is evidence that a single injection of bevacizumab lasts for 4 to 6 weeks. Deterioration of visual acuity and recurrence of macular edema are often seen again after 8 to 12 weeks (35).

Visual function recovery after bevacizumab treatment in the presence of macular ischemia is not as good as in the absence of ischemia. The foveal thickness may decrease after the injection, but this reduction does not correlate with an improvement in visual acuity (33).

A phase 2 randomized, multi-center clinical trial was conducted by the Diabetic Retinopathy Clinical Research Network (DRCR.net) at 36 clinical sites in the U.S. (36). The study was designed to provide data on the short-term effect of intravitreal bevacizumab for DME. The patients were assigned randomly to one of five groups: focal photocoagulation at baseline (N = 19, Group A), intravitreal injection of 1.25 mg bevacizumab at baseline and 6 weeks (N = 22, Group B), intravitreal injection of 2.5 mg bevacizumab at baseline and 6 weeks (N = 24, Group C), intravitreal injection of 1.25 mg bevacizumab at baseline and sham injection at 6 weeks (N = 22, Group D), or intravitreal injection of 1.25 mg bevacizumab at baseline and 6 weeks with photocoagulation at 3 weeks

**TABLE 36-1  BEVACIZUMAB FOR DME**

| Authors | Study | N° Cases | Doses | N° Injections | Follow-up | Previous treat | Results VA | ≥3 Lines |
|---------|-------|----------|-------|---------------|-----------|----------------|------------|----------|
| Haritoglou 2006 (32) | Prospective | 51 | 1.25 mg | ≥2 | 6 weeks | Yes | | 26% |
| PACORES 2007 (29) | Retrospective | 68 | 1.25 mg 2.5 mg | 1–3 | 6 months | Yes | | 55.1%[a] |
| Chung 2008 (33) | Pospective | 59 | 1.25 mg | ≥1 | 3 months | | | |
| | MIG | 18 | | | | | [b] | [b] |
| | N-MIG | 41 | | | | | [b] | |
| Kook D 2008 (34) | Prospective | 126 | 1.25 mg | >1 | 12 months | Yes | 1 line[c] | |

DME, diabetic macular edema; VA, visual acuity; MIG, macular ischemia group; N-MIG, nonmacular ischemia group.
[a]Improve of ≥2 lines.
[b]MIG 22% loss ≥3 lines and improve 16% ≥ 1 line.
N-MIG 5% loss ≥3 lines.
[c]Mean lines gain from baseline evaluation to last follow up.

(N = 22, Group E). Although about half of eyes demonstrated an initial positive response to intravitreal bevacizumab (exceeding an 11% reduction in retinal thickness compared with baseline at either the 3-week or 6-week visit), this response was similar to that observed in the laser group after more than 3 weeks. In addition, the magnitude of the response was not large for most subjects. Two doses of bevacizumab are being used: 1.25 mg and 2.5 mg. Both concentrations work in a similar way reducing macular edema and restoring visual acuity in DME. A combination of bevacizumab and laser photocoagulation was tested and no apparent short-term benefit or adverse outcomes were found (36). A large phase 3 randomized clinical trial is important to determine the value of bevacizumab in DME.

## MACULAR EDEMA IN VASCULAR OCCLUSIONS

Venous occlusions are the second most common retinal vascular disease after diabetic retinopathy. Vision loss in these cases is associated with macular edema and macular ischemia. Laser photocoagulation has been the only evidence-based treatment for patients with macular edema secondary to branch vein occlusions (BRVO) since 1984 when the BRVO Study (37) was published. The BRVO study showed that 63% of laser treated patients had improved ≥2 lines of vision compare with 36% of the control eyes with a mean gain in visual acuity of 1.3 lines in the treated group.

Laser photocoagulation proved not to be useful in macular edema secondary to central retina vein occlusion. The Central Vein Occlusion Study (38) found that initial visual acuity is the best prognostic factor for patients; patients with initial visual acuity of 20/40 or better often retain good vision, patients with initial visual acuity of 20/50 to 20/200 have a variable prognosis (20% may get better), and patients with initial visual acuity worse than 20/200 have a poor prognosis (80% remain 20/200 or worse).

Bevacizumab is being used for macular edema in branch and central occlusions with promising outcomes (Table 36-2) (Figs. 36-1 and 36-2). Investigators reported gain of 2 to 4.8 lines of vision after bevacizumab treatment in patients with macular edema secondary to vein occlusions (39–41). Around 67% of the patients gain 3 or more lines of visual acuity after treatment (40,42). The optimum dosing and sequence for treatment is still undetermined. The literature available seems to indicate that multiple injections are required to achieve better visual acuity and to maintain improvement. Two to three injections over the first 6 months appear to be the most common management strategy. (43). Visual improvement and reduction in macular thickness is reported as early as 1 week after treatment and remains stable or improves for up to 2 months after the injection (43,44). Three to four months after treatment visual acuity declined and macular thickness increased in some patients (44). To date no investigators have reported worsening of nonperfusion after treatment with bevacizumab, and some of them reported collateral vessel formation.

### Irvine-Gass Syndrome

Cataract surgery with intraocular lens implantation can be complicated by postoperative cystoid macular edema (Irvine-Gass Syndrome). The incidence of clinically significant cystoid macular edema (CME), defined as a snellen visual acuity of 20/40 or worse with petaloid perifoveal macular edema, was reported in between 0% and 13% (45,46). Postsurgical macular edema resolves spontaneously in nearly 75% of cases within 6 months. In other cases, where spontaneous resolution is not achieved, CME can be difficult to treat. Treatments used for Irvine-Gass syndrome include systemic, periocular, intravitreal, and topical corticosteroids; oral and topical nonsteroidal anti-inflammatory drugs (NSAIDs); oral and topical carbonic anhydrase inhibitors; and *pars plana* vitrectomy. Cases that are refractory to medical treatment with steroid and nonsteroid medication, and patients with contraindication for steroid use can be treated with anti-VEGF drugs.

## TABLE 36-2 BEVACIZUMAB FOR MACULAR EDEMA SECONDARY TO VASCULAR OCCLUSIONS

| Authors | Study ME | N° Cases | Doses | N° Injections | Follow-up | Previous treat | Results VA | ≥3 Lines |
|---|---|---|---|---|---|---|---|---|
| Iturralde 2006 (173) | Retrospective CRVO | 16 | 1.25 mg | ≥1 | 3 months | Yes | 87%[a] | |
| Costa 2007 (42) | Prospective CRVO/HRVO | 6 | 2 mg | 3 | 25 weeks | No | | 66.6% |
| Rabena 2007 (43) | Retrospective BRVO | 27 | 1.25 mg | 2–3 | 5.3 months | Yes | 44%[a] | |
| Ferrara 2007 (174) | Retrospective CRVO | 6 | 1.25 mg | 4–10 | 12 months | No | | 66.6% |
| Prigingler 2007 (41) | Prospective CRVO | 46 | 1.25 mg | 2–4 | 6 months | Yes | 2.7 lines[b] | |
| Kreutzer 2008 (175) | Prospective BRVO | 34 | 1.25 mg | 2–6 | 6 months | Yes | 3 lines[b] | 62%[c] |
| Kriechbaum 2008 (28) | Prospective CRVO BRVO | 29 8 21 | 1 mg | 3 | 6 months | No Yes | 2.4 lines[b] 3 lines[b] | |
| PACORES 2008 (40) | Retrospective BRVO | 45 | 1.25 mg 2.5 mg | 1–5 | 6 months | Yes | 4.8 lines[b] | 67% |
| Chung 2008 (176) | Retrospective BRVO | 50 | 1.25 | 1–3 | 3 months | Yes | | 56%[d] |
| Jaissle GB 2008 (39) | Prospective BRVO | 23 | 1.25 mg | 1.6 mean | 12 months | No | 3 lines[b] | |

CRVO, central retinal vein occlusion; HRVO, hemiretinal vein occlusion; BRVO, branch retinal vein occlusion; ME, macular edema; DME, diabetic macular edema; VA, visual acuity.
[a]Percentage of eyes experience a halving of the visual angle from baseline VA.
[b]Mean lines gain from baseline evaluation to last follow up.
[c]≥ 2 or more lines of visual acuity gain.
[d]≥ 1 line or more of visual acuity gain.

Intravitreal bevacizumab has been used in several cases of pseudophakic CME with positive results (27,47,48). The Pan-American collaborative Study Group (27) reported the largest series of patients with Irvine-Gass syndrome treated with bevacizumab. The report includes 28 eyes from 5 different institutions with CME after cataract surgery treated with primary intravitreal bevacizumab. The mean time from cataract surgery to treatment was 13 months (range 1–60). None of the eyes receive intravitreal treatments or had vitreous surgery previously. Seventy-one percent of patients gained 2 lines or more of visual acuity after bevacizumab treatment, with a mean significant reduction in central macular thickness.

A German group reported (49) 16 eyes with refractory macular edema after cataract surgery that received intravitreal bevacizumab. Interesting, none of the eyes experienced improved visual function despite multiple injections. Although central retinal thickness improved significantly in 81% of patients, the anatomical change was mild and did not translate into visual improvement in most of the cases. Patients in this study were heterogeneous with chronic and recalcitrant CME.

Eyes included in the study did not respond to previous treatment with NSAIDs, corticosteroids, or acetazolamide.

The difference in the characteristics of patients in both studies may explain the divergence in results. Treatment of postoperative CME remains controversial, especially in cases of chronic CME, which is often unresponsive to different therapies.

## IDIOPATHIC MACULAR TELANGIECTASIS

Idiopathic macular telangiectasias (IMT) are dilated capillaries that develop in the macula and perifoveolar areas without a known cause. In 1993, Gass and Blodi (50) established a classification of these entities with subgroups and stages. In type 2 (perifoveal telangiectasia) the telangiectatic blood vessel is limited to the perifoveolar area and is associated with leakage and cystic appearance of the fovea. Typical findings in fluorescein angiography are parafoveal ectatic capillaries and late

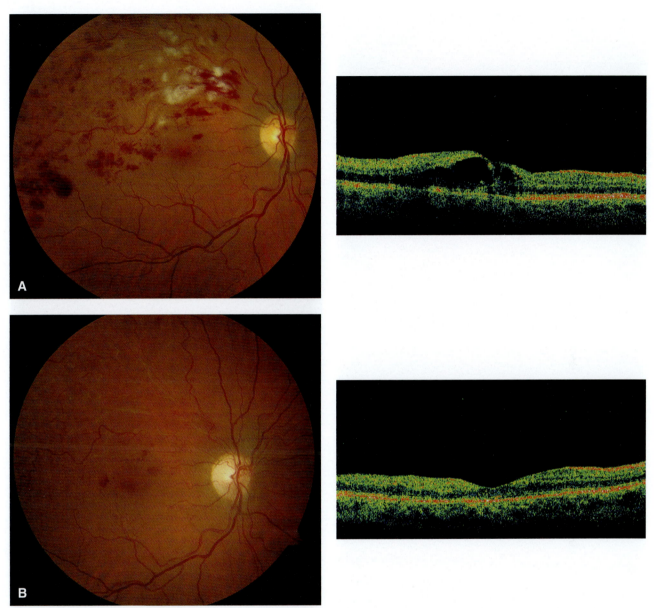

**Figure 36-1. A:** Fundus photo and OCT of right eye demonstrating Branch retinal vein occlusion and macular edema, AV 20/100. **B:** Fundus photo and OCT 6 months later after one Avastin treatment. Visual acuity (VA) 20/20 at 1-year follow-up.

diffuse leakage, mainly temporal to fovea. Yannuzzi et al. (51) have recently updated the classification scheme for IMT in which type 2 A is referred as perifoveal telangiectasia. This entity has been divided into two stages: nonproliferative, characterized by perifoveal telangiectasis, crystalline deposits, subretinal pigment plaques, right angle vessels, and inner lamellar cysts; and proliferative, which is defined by the presence of choroidal neovascularization.

Bevacizumab has been used in nonproliferative and proliferative type 2 telangiectasias with diverse results (52–58). Issa et al. (53) report a mean increase in visual acuity of 8 letters after intravitreal bevacizumab administration in 6 eyes with nonproliferative type 2 IMT; the 16 and 21-month follow up showed that VEGF inhibition resulted in an increase in mean visual acuity and decrease in parafoveal

leakage and central retinal thickness in all treated eyes. The authors conclude that the effect was temporary, with a rebound effect on parafoveal leakage and central retinal thickness about 3 to 4 months after treatment. The use of bevacizumab appears to be more advantageous in cases of proliferative disease (59).

## Uveitis

CME and choroidal neovascularization (CNV) are the two complications associated with uveitis that have been treated with intravitreal bevacizumab.

CME is one of the most common causes of significant visual loss in patients with intraocular inflammation. It is more often associated with intermediate uveitis, posterior uveitis,

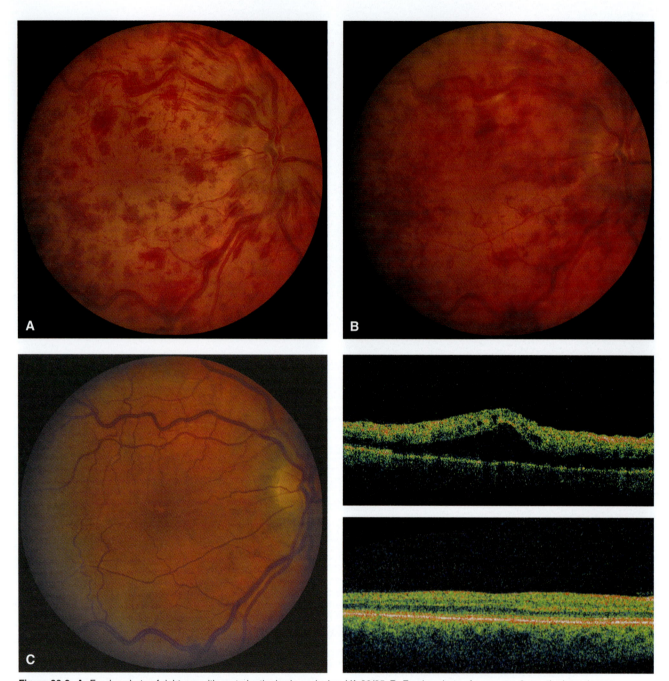

**Figure 36-2. A:** Fundus photo of right eye with central retinal vein occlusion, VA 20/25. **B:** Fundus photo of same eye 2 months later demonstrating increase in hemorrhage. OCT shows macular edema, VA 20/200. **C:** Fundus photo of same eye after four intravitreal bevacizumab treatments. OCT shows resolution of macular edema VA 20/25.

and panuveitis. Studies showed increased aqueous humor levels of VEGF in patients with uveitic macular edema (60). The classic approach to treat uveitic CME includes corticosteroids (topical, intravitreal or systemic), NSAIDs (topical and systemic), and systemic carbonic anhydrase inhibitors. Bevacizumab has been used for uveitic CME in an attempt to block VEGF and address CME from a different causative mechanism. Coma et al. (61) published the results of 13 eyes with recalcitrant CME secondary to uveitis treated with intra-

vitreal bevacizumab; more than a third of patients experienced improved visual acuity, and 46% had decrease foveal thickness after treatment. These results were similar to the results of Mackensen et al. (62) where 40% of eyes improved visual acuity after treatment.

CNV may occur in uveitic patients secondary to inflammation and/or ischemia. It is a rare complication and sometimes responds to systemic and local corticosteroids, photodynamic therapy (PDT), and more recently anti-VEGF treatment. Bevacizumab has been used to treat CNV (subfoveal, juxtafoveal, and peripapillary) secondary to uveitis with positive results (63–66). It is also being used in CNV secondary to multifocal choroiditis and chorioretinitis (67,68), toxoplasmosis (69,70), presumed ocular histoplasmosis (71,72), and punctate inner choroidopathy (73), with promising results.

## BEVACIZUMAB IN CHOROIDAL NEOVASCULARIZATION

CNV is an important cause of visual loss. The visual loss is mainly associated with intraretinal or subretinal fluid, hemorrhage, or fibrosis. CNV most commonly occurs in the setting of ARMD, but it may result from any retinal pigment epithelium and Bruch's membrane-complex perturbation. CNV may arise from more than 25 different ocular diseases including angioid streaks, multifocal choroiditis, myopia, and trauma.

The development of CNV has been shown to be associated with an alteration in the delicate balance of various growth factors involved in angiogenesis (74–76). VEGF is a powerful angiogenic factor and is essential for the development of CNV. On the other hand, pigment epithelium derived factor (PEDF) is known to be a strong inhibitor of neovascularization. In presence of bevacizumab, the VEGF level is reduced and PEDF level is increased; these changes are favorable for inhibition of CNV angiogenesis (77).

Bevacizumab has been used for CNV with good results after intravitreal treatment in age related macular degeneration, pathologic myopia, idiopathic CNV (78,79), CNV secondary to central serous retinopathy (78), to adult-onset vitelliform dystrophy and Best' disease (80,81), to angioid streaks (82–84), to pseudoxanthoma elasticum (85,86), and choroidal osteoma (87,88).

## AGE-RELATED MACULAR DEGENERATION

CNV is responsible for 80% to 90% of severe cases of vision loss in ARMD patients (89–92). Rosenfeld et al. were the first to report the use of bevacizumab in ARMD patients. Since then, clinical experience with bevacizumab has been published in retrospective and prospective studies, case series, and multiple personal experiences with unpublished data.

Bevacizumab has been tried in patients with subfoveal classic and occult membranes, in naïve and previously treated patients, in lesions with subretinal hemorrhage and with pigment epithelium detachment (Table 36-3) (Fig. 36-3) (93–103).

Patients considered treatment failures after intravitreal pegaptanib (Macugen) and PDT, and patients with chronic lesions with poor visual acuity show some visual gain from bevacizumab treatment (98,99,104,105).

The most commonly used dose is 1.25 mg in 0.05 cc; some reports compared 2.5 mg with the 1.25mg and did not observe statistically significant differences in changes of visual acuity, ocular coherence tomography (OCT) macular thickness, or number of reinjections needed (106). The optimal treatment schedule is unknown. Arias et al. (107) compared the scheme of loading dose (bevacizumab administered once a month for three months then prn versus Avastin × 1 with subsequent prn dosing) and found that patients did better when bevacizumab is administered in 3 doses once a month and then as needed. Retreatment is necessary to achieve and maintain visual gain;

## TABLE 36-3   BEVACIZUMAB FOR AMD

| Authors | Study ME | N° Cases | Doses | N° Injections | Follow-up | Loss ≥3 Lines | ≥1 Line | ≥3 Lines |
|---|---|---|---|---|---|---|---|---|
| Yoganathan 2006 (99) | Retrospective | 50 | 1.25 mg | 3.5 mean | 6.8 months | 0 | 71% | |
| | Naïve | | | | | | | 43% |
| | Pretreat | | | | | | | 17% |
| Aisenbrey 2007 (177) | Prospective | 30 | 1.25 mg | 1.6 mean | 3 months | 3.3% | 69.9 | 46.6% |
| | O S M | | | | | | | |
| Stifer 2007 (109) | Retrospective | 12 | 1 mg | 3.1 mean | 12 months | 0 | 38% | 9.5% |
| | S Hemorrhage | | | | | | | |
| PACORES 2008 (106) | Retrospective | 63 | 1.25 mg | 3.5 mean | 12 months | – | – | 47.6[a] |
| | S M naïve | | 2.5 mg | | | | | |
| Bashur 2008 (108) | Prospective | 51 | 2.5 mg | 3.4 mean | 12 months | 1% | – | 35.3% |
| | S all types | | | | | | | |
| Furino 2008 (178) | Prospective | 12 | 1.25 mg | 2.4 mean | 5.7 months | 0 | 91.6% | 42% |
| | OSM naïve | | | | | | | |

O, Occult; S, Subfoveal; M, Membrane.

[a]≥2 lines gain vision.

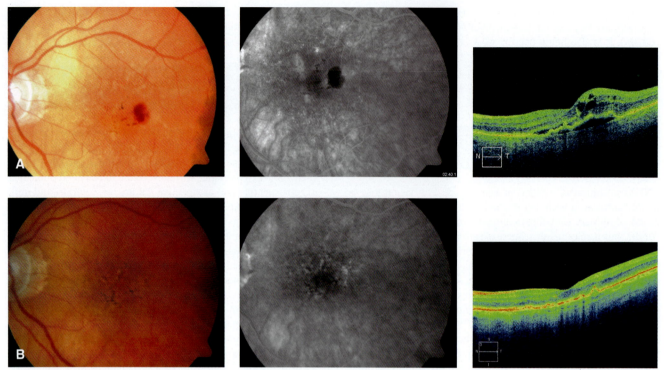

**Figure 36-3. A:** Fundus photo and IVFA of subfoveal CNVM with AMD. **B:** IVFA of the same eye demonstrating resolution of the leakage after 3 treatments with bevacizumab.

some investigators have reported a mean of 3 to 4 injections over 12 months (95,106,108,109). The need for chronic therapy is indicated by the recurrence of leakage from the CNV, defined as a decrease of visual acuity associated with an increase of subretinal fluid, macular edema on OCT and/or fluorescein angiography, that was observed after the initial treatment in almost all the patients in different reports.

The difference in safety and efficacy between ranibizumab and bevacizumab has been hotly debated. Currently, the CATT trial is designed to compare the visual outcomes and side effects between the two anti-VEGF agents. Additionally, regular versus prn dosing will be evaluated to determine if there is a difference in outcomes and side effects.

## Pathologic Myopia

Pathologic myopia accounts for approximately 60% of choroidal neovascularization in patients younger that 50 years of age. Nearly 10% of patients with degenerative retinal findings consistent with high myopia develop CNV. The long-term prognosis of myopic CNV is generally poor, with almost 100% of patients with CNV untreated having vision worse than 20/200 during five years of follow-up (110).

PDT with verteporfin has been shown to reduce the risk of visual loss, and is the only approve treatment for subfoveal CNV in myopia. At one-year follow up the VIP (The Verteporfin in Photodynamic Study) study showed that 72% of treated eyes compared with 44% of placebo eyes lost less than 8 letters. However, at the two-year follow up the trial failed to demonstrate a statistically significant benefit in the PDT-treated eyes (111). Moreover, in the VIP study less

than 25% of the patients improved one or more lines at 3 months.

In 2005, Nguyen et al. (112) reported the use of systemic bevacizumab for treatment of subfoveal CNV secondary to myopia. This article provided the first suggestion that VEGF is involved in promoting CNV in myopia. There are an increasing number of publications supporting the use of bevacizumab for CNV secondary to pathological myopia (Table 36-4). Difference in inclusion criteria and evaluation methods make comparison between these studies difficult. In general most investigators agree that intravitreal bevacizumab may result in better visual outcomes compared with PDT. The median visual improvements after PDT at 3- and 12-month visits were 0.0 line and 0.2 lines, respectively. This was considerably less than the mean improvement of 3.5, 3.6 and 2.9 lines observed by other investigators in bevacizumab treated eyes (113–115). Based on these findings, intravitreal bevacizumab seems to be a promising treatment for myopic CNV.

## BEVACIZUMAB IN RETINAL AND IRIS NEOVASCULARIZATION

Neovascularization of the retina and iris are highly correlated with retinal ischemia. It is well known that severe retinal ischemia increase VEGF levels (116,117). Intravitreal VEGF injection produces retina and iris neovascularization in several animal models. Inhibition of VEGF production is being proposed as a treatment for retinal-ischemia-induced neovascularization (Figs. 36-4 and 36-5).

## TABLE 36-4    BEVACIZUMAB IN CNV SECONDARY TO MYOPIA

| Authors | Study | N° Cases | Doses | Mean N° Injections | Follow-up | Mean visual improvement | ≥2 Lines |
|---------|-------|----------|-------|--------------------|-----------| ------------------------|----------|
| Chan WM 2008 (115) | Prospective | 29 | 1.25 mg | 3.6 | 12 months | 2.9 lines | 72.4% |
| Ikuno Y 2008 (179) | Retrospective | 63 | 1 mg | 2.4 | 12 months | | 40%[a] |
| Gharbiya 2008 (114) | Prospective | 20 | 1.25 mg | 4 | 12 months | 3.6 lines | 90% |
| Arias L 2008 (180) | Prospective | 17 | 1.25 mg | 1.1 | 6 months | 1.7 lines | 29% |
| Hernandez 2007 (181) | Prospective | 14 | 2.5 mg | ≥1 | 3 months | | 50%[b] |
| Mandal 2007 (182) | Prospective | 12 | 1.25 mg | ≥1 | 6 months | | 75%[c] |
| Yamamoto 2007 (113) | Retrospective | 11 | 1.25 mg | 1/2 | 5.5 months | 3.5 lines | 72% |
| Sakaguchi 2007 (183) | Prospective | 8 | 1 mg | 1/2 | 4.4 months | | 75% |
| Tewari 2006 (184) | Case Report | 1 | 1.25 mg | 2 | 6 months | 6 lines | 100% |

[a]40% of the patients gain ≥3 lines.
[b]50% of the patients gain 1 to 3 lines (snellen) of vision.
[c]75% of the patients gain ≥3 lines of vision.

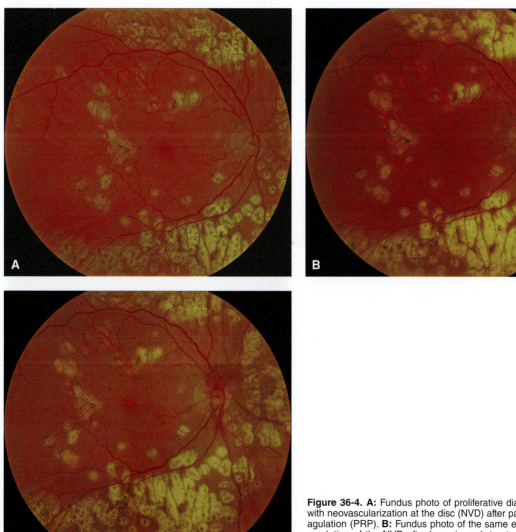

**Figure 36-4. A:** Fundus photo of proliferative diabetic retinopathy with neovascularization at the disc (NVD) after panretinal photocoagulation (PRP). **B:** Fundus photo of the same eye demonstrating resolution of the NVD after bevacizumab treatment without additional PRP. **C:** Fundus photo of the same eye with recurrence or rebound of the NVD.

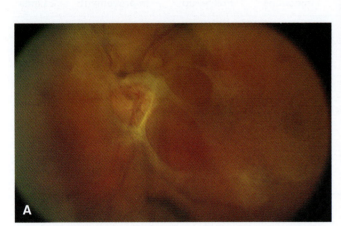
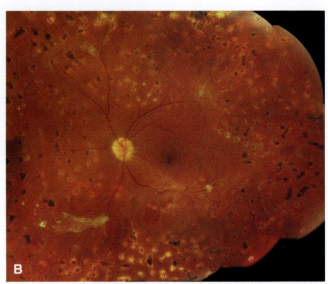

**Figure 36-5. A:** Fundus photo of right eye with proliferative diabetic retinopathy and tractional retinal detachment prior to treatment with bevacizumab. **B:** Fundus photo of the same eye a month after PPV demonstrating flat retina without traction.

Bevacizumab has been used in active neovascularization secondary to proliferative diabetic retinopathy and branch retinal occlusion with excellent outcomes (118–122). Moradian et al. (123) reported clearing of vitreous hemorrhage and regression of active fibrovascular tissue 1 week after treating 38 eyes with intravitreal bevacizumab. Some authors proposed the use of bevacizumab in combination with standard panretinal-photocoagulation (PRP) to prevent foveal thickness secondary to laser treatment (124,125).

Iris neovascularization (NVI) and neovascular glaucoma (NVG) associated with diabetic retinopathy and central retinal vein occlusion have been treated with bevacizumab (126–130). Reduction of intraocular pressure and regression of NVI have occurred as quickly as 48 hours after the treatment.

Jiang et al. (131) found regression of NVI in 26 (of 28) eyes treated with intravitreal bevacizumab. Regression was associated with decrease in intraocular pressure in 10 of the 11 eyes with pretreatment NVG. Similar results were found by Wakabayashi et al. (132) in their series. A rapid regression or disappearance of NVI was achieved in all eyes (41 eyes) with one bevacizumab injection. By six months, 44% of eyes had a recurrence of NVI that was resolved by repeated bevacizumab injections and additional photocoagulation. Marked regression of new vessels was evident in eyes with open and closed angle neovascular glaucoma; however, bevacizumab failed to lower the intraocular pressure (IOP) in the closed angle glaucoma group. These patients required glaucoma surgery to control intraocular pressure. A combination of photocoagulation with bevacizumab is being proposed to achieve a more rapid decrease of intraocular eye pressure and long standing NVI regression (133).

Other ischemic retinal diseases that involve vitreous hemorrhage and neovascularization have been treated with bevacizumab. Examples of these are neovascularization in patients with Eales disease (134,135), familial exudative vitreoretinopathy (136), and sickle cell retinopathy (137).

## BEVACIZUMAB IN RETINOPATHY OF PREMATURITY

Retinopathy of prematurity (ROP) is a leading cause of childhood blindness in industrialized and developing countries. Investigators have suggested that VEGF plays an important role in pathogenesis of ROP (138,139). Patients with stage 4 ROP have elevated vitreous concentrations of VEGF, especially eyes with active stage 4 compared with eyes with inactive stage 4 (140). Destruction of cellular elements that release VEGF in the peripheral retina and adjacent to extraretinal fibrovascular proliferation has proven to be effective (141). Laser therapy given earlier in the acute phase of ROP is currently recommended. Despite treatment and appropriated timing, zone I cases often have bad outcomes. Based on these observations and trying to address the zone I cases, some authors proposed the use of bevacizumab in premature births with zone I pathology.

Since 2007, several publications reported bevacizumab treatment for zone I (stage 3 and 4), and posterior zone II ROP (142–146). Authors perform one intravitreal injection of 0.4 mg to 0.75 mg of bevacizumab with or without laser photocoagulation, and with or without *pars plana* vitrectomy. In general, bevacizumab treatment showed decreased new vessel leakage, decreased venous dilatation and arteriolar tortuosity, decreased vitreous haze, and decreased iris vascular engorgement. Although new vessel regression may be achieved by laser photocoagulation alone, the prompt resolution of membranes suggests an effect of intravitreal bevacizumab. These observations strongly suggest that bevacizumab effectively reduces vascular activity in ROP.

Because ROP shows clinical and pathological features similar to those of proliferative diabetic retinopathy, they also may share the same risks. Honda et al. (144) showed an acute proliferative membrane contraction leading to traction retinal detachment 24 hours after an intravitreal injection of bevacizumab for advanced ROP. The development and progression of tractional detachment in this case is believed to be due to a rapid neovascular involution with accelerated fibrosis and posterior hyaloid contraction, as a response to decreased levels of VEGF and not to the natural course of aggressive ROP.

## Other Indications

Intravitreal bevacizumab has been used in radiation optic neuropathy and radiation maculopathy with improvement in visual acuity and resolution of the optic nerve swelling and macular edema (147–150). Retinal angiomatous proliferation, central serous retinopathy, and coadjutant in retina surgery are some of the other uses of intravitreal bevacizumab (151–155).

## SAFETY AND COMPLICATIONS WITH BEVACIZUMAB

Intravitreal bevacizumab has been associated to several ocular and systemic complications:

| Ocular Complications | Incidence |
|---|---|
| Retinal pigment epithelium tears in patients with AMD | 0.8%-6% (156–159) |
| Endophthalmitis | 0.019–0.16% (160,161) |
| Uveitis | 0.09% to 0.1% (161–163) |
| Tractional retinal detachment in patients with severe proliferative diabetic retinopathy | 0.16% to 5.2% (161–164) |
| Elevated intraocular pressure | 0.16% (161) |

| Systemic Complications | Incidence |
|---|---|
| Transient elevation in systemic blood pressure | 0.6% (161) |
| Cerebrovascular accidents and myocardial infarction | 0.5% and 0.4% (161) |

Hoskin et al. first described retinal pigment epithelium (RPE) tears as a complication of pigment epithelial detachments (PED) in the setting of wet ARMD (165). Clinically these tears are a well-demarcated area of bare choroid visible immediately adjacent to a hyperpigmented area, which represents the redundant, retracted RPE. The incidence of spontaneous RPE tears in eyes with ARMD-related PED over a 1-year follow up is 10% (although the authors of this study concede that this figure may underestimate the true incidence) (166). Tears of the RPE have been reported in association with all VEGF-modulating intravitreal therapies (ranibizumab, pegaptanib, or bevacizumab) for wet ARMD treatment (156–159,167,168). In general, all these eyes harbored a fibrovascular PED or PED associated with occult CNV and most tears occurred within weeks of the first or second intravitreal injection. RPE tears showed identical characteristics to spontaneous RPE rip. Whether anti-VEGF treatment has a causal role in the development of tears of

the RPE becomes an important question. Usually most rips occurred within days to weeks of the treatment, further raising suspicion for a precipitating role. Because RPE tears occur spontaneously in the setting of AMD, this temporal relationship may simply be coincidence. Because many of the RPE tears were asymptomatic, the timing of the detection may reflect the follow-up interval rather than the exact onset of the event.

Metrorrhagias in young women (incidence of 23.1%) (162,169), visual hallucinations (170), transient global amnesia (171), and skin eruption (172) have been reported.

## CONCLUSION

The utilization of intravitreal bevacizumab for age related macular degeneration, diabetic retinopathy, venous occlusive disease, retinopathy of prematurity and other VEGF mediated diseases has dramatically increased over the past few years. Despite a tremendous amount of clinical experience suggesting improvement in visual outcomes in these disorders, ongoing randomized controlled clinical trials remain necessary to determine if bevacizumab safety and efficacy compared to Lucentis. Further studies of the anti VEGF agents with longer follow up will increase our understanding of the long-term role of bevacizumab in the management of retinal diseases.

### References

1. Ehrlich P. On immunity with specific reference to cell life. *Proc R Soc London* 1900;66:429.
2. Malecaze F, Clamens S, Simorre-Pinatel V, et al. Detection of vascular endothelial growth factor messenger RNA and vascular endothelial growth factor-like activity in proliferative diabetic retinopathy. *Arch Ophthalmol* 1994;112:1476–1482.
3. Kvanta A, Algvere PV, Berglin L, et al. Subfoveal fibrovascular membranes in age-related macular degeneration express vascular endothelial growth factor. *Invest Ophthalmol Vis Sci* 1996;37:1929–1934.
4. Hurwitz H, Fehrenbacher L, Novotny W, et al. Bevacizumab plus irinotecan, fluorouracil, and leucovorin for metastatic colorectal cancer. *N Engl J Med* 2004;350:2335–2342.
5. Presta LG, Chen H, O'Connor SJ, et al. Humanization of an anti-vascular endothelial growth factor monoclonal antibody for the therapy of solid tumors and other disorders. *Cancer Res* 1997;57:4593–4599.
6. Ferrara N, Hillan KJ, Gerber HP, et al. Discovery and development of bevacizumab, an anti-VEGF antibody for treating cancer. *Nat Rev Drug Discov* 2004;3:391–400.
7. Chen Y, Wiesmann C, Fuh G, et al. Selection and analysis of an optimized anti-VEGF antibody: crystal structure of an affinity-matured Fab in complex with antigen. *J Mol Biol* 1999;293:865–881.
8. Hsei VC, Novotny WF, Margolin K, et al. Population pharmacokinetic (PK) analysis of bevacizumab (BV) in cancer subjects. *Proc Am Soc Clin Oncol* 2001;20(69a) (abstract 2 72).
9. Lu JF, Bruno R, Eppler S, et al. Clinical pharmacokinetics of bevacizumab in patients with solid tumors. *Cancer Chemother Pharmacol* 2008;62(5):779–786.
10. Bakri SJ, Snyder MR, Reid JM, et al. Pharmacokinetics of intravitreal bevacizumab (Avastin). *Ophthalmology* 2007;114(5):855–859.
11. Bakri SJ, Snyder MR, Reid JM, et al. Pharmacokinetics of intravitreal ranibizumab (Lucentis). *Ophthalmology* 2007;114(12):2179–2182.
12. Csaky KG, et al. IOVS 2007;48:ARVO E-Abstract 4936.
13. Krohne TU, Eter N, Holz FG, et al. Intraocular pharmacokinetics of bevacizumab after a single intravitreal injection in humans. *Am J Ophthalmol* 2008;146(4):508–512.
14. Zhu Q, Ziemssen F, Henke-Fahle S, et al. Vitreous levels of bevacizumab and vascular endothelial growth factor-A in patients with choroidal neovascularization. *Ophthalmology* 2008;115(10):1750–1755.

15. Heiduschka P, Fietz H, Hofmeister S, et al. Tübingen Bevacizumab Study Group. Penetration of bevacizumab through the retina after intravitreal injection in the monkey. *Invest Ophthalmol Vis Sci* 2007;48(6):2814–2823.

16. Shahar J, Avery RL, Heilweil G, et al. Electrophysiologic and retinal penetration studies following intravitreal injection of bevacizumab (Avastin). *Retina* 2006;26(3):262–269.

17. Feiner L, Barr EE, Shui YB, et al. Safety of intravitreal injection of bevacizumab in rabbit eyes. *Retina* 2006;26(8):882–888.

18. Manzano RP, Peyman GA, Khan P, et al. Testing intravitreal toxicity of bevacizumab (Avastin). *Retina* 2006;26(3):257–261.

19. Bakri SJ, Cameron JD, McCannel CA, et al. Absence of histologic retinal toxicity of intravitreal bevacizumab in a rabbit model. *Am J Ophthalmol* 2006;142(1):162–164.

20. Luthra S, Narayanan R, Marques LE, et al. Evaluation of in vitro effects of bevacizumab (Avastin) on retinal pigment epithelial, neurosensory retinal, and microvascular endothelial cells. *Retina* 2006;26(5):512–518.

21. Gerber HP, Ferrara N. Pharmacology and pharmacodynamics of bevacizumab as monotherapy or in combination with cytotoxic therapy in preclinical studies. *Cancer Res* 2005;65(3):671–680.

22. Peters S, Heiduschka P, Julien S, et al. Ultrastructural findings in the primate eye after intravitreal injection of bevacizumab. *Am J Ophthalmol* 2007;143(6):995–1002.

23. Carneiro A, Falcão M, Azevedo I, et al. Multiple effects of bevacizumab in angiogenesis: implications for its use in age-related macular degeneration. *Acta Ophthalmol* 2009;87(5):517-23 [Epub ahead of print 2008 Aug 20].

24. Moshfeghi AA, Rosenfeld PJ, Puliafito CA, et al. Systemic bevacizumab (Avastin) therapy for neovascular age-related macular degeneration: twenty-four-week results of an uncontrolled open-label clinical study. *Ophthalmology* 2006;113(11):2002.e1–2002.e12.

25. Shah MA, Ilson D, Kelsen DP. Thromboembolic events in gastric cancer: high incidence in patients receiving irinotecan- and bevacizumab-based therapy. *J Clin Oncol* 2005;23(11):2574–2576.

26. Saif MW, Mehra R. Incidence and management of bevacizumab-related toxicities in colorectal cancer. *Expert Opin Drug Saf* 2006;5(4):553–566.

27. Arevalo JF, Garcia-Amaris RA, Roca JA, et al. Pan-American Collaborative Retina Study Group. Primary intravitreal bevacizumab for the management of pseudophakic cystoid macular edema: pilot study of the Pan-American Collaborative Retina Study Group. *J Cataract Refract Surg* 2007;33(12):2098–2105.

28. Kriechbaum K, Michels S, Prager F, et al. Intravitreal Avastin for macular oedema secondary to retinal vein occlusion: a prospective study. *Br J Ophthalmol* 2008;92(4):518–522.

29. Arevalo JF, Fromow-Guerra J, Quiroz-Mercado H, et al. Pan-American Collaborative Retina Study Group. Primary intravitreal bevacizumab (Avastin) for diabetic macular edema: results from the Pan-American Collaborative Retina Study Group at 6-month follow-up. *Ophthalmology* 2007;114(4):743–750.

30. Melo GB, Farah ME, Aggio FB. Intravitreal injection of bevacizumab for cystoid macular edema in retinitis pigmentosa. *Acta Ophthalmol Scand* 2007;85(4):461–463.

31. Early Treatment Diabetic Retinopathy Study Research Group. Photocoagulation for diabetic macular edema. Early Treatment Diabetic Retinopathy Study report number 1. *Arch Ophthalmol* 1985;103:1796–1806.

32. Haritoglou C, Kook D, Neubauer A, et al. Intravitreal bevacizumab (Avastin) therapy for persistent diffuse diabetic macular edema. *Retina* 2006;26(9):999–1005.

33. Chung EJ, Roh MI, Kwon OW, et al. Effects of macular ischemia on the outcome of intravitreal bevacizumab therapy for diabetic macular edema. *Retina* 2008;28(7):957–963.

34. Kook D, Wolf A, Kreutzer T, et al. Long-term effect of intravitreal bevacizumab (avastin) in patients with chronic diffuse diabetic macular edema. *Retina* 2008;28(8):1053–1060.

35. Roh MI, Byeon SH, Kwon OW. Repeated intravitreal injection of bevacizumab for clinically significant diabetic macular edema. *Retina* 2008;28(9):1314–1318.

36. Scott IU, Edwards AR, Beck RW, et al. (Diabetic Retinopathy Clinical Research Network). A phase II randomized clinical trial of intravitreal bevacizumab for diabetic macular edema. *Ophthalmology* 2007;114(10):1860–1867.

37. The Branch Vein Occlusion Study Group. Argon laser photocoagulation for macular edema in branch vein occlusion. *Am J Ophthalmol* 1984;98(3):271–282.

38. The Central Vein Occlusion Study Group. Evaluation of grid pattern photocoagulation for macular edema in central vein occlusion. The Central Vein Occlusion Study Group M report. *Ophthalmology* 1995;102(10):1425–1433.

39. Jaissle GB, Leitritz M, Gelisken F, et al. One-year results after intravitreal bevacizumab therapy for macular edema secondary to branch retinal vein occlusion. *Graefes Arch Clin Exp Ophthalmol* 2008;247(1):27–33.

40. Wu L, Arevalo JF, Roca JA, et al. Comparison of two doses of intravitreal bevacizumab (Avastin) for treatment of macular edema secondary to branch retinal vein occlusion: results from the Pan-American Collaborative Retina Study Group at 6 months of follow-up. *Retina* 2008;28(2):212–219.

41. Priglinger SG, Wolf AH, Kreutzer TC, et al. Intravitreal bevacizumab injections for treatment of central retinal vein occlusion: six-month results of a prospective trial. *Retina* 2007;27(8):1004–1012.

42. Costa RA, Jorge R, Calucci D, et al. Intravitreal bevacizumab (avastin) for central and hemicentral retinal vein occlusions: IBeVO study. *Retina* 2007;27(2):141–149.

43. Rabena MD, Pieramici DJ, Castellarin AA, et al. Intravitreal bevacizumab (Avastin) in the treatment of macular edema secondary to branch retinal vein occlusion. *Retina* 2007;27(4):419–425.

44. Hsu J, Kaiser RS, Sivalingam A, et al. Intravitreal bevacizumab (avastin) in central retinal vein occlusion. *Retina* 2007;27(8):1013–1019.

45. Flach AJ. The incidence, pathogenesis and treatment of cystoid macular edema following cataract surgery. *Trans Am Ophthalmol Soc* 1998;96:557–634.

46. Mentes J, Erakgün T, Afrashi F, et al. Incidence of cystoid macular edema after uncomplicated phacoemulsification. *Ophthalmologica* 2003;217:408–412.

47. Barone A, Prascina F, Russo V, et al. Successful treatment of pseudophakic cystoid macular edema with intravitreal bevacizumab. *J Cataract Refract Surg* 2008;34(7):1210–1212.

48. Mason JO III, Albert MA Jr, Vail R. Intravitreal bevacizumab (Avastin) for refractory pseudophakic cystoid macular edema. *Retina* 2006;26(3):356–357.

49. Spitzer MS, Ziemssen F, Yoeruek E, et al. Efficacy of intravitreal bevacizumab in treating postoperative pseudophakic cystoid macular edema. *J Cataract Refract Surg* 2008;34(1):70–75.

50. Gass JD, Blodi BA. Idiopathic juxtafoveolar retinal telangiectasis: update of classification and follow-up study. *Ophthalmology* 1993;100:1536–1546.

51. Yannuzzi LA, Bardal AMC, Freund KB, et al. Idiopathic macular telangiectasia. *Arch Ophthalmol* 2006;124:450–460.

52. Maia OO Jr, Bonanomi MT, Takahashi WY, et al. Intravitreal bevacizumab for foveal detachment in idiopathic perifoveal telangiectasia. *Am J Ophthalmol* 2007;144(2):296–299.

53. Charbel Issa P, Finger RP, Holz FG, et al. Eighteen-month follow-up of intravitreal bevacizumab in type 2 idiopathic macular telangiectasia. *Br J Ophthalmol* 2008;92(7):941–945.

54. Charbel Issa P, Holz FG, Scholl HP. Findings in fluorescein angiography and optical coherence tomography after intravitreal bevacizumab in type 2 idiopathic macular telangiectasia. *Ophthalmology* 2007;114(9):1736–1742.

55. Mandal S, Venkatesh P, Abbas Z, et al. Intravitreal bevacizumab (Avastin) for subretinal neovascularization secondary to type 2 A idiopathic juxtafoveal telangiectasia. *Graefes Arch Clin Exp Ophthalmol* 2007;245(12):1825–1829.

56. Moon SJ, Berger AS, Tolentino MJ, et al. Intravitreal bevacizumab for macular edema from idiopathic juxtafoveolar retinal telangiectasis. *Ophthalmic Surg Lasers Imaging* 2007;38(2):164–166.

57. Gamulescu MA, Walter A, Sachs H, et al. Bevacizumab in the treatment of idiopathic macular telangiectasia. *Graefes Arch Clin Exp Ophthalmol* 2008;246(8):1189–1193.

58. Gamulescu MA, Walter A, Sachs H, et al. Bevacizumab in the treatment of idiopathic macular telangiectasia. *Graefes Arch Clin Exp Ophthalmol* 2008;246:1189–1193.

59. Kovach JL, Rosenfeld PJ. Bevacizumab (Avastin) therapy for idiopathic macular telangiectasia Type II. *Retina* 2008;29(1):27–32.

60. Fine HF, Baffi J, Reed GF, et al. Aqueous humor and plasma vascular endothelial growth factor in uveitis-associated cystoid macular edema. *Am J Ophthalmol* 2001;132:794–796.

61. Cordero Coma M, Sobrin L, Onal S, et al. Intravitreal bevacizumab for treatment of uveitic macular edema. *Ophthalmology* 2007;114(8):1574–1579.

62. Mackensen F, Heinz C, Becker MD, et al. Intravitreal bevacizumab (avastin) as a treatment for refractory macular edema in patients with uveitis: a pilot study. *Retina* 2008;28(1):41–45.

63. Kurup S, Lew J, Byrnes G, et al. Therapeutic efficacy of intravitreal bevacizumab on posterior uveitis complicated by neovascularization. *Acta Ophthalmol* 2008;87(3):349–352.

64. Mansour AM, Mackensen F, Arevalo JF, et al. Intravitreal bevacizumab in inflammatory ocular neovascularization. *Am J Ophthalmol* 2008;146(3):410–416.

65. Tran TH, Fardeau C, Terrada C, et al. Intravitreal bevacizumab for refractory choroidal neovascularization (CNV) secondary to uveitis. *Graefes Arch Clin Exp Ophthalmol* 2008;246(12):1685–1692.

66. Adán A, Mateo C, Navarro R, et al. Intravitreal bevacizumab (avastin) injection as primary treatment of inflammatory choroidal neovascularization. *Retina* 2007;27(9):1180–1186.

67. Fine HF, Zhitomirsky I, Freund KB, et al. Bevacizumab (Avastin) and ranibizumab (Lucentis) for choroidal neovascularization in multifocal choroiditis. *Retina* 2008;29(1):8–12.

68. Seth RK, Stoessel KM, Adelman RA. Choroidal neovascularization associated with West Nile virus chorioretinitis. *Semin Ophthalmol* 2007;22(2):81–84.

69. Guthoff R, Goebel W. Intravitreal bevacizumab for choroidal neovascularization in toxoplasmosis. *Acta Ophthalmol* 2009;87(6):688–690. [Epub ahead of print July 8, 2008]

70. Ben Yahia S, Herbort CP, Jenzeri S, et al. Intravitreal bevacizumab (Avastin) as primary and rescue treatment for choroidal neovascularization secondary to ocular toxoplasmosis. *Int Ophthalmol* 2008;28(4):311–316.

71. Adán A, Navarro M, Casaroli-Marano RP, et al. Intravitreal bevacizumab as initial treatment for choroidal neovascularization associated with presumed ocular histoplasmosis syndrome. *Graefes Arch Clin Exp Ophthalmol* 2007;245(12):1873–1875.

72. Schadlu R, Blinder KJ, Shah GK, et al. Intravitreal bevacizumab for choroidal neovascularization in ocular histoplasmosis. *Am J Ophthalmol* 2008;145(5):875–878.

73. Vossmerbaeumer U, Spandau UH, V Baltz S, et al. Intravitreal bevacizumab for choroidal neovascularisation secondary to punctate inner choroidopathy. *Clin Experiment Ophthalmol* 2008;36(3):292–394.

74. Ohno-Matsui K, Morita I, Tombran-Tink J, et al. Novel mechanism for age-related macular degeneration: an equilibrium shift between the angiogenesis factors VEGF and PEDF. *J Cell Physiol* 2001;189:323–333.

75. Tong JP, Yao YF. Contribution of VEGF and PEDF to choroidal angiogenesis: a need for balanced expressions. *Clin Biochem* 2006;39:267–276.

76. Tong JP, Chan WM, Liu DT, et al. Aqueous humor levels of vascular endothelial growth factor and pigment epithelium-derived factor in polypoidal choroidal vasculopathy and choroidal neovascularization. *Am J Ophthalmol* 2006;141:456–462.

77. Chan WM, Lai TY, Chan KP, et al. Changes in aqueous vascular endothelial growth factor and pigment epithelial-derived factor levels following intravitreal bevacizumab injections for choroidal neovascularization secondary to age-related macular degeneration or pathologic myopia. *Retina* 2008;28(9):1308–1313.

78. Chan WM, Lai TY, Liu DT, et al. Intravitreal bevacizumab (avastin) for choroidal neovascularization secondary to central serous chorioretinopathy, secondary to punctate inner choroidopathy, or of idiopathic origin. *Am J Ophthalmol* 2007;143(6):977–983.

79. Mandal S, Garg S, Venkatesh P, et al. Intravitreal bevacizumab for subfoveal idiopathic choroidal neovascularization. *Arch Ophthalmol* 2007;125(11):1487–1492.

80. Montero JA, Ruiz-Moreno JM, De La Vega C. Intravitreal bevacizumab for adult-onset vitelliform dystrophy: a case report. *Eur J Ophthalmol* 2007;17(6):983–986.

81. Leu J, Schrage NF, Degenring RF. Choroidal neovascularisation secondary to Best's disease in a 13-year-old boy treated by intravitreal bevacizumab. *Graefes Arch Clin Exp Ophthalmol* 2007;245(11):1723–1725.

82. Pedersen R, Soliman W, Lund-Andersen H, et al. Treatment of choroidal neovascularization using intravitreal bevacizumab. *Acta Ophthalmol Scand* 2007;85(5):526–533.

83. Rinaldi M, Dell'Omo R, Romano MR, et al. Intravitreal bevacizumab for choroidal neovascularization secondary to angioid streaks. *Arch Ophthalmol* 2007;125(10):1422–1423.

84. Teixeira A, Moraes N, Farah ME, et al. Choroidal neovascularization treated with intravitreal injection of bevacizumab (Avastin) in angioid streaks. *Acta Ophthalmol Scand* 2006;84(6):835–836.

85. Finger RP, Charbel Issa P, Ladewig M, et al. Intravitreal bevacizumab for choroidal neovascularisation associated with pseudoxanthoma elasticum. *Br J Ophthalmol* 2008;92(4):483–487.

86. Bhatnagar P, Freund KB, Spaide RF, et al. Intravitreal bevacizumab for the management of choroidal neovascularization in pseudoxanthoma elasticum. *Retina* 2007;27(7):897–902.

87. Narayanan R, Shah VA. Intravitreal bevacizumab in the management of choroidal neovascular membrane secondary to choroidal osteoma. *Eur J Ophthalmol* 2008;18(3):466–468.

88. Ahmadieh H, Vafi N. Dramatic response of choroidal neovascularization associated with choroidal osteoma to the intravitreal injection of bevacizumab (Avastin). *Graefes Arch Clin Exp Ophthalmol* 2007;245(11):1731–1733.

89. Age-Related Eye Disease Study Research Group. Potential public health impact of Age-Related Eye Disease Study results: AREDS report no. 11. *Arch Ophthalmol* 2003;121:1621–1624.

90. Klein R, Peto T, Bird A, et al. The epidemiology of age-related macular degeneration. *Am J Ophthalmol* 2004;137:486–495.

91. Eye Diseases Prevalence Research Group. Causes and prevalence of visual impairment among adults in the United States. *Arch Ophthalmol* 2004;122:477–485.

92. Eye Diseases Prevalence Research Group. Prevalence of age related macular degeneration in the United States. *Arch Ophthalmol* 2004;122:564–572.

93. Chen E, Kaiser RS, Vander JF. Intravitreal bevacizumab for refractory pigment epithelial detachment with occult choroidal neovascularization in age-related macular degeneration. *Retina* 2007;27(4):445–450.

94. Emerson MV, Lauer AK, Flaxel CJ, et al. Intravitreal bevacizumab (Avastin) treatment of neovascular age-related macular degeneration. *Retina* 2007;27(4):439–444.

95. Goff MJ, Johnson RN, McDonald HR, et al. Intravitreal bevacizumab for previously treated choroidal neovascularization from age-related macular degeneration. *Retina* 2007;27(4):432–438.

96. Jonas JB, Libondi T, Ihloff AK, et al. Visual acuity change after intravitreal bevacizumab for exudative age-related macular degeneration in relation to subfoveal membrane type. *Acta Ophthalmol Scand* 2007;85(5):563–565.

97. Chen CY, Wong TY, Heriot WJ. Intravitreal bevacizumab (Avastin) for neovascular age-related macular degeneration: a short-term study. *Am J Ophthalmol* 2007;143(3):510–512.

98. Melamud A, Stinnett S, Fekrat S. Treatment of neovascular age-related macular degeneration with intravitreal bevacizumab: efficacy of three consecutive monthly injections. *Am J Ophthalmol* 2008;146(1):91–95.

99. Yoganathan P, Deramo VA, Lai JC, et al. Visual improvement following intravitreal bevacizumab (Avastin) in exudative age-related macular degeneration. *Retina* 2006;26(9):994–998.

100. Lazic R, Gabric N. Intravitreally administered bevacizumab (Avastin) in minimally classic and occult choroidal neovascularization secondary to age-related macular degeneration. *Graefes Arch Clin Exp Ophthalmol* 2007;245(1):68–73.

101. Rich RM, Rosenfeld PJ, Puliafito CA, et al. Short-term safety and efficacy of intravitreal bevacizumab (Avastin) for neovascular age-related macular degeneration. *Retina* 2006;26(5):495–511.

102. Bashshur ZF, Bazarbachi A, Schakal A, et al. Intravitreal bevacizumab for the management of choroidal neovascularization in age-related macular degeneration. *Am J Ophthalmol* 2006;142(1):1–9.

103. Avery RL, Pieramici DJ, Rabena MD, et al. Intravitreal bevacizumab (Avastin) for neovascular age-related macular degeneration. *Ophthalmology* 2006;113(3):363–372.

104. Ehrlich R, Weinberger D, Priel E, et al. Outcome of bevacizumab (Avastin) injection in patients with age-related macular degeneration and low visual acuity. *Retina* 2008;28(9):1302–1307.

105. Spaide RF, Laud K, Fine HF, et al. Intravitreal bevacizumab treatment of choroidal neovascularization secondary to age-related macular degeneration. *Retina* 2006;26(4):383–390.

106. Arevalo JF, Fromow-Guerra J, Sanchez JG, et al. Primary intravitreal bevacizumab for subfoveal choroidal neovascularization in age-related macular degeneration: results of the Pan-American Collaborative Retina Study Group at 12 months follow-up. *Retina* 2008;28(10):1387–1394.

107. Arias L, Caminal JM, Casas L, et al. A study comparing two protocols of treatment with intravitreal bevacizumab (Avastin) for neovascular age-related macular degeneration. *Br J Ophthalmol* 2008;92(12):1636–1641.

108. Bashshur ZF, Haddad ZA, Schakal A, et al. Intravitreal bevacizumab for treatment of neovascular age-related macular degeneration: a one-year prospective study. *Am J Ophthalmol* 2008;145(2):249–256.

109. Stifter E, Michels S, Prager F, et al. Intravitreal bevacizumab therapy for neovascular age-related macular degeneration with large submacular hemorrhage. *Am J Ophthalmol* 2007;144(6):886–892.

110. Yoshida T, Ohno-Matsui K, Yasuzumi K, et al. Myopic choroidal neovascularization: a 10-year follow-up. *Ophthalmology* 2003;110:1297–1305.

111. Blinder KJ, Blumenkranz MS, Bressler NM, et al. Verteporfin therapy of subfoveal choroidal neovascularization in pathologic myopia: 2-year results of a randomized clinical trial—VIP Report No. 3. *Ophthalmology* 2003;110:667–673.

112. Nguyen QD, Shah S, Tatlipinar S, et al. Bevacizumab suppress choroidal neovascularization caused by pathological myopia. *Br J Ophthalmol* 2005;89:1368–1370.

113. Yamamoto I, Rogers AH, Reichel E, et al. Intravitreal bevacizumab (Avastin) as treatment for subfoveal choroidal neovascularisation secondary to pathological myopia. *Br J Ophthalmol* 2007;91(2):157–160.

114. Gharbiya M, Allievi F, Mazzeo L, et al. Intravitreal bevacizumab treatment for choroidal neovascularization in pathologic myopia: 12-month results. *Am J Ophthalmol* 2008;147(1):84–93.

115. Chan WM, Lai TY, Liu DT, et al. Intravitreal bevacizumab (Avastin) for myopic choroidal neovascularization: 1-year results of a prospective pilot study. *Br J Ophthalmol* 2008;93(2):150–154.

116. Tolentino MJ, Miller JW, Gragoudas ES, et al. Vascular endothelial growth factor is sufficient to produce iris neovascularization and neovascular glaucoma in a nonhuman primate. *Arch Ophthalmol* 1996;114:964–970.

117. Adamis AP, Shima DT, Tolentino MJ, et al. Inhibition of vascular endothelial growth factor prevents retinal ischemia associated iris neovascularization in a nonhuman primate. *Arch Ophthalmol* 1996;114:66–71.

118. Avery RL, Pearlman J, Pieramici DJ, et al. Intravitreal bevacizumab (Avastin) in the treatment of proliferative diabetic retinopathy. *Ophthalmology* 2006;113(10):1695.e1–1695.e15.

119. Jorge R, Costa RA, Calucci D, et al. Intravitreal bevacizumab (Avastin) for persistent new vessels in diabetic retinopathy (IBEPE study). *Retina* 2006;26(9):1006–1013.

120. Spaide RF, Fisher YL. Intravitreal bevacizumab (Avastin) treatment of proliferative diabetic retinopathy complicated by vitreous hemorrhage. *Retina* 2006;26(3):275–278.

121. Minnella AM, Savastano CM, Ziccardi L, et al. Intravitreal bevacizumab (Avastin) in proliferative diabetic retinopathy. *Acta Ophthalmol* 2008;86(6):683–687.

122. Ahmadieh H, Moradian S, Malihi M. Rapid regression of extensive retinovitreal neovascularization secondary to branch retinal vein occlusion after a single intravitreal injection of bevacizumab. *Int Ophthalmol* 2005;26:191–193.

123. Moradian S, Ahmadieh H, Malihi M, et al. Intravitreal bevacizumab in active progressive proliferative diabetic retinopathy. *Graefes Arch Clin Exp Ophthalmol* 2008;246(12):1699–1705.

124. Mason JO III, Yunker JJ, Vail R, et al. Intravitreal bevacizumab (Avastin) prevention of panretinal photocoagulation-induced complications in patients with severe proliferative diabetic retinopathy. *Retina* 2008;28(9):1319–1324.

125. Tonello M, Costa RA, Almeida FP, et al. Panretinal photocoagulation versus PRP plus intravitreal bevacizumab for high-risk proliferative diabetic retinopathy (IBeHi study). *Acta Ophthalmol* 2008;86(4):385–389.

126. Yazdani S, Hendi K, Pakravan M. Intravitreal bevacizumab (Avastin) injection for neovascular glaucoma. *J Glaucoma* 2007;16(5):437–439.

127. Vatavuk Z, Bencic G, Mandic Z. Intravitreal bevacizumab for neovascular glaucoma following central retinal artery occlusion. *Eur J Ophthalmol* 2007;17(2):269–271.

128. Iliev ME, Domig D, Wolf-Schnurrbursch U, et al. Intravitreal bevacizumab (Avastin) in the treatment of neovascular glaucoma. *Am J Ophthalmol* 2006;142(6):1054–1056.

129. Oshima Y, Sakaguchi H, Gomi F, et al. Regression of iris neovascularization after intravitreal injection of bevacizumab in patients with proliferative diabetic retinopathy. *Am J Ophthalmol* 2006;142(1):155–158.

130. Avery RL. Regression of retinal and iris neovascularization after intravitreal bevacizumab (Avastin) treatment. *Retina* 2006;26(3):352–354.

131. Jiang Y, Liang X, Li X, et al. Analysis of the clinical efficacy of intravitreal bevacizumab in the treatment of iris neovascularization caused by proliferative diabetic retinopathy. *Acta Ophthalmol.* 2009;87(7):736-40 [Epub ahead of print September 18, 2008]

132. Wakabayashi T, Oshima Y, Sakaguchi H, et al. Intravitreal bevacizumab to treat iris neovascularization and neovascular glaucoma secondary to ischemic retinal diseases in 41 consecutive cases. *Ophthalmology* 2008;115(9):1571–1580.

133. Ehlers JP, Spirn MJ, Lam A, et al. Combination intravitreal bevacizumab/panretinal photocoagulation versus panretinal photocoagulation alone in the treatment of neovascular glaucoma. *Retina* 2008;28(5):696–702.

134. Küçükerdönmez C, Akova YA, Yilmaz G. Intravitreal injection of bevacizumab in Eales disease. *Ocul Immunol Inflamm* 2008;16(1):63–65.

135. Kumar A, Sinha S. Rapid regression of disc and retinal neovascularization in a case of Eales disease after intravitreal bevacizumab. *Can J Ophthalmol* 2007;42(2):335–336.

136. Tagami M, Kusuhara S, Honda S, et al. Rapid regression of retinal hemorrhage and neovascularization in a case of familial exudative vitreoretinopathy treated with intravitreal bevacizumab. *Graefes Arch Clin Exp Ophthalmol* 2008;246(12):1787–1789.

137. Siqueira RC, Costa RA, Scott IU, et al. Intravitreal bevacizumab (Avastin) injection associated with regression of retinal neovascularization caused by sickle cell retinopathy. *Acta Ophthalmol Scand* 2006;84(6):834–835.

138. Pieh C, Agostini H, Buschbeck C, et al. VEGF-A, VEGFR-1, VEGFR-2 and Tie2 levels in plasma of premature infants: relationship to retinopathy of prematurity. *Br J Ophthalmol* 2008;92(5):689–693.

139. Smith LE. Pathogenesis of retinopathy of prematurity. *Growth Horm IGF Res* 2004;14(suppl A):S140–S144.

140. Sonmez K, Drenser KA, Capone A Jr, et al. Vitreous levels of stromal cell-derived factor 1 and vascular endothelial growth factor in patients with retinopathy of prematurity. *Ophthalmology* 2008;115(6):1065–1070.

141. Early Treatment for Retinopathy of Prematurity Cooperative Group. Revised indications for the treatment of retinopathy of prematurity: results of the Early Treatment for Retinopathy of Prematurity Randomized Trial. *Arch Ophthalmol* 2003;121:1684–1696.

142. Travassos A, Teixeira S, Ferreira P, et al. Intravitreal bevacizumab in aggressive posterior retinopathy of prematurity. *Ophthalmic Surg Lasers Imaging* 2007;38(3):233–237.

143. Chung EJ, Kim JH, Ahn HS, et al. Combination of laser photocoagulation and intravitreal bevacizumab (Avastin) for aggressive zone I retinopathy of prematurity. *Graefes Arch Clin Exp Ophthalmol* 2007;245(11):1727–1730.

144. Honda S, Hirabayashi H, Tsukahara Y, et al. Acute contraction of the proliferative membrane after an intravitreal injection of bevacizumab for advanced retinopathy of prematurity. *Graefes Arch Clin Exp Ophthalmol* 2008;246(7):1061–1063.

145. Mintz-Hittner HA, Kuffel RR Jr. Intravitreal injection of bevacizumab (avastin) for treatment of stage 3 retinopathy of prematurity in zone I or posterior zone II. *Retina* 2008;28(6):831–838.

146. Kusaka S, Shima C, Shimojyo H, et al. Efficacy of Intravitreal Injection of Bevacizumab for Severe Retinopathy of Prematurity: A Pilot Study. *Br J Ophthalmol* 2008;92(11):1450–1455.

147. Finger PT. Anti-VEGF bevacizumab (Avastin) for radiation optic neuropathy. *Am J Ophthalmol* 2007;143(2):335–338.

148. Ziemssen F, Voelker M, Altpeter E, et al. Intravitreal bevacizumab treatment of radiation maculopathy due to brachytherapy in choroidal melanoma. *Acta Ophthalmol Scand* 2007;85(5):579–580.

149. Finger PT, Chin K. Anti-vascular endothelial growth factor bevacizumab (avastin) for radiation retinopathy. *Arch Ophthalmol* 2007;125(6):751–756.

150. Gupta A, Muecke JS. Treatment of radiation maculopathy with intravitreal injection of bevacizumab (Avastin). *Retina* 2008;28(7):964–968.

151. Meyerle CB, Freund KB, Iturralde D, et al. Intravitreal bevacizumab (Avastin) for retinal angiomatous proliferation. *Retina* 2007;27(4):451–457.

152. Joeres S, Heussen FM, Treziak T, et al. Bevacizumab (Avastin) treatment in patients with retinal angiomatous proliferation. *Graefes Arch Clin Exp Ophthalmol* 2007;245(11):1597–1602.

153. Costagliola C, Romano MR, dell'Omo R, et al. Intravitreal bevacizumab for the treatment of retinal angiomatous proliferation. *Am J Ophthalmol* 2007;144(3):449–451.

154. Ghazi NG, Knape RM, Kirk TQ, et al. Intravitreal bevacizumab (avastin) treatment of retinal angiomatous proliferation. *Retina* 2008;28(5):689–695.

155. Yang CM, Yeh PT, Yang CH, et al. Bevacizumab pretreatment and long-acting gas infusion on vitreous clear-up after diabetic vitrectomy. *Am J Ophthalmol* 2008;146(2):211–217.

156. Spandau UH, Jonas JB. Retinal pigment epithelium tear after intravitreal bevacizumab for exudative age-related macular degeneration. *Am J Ophthalmol* 2006;142:1068–1070.

157. Ronan SM, Yoganathan P, Chien FY, et al. Retinal pigment epithelium tears after intravitreal injection of bevacizumab (avastin) for neovascular age-related macular degeneration. *Retina* 2007;27(5):535–540.

158. Chan CK, Meyer CH, Gross JG, et al. Retinal pigment epithelial tears after intravitreal bevacizumab injection for neovascular age-related macular degeneration. *Retina* 2007;27(5):541–551.

159. Gelisken F, Ziemssen F, Voelker K, et al. Retinal pigment epithelial tear following intravitreal bevacizumab injection for neovascular age related macular degeneration. *Acta Ophthalmol Scand* 2006;84(6):833–834.

160. Mason JO III, White MF, Feist RM, et al. Incidence of acute onset endophthalmitis following intravitreal bevacizumab (Avastin) injection. *Retina* 2008;28(4):564–567.

161. Wu L, Martínez-Castellanos MA, Quiroz-Mercado H, et al; Pan American Collaborative Retina Group (PACORES). Twelve-month safety of intravitreal injections of bevacizumab (Avastin(R)): results of the Pan-American Collaborative Retina Study Group (PACORES). *Graefes Arch Clin Exp Ophthalmol* 2008;246(1):81–87.

162. Shima C, Sakaguchi H, Gomi F, et al. Complications in patients after intravitreal injection of bevacizumab. *Acta Ophthalmol* 2008;86(4):372–376.

163. Arevalo JF, Maia M, Flynn HW Jr, et al. Tractional retinal detachment following intravitreal bevacizumab (Avastin) in patients with severe proliferative diabetic retinopathy. *Br J Ophthalmol* 2008;92(2):213–216.

164. Hoskin A, Bird AC, Sehmi K. Tears of detached retinal pigment epithelium. *Br J Ophthalmol* 1981;65:417–422.

165. Lee GKY, Lai TYY, Chan WM, et al. Retinal pigment epithelial tear following intravitreal ranibizumab injections for neovascular age-related macular degeneration. *Graefes Arch Clin Exp Ophthalmol* 2007;245(8):1225–1227.

166. Caswell AG, Kohen D, Bird AC. Retinal pigment epithelial detachments in the elderly: classification and outcome. *Br J Ophthalmol* 1985;69:397–403.

167. Carvounis PE, Kopel AC, Benz MS. Retinal pigment epithelium tears following ranibizumab for exudative age-related macular degeneration. *Am J Ophthalmol* 2007;143:504–505.

168. Singh RP, Sears JE. Retinal pigment epithelial tears after pegaptanib injection for exudative age-related macular degeneration. *Am J Ophthalmol* 2006;142:160–162.

169. Rodrigues EB, Shiroma H, Meyer CH, et al. Metrorrhagia after intravitreal injection of bevacizumab. *Acta Ophthalmol Scand* 2007;85(8):915–916.

170. Tan CS, Sanjay S, Eong KG. Charles Bonnet syndrome (visual hallucinations) after intravitreal avastin injection for age-related macular degeneration. *Am J Ophthalmol* 2007;144(2):330–331.

171. Byeon SH, Kwon OW, Lee SC. Transient global amnesia following intravitreal injection of bevacizumab. *Acta Ophthalmol* 2009;87(5):570 [Epub ahead of print June 5, 2008].

172. Amselem L, Diaz-Llopis M, Garcia-Delpech S, et al. Papulopustular eruption after intravitreal bevacizumab (Avastin®). *Acta Ophthalmol* 2008;87(1):110–111.

173. Iturralde D, Spaide RF, Meyerle CB, et al. Intravitreal bevacizumab (Avastin) treatment of macular edema in central retinal vein occlusion: a short-term study. *Retina* 2006;26(3):279–284.

174. Ferrara DC, Koizumi H, Spaide RF. Early bevacizumab treatment of central retinal vein occlusion. *Am J Ophthalmol* 2007;144(6):864–871.

175. Kreutzer TC, Alge CS, Wolf AH, et al. Intravitreal bevacizumab for the treatment of macular oedema secondary to branch retinal vein occlusion. *Br J Ophthalmol* 2008;92(3):351–355.

176. Chung EJ, Hong YT, Lee SC, et al. Prognostic factors for visual outcome after intravitreal bevacizumab for macular edema due to branch retinal vein occlusion. *Graefes Arch Clin Exp Ophthalmol* 2008;246(9):1241–1247.

177. Aisenbrey S, Ziemssen F, Völker M, et al. Intravitreal bevacizumab (Avastin) for occult choroidal neovascularization in age-related macular degeneration. *Graefes Arch Clin Exp Ophthalmol* 2007;245(7):941–948.

178. Furino C, Boscia F, Recchimurzo N, et al. Intravitreal bevacizumab for treatment-naïve subfoveal occult choroidal neovascularization in age-related macular degeneration. *Acta Ophthalmol* 2008;87(4):404–407.

179. Ikuno Y, Sayanagi K, Soga K, et al. Intravitreal Bevacizumab for Choroidal Neovascularization Attributable to Pathological Myopia: One-Year Results. *Am J Ophthalmol* 2008;147(1):94–100.

180. Arias L, Planas N, Prades S, et al. Intravitreal bevacizumab (Avastin) for choroidal neovascularisation secondary to pathological myopia: 6-month results. *Br J Ophthalmol* 2008;92(8):1035–1039.

181. Hernández-Rojas ML, Quiroz-Mercado H, Dalma-Weiszhausz J, et al. Short-term effects of intravitreal bevacizumab for subfoveal choroidal neovascularization in pathologic myopia. *Retina* 2007;27(6):707–712.

182. Mandal S, Venkatesh P, Sampangi R. Intravitreal bevacizumab (Avastin) as primary treatment for myopic choroidal neovascularization. *Eur J Ophthalmol* 2007;17:620–626.

183. Sakaguchi H, Ikuno Y, Gomi F, et al. Intravitreal injection of bevacizumab for choroidal neovascularisation associated with pathological myopia. *Br J Ophthalmol* 2007;91(2):161–165.

184. Tewari A, Dhalla MS, Apte RS. Intravitreal bevacizumab for treatment of choroidal neovascularization in pathologic myopia. *Retina* 2006;26(9):1093–1094.

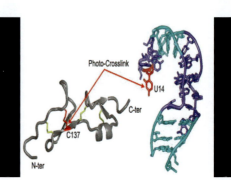

# The First Anti-VEGF Therapy: Pegaptanib Sodium

Anthony P. Adamis

## INTRODUCTION

Until recently, the treatment of ocular neovascular diseases such as age-related macular degeneration (AMD), diabetic retinopathy (DR), and retinal vein occlusion (RVO) has been restricted to ablative laser-based procedures and surgical interventions. More than a decade of research has identified a central role for vascular endothelial growth factor (VEGF) in the etiology of these diseases, resulting in revolutionary new treatments based on inhibiting VEGF. Two anti-VEGF agents are approved as intravitreal therapies for neovascular AMD. Pegaptanib sodium, the first approved agent, is an RNA aptamer that binds the VEGF$_{165}$ isoform while ranibizumab is a monoclonal antibody antigen-binding fragment that binds all VEGF isoforms. Bevacizumab, a related monoclonal antibody, also is being evaluated for the treatment of ocular neovascular diseases in off-label studies. This chapter will focus on the development and clinical application of pegaptanib.

## VEGF AS A THERAPEUTIC TARGET IN OCULAR NEOVASCULAR DISEASE

The importance of VEGF in ocular neovascular diseases stems from its key properties as a regulator of physiological and pathological angiogenesis (1) and as a potent promoter of vascular permeability (2). As such, it contributes to two proximate causes of vision loss: the growth of aberrant retinal vasculature and macular edema. Clinical studies established that vitreous levels of VEGF were elevated in a number of ocular neovascular conditions (3–6) while preclinical work with several animal model systems demonstrated that such elevations were both necessary and sufficient for the development of ocular neovascularization (7,8). Studies using animal models of diabetes also were important in establishing the role of VEGF in promoting the increased retinal leukostasis characteristic of DR believed to mediate much of the damage to the retinal vasculature associated with this disease (9).

Alternative splicing of the VEGF gene generates six principal isoforms (1,10) with VEGF$_{165}$ and VEGF$_{121}$ being the most common variants in normal eyes (11). Preclinical evidence suggests that VEGF$_{165}$ is especially pathogenic in that it was dramatically upregulated in a rodent model of ischemic neovascularization (12) and had more potent proinflammatory properties than VEGF$_{121}$

(13). Such properties included chemoattraction of monocytes (13), which amplifies neovascularization induced by ischemia (12) or laser wounding (14–16), and upregulation of retinal expression of intercellular cell adhesion molecule-1 (13), a mediator of retinal leukostasis in DR (9). These data suggested that specific inactivation of VEGF$_{165}$ could significantly ameliorate the effects of VEGF in ocular neovascular diseases. This concept was supported by two key preclinical observations in rodent models: not only was intravitreal pegaptanib as effective as a VEGF-receptor (R)-Fc fusion protein that binds all VEGF isoforms in suppressing ischemic ocular neovascularization (12) but it was also capable of reversing the diabetes-induced breakdown of the blood-retinal barrier (17).

VEGF exerts a wide range of actions both in the eye, where it is important in the maintenance of retinal neurons (18) and the choriocapillaris (19), and in the nervous system, kidney, bone, and liver (9,20,21). Furthermore, the aberrant neovasculature found in AMD and DR is especially permeable, increasing the potential for systemic exposure to intravitreal anti-VEGF agents (22), as evidenced by the detection of therapeutic effects in the fellow eyes following anti-VEGF therapies in DR (23) and AMD (24). The safety of nonselective versus selective anti-VEGF therapies will be explored in the clinical section of this review.

## DEVELOPMENT OF PEGAPTANIB AS AN ANTI-VEGF OCULAR THERAPEUTIC AGENT

Pegaptanib is an RNA aptamer that was developed through three applications (25–27) of the SELEX [systematic evolution of ligands by exponential enrichment] procedure (28,29) using VEGF$_{165}$ as a target. Chemical modifications of the constituent nucleotides were used to improve its nuclease resistance and affinity, and two 5' polyethylene glycol substituents were added to increase bioavailability (30). Pegaptanib was found to block the binding of VEGF$_{165}$ to endothelial cell receptors, to inhibit VEGF$_{165}$-mediated cell signaling and proliferation (31), and to reduce VEGF$_{165}$-induced vascular permeability (27,32) while not affecting responses to VEGF$_{121}$ (31). Pegaptanib's selectivity for VEGF$_{165}$ derives from its interaction with the heparin-binding domain of VEGF$_{165}$ (33), which is not present in VEGF$_{121}$ (10). The predicted secondary structure of pegaptanib and its interaction with the heparin-binding domain of VEGF$_{165}$ are shown in Figure 37-1 (30).

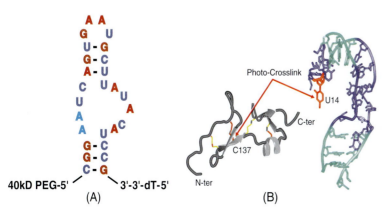

**Figure 37-1. A:** The sequence and predicted secondary structure of pegaptanib with 2'-O-methylated purines shown in red, 2'-fluorine-modified pyrimidines shown in blue, and unmodified ribonucleotides shown in black. The nucleotide modifications were made to increase bioavailability. The site of attachment of a 40 kDa polyethylene glycol (PEG) moiety is shown. **B:** The interaction between the 55 amino acid heparin-binding domain of VEGF$_{165}$ and pegaptanib. The free heparin-binding domain of VEGF$_{165}$ is shown in gray with disulfide bonds in yellow. Pegaptanib is shown in teal, with the interaction between cysteine-137 of VEGF$_{165}$ and uridine-14 of the aptamer indicated in red. (Reproduced from Ng EW, Shima DT, Calias P, et al. Pegaptanib, a targeted anti-VEGF aptamer for ocular vascular disease. *Nat Rev Drug Discov* 2006;5:123–132, with permission.).

Initial pharmacokinetic studies of pegaptanib performed in monkeys found mean half-lives after intravitreal and intravenous administration of 94 hours and 9.3 hours, respectively, suggesting that clearance from the eye is rate-limiting; pegaptanib remained fully active in VEGF-binding assays 28 days after intravitreal injection (34). A subsequent clinical study of pegaptanib pharmacokinetics following intravitreal injection evaluated 147 patients with neovascular AMD who received either 1 mg or 3 mg every 6 weeks for 54 weeks (35). Mean maximal plasma concentrations in the 1 mg group ranged from 20 to 24 ng/ml; pegaptanib remained above the level of detection (8 ng/ml) for 1 week with a plasma mean terminal half-life of 10 days. Repeat injections did not result in any plasma accumulations nor were there detectable serum antibodies to pegaptanib (35).

## Efficacy and Safety of Pegaptanib in the Treatment of Neovascular AMD

The efficacy and safety of pegaptanib for the treatment of neovascular AMD was established in the pivotal V.I.S.I.O.N. (VEGF Inhibition Study in Ocular Neovascularization) phase 2/3 trials (36). These two concurrent, multicenter, randomized, sham-controlled, dose-ranging trials enrolled subjects with all angiographic subtypes of neovascular AMD and lesions ≤12 disk areas. Subjects were randomized to receive intravitreal pegaptanib (0.3, 1, or 3 mg) or sham injections every 6 weeks for 54 weeks. For subjects with predominantly classic lesions, photodynamic therapy (PDT) with verteporfin was administered at the investigator's discretion. The primary endpoint was the proportion of subjects losing <15 letters of visual acuity (VA); secondary endpoints included proportions gaining ≥0, ≥5, ≥10, or ≥15 letters, proportions losing ≥30 letters, mean changes in VA, and proportions progressing to legal blindness (VA 20/200 or worse) in the study eye. Of 1208 subjects enrolled, 1186 (98%) received at least one treatment (mean: 8.5 of a possible 9 injections) and were evaluated at week 54.

## Efficacy of Pegaptanib

All pegaptanib doses proved superior to sham according to the primary endpoint. Compared to 55% of sham subjects, proportions losing <15 letters for the 0.3 mg, 1 mg, and 3 mg groups were 70% ($p < .001$), 71% ($p < .001$), and 65% ($p < .03$), respectively (36). As no further benefit accrued to higher doses, further analysis was restricted to the 0.3 mg dose. Pegaptanib was superior to sham for all secondary endpoints as well, including proportions losing ≥30 letters (10% vs. 22%, respectively; $p < .001$) or progressing to legal blindness (38% vs. 56%, respectively; $p < .001$), mean change in VA ($-7.95$ vs. $-15.05$ letters, respectively; $p < .05$), and gaining ≥0, ≥5, ≥10, or ≥15 letters ($p < .05$ for each comparison) as depicted in Figure 37-2 (37). Subgroup analysis revealed that the treatment benefit was conferred irrespective of baseline VA, lesion size, angiographic subtype, sex, age, race, or iris color.

In the second year of the study, 1053 subjects were rerandomized for an additional 48 weeks, with 943 (90%) being evaluated at week 102 (38). Subjects receiving pegaptanib in year 1 were randomized either to the same dose or to discontinue treatment, while sham subjects from year 1 were randomized either to continue or discontinue sham or to switch to one of the three drug doses. Compared to those receiving sham for 2 years (including those discontinuing sham), subjects continuing 0.3 mg pegaptanib for 2 years received significant clinical benefit according to the primary endpoint (45% losing <15 letters vs. 59%, respectively; $p < .05$). Subjects receiving 0.3 mg pegaptanib also had superior outcomes in terms of mean VA, likelihood of progressing to legal blindness, and proportions gaining vision compared to subjects receiving usual care. Moreover, a higher proportion of those continuing treatment for 2 years had a <15 letter loss compared to those who discontinued treatment in year 2 (38).

A further exploratory subgroup analysis of the V.I.S.I.O.N. data was also conducted to assess whether pegaptanib had benefits in treating earlier stage lesions (39). Two subgroups were defined as exemplifying early disease based on criteria such as baseline lesion size, lack of prior PDT, absence of classic lesions, and absence of lipid. For these two groups, proportions losing <15 letters were 76% and 80% among subjects receiving 0.3 mg pegaptanib compared with 50% and 57% for the sham group ($p = .03$ and $p = .05$, respectively); in addition, sham-treated subjects were approximately 10 times more likely to progress to legal blindness. Despite the relatively small size of the subgroups included in this analysis, these results suggest that earlier treatment of AMD with pegaptanib

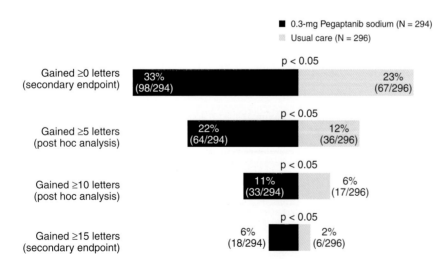

**Figure 37-2.** The proportion of subjects who maintained or gained visual acuity at 54 weeks in the V.I.S.I.O.N. (VEGF Inhibition Study in Ocular Neovascularization) trials. (Reproduced from Ng EW, Adamis AP. Targeting angiogenesis, the underlying disorder in neovascular age-related macular degeneration. *Can J Ophthalmol* 2005;40:352–368, with permission.)

may result in superior vision outcomes (39). Very similar conclusions recently were reported from a retrospective study of 90 subjects receiving pegaptanib as primary therapy, where the proportion of subjects losing <15 letters was 90% (40).

Data from the ranibizumab phase 3 trials in neovascular AMD strongly suggested that blockade of all VEGF-A isoforms is more effective than $VEGF_{165}$ blockade alone. Where pegaptanib showed good efficacy was in preclinical models manifesting retinal ischemia and neovascularization, where $VEGF_{165}$ was the predominant isoform. Thus, pegaptanib may show greater efficacy in DR and RVO. Conversely, retinal ischemia does not appear to be an important driver of choroidal neovascularization.

## Safety of Pegaptanib

The long-term safety of pegaptanib has been established in more than 4 years of follow-up in the V.I.S.I.O.N. trials (36,41–43). Injection-related events such as endophthalmitis, cataract, and retinal detachment were rare, and prolonged treatment with pegaptanib was not found to have detrimental effects on the retinal pigment epithelium (RPE) or on retinal neurons (44). In a separate dedicated systemic safety trial, 147 subjects with neovascular AMD received 1 mg or 3 mg pegaptanib every 6 weeks for 54 weeks (3 to 10 times the clinical dose), and no systemic safety signals were detected (35). There have been occasional postmarketing reports of RPE tears with pegaptanib (45). A recent review found that reports of RPE tears following the administration of all three anti-VEGF agents occurred primarily in eyes with existing RPE detachments (46). There also have been rare instances of anaphylactoid reactions with pegaptanib therapy (47).

Since inactivation of VEGF has the potential for interfering with a wide range of physiological processes, there are concerns about the potential systemic effects resulting from intravitreally administered anti-VEGF agents. An analysis of data from the ranibizumab trials, which for the first time demonstrated a mean increase in vision for AMD subjects in a trial of anti-VEGF therapy (48,49), found a significantly greater incidence of nonocular hemorrhage in those receiving ranibizumab (50). In addition, a preliminary analysis of the ongoing SAILOR trial has identified a significantly greater incidence of stroke (1.2% vs. 0.3%, respectively; $p = .02$) between the 0.3 mg and 0.5 mg doses, prompting a physician advisory letter from the manufacturer (51). A subsequent analysis of the final 1-year SAILOR data (52) revealed, though, that while the stroke incidence was still higher in the 0.5 mg group (1.2% vs. 0.7%), this difference was no longer statistically significant. It remains to be established whether there is any trade-off between the greater efficacy of agents that inactivate all VEGF isoforms, such as ranibizumab, and the safety in selectively targeting $VEGF_{165}$ with pegaptanib.

## INVESTIGATIONAL STUDIES INVOLVING PEGAPTANIB

Pegaptanib is being investigated as a treatment for ocular diseases other than neovascular AMD, including diabetic macular edema (DME) and proliferative diabetic retinopathy (PDR), as well as macular edema secondary to central retinal vein occlusion (CRVO) and branch retinal vein occlusion (BRVO). Pegaptanib also is being evaluated for use in alternate approaches, such as pegaptanib maintenance therapy following induction with a nonselective anti-VEGF agent or in combination with other treatments.

## DIABETIC MACULAR EDEMA AND PROLIFERATIVE DIABETIC RETINOPATHY

Photocoagulation until recently has been the standard of care for DME and PDR (9), with pars plana vitrectomy being used for those with serious complications of progressive retinopathy (53). However, the importance of VEGF in PDR pathogenesis was highlighted in a recent study in which high vitreous levels of VEGF were found to be a significant predictor of progression of PDR following vitreous surgery (54), supporting the investigation of pegaptanib for the treatment of ocular complications of diabetes.

The use of pegaptanib in the treatment of DME was evaluated in a phase 2, double-masked, multicenter, randomized controlled trial (55) in which 172 subjects with DME received intravitreal pegaptanib (0.3 mg, 1 mg, or 3 mg) or sham injections at baseline and at 6 and 12 weeks; additional injections, including the option of photocoagulation, were given through week 30 as needed, with final assessments at 36 weeks. Compared with sham, 0.3 mg pegaptanib resulted in significant clinical benefit according to all three prespecified endpoints, median VA (20/50 vs. 20/63, respectively; $p = .04$), mean change in retinal thickness on optical coherence tomography (OCT) ($-68$ $\mu$m vs. $+4$ $\mu$m, respectively; $p = .02$), and proportions requiring photocoagulation therapy (25% vs. 48%, respectively; $p = .04$) (55).

Among subjects in the DME trial (56), there were 16 evaluable subjects with retinal neovascularization at the study entry; eight of 13 (62%) eyes receiving pegaptanib had complete regression of neovascularization at 36 weeks as assessed by fundus photographs, absence of leakage on fluorescein angiography or both. Cessation of treatment led to recurrence of the neovascularization in three of these eyes. Figure 37-3 shows an example of a case where regression of retinal neovascularization at week 36 was followed by the reappearance of neovascularization at week 52. There was no regression in any of the three sham-treated eyes with baseline neovascularization or in the four fellow eyes with neovascularization of subjects treated with pegaptanib. Similarly, in a pilot study of patients with PDR given pegaptanib every 6 weeks or panretinal photocoagulation (PRP) for 30 weeks with a final assessment at 36 weeks, eight of eight (100%) pegaptanib-treated patients showed complete regression of neovascularization (56). In contrast, only three of eight (38%) eyes treated with PRP had regression, with one eye developing vitreous hemorrhage and four of eight (50%) continuing to have active neovascularization at week 36 (57). The presence of retinal cysts did not appear to affect responses to pegaptanib, with similar improvements in VA and in center point thickness at week 12 or week 36 in patients with or without retinal cysts (58).

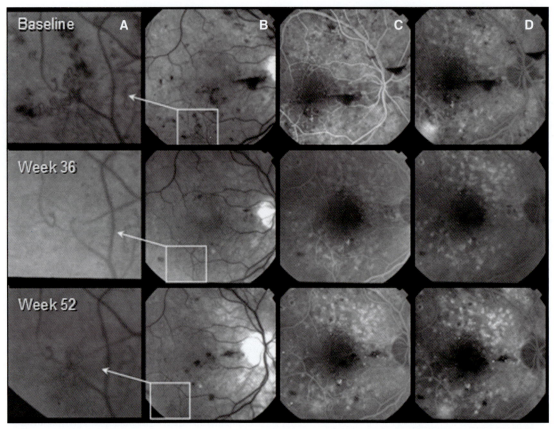

**Figure 37-3.** Subject 10. **First row:** Baseline visit shows a magnification of retinal neovascularization elsewhere (NVE) **(A)**, the location of the neovascularization along the inferotemporal arcade (red-free photograph) **(B)**, areas of capillary nonperfusion in the early-phase frame (fluorescein angiogram) **(C)**, and leakage from the NVE in the late-phase frame (fluorescein angiogram) **(D). Second row:** At week 36, after six periodic pegaptanib injections and 6 weeks since the most recent injection, regression of NVE is seen on red-free photographs **(A, B)**, lessening of apparent microaneurysms in the early phase **(C)**, and regression of leakage from NVE in the late phase **(D). Third row:** Fifty-two weeks after study entry and 22 weeks since the last pegaptanib injection, the reappearance of NVE is seen on red-free photographs **(A, B)** as well as the reappearance of leakage from NVE in the early- and late-phase frames **(C, D)**. (Reproduced from Adamis AP, Altaweel M, Bressler NM, et al. Changes in retinal neovascularization after pegaptanib (Macugen) therapy in diabetic individuals. *Ophthalmology* 2006;113:23–28, with permission.)

## MACULAR EDEMA SECONDARY TO CRVO AND BRVO

Various surgical procedures have been proposed for the treatment of RVO such as vitrectomy, internal limiting membrane peeling, and radial optic neurotomy, yet there is limited support for these approaches (59). Furthermore, while PRP is recommended for those with neovascularization related to ischemic CRVO, there is no proven approach for the treatment of macular edema associated with RVO (59). The use of pegaptanib has been evaluated for the treatment of CRVO-associated macular edema in a prospective, multicenter, double-masked, sham-controlled, phase 2 trial in which 98 subjects with CRVO of ≤6 months' duration were randomized to pegaptanib (0.3 mg or 1 mg) or sham injection given every 6 weeks for 24 weeks, with main endpoints assessed at week 30 and follow-up to 52 weeks (60,61). PRP was permitted for subjects developing ocular neovascularization. At 30 weeks, the mean VA change from baseline was +7.1, +9.9, and −3.2 letters for 0.3 mg, 1 mg, and sham, respectively ($p = .09$ for 0.3 mg and $p = .02$ for 1 mg vs. sham). Mean reductions in retinal thickness at the center point and at the center subfield from base-

line to week 30 were 95 μm and 112 μm lower, respectively, in the 0.3 mg pegaptanib group compared with sham ($p = .13$ and $p = .06$, respectively) (61). At 52 weeks, pegaptanib conferred significant clinical benefit over sham according to the proportion of subjects losing ≥15 letters (6% vs. 31%, $p = .05$) (62) and according to mean change in retinal thickness at the center subfield ($−291$ μm vs. $−168$ μm, respectively; $p = .05$) (59). In the BRVO study (63), an open-label trial, pegaptanib was administered every 6 weeks for up to 54 weeks at investigator discretion; interim results showed improvements from baseline in terms of mean VA and reductions in macular edema within 1 week.

## NONSELECTIVE INDUCTION AND PEGAPTANIB MAINTENANCE THERAPY

To address concerns regarding the safety of prolonged inhibition with nonselective VEGF antagonists, 20 patients with neovascular AMD were treated with an initial injection of 1.25 mg bevacizumab followed by 0.3 mg pegaptanib every 6 weeks for a total of nine injections. Four patients received a second bevacizumab booster injection (64). At 54 weeks, 19 patients (95%) had gained ≥1 line of VA and nine patients (45%) had gained ≥ 3 lines, with all patients having decreased retinal thickness. In a similar study involving 17 eyes with neovascular AMD that initially were treated with pegaptanib (mean: 7.8 injections) and boosted with bevacizumab (mean: 1.4 injections) or ranibizumab (mean: 0.9 injections), 47% of eyes gained ≥3 lines of VA and 76% gained ≥0 lines of VA over a mean follow-up of 12 months (65). Positive outcomes have also been reported from other studies involving similar protocols using induction with bevacizumab (66,67), ranibizumab (68), or either agent (69). The most extensive of these was an open-label study in which subjects received induction with either bevacizumab, ranibizumab, or both followed by pegaptanib maintenance injections every 6 weeks (69). In an interim analysis of the first 211 subjects completing a 36-week follow-up, this regimen resulted in a mean VA gain of 12.2 letters; VA gains of ≥0 and ≥3 lines occurred in 75% and 43% of subjects, respectively, and 90% of subjects lost <3 lines of VA. No booster treatment was given to 59% of subjects while 60% of those needing booster injections required only one treatment. Safety was excellent with no ocular or systemic signals noted (69).

## CONCLUSIONS

The development and success of anti-VEGF therapies has validated the concept of targeting the underlying molecular mechanisms of ocular neovascular diseases while the availability of several anti-VEGF agents further increases the flexibility of ophthalmologists in developing treatment strategies. Pegaptanib has shown favorable efficacy in neovascular AMD and has had promising results in treating other ocular neovascular diseases as well. In addition, protocols using induction with a nonselective agent followed by pegaptanib maintenance seek to take advantage of the proven long-term safety profile of pegaptanib.

## References

1. Ferrara N. Vascular endothelial growth factor: basic science and clinical progress. *Endocr Rev* 2004;25:581–611.
2. Senger DR, Connolly DT, Van de Water L, et al. Purification and NH2-terminal amino acid sequence of guinea pig tumor-secreted vascular permeability factor. *Cancer Res* 1990;50:1774–1778.
3. Aiello LP, Avery RL, Arrigg PG, et al. Vascular endothelial growth factor in ocular fluid of patients with diabetic retinopathy and other retinal disorders. *N Engl J Med* 1994;331:1480–1487.
4. Adamis AP, Miller JW, Bernal MT, et al. Increased vascular endothelial growth factor levels in the vitreous of eyes with proliferative diabetic retinopathy. *Am J Ophthalmol* 1994;118:445–450.
5. Lashkari K, Hirose T, Yazdany J, et al. Vascular endothelial growth factor and hepatocyte growth factor levels are differentially elevated in patients with advanced retinopathy of prematurity. *Am J Pathol* 2000;156:1337–1344.
6. Tripathi RC, Li J, Tripathi BJ, et al. Increased level of vascular endothelial growth factor in aqueous humor of patients with neovascular glaucoma. *Ophthalmology* 1998;105:232–237.
7. Ambati J, Ambati BK, Yoo SH, et al. Age-related macular degeneration: etiology, pathogenesis, and therapeutic strategies. *Surv Ophthalmol* 2003;48:257–293.
8. Ng EW, Adamis AP. Anti-VEGF aptamer (pegaptanib) therapy for ocular vascular diseases. *Ann N Y Acad Sci* 2006;1082:151–171.
9. Starita C, Patel M, Katz B, et al. Vascular endothelial growth factor and the potential therapeutic use of pegaptanib (Macugen) in diabetic retinopathy. *Dev Ophthalmol* 2007;39:122–148.
10. Robinson CJ, Stringer SE. The splice variants of vascular endothelial growth factor (VEGF) and their receptors. *J Cell Sci* 2001;114:853–865.
11. Kim I, Ryan AM, Rohan R, et al. Constitutive expression of VEGF, VEGFR-1, and VEGFR-2 in normal eyes. *Invest Ophthalmol Vis Sci* 1999;40:2115–2121.
12. Ishida S, Usui T, Yamashiro K, et al. VEGF164-mediated inflammation is required for pathological, but not physiological, ischemia-induced retinal neovascularization. *J Exp Med* 2003;198:483–489.
13. Usui T, Ishida S, Yamashiro K, et al. VEGF164(165) as the pathological isoform: differential leukocyte and endothelial responses through VEGFR1 and VEGFR2. *Invest Ophthalmol Vis Sci* 2004;45:368–374.
14. Tsutsumi C, Sonoda KH, Egashira K, et al. The critical role of ocular-infiltrating macrophages in the development of choroidal neovascularization. *J Leukoc Biol* 2003;74:25–32.
15. Espinosa-Heidmann DG, Suner IJ, Hernandez EP, et al. Macrophage depletion diminishes lesion size and severity in experimental choroidal neovascularization. *Invest Ophthalmol Vis Sci* 2003;44:3586–3592.
16. Sakurai E, Anand A, Ambati BK, et al. Macrophage depletion inhibits experimental choroidal neovascularization. *Invest Ophthalmol Vis Sci* 2003;44:3578–3585.
17. Ishida S, Usui T, Yamashiro K, et al. VEGF164 is proinflammatory in the diabetic retina. *Invest Ophthalmol Vis Sci* 2003;44:2155–2162.
18. Nishijima K, Ng YS, Zhong L, et al. Vascular endothelial growth factor-A is a survival factor for retinal neurons and a critical neuroprotectant during the adaptive response to ischemic injury. *Am J Pathol* 2007;171:53–67.
19. Blaauwgeers HG, Holtkamp GM, Rutten H, et al. Polarized vascular endothelial growth factor secretion by human retinal pigment epithelium and localization of vascular endothelial growth factor receptors on the inner choriocapillaris. Evidence for a trophic paracrine relation. *Am J Pathol* 1999;155:421–428.
20. Kamba T, McDonald DM. Mechanisms of adverse effects of anti-VEGF therapy for cancer. *Br J Cancer* 2007;96:1788–1795.
21. Verheul HM, Pinedo HM. Possible molecular mechanisms involved in the toxicity of angiogenesis inhibition. *Nat Rev Cancer* 2007;7:475–485.
22. van Wijngaarden P, Coster DJ, Williams KA. Inhibitors of ocular neovascularization: promises and potential problems. *JAMA* 2005;293:1509–1513.
23. Avery RL, Pearlman J, Pieramici DJ, et al. Intravitreal bevacizumab (Avastin) in the treatment of proliferative diabetic retinopathy. *Ophthalmology* 2006;113:1695–1705.
24. Kiernan DF, Hariprasad SM, Praley A, et al. Injected anti-VEGF drugs exert an effect on visual acuity in the fellow eye. *Invest Ophthalmol Vis Sci* 2007;48:E-Abstract 4938.
25. Jellinek D, Green LS, Bell C, et al. Inhibition of receptor binding by high-affinity RNA ligands to vascular endothelial growth factor. *Biochemistry* 1994;33:10450–10456.
26. Green LS, Jellinek D, Bell C, et al. Nuclease-resistant nucleic acid ligands to vascular permeability factor/vascular endothelial growth factor. *Chem Biol* 1995;2:683–695.
27. Ruckman J, Green LS, Beeson J, et al. 2'-Fluoropyrimidine RNA-based aptamers to the 165-amino acid form of vascular endothelial growth factor (VEGF165). Inhibition of receptor binding and VEGF-induced vascular permeability through interactions requiring the exon 7-encoded domain. *J Biol Chem* 1998;273:20556–20567.
28. Ellington AD, Szostak JW. In vitro selection of RNA molecules that bind specific ligands. *Nature* 1990;346:818–822.
29. Tuerk C, Gold L. Systematic evolution of ligands by exponential enrichment: RNA ligands to bacteriophage T4 DNA polymerase. *Science* 1990;249:505–510.
30. Ng EW, Shima DT, Calias P, et al. Pegaptanib, a targeted anti-VEGF aptamer for ocular vascular disease. *Nat Rev Drug Discov* 2006;5:123–132.
31. Bell C, Lynam E, Landfair DJ, et al. Oligonucleotide NX1838 inhibits VEGF165-mediated cellular responses in vitro. *In Vitro Cell Dev Biol Anim* 1999;35:533–542.
32. Eyetech Study Group. Preclinical and phase 1. A clinical evaluation of an anti-VEGF pegylated aptamer (EYE001) for the treatment of exudative age-related macular degeneration. *Retina* 2002;22:143–152.
33. Lee JH, Canny MD, De Erkenez A, et al. A therapeutic aptamer inhibits angiogenesis by specifically targeting the heparin binding domain of VEGF165. *Proc Natl Acad Sci USA* 2005;102:18902–18907.
34. Drolet DW, Nelson J, Tucker CE, et al. Pharmacokinetics and safety of an anti-vascular endothelial growth factor aptamer (NX1838) following injection into the vitreous humor of rhesus monkeys. *Pharm Res* 2000;17:1503–1510.
35. Apte RS, Modi M, Masonson H, et al. Pegaptanib 1-year systemic safety results from a safety-pharmacokinetic trial in patients with neovascular age-related macular degeneration. *Ophthalmology* 2007;114:1702–1712.
36. Gragoudas ES, Adamis AP, Cunningham ET Jr, et al. Pegaptanib for neovascular age-related macular degeneration. *N Engl J Med* 2004;351:2805–2816.

37. Ng EW, Adamis AP. Targeting angiogenesis, the underlying disorder in neovascular age-related macular degeneration. *Can J Ophthalmol* 2005;40:352–368.

38. Chakravarthy U, Adamis AP, Cunningham ET Jr, et al. Year 2 efficacy results of 2 randomized controlled clinical trials of pegaptanib for neovascular age-related macular degeneration. *Ophthalmology* 2006;113:1508–1521.

39. Gonzales CR. Enhanced efficacy associated with early treatment of neovascular age-related macular degeneration with pegaptanib sodium: an exploratory analysis. *Retina* 2005;25:815–827.

40. Quiram PA, Hassan TS, Williams GA. Treatment of naive lesions in neovascular age-related macular degeneration with pegaptanib. *Retina* 2007;27:851856.

41. D'Amico DJ, Masonson HN, Patel M, et al. Pegaptanib sodium for neovascular age-related macular degeneration: two-year safety results of the two prospective, multicenter, controlled clinical trials. *Ophthalmology* 2006;113:992–1001.

42. Singerman LJ, Masonson H, Patel M, et al. Pegaptanib sodium for neovascular age-related macular degeneration: third-year safety results of the V.I.S.I.O.N. trial [Epub ahead of print, 2008]. *Br J Ophthalmol*, doi:10.1136/bjo.2007.132597.

43. Marcus D, VEGF Inhibition Study in Ocular Neovascularization Clinical Trial Group. Four-year safety of pegaptanib sodium in neovascular age-related macular degeneration (AMD): Results of the V.I.S.I.O.N. trial. *Invest Ophthalmol Vis Sci* 2008;49:E-Abstract 5069.

44. Altaweel MM, VEGF Inhibition Study in Ocular Neovascularization Clinical Trial Group (V.I.S.I.O.N.) Study Group. Effects of intravitreal injection of pegaptanib on the retinal pigment epithelium and optic nerve. *Invest Ophthalmol Vis Sci* 2007;48:E-Abstract 3369.

45. Chang LK, Flaxel CJ, Lauer AK, et al. RPE tears after pegaptanib treatment in age-related macular degeneration. *Retina* 2007;27:857–863.

46. Chang LK, Sarraf D. Tears of the retinal pigment epithelium: an old problem in a new era. *Retina* 2007;27:523–534.

47. Steffensmeier AC, Azar AE, Fuller JJ, et al. Vitreous injections of pegaptanib sodium triggering allergic reactions. *Am J Ophthalmol* 2007;143:512–513.

48. Brown DM, Kaiser PK, Michels M, et al. Ranibizumab versus verteporfin for neovascular age-related macular degeneration. *N Engl J Med* 2006;355:1432–1444.

49. Rosenfeld PJ, Brown DM, Heier JS, et al. Ranibizumab for neovascular age-related macular degeneration. *N Engl J Med* 2006;355:1419–1431.

50. Gillies MC, Wong TY. Ranibizumab for neovascular age-related macular degeneration. *N Engl J Med* 2007;356:748–749; author reply 749–750.

51. Genentech. Dear Health Care Provider. http://www.gene.com/gene/products/information/pdf/healthcare-provider-letter.pdf. Accessed July, 2008.

52. Boyer DS. SAILOR safety outcomes at one year: Does ranibizumab increase the risk of thromboembolic events? Paper presented at: The Bascom Palmer Eye Institute Angiogenesis, Exudation and Degeneration Meeting; February 23, 2008; Key Biscayne, Fla.

53. Smiddy WE, Flynn HW Jr. Vitrectomy in the management of diabetic retinopathy. *Surv Ophthalmol* 1999;43:491–507.

54. Funatsu H, Yamashita H, Mimura T, et al. Risk evaluation of outcome of vitreous surgery based on vitreous levels of cytokines. *Eye* 2007;21:377–382.

55. Cunningham ET Jr, Adamis AP, Altaweel M, et al. A phase II randomized double-masked trial of pegaptanib, an anti-vascular endothelial growth factor aptamer, for diabetic macular edema. *Ophthalmology* 2005;112:1747–1757.

56. Adamis AP, Altaweel M, Bressler NM, et al. Changes in retinal neovascularization after pegaptanib (Macugen) therapy in diabetic individuals. *Ophthalmology* 2006;113:23–28.

57. Gonzalez VH, Vann VR, Banda GP, . Pegaptanib sodium (Macugen®) versus panretinal photocoagulation (PRP) for the regression of proliferative diabetic retinopathy. *Invest Ophthalmol Vis Sci* 2007;48:E-Abstract 4030.

58. Goldbaum M, Csaky KG. Impact of retinal cysts on outcomes in patients with diabetic macular edema treated with pegaptanib. *Invest Ophthalmol Vis Sci* 2008;49:E-Abstract 3465.

59. Mohamed Q, McIntosh RL, Saw SM, et al. Interventions for central retinal vein occlusion: an evidence-based systematic review. *Ophthalmology* 2007;114:507–519, 524.

60. Patel SS, Macugen in CRVO Study Group. Pegaptanib sodium for the treatment of macular edema following central retinal vein occlusion (CRVO): anatomical outcomes. *Invest Ophthalmol Vis Sci* 2007;48:E-Abstract 311.

61. Wells JA III, Pegaptanib in Central Retinal Vein Occlusion Study Group. Pegaptanib sodium for treatment of macular edema secondary to central retinal vein occlusion (CRVO). *Invest Ophthalmol Vis Sci* 2006;47:E-Abstract 4279.

62. Wells JA III, Wroblewski JJ, Macugen in CRVO Study Group. Pegaptanib sodium for the treatment of macular edema following central retinal vein occlusion (CRVO): functional outcomes. *Invest Ophthalmol Vis Sci* 2007;48:E-Abstract 1544.

63. Wroblewski JJ, Wells JA, Gonzales W, et al. Open label pegaptanib for the treatment of macular edema secondary to branch retinal vein occlusion (BRVO). *Invest Ophthalmol Vis Sci* 2007;48:E-Abstract 310.

64. Hughes MS, Sang DN. Safety and efficacy of intravitreal bevacizumab followed by pegaptanib maintenance as a treatment regimen for age-related macular degeneration. *Ophthalmic Surg Lasers Imaging* 2006;37:446–454.

65. Farah SE. Treatment of neovascular age-related macular degeneration with pegaptanib and boosting with bevacizumab or ranibizumab as needed. *Ophthalmic Surg Lasers Imaging* 2008;39:294–298.

66. Barnes CH. Efficacy and safety of intravitreal (IVT) bevacizumab induction and pegaptanib sodium maintenance in patients with neovascular age-related macular degeneration (NV-AMD). *Invest Ophthalmol Vis Sci* 2007;48:E-Abstract 3371.

67. Offermann I, Hoer M, Tan M, et al. Pegaptanib-enhancement of intravitreal bevacizumab therapy for choroidal neovascularization. *Invest Ophthalmol Vis Sci* 2007;48:E-Abstract 4546.

68. Sang DN, Hughes MS, Chin C. Induction/maintenance therapy with ranibizumab (Lucentis) followed by pegaptanib (Macugen) intravitreal injections in the treatment of age-related macular degeneration. *Invest Ophthalmol Vis Sci* 2007;48:E-Abstract 1795.

69. Friberg TR, LEVEL Study Group. Evaluation of efficacy and safety in maintaining visual acuity with sequential treatment of neovascular AMD: the LEVEL Study. *Invest Ophthalmol Vis Sci* 2007;48:E-Abstract 4568.

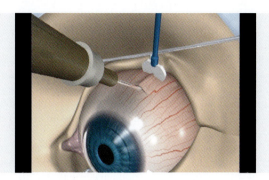

# Periocular Steroids

Beatriz S. Takahashi ■ Jason S. Slakter ■ Howard F. Fine

# INTRODUCTION

Periocular steroids were first used clinically in the 1950s. Delivering the medication locally maximizes the effect of the drug while minimizing systemic side effects. There are different ways of delivering periocular corticosteroids (1):

- Subconjunctival injection: the drug is introduced between the conjunctiva and Tenon's capsule. The procedure is simple and safe to perform, but less of the drug is absorbed.
- Anterior sub-Tenon's injection: the drug is injected between Tenon's capsule and the sclera. This can be performed in any quadrant; the drug is visible after delivery.
- Posterior sub-Tenon's injection: the drug is injected in a similar fashion to an anterior sub-Tenon's injection, with the patient looking away from the quadrant chosen to allow more posterior access. The drug typically cannot be visualized, and the minor risk of accidental globe perforation increases slightly.
- Retrobulbar injection: a standard retrobulbar injection with a shorter needle is performed.

# TRIAMCINOLONE ACETONIDE

Triamcinolone acetonide (TA), or $9\alpha$-fluoro-$16\alpha$-hydroxyprednisolone, is an intermediate-acting corticosteroid. It is supplied as a crystalline suspension (Bristol-Myers Squibb, Princeton, NJ), which allows it to dissolve in and around the eye in a sustained-release fashion. The intravitreal use of triamcinolone is a well-established procedure (2–4).

As with other corticosteroids, the use of periocular TA has also been associated with local sequelae including sterile conjunctival ulceration (5), intraocular pressure rise and cataracts (6,7), central serous chorioretinopathy (8), as well as ptosis and orbital fat prolapsed (9–11), cutaneous hypopigmentation (12) and periocular abscess (13). The location of the drug and its proximity to the macular area is important for the outcome. When sub-Tenon's injection is performed, a superiotemporal procedure is typically preferred (14).

Cytotoxicity *in vitro* has been reported (15,16). The preservation vehicle used for triamcinolone (0.99% benzyl alcohol, 0.75% carboxymethylcellulose, 0.04% polysorbate 80) has also been studied for toxicity to human retinal pigment epithelium cells (ARPE19). The viability of the cells was the greatest in preservative free formulations, followed by the vehicle alone and then by the trade formulation (17). The vehicle used with TA has also been showed to have toxicity to the retina and to the lens after intravitreal injection in an animal model (18).

TA was shown to reduce the expression of ICAM-1 when modulated by phorbol 12-myristate 13-acetate in a human bladder carcinoma-derived epithelial cell line *in vitro* (19) as well as to inhibit choroidal endothelial cells migration and permeability in a dose dependant manner (20). Another experiment with oxygen-induced retinopathy in rats showed decreased vascular leakage with 20 mg/ml triamcinolone (21), a smaller area of neovascularization, a lower concentration of vascular endothelial growth factor (VEGF) and blockage of

upregulation of proinflammatory factors such as TNF$\alpha$, IL-1$\beta$, ICAM-1, p-p38 MAPK, p-JNK MAPK, p-ERK MAPK, p-IkB, NFkB, HIF-$\alpha$ (22). Neovascularization has a dose dependant response to TA. Other experiments with triamcinolone showed less leukocyte accumulation in ischemia induced eyes (23), smaller retinal endothelial cell nuclei counts compared to controls in a rat model of retinopathy of prematurity (24), inhibition of corneal neovascular response after subconjunctival injection of the corticosteroid (25), degenerative changes on fibroblasts, and more macrophages within as well as adjacent to an area where the drug was injected subconjunctivally before glaucoma surgery (26).

In an experimental study with laser treated rats, 2 mg or 0.5 mg of posterior sub-Tenon's triamcinolone was administered (27). Animals treated with 2 mg of triamcinolone showed statistically significantly lower leakage than 0.5 mg treated and controls. When treatment was given, the choroidal neovascularization (CNV) membranes were thinner than the control eyes. Similar results were observed in laser treated models (28).

Periocular triamcinolone has been successfully used to treat macular edema secondary to branch vein occlusion associated with retinal arteriovenous malformation (29). Changes in the central retinal thickness were also observed in patients treated for refractory cystoid macular edema for diabetic retinopathy with retrobulbar triamcinolone. In those patients, intraocular pressure elevation was observed, but all cases could be controlled with topical glaucoma medications (30).

A prospective study evaluating the subconjunctival injection of triamcinolone demonstrated the successful treatment of 10 patients with recalcitrant anterior scleritis; six of those patients were able to discontinue systemic therapy. The symptoms of pain, redness, and scleral inflammation resolved in all but one patient. One patient developed high intraocular pressure which was stabilized with topical medication and another had subconjunctival hemorrhage (31). Nonnecrotizing anterior scleritis could also be controlled with subconjunctival triamcinolone (32,33).

In a clinical trial comparing posterior sub-Tenon's injection of triamcinolone and orbital floor methylprednisolone for noninfectious posterior uveitis with cystoid macular edema and/or vitritis, improvement rates were not statistically different between groups. Both groups enjoyed a statistically significant improvement in visual acuity at 6 weeks and at 3 months. Of 30 eyes that received sub-Tenon triamcinolone, 2 patients in the triamcinolone group had lid ptosis and another 2 developed raised intraocular pressure (34–38).

Posterior sub-Tenon's triamcinolone was used in a prospective case control study to evaluate its effects before panretinal photocoagulation in diabetic retinopathy (34). Eyes treated with triamcinolone had less increase in their retinal thickness and better final visual acuity than eyes not treated with the steroids one week before the laser procedure. Pretreatment of diabetic macular edema with sub-Tenon's triamcinolone before grid pattern laser photocoagulation showed that foveal thickness at 24 weeks was thinner in treated patients than in controls, but no difference was observed in vision (35). Another randomized study showed no advantage on ocular coherence tomagraphy (OCT) thickness or final visual acuity in patients treated with peribulbar TA with and

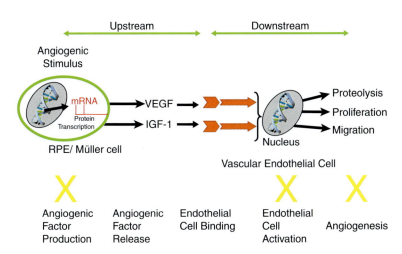

**Figure 38-1.** Anecortave acetate inhibits the angiogenic proteolytic cascade by inhibiting the expression of urokinase plasminogen activator and matrix metalloproteinases and up-regulating the expression of the urokinase plasminogen activator inhibitor plasminogen activator inhibitor-1. In addition, anecortave acetate inhibits vascular endothelial cell proliferation and migration. IGF, insulin-like growth factor; VEGF, vascular endothelial growth factor. (Adapted from Slakter JS. Anecortave acetate for treating or preventing choroidal neovascularization. *Ophthalmol Clin North Am* 2006;19(3):373–380.)

without focal laser; all randomized groups showed reduction in retinal thickening and no benefit on visual acuity (36).

Intravitreal triamcinolone (IVTA) was compared to posterior sub-Tenon's triamcinolone in a study for diffuse diabetic macular edema by Cardillo. Central macular thickness of eyes treated with IVTA was statistically thinner than eyes treated with posterior sub-Tenon's triamcinolone at 1 month and 3 months, but the difference not confirmed at 6 months. For visual acuity, both treatments raised the acuity, but IVTA was statistically better at 3 months, again not statistically significant at 6 months. None of the study eyes, previously treated with topical 1% prednisolone, showed increase in intraocular pressure (IOP) (39). Another randomized clinical trial for refractory diabetic macular edema showed statistically significant results only in eyes treated with intravitreal triamcinolone both for thickness of the retina and visual acuity (40). Eyes treated with sub-Tenon's triamcinolone for diabetic macular edema that did not respond to this approach can still respond when the same corticosteroid is injected intravitreal (41). Similar responses for visual acuity and retinal thickness were observed in groups treated with sub-Tenon's and with intravitreal injections (42).

A comparison between sub-Tenon's injection of TA and prednisolone acetate 1% eye drops for controlling inflammation after vitrectomy was reported and no differences in symptoms nor in observable inflammation was seen (37). A case of benign lymphoid hyperplasia was successfully treated with 20 mg/0.5 ml subconjunctival injection of triamcinolone close to a salmon patch area (43).

## ANECORTAVE ACETATE

Anecortave acetate 15 mg (RETAANE®; Alcon, Forth Worth, TX, USA) is an angiostatic cortisone that inhibits pathologic neovascularization at multiple steps within the angiogenic cascade, and does not show typical ocular glucocorticoid-induced side-effects such as cataract formation and increased intraocular pressure. Anecortave acetate can suppress (a) the expression of some extracellular proteinases (44), (b) endothelial cell proliferation and differentiation, and (c) the synthesis of proangiogenic growth factors and their receptors (Fig. 38-1).

Preclinical efficacy pharmacology studies showed that anecortave acetate significantly inhibited corneal, retinal, and choroidal neovascularization as well as tumor growth in various species (44,45–51). Moreover, it inhibited the growth of the pathologic newly forming vessels, and did not affect preexisting normal vessels. In order to maintain its angiostatic activity and eliminate typical untoward glucocorticoid effects, a hydroxyl group in cortisol was replaced by a double bond at the C9–11 position, and a 21-acetate was added to enhance drug penetration and prolong duration of the depot (Fig. 38-2) (45). Anecortave acetate has one major active metabolite, anecortave desacetate (AL-4940); this metabolite is formed by the deacetylation of the parent molecule. Because anecortave desacetate binds only moderately to plasma proteins and does not inhibit human hepatic cytochrome P-450 isozymes, it is unlikely to participate in drug-drug interactions (46). Genotoxicity, carcinogenicity, and reproductive toxicity studies *in vivo* revealed no significant ocular or systemic toxicities (47). During clinical trials, the drug was safe and well tolerated both as a primary therapy and as adjunctive therapy to VISUDYNE® photodynamic therapy (PDT) (48).

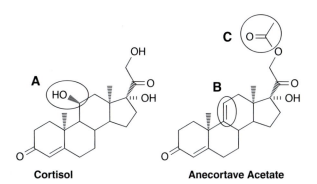

**Figure 38-2.** Three modifications made to cortisol to generate anecortave acetate. The 11B-hydroxyl group, which is essential for glucocorticoid activity, was removed from cortisol. A double bond between C9 and C11 was added to prevent in vivo enzymatic rehydroxylation at C11, and acetate group was added at C21 to enhance ocular penetration and provide ideal physical-chemical properties for administration of a slow-release depot. (Adapted from Slakter JS. Anecortave acetate for treating or preventing choroidal neovascularization. *Ophthalmol Clin North Am* 2006; 19(3):373–380.)

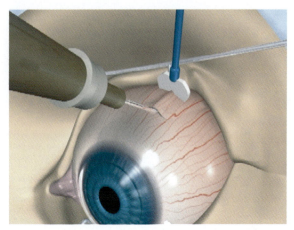

**Figure 38-3.** Anecortave acetate is delivered as a periocular juxtascleral depot using a specially designed blunt-tipped cannula to deliver the drug onto the outer surface over the macula. (Adapted from Slakter JS. Anecortave acetate for treating or preventing choroidal neovascularization. *Ophthalmol Clin North Am* 2006;19(3):373–380.)

Anecortave acetate 15 mg is delivered as a posterior juxtascleral depot (PJD) to the superotemporal quadrant of the eye. During the PJD administration procedure, the patient is placed in a supine or reclined chair. After topical anesthesia and administration of ophthalmic 5% povidone-iodine, a 1 to 1.5 mm incision is made through the conjunctiva and Tenon's capsule. A specially designed blunt-tipped cannula is used to deliver the drug on to the bare sclera overlying the macular area, and a counter pressure device is used to minimize reflux of the suspension (Fig. 38-3) (52). This unique delivery system helps to avoid the risks of intraocular damage, endophthalmitis, and retinal detachment associated with intraocular delivery procedures. Although there is a theoretical risk of damaging the optic nerve or posterior ciliary arteries with PJD approach, no cases of such complications have been reported.

As of October 2007, following more than 12,500 PJD administrations of Anecortave acetate or vehicle, six clinically relevant procedure-related adverse events have been reported. One of the six events was a globe perforation in a patient receiving their seventh PJD administration. The treating physician suspected that the perforation may have been related to the presence of scar tissue resulting from previous PJD administration procedures. Based upon a review of these cases, the Independent Safety Committee overseeing the anecortave acetate studies recommended that all ongoing anecortave acetate PJD clinical studies continue without changes to the clinical protocols or PJD procedure. Overall, these events occurred at an incidence of less than 0.05% and are not unexpected, since conjunctival incisions or periocular injections have been associated clinically with such outcomes.

The correct location of the drug is essential for anecortave acetate's efficacy as it affects the bioavailability in the retina and choroid. A study performed in rabbits using both magnetic resonance imaging and ultrasonography showed that the correct location of the drug behind the posterior pole was achieved using the special cannula, where the depot remained up to 4 weeks after the procedure (48,53,54). The same optimum location in humans was not achieved if a corticosteroid

was injected without the specialized cannula (14). In Cynomolgus monkeys, amounts of anecortave acetate decrease early after PJD administration, but the drug can still be found in substantial concentrations within the sclera supporting a retreatment interval of 6 months (46). In an Alcon-sponsored study comparing different doses of anecortave acetate suspension versus vehicle in patients with exudative AMD, patients had their blood analyzed for drug levels following the PJD administration procedure. The highest detectable concentrations of anecortave desacetate in the blood were observed at 1 to 2 days postprocedure but decreased below detectable levels within 2 weeks of the injection; based on these observations, this drug is not expected to accumulate in plasma.

In the same Alcon-sponsored study described above, anecortave acetate 15 mg was statistically superior to vehicle in a monotherapy trial involving patients with exudative AMD. The majority of the CNV lesions in this study were predominantly classic lesions and patients received drug or vehicle every 6 months for 24 months (55,56). When compared to 3 mg and 30 mg, anecortave acetate 15 mg was statistically superior to placebo and numerically superior to the other two dosages in maintaining vision at 12 and 24 months. At 12 months, anecortave acetate 15 mg was statistically superior to placebo comparing mean change in visual acuity from baseline, stabilization of visual acuity and prevention of severe vision loss. Subgroup analysis of predominantly classic lesions showed the same pattern (57). A positive result was also observed in a combination therapy trial with PDT. More eyes treated with both PDT and anecortave acetate 15 mg or 30 mg maintained vision at 6 months. Seventy-eight percent of the eyes treated with the combination did not demonstrate severe vision loss compared to 68% of eyes receiving PDT alone; however, this result was not statistically significant (48). During a large comparison study of anecortave acetate 15 mg versus PDT, anecortave acetate 15 mg was clinically equivalent to PDT for reducing the risk of moderate loss of vision in patients with predominantly classic CNV (58); however, the results failed to meet the primary endpoint of statistical noninferiority. In these studies, reflux of the drug during or immediately after administration of the drug and treatments administered outside of the defined treatment window were identified as potentially controllable factors associated with lower efficacy (56). Anecortave acetate 15 mg remains to be approved by the Food and Drug Administration (FDA) for the treatment of exudative age-related macular degeneration (AMD) in the United States, but it has obtained regulatory approval for use in Australia, South Africa, Venezuela, and Mexico.

The Anecortave Acetate Risk Reduction Trial (AART) is a ground-breaking study evaluating the safety and efficacy of anecortave acetate for reducing the risk of progression to exudative AMD in at risk patients with nonexudative disease. The trial began in early 2004, and enrolment finished in January 2006 (58). In order to enter this 4-year study, patients were required to have a diagnosis of exudative AMD in the nonstudy eye and 5 or more intermediate or large soft drusen, confluent drusen within 3000 μm of the fovea and hyperpigmentation in the study eye. This trial will provide data to determine the value of anecortave acetate in reducing the risk of CNV development and its long-term effect on vision in this patient population (59).

# CONCLUSIONS

Based on the complex pathophysiology of most retinal diseases, the most effective treatment paradigms may require a variety of pharmacologic agents used in combination to target different steps along the angiogenic and/or inflammatory signalling pathways. Both traditional steroids like triamcinolone as well as modified corticosteroids, such as anecortave acetate, have potential to play a role in managing these diseases. Even in the treatment of exudative AMD, where intravitreal anti-VEGF therapies, such as LUCENTIS® and off-label AVASTIN® (Genentech), have provided a substantial step forward in therapeutic benefit and have become the current standard of care, the majority of patients do not obtain significant visual improvement over a course of two years of therapy. Consequently, opportunities remain for providing increased patient benefit in this and other visually devastating retinal diseases.

## References

1. Nozik RA. Periocular injection of steroids. *Trans Am Acad Ophthalmol Otolaryngol* 1972;76(3):695–705.
2. Spaide RF, Sorenson J, Maranan L. Combined photodynamic therapy with verteporfin and intravitreal triamcinolone acetonide for choroidal neovascularization. *Ophthalmology* 2003;110(8):1517–1525.
3. Jonas JB, Kreissig I, Hugger P, et al. Intravitreal triamcinolone acetonide for exudative age-related macular degeneration. *Br J Ophthalmol* 2003;87:462–468.
4. Ranson NT, Danis RP, Ciulla TA, et al. Intravitreal triamcinolone in subfoveal recurrence of choroidal neovascularization after laser treatment in macular degeneration. *Br J Ophthalmol* 2002;86:527–529.
5. Agrawal S, Agrawal J, Agrawal TP. Conjunctival ulceration following triamcinolone injection. *Am J Ophthalmol* 2003;136(3):539–540.
6. Iwao K, Inatani M, Takahiro K, et al. Frequency and risk factors for intraocular pressure elevation after posterior sub-tenon capsule triamcinolone acetonide injection. *J Glaucoma* 2007;16(2):251–256.
7. Jonas JB, Kreissig I, Degenring R. Intraocular pressure after intravitreal injection of triamcinolone acetonide. *Br J Ophthalmol* 2003;87:24–27.
8. Baumal CR, Martidis A, Truong SN. Central Serous Chorioretinopathy associated with periocular corticosteroid injection treatment for HLA-B27 associated iritis. *Arch Ophthalmol* 2004;122:926–928.
9. Dal Canto AJ, Downs-Kelly E, Perry JD. Ptosis and orbital fat prolapsed after posterior sub-Tenon's capsule triamcinolone injection. *Ophthalmology* 2005;112(6):1092–1097.
10. Smith JR, George RK, Rosenbaum JT. Lower eyelid herniation of orbital fat may complicate periocular corticosteroid injection. *Am J Ophthalmol* 2002;133(6):845–847.
11. Song A, Carter KD, Nerard JA, et al. Steroid-induced ptosis: case studies and histopathologic analysis [Epub ahead of print, 2007]. *Eye*; doi:10.1038/sj.eye.6702667.
12. Gallardo MJ, Johnson DA. Cutaneous hypopigmentation following a posterior sub-tenon triamcinolone injection. *Am J Ophthalmol* 2004;137(4):779–780.
13. Oh IK, Baek S, Huh K, et al. Periocular abscess caused by Pseudallescheria boydii after a posterior subtenon injection of triamcinolone acetonide. *Graefe's Arch Clin Exp Ophthalmol* 2007;245:164–166.
14. Freeman WR, Green RL, Smith RE. Echographic localization of corticosteroids after periocular injection. *Am J Ophthalmol* 1987;103(3 Pt 1):281–288.
15. Yeung CY, Chan KP, Chiang SWY, et al. The toxic and stress responses of cultured human retinal pigment epithelium (ARPE19) and human glial cells (SVG) in the presence of triamcinolone. *Invest Ophthalmol Vis Sci* 2003;44(12):5293–5300.
16. Narayanan R, Mungcal JK, Kenney MC, et al. Toxicity of triamcinolone acetonide on retinal neurosensory and pigment epithelial cells. *Invest Ophthal Vis Sci* 2006;47(2):722–728.
17. Shaikh S, Ho S, Engelmann LA, et al. Cell viability effects of triamcinolone acetonide and preservative vehicle formulations. *Br J Ophthalmol* 2006;90:233–236.
18. Kai W, Yanrong J, Xiaoxin L. Vehicle of triamcinolone acetonide is associated with retinal toxicity and transient increase of lens density. *Graefe's Arch Clin Exp Ophthalmol* 2006;244:1152–1159.
19. Penfold PL, Wen L, Madigan MC, et al. Triamcinolone Acetonide modulates permeability and intercellular adhesion molecule-1 (ICAM-1) expression of the ECV304 cell line: implications for macular degeneration. *Clin Exp Immunol* 2000;121:458–465.
20. Wang Y, Friedrichs U, Eichler W, et al. Inhibitory effects of triamcinolone acetonide on bFGF-induced migration and tube formation in choroidal microvascular endothelial cells. *Graefe's Arch Clin Exp Ophthalmol* 2002;240:42–48.
21. Kim YH, Chung IY, Choi MY, et al. Triamcinolone suppresses retinal vascular pathology via a potent interruption of proinflammatory signal-regulated activation of VEGF during a relative hypoxia. *Neurobiol Dis* 2007;26(3):569–576.
22. Hartnett ME, Martiniuk DJ, Saito Y, et al. Triamcinolone reduces neovascularization, capillary density and IGF-1 receptor phosphorylation in a model of oxygen-induced retinopathy. *Invest Ophthalmol Vis Sci* 2006;47(11):4975–4982.
23. Mizuno S, Nishiwaki A, Morita H, et al. Effects of Periocular administration of triamcinolone acetonide on leukocyte-endothelium interactions in the ischemic retina. *Invest Ophthalmol Vis Sci* 2007;48(6):2831–2836.
24. Akkoyun I, Yilmaz G, Oto S, et al. Impact of triamcinolone acetonide on retinal endothelial cells in a retinopathy of prematurity mouse model [Epub ahead of print, 2007]. *Acta Ophthalmol Scand*; doi:10.1111/j.1600-0420.2007.00945.x.
25. Murata M, Shimizu S, Horiuchi S, et al. Inhibitory effect of triamcinolone acetonide on corneal neovascularization. *Graefe's Arch Clin Exp Ophthalmol* 2006;244:205–209.
26. Giangiacomo J, Dueker DK, Adelstein EH. Histopathology of triamcinolone in the subconjunctiva. *Ophthalmology* 1987;94(2):149–153.
27. Kato A, Kimura H, Okabe K, et al. Suppression of laser-induced choroidal neovascularization by posterior sub-tenon administration of triamcinolone acetonide. *Retina* 2005;25(4):503–509.
28. Ciulla TA, Criswell MH, Danis RP, et al. Intravitreal triamcinolone acetonide inhibits choroidal neovascularization in a laser-treated rat model. *Arch Ophthalmol* 2001;119:399–403.
29. Federici T, Batlle I. Periocular triamcinolone acetonide as treatment for macular edema secondary to branch vein occlusion associated with retinal arteriovenous malformation. *Retina* 2006;26:1079–1080.
30. Koga T, Mawatari Y, Inumaru J, et al. Trans-tenon's retrobulbar triamcinolone acetonide infusion for refractory diabetic macular edema after vitrectomy [Epub ahead of print 2005]. *Graefes Arch Clin Exp Ophthalmol* 2005;243(12):1247–1252.
31. Zamir E, Read RW, Smith RE, et al. A Prospective evaluation of subconjunctival injection of triamcinolone acetonide for resistant anterior scleritis. *Ophthalmol* 2002;109(4):798–805.
32. Sen HN, Ursea R, Nussenblatt RB, et al. Subconjunctival corticosteroid injection for the treatment of non-necrotising anterior scleritis. *Br J Ophthalmol* 2005;89:917–918.
33. Albini TA, Zamir E, Read RW, et al. Evaluation of subconjunctival triamcinolone for nonnecrotizing anterior scleritis. *Ophthalmology* 2005;112(10):1814–1820.
34. Shimura M, Yasuda K, Shiono T. Posterior sub-tenon's capsule injection of triamcinolone acetonide prevents panretinal photocoagulation-induced visual dysfunction in patients with severe diabetic retinopathy and good vision. *Ophthalmology* 2006;113(3):381–387.
35. Shimura M, Nakazawa T, Yasuda K, et al. Pretreatment of posterior subtenon injection of triamcinolone acetonide has beneficial effects for grid pattern photocoagulation against diffuse diabetic macular oedema. *Br J Ophthalmol* 2007;91:449–454.
36. Diabetic Retinopathy Clinical Research Network et al. randomized trial of peribulbar triamcinolone acetonide with and without focal photocoagulation for mild diabetic macular edema. A pilot study. *Ophthalmol* 2007;114(6):1190–1196.
37. Paccola L, Jorge R, Barbosa JC, et al. Anti-inflammatory efficacy of a single posterior subtenon injection of triamcinolone acetonide versus prednisolone acetate 1% eye drops after pars plana vitrectomy [Epub ahead of print, 2007]. *Acta Ophthalmol Scand*; doi:10.1111/j.1600-0420.2007.00923.x/.
38. Ferrante P, Ramsey A, Bunce C, et al. Clinical trial to compare efficacy and side-effects of injection of posterior sub-Tenon triamcinolone versus orbital floor methylprednisolone in the management of posterior uveitis. *Clin Experiment Ophthalmol* 2004;32(6):563–568.
39. Cardillo JA, Melo LAS, Costa RA, et al. Comparison of intravitreal versus posterior sub-Tenon's capsule injection of triamcinolone acetonide for diffuse diabetic macular edema. *Ophthalmol* 2005;112(9):1557–1563.
40. Bonini Filho MA, Jorge R, Barbosa JC, et al. Intravitreal injection versus sub-tenon's infusion of triamcinolone acetonide for refractory diabetic macular edema: a randomized clinical trial. *Invest Ophthalmol Vis Sci* 2005;46(10):3845–3849.
41. Ozdek S, Bahceci UA, Gurelik G, et al. Posterior subtenon and intravitreal triamcinolone acetonide for diabetic macular edema. *J Diabetes Complications* 2006;20(4):246–251.
42. Choi YJ, Oh IK, Oh JR, et al. Intravitreal versus posterior subtenon injection of triamcinolone acetonide for diabetic macular edema. *Korean J Ophthalmol* 2006;20(4):205–209.
43. Telander DG, Lee TZ, Pambuccian SE, et al. Subconjunctival corticosteroids for benign lymphoid hyperplasia. *Br J Ophthalmol* 2005;89:770–787.

44. Penn JS, Rajaratnam VS, Collier RJ, et al. The effect of an angiostatic steroid on neovascularization in a rat model of retinopathy of prematurity. *Invest Ophthalmol Vis Sci* 2001;42(1):283–290.

45. Clark AF. Mechanism of action of the angiostatic cortisene Anecortave Acetate. *Surv Ophthalmol* 2007;52(Suppl 1):S26–S34.

46. Dahlin DC, Rahimy MH. Pharmacokinetics and metabolism of anecortave acetate in animals and humans. *Surv Ophthalmol* 2007;52(Suppl 1):S49–S61.

47. Heaton J, Kastner P, Hackett R. Preclinical safety of Anecortave Acetate. *Surv Ophthalmol* 2007;52(Suppl 1):S35–S40.

48. Regillo CD, D`Amico DJ, Mieler WF, et al. Clinical safety profile of posterior juxtascleral depot administration of Anecortave Acetate 15 mg suspension as primary therapy or adjunctive therapy with Photodynamic therapy for treatment of wet age-related macular degeneration. *Surv Ophthalmol* 2007;52(Suppl 1):S70–S78.

49. Clark AF, Mellon J, Li XY, et al. Inhibition of intraocular tumor growth by topical application of the angiostatic steroid anecortave acetate. *Invest Ophthalmol Vis Sci* 1999;40(9):2158–2162.

50. Jockovich M, Murray TG, Escalona-Benz E, et al. Anecortave Acetate as single and adjuvant therapy in the treatment of retinal tumors of LH (BETA) T(AG) mice. *Invest Ophthalmol Vis Sci* 2006;47(4):1264–1268.

51. Clark AF. Preclinical efficacy of anecortave acetate. *Surv Ophthalmol* 2007;52(Suppl 1):S41–S48.

52. Kaiser PK, Goldberg MF, Davis AA, et al. Posterior Juxtascleral Depot Administration of Anecortave Acetate. *Surv Ophthalmol* 2007;52(Suppl 1):S62–S69.

53. Augustin AJ, D`Amico DJ, Mieler WF, et al. Safety of posterior juxtascleral depot administration of the angiostatic cortisone anecortave acetate for treatment of subfoveal choroidal neovascularization in patients with age-related macular degeneration. *Graefes Arch Clin Exp Ophthalmol* 2005;243(1):9–12.

54. Jockovich ME, Murray TG, Clifford PD, et al. Posterior juxtascleral injection of anecortave acetate: magnetic resonance and echographic imaging and localization in rabbit eyes. *Retina* 2007;27(2):247–252.

55. D`Amico DJ, Goldberg MF, Hudson H, et al. Anecortave Acetate as monotherapy for treatment of subfoveal lesions in patients with exudative age-related macular degeneration (AMD): Interim (Month 6) Analysis of clinical safety and efficacy. *Retina* 2003;23(1):14–23.

56. Russel SR, Hudson HL, Jerdan JA, and Anecortave Acetate Clinical Study Group. Anecortave Acetate for the treatment of exudative age-related macular degeneration– a review of clinical outcomes. *Surv Ophthalmol* 2007;52(Suppl 1):S79–S90.

57. D`Amico DJ, Goldberg MF, Hudson H, et al. The Anecortave Acetate Clinical Study Group. Anecortave Acetate as monotherapy for treatment of subfoveal neovascularization in age-related macular degeneration. Twelve-month clinical outcomes. *Ophthalmol* 2003;110(12):2372–2383.

58. Slakter JS, Bochow T, D`Amico DJ, et al. Anecortave Acetate (15 milligrams) versus Photodynamic Therapy for treatment of subfoveal neovascularization in age-related macular degeneration. *Ophthalmol* 2006;113:3–13.

59. Slakter JS. Anecortave acetate for treating or preventing choroidal neovascularization. *Ophthalmol Clin N Am* 2006;19:373–380.

# 39

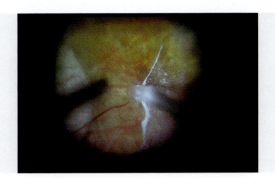

# Intravitreal Triamcinolone

Francisco Gómez-Ulla ■ Javier Ferro
Maria José Blanco ■ Maximino Abraldes

## BACKGROUND

Glucocorticosteroids are synthetic analogs of hormones produced by the suprarenal gland. Traditionally these drugs have been used for their anti-inflammatory properties and as immunosuppressants, for their ability to inhibit the activities of different cells types including lymphocytes, macrophages, neutrophiles, basophiles, endothelial vascular cells, and fibroblasts. The inhibitory effect of corticoids on fibroblast proliferation and endothelial vascular cells (1) had been observed *in vitro* and given rise to numerous possible therapeutic applications. However, these therapies were initially hindered by the inability to obtain sufficiently high doses of intraocular glucocorticoids using traditional topical or systemic administrations (2). In 1970, Machemer et al. (3) were the first to use intravitreal steroids in an animal model with retinal detachment. Intravitreal injections of triamcinolone were administered to obtain sufficient concentrations of intraocular corticoids inside the eye to prevent the development of proliferative vitreoretinopathy (PVR) after surgery. Other experimental models appeared later, evaluating the therapeutic effects of corticoid injections into the vitreous cavity (4,5).

Corticosteroids are known to reduce inflammation and tissue edema. Clinical studies suggest that intravitreal injections of steroids after the vehicle is removed may be an appropriate treatment for intraocular neovascular or edematous diseases (6–9). Steroids have been found to be potent inhibitors of vascular endothelial growth factor (VEGF) and may reduce the leakage of fluid from compromised capillaries in patients with maculopathy as well as inhibit neovascularization.

Triamcinolone acetonide (TA) is a corticosteroid with practically no water solubility which prolongs its presence in the vitreous nearly five times as compared to hydrocortisone (10). This increased media life makes it a useful alternative for the treatment of inflammatory ocular pathologies or other proliferative intraocular diseases.

Since the 1970s, many articles have been published evaluating the pharmacological effects of intraocular triamcinolone, as well as determining its safety and therapeutic effectiveness for a wide range of ophthalmologic pathologies (11–16).

In 1977, Perry et al. (17) published an article describing the apparent safety of an accidental intravitreal injection. A similar situation was described in 1993 by Gomez-Ulla et al. (18), when paramethasone acetate was inadvertently injected into the vitreous cavity during a subtenon's placement of the medication; side effects were not noted. These incidents preceded planned intravitreal corticoid injection. The first intentional intraocular injections of triamcinolone in humans were administered in 1993 and 1994 by Dominguez et al. (19,20) for the treatment of pathologies like macular edema and choroidal neovascularization and in 1995 by Pendfold et al. (21) to treat 28 patients with exudative or wet age-related macular degeneration.

## INTRAVITREAL STEROIDS IN DIABETIC RETINOPATHY

Intravitreal triamcinolone acetonide (IVTA) has been applied with an exponentially increasing frequency for various intraocular neovascular and edematous diseases, including diabetic macular edema (DME), proliferating diabetic retinopathy, and neovascular glaucoma due to proliferative diabetic retinopathy (PDR).

In DME, the edema may almost completely resolve, and visual acuity may increase as much as macular ischemia and the tissue destruction by the diabetic process may allow. For PDR and neovascular glaucoma, investigations have suggested an antiangiogenic effect of IVTA (22). The use of other steroids like intravitreal dexamethasone and slow release device such as sustained release fluocinolone intravitreal implant, are also areas of active research.

IVTA is a promising therapeutic method for DME that fails to respond to conventional laser photocoagulation (23–28).

Different techniques (nonfilter and filter techniques) applied to reduce the solvent agent benzyl alcohol (9.9 mg/ml) from a commercially prepared TA suspension were made (29).

Two different nonfilter techniques were used: sedimentation and centrifugation. Commercially prepared TA suspension was allowed to sediment overnight and 0.9 ml of the supernatant was extracted with a tuberculin syringe. The pellet was resuspended with 0.9 or 0.5 ml of balanced salt solution (BSS). In the other nonfilter technique, the commercial suspension was centrifuged at $3000 \times g$ for 5 minutes; 0.9 ml of the supernatant was extracted with a tuberculin syringe and the pellet resuspended with 1 ml of BSS.

Filtered triamcinolone has been prepared by taking 0.62 ml from the commercial TA ampoule, following the technique described by Jonas (8,9). The extracted volume was placed in a tuberculin syringe (1 ml) filled with Ringer lactate solution. Two different syringe driven filter units were evaluated: a Millipore filter and a Pall filter. The selected filter was placed on the top of the syringe and most of the contents of the syringe were pressed through the filter, with the triamcinolone crystals remaining in the syringe. The syringe was refilled with Ringer lactate solution and the same procedure was repeated three times. In the end, 0.2 ml of the solution was left in the syringe.

Intravitreal injection of triamcinolone effectively reduces macular thickening due to diffuse DME, at least in the short term. However, in this chronic disease, the need to repeat intravitreal injections every 4 to 6 months will increase the risk of injection-related complications and may not be tolerated by the patients.

The injection technique is as follows. Topical anesthesia is applied to the ocular surface followed by preparation with 5% povidone iodine. A cotton-tipped applicator soaked in povidone iodine is then applied to the injection site, 3.5 mm posterior to the limbus in pseudophakic eyes and 4.0 mm posterior to the limbus in phakic eyes. TA is injected through the inferior pars plana at a dose of 4 mg (0.1 ml). A 30-gauge needle is used. Indirect ophthalmoscopy is used to confirm proper intravitreal localization of the suspension and perfusion of the optic nerve head (30).

The complications of IVTA include secondary ocular hypertension in about 40% of the eyes, medically uncontrollable high intraocular pressure (IOP) leading to antiglaucomatous surgery in about 1% to 2% (31,32), posterior subcapsular cataract and nuclear cataract leading to cataract surgery in about 15% to 20%, especially in elderly patients within 1 year after injection (22,33), postoperative infectious endophthalmitis with a rate of about 1:500 or 1:1000 (34–36), noninfectious endophthalmitis (36,37), and pseudo-endophthalmitis (38), which can recur even after successive injections (39). IVTA can be combined with other intraocular surgeries including cataract surgery (40), particularly in eyes with iris neovascularization due to diabetic retinopathy.

Pars plana vitrectomy (PPV) with or without internal limiting membrane (ILM) peeling has also been advocated for the treatment of diabetic maculopathy (41), the reasons being mainly to relieve anteroposterior vitreomacular traction, tangential traction, as well as to remove interleukin 6 (IL-6), VEGF and other vasopermeable factors from the vitreous, improve microcirculation, and improve oxygenation (42–45). The benefit of ILM peeling is that it ensures that all posterior hyaloidal traction has been removed (46). When laser photocoagulation and TA treatment is not effective for diabetic maculopathy, vitrectomy with the complete removal of the posterior hyaloid face, including possible removal of the ILM, should be considered (47–49). TA greatly improves the visualization of the ILM. TA is used during vitrectomy to visualize the hyaloid. After the posterior hyaloid is surgically separated from the optic nerve head and posterior retina, TA suspension is injected over the posterior pole and an intraocular forceps is used to peel the ILM in a circumferential manner. The peeled area is seen as an area lacking white specks.

Several complications of advanced diabetic retinopathy can be treated surgically. Vitrectomy can clear media opacities, relieve traction on the retina, and make adequate laser treatment of the retina possible. IVTA may be an additional tool in PPV for PDR (50). After a core PPV, a little quantity of TA aqueous suspension (40 mg/ml) is injected into the mid vitreous cavity (51). This suspension is very useful to delaminate and remove the fibrovascular proliferation and to visualize the posterior hyaloid, thus allowing a complete posterior hyaloid separation and removal. After surgery, 0.1 to 0.2 ml of TA is left in the vitreous cavity to help the reabsorption of macular edema and control intraocular inflammation (Figs. 39-1 to 39-3).

## Triamcinolone Acetonide Used as an Aid to Visualization of the Vitreous and the Posterior Hyaloid during Pars Plana Vitrectomy

The interaction between the posterior vitreous cortex and the retinal surface plays a key role in the pathogenesis of several ocular diseases. An attached or incompletely separated posterior hyaloid can provide a source of traction in conditions such as macular hole (MH), vitreomacular traction syndrome, and PVR or serve as a scaffold for fibrovascular proliferation in PDR.

Although a complete removal of the vitreous and posterior hyaloid membrane is an important surgical goal when a PPV is used to treat the above mentioned diseases, a layer of posterior vitreous cortex often remains on the retinal surface after an apparent vitreous detachment during surgery. Consequently, in spite of the development of different surgical techniques for creating a surgical PVD using cannulas (silicone tipped or hard) and forceps with active or passive suction, the

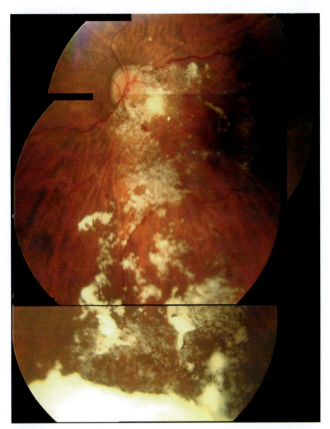

**Figure 39-1.** Intraocular triamcinolone crystals following vitrectomy for diabetic macular edema.

surgeon cannot be certain that the posterior hyaloid separation and complete vitrectomy have been successful because of the transparency of these structures.

In 2000, Peyman et al. (52) first described the use of IVTA as an aid to improve the visualization of the posterior hyaloid and thus assist in its separation during PPV. The IVTA-assisted PPV permits the observation of the residual vitreous cortex left on the retina as small islands which can be removed using vitreal forceps. Similarly, the use of IVTA enables the visualization of all the epiretinal membranes (ERMs) by showing a clear contrast with the unstained retina. IVTA suspension particles trapped in the peripheral vitreous also enable a clear visualization of the vitreous base, which permits its complete removal (53).

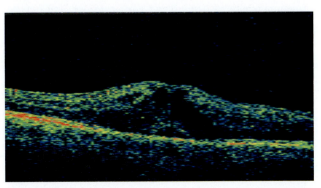

**Figure 39-2.** The optical coherence tomography scan obtained through the fovea revealed loss of the normal foveal contour, diffuse macular thickening, intraretinal cysts, and fluid accumulation.

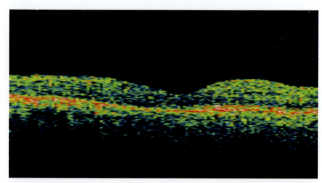

**Figure 39-3.** Optical coherence tomography done 3 months after vitrectomy and intravitreal triamcinolone acetonide showed a decrease of foveal thickness, complete resolution of intraretinal cysts and a normal macular anatomical architecture.

It is not surprising to suggest that the intraoperative use of intravitreal TA has at least three advantages: the provision of certainty during the surgical maneuver by improving the visualization of the hyaloid, the detection of a very thin hyaloid cortex as well as ERM's remaining on the retinal surface and the reduction of postoperative inflammation, which is a major cause of postoperative complications, like PVR. We must remember that PVR is the most common cause of rhegmatogenous retinal detachment surgery failure and it is responsible for recurrent retinal detachments in 5% to 10% of eyes. In the surgical repair of rhegmatogenous retinal detachment complicated with PVR, the major goals are the removal of vitreous scaffolding and tractional membranes and the use of IVTA facilitates the visualization and delineation of both.

Different authors have carried out a TA-assisted PPV in several diseases such as DME, PDR, and PVR (52–58) stressing good vitreous visualization, the absence of retinal toxicity, and the possibility of preventing fibrin syndrome and PVR after surgery. Sakamoto et al. used IVTA to improve the visibility of the hyaloid during PPV in 13 eyes with PVR and found favorable anatomic and functional results. By use a laser flare meter, they also found a significantly lower postoperative blood-ocular barrier breakdown in the eyes treated with IVTA-assisted PPV than in those treated without IVTA. Enaida et al. (55) found that the number of reoperations due to preretinal fibrous membrane formation decreased in TA-assisted PPV for all cases and especially in those with PDR, with a significant statistical difference.

Although Hida et al. (59) have suggested that the vehicle of commercially available depot corticosteroid, and not the crystalline itself, could be toxic to intraocular tissue, no relevant postoperative complications in terms of retinal toxicity were observed in these studies. The absence of toxic effects of commercially available IVTA may be explained by the low dose injected and by the fast removal of TA from the vitreous cavity. The same reason could explain why pathologically increased IOP which is one of the most common postoperative complications of intravitreal triamcinolone (31), has not been found.

## Triamcinolone Acetonide-Assisted Peeling of the Internal Limiting Membrane

The peeling of the ILM has been recommended as an effective means of reducing tangential traction on the retina surface in many macular diseases, especially in idiopathic MHs (60,61), cellophane maculopathy or macular pucker, and diabetic retinopathy. Many reports suggest that ILM peeling increases the rate of anatomic closure of the MH and may decrease late reopening (62). However, the removal of the ILM is very complex because of the difficulty in its visualization and consequent risk of incomplete peeling or retinal damage.

Recently, the concept of staining the ILM has been introduced. Indocyanine green (ICG) was first used to enhance visualization and removal of the ILM (63), however, concerns regarding its toxicity persist (64,65). Trypan blue and TA were subsequently reported to have similar effects (56,66,67). While ICG stains all layers of the ILM and alters the cleavage plane between the ILM and the innermost retinal layers, TA does not stain the ILM selectively and does not behave like a stainer. It forms a thin layer with white specks on the surface of the ILM, which not only assists in the initial picking-up of the ILM, but also helps in identifying the margins of the unpeeled ILM, which are sometimes missed during the ILM peeling without an adjuvant.

Although the preservative in TA suspension may cause toxic effects on the retina (59), TA itself may not be toxic because submacular deposition of the substance has reportedly shown no apparent adverse effects (68). In MH surgery one must take special care not to leave any intraocular deposit, because this is thought to be the responsible for the hole closure failure.

## TRIAMCINOLONE ACETONIDE-ASSISTED PARS PLANA VITRECTOMY IN HIGH MYOPIA

It is well known that the vitreous gel of patients with high myopia differs from emmetropic subjects. Synchisis and syneresis of the vitreous are common findings in young myopic patients. It is also conceivable that the vitreoretinal adhesion may be weaker in those patients explaining why posterior vitreous detachment (PVD) appears to develop nearly 10 years earlier in high myopia (> −6 diopters) than in emmetropia (69).

Diagnosing PVD in high myopia is more difficult than in nonmyopia. It can be commonly misdiagnosed with large lacuna formation or extensive vitreous liquefaction, because the posterior hyaloid membrane is thin and delicate. The thinness of the posterior cortex can explain the difficulty in assessment preoperatively as well as during surgery. It could also explain the interesting occurrence of a PVD in some previously vitrectomized eyes in which the posterior hyaloid membrane has been left in place with or without a thin sheet of cortical gel. TA (52) is the best tool to assess and map the relationship between the posterior hyaloid and its retinal surface.

In nonmyopic eyes without PVD, the premacular liquefied space usually seems to lose the construction of gel and forms only a thin layer of vitreous cortex that becomes clearly visualized as a white structure after injection of TA. Another liquefied space with a similar appearance is confirmed on the optic disk adjacent to the premacular area (Fig. 39-4). Both liquefied

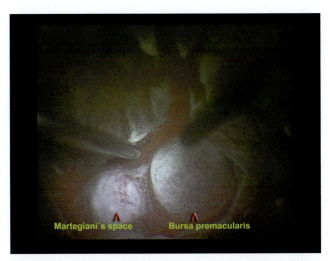

**Figure 39-4.** Normal appearance of the triamcinolone stained vitreous highlighting the premacular bursa and Martegiani's space in nonmyopic eyes at the time of vitreous surgery.

areas are separated by a "wall" of thick vitreous cortex with few TA crystals accumulated at that point, and correspond to previous autopsy findings called bursa premacularis or posterior vitreous pocket, and Martegiani's space respectively. In highly myopic eyes without PVD however, these structures cannot be individualized after TA injection. We speculate that the main cause for this phenomenon is the lack of thick vitreous surrounding both the prepapillary and the premacular spaces.

True complete PVD represents the total separation not only of cortical gel but also of the posterior hyaloid membrane from the retinal surface, whereas partial PVD is defined as the detachment of only a part of the cortical gel and the posterior hyaloid membrane (70). The classic approach to partial PVD would suggest that both the detached and undetached posterior hyaloid membranes would remain connected with a variable amount of tractional force transmitted between them. However, this was not found to be true in every case. During TA-assisted PPV in highly myopic eyes, residual undetached cortical vitreous (RCV) can be observed directly after the steroid particles adhere to the vitreous fibers. In those patches of residual cortex, the undetached posterior hyaloid becomes isolated while the rest of the vitreous separates away. In these areas, the adherence between hyaloid membrane and the retina could be stronger than its cohesive strength at the time of the detachment of the posterior hyaloid, thus resulting tearing and isolation. The posterior hyaloid, in the form of a fragile membrane, is usually difficult to be separated from the retina in a continuous manner in cases of high myopia. This phenomenon of hyaloid rupture can also occur in eyes without myopia, especially in the foveal area, but seems to be more prominent and ubiquitous in highly myopic eyes. Kishi and Shimizu (71) postulated that it is the posterior wall of the liquefied space in the premacular vitreous (bursa premacularis) that remains attached to the retina during PVD. This is similar to what we have frequently observed in highly myopic patients, but in this case most of the vitreous seems to behave as a giant liquefied bursa in front of the retina.

The location, size, and number of RCV patches are variable and appear in 83% of high myopic patients who underwent

vitrectomy for rhegmatogenous retinal detachment (72). The most frequent locations for these vitreous "islands" are the macula and optic disc. This "patched" form is not well defined with the classification of PVD into partial and complete.

We use TA as a marker in all highly myopic eyes undergoing vitrectomy, except in those cases with MH in order to prevent the crystals from getting into contact with the retinal pigment epithelium. Without the use of TA, many cases would have been misdiagnosed as complete PVD during vitrectomy. For example, in eyes with optically empty vitreous and negative fish-strike sign, which showed variable amounts of TA crystals adhered to one or more retinal areas, back-flush maneuvers were used to check whether the crystals can be mobilized or not. In the latter case, it is diagnosed as RCV instead of PVD. Matsumoto et al. (73) observed, using transmission electron microscopy, that eyes that did not have any TA granules adherent to the retinal surface intraoperatively did not have any residual posterior hyaloid on ILM. We prefer not to perform active aspiration over the area with retained crystals, where the residual cortex is very thin, in order to avoid direct transmission of the aspiration force over the adjacent retina and its subsequent incarceration in the extrusion needle. Therefore, we prefer to perform RCV removal by gentle and careful sweeping maneuvers with a silicone tip and no aspiration at the site with retained TA crystals. The remaining posterior hyaloid membrane characteristically rolls up (Fig. 39-5) while the adhered crystals enhance the maneuver. The separated complex can be then easily removed with an intraocular forceps. On the other hand, we consider active aspiration to be a good method for detaching the posterior hyaloid in eyes without high myopia where the thick cortex that remains attached to the retina allows uniform distribution of the aspiration force in front of the needle and prevents retinal incarceration. By using active aspiration, surgical PVD is easily expanded up to the equator in emmetropic patients. In highly myopic eyes, however, true complete PVD can be difficult or even impossible to achieve in many cases.

Uchino et al. (74) observed that optical coherence tomography (OCT) can be used to assess the clinical condition of the posterior vitreoretinal interface, but due to instrument limitations

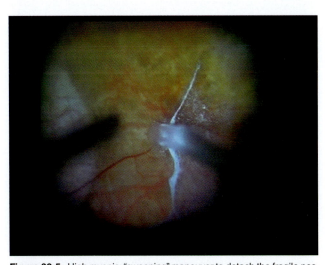

**Figure 39-5.** High myopia: "sweeping" maneuver to detach the fragile posterior vitreous cortex and hyaloid.

about 9% of normal eyes remain not recognizable. In the same study, authors found that all eyes with complete PVD showed Weiss's ring on biomicroscopy. These observations are not consistent with those 7% of eyes with PVD presenting a hole instead of a complete or partial Weiss's ring in the posterior hyaloid on biomicroscopy or scanning laser ophthalmoscope (75). During vitrectomy in highly myopic eyes, we have frequently observed both the peripapillary glial tissue (Weiss's ring) and its surrounding hyaloid membrane remaining attached to the optic nerve while the rest of the posterior hyaloid has been intentionally detached from the retina. Recently, OCT with 3-$\mu$m axial resolution was shown to be useful for PVD detection with persistent vitreofoveal attachment and subtle irregular foveal contour in patients with visual distortion (76). There is still, however, no clinical way to recognize isolated RCV and they cannot be clearly visualized during vitrectomy without using TA suspension.

Even though some studies suggest that RCV may be related to the development of idiopathic premacular fibrosis (71,77), at present, it is unclear whether the residual vitreous cortex should be removed, except in those cases where there is a traction over the retina. In some myopic eyes, anomalous strands of vitreous attached to the posterior pole can also be clearly individualized with TA. Those unions have to be carefully removed specially in cases with retinal detachment over staphylomata or with macular retinoschisis.

In summary, the use of TA suspension and specific surgical maneuvers, like backflushing and sweeping of the crystals, greatly improve the visibility of the posterior vitreous cortex in highly myopic eyes, allowing for a better comprehension of its vitreoretinal relationship.

## CONCLUSIONS

IVTA could be a useful therapy for some ocular diseases that are accompanied by macular edema not responsive to other treatments as is the case of DME refractory to photocoagulation. However, sometimes it is necessary to repeat the injections to prevent loss of efficiency over time and the relapse of the edema. It is important to point out that some complications such as the development of cataracts, ocular hypertension, and glaucoma can occur with this technique, and surgery may be necessary (see Chapter Complications of Pharmacotherapy).

IVTA has become quite widespread as an adjuvant to conventional surgery with the aim to prevent short-term postoperative inflammation control, reduce risk of re-proliferation, and distinguish vitreal remains during the surgery. This surgical method allows one to perform a complete vitrectomy and improve the extraction of posterior hyaloid, vitreal membranes and even ILM. The technique is especially useful in patients with complex anatomosurgical structures, such as highly myopic eyes.

### References

1. Ruhmann AG, Berliner DL. Effect of steroids on growth of mouse fibroblasts *in vitro*. *Endocrinology* 1965;76:916–927.
2. Rozen V, Chernin L. Effect of different doses of glucocorticoids on growth of monolayer cultures of connective tissue. *Fed Proc* 1974;24:861.
3. Machemer R, Sugita G, Tano Y. Treatment of intraocular proliferation with intravitreal steroids. *Tr Am Ophth Soc* 1979;77:177–178.
4. Tano Y, Sugita G, Abrams G, et al. Inhibition of intraocular proliferations with intravitreal corticosteroids. *Am J Ophthalmol* 1980;89(1):131–136.
5. Tano Y, Chandler DB, McCuen BW, et al. Glucocorticosteroid inhibition of intraocular proliferation after injury. *Am J Ophthalmol* 1981;91(2):184–189.
6. Danis RP, Ciulla TA, Pratt LM, et al. Intravitreal triamcinolone acetonide in exudative age-related macular degeneration. *Retina* 2000;20:244–250.
7. Greenberg PB, Martidis A, Rogers AH, et al. Intravitreal triamcinolone acetonide for macular oedema due to central retinal vein occlusion. *Br J Ophthalmol* 2002;86:247–248.
8. Jonas JB, Hayler JK, Söfker A, et al. Intravitreal injection of crystalline cortisone as adjunctive treatment of proliferative diabetic retinopathy. *Am J Ophthalmol* 2001;131:468–471.
9. Jonas JB, Söfker A. Intraocular injection of crystalline cortisone as adjunctive treatment of diabetic macular edema. *Am J Ophthalmol* 2001;132:425–427.
10. Schimmer BP, Parker KL Adrenocorticotropic Hormone; Andrenocortical Steroids and Their Synthetic Analogs; Inhibitors of the Synthesis and Actions of Adrenocortical Hormones. In: Goodman & Gilman's The Pharmacological Basis of Therapeutics. MeGraw-Hill 2001:1649–1678.
11. Tano Y, Chandler D, Machemer R. Treatment of intraocular proliferation with intravitreal injection of triamcinolone acetonide. *Am J Ophthalmol* 1980;90(6):810–816.
12. Ishibashi T, Miki K, Sorgente N, et al. Effects of intravitreal administration of steroids on experimental subretinal neovascularization in the subhuman primate. *Arch Ophthalmol* 1985;103:708–711.
13. Ciulla TA, Criswell MH, Danis RP, et al. Intravitreal triamcinolone acetonide inhibits choroidal neovascularization in a laser-treated rat model. *Arch Ophthalmol* 2001;119(3):399–404.
14. Ciulla TA, Criswell MH, Danis RP, et al. Choroidal neovascular membrane inhibition in a laser treated rat model with intraocular sustained release triamcinolone acetonide microimplants. *Br J Ophthalmol* 2003;87(8):1032–1037.
15. Antoszyk AN, Gottlieb JL, Machemer R, et al. The effects of intravitreal triamcinolone acetonide on experimental pre-retinal neovascularization. *Graefes Arch Clin Exp Ophthalmol* 1993;231(1):34–40.
16. Danis RP, Bingaman DP, Yang Y, et al. Inhibition of preretinal and optic nerve head neovascularization in pigs by intravitreal triamcinolone acetonide. *Ophthalmology* 1996;12:2099–2104.
17. Perry HT, Cohn BT, NAuheim JS. Accidental intraocular injection with a Dermojet syringe. *Arch Dermatol* 1977;113(8):1131.
18. Gómez-Ulla F, Gonzalez F, Ruiz-Fraga C. Unintentional intraocular injection of corticosteroids. *Acta Ophthalmol Scan* 1993;71:419–421.
19. Dominguez A, Quiroga P, Jareño M. El tratamiento de enfermedades médicas con triamcinolona intravítrea. *Arch Soc Esp Oftalmol* 1993;65:491–508.
20. Dominguez Collazo A. Devices and drugs introduced intraocularly for the treatment of eye diseases "in the office". *An R Acad Nac Med (Madr)* 1994;111(2):377–385.
21. Penfold PL, Gyory JF, Hunyor AB, et al. Exudative macular degeneration and intravitreal triamcinolone. A pilot study. *Aust N Z J Ophthalmol* 1995;23(4):293–298.
22. Jonas JB. Intravitreal triamcinolone acetonide for diabetic retinopathy. *Dev Ophthalmol* 2007;39:96–110.
23. Sutter FK, Simpson JM, Gillies MC. Intravitreal triamcinolone for diabetic macular edema that persists after laser treatment: three-month efficacy and safety results of a prospective, randomized, double-masked, placebo-controlled clinical trial. *Ophthalmology* 2004;111:2044–2049.
24. Negi AK, Vernon SA, Lim CS, et al. Intravitreal triamcinolone improves vision in eyes with chronic diabetic macular oedema refractory to laser photocoagulation. *Eye* 2005;19(7):747–751.
25. Er H, Yilmaz H. Intravitreal cortisone injection for refractory diffuse diabetic macular edema. *Ophthalmologica* 2005;219(6):394–400.
26. Gibran SK, Cullinane A, Jungkim S, et al. Intravitreal triamcinolone for diffuse diabetic macular oedema. *Eye* 2006;20(6):720–724.
27. Selim Kocabora M, Kucuksahin H, Gulkilik G, et al. Treatment of diabetic macular edema with intravitreal triamcinolone acetonide injection: functional and anatomical outcomes. *J Fr Ophthalmol* 2007;30(1):32–38.
28. Gillies MC, Islam A, Zhu M, et al. Efficacy and Safety of Multiple Intravitreal Triamcinolone Injections for Refractory Diabetic Macular Oedema. *Br J Ophthalmol* 2007;91(10):1323–1326.
29. Garcia-Arumi J, Boixadera A, Giralt J, et al. Comparison of different techniques for purification of triamcinolone acetonide suspension for intravitreal use. *Br J Ophthalmol* 2005;89:1112–1114.
30. Gomez-Ulla F, Marticorena J, Alfaro V, et al. Triamcinolona intravítrea y edema macular diabético. In: Alfaro V, Gómez-Ulla F, Quiroz-Mercado H, Figueroa MS, Villalva SJ (eds). *Retinopatía Diabética. Tratado médico quirúrgico.* Mac Line, S. L, 2006:179–198.
31. Jonas JB, Kreissig I, Degenring R. Intraocular pressure after intravitreal injection of triamcinolone acetonide. *Br J Ophthalmol* 2003;87:24–27.
32. Massin P, Audren F, Haouchine B, et al. Intravitreal triamcinolone acetonide for diabetic diffuse macular edema: preliminary results of a prospective controlled trial. *Ophthalmology* 2004;111:218–224.

33. Jonas JB, Kreissig I, Sofker A, et al. Intravitreal injection of triamcinolone for diffuse diabetic macular edema. *Arch Ophthalmol* 2003;121:57–61.

34. Jonas JB, Kreissig I, Degenring RF. Endophthalmitis after intravitreal injection of triamcinolone acetonide. *Arch Ophthalmol* 2003;121:1663–1664.

35. Moshfeghi DM, Kaiser PK, Scott IU, et al. Acute endophthalmitis following intravitreal triamcinolone acetonide injection. *Am J Ophthalmol* 2003;136: 791–796.

36. Nelson ML, Tennant MT, Sivalingam A, et al. Infectious and presumed noninfectious endophthalmitis after intravitreal triamcinolone acetonide injection. *Retina* 2003;23:686–691.

37. Roth DB, Chieh J, Spirn MJ, et al. Noninfectious endophthalmitis associated with intravitreal triamcinolone injection. *Arch Ophthalmol* 2003;121:1279–1282.

38. Sutter FK, Gillies MC. Pseudo-endophthalmitis after intravitreal injection of triamcinolone. *Br J Ophthalmo* 2003;87:972–974.

39. Marticorena J, Gomez-Ulla F, Romano MR, et al. Repeated pseudoendophthalmitis after combined photodynamic therapy and intravitreal triamcinolone available. *Graefes Arch Clin Exp Ophthalmol* 2007;245(9):1403–1404.

40. Habib MS, Canon PS, Steel DH. The combination of intravitreal triamcinolone and phacoemulsification surgery in patients with diabetic foveal oedema and cataract. *BMC Ophthalmol* 2005;22:5–15.

41. Yamamoto T, Hitani K, Sato Y, et al. Vitrectomy for diabetic macular edema with and without internal limiting membrane removal. *Ophthalmologica* 2005;219:206–213.

42. Lewis H, Abrams GW, Blumenkranz MS, et al. Vitrectomy for diabetic macular oedema associated with posterior hyaloidal traction. *Ophthalmology* 1992;99:753–759.

43. Harbour JW, Smiddy WE, Flynn HW Jr, et al. Vitrectomy for diabetic macular oedema associated with a thickened and taut posterior hyaloid membrane. *Am J Ophthalmol* 1996;121:405–413.

44. Pendergast SD, Hassan TS, Williams GA, et al. Vitrectomy for diffuse macular oedema associated with a taut premacular posterior hyaloid. *Am J Ophthalmol* 2000;130:178–186.

45. Kaiser PK, Riemann CD, Sears JE, et al. Macular traction detachment and diabetic macular oedema associated with posterior hyaloidal traction. *Am J Ophthalmol* 2001;131:44–49.

46. Gandorfer A, Messmer EM, Ulbig MW, et al. Resolution of diabetic macular oedema after surgical removal of the posterior hyaloid and inner limiting membrane. *Retina* 2000;20:126–133.

47. Higuchi A, Ogata N, Jo N, et al. Pars plana vitrectomy with removal of posterior hyaloid face in treatment of refractory diabetic macular edema resistant to triamcinolone acetonide. *Jpn J Ophthalmol* 2006;50:529–531.

48. Mochizuki Y, Hata Y, Enaida H, et al. Evaluating adjunctive surgical procedures during vitrectomy for diabetic macular edema. *Retina* 2006;26:143–148.

49. Rosenblatt BJ, Shah GK, Sharma S, et al. Pars plana vitrectomy with internal limiting membranectomy for refractory diabetic macular edema without a taut posterior hyaloid. *Graefes Arch Clin Exp Ophthalmol* 2005;243:20–25.

50. Jonas JB, Söfker A, Degenring R. Intravitreal triamcinolone acetonide as an additional tool in pars plana vitrectomy for proliferative diabetic retinopathy. *Eur J Ophthalmol* 2003;13:468–473.

51. Zheng Y, Sun N, Xiong Q, et al. Triamcinolone-assisted pars plana vitrectomy for retinal disease. *Yan Ke Xue Bao* 2005;21:142–146.

52. Peyman GA, Cheema R, Conway MD, et al. Triamcinolone acetonide as an aid to visualization of the vitreous and posterior hyaloid during pars plana vitrectomy. *Retina* 2000;20:554–555.

53. Furino C, Ferrari TM, Boscia F, et al. Triamcinolone-assisted pars plana vitrectomy for proliferative vitreoretinopathy. *Retina* 2003;23:771–776.

54. Sakamoto T, Miyazaki M, Hisatomi T, et al. Triamcinolone-assisted pars plana vitrectomy improves the surgical procedures and decreases the postoperative blood-ocular barrier breakdown. *Graefe's Arch Clin Exp Ophthalmol* 2002;240:423–429.

55. Enaida H, Hata Y, Ueno A, et al. Possible benefits of triamcinolone-assisted pars plana vitrectomy for retinal diseases. *Retina* 2003;23:764–770.

56. Kimura H, Kuroda S, Nagata M. Triamcinolone acetonide-assisted peeling of the internal limiting membrane. *Am J Ophthalmol* 2004;137:172–173.

57. Sonoda KH, Sakamoto T, Enaida H, et al. Residual vitreous cortex after surgical posterior vitreous separation visualized by intravitreous triamcinolone acetonide. *Ophthalmology* 2004;111:226–230.

58. Doi N, Uemura A, Nakao K, et al. Vitreomacular adhesion and the defect in posterior vitreous cortex visualized by triamcinolone-assisted vitrectomy. *Retina* 2005;25:742–745.

59. Hida T, Chandler D, Arena JE, et al. Experimental and clinical observation of the intraocular toxicity of commercial corticosteroid preparations. *Am J Ophthalmol* 1986;101:190–195.

60. Gass JDM. Idiopathic senile macular hole. Its early stages and pathogenesis. *Arch Ophthalmol* 1988;196:629–39.

61. Park DW, Sipperley JO, Sneed SR, et al. Macular hole surgery with internal limiting membrane peeling and intravitreous air. *Ophthalmology* 1999;106:1392–1397.

62. Brooks HL. Macular hole surgery with and without internal limiting membrane peeling. *Ophthalmology* 2000;107:1939–1948.

63. Da Mata AP, Burk SE, Riemann CD, et al. Indocyanine green-assisted peeling of the retinal internal membrana during vitrectomy surgery for macular hole repair. *Ophthalmology* 2001;108:1187–1192.

64. Engelbrecht NE, Freeman J, Sternberg P, et al. Retinal pigment changes after macular hole surgery with indocyanine green-assisted internal limiting membrane peeling. *Am J Ophthalmol* 2002;133:89–94.

65. Marcin PC, McCuen BW II, Cummings TJ, et al. Effects of indocyanine green on the retina and retinal pigment epithelium in a porcine model of retinal hole. *Retina* 2004;24:275–282.

66. Vote BJ, Russell MK, Joondeph BC. Trypan blue-assisted vitrectomy. *Retina* 2004;24:736–738.

67. Fraser EA, Cheema RA, Roberts MA. Triamcinolone acetonide-assisted peeling of retinal internal limiting membrane for macular surgery. *Retina* 2003;23:883–884.

68. Enaida H, Sakamoto T, Ueno A, et al. Submacular deposition of triamcinolone acetonide after triamcinolone-assisted vitrectomy. *Am J Ophthalmol* 2003;135:243–246.

69. Akiba J. Prevalence of posterior vitreous detachment in high myopia. *Ophthalmology* 1993;100:1384–1388.

70. Ang A, Poulson A, Snead DR, et al. Posterior vitreous detachment: current concepts and management. *Compr Ophthalmol Update* 2005;6(4):167–175.

71. Kishi S, Shimizu K. Oval defect in detached posterior hyaloid membrane in idiopathic preretinal macular fibrosis. *Am J Ophthalmol* 1994;118:451–456.

72. Kakehashi A, Schepens CL, Trempe CL. Vitreomacular observations: vitreomacular adhesion and hole in the premacular hyaloid. *Ophthalmology* 1994;101:1515–1521.

73. Matsumoto H, Yamanaka I, Hisatomi T, et al. Triamcinolone acetonide-assisted pars plana vitrectomy improves residual posterior vitreous hyaloid removal: Ultrastructural analysis of the inner limiting membrane. *Retina* 2007;27(2):174–179.

74. Uchino E, Akinori U, Norio O. Initial stages of posterior vitreous detachment in healthy eyes of older persons evaluated by optical coherence tomography. *Arch Ophthal* 2001;119(10):1475–1479.

75. Akiba J, Ishiko S, Yoshida A. Variations of Weiss's ring. *Retina* 2001;21(3):243–246.

76. Witkin A, Ko T, Fujimoto J, et al. Vitreofoveal attachment causing metamorphopsia: an ultrahigh-resolution optical coherence tomography finding. *Retina* 2006;26(9):1085–1087.

77. Hikichi T, Takahashi M, Trempe CL, et al. Relationship between premacular cortical vitreous defects and idiopathic premacular fibrosis. *Retina* 1995;15(3):413–416.

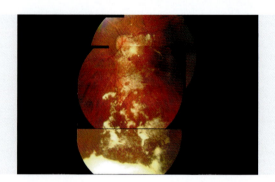

# Implications of the Off-Label Use of Medications in Vitreoretinal Surgery

Chirag C. Patel ■ Scott C. N. Oliver ■ Naresh Mandava
Jeffrey L. Olson ■ Hugo Quiroz-Mercado

## INTRODUCTION

In the United States, the "off-label" use of a medication means that it is being used for an indication that has not been approved by the Food and Drug Administration (FDA). The off-label use of medications is much more common than one may think. An estimated 20% of all medications prescribed in the United States are prescribed off-label (1). In certain specialties such as cardiology, psychiatry, and pediatrics, the rate of off-label drug use is even higher. Off-label prescribing is most commonly done with older medications that have found new uses but have not been subjected to the formal and often costly clinical trials required by the FDA to officially approve a drug for new indications. However, there is usually evidence in the medical literature to support and justify the off-label use.

The issue of off-label drug use has become more prominent recently in vitreoretinal surgery with the advent of vascular endothelial growth factor antagonists (VEGF-A), or anti-VEGF agents. Bevacizumab (Avastin, Genentech, south San Francisco, CA) was the first clinically available angiogenesis inhibitor in the United States. It was initially approved in 2004 for the treatment of metastatic colon and nonsmall cell lung cancer (2). In 2005, bevacizumab was first injected into a human eye. Two case reports resulted, one showing benefit in a patient with choroidal neovascularization from age-related macular degeneration (AMD) (3) and another showing improvement in macular edema in a patient with a central retinal vein occlusion (4). Despite the subsequent plethora of studies demonstrating safety and efficacy in treating a variety of ophthalmic conditions with intravitreal injections of bevacizumab, there is still no prospective, randomized, long-term, adequately powered safety and efficacy information for intravitreal bevacizumab. Also absent are rigorous dose escalation or dose frequency studies. There is, therefore, no scientifically determined optimal dose or dosing frequency.

In July 2006, ranibizumab (Lucentis, Genentech, south San Francisco, CA) was approved by the FDA for treatment of AMD by intravitreal injection. Ranibizumab is a Fab molecule derived from its parent molecule bevacizumab and works in a similar fashion by binding to VEGF-A (5). Despite FDA approval, many vitreoretinal surgeons have resisted using ranibizumab because bevacizumab is significantly cheaper. In the United States, a single dose of ranibizumab can cost about $2000 compared to $40 for a single dose of bevacizumab (6). There is also no compelling evidence that one works any better than the other. A small prospective study supports this conclusion (6), and there is currently an ongoing head to head clinical trial comparing the two drugs (7). Unless evidence surfaces that ranibizumab is a more effective drug, or until a more effective drug is developed, Avastin will likely continue to be used as a popular off-label drug by the vitreoretinal surgeon.

## OFF-LABEL DRUG USE IN VITREORETINAL SURGERY

Although the issue of the off-label use of medications has become popularized with the advent of bevacizumab, the reality is that a large number of medications injected intravitreally or used intraoperatively in vitreoretinal surgery are not FDA approved for that purpose. Examples include intravitreal injection of triamcinolone acetonide and antibiotics, and the intraoperative use of indocyanine green (ICG), and intraocular gases (e.g., $C_3F_8$ and $SF_6$).

Like Avastin, triamcinolone acetonide (Kenalog, Bristol-Myers Squibb, Princeton, NJ) has a counterpart that is FDA approved for intravitreal injection. Triamcinolone acetonide injectable suspension (Triesence, Alcon Laboratories, Ft. Worth, TX) is a preservative-free formulation that was developed specifically for intravitreal use and was FDA approved in 2007 for intravitreal injection for treatment of ocular inflammation and for intraoperative visualization of vitreous during vitrectomy. Kenalog had been used for many years prior to this, and has been shown to be useful for these purposes as well. A major difference between the two drugs is that a single dose of Kenalog in the United States costs about $10 while a dose of Triesence costs about $150. Despite the cost difference, there is little evidence that one works better than the other, and some studies have suggested that Kenalog may work better intraoperatively to stain vitreous than Triesence (8). This again raises the question of whether an off-label option maybe more sensible than its FDA approved counterpart.

For many drugs used by the vitreoretinal surgeon, there are no comparable FDA approved counterparts. Examples include antibiotics used for intravitreal injection for treatment of endophthalmitis, stains such as ICG which are used to highlight the internal limiting membrane to assist with membrane peeling, and intraocular gases used for retinal tamponade. These agents will likely never become FDA approved because it does not make financial sense for drug companies to sponsor the costly clinical trials to approve a drug for these indications. Nevertheless, one does not have to think twice when using such medications because they have been used consistently by vitreoretinal surgeons and their use has been established as the standard of care. Furthermore, there is reasonable evidence in the medical literature to justify the use of these off-label medications.

## LEGAL IMPLICATIONS OF OFF-LABEL USE

New drugs in the United States are generally tested through three phases of clinical trials. If the FDA is satisfied that the drug is safe and works for a specific indication based on these trials, it then approves the drug for use for that indication. However, once a drug is approved, the FDA has no authority to regulate the practice of medicine, and a physician can legally prescribe this medication off-label (for an indication other than that approved by the FDA). Therefore, once a drug is approved by the FDA, its off-label use by a physician is not regulated, and the off-label use is completely legal. A physician can use this drug for any purpose that they feel medically appropriate. This is true not only in the United States but in many countries worldwide.

Despite this lack of regulation, medications used off-label must be prescribed responsibly. There is always a delicate balance between patient safety and the physician's prerogative to use a medication that he or she feels will be of most benefit to the patient. If a medicine is used off-label, there should be adequate published literature or presentations and peer lectures at conferences supporting its use. One must also keep in mind that prospective, objectively corroborated information regarding side effects and dosage has not been formally established for off-label medications. Furthermore, anecdotal evidence or conclusions made from retrospective studies or small prospective studies are not equivalent to those based on the large prospective controlled trials used by the FDA to approve drugs. Physicians need to therefore be very vigilant of adverse effects when using medications off-label.

Medical–legal questions may arise when an adverse effect occurs after the off-label use of a medication. Generally, a patient may successfully sue the practitioner if it can be proven that in that circumstance the off-label use of the medication was negligent, especially if harm was reasonably foreseeable and preventable. However, if the off-label use of a medication has taken place regularly and openly and colleagues have also been using it over a period of time, with a reasonable degree of success and without patients being harmed, then this can be considered standard of care. In this setting, it would be almost impossible for a prospective claimant to establish that harm was reasonably foreseeable (9).

Given the greater risks involved when using a drug off-label, it is important that a physician obtain an informed consent after thoroughly discussing the risks and benefits of an off-label medication prior to prescribing or administering it to the patient.

## CONCLUSIONS

The off-label use of medications is common in vitreoretinal surgery. However, it is always important to remember that a drug used off-label does not have the backing of scientific rigor from prospective, randomized controlled trials for a specific indication. There is always a higher risk for both the patient and practitioner with off-label drug use, and extra care should be taken. Although a drug can be used legally by a physician for any indication after it is approved by the FDA, one should not use this freedom haphazardly. Generally, there should be some evidence in the medical literature supporting the off-label use of a medication. The more widespread and common the off-label use of a drug is, the safer it is for a physician in the event of an adverse or unexpected reaction of the medication. In contrast, if an adverse reaction occurs with the off-label use of a drug that is not used widely by colleagues and that has limited support in the medical literature for a certain indication, then a physician would be placing him or herself at legal risk.

In general, whenever prescribing a medication, and especially an off-label medication, it is important to communicate effectively with the patient so that the risks and benefits of taking medication are clearly understood, and so that there are no surprises for anyone in the unfortunate event of an adverse reaction.

### References

1. Radley DC, Finkelstein SN, Stafford RS. Off-label prescribing among office-based physicians. *Arch Intern Med* 2006;166(9):1021–1026.
2. Shih T, Lindley C. Bevacizumab: an angiogenesis inhibitor for the treatment of solid malignancies. *Clin Ther* 2006;28(11):1779–1802.
3. Rosenfeld PJ, Moshfeghi AA, Puliafito CA. Optical coherence tomography findings after an intravitreal injection of Bevacizumab (Avastin) for neovascular age-related macular degeneration. *Ophthalmic Surg Lasers Imaging* 2005;36:270–271.
4. Rosenfeld PJ, Fung AE, Puliafito CA. Optical coherence tomography findings after an intravitreal injection of Bevacizumab (Avastin) for macular edema from central retinal vein occlusion. *Ophthalmic Surg Lasers Imaging* 2005;36:336–339.
5. Gaudreault J, Fei D, Rusit J, et al. Preclinical pharmacokinetics of Ranibizumab (rhuFabV2) after a single intravitreal administration. *Invest Ophthalmol Vis Sci* 2005;46(2):726–733.
6. Subramanian ML, Ness S, Abedi G, et al. Bevacizumab vs ranibizumab for age-related macular degeneration: early results of a prospective double-masked, randomized clinical trial. *Am J Ophthalmol* 2009;148(6):875–882.
7. Comparison of AMD Treatments Trial (CATT): Lucentis—Avastin Trial (Ongoing). http://www.nei.nih.gov/catt. Accessed September 15, 2010
8. Moshfeghi AA, Nugent AK, Nomoto H, et al. Triamcinolone acetonide preparations: impact of crystal size on in vitro behavior. *Retina* 2009;29(5):689–698.
9. Strauss SA. 'Off-label' use of medicine: some legal and ethical implications. *SA Practice Management* 1998;19(1):12–19.

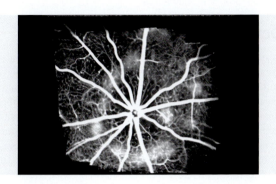

# Laser Treatment of Choroidal Neovascularization

Marc J. Spirn ■ Carl Regillo

The word "laser" is an acronym that stands for "light amplification by stimulated emission of radiation." Lasers concentrate high amounts of energy into a narrow beam of monochromatic electromagnetic radiation. In doing so, lasers play an important diagnostic and therapeutic role in present day ophthalmology, enabling ophthalmologists to lower intraocular pressure, remove lesions of the skin, and even perform refractive surgery. Vitreoretinal specialists rely heavily on lasers to treat a number of neovascular problems.

Choroidal neovascularization (CNV) underlies a number of visually debilitating eye conditions, including age-related macular degeneration (AMD), ocular histoplasmosis syndrome, pathologic myopic, and posttraumatic choroidal rupture, among others. The untreated natural history of CNV typically involves fibrosis, and if the lesion involves the fovea, concomitant vision loss occurs.

The Macular Photocoagulation Study (MPS) was initiated in 1979 to determine the effect of laser photocoagulation on CNV secondary to AMD, ocular histoplasmosis syndrome, and idiopathic lesions. The MPS was a series of randomized controlled clinical trials sponsored by the National Eye Institute. Between 1979 and 1994, the MPS evaluated extrafoveal, juxtafoveal, and subfoveal lesions, comparing laser photocoagulation to observation.

## LESION CLASSIFICATION

Historically, CNV has been classified by its location relative to the foveal avascular zone (FAZ), as determined by fluorescein angiogram. Extrafoveal lesions, which are located between 200 and 2500 microns from the FAZ, cause the least visual disturbance. Juxtafoveal lesions, which are 1 to 199 microns from the FAZ, and subfoveal lesions, which involve the FAZ, cause more profound visual complaints.

## EXTRAFOVEAL LESIONS

### Senile Macular Degeneration Study

In patients over the age of 55, AMD is the leading cause of legal blindness in the developed world. While only approximately 10% of AMD patients have exudative AMD, i.e., which is associated with CNV, 90% of vision loss in AMD patients occurs secondary to CNV. The first MPS study was the Senile Macular Degeneration Study (SMDS). This study was designed to answer the question "Is argon laser photocoagulation useful in preventing severe vision loss in eyes with evidence of senile macular degeneration and a choroidal neovascular membrane outside the fovea?" (1). To be eligible for this study, patients had to exhibit extrafoveal AMD-related CNV and visual acuity of 20/100 or better. Extrafoveal lesions were defined as being 200 to 2500 microns from the center of the FAZ.

At 18 months, 60% of untreated eyes versus 25% of treated eyes experienced severe vision loss, defined as a loss of six or more lines of visual acuity. Because of this marked discrepancy between treatment and observation, recruitment was terminated after 18 months. The initial cohort was, however, followed over time. By 5 years of follow up, 46% of treated eyes and 64% of untreated eyes had lost six or more lines of visual acuity (2–4), suggesting a significant advantage to undergoing laser photocoagulation for extrafoveal lesions. After 5 years, however, 54% of laser treated eyes developed recurrent neovascularization either contiguous to or independent from the original lesion. Despite this high recurrence rate, the SMDS showed that laser treatment to AMD-related CNV at least 200 microns from the center of the FAZ reduced the risk of severe visual loss.

## Ocular Histoplasmosis Study

In ocular histoplasmosis syndrome, CNV may emanate from previous areas of chorioretinal atrophy. When CNV encroaches on the foveal center, vision loss may occur. The ocular histoplasmosis study (OHS) was initiated to evaluate whether argon laser photocoagulation prevents vision loss in patients with extrafoveal CNV from ocular histoplasmosis syndrome. At 5 years, 10% of treated eyes lost six or more lines of visual acuity compared to 41% of untreated eyes (4). At 5 years, the rate of recurrence was 26%. This rate of recurrence was lower than that in treated patients with AMD and with idiopathic causes. As with AMD patients, laser photocoagulation of ocular histoplasmosis-related extrafoveal lesion was shown to decrease the risk of vision loss.

## Idiopathic Neovascularization Study

The idiopathic neovascularization study (INVS) was a separate arm of the MPS study that evaluated the effect of argon laser photocoagulation in eyes with extrafoveal CNV secondary to an unknown disease process (i.e., idiopathic). Like the SMDS and OHS, the INVS evaluated whether argon photocoagulation prevented severe vision loss compared to observation in eyes with idiopathic lesions (3). The small number of patients in the INVS precluded subgroup analysis. Despite a small patient population, however, the results suggested a treatment benefit from laser compared to observation. At one year, 40% of untreated patients compared to 18% of treated patients had experienced a loss of six lines of vision. As with the AMD and ocular histoplasmosis subgroups, recurrence was common. By 5 years, 34% of patients had recurrence.

## PROGNOSIS

Based on the results of the SMDS, OHS, and INVS studies, it appeared that patients with ocular histoplasmosis syndrome-related extrafoveal CNV responded better to laser than patients with idiopathic or AMD related lesions. Patients with ocular histoplasmosis had lower rates of severe visual loss and lower rates of recurrence compared to patients with idiopathic CNV and AMD patients. Although the sample size was small for idiopathic lesions, these patients seemed to have an intermediate prognosis between ocular histoplasmosis-related and AMD-related extrafoveal lesions. While AMD patients seemed to do the worst among these three subgroups, they still did significantly better with laser photocoagulation than with observation alone.

## TREATMENT PROTOCOL FOR EXTRAFOVEAL LESIONS

In patients who met eligibility criteria, treatment was carried out as soon as possible after the initial diagnosis. Two essential elements of the treatment protocols in SMDS, OHS, and INVS included a fluorescein angiogram within 72 hours of treatment and retrobulbar anesthesia to ensure akinesia of the globe and to facilitate treatment. Using argon blue green laser, the goal of treatment was to treat and obliterate the neovascular complex in its entirety. Treatment consisted of uniform white overlapping laser burns. The parameters were set such that each burn was 200 microns in size and 0.5 seconds in duration. The burns extended 100 to 125 microns beyond the CNV on all sides. If the CNV was within 350 microns of the FAZ, burn size and duration were reduced to 100 microns and 0.2 seconds to reduce the probability of treating the FAZ. When blood, pigmentation, or blocked fluorescence was present, photocoagulation was extended 100 to 125 microns beyond these areas. In treated patients, follow up was arranged between 3 and 9 weeks after photocoagulation, followed by visits at 3 months, 6 months, and then every 6 months if treatment effect persisted. A fluorescein angiogram was performed at each follow up, and any sign of recurrence was promptly retreated with laser photocoagulation.

## JUXTAFOVEAL LESIONS

### Age-Related Macular Degeneration Study–Krypton Laser, Ocular Histoplasmosis Study–Krypton Laser, and Idiopathic Neovascularization Study–Krypton Laser

After the initial success of treating extrafoveal lesions with laser photocoagulation, the MPS turned its attention to treating juxtafoveal lesions, which were located between 1 and 199 microns from the FAZ. As with extrafoveal lesions, juxtafoveal lesions were divided into AMD-related, ocular histoplasmosis-related, and idiopathic. Patients deemed eligible underwent krypton laser photocoagulation with the hope of obliterating the CNV and preventing vision loss.

As with extrafoveal lesions, laser photocoagulation decreased the risk of severe vision loss when applied to juxtafoveal lesions. The results, however, were tempered by higher rates of severe vision loss and higher rates of recurrence. At the five follow-up point, 61% of untreated eyes versus 52% of treated eyes lost six or more lines of visual acuity in patients with AMD. In patients with ocular histoplasmosis at five years, 28% of untreated eyes lost six lines of visual acuity compared to 10% of treated eyes. Similarly, among idiopathic lesions, 28% of untreated lesions versus 20% of treated lesions sustained severe vision loss at five years.

Initially, there was hesitancy to treat juxtafoveal lesions because of their close proximity to the fovea and the fear of inducing vision loss. These factors may have contributed to the high rates of persistence in juxtafoveal lesions. For example in the Age-Related Macular Degeneration Study–Krypton Laser (AMDS-K) study, 32% of patients had persistent neovascularization and 47% had recurrence over 5 years. This is compared to 10% persistence and 47% recurrence of extrafoveal lesions at 5 years. Thus, most of the difference between juxtafoveal and extrafoveal lesions was with persistence rather than recurrence, suggesting a possibility of inadequate initial treatment.

As with the other MPS related studies, patients enrolled in the AMDS-K, Ocular Histoplasmosis Study–Krypton Laser (OHS-K), and Idiopathic Neovascularization Study–Krypton Laser (INVS-K) were questioned about their medical history. During subgroup analysis it was determined that for juxtafoveal lesions in patients with AMD, normotensive patients experienced a greater benefit from laser treatment than did patients with a history of hypertension. In fact, AMD patients with hypertension and juxtafoveal lesions did not appear to gain a significant benefit from treatment.

As mentioned previously, the recurrence rate for extrafoveal lesions was high. Given the location of juxtafoveal lesions closer to the FAZ, one might expect the recurrence and persistence rates to be higher on the foveal side, since treatment may be impeded by the FAZ. In fact, this was the case. At five years, 78% of AMD patients had recurrence or persistence of the lesion, and 33% of ocular histoplasmosis patients had recurrence or persistence. Because the sample size for the idiopathic group was small, recurrence rates could not be reliably reported. As with extrafoveal lesions, therefore, patients with ocular histoplasmosis did best, with the lowest rates of recurrence, persistence and visual loss.

## TREATMENT PROTOCOL FOR JUXTAFOVEAL LESIONS

To be included, patients had to have AMD-related, ocular histoplasmosisñrelated, or idiopathic CNV located within 199 microns but not closer than 1 micron from the FAZ. Patients had to have a fluorescein angiogram within 72 hours of treatment, and retrobulbar anesthesia was administered to facilitate treatment by ensuring immobility of the globe. Pretreatment visual acuity had to be better than or equal to 20/400. Krypton laser photocoagulation was then performed with the goal of completely obliterating the lesion by producing a uniform whitening of the overlying retina. Treatment was aimed to cover the entire CNV plus an additional 100 microns beyond the edge of hyperfluorescence (on the side away from the FAZ or if the foveal edge was greater than 100 microns from the FAZ). If areas of blocked fluorescence were present, for example from blood or pigment, the laser was extended 100 microns into the area of blocked fluorescence. Treated patients were re-evaluated at 2 weeks, 4 weeks, 6 weeks, 3 months, and then every 6 months after treatment. If persistence or recurrence was noted, retreatment was performed.

## SUBFOVEAL LESIONS

Given the relative success of treating juxtafoveal and extrafoveal lesions, the MPS turned its attention to subfoveal CNV. To be eligible for these trials, patients had to have new blood vessels under the geometric center of the fovea as determined by fluorescein angiogram. Eyes with CNV under the fovea were known to have a poor natural history, and the hope was that performing laser photocoagulation might improve outcomes by decreasing the visual loss compared to the natural history (5,6). Patients with subfoveal CNV were divided into two groups, those with new choroidal neovascular lesions and those with recurrent lesions which had previously treatment for extrafoveal or juxtafoveal lesions.

Patients with new lesions that met inclusion criteria and who were willing to participate in the study were randomized to receive either argon green laser, krypton red laser, or no treatment. Ninety-seven patients underwent argon green laser, 92 patients underwent krypton red laser, and 184 patients were randomized to no treatment. Initially, treated patients were more likely to lose vision than untreated patients, because administering laser to the FAZ diminished vision. At 3 months, 20% of treated patients and 11% of untreated patients lost 6 or more lines of visual acuity. Yet, over time, treated patients were less likely to continue losing vision, while untreated patients were more likely to lose vision. At 24 months, 20% of treated patients and 37% of untreated patients had lost 6 or more lines of visual acuity. In fact, at 24 months, laser treated eyes lost an average of 3 lines of visual acuity, while untreated eyes lost an average of 4 lines of visual acuity. Laser treated eyes also retained better contrast sensitivity and reading speed than did eyes that were observed. Thus, in treated eyes, there was a higher likelihood of losing vision in the short term, but in the long run on average did better with laser than with observation. This study did not show any reason to favor argon green versus krypton red wavelength laser.

The results of the recurrent subfoveal laser photocoagulation study were similar to those for patients with new subfoveal CNV. As with patients with new lesions, there was an immediate decline in vision in laser treated eyes followed by stabilization as time progressed. At 24 months, 9% of treated and 28% of untreated eyes had lost 6 or more lines of visual acuity. As with to patients with new lesions, contrast sensitivity and reading speed were maintained better in the laser treated group than in the observation group. Because of the similarity between recurrent and new lesion study groups, the recurrent lesion study was halted prior to target enrollment.

## TREATMENT PROTOCOL FOR SUBFOVEAL LESIONS

Patients had to have a fluorescein angiogram within 96 hours of treatment. Fluorescein angiogram had to document a well-demarcated lesion, less than or equal to 3.5 standard disk areas (where 1 disk area was equal to $1.77$ mm$^2$) with vessels under the geometric center of the FAZ. Patients could not currently be using or previously have used systemic steroids and had to

be available for follow up for 5 years. In the new lesion study, patients could not have had prior photocoagulation. In the recurrent lesion study, patients could have prior laser photocoagulation, but laser had to have been outside the FAZ. The best corrected vision had to be between 20/40 and 20/320. If patients met these criteria, they were randomized to either krypton red or argon green laser or no treatment at all. Photocoagulation was performed according to the standard protocol, causing intense white burns and extending 100 microns beyond the perimeter of the lesion. In recurrent lesions, the laser burns were extended 300 microns into the old treatment scar, and whenever a feeder vessel could be identified, the feeder vessel was obliterated with burns 100 microns beyond the vessel on both sides and 300 microns beyond the base. Retrobulbar anesthesia was recommended in these patients, but unlike in the juxtafoveal and extrafoveal studies, it was not mandatory. In treated patients, follow up was arranged at 3 and 6 weeks post treatment, where fluorescein angiography was performed, then at 3 months, 6 months, and annually unless symptoms developed.

## CHOOSING WAVELENGTH OF LIGHT

Ideally, laser photocoagulation of CNV should pinpoint the neovascular complex, destroy it, and minimize collateral damage. Because the CNV is located subretinally, optimal laser photocoagulation should penetrate and bypass the retina without destroying any retinal tissue en route to the CNV. Where blood is present, the laser should penetrate the blood while being absorbed by the underlying vascular complex. Although many of these characteristics have been met with photodynamic therapy with verteporfin (vPDT), with "hot" laser there is no perfect wavelength that fits all of the above criteria. Until 2000, when vPDT became available, much effort and discussion went into determining optimal wavelength for laser photocoagulation.

It is important to note that certain retinal elements are more prone to destruction by different wavelengths of light. For example, blue light is highly absorbed by xanthophyll pigment in the inner and outer plexiform layers (7,8). Due to higher absorption in these layers, argon blue laser preferentially damages these retinal layers during photocoagulation. This may promote visual loss, and it destroys retinal tissue superficial to the neovascular complex. In addition, blue laser is also highly absorbed by the parafoveal vessels, making these vessels susceptible to damage when blue light is used. Conversely, red, green, and yellow wavelengths are minimally absolved by xanthophyll, making them more suitable choices for treatment close to the FAZ. Red wavelengths also have the advantage of penetrating blood, which is frequently part of the neovascular complex, as well as penetrating nuclear sclerosis which is commonly found in older patients, e.g., AMD patients. Although red penetrates well, it is not absorbed as well as other wavelengths by the hemoglobin found in the vasculature, including the neovascular complex, thereby making it somewhat suboptimal. Conversely, green and yellow wavelengths are well taken up by hemoglobin in the vasculature and they penetrate well into the subretinal space with little superficial damage to the xanthophylls containing layers (9). The disadvantage of these wavelengths is that they do not penetrate blood very well and thus are limited when subretinal blood is present.

Partly due to the above mentioned concerns around blue light, argon blue-green was abandoned in the juxtafoveal and subfoveal trials. By that time, preliminary studies were suggesting that using wavelengths other than argon blue-green may be advantageous especially as one treats closer to the FAZ (10–15). Krypton red was ultimately settled upon as the wavelength of choice in the MPS juxtafoveal trials, while the subfoveal trials included subgroups treated with both krypton red laser as well as groups with argon green laser. In those trials there was no discernible difference between the two wavelengths.

## FEEDER VESSEL TREATMENT

In certain neovascular complexes, a feeder vessel may be present. Feeder vessels are afferent vessels that perfuse the CNV from the choroidal vasculature. In theory, ablating the feeder vessel could diminish the inflow to the CNV and, by obliterating its vascular supply source, theoretically the CNV could be shut down. The first study to acknowledge the importance of feeder vessel treatment was the recurrent subfoveal MPS trial. In that study, feeder vessels were targeted (in addition to the neovascular complex) when they could be identified. However, identification was difficult with fluorescein angiography alone, likely leaving many feeder vessels untreated or under treated.

With the introduction of indocyanine green imaging, feeder vessel observation and treatment improved. In 1997, Shiraga et al. described feeder vessel treatment of AMD related subfoveal CNV (16). In their study, they utilized indocyanine green (ICG) guided videoangiography (vICG) to localize the feeder vessel for new subfoveal lesions. Of 170 patients, 37 (22%) met the eligibility criteria, which included identification of the feeder vessel on vICG. Yellow and red dye laser photocoagulation was then performed covering the entire feeder vessel and 300 microns on all sides with intense white burns. Importantly, the laser burns avoided the FAZ. Anatomic closure of CNV was achieved in 70% of patients, while 30% persisted or worsened. Preoperative visual acuity correlated positively with post treatment visual acuity and the authors concluded from this small study that feeder vessel should be considered as a treatment option for subfoveal CNV secondary to AMD. Feeder vessel treatment with ICG was short lived, however, because after a short time, vPDT came to market, followed shortly after by pegaptanib, ranibizumab, and bevacizumab. Furthermore, because of these new treatments, feeder vessel treatment was never formally put to the test in a large, prospective, controlled clinical trial and, therefore, its efficacy remains uncertain.

### Non-MPS Laser Treatment

Although the MPS looked at CNV in AMD, ocular histoplasmosis, and idiopathic situations, CNV can occur in a number of other disease states including angioid streaks, myopia, post inflammation (e.g., after punctuate inner choroidopathy), and

post trauma among others. Although large multicenter randomized clinical trials were not performed to back up such recommendations, many clinicians advocated treating these lesions with thermal laser, particularly when CNV was juxtafoveal or extrafoveal.

## LASER COMPLICATIONS/ CONSIDERATIONS

Laser photocoagulation may lead to several complications including inadvertent treatment of the foveola, secondary subretinal neovascularization, hemorrhage, contraction of the internal limiting membrane (17), rips of the retinal pigment epithelium (18), and choroidal ischemia (19). One of the most feared complications is inadvertent laser to the foveola. In the MPS studies, this was minimized by use of retrobulbar anesthesia to promote akinesia when treating juxtafoveal and extrafoveal lesions. When treating subfoveal lesions in the MPS studies, retrobulbar anesthesia was optional in part because treating the foveola was necessary so akinesia was less important.

Laser burn growth or "creep" is another manner in which laser treatment can deleteriously affect vision. Laser scars have been found to increase in size over time. If the original treatment is close to the foveola, e.g., with a juxtafoveal CNV, growth of the scar can creep into the foveola and diminish vision. Expansion of the scar may occur in both myopic degeneration as well as in nonmyopic disease entities. Morgan and Schatz (20) reviewed patients who had undergone successful thermal laser treatment for neovascular AMD. When followed for 2 to 81 months, they found that 70% of patients demonstrated an increase in laser burn size, with a mean growth of 290 microns. Similarly, Broncato et al. noted scar expansion in 97% of pathologic myopes over 12 months after successful thermal laser treatment (21). Over the first year, the mean enlargement was 103% with the greatest enlargement occurring in the same direction as the maximal extension of the myopic peripapillary crescent.

Another potential complication of laser photocoagulation is secondary CNV. Because laser photocoagulation disrupts Bruch's membrane, laser photocoagulation can provide a conduit for choroidal vessels to grow into the subretinal space. This may be one mechanism of recurrent disease, although this is a rare complication.

A rare complication was described by Iranmanesh et al., who reported a patient who developed a macular hole three years after thermal laser photocoagulation for an extrafoveal CNV. They postulated that contraction of the scar caused tangential traction on the fovea leading to a macular hole formation.

### Laser to Prevent Choroidal Neovascularization

Some preliminary studies suggested that applying laser prophylactically to the retina may reduce the risk of vision loss in eyes with high-risk dry AMD. However, results from different studies conflicted. Given the interest in preventing vision loss from neovascular AMD, the leading cause of vision loss in adults over 55 years old in the western world, the Complications of Age-related Macular Degeneration trial (CAPT) was initiated. The CAPT trial was a multicenter, randomized, National Eye Institute-sponsored clinical trial that sought to determine whether applying prophylactic photocoagulation prevented vision loss in patients at risk for developing neovascular AMD.

Patients underwent laser photocoagulation upon randomization and again at 12 months if drusen had sufficiently resolved. Using argon green laser (whenever possible) typical treatment consisted of 60 burns in a grid pattern using 100 mw burns of 0.1 second duration within an annulus of 1500 to 2500 microns from the foveal center. The intensity of the burns was desired to be barely visible, and 15 burns were applied in each quadrant without aiming for specific drusen. The results demonstrated no treatment advantage for eyes undergoing laser treatment: low-intensity treatment did not demonstrate any clinically significant vision benefit in patients with bilateral large drusen.

## NEW TREATMENTS

Although laser photocoagulation was a giant leap forward in the treatment of CNV, high rates of CNV recurrence and vision loss left clinicians hoping for more advances. In 2000, photodynamic therapy with verteporfin was introduced, allowing physicians to treat subfoveal (or juxtafoveal) CNV with less collateral damage. Shortly after, intravitreal pegaptanib, an inhibitor of vascular endothelial growth factor (VEGF) isomer 165, was introduced. Most recently intravitreal bevacizumab and intravitreal ranibizumab became available to treat CNV, the latter of which was FDA approved for intraocular use. For the first time a significant percentage of patients with neovascular AMD gained vision with treatment, while most patients at least maintained vision. In the current treatment environment, the role of thermal laser is minimal. Given the impressive results with ranibizumab and bevacizumab, one could argue that thermal laser should not be applied to any subfoveal or juxtafoveal lesions, regardless of etiology. The only situation in which thermal laser still maintains some utility is in the treatment of extrafoveal lesions. Yet, given its high recurrence rate even in these lesions (54% in AMD, 26% in OHS, and 34% in idiopathic), patients that undergo thermal laser must be followed closely. At the earliest sign of recurrence or persistence, clinicians should consider treatment with alternative agents.

## SUMMARY

In conclusion, laser photocoagulation was a tremendous advance in the treatment of CNV, which previously had no effective treatment. Despite vigilant follow up, patients who underwent laser photocoagulation had high recurrence rates and high rates of visual loss. Yet, patients who underwent laser photocoagulation for AMD, ocular histoplasmosis syndrome, and idiopathic lesions did better on average than did patients who were only observed. In the current environment, however, the role of laser photocoagulation for CNV is limited to extrafoveal lesions.

## References

1. Macular Photocoagulation Study Group. Argon laser photocoagulation for senile macular degeneration: results of a randomized clinical trial. *Arch Ophthalmol* 1982;100:912–918.
2. Macular Photocoagulation Study Group. Argon laser photocoagulation for ocular histoplasmosis: results of a randomized clinical trial. *Arch Ophthalmol* 1983;101:1347–1357.
3. Macular Photocoagulation Study Group. Argon laser photocoagulation for idiopathic neovascularization: results of a randomized clinical trial. *Arch Ophthalmol* 1983;101:1358–1361.
4. Macular Photocoagulation Study Group. Argon laser photocoagulation for neovascular maculopathy: five-year results from randomized clinical trials. *Arch Ophthalmol* 1991;109:1109–1114.
5. Bressler SB, Bressler NM, Fine SL, et al. Natural course of choroidal neovascular membranes within the foveal avascular zone in senile macular degeneration. *Am J Ophthalmol* 1982;93:157–163.
6. Guyer DR, Fine SL, Maguire MG, et al. Subfoveal choroidal neovascular membranes in age-related macular degeneration: visual prognosis in eyes with relatively good visual acuity. *Arch Ophthal* 1986;104:702–705.
7. Marshall J, Hamilton AM, Bird AC. Intra-retinal absorption of argon laser irradiation in human and monkey retinae. *Experientia* 1974;30:1335–1337.
8. Delori FC, Pomerantzeff O. Monochromatic light for treatment and diagnosis: Physical principles. In: Freeman HM, Hirose T, Schepens CL (eds). *Vitreous surgery and advances in fundus diagnosis and treatment.* New York: Appleton-Century-Crofts, 1977;587–597.
9. Trempe CL, Mainster MA, Pomerantzeff O, et al. Macular photocoagulation: optimal wavelength selection. *Ophthalmology* 1982;89:721–728.
10. Singerman LJ. Red krypton laser therapy of macular and retinal vascular diseases. *Retina* 1982;2:15–28.
11. Yannuzzi LA. Krypton red laser photocoagulation for subretinal neovascularization. *Retina* 1982;2:29–46.
12. Sabbates FN, Lee KY, Ziemianski MC. A comparative study of argon and krypton laser photocoagulation in the treatment of presumed ocular histoplasmosis syndrome. *Ophthalmology* 1982;89:729–734.
13. Singerman LJ. Total argon versus krypton versus partial laser photocoagulation for choroidal neovascularization in the presumed ocular histoplasmosis syndrome. *Int Ophthalmol Clin* 1983;23:83–100.
14. Bird AC, Grey RHB. Photocoagulation of disciform macular lesions with krypton laser. *Br J Ophthalmol* 1979;63:669–673.
15. Yassur Y, Axer-Siegal R, Cohen S, et al. Treatment of neovascular senile maculopathy at the foveal capillary free zone with red krypton laser. *Retina* 1982;2:127–133.
16. Shiraga F, Ojima Y, Matsuo T, et al. Feeder vessel photocoagulation of subfoveal choroidal neovascularization secondary to age-related macular degeneration. *Ophthalmology* 1998;105:662–669.
17. Avila MP, Weiter JJ, Jalkh AE, et al. Natural history of choroidal neovascularization in degenerative myopia. *Ophthalmology* 1984;91:1573–1581.
18. Cutler S, Ederer F. Maximum utilization of the life table method in analyzing survival. *J Chron Dis* 1958;8:699–712.
19. Shah SS, Schachat AP, Murphy RP, et al. The evolution of argon laser photocoagulation scars in patients with the ocular histoplasmosis syndrome. *Arch Ophthalmol* 1988;106:1533–1536.
20. Morgan CM, Schatz H. Atrophic creep of the retinal pigment epithelium after focal macular photocoagulation. *Ophthalmology* 1989;96:96–103.
21. Brancoato R, Pece A, Avanza P, et al. Photocoagulation scar expansion after laser therapy for choroidal neovascularization in degenerative myopia. *Retina* 1990;10:239–243.

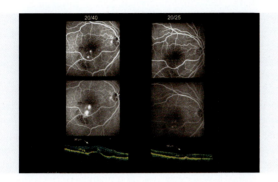

# Combination Therapy in the Treatment of Choroidal Neovascularization due to Age-Related Macular Degeneration

Albert J. Augustin

## INTRODUCTION

Over the past decade, many new treatment options are available for the management of choroidal neovascularization (CNV) secondary to age-related macular degeneration (AMD). These treatments help delay the progress of CNV, offering a temporary slowing, or even some reversal, of the new blood vessel growth. Some provide improvements in visual acuity (VA). The difficulty in finding a more robust and lasting treatment for this condition is multifactorial; it may be due, in part, to the fact that no single action or chain of events is responsible for the damage to the retina. Multiple pathways or factors are involved, and treatments must address each of these pathways in order to be efficacious. At the same time, care must be taken not to harm the normal vasculature of the retina in any way. For these reasons, it may be that combination therapies that target two or more of these factors could be the most ideal way to treat CNV.

## NEOVASCULARIZATION AND THE ANGIOGENIC CASCADE

In normal, healthy humans, angiogenesis plays a crucial physiological role in tissue and organ growth, wound healing, and many other processes. However, the irregular and uncontrolled proliferation of new blood vessels can manifest itself as cancerous tumors in many parts of the body. In the context of eye disease, this proliferation presents as CNV.

As the human eye ages, choroidal vascular atrophy leads to a metabolic breakdown where the choriocapillaris underlying the retinal pigment epithelium lose their ability to transfer oxygen and nutrients to the surrounding cells (1,2). The resulting oxidative stress and hypoxia cause local inflammation beneath the retinal pigment epithelium (RPE), and trigger the upregulation of vascular endothelial growth factor (VEGF), a proangiogenic protein that stimulates the formation of new blood vessels (3). VEGF also upregulates the production and release of matrix metalloproteinases (MMP) 2 and 9 which degrade the extracellular matrix and lead to endothelial leakage, and vascular endothelial cell migration and proliferation. Plasma proteins are expelled from the vessels and form an inviting bed, on, or around the perimeter of the vessels, where additional new endothelial growth (i.e., lumen and vascular formation) can take place (4,5).

These newly formed vessels extend into the RPE and Bruch's membrane, where they create edema and scarring (6) of the retina which can lead to permanent central vision loss.

Other proangiogenic factors that are upregulated and which trigger a strong neovascular response include transforming growth factors-α (acidic) and β (basic), and insulin-like growth factor 1 (7). These factors are not found at detectable levels in the normal RPE, but are expressed in the tissue of newly formed blood vessels.

## CAUSES OF NEOVASCULARIZATION

Although VEGF is the most important growth factor in causing new vessel growth, it is not the initiating factor. After normal aging, smoking (8) is one of the most significant contributing factors in the development of AMD because it induces oxidative stress in the retinal vasculature. Other risk factors known to induce trauma or stress in the blood vessels include high body mass index, waist circumference, lack of physical exercise, (9) elevated systolic blood pressure and subclinical atherosclerosis (10). Evidence from epidemiological and observational studies has been inconsistent, but the majority of studies suggest that a diet high in polyunsaturated, monounsaturated, and vegetable fats may be protective against AMD (11).

Importantly, it must also be noted that VEGF expression occurs as an epi-phenomenon secondary to other processes which have different triggers. It has been shown, for example, that the expression of VEGF is upregulated in the endothelial layer of the choriocapillaries as well as in larger choroidal vessels in eyes that have undergone photodynamic therapy. This expression of VEGF was not seen in areas of the same eye that had not been exposed to photodynamic therapy (PDT), or in the eyes of age-matched controls (12). Thus, a procedure that is widely used to treat CNV on one hand, also stimulates additional CNV on the other. Also, CNV itself triggers inflammation in the adjoining tissue, and this again, upregulates the expression of VEGF.

## TREATMENT OPTIONS AND THEIR LIMITATIONS

### Anti-VEGF Drugs

In the therapeutic setting, treating CNV is not as simple as targeting the angiogenic cascade or any one of its stages. Three antiangiogenic therapies are now widely available: the VEGF aptamer pegaptanib sodium, and the monoclonal antibodies ranibizumab and bevacizumab. Each of these acts by inhibiting the formation of new blood vessels, and has shown some efficacy in reducing CNV.

Rosenfeld et al. (13) showed that ranibizumab could reverse some of the loss in vision caused by CNV, with VA improving in one-quarter to one-third of patients who received monthly intravitreal injections. Gragoudas et al. (14) showed that loss of VA could be slowed with injections of intravitreal pegaptanib every six weeks, and that approximately 20% of patients had a gain of at least 5 ETDRS letters.

Bevacizumab is also widely used to slow or reverse the progress of CNV, although at present, it has not been approved for this purpose by the Food and Drug Administration in the United States, or by any other licensing authorities worldwide. An attractive feature of bevacizumab is that in small studies, it appeared to reverse CNV and led to an improvement in VA with one to three injections, sustained over several months.

But while anti-VEGF monotherapy appears useful for blocking new blood vessel formation, recent research has suggested that it also stimulates the release of compensatory proangiogenic factors which counteract its anti-VEGF activity, and induce new blood vessel formation. This compensatory reaction was not seen in laboratory animals that received a combination therapy involving three elements: anti-VEGF, an integrin-antagonist, and an antagonist of vascular-endothelial cadherin-mediated adhesion. It was observed in animals treated with anti-VEGF monotherapy (15).

This means that not only will the effectiveness of anti-VEGF therapies be limited when they are used as monotherapy, but that also, whatever role they do play may be temporary. Anti-VEGF will antagonize the CNV, reduce or stop vessel leakage and alleviate the edema, but this effect lasts only as long as the anti-VEGF itself. Once the anti-VEGF effect has worn off, leakage and edema recur. This will happen because the compensatory action of releasing new VEGF will continue to stimulate neovascular growth, even as the anti-VEGF treatment blocks the formation of abnormal vasculature. Patients could be required to undergo anti-VEGF treatments for an unlimited, and unknowable length of time. Furthermore, in view of the upregulation of proangiogenic factors in response to anti-VEGF treatment, this could suggest a rebound effect, should the patient ever discontinue anti-VEGF therapy (16). Therefore, controlling or antagonizing the upregulation of VEGF in any of its isoforms is now thought to be only one of the processes involved in treating CNV.

## Photodynamic Therapy

A second aspect of treating CNV is the eradication of the existing neovascularization. No matter how effective an antiangiogenic drug may be at preventing the sprouting of new blood vessels in the retina, it does nothing to address the issue of new vessel growth that is already established. Laser photocoagulation therapy has been used for many years in treating some forms of cancer, but its efficacy in treating CNV related to AMD has been limited. On one hand, the procedure uses a precise and focused laser beam, but the CNV is usually somewhat diffuse. The risk of destroying surrounding tissue, especially the photoreceptors lying on top of the neovascularization, is considerable. Also, the procedure can only be used for extrafoveal lesions, not subfoveal or juxtafoveal lesions. Finally, laser photocoagulation generally has a high recurrence rate. PDT was approved as a treatment for CNV in 1999 and offers a complementary action to that seen with anti-VEGF agents. While anti-VEGF drugs arrest, or slow the development of new blood vessels, PDT eradicates the CNV that has already taken place.

PDT entails the intravenous infusion of verteporfin (benzoporphyrin derivative), which is a red laser activated monoacid. The photosensitizer, once exposed to the laser light, releases highly reactive short-lived singlet oxygen and other reactive oxygen intermediates which lead to cellular endothelial damage, which then destroys the abnormal blood vessels. There is also further release of vasoactive and thrombogenic signaling molecules, which cause acute thrombosis of the capillaries, followed by decreased vessel leakage. Contrary to laser photocoagulation, only the vessels which have taken up the verteporfin are affected, and therefore, the surrounding tissue is not harmed.

Numerous studies worldwide have now demonstrated the benefit of PDT therapy in patients with classic subfoveal, predominantly classic, and occult CNV (Table 42-1). Most trials with PDT as monotherapy demonstrate a reduction or slowing in vision loss rather than an improvement in VA. Significant improvement of VA in large number of patients has not been seen in any of the major PDT monotherapy trials. The procedure mainly benefits patients with minimally classic CNV or mixed lesions. Smaller lesions respond better to treatment than larger lesions (Table 42-1).

In recent years, certain drawbacks to PDT monotherapy have been identified. First, the therapy requires additional treatments as new CNV arises. Past studies have reported patients receiving an average of 3.1 treatments over 12 months (17) and an average of 5.6 treatments over 24 months (18). Secondly, a small study (12) in elderly patients who had been treated with PDT showed overexpression of VEGF in the endothelial layer of choriocapillaries as well as within larger vessels. Overexpression of VEGF was not evident in eyes that had not been treated with PDT. The same sites showed positive upregulation of vascular endothelial growth factor receptor 3 (VEGFR-3) and pigment epithelium derived growth factor (PEDF). Thus, like anti-VEGF when used as monotherapy, PDT also stimulates VEGF expression, which could, in turn, lead to more neovascular proliferation. Furthermore, PDT is known to cause inflammation which exacerbates the cycle of VEGF upregulation and can trigger neovascularization.

Finally, an *in vitro* study has demonstrated that PDT resulted in a morphologically and functionally detectable breakdown of the outer blood-retinal barrier function of the RPE, although there was no damage to the RPE cells. Increasing the concentration of verteporfin however, can result in RPE cell damage (19).

## STEROIDS

The use of intravitreal corticosteroids has also been proposed as a treatment for CNV. There are several reasons for this. The steroid triamcinolone acetonide has anti-inflammatory properties and so could be beneficial in combating the inflammation that results from both oxidative stress and from PDT. All inflammatory cells are known to make and release VEGF (20), therefore, triamcinolone, and other steroids which have antiangiogenic properties could conceivably be used to block this VEGF expression. Steroids also have antifibrotic and antipermeability characteristics which help maintain the blood-retinal barrier. The results from several studies that have used triamcinolone as monotherapy have produced mixed results and were far from conclusive. However, when used in combination with PDT, triamcinolone seems to offer a synergistic action (21).

A significant drawback to the use of intravitreal triamcinolone is that it dramatically increases intraocular pressure (IOP) (22). Such increases in IOP can be deleterious for patients who either have, or are at risk of primary open-angle glaucoma, since the increases may exacerbate the trauma to the optic nerve head. Such increases in IOP have been known

**TABLE 42-1  RESULTS FROM MAJOR STUDIES IN THE TREATMENT OF AGE-RELATED MACULAR DEGENERATION**

| Studies | No. of patients | Treatment | Study design/ follow-up | Major outcomes |
|---|---|---|---|---|
| TAP-1[a] | 609 | Verteporfin PDT vs Pbo | 12-month randomized controlled study | 61% of patients treated with PDT lost ≤15 letters vs. 46% in placebo arm. |
| TAP-2[b] | 529 | Verteporfin PDT vs Pbo | 24-month. Continuation of TAP-1 | 53% of patients in PDT group lost ≤15 letters vs. 38% in placebo group: 82% of PDT-treated patients and 70% of Pbo-treated patients lost ≤6 lines. |
| VIP-2[c] | 339 | Verteporfin PDT vs sham | 24-month placebo-controlled (sham) randomized trial | 46% of PDT-treated patients lost ≤3 lines vs. 33% in Pbo group. 71% of PDT-treated patients lost ≤6 lines vs. 53% in the placebo group. Outcomes favored patients with lesions ≤4 DA dia. and/or visual acuity 20/50 or better. |
| VISION[d] | 1186 | Pegaptinib | 54-week randomized dose-ranging study | 70% of patients treated with 0.3 mg pegaptinib lost ≤15 letters vs. 55% in control group. 22% of patients in control group lost ≥6 lines vs. 10% in pegaptinib group. |
| MARINA[e] | 716 | Ranibizumab 0.3 or 0.5 mg | 24-month sham-controlled rolled, randomized study | At 12 months ~95% of patients lost ≤15 letters vs. 5% in sham treatment, arm. Patients in study group gained, on average, 7 letters over baseline vs. a lose of 10 letters in patients receiving sham treatment. |
| PIER[f] | 184 | Ranibizumab vs sham | 24-month. Ranibizumab monthly for first 3 months, then quarterly | Patients treated with ranibizumab had a mean loss of 0.2 ETDRS letters vs. 16.3 letters in patients treated with a sham. |
| ANCHOR[g] | 423 | Ranibizumab vs. PDT and/or PDT sham | 24-month sham controlled | At 12 months ~95% of ranibizumab-treated patients lost ≤15 letters vs. 64% in the PDT-treated arm. 36%–40% of ranibizumab-treated patients gained ≥15 letters vs. 6% in the PDT-treated arm. |
| PrONTO[h] | 40 | Ranibizumab monthly for first 90 days, then as needed for next 24 months | 24-month prospective nonrandomized case study | VA improved 10.7 letters and retinal thickness decreased 215 microns. Values returned to baseline in ~60% of patients. Mean number of treatments was 9.9 over 24 months. |
| Augustin et al.[i] | 41 | Verteporfin PDT Plus intravitreal Triamcinolone | 24-month interventional case series | VA at baseline = 20/133. VA at 12 months = 20/84. VA at 24 months = 20/81. 31.7% of patients had improvement in VA of ≥3. |
| Augustin et al.[j] | 184 | Verteporfin PDT Plus intravitreal triamcinolone | Noncomparative interventional case study | Visual acuity at baseline 20/125. Improvement in VA from baseline 1.22 lines on Snellen chart; 1.43 lines on laser interferometry. |
| Augustin et al.[k] | 104 | Verteporfin PDT, intravitreal dexamethasone, and bevacizumab | 40-week noncomparative interventional case series | At 40 weeks follow-up VA improved from 20/126 to 20/85. Mean retinal thickness decreased from 463.5 microns to 281 microns. |
| Dhalla et al.[l] | 24 | Verteporfin PDT plus IV bevacizumab | Retrospective case series | At 7 months follow-up, 20 of 24 patients had no loss or a gain in VA. Mean improvement in VA was 2.04 Snellen lines. |
| Ahmadieh et al.[m] | 17 | Verteporfin PDT, bevacizumab, and intravitreal triamcinolone | Prospective interventional case series | BCVA improved from 0.74 logMAR at baseline to 0.52 log MAR at 12 weeks, and 0.41 at 24 weeks. Retinal thickness decreased from 395 to 221 microns. |
| Focus[n] | 162 | Ranibizumab vs verteporfin PDT plus ranibizumab | 12-month safety and efficacy study | ~90% of patients receiving ranibizumab/PDT lost ≤15 letters. 11.4% of patients receiving dual therapy developed serious ocular inflammation. ~2% developed endophthalmitis. |
| Lazic[o] | 165 | PDT and bevacizumab in combination vs. each treatment as monotherapy | 3-month randomized pilot study | log MAR changes from baseline at 3 months' follow-up were +0.079, +0.223, and −0.012 for bevacizumab, combo therapy, and PDT, respectively (all <0.0001). |

BCVA, best-corrected visual acuity; ETDRS, early treatment diabetic retinopathy study; logMAR, logarithm of the minimum angle of resolution; Pbo, placebo; PDT, photodynamic therapy; TAP. study treatment of age-related macular degeneration with photodynamic therapy study; VA, visual acuity.

[a]*Arch Ophthalmol* 1999;117(10):1329–1345.
[b]*Arch Ophthalmol* 2001;119(2):198–207.
[c]*Am J Ophthalmol* 2001;13(5):541–560.
[d]*N Engl J Med* 2004;351 (27): pg 2805.
[e]*N Engl J Med* 2006;355(14):1419–1431.
[f]Genentech press release concerning PIER study: http://www.gene.com/gene/news/press-releases/display. do?method=detail&id=9747. Accessed December 28, 2007.
[g]*N Engl J Med* 2006;355(14):1432–1444.
[h]*Am J Ophthalmol* 2007;143(4):566–583.
[i]*Am J Ophthalmol* 2006;141:638–645.
[j]*Ophthalmology* 2006;113:14–22.
[k]*Retina* 2007;27(2):113–140.
[l]*Retina* 2006;26(9):988–993.
[m]*BMC Ophthalmol* 2007;7:10.
[n]*Arch Ophthalmol* 2006;124(11):1532–1542.
[o]*Ophthalmology* 2007;114:1179–1185.

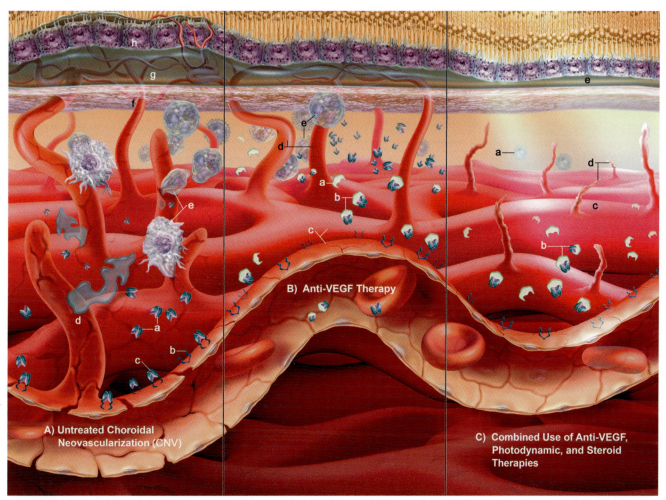

**Figure 42-1.**
(A) Untreated Choroidal Neovascularization (CNV)
    (a) Vascular Endothelial Growth Factor (VEGF)
    (b) VEGF receptor
    (c) VEGF binds to VEGF receptors
    (d) VEGF promotes neovascularization and leakage in capillaries
    (e) Inflammatory cells
    (f) Neovasculature penetrates Bruch's membrane and into sub-RPE space
    (g) Subretinal Pigment Epithelium edema
    (h) Retinal Pigment Epithelium (RPE)
(B) Anti-VEGF Therapy
    (a) Anti-VEGF
    (b) Anti-VEGF blocks the effect of VEGF
    (c) Anti-VEGF therapy tightens gaps in choroidal vessel walls and reduces leakage, inflammation, and angiogenesis
    (d) Existing CNV remains
    (e) Lingering inflammation
(C) Combined use of anti-VEGF, photodynamic, and steroid therapies
    (a) Steroid therapy minimizes inflammation from photodynamic therapy (PDT)
    (b) Anti-VEGF therapy deters further choroidal angiogenesis
    (c) CNV eliminated. Choroidal capillary walls return to normal
    (d) PDT eradicates existing CNV
    (e) Sub-RPE and sub-retinal edema subsides

to last for several months (23), and in extreme cases have required paracentesis to alleviate the IOP. A second steroid, dexamethasone, has also been proposed as a useful treatment. It offers much the same benefit as triamcinolone in terms of its angiostatic action, but has fewer side effects as compared to triamcinolone. Dexamethasone is a short-acting steroid, and has the advantage of being administered in solution form, rather than as a suspension; therefore it is cleared from the vitreous much faster than triamcinolone. Dexamethasone also exerts little action on the trabecular meshwork

and therefore is not associated with the spikes in IOP that are seen with triamcinolone use.

## RATIONALE FOR TRIPLE THERAPY

Each of these treatments, when used as monotherapy, seems to have its own benefits in terms of attacking certain

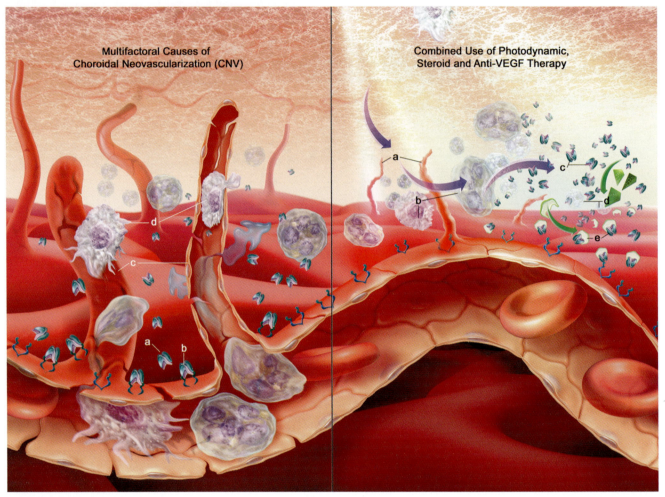

**Figure 42-2.** Multifactoral causes of choroidal neovascularization (CNV)
(a) Vascular Endothelial Growth Factor (VEGF)
(b) VEGF bound to VEGF receptor
(c) Formation of neovasculature
(d) Extravasation of inflammatory cells
Combined use of photodynamic, steroid and anti-VEGF therapies
(a) Photodynamic therapy (PDT) eradicates neovasculature
(b) PDT causes an inflammatory reaction that affects adjoining tissues
(c) Inflammation triggers new additional expression of VEGF
(d) Steroid therapy reduces the inflammation
(e) Anti-VEGF competitively inhibits the binding of VEGF, thus preventing formation of new vasculature

aspects of the angiogenic cascade. Each one has its drawbacks as well: PDT leads to inflammation which also stimulates VEGF expression; anti-VEGF drugs stimulate compensatory VEGF expression on their own; steroids increase IOP and the risk of cataracts. With that in mind, it is reasonable to propose that a combination therapy involving each of these treatments used concomitantly might offer some level of synergistic action. Dorrell et al. (15) conducted a study in the animal model using monotherapy, and combination therapies consisting of an anti-VEGF agent, an integrin-antagonist, and an antagonist of vascular-endothelial cadherin-mediated adhesion. The data showed that certain combinations were more efficacious than monotherapy, even when used at doses 100 fold less than what was used in the monotherapy arms.

Augustin et al. have suggested that when these treatments are used in combination, each will impart its own particular

beneficial mechanism of action: PDT will eradicate existing CNV; intravitreal steroids will combat the inflammation that is caused by PDT and other proinflammatory events; anti-VEGF will prevent the formation of new blood vessels (16).

Augustin et al. (24,25) treated a total of 225 patients having all forms of CNV lesions with the dual therapy of verteporfin PDT and triamcinolone. They reported that after one treatment, a majority of patients had significant ($p < .0001$) and sustained improvements in VA, and that for many patients, such improvements lasted throughout 40 weeks to two years of follow-up.

These study results show that combination therapy with verteporfin PDT and intravitreal triamcinolone is more effective than when either agent is used as monotherapy. However, the fact that retreatments were needed suggests that PDT/steroid therapy still is not entirely adequate. To address this issue, Augustin et al. (24,25) proposed that,

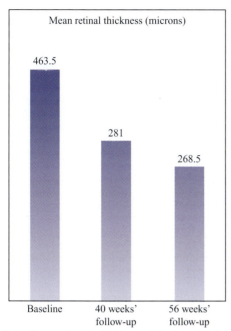

Mean retinal thickness (microns)

**Figure 42-3.** Changes in retinal thickness following triple therapy.

fewer treatments, and/or produce fewer adverse side effects (Fig. 42-1 and Fig. 42-2).

In an interventional case series (16), 104 patients with all types of CNV were treated with verteporfin PDT, intravitreal dexamethasone, and bevacizumab and followed for 56 weeks. The antiangiogenic bevacizumab was chosen over ranibizumab because bevacizumab, in a previous study, was found to improve VA by as much as 38%, and that this improvement lasted approximately 90 days, following a single injection (26). Ranibizumab requires an unlimited number of treatments, one month apart, which is costly and inconvenient for the patient. One of the endpoints of this investigation was to determine whether comparable sustained improvements in VA could be achieved with a single treatment.

The results of this investigation showed a mean improvement in VA from 20/126 at baseline, to 20/85 at 40 weeks follow-up, which corresponds to an improvement of 1.8 ETDRS lines. VA at 56 weeks follow-up was 20/79. There was also a significant decrease in retinal thickness, from 463.5 microns at baseline, to 281 microns at 40 weeks follow-up, and 268.5 microns at 56 weeks follow-up. This indicates that both functional and anatomical improvements were seen with this triple therapy (Fig. 42-1, Fig. 42-2, and Fig. 42-3).

Figure 42-4 shows both, angiography and optical coherence tomography (OCT's) of a patient from this series who suffered from a double retinal angiomatus proliferation (RAP)-lesion treated with one triple-therapy cycle. After 10 months the lesion is still inactive, OCT shows nearly physiological retinal shape and VA increased to 20/25.

owing to the entirely different but complementary mechanisms of actions among verteporfin PDT, steroids, and antiangiogenic drugs, a combination therapy involving each of these options could potentially improve VA. This improvement could be sustained for longer periods of time, entail

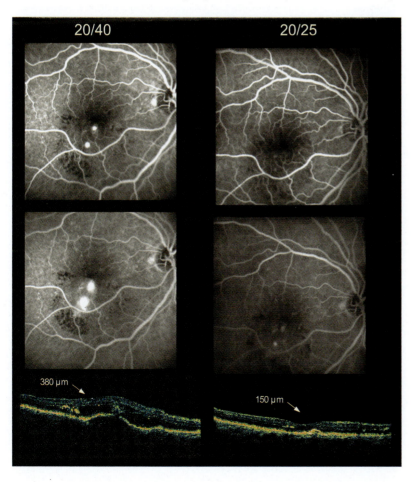

**Figure 42-4.** Early and late phase angiogram and optical coherence tomography (OCT) of a double retinal angiomatous proliferation lesion treated with one triple-therapy cycle. Left: Before treatment. Right: Ten months after treatment. The lesion is inactive; OCT shows nearly physiological retinal shape and visual acuity increased to 20/25.

One aspect of this particular triple therapy regimen which requires further study is the appropriate fluence rate for the treatment. PDT typically entails exposure to red light laser at 693 nanometers delivered at 50 J/cm$^2$ for 83 seconds. However, in this study, the fluence rate was reduced to 42 J/cm$^2$ and the time of exposure was reduced from 83 seconds to 70 seconds. This was done with the aim of limiting potential damage to the choroidal tissue. Other studies have also evaluated the use of reduced fluence regimens (27,28), but the results have been inconclusive and suggest that there is no advantage in safety or efficacy arising from reduced fluence or irradiation.

## CONCLUSION

Numerous treatments for CNV associated with AMD are available at this time, but there are limitations to almost all of these treatments when they are used individually. PDT eradicates existing neovascularization, but produces inflammation, which triggers the release of VEGF. Triamcinolone, used to treat inflammation, has some limited antiangiogenic potential, but not enough to arrest all angiogenesis. Therefore, neovascularization continues. This necessitates the use of an antiangiogenic agent. But antiangiogenics themselves induce the compensatory expression of VEGF and other proangiogenic proteins. Furthermore, the antiangiogenics which are currently available require regular treatments, either at monthly, or at 6 week intervals. Such treatments are costly, inconvenient, and may be traumatic to patients with macular degeneration, most of whom are elderly. Therefore, one drug or treatment will not address every link in this chain of events. Different drugs, and different procedures, used concomitantly will be needed to counteract each separate process in the cascade. Evidence at this time suggests that such combination therapies are superior in every way to monotherapy. Moreover, these therapies seem to have functional as well as anatomic benefits, and may achieve comparable end results such as improved VA, thinning of the retina and regression of the angiogenesis, with fewer treatments which have more lasting benefits.

### References

1. Penfold PL, Madigan MC, Gilles MC, et al. Immunological and Aetiological Aspects of Macular Degeneration. *Prog Retin Eye Res* 2001;20(3):385–414.
2. Beatty S, Koh H, Phil M, et al. The Role of oxidative stress in the pathogenesis of age-related. macular degeneration. *Surv Ophthalmol* 2000;45:115–134.
3. Kannan R, Zhang N, Sreekumar PG, et al. Stimulation of apical and basolateral VEGF-A and VEGF-C secretion by oxidative stress in polarized retinal pigment epithelial cells. *Mol Vis* 2006;12:1649–1659.
4. Ka T. Vascular endothelial growth factor: a potent and selective angiogenic agent. *J Biol Chem* 1996;271:603–606.
5. Steen B, Sejersen S, Berglin L. Matrix metalloproteinases and metalloproteinase inhibitors in choroidal neovascular membranes. *Invest Ophthalmol Vis Sci* 1998;39(11):2194–2000.
6. Ryan SJ, Mitti RN, Maumenee AE. The Disciform Response; an historical prospective. *Albrecht von Graefe's Arch Klin Exp Ophthalmol* 1980;215(1):1–20.
7. Ferrara N, Gerber HP, LeCouter J. The biology of VEGF and its receptors. *Nat Med* 2003;9(6):669–676.
8. Smith W, Mitchell P, Leeder SR. Smoking and age-related maculopathy. The Blue Mountains Eye Study. *Arch Ophthalmol* 1996;114(12):1518–1523.
9. Seddon JM, Cote J, Davis N. Progression of age-related macular degeneration: Association with body mass index, waist circumference, and waist-hip ratio. *Arch Ophthalmol* 2003;121(6):785–792.
10. van Leeuwen R, Ikram MK, Vingerling JR. Blood pressure, atherosclerosis, and the incidence of age-related maculopathy: the Rotterdam Study. *Invest Ophthalmol Vis Sci* 2003;44(9):3771–3777.
11. Seddon JM, Cote J, Rosner B. Progression of age-related macular degeneration: association with dietary fat, transunsaturated fat, nuts, and fish intake. *Arch Ophthalmol* 2003;121(12):1728–1737.
12. Schmidt-Erfurth U, Schlötzer-Schrehard U, Cursiefen C. Influence of photodynamic therapy on expression of vascular endothelial growth factor (VEGF), VEGF receptor 3, and pigment epithelium-derived factor. *Invest Ophthalmol Vis Sci* 2003;44(10):4473–4480.
13. Rosenfeld PJ, Brown DM, Heier JS. Ranibizumab for neovascular age-related macular degeneration. *N Engl J Med* 2006;355(24):1419–1431.
14. Gragoudas ES, Adamis AP, Cunningham ET. Pegaptanib for neovascular age-related macular degeneration. *N Engl J Med* 2004;351(27):2805–2817.
15. Dorrell MI, Aguilar E, Scheppke L, et al. Combination angiostatic therapy completely inhibits ocular and tumor angiogenesis. *Proc Natl Acad Sci U S A* 2007;104(3):967–972.
16. Augustin AJ, Puls S, Offermann I, et al. Triple therapy for choroidal neovascularization due to age-related macular degeneration: verteprofin PDT, bevacizumab, and dexamethasone. *Retina* 2007;27(2):113–140.
17. Verteporfin in Photodynamic Therapy study group. Verteporfin therapy of subfoveal choroidal neovascularization in age-related macular degeneration: two-year results of a randomized clinical trial including lesions with occult with no classic choroidal neovascularization–verteporfin in photodynamic therapy report 2. *Am J Ophthalmol* 2001;131:541–560.
18. Bressler NM. Treatment of age-related macular degeneration with photodynamic therapy (TAP) study group. Photodynamic therapy of subfoveal choroidal neovascularization in age-related macular degeneration with verteporfin: two-year results of 2 randomized clinical trials-tap report 2. *Arch Ophthalmol* 2001;119(2):198–207.
19. Mennel S, Peter S, Meyer CH, et al. Effect of photodynamic therapy on the function of the outer blood-retinal barrier in an in vitro model. *Graefes Arch Clin Exp Ophthalmol* 2006;244(8):1015–1021.
20. Möhle R, Green D, Moore MA. Constitutive production and thrombin-induced release of vascular endothelial growth factor by human megakaryocytes and platelets. *Proc Natl Acad Sci U S A* 1997;94:663–668.
21. Spaide RF, Sorenson J, Maranan L. Photodynamic therapy with verteporfin combined with intravitreal injection of triamcinolone acetonide for choroidal neovascularization. *Ophthalmology* 2005;112(2):301–304.
22. Jonas JB, Degenring RF, Kreissig I. Intraocular pressure elevation after intravitreal triamcinolone acetonide injection. *Ophthalmology* 2005;112:593–598.
23. Rhee DJ, Peck RE, Belmont J. Intraocular pressure alterations following intravitreal triamcinolone acetonide. *Br J Ophthalmol* 2006;90(8):999–1003.
24. Augustin AJ, Schmidt- Erfurth U. Verteprofin therapy combined with intravitreal triamcinolone in all types of choroidal neovascularization due to age-related macular degeneration. *Ophthalmology* 2006;113:14–22.
25. Augustin AJ, Schmidt- Erfurth U. Verteporfin and intravitreal triamcinolone acetonide combination therapy for occult choroidal neovascularization in age-related macular degeneration. *Am J Ophthalmol* 2006;141:638–645.
26. Spaide RF, Laud K, Fine HF, et al. Intravitreal bevacizumab treatment of choroidal neovascularization secondary to age-related macular degeneration. *Retina* 2006;26(4):383–390.
27. Azab M, Boyer DS, Bressler NM, et al. Verteporfin therapy of subfoveal minimally classic choroidal neovascularization in age-related macular degeneration: 2-year results of a randomized clinical trial. *Arch Ophthalmol* 2005;123(4):448–457.
28. Miller JW, Update on PDT. Oral presentation at American Academy of Ophthalmology meeting. Chicago, USA: 2005:14–18.

# Infectious Diseases of the Macula, Pediatrics, and Trauma

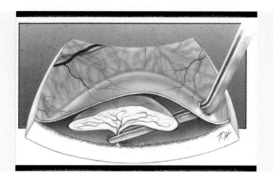

# Submacular Surgery

Nancy Holekamp

## INTRODUCTION

Submacular surgery evolved during the 1990s in an attempt to offer patients with subfoveal choroidal neovascularization (CNV) an alternative treatment to observation or laser photocoagulation. With the advent of intravitreal anti-vascular endothelial growth factor (anti-VEGF) injections for the treatment of CNV, submacular surgery is rarely used. Nevertheless, the surgical techniques of submacular surgery have refined and they are now an established part of the vitreoretinal surgeon's armamentarium. Submacular surgical techniques can be used to access the subretinal space to remove many types of CNV: subfoveal, juxtafoveal, extrafoveal, peripapillary, occult, and hemorrhagic. They can also be used to address other subretinal pathology such as fibrosis, parasites, and intraocular foreign bodies. The surgical techniques and their application in the treatment of submacular CNV are discussed in this chapter.

## SURGICAL TECHNIQUE

Submacular surgery begins with a standard 20-gauge three-port pars plana vitrectomy (PPV). The trocars used in small-gauge transconjunctival sutureless vitrectomy surgery do not allow the angled instruments required for submacular surgery. According to the surgeon's preference, a combination of 20-gauge and small-gauge vitrectomy may be used. The locations of the right- and left-handed sclerotomies are chosen to provide comfortable access to submacular pathology. It is helpful to have a preoperative angiogram available when choosing sclerotomy sites in cases of CNV. A sclerotomy site should provide straight line access to the retinotomy site and thus to the underlying subretinal pathology. In selective cases, it may be helpful to rotate away from the conventional 12' o clock surgeon's position so that direct access avoids previous laser scars, the papillomacular bundle, and the optic nerve (1).

After a core vitrectomy, the posterior hyaloid membrane is stripped from the retinal surface out to the equator in eyes without a posterior vitreous detachment (PVD). This may be accomplished with a vitrectomy probe or soft-tipped silicone cannula using active aspiration (2) over the optic nerve (Fig. 43-1) or with a 130-degree angled flat-tipped pick, a "hyaloid lifter" (3) (Fig. 43-2). Triamcinolone acetonide (TA) may also be used as an adjunct to vitrectomy to visualize the posterior vitreous cortex and assist with surgical separation of posterior hyaloid from retina (4). A Weiss ring should be seen to confirm the surgical PVD. This step is necessary because macular retinotomies are not treated with laser photocoagulation.

After a peripheral vitrectomy, the retinotomy site is chosen. Its location should provide straight line access to the subretinal pathology from the dominant-hand sclerotomy, avoid major vessels and be as far away from the foveal center but still within reaching distance of the submacular CNV. Small retinotomies near the papillomacular bundle do not cause postoperative visual-field loss (5). Therefore, a right handed surgeon operating on a left eye can use a retinotomy superior nasal to the fovea for subfoveal CNV access. A commonly selected retinotomy site may be the area temporal to the fovea near the

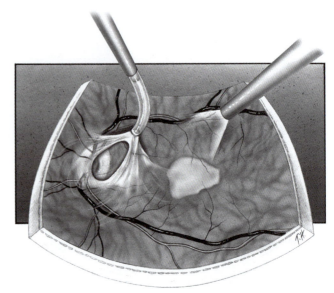

**Figure 43-1.** A soft-tipped silicone cannula is used to separate the posterior hyaloid from the retinal surface.

horizontal raphe (6). The retinotomy can be made by using a 36-gauge 130-degree angled subretinal pick to perforate neurosensory retina (Fig. 43-3). Care must be taken not to scrape underlying retinal pigment epithelium (RPE) or choroid to avoid bleeding or subsequent development of CNV (7). A 36-gauge angled pick creates a small, almost imperceptible access site to the subretinal space. It is ideal for small subfoveal CNV. Alternatively intraocular diathermy can be lightly applied to the edge of a large of extrafoveal membrane to create the retinotomy site. In this fashion, a retinotomy can be performed through the area of diathermy with a myringotomy blade (8). This creates a larger, more visible access site to the subretinal space. Any retinal capillary hemorrhages can be easily controlled by temporarily raising intraocular pressure to 100 mm Hg pressure. If utilizing the first technique, attention must be paid to the precise location of the small, almost imperceptible retinotomies, so that other instruments can be introduced in

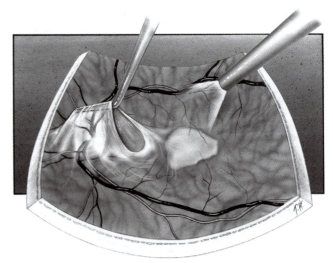

**Figure 43-2.** A "hyaloid lifter" is used to hook a Weiss' ring and create a surgical posterior vitreous detachment.

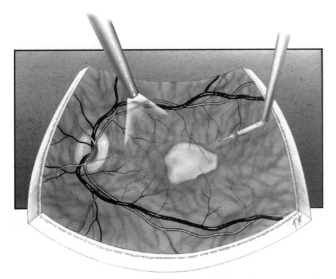

**Figure 43-3.** A 36-gauge angled subretinal pick is used to create a retinotomy.

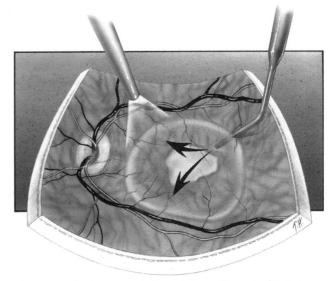

**Figure 43-4.** A 33-gauge angled cannula is used to create a limited neurosensory retinal detachment.

the subretinal space at the same site. If necessary, a retinotomy can be carefully lengthened with vertical scissors (6).

A shallow, limited neurosensory detachment is created to provide working space under the retina and to gain access to the submacular CNV. A 130-degree angled 33-gauge cannula is introduced through the retinotomy, and a trace amount of balanced salt solution is infused in a slow controlled manner into the subretinal space by the surgical assistant (Fig. 43-4). A vigorous infusion can blow a hole through the fovea or create a retinal dehiscence at points of retinal-subretinal adhesion. The angled 33-gauge cannula and concomitant hydrodissection can

be used to separate the overlying retina from the underlying subretinal pathology gently. Scars from previous laser surgery, fibrotic CNV, chronic lipid from the CNV, and chorioretinal anastomoses can prove particularly adherent. It is important to release all attachments to the neurosensory retina so that removal of CNV will not result in macular tears. There is also a 36-gauge microcannula available for subretinal use (9).

The 130-degree angled subretinal pick is used through the retinotomy to bluntly dissect the CNV from the surrounding tissue (Fig. 43-5). If the CNV lies anterior to the RPE, as in the case of a membrane secondary to ocular histoplasmosis,

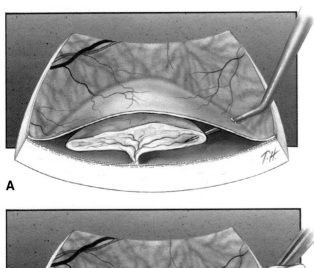

**A**

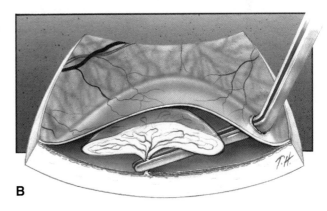

**B**

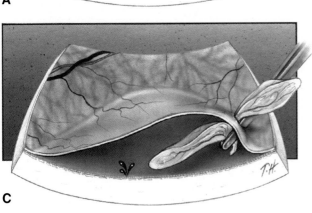

**C**

**Figure 43-5.** The angled subretinal pick is used to bluntly dissect the choroidal neovascularization from surrounding tissue. The edge of the membrane can then be grabbed with horizontal subretinal forceps. Hemorrhage at the vascular ingrowth stalk is prevented by raising the intraocular pressure.

the pick can be used to lift the edges of the CNV off the underlying sheet of RPE. There is a rim of fibrin that may also be elevated. All edges of the CNV can be dissected off the RPE, so that only the vascular ingrowth stalk remains attached to the choroid. If the CNV lies beneath or within the RPE layer as in membranes secondary to AMD, the pick can be used to dissect the CNV free from surrounding tissues and limit the area of RPE lost with extraction of the CNV. Pick dissection is carried out under normal intraocular pressure, but pressure is elevated quickly at the first sign of hemorrhage. If necessary, the endolaser probe can be placed behind the retina to achieve hemostasis by photocoagulation (6). After dissection and separation of the CNV, the 130-degree angled horizontal forceps are introduced through the retinotomy to grasp and slowly remove the CNV (Fig. 43-5). When the CNV has been dissected free except for the vascular ingrowth stalk, the tissue is extracted easily, leaving behind intact RPE. It is important to raise the intraocular pressure for hemostasis prior to disconnecting the vascular ingrowth stalk. Intraocular pressure is lowered slowly, with careful observation for any bleeding. When being pulled out from the subretinal space, CNV complexes usually fit easily through small retinotomies and can then be aspirated with the vitrector. Alternatively, the CNV complex can be removed from the eye through the pars plana, if histopathologic examination is desired. Occasionally, the tissue may be so fibrotic that it cannot be cut by the vitrector and may require enlargement of the sclerotomy and extraction through the pars plana. If the retinotomy is enlarged, additional endothermy may be applied at the edges sufficient to visualize the edges of the retinal defect (6). It may be desirable to laser large, irregular retinotomies if they are well extrafoveal.

In cases in which the RPE will probably be extracted along with the CNV, one must watch carefully for the cleavage point of the RPE. If it appears as though a large area of healthy RPE need to be removed, horizontal subretinal scissors can be used to cut healthy RPE from the diseased tissue. This can also be done to cleave CNV from adherent laser scars.

Indirect ophthalmoscopy is carried out to confirm that no iatrogenic retinal tears have occurred from passing sharp, angled instruments into the eye. If tears are seen they can be treated with cryopexy or laser followed by gas tamponade. If a large tear is visualized, then a buckle may also be placed. The retinotomy site is usually not treated with laser photocoagulation due to its macular location. Laser may be considered for certain circumstances such as large retinotomy, extensive subretinal blood or extramacular location. A complete air-fluid exchange is carried out, aspirating over the optic nerve head with a soft-tipped extrusion cannula. A 33-gauge cannula can be used to aspirate at the retinotomy, removing any residual subretinal fluid or hemorrhage. In uncomplicated cases, fluid may be reintroduced into the vitreous cavity with a soft-tipped cannula pointing away from the macula and retinotomy until only a 10% to 15% gas bubble remains. A full air or gas fill may be indicated in patients who cannot maintain face-down positioning after surgery. Postoperatively, the patient is instructed to remain strictly face-down overnight so that the air bubble can seal the retinotomy. A surgeon may use a nonexpansile concentration of

| TABLE 43-1 | SUMMARY OF SURGICAL RESULTS |
| --- | --- |
| Better surgical results in focal disease[a] | Poor surgical results on diffuse disease[b] |
| Ocular histoplasmosis | Age-related macular degeneration |
| Idiopathic | High myopia |
| Multifocal choroiditis | Angioid streaks |

[a]Often subfoveal retinal pigment epithelium is preserved.
[b]Usually subfoveal retinal pigment epithelium is lost.

perfluoropropane gas ($C_3F_8$) in aphakic or pseudophakic eyes to eliminate the need for prone positioning or to achieve prolonged gas tamponade. In phakic eyes, sulfur hexafluoride gas may be used. In cases of a large retinotomy or inability to position, silicone oil may be rarely employed (6).

## ANATOMICAL FINDINGS IN SUBMACULAR SURGERY

Submacular surgery was pioneered for the removal of subfoveal CNV resulting from a number of causes including AMD, ocular histoplasmosis, multifocal choroiditis, high myopia, angioid streaks, and idiopathic causes. With the advent of therapy utilizing agents targeting VEGF submacular surgery is less commonly used.

Surgical success after removing subfoveal CNV depends on the underlying disease. Eyes with subfoveal CNV caused by focal disease of the RPE-Bruch's membrane-choriocapillaris complex have a good chance for better postoperative visual acuity (VA) (10) (Table 43-1). Postoperative VA of 20/40 or better, in 30% to 40% of eyes with subfoveal CNV caused by ocular histoplasmosis, multifocal choroiditis or idiopathic causes have been observed in several retrospective series (11–16). With focal disease, the CNV membrane lies anterior to the RPE (Fig. 43-6). If the CNV is removed surgically, the subfoveal RPE is preserved. In contrast, eyes with subfoveal CNV

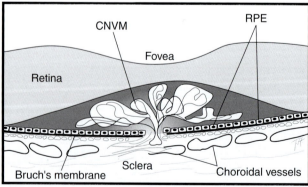

**Figure 43-6.** If the choroidal neovascularization has a single ingrowth stalk and lies anterior to the retinal pigment epithelium, there is a favorable surgical prognosis.

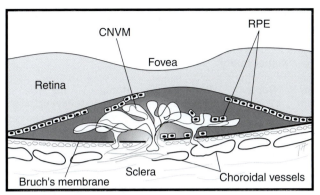

**Figure 43-7.** If the choroidal neovascularization has multiple ingrowth sites and lies beneath or within the disrupted retinal pigment epithelium, then the surgical outlook is guarded.

caused by diffuse degenerative diseases of the RPE-Bruch's membrane-choriocapillaris complex have little chance for better postoperative VA (10) (Table 43-1). Examples of diffuse degenerative disease of the RPE-Bruch's membrane-choriocapillaris complex include age-related macular degeneration, angioid streaks, and myopic degeneration. In cases of CNV secondary to degenerative disease, the CNV lies under or within the RPE (Fig. 43-7), when the CNV is removed, subfoveal RPE is removed as well. Following submacular surgery, intact native RPE is critical to foveal photoreceptor function and return of good VA (16).

## Surgical Case Selection for Subfoveal Choroidal Neovascularization

Case selection is important. Current techniques allow for the removal of subfoveal neovascular membranes, but do not adequately treat the underlying disease or degeneration of the subfoveal RPE-Bruch's membrane-choriocapillaris complex. Factors that describe subfoveal CNV with a favorable surgical prognosis are listed in Table 43-2 (10).

| TABLE 43-2 | CHARACTERISTICS OF SUBFOVEAL CHOROIDAL NEOVASCULARIZATION (CNV) WITH A FAVORABLE SURGICAL PROGNOSIS |
|---|---|

Patient younger than 50 years

Subretinal pigmented halo around the CNV

Sharply defined borders and plaquelike elevation to the CNV

No biomicroscopic or stereoscopic angiography evidence of retinal pigment epithelial elevation

Fellow eye normal

Good visual potential (i.e., no prior subfoveal laser)

Short duration of foveal involvement

Origin of CNV away from the foveal center

Few adhesions of CNV to retina or adjacent scars

## Complications of Submacular Surgery for Subfoveal Choroidal Neovascularization

Vitrectomy surgery to remove subfoveal CNV is prone to the same complications as other types of vitrectomy surgery. There is a small risk of endophthalmitis (less than 1%), retinal tear, and detachment (both less than 5%). There is also a risk of progressive nuclear cataract. In one study, the risk approached 80%, 2 years after vitrectomy in individuals older than 50 years. The risk was less than 10% in individuals younger than 50 years of age (11–17).

Other types of complications are specific to submacular surgery. There is an active blood vessel that is severed which may cause small postoperative hemorrhage. This hemorrhage usually clears spontaneously in a vitrectomized eye. Problems may occur with the retinotomy. If the patient does not position correctly in a face-down position, there may be a persistent neurosensory detachment of the macula. Particularly in children, positioning may be difficult and a full air fill is required. The retinotomy is usually invisible one month after surgery, but may remain open in cases of a second submacular surgery. Mild epiretinal tissue may be present at the retinotomy site. CNV has been reported to occur at the retinotomy site (18). CNV formation may be secondary to scraping the RPE with the 36-gauge pick. An extrafoveal CNV at the retinotomy site can be photocoagulated or may possibly be treated with photodynamic therapy (PDT) or anti-VEGF agents. Finally, peripheral visual-field loss after vitrectomy with the removal of subretinal CNV has been described (19).

The most common complication of submacular surgery is recurrent CNV. Depending on the underlying cause of the CNV, recurrent neovascularization can occur in 18% to 100% of eyes (Table 43-3). In a study of 117 eyes that underwent submacular surgery for subfoveal CNV resulting from ocular histoplasmosis, 44% of eyes developed recurrent CNV with a median follow-up of 13 months (20). Median time to recurrence was 3 months. In ocular histoplasmosis, recurrences occur at the original ingrowth site. If detected early, when still nonsubfoveal, recurrences can be treated with laser, PDT or with anti-VEGF agents. In fact, patients with laser-eligible recurrences did well visually in a small retrospective series (20). Because recurrent CNV following submacular surgery is common, routine postoperative care includes frequent fluorescein angiography to detect and treat early/recurrent neovascularization.

## SUBMACULAR SURGERY FOR NONSUBFOVEAL CHOROIDAL NEOVASCULARIZATION

The techniques used in subfoveal CNV removal may be applied to the removal of any CNV including: juxtafoveal, extrafoveal, peripapillary, occult, and hemorrhagic. However, anti-VEGF agents are also useful for these types of CNV, making submacular surgery a rarity. A few notable exceptions exist. It may be useful to consider submacular surgery for very large fibrotic nonsubfoveal membranes that create an elevation of the retina

**TABLE 43-3   SURGICAL RESULTS: A SINGLE SURGEON'S EXPERIENCE IN 247 CASES**

| Diseases | Postoperative visual acuity, % | | | Postoperative change in visual acuity | | | Recurrence rate | Mean follow-up, mo |
|---|---|---|---|---|---|---|---|---|
| | ≥20/40 | 20/50–20/100 | ≤20/200 | Better ≥3 lines | Same ±2 lines | Worse ≤3 lines | | |
| Ocular histoplasmosis (n = 120) | 35 | 30 | 35 | 40 | 44 | 16 | 42 | 13 |
| Multifocal choroiditis (n = 17) | 59 | 29 | 12 | 65 | 29 | 6 | 18 | 8 |
| Idiopathic (n = 19) | 21 | 26 | 53 | 42 | 53 | 5 | 37 | 10 |
| Age-related macular degeneration (n = 60) | 3 | 13 | 84 | 15 | 65 | 20 | 32 | 13 |
| High myopia (n = 17) | 12 | 41 | 47 | 12 | 65 | 23 | 53 | 10 |
| Angioid streaks (n = 5) | 0 | 20 | 80 | 0 | 100 | 0 | 100 | 6 |

and disturb visual function. Submacular surgery can serve to de-bulk such lesions. Another example would be poorly defined extrafoveal CNV that creates a very large exudative macular detachment. In one such case reported in the literature, VA improved from 20/200 to 20/25 with 18 months of follow-up after submacular surgery (21).

## EVIDENCE-BASED EVALUATION OF SUBMACULAR SURGERY

In the mid 1990's a randomized, multi-centered prospective clinical trial sponsored by the National Institute of Health was initiated to evaluate submacular surgery for CNV due to AMD, hemorrhagic AMD, and ocular histoplasmosis or idiopathic causes. These trials were called the Submacular Surgery Trials or SST. The SST Research Group was unable to demonstrate any benefit either from surgery for subfoveal CNV or for hemorrhagic CNV lesions compared to observation with respect to VA, reading speed, or contrast threshold in eyes with AMD (22–25). However, the trial found that removal of subfoveal hemorrhagic CNV lesions was able to prevent severe VA loss (26) for AMD patients with low preoperative VA due to large hemorrhagic or fibrotic membranes (26,27). In particularly large or thick cases of submacular hemorrhage, surgery allowed postoperative fluorescein angiography testing and if necessary, subsequent treatments (28,29). Thus, the conclusion from the SST for eyes with AMD was that submacular surgery was not recommended for CNV without hemorrhage, but it could be considered as salvage therapy for eyes with poor vision and hemorrhagic CNV. The Submacular Surgery Trial for eyes with CNV due to ocular histoplasmosis or idiopathic causes found a slight benefit for eyes with VA of 20/200 or worse at baseline (30).

In 2009, a systematic Cochrane review of submacular surgery for CNV secondary to age-related macular degeneration disclosed no benefit of submacular surgery in most people with subfoveal CNV toward preventing visual loss (31). Complica-

tions such as cataract and retinal detachment were deemed to be a significant consequence of the procedure.

## OTHER AVENUES FOR SUBMACULAR RESEARCH/ SURGERY

Submacular surgery is a particularly useful skill in the armamentarium of the researcher as well as the surgeon. Research regarding AMD and subfoveal CNV is ongoing as is demonstrated through the use of autologous transplantation of the RPE and choroid (32). Human photoreceptor transplantation has been performed in retinitis pigmentosa through the use of submacular surgery (33).

Submacular surgery also lends itself to hemorrhages associated with macroaneurysms and hard exudates associated with diabetic macular edema.

There are reports of visual improvement in submacular surgery with tissue plasminogen activator-assisted thrombolysis in hemorrhages involving the center of the fovea connected with retinal arterial macroaneurysms (34,35). Diabetic hard exudates and macular edema are difficult to manage. There are some reports indicating that submacular surgery was effective and safe in removing macular hard exudates from diabetic patients (36).

Finally, submacular surgical technique may be particularly useful in the removal of subretinal nematodes and parasites (37,38).

### References

1. Jacobi FK, Pavlovic S. Temporal pars plana surgery for submacular surgery. *Retina* 1998;18:70.
2. Mein CE, Flynn HW Jr. Recognition in removal of the posterior cortical vitreous during vitreoretinal surgery for impending macular hole. *Am J Ophthalmol* 1991;112:611.
3. Holekamp NM, Thomas MA. Surgical removal of choroidal neovascular membranes. In: Peyman GA, Meffert SA, Chou F, et al. (eds). *Advanced vitreoretinal surgical techniques*. London: Martin Dunitz, 2000.

4. Sakamoto T, Ishibashi T. Visualizing vitreous in vitrectomy by triamcinolone *Graefes Arch Clin Exp Ophthalmol.* 2009;247(9):1153–1163. DOI:10.1007/s00417-009-1118-2.

5. Holekamp NM, Thomas MA. Subretinal surgery. In: Guyer DR, Yanuzzi LA, Chang S, et al. (eds). *Retina-vitreous-macula.* Philadelphia, PA: WB Saunders, 1998.

6. Thomas MA, Williams DF, Gilbert M. Surgical removal of submacular hemorrhage and subfoveal choroidal neovascular membranes. *Int Ophthalmol Clin* 1992;32(2):173–188.

7. McCannel CA, Syrquin MG, Schwartz SD. Submacular surgery complicated by a choroidal neovascular membrane at the retinotomy site. *Am J Ophthalmol* 1996;122:737.

8. Berger AS, Conway M, Del Priore LV, et al. Submacular surgery for subfoveal choroidal neovascular membranes in patients with presumed ocular histoplasmosis. *Arch Ophthalmol* 1997;115(8):991–996.

9. Thomas MA, Halperin LS. Subretinal endolaser treatment of a choroidal bleeding site. *Am J Ophthalmol* 1990;109:742–744.

10. Gass JDM. Biomicroscopic and histopathologic considerations regarding the feasibility of surgical excision of subfoveal neovascular membranes. *Am J Ophthalmol* 1994;118:285.

11. Thomas MA, Kaplan HJ. Surgical removal of subfoveal neovascularization in the presumed ocular histoplasmosis syndrome. *Am J Ophthalmol* 1991; 111(1):1–7.

12. Holekamp NM, Thomas MA, Dickinson JD, et al. Surgical Removal of subfoveal choroidal neovascularization in the presumed ocular histoplasmosis: stability of early visual results. *Ophthalmology* 1997;104:22.

13. Berger AS, Conway M, Del Priore LV, et al. Submacular surgery for subfoveal choroidal neovascular membranes in presumed ocular histoplasmosis. *Arch Ophthalmol* 1997;115:991.

14. Berger AS, Kaplan HJ. Clinical experience with the surgical removal of subfoveal neovascular membranes: short term post-operative results. *Ophthalmology* 1994;101:1384.

15. Thomas MA, Grand MG. Williams DF, et al. Surgical management of subfoveal choroidal neovascularization. *Ophthalmology* 1992;99:952.

16. Thomas MA, Dickinson JD, Melberg NS, et al. Visual results after surgical removal of subfoveal choroidal neovascular membranes. *Ophthalmology* 1994;101:1384.

17. Melberg NM, Thomas MA. Nuclear sclerotic cataract after vitrectomy in patients younger than 50 years of age. *Ophthalmology* 1995;15:1466.

18. McCannel CA, Syrquin MG, Schwartz SD. Submacular surgery complicated by a choroidal neovascular membrane at the retinotomy site. *Am J Ophthalmol* 1996;122:737.

19. Melberg NS, Thomas MA. Visual field loss after pars plana vitrectomy with air-fluid exchange. *Am J Ophthalmol* 1995;120:386.

20. Melberg NS, Thomas MA, Dickinson JD, et al. Managing recurrent neovascularization after subfoveal surgery in POHS. *Ophthalmology* 1996;103(7):1064–1067.

21. Connor TB, Wolf MD, Arrindell EL, et al. Surgical removal of an extrafoveal fibrotic choroidal neovascular membrane with foveal serous detachment in age-related macular degeneration. *Retina* 1994;14:125.

22. Submacular Surgery Trials (SST) Research Group. Surgery for hemorrhagic choroidal neovascular lesions of age-related macular degeneration: ophthalmic findings. SST report no. 13. *Ophthalmology* 2004;111:1993–2006.

23. Submacular Surgery Trials (SST) Research Group. Surgery for hemorrhagic choroidal neovascular lesions of age-related macular degeneration: quality-of-life findings. SST report no. 14. *Ophthalmology* 2004;111:2007–2014.

24. Submacular Surgery Trials (SST) Research Group. Surgery for subfoveal choroidal neovascularization in age-related macular degeneration: ophthalmic findings. SST report no. 11. *Ophthalmology* 2004;111:1967–1980.

25. Submacular Surgery Trials (SST) Research Group. Surgery for subfoveal choroidal neovascularization in age-related macular degeneration: quality-of-life findings. SST report no. 12. *Ophthalmology* 2004;111:1981–1992.

26. Falkner CI, Leitich H, Frommlet F, et al. The end of submacular surgery for age-related macular degeneration? A meta-analysis. *Graefes Arch Clin Exp Ophthalmol* 2007;245(4):490–501. Epub 2006 May 4.

27. Thompson JT, Sjaarda RN. Vitrectomy for the treatment of submacular hemorrhages from macular degeneration: a comparison of submacular hemorrhage/membrane removal and submacular tissue plasminogen activator-assisted pneumatic displacement. *Trans Am Ophthalmol Soc* 2005;103: 98–107; discussion 107.

28. Shah SP, Hubschman JP, Gonzales CR, et al. Submacular combination treatment for management of acute, massive submacular hemorrhage in age-related macular degeneration. *Ophthalmic Surg Lasers Imaging* 2009; 40(3):308–315.

29. Haupert CL, McCuen BW II, Jaffe GJ, et al. Pars plana vitrectomy, subretinal injection of tissue plasminogen activator, and fluid-gas exchange for displacement of thick submacular hemorrhage in age-related macular degeneration. *Am J Ophthalmol* 2001;131(2):208–215.

30. Hawkins BS, Bressler NM, Bressler SB, et al. Surgical removal vs observation for subfoveal choroidal neovascularization, either associated with the ocular histoplasmosis syndrome or idiopathic: I. Ophthalmic findings from a randomized clinical trial: Submacular Surgery Trials (SST) Group H Trial: SST Report No. 9. *Arch Ophthal* 2004;122(11):1597–1611.

31. Giansanti F, Eandi CM, Virgili G. Submacular surgery for choroidal neovascularisation secondary to age-related macular degeneration. *Cochrane Database of Systematic Reviews* 2009, Issue 2. Art. No.: CD006931. DOI:10.1002/14651858.CD006931.pub2

32. MacLaren RE, Uppal GS, Balaggan KS, et al. Autologous transplantation of the retinal pigment epithelium and choroid in the treatment of neovascular age-related macular degeneration. *Ophthalmology* 2007;114(3):561–570.

33. Kaplan HJ, Tezel TH, Berger AS, et al. Human photoreceptor transplantation in retinitis pigmentosa. A safety study. *Arch Ophthalmol* 1997;115(9):1168–1172.

34. Humayun M, Lewis H, Flynn HW Jr, et al. Management of submacular hemorrhage associated with retinal arterial macroaneurysms. *Am J Ophthalmol* 1998;126(3):358–361.

35. Oie Y, Emi K. Surgical excision of retinal macroaneurysms with submacular hemorrhage. *Jpn J Ophthalmol* 2006;50(6):550–553. DOI:10.1007/s10384-006-0369-2.

36. Naito T, Matsushita S, Sato H, et al. Results of submacular surgery to remove diabetic submacular hard exudates. *J Med Invest* 2008;55(3–4):211–215.

37. Yamamoto S, Hayashi M, Takeuchi S. Surgically removed submacular nematode. *Br J Ophthalmol* 1999;83(9):1088.

38. Lerdvitayasakul R, Lawtiantong T. Removal of submacular cysticercosis: a case report. *J Med Assoc Thai* 1991;74(12):675–678.

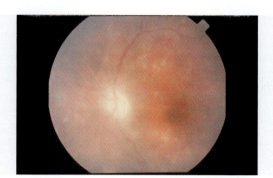

# Ocular Parasitic Disease

Rafael Cortez ■ Gema Ramirez ■ Lucienne Collet

In 1950, Wilder reported the first cases of larval forms of nematodal intestinal roundworms causing intraocular disease (1). This chapter focuses on two disorders associated with parasitic infections: ocular toxocariasis and diffuse unilateral subacute neuroretinitis (DUSN).

## OCULAR TOXOCARIASIS

Human infection by toxocara, the common roundworms of dogs and cats, can take one of two forms: visceral larva migrans (VLM) (2) and ocular toxocariasis (OT) (1,3). The form of the infection depends on the amount of parasites, site of infection, migratory behavior, and the host immunological response (4,5).

VLM is a generalized systemic involvement due to migration of *T. canis* second stage larvae. The patient with VLM is typically a child 6 months to 5 years of age, generally the course of the disease is subclinical, but it can be characterized by self-limited fever, malaise, irritability, pallor, anorexia, hepatomegaly, pulmonary signs, and marked eosinophilia (6–9).

OT appears in patients older than those with VLM, with an average age of 7.5 to 8.6 years and rarely have a history of pica (4,5). Toxocara and other VLM were found to be the cause of intraocular inflammation in 9.4% of all pediatric uveitis cases (10,11). Rarely, a patient presents with VLM and OT at the same time or at later times (4).

### Epidemiology and Life Cycle of *Toxocara Canis*

The adult dog usually acquires *T. canis* infection by eating eggs or second stage larva found in contaminated soil or infected meat or feces. The larva encysts, and if the animal becomes pregnant some of the larvae may reactivate, at that time they can infect the fetal puppies in the uterus. Following birth the larvae migrate to the puppy's lungs, then pass through the bronchioles to the trachea and pharynx where they are swallowed, and finally grow to become egg-producing adult worms in the gastrointestinal tract. The eggs begin to be excreted about four weeks after birth (12). Toxocara eggs are found in soil throughout tropical and temperate climates. In the United States and Western Europe samples taken from parks and other public places have yielded 10% to 30% contamination rate (13).

Humans are infected primarily from ingestion of soil (pica) contaminated with *T. canis* larvae or ingestion of contaminated foods (14). Humans are not natural hosts of toxocara.

After humans ingest eggs from the parasite, they develop into second stage larvae in small intestine, enter the portal circulation, hematogenous and lymphatic routes and encyst in tissues (15). Afterwards the parasites reach the eye through the retinal, ciliary and choroidal circulation.

### Clinical Presentation

Patients with OT present with unilateral decreased vision, strabismus or leukocoria. The disease is typically unilateral, cases with bilateral involvement are extremely rare (16). Youngest children do not report visual changes, even if visual acuity is deeply affected, parents may seek attention only when signs become striking. Consequently, diminished visual acuity is frequently detected on routine examination (17–19).

Several ocular presentations have been recognized. Probably the most common presentation is a granuloma either on posterior pole or periphery (14,17,18). In some cases the child may develop overt signs of ocular inflammation. In others inflammation may have resolved (19). Some patients may present with a more marked chronic inflammation in the retina and vitreous known as nematode endophthalmitis.

### Posterior Pole Granuloma

In the acute stage, retinochoroiditis appears clinically as a hazy, ill defined white lesion with overlaying inflammatory cells in the vitreous. As the acute inflammatory reaction subsides the lesion appears as a well-defined elevated mass ranging from one-half to four disc diameters in size (19,20). In some cases traction bands may extend from the lesion to the optic disc or macular area. In chronic granuloma large retinal vessels may enter the mass and disappear into its substance, probably representing retinochoroidal anastomosis (21) (Fig. 44-1).

### Peripheral Granuloma

OT can occur as an acute inflammatory process in the peripheral retina and ciliary body region (22). It may be preceded by a mild acute inflammation in anterior or posterior segment, or the eye may be quiet. The peripheral granuloma appears as a hazy, white, elevated reaction in the peripheral fundus, associated with retinal folds from the peripheral mass to the optic nerve head or to other areas of the fundus. In some cases the traction may lead to macular ectopia and severe vision loss (Fig. 44-2A and B). Wilkinson and Welch described peripheral

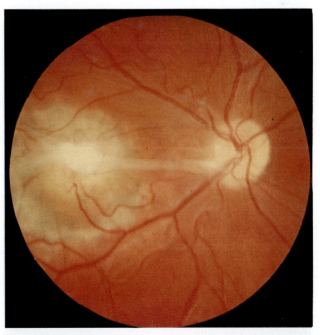

**Figure 44-1.** Posterior pole toxocara granuloma. Note a traction band extending from the lesion to the optic disc, and retinochoroidal anastomosis.

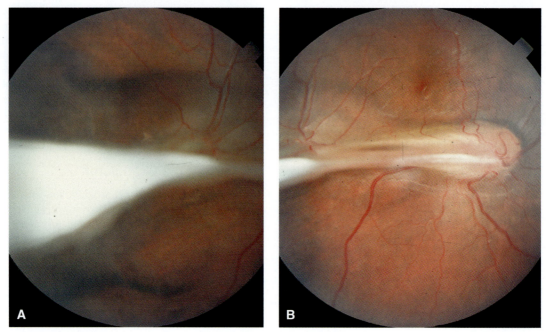

**Figure 44-2. A** and **B:** Toxocara peripheral granuloma with retinal fold extending to the optic nerve and macular ectopia.

involvement in 44% of eyes with OT (17). It is likely that many cases of "congenital" retinal folds are acquired in peripheral *T. canis* retinal granulomas (21).

## Chronic Endophthalmitis

These cases are usually associated with a cyclitic membrane, retinal detachment, low grade anterior uveitis, posterior synechiae (Fig. 44-3). The cyclitic membrane begins in the

quadrant of the most intense peripheral fundus inflammation and progresses across the posterior surface of the lens (21) (Fig. 44-4). Severe vitreitis may manifest as leukocoria (1). The clinician may observe through the hazy vitreous a yellow white mass, usually in the peripheral retina, which may resemble an endophytic retinoblastoma (21). Toxocara endophthalmitis does not produce much pain or photophobia and external ocular examination reveals only minimal signs of inflammation, usually with no ciliary flush (21) though hypopyon may develop

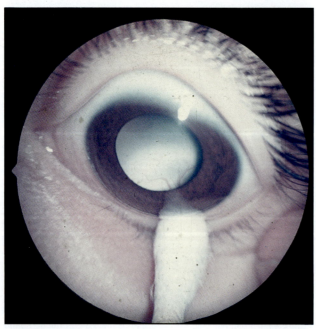

**Figure 44-3.** Cicatricial peripheral inflammatory mass and cyclitic membrane in a child with ocular toxocariasis.

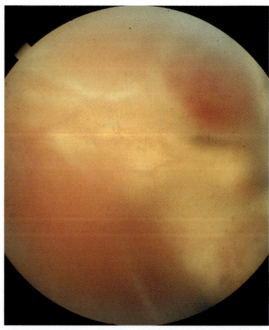

**Figure 44-4.** Toxocara chronic endophthalmitis with partial retinal detachment.

in severe cases (23). The cicatricial stage is characterized by tractional bands that may pull retina and ciliary body. Patients with endophthalmitis are usually younger than patients with posterior pole granuloma.

## Atypical Presentation

OT atypical presentations may include: optic nerve granuloma (24), papillitis (25), inflammatory iris mass, intracorneal larvae (26–33), motile larvae in the vitreous and retina (25), and scleritis (18). We evaluated two cases with vitreous hemorrhage; and after the hemorrhage cleared, typical fundus changes of a posterior pole granuloma were detected.

## Differential Diagnosis

Toxocara endophthalmitis may closely resemble an endophytic retinoblastoma (RB). Shields et al. found that 42% of patients with presumed RB had pseudoretinoblastoma, and among them 16% had OT (26). There are several clinical features that may help differentiate both entities. The mean age at presentation for RB is 22 to 23 months, while for OT is 7.5 to 8.9 years (4,5). RB show tumor growth. Finally, RB does not cause inflammation.

In OT cases there is vitreoretinal traction and signs of inflammation, and a posterior subcapsular cataract, which is unusual in patients with RB. In cases in which the differential diagnosis is relatively difficult, ultrasonography and computed tomography are valuable in demonstrating intraocular tumor and calcium (17).

Additionally, OT may present with eosinophils in the vitreous or aqueous humor without evidence of malignant cells and normal levels of dehydrogenase lactate and phosphoglucose isomerase (27). Other entities to be excluded are toxoplasmic retinochoroiditis, pars planitis, retinopathy of prematurity, familial exudative vitreoretinopathy, persistent fetal vasculature, Coat's disease, and organized vitreous hemorrhage.

## Diagnosis

The current test of choice to document systemic or ocular infection with *Toxocara canis* is the ELISA test (17,21) with 90% of sensitivity and specificity. Although the Center for Disease Control and Prevention consider serum ELISA titers less than 1:32 to be insignificant in the diagnosis of systemic toxocariasis (17), others have stated that a serum titer of 1:8, or even lower is sufficient to support the diagnosis of OT if the patient has signs and symptoms compatible with that disorder (17). However a positive serum titer cannot be used to absolutely confirm the diagnosis of OT, although the absence of serologic evidence of toxocara infestation may assist in reducing the odds of this organism as being the cause of ocular disease (17). Authors have found that 31.8% of 333 children without sings of OT exhibited a serum titer ≥1:16. Elisa testing of intraocular fluids has demonstrated to be of great value in diagnosing OT (19).

## Treatment

Treatment depends primarily on the stage of inflammation initially observed and the secondary structural changes in the vitreous and retina associated with this infestation (17). In most cases of severe nematode endophthalmitis, the natural course of the disease is characterized by numerous complications which frequently result in total blindness. Therefore, prompt treatment in cases of severe endophthalmitis is justified (19).

## Medical Treatment

In OT the treatment objective is to reduce inflammation in order to prevent the formation of membranes that consequently can affect intraocular structures (28). Periocular and systemic steroids (0.5 to 1 mg/kg prednisone daily) are the mainstays for eyes with active vitreitis. Cycloplegic agents should be employed when signs of anterior segment involvement are present (17). In OT patients treated with antihelmintic agents, clinical improvement have been reported. Thiabendazole (25 mg/kg twice daily for 5 days with a maximum of 3 g/day), albendazole (800 mg twice daily for 6 days), or mebendazole (100 to 200 mg twice daily for 5 days) (28,29). Although it has been suggested that antihelmintic treatment may initiate an intraocular inflammation due to a hypersensitivity response to the dead larvae (30) clinical and experimental evidence indicate that this is not the case (28,31). The ultimate utility of antihelmintic therapy remains an open question (19,28).

## Surgical Treatment

Surgery is saved for post-inflammatory complications such as persistent vitreous opacification, retinal detachment, epiretinal membrane formation with vitreomacular or optic nerve traction, vitreous opacification. (Fig. 44-5A and B) The most common surgical indication in OT is retinal detachment (32–35). Studies have shown that the retina can be reattached in 71% to 88% of the cases, with visual improvement in most patients (34).

## DIFFUSE UNILATERAL SUBACUTE NEURORETINITIS

DUSN was first described by Gass and Scelfo in 1978 (36). They reported 29 patients between the ages 5 and 22 years, with severe visual loss in one eye, vitreitis, mild papillitis, and recurrent crops of evanescent, gray-white lesions affecting the outer retina and retinal pigment epithelium (RPE). These lesions are followed by progressive loss of visual field, optic atrophy, narrowing of the major retinal vessel, diffuse as well as focal RPE depigmentation throughout the fundus, and a moderate to marked reduction of the b-wave amplitude in the multifocal electroretinogram (mfERG). Previously this condition was described as "unilateral wipe-out syndrome" (37). In a later report, 12 additional patients were described, and in two of them a motile subretinal nematode was observed (38).

DUSN is prevalent in southeastern USA and the Caribbean, although some cases have been reported in the upper midwestern USA, Canada, the Caribbean, the northern part of South America, Europe, and China (39–41). In the United States, DUSN probably is caused by at least two different nematodes. The smaller one measures between 400 and 1000 um in length, and has a diameter of approximately one twentieth of its length

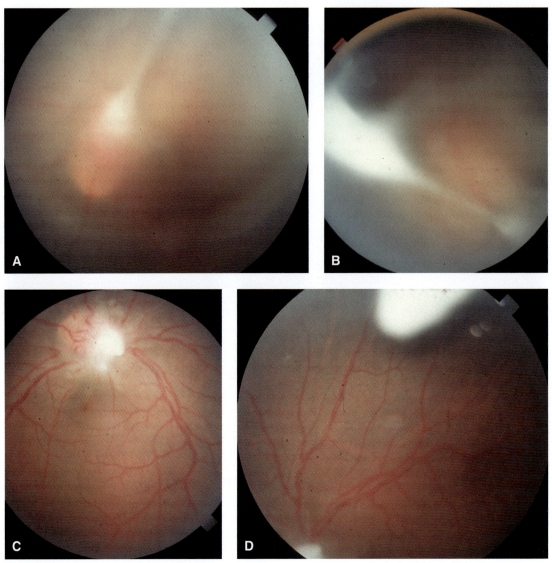

**Figure 44-5.** **A**1 and **B**1: Toxocara peripheral granuloma with tractional fibrotic band extending to the optic nerve. **A**2 and **B**2: Same case as **A**1 and **B**1 after pars plana vitrectomy.

(39,41). It is found in patients mainly from the southeastern US, the Caribbean, and the northern part of South America (39–41). A larger nematode, 1500 to 2000 um in length, is responsible for DUSN in patients in the northern midwestern USA, and in some patients from Brazil, however one case was reported in Brazil caused by a large nematode (41–43).

## Clinical Manifestations

Ocular findings in DUSN have been well described by Gass and associates (36,38,39). Most patients are young and healthy, ranging in age from 11 to 65 years (mean 24 years) at the time of the initial examination. It is for the most part, a unilateral condition; bilateral cases have been described even though it is not common (41,43–45).

Many patients, particularly children, may be asymptomatic until visual loss is discovered in a routine eye examination. Other patients may present with acute onset of multiple rapidly

changing paracentral or central scotoma, photopsias or vision loss in one eye (38,46). In the early stages, inflammation in the anterior segment is uncommon, though in one patient keratic precipitates and hypopyon were observed and reported (38). Visual acuity may be reduced moderately if the condition is detected early, but usually it is markedly decreased at the time of presentation.

The fundus changes, which are the most prominent feature of this syndrome, have been divided into early and late findings (38). Onset of DUSN is subtle and progressive (36). Patients in the early stages of the disease may present with low vision in the affected eye, mild to moderate vitreitis, optic-disc swelling, and recurrent crops of evanescent, multifocal gray-white lesions at the level of the outer retina. The lesions typically are clustered in one segment of the fundus, and successive crops of these lesions may recur in close proximity to previously affected areas. The nematode, which often assumes an S-shape or coiled configuration, should be sought in the

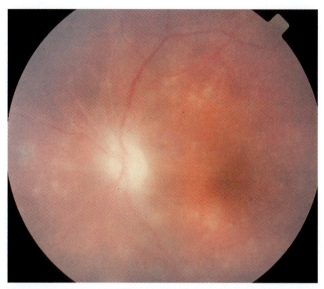

**Figure 44-6.** Early-stage diffuse unilateral subacute neuroretinitis: vitre-itis, optic disc swelling, and crops of multifocal gray-white lesions.

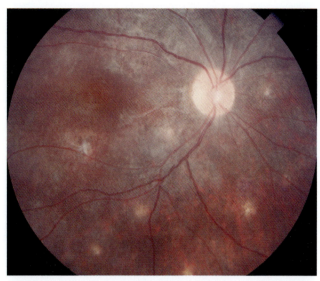

**Figure 44-8.** Late-stage diffuse unilateral subacute neuroretinitis. Diffuse as well as focal changes of retinal pigment epithelium. Narrowing of retinal arterioles and mild optic nerve pallor.

vicinity of the active lesions. In the absence of these white lesions there are not clues of the location of the worm. Nematodes (47,48) propel themselves by series of slow coiling and uncoiling movements, or some times by slithering, snake-like movements. The examining light seems to stimulate movements in the nematode and makes it move deeper into the subretinal space, consequently the clinician looses the possibility to identify it; in these cases the light should be turned off and wait for several seconds until the worm re-appears and rises from deep structures (36,38,47).

Occasionally, perivenous exudation and sheathing, cystoid macular edema, intraretinal and subretinal hemorrhages, retinal exudation, and neovascularization might be found during the early stages of the disease (38,48) (Figs. 44-6 and 44-7A and B).

Over a period of weeks to months late onset manifestations gradually appear (37). The changes are usually less prominent in the central area, characterized as diffuse and focal RPE depigmentation, however pigment spicule formation is uncommon. There is a gradual narrowing of the retinal vessels and increasing optic disc pallor, in consequence it is frequent to observe an afferent pupillary defect. In general, the degree of optic disc pallor and retinal vessels narrowing parallel that of central visual loss, but striking exceptions occur (36,38) (Figs. 44-8 and 44-9).

Fluorescein angiography (FA) shows hypofluorescent lesions that turn hyperfluorescent in the late stages of the study, as well as leakage of the dye at the level of optic nerve and active lesions, and petaloid hyperfluorescence in cases with cystoid macular edema. In more advanced stages of the

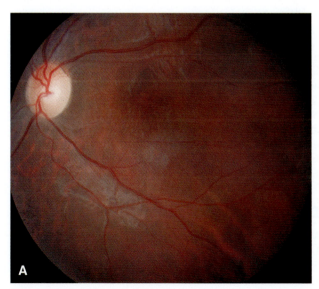

**Figure 44-7. A** and **B:** Early-stage diffuse unilateral subacute neuroretinitis. The parasite was visualized in an area of slight retinal changes.

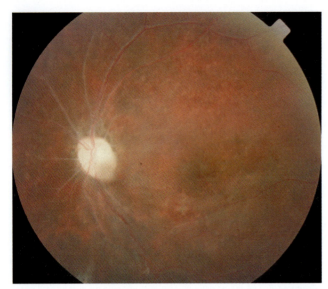

**Figure 44-9.** Late-stage diffuse unilateral subacute neuroretinitis. Optic nerve atrophy, diffuse changes of retinal pigment epithelium, narrowing of retinal vessels.

disease, FA may show multiple hyperfluorescent lesions due to window defects secondary to RPE alterations together with a delay in the retinal circulation time (38).

In Venezuela evaluation of 78 patients showed in most cases the typical fundoscopic late changes described by Gass et al. (39,41). The mean age of these patients was 16.7 years, the presenting visual acuity was 20/400 or worse in 69 patients (84.1%). Additionally the subretinal nematode was identified in 33 eyes (40.2%), all the nematodes were small, measuring approximately 400 um in length.

## Diagnosis

Frequently, patients with DUSN have progressive loss of vision, and seek for medical attention in the late stages of the disease. Consequently, the clinician should focus on the early recognition of this syndrome, because treatment may prevent further deterioration of visual function and occasionally is followed by visual improvement (38). In suspicious patients we suggest first an evaluation with indirect ophthalmoscopy using a 20-diopter lens (or in some cases a 14-diopter lens) in order to locate the crops of evanescent white lesions and seek for the nematode near these areas. Subsequent biomicroscopy with a 78-diopter lens in that area allows the examiner to definitely identify the nematode (37,39,49). In the absence of white lesions, a careful biomicroscopic search of the entire fundus is necessary to find the worm, and some patients may require multiple visits. It is also possible to identify the parasite by careful examination of fundus photographs that include the suspicious areas (49).

FA is not helpful locating the nematode (39). Scanning laser ophthalmoscope using a blue light can help identify the worm due to its property of enhancing contrast, improving visualization, and recording a videography of the worms' movements (50).

MfERG is subnormal in the affected eye during all the stages of the disease, with b-wave being more affected than a-wave. Rarely mfERG is extinguished (37,39). Serologic studies, stool examination, and peripheral blood smears are of little value in the diagnosis of DUSN (38). *Toxocara* and *Baylisascaris procyonis* antibody titers have been suggested as diagnostic tools to try to characterize which nematode is producing the disease (51). No serologic test is currently available for *Ancylostoma*. Because of the possibility of commonly shared antigens by different nematodes, or seropositivity unrelated to the actual infesting nematode, interpretation of serologic testing is subject to some error (48).

## Etiology and Pathogenesis

There is no agreement on the identification of the subretinal nematode frequently found in DUSN syndrome. Reports suggest *Baylisascaris procyonis* (52), *Ancylostoma caninum* (53), *Dirofilaria* (54) and a larval form of *Toxocara canis* (55) as possible infectious agents involved in DUSN. However, the larval form of *T. canis* is smaller than the worm causing DUSN, and also there is lack of serologic evidence; the fundoscopic manifestations are different from those associated with other forms of ocular toxocariasis; and the prevalence of *T. canis* is not related with the few number of DUSN cases (39).

*A. caninum*, which is a common nematode that parasites dogs, is a suspect of causing DUSN because it frequently causes cutaneous larva migrans and it has been observed that some cases of cutaneous larva migrans later develop signs of DUSN. The worm can survive for months, even years without changing shape and its infective larva measures approximately 650 microns which corresponds with the agent described in DUSN (37). Scanning electron microscopic examination of a nematode excised from a case of DUSN by means of an eye wall biopsy was compatible but not diagnostic for *A. caninum* (53).

*Baylisascaris procyonis* is an intestinal nematode that infects raccoons and skunks, the larva measures between 300 to 2000 microns, and it has been proposed as the larger nematode causing DUSN (51,52). The infrequent history of exposure to raccoons or shunks, and the absence of central nervous system involvement make *B. procyonis* a highly unlikely cause of DUSN.

The pathogenesis of DUSN appears to involve a mechanical disruption and inflammation of the outer retina, as well as a local toxic effect on the outer retina caused by bioproducts left in the worm's wake, and a more diffuse toxic reaction affecting both the inner and outer retinal tissues (39,53)

Histopathologic study of an eye from a patient believed to be affected by DUSN, revealed a nongranulomatous vitreitis and retinitis, as well as retinal and optic nerve perivasculitis, extensive degeneration of the posterior retina, mild optic atrophy, mild degenerative changes in RPE, and a low-grade, patchy, nongranulomatous choroiditis (38).

## Differential Diagnosis

Many inflammatory conditions may mimic the early stages of DUSN such as posterior multifocal placoid pigment epitheliopathy (AMPPE), multiple evanescent white-dot syndrome (MEWDS), multifocal choroiditis (MC). In the early stages it may mimic toxoplasmosis, cytomegalovirus, bacterial abscess which all affect inner retina and leave a scar in the area of retinitis. Additionally, serpiginous choroiditis and AMPPE may resemble DUSN but in these cases patients may present with loss of vision if the lesions affect the center of the macular area with subsequent RPE defects. MEWDS can be distinguished from DUSN because MEWDS is accompanied by history of flu-like symptoms and photophobia, wreathlike hyperfluorescent dots in the FA, blind spot enlargement, multiple gray or whitish outer retinal lesions, mfERG decreased recordings and visual acuity may return even to normal levels in some cases after several weeks or months. On FA the white lesions in DUSN block the fluorescence in the early phases while in MEWDS the lesions are hyperfluorescent since the early stages of the angiogram. Additionally, DUSN may look like sarcoidosis in cases that show candle wax dripping exudate or subretinal exudates (53).

Due to the appearance of focal chorioretinal scars scattered throughout the fundus, sometimes DUSN may be mistaken with presumed ocular histoplasmosis syndrome (POHS), and MC, but what differentiates these entities from DUSN is the absence of optic atrophy, vitreitis, vessel attenuation, presence of normal looking RPE between punched out lesions. Eyes with central artery occlusion may show some characteristics that look like DUSN. Also, the late stages of DUSN may be confused with retinitis pigmentosa, secondary bone-spicule migration and posterior subcapsular opacification, but unilaterality it is characteristically a DUSN feature. Trauma may show some DUSN characteristics such as RPE changes, and optic atrophy.

# Treatment

Photocoagulation of the parasite, when it is localized, using 200 to 500 um, 0.2 to 0.5 s of thermal laser application is the treatment of choice. It causes no post-treatment exacerbation of inflammation, and it is successful in causing prompt and permanent inactivation of the disease. Visual acuity does not improve significantly unless the worm is killed soon after onset of visual loss (48).

One study showed that the use of the antihelmintic agents, such as thiabendazole and diethylcarbamazine in the treatment of patients with DUSN did not affect the vitality of the worm (39). It was concluded that in most patients the drug did not cross the blood- retina barrier in adequate concentration in order to affect the subretinal nematode (47). It has been suggested that if the worm cannot be found in a patient with vitreitis associated with a breakdown in the blood retinal barrier, another option is to perform a scatter pattern of laser burns in the vicinity of the multifocal active lesions to alter the blood-retinal barrier, before the administration of thiabendazole (22 mg/kg) administrated twice daily for 2 to 4 consecutive days (47,53,56). Additionally albendazole has been used to treat 6 patients with DUSN, during a 10 days course of 200 mg orally 3 times daily (41). The nematode was killed and was slowly reabsorbed in three of them. Adverse effects of a short term of albendazole are rare (41). Findings such as bilateral cases of DUSN, and the presence of a nematode in a patient who has undergone successful photocoagulation have been described. In light of these findings we recommend a course of systemic therapy in each patient with DUSN (41).

# References

1. Wilder HC. Nematode endophthalmitis. *Trans Am Acad Ophthalmol Otolaryngol* 1950;55:99–109.
2. Beaver PC, Snyder CH, Carrera GM, et al. Chronic eosinophilia due to visceral larva migrans. *Pediatrics* 1952;9:7–19.
3. Nichols RL. The etiology of visceral larva migrans I. Diagnostic morphology of infective second stage Toxocara Larvae. *J Parasitol* 1956;42:349–362.
4. Brown D. Ocular toxocara canis II. *J Pediatr Ophthalmol* 1970;7:182–191.
5. Schantz P, Meyer D, Glickman L. Clinical, serologic and epidemiologic characteristics of ocular toxocariasis. *Am J Trop Med Hyg* 1980;70:1269–1972.
6. Huntley CC, Costas MC, Lyerly A. Viscerla larva migrans syndrome: clinical characteristics and immunologic studies in 51 patients. *Pediatrics* 1965;36:532–536.
7. Zinkman WH. Systemic visceral larval migrans. In: Ryan S, Smith RE (eds). *Selected topics on the eye in systemic disease*, New York: Grune Straton, 1974.
8. Shantz PM, Glickman LT. Toxocaral visceral larva migrans. *N Eng J Med* 1978;298:436–439.
9. Schantz P, Glickman L. Current concepts in parasitology: toxocaral visceral larva migrans. *N Engl J Med* 1978;298:436–439.
10. BenEzra D, Cohen E, Maftzir G. Patterns of inflammation in children. *Bull Soc Belg Ophthalmol* 2001;279:35–38.
11. Shantz D, Myer D, Glickman T. Clinical, serological, and epidemiologic characteristics of ocular toxocariasis. *Am J Trop Med Hyg* 1979;28:24–28.
12. Walker JD. Posterior parasitic uveitis. In: Yanoff M, Duker J (eds). *Ophthalmology*, St. Louis: Mosby, 2002:1172.
13. Parke D, Shaver R. Toxocariasis. In: Pepose J, Holland G, Wilhelmus K (eds). *Ocular infection and immunity*, St. Louis: Mosby, 1996:1225–1235.
14. Maguire A. Ocular toxocariasis. In: Guyer D, Yanuzzi L, Chang S (eds). *Retina vitreous macula*, Philadelphia: WB Saunders, 1999:697–708.
15. Sprent J. The life cycles of nematodes in the family ascaridida. *J Parasitol* 1954;40:608–617.
16. Benitez del Castillo J, Herreros G, Guillen J. Bilateral ocular toxocariasis demonstrated by aqueous humor ELISA. *Am J Ophthalmol* 1995;119:514–516.
17. Wilkinson CP. Ocular toxocariasis. In: Ryan S, Schachat AP (eds). *Retina*, 4th ed, vol II. Philadelphia: Elsevier Mosby, 2006:1597–1604.
18. Gillespie SH, Dinning WJ, Voller A, et al. The spectrum of ocular toxocariasis. *Eye* 1993;7:415.
19. Shields JA. Ocular Toxocariasis: a review. *Surv Ophthalmol* 1984;28:361.
20. Ashton N. Larval granulomatosis of the retina due to toxocara. *Br J Ophthalmol* 1960;44:129–148.
21. Parke DW II, Shaver RP. Toxocariasis. In: Pepose JS, Holland GN, Wilhelmus KR (eds). *Ocular infection and immunology*. St Louis: Mosby-Year Book, 1996:1225.
22. Hogan MJ, Kimura SJ, Spencer WH. Visceral larva migrans and peripheral retinitis. *J Am Med Assoc* 1965;194:1345–1347.
23. Smith PH, Greer CH. Unusual presentation of ocular Toxocara infestation. *Br J Ophthalmol* 1971;55:317.
24. Bird A, Smith J, Curtin V. Nematode optic neuritis. *Am J Ophthalmol* 1970;69:72–77.
25. Phillips C, Mackenzie A. Toxocara larva papillitis. *Br Med Jr* 1973;1:154–155.
26. Shields JA, Parsons HM, Shields CL, et al. Lesions simulating retinoblastoma. *J Pediatr Ophthalmol Strabismus* 1991;28:338–340.
27. Romero-Rangel T, Foster C. Ocular toxocariasis. In: Foster C, Vitale A (eds). *Diagnosis and treatment of uveitis*. Philadelphia: WB Saunders, 2001:428–436.
28. Vitale A, Foster CS. Uveitis affecting infants and children. In: Harnett M, Trese M, Capone A Jr, Keats B, Steidl S (eds). *Pediatric retina*. Philadelphia: Lippincoptt Williams and Wilkins, 2005.
29. Dinning W, Gillespie S, Cooling R. Toxocariasis a practical approach to management of ocular disease. *Eye* 1988;2:580–582.
30. Byers B, Kimura S. Uveitis after death of larva in the vitreous cavity. *Am J Ophthalmol* 1974;77:63–66.
31. Watzke RC, Oaks JA, Folk JC. Toxocara canis infection in the eye. Correlation of clinical observations with developing pathology in the primate model. *Arch Ophthalmol* 1984;102:282–291.
32. Belmont J, Irvine A, Benson W. Vitrectomy in ocular toxocariasis. *Arch Ophthalmol* 1982;100:1912–1915.
33. Amin H, McDonald H, Han D. Vitrectomy update for macular traction in ocular toxocariasis. *Retina* 2000;20:80–85.
34. Small K, McCuen B, deJuan E. Surgical management of retinal traction caused by toxocariasis. *Am J Ophthalmol* 1989;108:10–14.
35. Hagler WS, Pollard ZF, Jarret WH, et al. Results of surgery for ocular toxocara canis. *Ophthalmology* 1981;88:1081–1086.
36. Gass JDM, Scelfo R. Diffuse unilateral subacute neuroretinitis. *J R Soc Med* 1978;71:95–111.
37. Gass JDM. *Stereoscopic atlas of macular disease: diagnosis and treatment*, 2nd ed, St. Louis: Mosby, 1977:226.
38. Gass J, Gilbert W, Guerry R, et al. Diffuse unilateral subacute neuroretinitis. *Ophthalmol* 1978;85:521–545.

39. Gass JDM, Braunstein RA. Further observations concerning the diffuse unilateral subacute neuroretinitis syndrome. *Arch Ophthalmol* 1983;101:1689–1697.

40. Cunha De Souza E, Lustosa da Cunha S, Gass JDM. Diffuse unilateral subacute neuroretinitis in South America. *Arch Ophthalmol* 1992;110:1261–1263.

41. Cortez R, Denny J, Muci-Mendoza R, et al. Diffuse unilateral subacute neuroretinitis in Venezuela. *Ophthalmology* 2005;112:2110–2114.

42. Cialdini AP, de Souza EC, Avilas MP. The first South America case of diffuse unilateral subacute neuroretinitis caused by a large nematode. *Arch Ophthalmol* 1999;117(10):1431–1432.

43. DeSouza EC, Lustosa da Cunha S, Gass JDM. Diffuse unilateral subacute neuroretinitis in South America. *Arch Ophthalmol* 1992;110:1261–1263.

44. DeSouza EC, Abujamra S, Nakashima Y, et al. Diffuse bilateral subacute neuroretinitis: first patient with documented nematodes in both eyes. *Arch Ophthalmol* 1999;117:1349–1351.

45. Harto MA, Rodriguez-Salvador V, Avino JA, et al. Diffuse unilateral subacute neuroretinitis in Europe. *Eur J Ophthalmol* 1999;9:58–62.

46. Carney M, Combs J. Diffuse unilateral subacute neuroretinitis. *Br J Ophthalmol* 1991;75:633–635.

47. Gass J, Callanan D, Bowman C. Successful oral therapy for diffuse unilateral subacute neuroretinitis. *Trans Am Ophthalmol Soc* 1991;89:97–112.

48. Davis J, Gass JDM, Olsen K. In: Ryan S, Shachat AP (eds). *Retina*, 4th ed, vol 2. Philadelphia, PA: Elsevier Inc, 2006:1721.

49. Cortez R, Pulido J. Diffuse unilateral subacute neuroretinitis. In: Quiroz-Mercado H, Alfaro DV III, Ligget P, Tano Y, Dejuan E (eds). *Macular surgery*, Philadelphia: Lippincott, Williams and Wilkins, 2000:287.

50. Moraes L, Cialdini A, Avila M, et al. Identifying live nematodes in diffuse unilateral subacute neuroretinitis by using the scanning laser ophthalmoscope. *Arch Ophthalmol* 2002;120:135–138.

51. Kazacos KR, Raymnond LA, Kazacos EA, et al. The raccoon ascarid. A probable cause of human ocular larva migrans. *Ophthalmology* 1985;92:1735–1744.

52. Kazacos KR, Vestre WA, Kazacos EA, et al. Diffuse unilateral subacute neuroretinitis syndrome: probable cause. *Arch Ophthalmol* 1984;102:967–968.

53. Gass JDM. *Stereoscopic atlas of macular diseases: diagnosis and treatment*, vol. 4. St. Louis: Mosby, 1997:622–628.

54. Parsons HE. Nematode chorioretinitis: report of a case. *Arch Ophthalmol* 1952;47:799–800.

55. Cunha de Souza E, Nakashima Y. DUSN: report of transvitreal surgical removal of a subretinal nematode. *Ophthalmology* 1995;102:1183–1186.

56. Maguire A, Zarbin M, Conner T, et al. Ocular penetration of thiabendazole. *Arch Ophthalmol* 1990;108:1675.

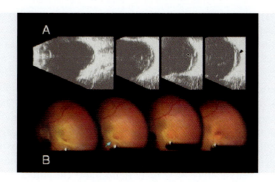

# Congenital Optic Disc Pits, Morning Glory Disc Anomaly, Optic Nerve Coloboma, and Peripapillary Staphyloma

Dolores Berger ■ John B. Kerrison ■ Arthur Korotkin

# CONGENITAL OPTIC DISC PITS

Congenital pits of the optic nerve head are rare congenital anomalies. Although the pathogenesis of optic disc pits is unclear, the great majority of reports in the literature describes optic disc pits as being the mildest variants in the spectrum of optic nerve head colobomas, which are attributed to imperfect closure of the upper end of the embryonic fissure (1). They appear as localized depressions typically measuring from one to several diopters in depth, with a mean of 5 diopters (2). They can be yellow-white, gray, or black in color (Fig. 45-1). It has been suggested that optic disc pits are the mildest manifestation in the spectrum of colobomas involving failure of closure of the embryonic fissure. There are several observations that are inconsistent with this hypothesis. While many colobomas are bilateral and often associated with other abnormalities, optic nerve pits are more typically unilateral and not associated with other findings. The vast majority of pits are solitary, but as many as three pits have been reported in the same optic nerve. There is no known teratogen or genetic inheritance described. Congenital optic disc pits have been associated with trisomy 18 and Alagille syndrome (3).

Optic disc pits were first described in 1882 by Wiethe (4). Although these lesions also were called crater-like holes, cavities, and congenital holes of the optic nerve head, the term "optic disc pit" has become widely accepted (5).

Macular detachment is the most common complication (Fig. 45-2A and B). Kranenburg (6) reviewed the world literature in 1960 and discovered 123 cases of optic disc pit, of which 25% had various types of macular lesions. Additional reports have described serous detachment of the macula secondary to congenital optic disc pits (2,6–9); however, the source of the subretinal fluid is still uncertain. The detachment typically extends from the retina adjacent to the optic disc pit into the macula, where it may remain asymptomatic or cause visual field defects and diminished central acuity. This typically occurs within the 2nd to 4th decade, although detachments have been reported in children as young as 6 years old (7). Detachments have been primarily associated with optic disc pits that are adjacent to the rim. The detachment is typically not associated with a posterior vitreous detachment and usually involves the macula within the boundaries of the temporal arcades.

## Clinical Features

Optic disc pits are considered by most authors to be on the spectrum of embryological anomalies that ranges from small asymptomatic pits to morning glory disc syndrome. Brown and Tasman (5) estimated the incidence of optic disc pits to be approximately one per 10,000 people in the general population, although there is considerable variance among studies (8). Men and women are equally affected. The defect generally ranges in size from 0.25 to 0.40 disc diameters (5). More than 50% are located on the temporal aspect of the disc, but approximately one-third are situated centrally; the remainder are found inferiorly, superiorly, and nasally (5,10–15). It is rare to find more than one pit, but as many as three have been reported in the same eye (6,16). Optic disc pits are unilateral in approximately 85% of patients, and the affected disc is larger than the unaffected disc in about 80% of cases (15).

Patients may be asymptomatic or have a visual field defect. With macular involvement, patients may present with loss of central vision. Visual acuity may vary depending on the extent of macular involvement. Visual field defects tend to be located superiorly and temporally as most pits are located inferiorly and nasally in the optic nerve. Arcuate scotomas, Bjerrum-type scotomas, altitudinal defects, paracentral scotomas, enlarged blind spot, generalized scotomas, nasal and temporal steps have all been documented (7). Natural history of pits with symptomatic retinal detachment tends to be that of progressive loss of vision with persistent submacular fluid.

The incidence of posterior vitreous detachment associated with optic disc pits has not been determined (10,17–21).

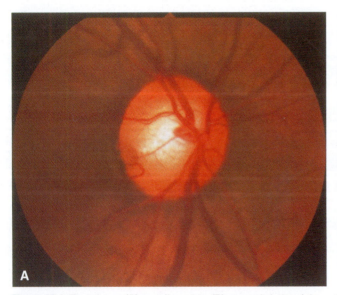
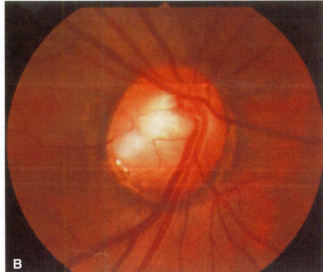

**Figure 45-1.** Round gray **(A)** or yellow-white **(B)** congenital pits of the optic nerve head are present on the temporal aspect of the disc. Peripapillary pigmentary changes and enlarged disc are found.

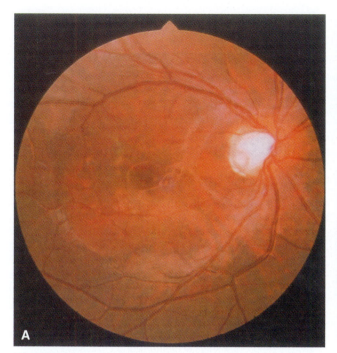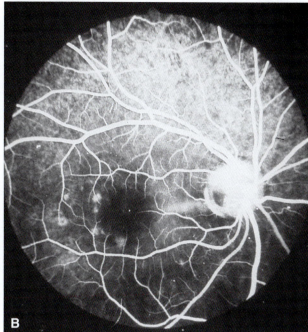

**Figure 45-2. A:** Color fundus photograph with an optic nerve pit showing subretinal fluid with macular detachment. **B:** Fluorescein angiogram reveals hypofluorescence of the optic disc pit in the early stage.

Brown and Tasman (6) observed posterior vitreous separation in 81%. Vitreous strands are observed occasionally extending from the pit into the vitreous gel. Bonnet (18) reported that 25 eyes with macular detachments associated with optic disc pits did not have posterior vitreous detachments at presentation, and two eyes had spontaneous reattachment of the macula following development of posterior vitreous detachment. Akiba et al. (19) demonstrated posterior vitreous detachments in only two (12%) of 17 eyes with optic disc pits and serous detachments of the macula.

Peripapillary retinal pigment epithelial disturbances usually are seen in eyes with optic disc pits along the rim of the disc (20). These peripapillary changes may develop over time with or without central serous retinal detachment.

Macular lesions, such as macular detachment, cystoid degeneration, macular edema, and schisis-like changes, occur in 30% to 50% of eyes with a congenital optic disc pit (6,15). Among them, serous retinal detachment that may mimic central serous chorioretinopathy is known to be a common complication.

Approximately 40% of eyes have an associated or previous serous detachment of the sensory retina (15). The serous detachment communicates with the optic disc (Figs. 45-2A and B and 45-3). Most of the retinal detachments are temporal

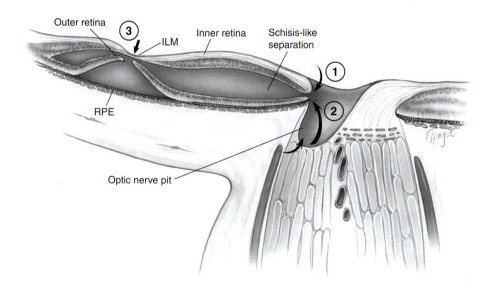

**Figure 45-3.** Schematic drawing of an axial view of the optic nerve head and surrounding tissues. Various theories describe the mechanism by which fluid enters into the intraretinal space to produce a schisis-like splitting of the neurosensory retina from the vitreous (1) or the cerebrospinal fluid (2). As a late complication, a true macular hole may develop (3). ILM, internal limiting membrane; RPE, retinal pigment epithelium.

to the disc and confined between the superior and inferior vascular arcades. If the pit is present on the nasal side of the disc, a serous retinal detachment is located outside the arcuates. The serous macular detachment generally is shallow (less than 1.0 mm in height) (20). Cystic changes within the detached macula are found in two thirds of cases, and a macular hole develops in about 25%.

A splitting of the retinal layers also has been described in eyes with congenital optic disc pits and retinal detachment (14,21). Although most authors have assumed that macular detachments are a result of fluid entering directly into the subretinal space, Lincoff et al. (14) proposed that the primary macular lesion is frequently a retinal schisis-like separation that communicates with the optic disc pit. In such eyes, true retinal detachment is regarded as a secondary phenomenon, typically localized to the central macula without connection to the pit. The fluid beneath the photoreceptors is more opaque than the relatively transparent zone of the elevation owing to the schisis-like cavity. Studies by Rutledge et al. (10), using optical coherence tomography (OCT), supported the concept of a bilaminar structure, in which a macular detachment develops secondarily to a pre-existing schisis-like lesion consisting of severe outer retinal edema.

The age of onset of the retinal detachment is variable, with the mean age being about 30 years (15). It has been seen in children within the first decade of life. Centrally located optic nerve head pits generally are not associated with detachment; retinal detachment is seen more commonly with larger, temporally located pits and usually involves the macula (15).

Tiny subretinal precipitates are visible in about one-third of eyes (5). In contrast to most lamellar holes, in which absence of the inner retinal layers is observed, the macular holes noted in conjunction with optic nerve head pits tend to involve the outer retina, giving the appearance that the internal limiting membrane is intact.

## Fluorescein Angiography

Fluorescein angiography has shown a variety of findings in patients (17). The optic nerve pit typically appears hypofluorescent in the early phase of the angiogram (Fig. 45-2B), with staining occurring later in the study. It was thought that blood vessels in this area leaked the fluid that entered into the subretinal space (22–25). Brown et al. (5,15) observed apparent leakage of dye into the subretinal fluid in three eyes with macular detachments and reported a higher incidence of pits in eyes with serous detachments than in eyes without subretinal fluid. There is usually no evidence, however, of dye passing from the pit into the adjacent subretinal fluid in the majority of cases (17).

## Visual Field Defects

The optic disc pit can be associated with visual field defects. The most common type of visual field defect is an arcuate scotoma, which occurs in about 25% of cases (2). Arcuate scotomas probably reflect the absence of the wedge of nerve fibers displaced by the optic disc pit. Larger pits may be associated with large Bjerrum-type scotomas or even altitudinal visual field defects. Paracentral scotomas, generalized and peripheral

localized constrictions, sector defects extending from the disc, and nasal or temporal steps also may be seen (15).

Central and paracentral scotomas can result from serous macular detachment or retinoschisis (21). Central field loss associated with pure retinoschisis is relatively mild, presumably because many neural pathways remain intact (21). Bridging retinal elements were proposed to explain why an absolute scotoma is not produced by the schisis-like elevation (14,20).

## Optical Coherence Tomography Findings

OCT significantly increased our understanding of ultrastructural features of pit-associated neurosensory detachments. One of the earliest reports by Linkoff et al. (9) demonstrated a division between outer and inner layers of the retina connected to the optic disc pit, which subsequently resolved after pneumatic displacement. Detachment may be associated with retinal edema and cystic degeneration imaged by OCT. The most prominent edema is present in the outer retina at the level of the outer plexiform layer, mimicking a true retinoschisis cavity (10). By OCT, the schisis-like cavity or edematous retina communicates with the optic disc. While some studies report no direct communicant between the optic pit and the subretinal space (10), other studies report that such a communication exists (11).

## Systemic Association

In general, systemic abnormalities have not been observed in association with congenital optic disc pits. Nevertheless, basal encephalocele and agenesis of the corpus callosum have been reported (22,23). A hereditary pattern is not usually present, although an autosomal dominant inheritance that is not associated with mutation in the PAX2 gene has been noted (24).

Many reports in the literature suggest that the pathogenesis of pits of the optic nerve head involves incomplete closure of the embryonic fissure and represents the mildest variant in the spectrum of optic disc colobomas (1). Clinical evidence, however, including the fact that there are few systemic associations, is inconsistent with this hypothesis (1):

■ Optic disc pits are usually unilateral, sporadic, and not associated with systemic anomalies. In contrast, colobomas are bilateral as often as they are unilateral and may be associated with a variety of systemic anomalies.
■ More than 50% of optic nerve head pits are located on the temporal aspect of the disc, and one third are at the center of the disc, locations that are unrelated to the embryonic fissure.

On the other hand, congenital optic disc pits sometimes are seen in combination with optic nerve colobomas. Furthermore, one or more cilioretinal arteries emerge from the majority of pits. These observations suggest that congenital pits of the optic nerve head may be pathologically related to colobomas of the optic nerve head, despite uncertainty regarding their respective pathogeneses.

## Pathogenesis of Serous Detachment

The pathogenesis and pathologic nature of the associated macular lesions and the origin of subretinal fluid remain controversial.

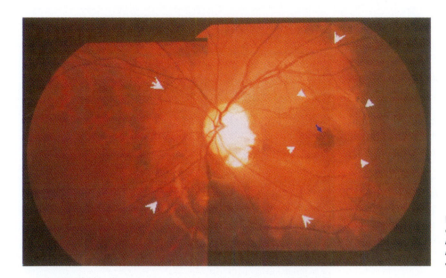

**Figure 45-4.** Fundus photograph demonstrating an optic disc pit, an inner-layer separation (*large arrowheads*), an outer-layer macular hold (*open arrowhead*), and an outer-layer sensory detachment (*small arrowheads*).

Although evidence in a model using collie dogs suggests that subretinal fluid originates from the vitreous cavity (26), no firm evidence for such a communication in humans has been found (5). There are several reports suggesting the existence of direct communication between the vitreous cavity and subretinal space. Sugar (12) proposed that fluid from the vitreous cavity leaks through the optic nerve head pit to fill the subretinal space (subretinal channel). Bonnet (18) found that none of their patients with macular detachments associated with optic nerve head pits had posterior vitreous detachments, and they observed a small hole in the roof of the pit in several cases. A small bubble of gas was observed to pass from the vitreous cavity into the subretinal space *via* the optic nerve head pit in a patient who underwent vitrectomy and gas injection without photocoagulation. Thus, Bonnet concluded that macular detachment combined with an optic disc pit has a rhegmatogenous component associated with vitreous traction.

Other possible sources of subretinal fluid in humans include cerebrospinal fluid from the subarachnoid space, leakage from choroidal vessels, leakage from small vessels located at the base of the pit into subretinal space (15), and entrance of fluid from the vitreous cavity through a secondary macular hole (27,28). Because an increase in vascular permeability is not observed by fluorescein angiography in many cases, most authors agree that the subretinal fluid originates from either the vitreous or cerebrospinal fluid (1) (Fig. 45-3).

Subretinal fluid accumulation resulting from leakage of cerebrospinal fluid through the optic disc pit first was noted by Regenbogen et al. (29). Neither experimental studies nor histopathologic evaluations, however, have demonstrated such a pathway. Intrathecal injections of fluorescein in humans and animals have not shown passage of dye into the subretinal fluid (26,30). Such a communication was demonstrated, however, by Chang et al. (31) in an eye with a retinal detachment associated with morning glory anomaly. Irvine and associates (32) demonstrated communication between the vitreous cavity and the orbit *via* a morning glory disc anomaly and the subarachnoid space of the optic nerve. During surgery, gas injected into the vitreous cavity escaped from the eye through a surgical window in the optic nerve sheath.

Regardless of the presumed source of fluid, most authors have assumed that macular detachments were the result of fluid entering directly into the subretinal space at the site of the optic disc pit. Macular edema, cystoid degeneration, and schisis-like changes were considered to be secondary effects from longstanding macular detachment (2). Recent data, however, have suggested the converse. Lincoff and associates (14), using stereoscopic examination of the macula in conjunction with kinetic perimetry, suggested that the macular elevation in the early stage of the disease is a separation of the inner retinal layers to produce a schisis-like splitting of the neurosensory retina, which emanated from the optic disc pit. At a later stage, an outer-layer macular hole and an outer-layer retinal detachment would develop (Fig. 45-4).

## Pathology

Peterson (33) reported that marked edema of the temporal lesion from the optic disc, particularly in the outer plexiform layer, was observed histopathologically, although a macular lesion was not identified clinically. Ferry (8) examined histologically two eyes that had been enucleated for the suspected clinical diagnosis of choroidal malignant melanoma. Both eyes had retinal detachments temporal to the optic disc. He showed herniation of dysplastic retina through a defect in the lamina cribrosa into a collagen-lined pocket. The progressive gliosis and "contraction of the retinal elements" contained in the pit may have produced a traction detachment of the macula. There were patchy photoreceptor degeneration, depigmentation of the retinal pigment epithelium, edema, and cystoid degeneration. Gass (2) noted cystic degeneration, partial splitting of the outer plexiform layer in the perifoveal area, and dysplastic tissue encapsulated in a multiloculated space that was separated from the subretinal space by multiple thin septa.

These reports demonstrate varying degrees of edema and cystic changes in the retina adjacent to the optic disc pit with or without retinal detachment. These findings are not contradictory to the concept of a bilaminar macular structure, as proposed by Lincoff et al. (14) or suggested by studies using OCT (10,11).

## Natural Course

The natural course of retinal detachment associated with optic disc pits is variable (1,17). The patient usually presents with symptoms of blurred vision and metamorphopsia secondary to foveal involvement. Sobol et al. (34) followed 15 eyes with optic nerve head pits and macular detachments for an average of 9 years and found that most patients with optic nerve head pits presented with visual acuities of about 20/40 to 20/60, with each patient losing three or more lines of vision within the next 6 months.

The subretinal fluid may be absorbed and then recur after a prolonged time. Chronic or intermittent macular detachment may be associated with long-term macular changes including full-thickness or outer-layer macular holes, cystic degeneration, retinoschisis with or without an outer-layer macular hole, and retinal pigment epithelial changes that reduce visual acuities (20,35).

Sobol et al. (34) found that 80% of 15 eyes lost vision to 20/200 or worse at the time of the last evaluation. The visual loss was generally complete within 6 months of presentation. Subretinal fluid absorbed spontaneously in four eyes (27%). Brown and Tasman (5) reported that among 20 untreated eyes followed for at least 1 year, the visual acuity was 20/100 or worse in 55%. The mean visual acuity at the end of the evaluation was about 20/80. They noted that, although some detachments resolved spontaneously, others persisted for years. After 5 years, most patients still had some subretinal fluid present.

## Treatment

Multiple treatment options are available for the retinal detachment associated with an optic disc pit. Detachments that do not involve the macula and those that do involve the macula and not the fovea can be observed without intervention. Macular detachments have been reported to resolve spontaneously up to 25% of the time.

If vision is decreased because of serous macular retinal detachment, laser treatment along the edge of the pit has been recommended to induce reattachment of the retina to the underlying retinal pigment epithelium and subsequent resorption of the subretinal fluid (Fig. 45-5). A few reports have documented a favorable response with such treatment, although some cases require multiple sessions (13,14,36–38). Laser treatment sometimes is performed with the krypton laser to minimize damage to the inner retinal layers (37). This may be followed by bedrest and bilateral eye patching. The difference in final visual outcome between treated and untreated groups, however, was not pronounced (15). Brown and Tasman (5) concluded that laser therapy is effective for flattening the retinal detachment but not for improving final visual outcome.

In eyes with severe visual loss that do not respond to laser therapy, the possibility of repeat laser treatment in conjunction with either injection of a long-acting gas into the vitreous cavity or pars plana vitrectomy with fluid-gas exchange may be considered (14,38,39). Yanyali and Bonnet (40) discussed their therapeutic results in 19 eyes with serous macular detachments associated with optic disc pits. Photocoagulation of the temporal margin of the nerve head was combined with

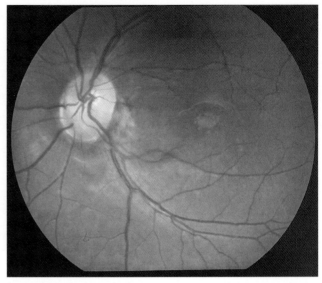

**Figure 45-5.** Fundus photograph showing photocoagulation scars along the edge of a pit.

intravitreal gas injection. Eight eyes (42%) required more than one procedure. At last examination, the macula was reattached in 17 (94%) of the 18 eyes with adequate follow-up, and visual acuity improved in 12 eyes (67%). Persistent subretinal fluid not involving the central macula was evident following successful surgery in three (17%) of the 18 patients. In 1995, Brown and Brown (39) described treatment outcomes in four cases in which laser therapy alone did not cure retinal detachments associated with optic disc pits. *Pars plana* vitrectomy, fluid-gas exchanges, and additional laser treatments were successful in reattaching the retina in all four eyes, although 7 months were required for complete resolution of subretinal fluid in one case.

Displaced and persistent subretinal fluid following intraocular gas tamponade was observed by Lincoff et al. (21). In this series, subretinal fluid was displaced inferior to the central macula, where it remained for 3 to 36 months, in seven of nine cases. The displacement of subretinal fluid was associated with a change in the location of the associated scotoma in all seven cases and improvement in vision in six cases, despite a persistence of inner retinal separation. In our institute, treatment of four patients with pars plana vitrectomy involving induction of posterior vitreous detachment and fluid-gas exchange, without any laser treatments, was successful in reattaching the retina, although several months were required for complete resolution of subretinal fluid, and unusual peripheral visual-field defects occurred in three of four cases (41).

Theodossiadis (42) treated nine consecutive patients who had unilateral maculopathy associated with optic disc pit with a macular buckling procedure. In eight of nine patients, the macular elevation included a schisis-like splitting in the internal layers of the neurosensory retina. A scleral sponge was fixed at the posterior pole, corresponding to the macula along the vertical axis. In all nine eyes, complete disappearance of subretinal and intraretinal fluid in the macula and in the surrounding area was noted without any additional treatment. The absorption of macular fluid started immediately after the

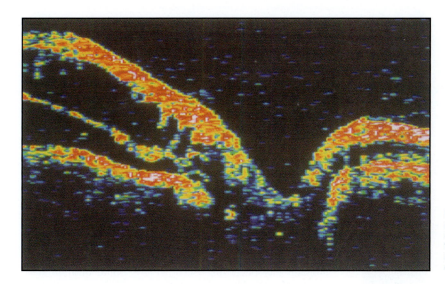

**Figure 45-6.** A horizontal optical coherence tomographic scan through the pit discloses a bilaminar structure in the neurosensory retina. A large, nonreflective space (schisis cavity) emanates from the optic never head pit. Tissues bridging the two separated layers are present.

operation and was complete after 5 to 6 months. Macular buckling may be an effective technique for the treatment of optic disc pit maculopathy, even though the source of the subretinal fluid is unknown.

Overall, the response to therapy has been variable and not correlated with the clinical appearance of the macula previously noted. According to the concept of a bilaminar structure, in which a macular detachment develops secondarily to a preexisting schisis-like lesion consisting of severe retinal edema, the prolonged course of fluid absorption (36,43,44), the occurrence of redetachment (13,44), and the frequency of treatment failure (2,36,38) after photocoagulation of the juxtapapillary retina may relate to an incomplete closure of a fistula that exists into the retinal stroma and not into the subretinal space (10).

Several reports (10,11) have demonstrated that OCT is a useful tool for studying the macular pathology associated with optic nerve head pits (Fig. 45-6). Additional studies using this tool may provide better understanding of the pathogenesis and lead to development of appropriate treatment of retinal detachment associated with optic disc pits.

## MORNING GLORY ANOMALY

In 1970, Kindler (45) reported on 10 patients with a unilateral, congenital optic nerve head anomaly that resembled the morning glory flower. The clinical appearance is characterized by an enlarged, excavated, funnel-shaped optic nerve head; a central core of white tissue; a peripapillary annulus of variably pigmented subretinal tissue; and retinal vessels that enter and exit from the borders of the defect (Fig. 45-7). The retinal vessels frequently are sheathed and straightened. The disc anomaly has been associated with retinal detachment (46), other ocular abnormalities (5,47,48), and congenital systemic anomalies (23).

### Clinical Features

Most cases of morning glory disc anomaly are unilateral, although bilateral cases have been reported. The visual acuity

in eyes with morning glory optic disc anomaly and no retinal detachment can range from near normal to hand motions (5). Strabismus may be associated. In unilateral cases, the possibility of concomitant strabismic amblyopia should be considered (49). The condition is twice as frequent in females as in males (5).

The optic nerve head is enlarged and excavated. There is a characteristic central core of white tissue and a peripapillary ring of pale subretinal tissue with pigmentary changes (50). The retinal vessels appear to enter and exit near the margin of the nerve head, because epipapillary connective tissue obscures the central area. The retinal vessels frequently are sheathed and straightened with anomalous branching.

Retinal detachment frequently is associated with the morning glory disc anomaly (31,32,45,51–55) (Fig. 45-8).

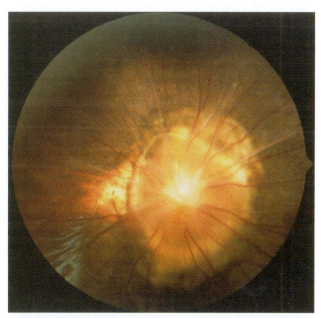

**Figure 45-7.** Fundus photograph showing a morning glory disc anomaly. The optic cup is covered by glial tissue. Peripapillary chorioretinal atrophy and without pigmentary changes also are seen.

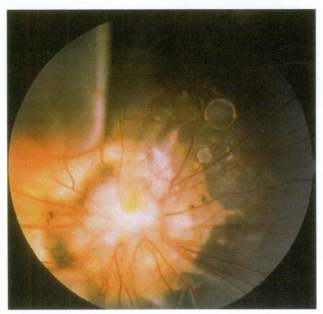

**Figure 45-8.** Bullous inferior retinal detachment in an eye with morning glory optic disc anomaly.

Among congenital anomalies of the optic nerve head, such as optic nerve coloboma or optic disc pits, the morning glory disc anomaly is most commonly associated with retinal detachment, which may result from a rhegmatogenous mechanism. Retinal detachment limited to the peripapillary retina or posterior pole is very common. The detachment occasionally extends to the periphery and becomes an extensive bullous retinal detachment.

## Systemic Anomalies

The morning glory disc anomaly does not occur as part of a multisystem genetic disorder, although the association of morning glory disc anomaly with the trans-sphenoidal form of basal encephalocele is well reported (23,49). Therefore, infants with the morning glory disc anomaly should be considered at increased risk for respiratory, endocrinologic, and neurologic problems (1). Patients with trans-sphenoidal encephalocele usually display a characteristic malformation complex of midfacial congenital anomalies, including hypertelorism, depressed nasal bridge, and cleft palate. Other congenital optic disc abnormalities including optic disc pit, coloboma, and megalopapilla also have been reported with basal encephalocele (5). The condition is almost always nonfamilial (56).

## Pathology

The histopathologic features of the morning glory disc anomaly are similar to those of congenital optic disc pits (32). Eyes with morning glory disc anomaly have a more extensive scleral defect, and retinal tissue usually extends posteriorly around the entire circumference of the optic nerve (32). This staphylomatous herniation may be demonstrated by computed tomography, magnetic resonance imaging, or ultrasonography (32).

Pedler (57) described the histopathologic features of an unusual coloboma of the optic nerve head that was similar to

the morning glory disc anomaly. Aberrant retinal tissue was displaced centrally and covered a portion of the nerve head. Retinal tissue also prolapsed posteriorly through an enlarged posterior scleral foramen. There was an annular proliferation of glial tissue in the subretinal space at the edge of the optic nerve head, and the lamina cribrosa was displaced posteriorly.

Cogan (58) reported similar histopathologic features in a specimen with vascularized connective tissue within the optic cup. The peripapillary cupping was so extensive as to pull the retina into the disc, resulting in traction from the abnormal papilla. The distortion of the peripapillary retina resulting from traction by epipapillary tissue, an enlarged scleral canal with absent lamina cribrosa, and proliferation of glial and retinal pigment epithelial cells surrounding the optic nerve head were found.

The embryologic defect leading to the morning glory disc anomaly has been discussed widely. Some authors have hypothesized that the morning glory disc anomaly results from incomplete closure of the embryonic fissure. Others have suggested that a primary mesenchymal abnormality is responsible, because of the clinical findings of a central glial tuft, vascular anomalies, and a scleral defect, together with the histologic findings of adipose tissue and smooth muscle within the peripapillary sclera in presumed cases of morning glory disc anomaly (1,50,58).

## Retinal Detachment

The development of retinal detachment has been well-recognized in association with morning glory disc anomaly, although its pathogenic mechanism remains unclear. Various explanations for the origin of the subretinal fluid include leakage from abnormal vasculature within the excavated area (45,50), traction from abnormal tissue within the excavated area (59), communication between the subarachnoid space and the subretinal space (2), and retinal breaks within the excavated area permitting fluid from the vitreous cavity to enter the subretinal space (12,55,53).

Several authors have reported that the detachment is nonrhegmatogenous, with subretinal fluid not extending to the ora serrata (4,45,59,60). Haik and associates (60) found that four eyes had spontaneous resolution of subretinal fluid and reattachment of the retina. Chang et al. (31) demonstrated an apparent communication between the subarachnoid and subretinal spaces. Metrizamide dye was injected into the subarachnoid space and subsequently appeared in the subretinal space, as viewed by computed tomographic scanning of the orbit.

A rhegmatogenous mechanism for the retinal detachment has been observed in other cases. von Fricken and Dhungel (53) identified a small retinal tear in the fovea in an eye with retinal detachment and morning glory disc anomaly. Peripapillary retinal breaks as the causes of retinal detachment were found in other cases (55,54). In our institute, we have followed nine eyes with extensive retinal detachment associated with morning glory disc anomaly over the past 8 years (unpublished data). Retinal breaks were present inside the peripapillary excavation in all but one eye. Retinal breaks were detected by slit lamp examination or after removal of peripapillary

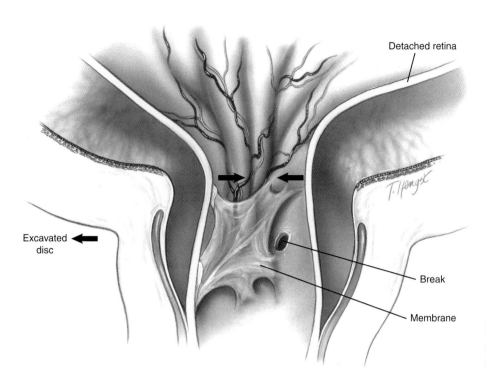

Figure 45-9. Schematic drawing or retinal detachment in an eye with morning glory disc anomaly. Retinal breaks can be detected under the peripapillary fibroglial tissue during vitrectomy in some cases with extensive retinal detachments.

fibroglial tissue during the vitreous surgery (Fig. 45-9). The peripapillary retinal breaks may be caused by tangential traction from the epipapillary tissue. Beyer et al. (49) evaluated 10 eyes and noted progressive tangential traction on the peripapillary retina in two of the eyes.

## Treatment

If retinal detachments result either from vitreoretinal traction, vitreoprepapillary traction, or a retinal break, techniques that are similar to those used in eyes with choroidal colobomas complicated by retinal detachment might provide favorable results (53). After the vitreous gel is excised, transvitreal removal of subretinal fluid is performed through the break. It is very difficult, however, to evacuate subretinal fluid through an original break in the excavated disc area in many cases, and a drainage retinotomy may be created outside of the excavated area. A long-lasting bubble is used to tamponade the break. Peripapillary laser therapy in conjunction with vitrectomy and fluid–gas exchange can be of benefit for flattening the retina in some cases (39). Harris and associates (54) reported that vitrectomy, fluid–gas exchange, and postoperative confluent krypton laser photocoagulation around the optic disc resulted in successful reattachment in an eye with a tiny slit-like retinal break and adjacent vitreous traction. They suggested that this treatment also might be successful if no retinal break is present and subretinal fluid originates from the subarachnoid space.

Because it is impossible to coagulate the retinal break inside the excavation during vitreous surgery, we tried cyanoacrylate glue retinopexy in nine eyes (unpublished data). The application of glue was particularly difficult in these eyes, however, because the breaks were present on the slope of the excavation, and it was hard to keep this area dry during glue application. Displacement of polymerized glue or the development of new retinal breaks at the edge of the glued area occurred with high incidence as a late complication following vitreous surgery. Multiple operations, including reapplication of glue, were required in many eyes. Six of nine eyes achieved final retinal reattachment. Unsuccessful procedures all were in patients younger than 10 years of age. In young patients, the peripapillary excavation is more prominent (Fig. 45-10), and this may be related to the severity of the malformation and to the difficulty in surgical treatment.

Involuntary or contractile movement of the peripapillary excavation has been reported in some cases (1,61). We also found retinal distortion around the excavated area in some

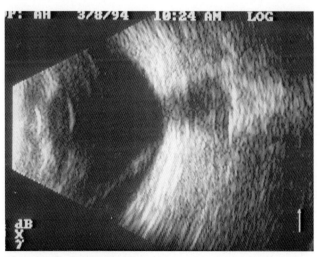

Figure 45-10. B-scan echography of the eye of a 4-year-old boy showing the marked excavation of the disc.

patients if the globe was tilted during vitreous surgery. These movements and distortions may cause displacement of glue or tearing of the retina at the edge of the glue, resulting in redetachment of the retina after vitrectomy.

Overall, particularly in young patients, it is very difficult to flatten the retina. Silicone oil injection combined with vitrectomy, with or without peripapillary photocoagulation, is an alternative surgical technique to provide semipermanent tamponade of the retinal break within the optic nerve head anomaly. The use of silicone oil injection in conjunction with vitrectomy is controversial, however, because it is not possible to rule out a connection between the nerve-head defect and the subarachnoid space, a finding observed in some cases of optic disc pits and optic nerve colobomas (32,50). Coll et al. (62) reported a case in which silicone oil used for tamponade migrated into the subretinal space. We also have experienced this complication in our series (unpublished). Regardless, consideration should be given to the possibility that certain retinal detachments associated with morning glory disc anomaly also may be rhegmatogenous in nature.

## Optic Nerve Coloboma

Colobomas of the optic disc result from incomplete or abnormal closure of the proximal end of the embryonic fissure (63). The embryonic fissure usually closes by approximately 5 or 6 weeks of gestation. Closure of the fissure starts in mid position and is said to extend anteriorly and posteriorly by the 10-mm stage (64). By the 18-mm stage (approximately 6 weeks of gestation), all except the most proximal portion is closed. Teratogenic insults in the later stages are likely to affect only the anterior- or posterior-most parts of the fissure, leading to iris or ciliary body defects or disc colobomas. The area of the defect also may contain a typical optic disc pit.

In optic disc coloboma, a sharply delimited, glistening white, bowl-shaped excavation occupies an enlarged optic disc (1) (Fig. 45-11). The excavation is decentered inferiorly, reflecting the position of the embryonic fissure relative to the primitive

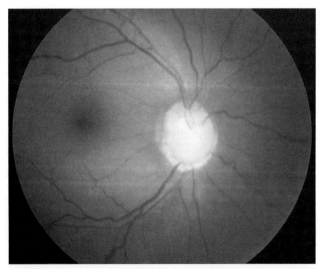

**Figure 45-11.** Coloboma of the optic disc. The disc is enlarged. A deep white excavation occupies half of the disc but spares the superior aspect.

epithelial papilla (1). The area of defect may extend further inferiorly to involve the adjacent retina and choroid, in which case microphthalmia is frequently present. There are several characteristic features, including partial or total excavation of the disc (inferiorly decentered); enlargement of the papillary area; a glistening white excavation; retinal blood vessels entering and exiting the nerve head from the border of the defect; and minimal peripapillary pigmentary disturbance (1,65).

Although the phenotypic profiles of optic disc coloboma and morning glory disc anomaly occasionally overlap, the ophthalmoscopic features of optic disc coloboma are most consistent with a primary structural dysgenesis involving the proximal embryonic fissure, as opposed to an anomalous dilatation confined to the distal optic stalk in the morning glory disc anomaly (1).

## Clinical Features

Colobomas of the optic nerve head are characterized by enlargement and partial or total excavation of the optic disc. The nerve head is usually about 50% larger than normal, but the size can vary by up to 2.5 times the width of the nerve head in the fellow eye (5). The depth of colobomatous defects ranges from minimal to 50 diopters (5). Peripapillary retinal pigment epithelial alterations are common.

Bilateral involvement is more common with isolated optic nerve head colobomas than with optic disc pits or the morning glory disc anomaly (5). Gopal and associates (66) examined 67 eyes of 40 patients with choroidal coloboma, of which 63% had optic disc involvement. They found that 87% of their patients with optic disc coloboma had bilateral involvement, supporting the theory that the embryonic insult during the second month of gestation is not focal but rather a manifestation of a more generalized insult. This seems reasonable if one considers that ocular colobomatous defects often are associated with systemic abnormalities as well (5). They also showed increased prevalence of microphthalmos with increased severity of the colobomatous defect.

Visual acuity, which depends primarily upon the integrity of the papillomacular bundle, is variable and has been noted to range from normal to no light perception (67). In patients with unilateral involvement, there may be a superimposed amblyopic component in affected eyes that may be responsive to occlusion therapy, as is the case with the morning glory disc anomaly (49).

Concomitant retinochoroidal or iris colobomatous defects may be present (Fig. 45-12). Like choroidal colobomas, optic disc colobomas may arise sporadically or be inherited (67,68).

Eyes with isolated optic disc colobomas are likely to develop serous macular detachments, in contrast to the rhegmatogenous retinal detachments that are seen with retinochoroidal colobomas (1).

## Systemic Anomalies

Multiple systemic abnormalities have been reported in conjunction with colobomatous defects in the eye (5), including diseases of the cardiovascular, central nervous, dermatologic, gastrointestinal, genitourinary, nasopharyngeal, and musculoskeletal systems, as well as combined conditions such as the CHARGE syndrome (coloboma, heart disease, atresia choanae,

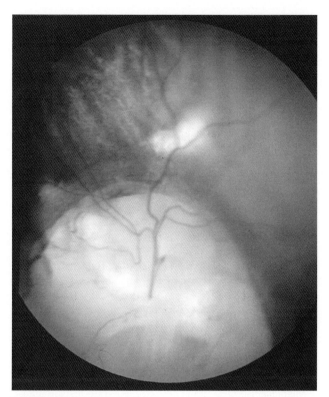

**Figure 45-12.** Retinal detachment in an eye with retinochoroidal coloboma involving the optic nerve head.

retarded growth, genital hypoplasia, ear anomalies, and/or deafness) (69), Walker-Warburg syndrome, Aicardi syndrome, and Goldenhar-Gorlin syndrome (1). Rarely, large orbital cysts can occur in cases associated with atypical excavations of the disc (1). Infants and young children with colobomatous defects should undergo general physical examinations to rule out the possibility of coexistent systemic abnormalities.

Recently, the genes responsible in several congenital anomalies have been identified. Paired box (PAX) genes are known to play a critical role in human development and disease. PAX2 encodes a transcription factor of the paired-box class of DNA-binding proteins, important for the development of the urogenital tract, optic nerve and adjacent retina, inner ear, and central nervous system. Some investigators have found that PAX2 is required for normal kidney and eye development, with a PAX2 defect leading to renal coloboma syndrome (70,71). It is unlikely, however, that PAX2 defects are common in patients with ocular colobomas in isolation (71).

## Pathology

Histopathologic examination has demonstrated up to 7 mm of widening of the perineural scleral canal (68). The optic nerve is present within the colobomatous defect, but it is sometimes atrophic or poorly developed. The lamina cribrosa may be displaced posteriorly or may be absent. A proliferation of glial tissue in the central depression has been described, and both adipose tissue and smooth muscle have been found surrounding the nerve (72,73). This pathologic finding accounts for the contractility of the optic disc seen on occasion in optic disc coloboma (1,74).

There is often an associated retinochoroidal coloboma, which typically does not contain choroid, retinal pigment epithelium, or normal retinal tissue. A white glial membrane is often present on the inner surface of the retinochoroidal coloboma, representing rudimentary retinal tissue derived from the inner layer of the optic cup (5). Retinal blood vessels may be present on the surface of the membrane. Other studies have indicated the presence of a schisis-like split in the retina at the margin of the coloboma, with the outer retinal layers not entering the coloboma (75).

## Retinal Detachment

Retinal detachment may be seen in association with optic nerve colobomas (63,67,76). The detachment most often occurs in the second or third decade of life and tends to be larger than those associated with optic disc pits (63). There is a direct correlation between the size of the coloboma and the prevalence of retinal detachment.

The source of the subretinal fluid is uncertain, but it is most likely derived from liquefied vitreous or from cerebrospinal fluid *via* a connection between the coloboma and the subarachnoid space. In a clinicopathologic study of an optic disc coloboma with associated macular detachment in a rhesus monkey, Lin and associates (77) noted disruption of the intermediary tissue of Kuhnt with diffusion of retrobulbar fluid from the orbit into the subretinal space. A case of retinoschisis combined with retinal detachment complicating optic nerve coloboma was reported (77). Spontaneous reattachment of the retina in an eye with optic nerve head coloboma and retinal detachment also has been described (78,79).

Concomitant retinochoroidal or iris colobomatous defects also may be present (Fig. 45-12). Retinal detachments associated with colobomas of the choroid and retina are usually rhegmatogenous (79,80–82). In some cases, retinal detachments may result from typical retinal breaks not associated with the coloboma, although the retinal breaks usually occur within the coloboma or along its edge (79,80–82) (Fig. 45-13).

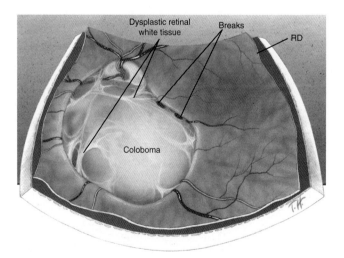

**Figure 45-13.** Schematic drawing of retinal detachment associated with choroidal coloboma involving the disc. The majority of breaks is located along the edge of the coloboma. Inside the coloboma, there are diaphanous sheets or bridges of incomplete retinal tissues.

Gopal et al. (82) examined 36 eyes and demonstrated that the breaks commonly were seen at the edge of the retinal detachment inside the coloboma or as oval breaks within the detached diaphanous tissue. The macula, if involved in the coloboma, occasionally harbors a retinal break (82). Preoperative identification of these breaks is difficult, however, for several reasons. The patients may have nystagmus. Furthermore, the lack of contrast because of the absence of retinal pigment epithelium and choroid contributes greatly to the difficulty in finding the breaks. Previously undetected breaks over the colobomas have been discovered at the time of vitrectomy (79,80–82).

## Treatment

Several treatments, including eye patching, bedrest, corticosteroids, vitrectomy, scleral buckling surgery, fluid–gas exchange, and photocoagulation have been used for sensory retinal detachments associated with optic nerve coloboma (1,13). Because spontaneous reattachment of a total retinal detachment in an infant with microphthalmos and optic-nerve coloboma has been reported (79), Schatz and McDonald (13) have advocated waiting 3 months before treatment. Peripapillary laser therapy in association with *pars plana* vitrectomy and fluid–gas exchange has been used successfully to flatten the retina (39). Nagano et al. (65) reported that pars plana vitrectomy and fluid–gas exchange without laser therapy flattened the macula in one case of retinal detachment with schisis-like separation associated with optic nerve coloboma.

Optic nerve coloboma often is associated with choroidal coloboma. In these eyes, retinal detachments can result from a rhegmatogenous mechanism. These detachments typically result from one or more breaks in the intercalary membrane, the thin, diaphanous sheet over the coloboma that is continuous with the sensory retina (82). These breaks are difficult to visualize because of the lack of contrast resulting from the absence of choroid and retinal pigment epithelium. A chorioretinal adhesion cannot be created within the coloboma, because of the absence of underlying choroidal tissue and pigment epithelium. Various methods have been used to create chorioretinal adhesions surrounding colobomas. Successful results have been reported after applying penetrating diathermy or photocoagulation to the edge of the coloboma (83), and after creating a radial scleral buckle along the margin of the coloboma (84). In their review of the literature, Wang and Hilton (84) concluded that vitrectomy with intraocular gas tamponade and creation of a chorioretinal adhesion along the edge of the coloboma without a scleral buckle is now the preferred technique. In more recent reports, anatomic success was obtained in over 90% of cases (80,81,85).

To treat rhegmatogenous retinal detachments associated with chorioretinal coloboma, vitrectomy is performed with the anomalous retinal tissue within the coloboma inspected to try to identify any specific breaks. Sometimes a small round or slit-like defect is found along the edge of the coloboma (Fig. 45-13). Some breaks are obscured by surrounding incomplete sheets or bridges of retinal tissue within the coloboma. A thin, blunt-tipped needle on a flute handle is used to search for a defect within the coloboma through which subretinal fluid can be evacuated (85). The breaks are seen intraoperatively in some eyes, based on the behavior of the retina during fluid–air exchange. The majority of breaks are located within two disc diameters of the colobomatous margin (82). In some cases, the subretinal fluid can be removed readily to flatten the retina. In many cases, however, no subretinal fluid can be withdrawn through the coloboma. Trans-scleral drainage or drainage through a retinotomy is performed in those cases (85). Drainage of subretinal fluid is desirable even though an intravitreal gas bubble is used later, because the detachment is often chronic and the subretinal fluid is viscous. If the retina settles properly, photocoagulation or trans-scleral cryotherapy is applied around the edge of the coloboma. A long-acting gas is preferred for effective intraocular tamponade. A large bubble is also desirable because of the inferior location of the coloboma (85). Silicone oil has been used for temporary tamponade (80,81), but this is rarely necessary (85).

If the coloboma surrounds the optic nerve head, the peripapillary portion of the coloboma is not coagulated intraoperatively, to avoid excessive damage to the nerve fiber layer. The margin of the coloboma around the nerve head is treated postoperatively with krypton laser (85). Depending on the size and location of the coloboma, cyanoacrylate glue retinopexy to directly close breaks may be of benefit to avoid damaging the nerve-fiber layer in the papillomacular area (80).

## Peripapillary Staphyloma

Peripapillary staphyloma is an extremely rare, usually unilateral, congenital anomaly characterized by a relatively normal-appearing optic disc located at the base of a staphylomatous excavation (5) (Fig. 45-14). Atrophic changes of the choroid and retinal pigment epithelium usually are seen within the walls of the defect. Unlike the morning glory disc anomaly, there is no central glial tuft overlying the disc, and the retinal vascular pattern remains normal, apart from reflecting the

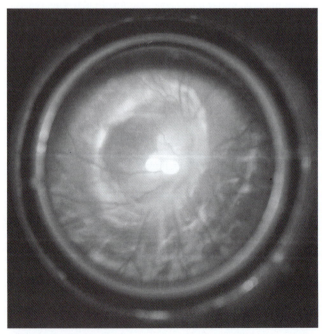

**Figure 45-14.** Peripapillary staphyloma. This is a relatively normal disc, with absence of central glial tissue and vascular anomalies in the deep peripapillary excavation.

essential contour of the lesion (1). The staphylomatous excavation in peripapillary staphyloma is also notably deeper than that seen in the morning glory disc anomaly (1). Although the depth of the optic disc often ranges from 8 to 20 diopters (approximately 3 to 8 mm) (5), the macula is usually within 1 to 2 diopters of emmetropia. Several cases of contractile peripapillary staphyloma have been noted (86,87).

The visual acuity can be normal in mild cases, but severe loss of vision generally is seen with more pronounced defects (5,88). Peripapillary staphyloma generally has not been associated with other ocular or systemic congenital defects, and no evidence is available to suggest a hereditary factor (5).

The relatively normal appearance of the optic disc suggests that the development of this structure is complete prior to the onset of the staphylomatous process. Pollock has argued that the clinical features of peripapillary staphyloma are most consistent with diminished peripapillary structural support, perhaps resulting from incomplete differentiation of the sclera from posterior neural crest cells in the fifth month of gestation. Staphyloma formation presumably occurs if establishment of normal intraocular pressure leads to herniation of unsupported ocular tissues through the defect. According to this concept of pathogenesis, peripapillary staphyloma and the morning glory disc anomaly may be pathologically distinct, both in the timing of the insult (fifth month versus fourth week of gestation) and in the embryologic site of structural dysgenesis (posterior sclera versus distal optic stalk) (1).

Most reports in the literature have described attached retina at the base of the staphyloma. Limited retinal detachments within the staphyloma have also been reported, however, most of which have spontaneous contractions of the walls of larger staphylomas (86,87). Diagnostic ultrasonography (B-scan) is useful to demonstrate retinal detachment within a large peripapillary staphyloma. There can be extensive retinal pigment epithelial and choroidal pigmentary atrophy beyond the immediate peristaphyloma retina, representing resolved anterior retinal detachment with secondary pigment alterations (88).

If a limited retinal detachment enlarges subsequent to occurrence of a retinal break within the staphyloma, vitrectomy may be indicated to reattach the retina. The techniques used are similar to those used in eyes with morning glory disc anomaly complicated by retinal detachment.

## References

1. Brodsky MC. Congenital optic disk anomalies. *Surv Ophthalmol* 1994; 39:89.
2. Gass JDM. Serous detachment of the macula: secondary to congenital pit of the optic nervehead. *Am J Ophthalmol* 1969;67:821.
3. Fea A, Grosso A, Rabbione M, et al. Alagille syndrome and optic pit. *Graefes Arch Clin Exp Ophthalmol* 2007;245(2):315–317.
4. Wiethe T. Ein fall von angeborener feformitat der sehnervenpapille. *Arch Augenheilkd* 1882;11:14.
5. Brown GC, Tasman WS. Excavated and colobomatous defects. In: Brown GC, Tasman WS (eds). *Congenital anomalies of the optic disc*, New York: Grune & Stratton, 1983:97–215.
6. Kranenburg EW. Crater-like holes in the optic disc and central serous retinopathy. *Arch Ophthalmol* 1960;64:912.
7. Sadun AA. Optic disc pits and associated serous macular detachment. In: Ryan SJ, Schachat AP (eds). *Retina*, 4th ed. St. Louis: Mosby, 2001.
8. Ferry AP. Macular detachment associated with congenital pit of the optic nerve head: pathologic findings in two cases simulating malignant melanoma of the choroid. *Arch Ophthalmol* 1963;70:346.
9. Lincoff H, Schiff W, Krivoy D, et al. Optic coherence tomography of optic disk pit maculopathy. *Am J Ophthalmol* 1996;122(2):264–266.
10. Rutledge BK, Puliafito CA, Duker JS, et al. Optical coherence tomography of macular lesions associated with optic nerve head pits. *Ophthalmology* 1996;103(7):1047–1053.
11. Krivoy D, Gentile R, Liebmann JM, et al. Imaging congenital optic disc pits and associated maculopathy using optical coherence tomography. *Arch Ophthalmol* 1996;114(2):165–170.
12. Sugar HS. Congenital pits in the optic disc and their equivalents (congenital colobomas and colobomalike excavations) associated with submacular fluid. *Am J Ophthalmol* 1967;63:298.
13. Schatz H, McDonald HR. Treatment of sensory retinal detachment associated with optic nerve pit or coloboma. *Ophthalmology* 1988;95:178.
14. Lincoff H, Lopez R, Kreissig I, et al. Retinoschisis associated with optic pits. *Arch Ophthalmol* 1988;106:61.
15. Brown GC, Shields JA, Goldberg RE. Congenital pits of the nerve head: II. Clinical studies in humans. *Ophthalmology* 1980;87:51.
16. Henkind P. Craterlike holes of the optic nerve. *Am J Ophthalmol* 1963; 55:613.
17. Gass JDM. Optic nerve diseases that may masquerade as macular diseases. In: Gass JDM (ed). *Stereoscopic atlas of macular diseases: diagnosis and treatment*, 3rd ed, vol 2. St Louis: Mosby–Year Book, 1987:728.
18. Bonnet M. Serous macular detachment associated with optic nerve pits. *Graefes Arch Clin Exp Ophthalmol* 1991;229:526.
19. Akiba J, Kakehashi A, Hikichi T, et al. Vitreous findings in cases of optic nerve pits and serous macular detachment. *Am J Ophthalmol* 1993;116:38.
20. Sadun AA. Optic disc pits and associated serous macular detachment. In: Ryan SJ, Schachat AP, Murphy RP (eds). *Retina*, vol 2. St. Louis: Mosby–Year Book, 1994:1829.
21. Lincoff H, Yannuzzi L, Singerman L, et al. Improvement in visual function after displacement of the retinal elevations emanating from optic pits. *Arch Ophthalmol* 1993;111:1071.
22. Van Nouhuys JM, Bruyn GW. Nasopharyngeal transsphenoidal encephalocele, craterlike hole in the optic disc and agenesis of the corpus callosum, pneumoencephalographic visualization in a case. *Psychiatry Neurol Neurochir* 1964;67:243.
23. Pollock JA, Newton TH, Hoyt WF. Transsphenoidal and transethmoidal encephaloceles. *Radiology* 1968;90:442.
24. Stefko ST, Campochiaro P, Wang P, et al. Dominant inheritance of optic pits. *Am J Ophthalmol* 1997;124:112.
25. Gordon R, Chatfield RK. Pits in the optic disc associated with macular degeneration. *Br J Ophthalmol* 1969;53:481.
26. Brown GC, Shields JA, Patty BE, et al. Congenital pit of the optic nerve head: I. Experimental studies in collie dogs. *Arch Ophthalmol* 1979;97:1341.
27. Sugar HS. An explanation for the acquired macular pathology associated with congenital pits of the optic disc. *Am J Ophthalmol* 1964;57:833.
28. Theodossiadis GP, Koutsandrea C, Theodossiadis PG. Optic nerve pit with serous macular detachment resulting in rhegmatogenous retinal detachment. *Br J Ophthalmol* 1993;77:385.
29. Regenbogen L, Stein R, Lazar M. Macular and juxtapapillary serous retinal detachment associated with pit of the optic disk. *Ophthalmologica* 1964;148:247.
30. Kalina RE, Conrad WC. Intrathecal fluorescein for serous macular detachment. *Arch Ophthalmol* 1976;94:1421.
31. Chang S, Haik BJ, Ellsworth RM, et al. Treatment of total retinal detachment in morning glory syndrome. *Am J Ophthalmol* 1984;97:596.
32. Irvine AR, Crawford JB, Sullivan JH. The pathogenesis of retinal detachment with morning glory disc and optic pit. *Trans Am Ophthalmol Soc* 1986;84:280.
33. Peterson AP. Pits or crater-like holes in the optic disc. *Acta Ophthalmol* 1958;36:435.
34. Sobol WM, Blodi CF, Folk JC, et al. Long-term visual outcome in patients with optic nerve pit and serous retinal detachment of the macula. *Ophthalmology* 1990;97:1539.
35. Wilkinson CP, Rice TS. Optic nervehead pit. In: Wilkinson CP, Rice TS (eds). *Michels retinal detachment*, 2nd ed, St. Louis: Mosby–Year Book, 1997:149.
36. Theodossiadis GP. Evolution of congenital pit of the optic disk with macular detachment in photocoagulated and nonphotocoagulated eyes. *Am J Ophthalmol* 1977;84:620.
37. Annesley W, Brown G, Bolling J, et al. Treatment of retinal detachment with congenital optic pit by krypton laser photocoagulation. *Graefes Arch Clin Exp Ophthalmol* 1987;2215:311.
38. Cox MS, Witherspoon CD, Morris RE, et al. Evolving techniques in the treatment of macular degeneration caused by optic nerve pits. *Ophthalmology* 1988;95:889.
39. Brown GC, Brown MM. Treatment of retinal detachment associated with congenital excavated defects of the optic disc. *Ophthalmic Surg* 1995;26:11.
40. Yanyali A, Bonnet M. Treatment of macular detachment complicating optic disk coloboma pits: long-term results of the photocoagulation-gas combination. *J Fr Ophthalmol* 1993;16:523.
41. Hirakata A, Hida T, Shinoda K, et al. Remarkable visual field loss after closed vitrectomy of optic nerve pit maculopathy [abstract]. Presented at the Centennial Annual Meeting of the American Academy of Ophthalmology; 1996; Chicago, Illinois.

42. Theodossiadis GP. Treatment of maculopathy associated with optic disk pit by sponge explant. *Am J Ophthalmol* 1996;121:630.

43. Chan CK, Wessels IF. Delayed subretinal fluid absorption after pneumatic retinopexy. *Ophthalmology* 1989;96:1691.

44. Brockhurst RJ. Optic pits and posterior retinal detachment. *Trans Am Ophthalmol Soc* 1976;73:264.

45. Kindler P. Morning glory syndrome: unusual congenital optic disc anomaly. *Am J Ophthalmol* 1970;69:376.

46. Steinkuller PG. The morning glory disc anomaly: case report and literature review. *J Pediatr Ophthalmol* 1980;17:81.

47. Traboulsi EI, O'Neill JF. The spectrum in the morphology of the so-called "morning glory disc anomaly." *J Pediatr Ophthalmol Strabismus* 1988;25:93.

48. Duvall J, Miller SL, Cheatle E, et al. Histopathologic study of ocular changes in a syndrome of multiple congenital anomalies. *Am J Ophthalmol* 1987; 103:701.

49. Byer WB, Quencer RM, Osher RH. Morning glory syndrome: a functional analysis including fluorescein angiography, ultrasonography, and computerized tomography. *Ophthalmology* 1982;100:1361.

50. Wilkinson CP, Rice TS. Morning glory disc anomaly. In: Wilkinson CP, Rice TS (eds). *Michels retinal detachment*, 2nd ed, St. Louis: Mosby–Year Book, 1997:154.

51. Bartz-Schmidt KU, Heimann K. Pathogenesis of retinal detachment associated with morning glory disc. *Int Ophthalmol* 1995;19:35.

52. Haik BG, Greenstein SH, Smith ME, et al. Retinal detachment in the morning glory anomaly. *Ophthalmology* 1984;91:1638.

53. von Fricken MA, Dhungel R. Retinal detachment in the morning glory syndrome: pathogenesis and management. *Retina* 1984;4:97.

54. Harris MJ, de Bustros S, Michels RG, et al. Treatment of combined traction-rhegmatogenous retinal detachment in the morning glory syndrome. *Retina* 1984;4:259.

55. Akiyama K, Azuma N, Hida T, et al. Retinal detachment in the morning glory syndrome. *Ophthalmic Surg* 1984;15:841.

56. Traboulsi EI. Morning glory disc anomaly or optic nerve coloboma? *Arch Ophthalmol* 1994;112:153.

57. Pedler C. Unusual coloboma of the optic nerve entrance. *Br J Ophthalmol* 1978;45:803.

58. Cogan DG. Coloboma of optic nerve with overlay of peripapillary retina. *Br J Ophthalmol* 1978;62:347.

59. Hamada S, Ellsworth RM. Congenital retinal detachment and the optic disc anomaly. *Am J Ophthalmol* 1969;67:821.

60. Haik BG, Greenstein SG, Smith ME, et al. Retinal detachment in the morning glory syndrome. *Ophthalmology* 1983;90(suppl):76.

61. Wise JB, MacLean JL, Gass JDM. Contractile peripapillary staphyloma. *Arch Ophthalmol* 1966;75:626.

62. Coll GE, Chang S, Flynn TE, et al. Communication between the subretinal space and the vitreous cavity in the morning glory syndrome. *Graefes Arch Clin Exp Ophthgalmol* 1995;233:441.

63. Lyle DJ. Coloboma of the optic nerve. *Am J Ophthalmol* 1932;15:347.

64. Pagon RA, Spaeth GL. Congenital malformation of the eye. In: Tasman W, Jaeger EA (eds). *Duane's foundations of clinical ophthalmology*, (revised ed), vol 1. Philadelphia, PA: Lippincott–Raven Publishers, 1995.

65. Nagano E, Hirakata A, Oshitari K, et al. A surgically treated case of choroidal coloboma with retinoschisis and macular detachment. *Jpn J Clin Ophthalmol* 1999;53:1261–1263.

66. Gopal L, Badrinath SS, Kumar KS, et al. Optic disc in fundus coloboma. *Ophthalmology* 1996;103:2120.

67. Savell J, Cook JR. Optic nerve colobomas of autosomal-dominant heredity. *Arch Ophthalmol* 1976;94:395.

68. Wilkinson CP, Rice TS. Optic nervehead colobomas. In: Wilkinson CP, Rice TS (eds). *Michels retinal detachment*, 2nd ed, St. Louis: Mosby–Year Book, 1997:156.

69. Pagon RA, Graham JM, Zonana J, et al. Coloboma, congenital heart disease, and choanal atresia with multiple anomalies: CHARGE association. *J Pediatr* 1981;99:223.

70. Sanyanusin P, Schimmenti LA, McNoe LA, et al. Mutation of the PAX2 gene in a family with optic nerve colobomas, renal anomalies and vesicoureteral reflux. *Nat Genet* 1995;9:358.

71. Cunliffe HE, McNoe LA, Ward TA, et al. The prevalence of PAX2 mutations in patients with isolated colobomas or colobomas associated with urogenital anomalies. *J Med Genet* 1998;35:806.

72. Font RL, Zimmerman LE. Intrascleral smooth muscle in coloboma of the optic disc. *Am J Ophthalmol* 1971;72:452.

73. Willis R, Zimmerman LE, O'Grady R, et al. Heterotopic adipose tissue and smooth muscle in the optic disc, association with isolated colobomas. *Arch Ophthalmol* 1972;88:139.

74. Foster JA, Lam S. Contractile optic disc coloboma. *Arch Ophthalmol* 1991;109:472.

75. Schubert HD. Schisis-like rhegmatogenous retinal detachment associated with choroidal colobomas. *Graefes Arch Clin Exp Ophthalmol* 1995; 233:74.

76. Goldberg RE. Optic nerve pit and associated coloboma with serous detachment. *Arch Ophthalmol* 1974;97:160.

77. Lin CCL, Tso MOM, Vygantas CM. Coloboma of the optic nerve associated with serous maculopathy: a clinicopathological correlative study. *Arch Ophthalmol* 1984;102:1651.

78. Hotta K, Hirakata A, Hida T. Retinoschisis associated with disc coloboma. *Br J Ophthalmol* 1999;106:124.

79. Bochow TW, Olk RJ, Knupp JA, et al. Spontaneous reattachment of a total retinal detachment in an infant with microphthalmos and an optic nerve coloboma. *Am J Ophthalmol* 1991;112:347.

80. Hanneken A, deJuan E, McCuen BW. The management of retinal detachments associated with choroidal colobomas by vitreous surgery. *Am J Ophthalmol* 1991;111:271.

81. McDonald HR, Lewis H, Brown G, et al. Vitreous surgery for retinal detachment associated with choroidal coloboma. *Arch Ophthalmol* 1991;109:1399.

82. Gopal L, Badrinath SS, Sharma T, et al. Pattern of retinal breaks and retinal detachments in eyes with choroidal coloboma. *Ophthalmology* 1995; 102:1212.

83. Sakai T. Three cases of retinal detachment associated with congenital coloboma of the choroid. *Folia Ophthalmol Jap* 1968;19:808.

84. Wang K, Hilton GF. Retinal detachment associated with coloboma of the choroid. *Trans Am Ophthalmol Soc* 1985;83:49.

85. Wilkinson CP, Rice TS. Retinal detachment and choroidal coloboma. In: Wilkinson CP, Rice TS (eds). *Michels retinal detachment*, 2nd ed, St. Louis: Mosby–Year Book, 1997:733.

86. Sugar H, Beckman H. Peripapillary staphyloma with respiratory pulsation. *Am J Ophthalmol* 1969;68:895.

87. Kral K, Svarc D. Contractile peripapillary staphyloma. *Am J Ophthalmol* 1971;71:1090.

88. Gottlieb JL, Prieto DM, Vander JF, et al. Peripapillary Staphyloma. *Am J Ophthalmol* 1997;124:249.

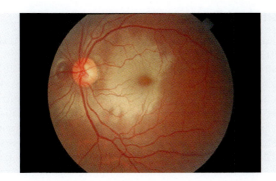

# Macular Trauma

Reinaldo A. Garcia Arismendi ■ D. Virgil Alfaro, III, ■ J. Fernando Arevalo
Oria Veronica ■ Gomez Ulla ■ Giora Treister

Eye injury is a significant disabling American health problem. The National Research Council reported that "injury is probably the most under-recognized mayor health problem facing the nation today. The study of injury presents unparalleled opportunities for reducing morbidity and for realizing significant savings in both financial and human terms." Data from the National Center for Health Statistics' Health Interview Survey, conducted in 1977, estimated that nearly 2.4 million eye injuries occur in the United States annually. This report calculated that nearly one million Americans have permanent significant visual impairment due to injury, with more than 75% of these individuals being monocularly blind. Eye injury is a leading cause of monocular blindness in the United States, and is second only to cataract as the most common cause of visual impairment. A wide variety of direct and indirect closed-globe trauma can affect the posterior segment. In this chapter we will talk about the most important conditions that can affect the posterior segment and the macula.

## TRAUMATIC MACULAR HOLE

The first published case of macular hole (MH) in a young man with an eye trauma appeared in 1869 by Knapp (1). In our days traumatic MH formation is a relatively common posterior segment complication of severe contusion injury; trauma itself accounts for up to 9% of eyes that develop full-thickness MHs (2). However, the etiology by which traumatic holes occur is not well understood and despite the large number of publications related to this topic, the cause of MH remains controversial.

### Pathogenesis

In the setting of idiopathic MHs, the vitreous is believed to have a crucial role in the pathogenesis. Recent findings suggest that full thickness MHs develop in a situation where there is failure of normal age related separation of the vitreous cortex from the posterior pole as a result of an abnormally tenacious attachment to the fovea. The formation of an idiopathic MH typically occurs over weeks to months. Although some traumatic MHs also occur weeks or months following the trauma, traumatic MHs are typically not associated with a gradual onset.

Many mechanisms such as contusion necrosis, subfoveal hemorrhage, mechanical deformity, and vitreous traction have been considered as possible causes of traumatic MHs, and Ho and associates outlined in 1998 four basic historical theories regarding its cause: the traumatic theory, the cystic degeneration theory, the vascular theory, and the vitreous theory (1). We as others (3–5) believe that in those cases in which the traumatic MH is not present initially but develops weeks to months following the incident the mechanism is probably similar to that of idiopathic MHs seen in elderly patients and the contusion and post-traumatic inflammation probably initiates and potentiates the abnormal epiretinal and vitreoretinal contraction. In the case of the MH that forms immediately following contusion injury, rapid changes in the shape of the eye with shortening in the anterior–posterior dimension with equatorial elongation and rebound may result in the rapid creation of

anterior–posterior and tangential vitreoretinal traction in the area of the fovea. This acute event in a young patient with an attached posterior hyaloid and rigid internal limiting membrane (ILM) may lead to a small dehiscence of the fovea after trauma (4). Then, the acute transient nature of tangential traction and tissue proliferation, possibly by glial cells or retinal pigment epithelium (RPE) cells, may play an important role in MH closure and may explain the more frequent occurrence of spontaneous reapproximation of the edges of the hole in some cases.

### Clinical Presentation

Patients with traumatic MHs tend to be young, and posterior vitreous detachment is typically absent in these eyes. Clinically, visual acuity is usually reduced to 20/80 to 20/400, and biomicroscopic examination typically shows a round, sharply defined hole measuring about 300 to 500 μm with a surrounding cuff of neurosensory detachment; however, in some instances the hole may be larger or show irregular margins (2) (Fig. 46-1). Traumatic damage of the RPE can be associated with traumatic MHs; it is usually manifested as a mottling of the RPE near or within the center of the macula. This potentially has significant importance for vision recovery after trauma and surgical repair (5).

### Management

*Pars plana* vitrectomy (PPV) has demonstrated efficacy and safety for patients with idiopathic MHs however there is no consensus on the operative treatment for this disease, because some cases demonstrate spontaneous closure of the MH and improved visual acuity. Mitamura et al. (6) and Yamashita et al. (7) published the largest series of eleven and eighteen traumatic MHs with spontaneously resolution in 64% and 44% respectively. This result suggests that the spontaneous closure rate is much greater in traumatic MH than in idiopathic MH, although the number of cases reported was small. Common features of patients with spontaneous closure of traumatic MH

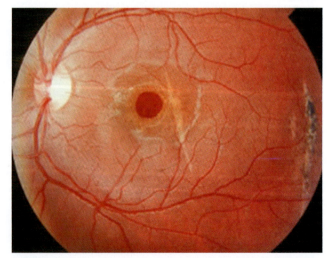

**Figure 46-1.** Sharply defined hole measuring about 1000 μm with a surrounding cuff of neurosensory detachment, traumatic damage of the retinal pigment epithelium manifested as a less pigment mottling of the RPE surrounding the macular hole. See a gliotic scar from an associate choroidal rupture temporal to the macular hole. (Courtesy of Jose Dalma, MD.)

were young age, small size of MH, no fluid cuff and no posterior vitreous detachment. Several authors (6,7,8) reported that they observed spontaneous MH closure through 1 week to 4 to 6 months after injury. Then, some authors support that an observation for a period of up to four months may be a management of choice for traumatic MH. However, still it is very difficult to decide when to perform vitrectomy, because the longer the delay, the more likely it is that the photoreceptor cells will be damaged. Because vitreous surgery can lead to hole closure with visual improvement in most eyes and the favorable results may probably be related to the younger age of the patients and the shorter duration of the MH, others (9) believe that an observation is probably a dubious initial treatment option, since a conservative approach may lessen the chance of a good anatomical and functional recovery.

## Surgical Technique

The surgical technique for traumatic MHs does not differ significantly from the idiopathic hole; however, since most of the patients with traumatic holes are younger, additional considerations are necessary. First, the posterior hyaloid may be more difficult to remove, requiring added manipulations. A few investigators have suggested enzyme assistance using plasmin for these patients (10). Younger patients tend to have more significant intraocular proliferation following trauma or retinal detachment. With this in mind, some authors (3,9) suggests epiretinal dissection or ILM removal in addition to posterior hyaloidal separation. Removal of the ILM surrounding the hole is the only way to ensure complete removal of significant epiretinal proliferation; then ILM removal may be considered as a prophylactic measure against MH reopening. Then, peeling of the inelastic ILM has proven effective and appears indicated for traumatic MHs (3,9) however, aggressive attempts to remove the ILM may result in iatrogenic injury. To facilitate and expedite removal, a dilute concentration if indocyanine green (ICG) dye may be used. Some controversy exists as to the safety of ICG in the posterior segment. Finally, silicone oil has been reported as an alternative to intraocular gas primarily because of the hypothesis that face-down positioning is less important with oil due to its prolonged, complete tamponade effect and secondarily because many of the patients are young and cannot tolerate face down positioning. However, its use does require an additional surgery for subsequent oil removal and may not provide the same efficacy as gas. Some authors believe that the silicone oil may provide less tamponade effect as the MH closes and the foveal region begins to recover the normal foveal depression (11).

In general, the success of surgical treatment in terms of anatomical closure of the traumatic hole and improvement of vision varies by study, but overall appears to be similar to idiopathic MHs (3).

## TRAUMATIC MACULAR HOLE–RELATED RETINAL DETACHMENT

The role of vitrectomy surgery for MH-related retinal detachment caused by blunt ocular injury is not well established because of the rarity of the condition. Chen et al. (12) reported eight patients with traumatic MH-related retinal detachment treated with a standard three-port PPV combined with gas tamponade initially or subsequently. Because of the high incidence of peripheral retinal breaks (50%) and in order to avoid any missing breaks and mild anterior proliferative vitreoretinopathy they performed encircling scleral buckle in six selective cases; ILM peeling was done in only two cases. They reported successful retinal re-attachment in seven eyes (87.5%), and the MH was successfully closed in all eyes (100%). They concluded that extent of retinal detachment and presence of peripheral retinal breaks, vitreous hemorrhage, or hyphema had no discernible significant influence on retinal re-attachment rate in patients with MH-related retinal detachment.

## COMMOTIO RETINAE (BERLIN'S EDEMA)

The term Commotio Retinae has been used since 1873, when Berlin described a transient whitening of the retina after blunt trauma to the globe and invoked the Latin term for retinal contusion, Commotion Retinae (13). This condition is typically characterized by transient gray-white discoloration or opacification of the outer sensory retina. The opacification may be confined to the macular area, in which case is referred to as Berlin's edema, or it can occur peripherally. The symptoms are determined by the location of the lesion. If only the peripheral retina is involved the patient may have no visual complaints. If the posterior pole is affected the patient may report decreased vision but sometimes the lesion may take several hours to be visible ophthalmoscopically. If the entire posterior pole is involved, a pseudo cherry-red spot may be present (Fig. 46-2). As the retinal opacification resolves, vision may return to normal and there may be no ophthalmoscopic findings after the resolution. With more severe blunt trauma, visual loss may persist, and the opacification may be replaced by mottling of the RPE (14).

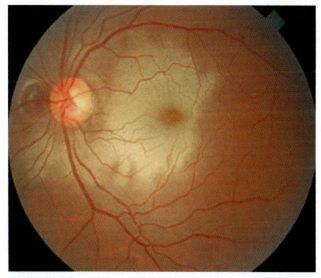

**Figure 46-2.** Transient gray-white discoloration or opacification of the outer sensory retina. If the entire posterior pole is involved, a pseudo cherry red spot may be present. (Courtesy of Jose Dalma, MD.)

## Pathogenesis

Berlin postulated (13) that extracellular edema resulted in the loss of retinal transparency, and the condition became known as Berlin's edema. Subsequent histopathologic studies in animals revealed a different pathogenesis. Blight and Hart described marked intracellular edema of the retinal glial elements after trauma induced retinal whitening in pigs. They also found receptor outer segment fragmentation and marked intracellular edema of the RPE using the same pig model (15,16). Sipperly et al. (17) detected disruption of only the photoreceptor outer segment in an owl monkey model. Kohno et al. (18) demonstrated disruption of photoreceptor outer segment in addition to intracellular edema in Muller cells, retinal pigment epithelial cells, nerve fibers, and the outer plexiform layer axons of photoreceptor cells. Mansour et al. (19) in the histopathologic analysis of a single human eye showed the development of clinical commotion retinae within 24 hours of moderately severe blunt trauma. Photoreceptor outer segment disruption and damage to the RPE were noted. These findings, in addition to the aforementioned animal studies, suggest the mechanical disruption at the photoreceptor outer segment-RPE interface is most likely responsible for the gray-white appearance of the retina in commotion retinae. Although some pathology reports of commotio retinae have noted the appearance of fluid-filled spaces in the outer retinal layers, evidence of extracellular edema in commotion retinae has not been consistently found. Finally, Monsour et al. (19) attributed the susceptibility of the outer segments to the architecture of the retina, particularly the Muller cell skeletal system because Muller cells occupy the retina from the ILM to the photoreceptor inner segment and support all cellular layers except the photoreceptor outer segments.

## Management

There is no treatment of proven benefit for Commotio Retinae, Visual acuity tends to recover in 60% of cases however forty percent of patients with severe macular involvement may have permanent macular damage and varying degrees of visual loss (20).

## CHOROIDAL RUPTURE

This condition was first described by von Graefe (21) in 1854, in our days is a common complication of blunt ocular trauma and the indirect form can be seen in 5% to 10% of blunt ocular injuries (22). Choroidal rupture are tears of the choroids, Bruch's membrane and RPE and may be classified as direct or indirect.

## Pathogenesis

The choroidal rupture in contusion trauma is probably caused by a rapid shortening of the globe's anteroposterior diameter and its expansion in the frontal plane. (22) With blunt trauma the distensible retina and the dense sclera are relatively resistant to rupture however, Bruch's membrane, its adjacent RPE and its adherent choriocapillaris are relatively inelastic and rupture more easily (23).

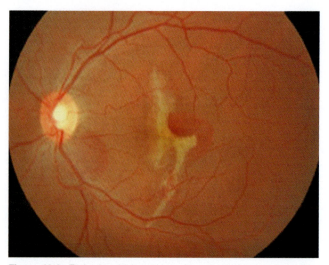

**Figure 46-3.** Early choroidal ruptures with subretinal hemorrhage. The crescent-shape lesion may not become visible ophthalmoscopically until the overlying hemorrhage resolves. As the subretinal hemorrhage and edema resorb, choroidal tear may become evident appearing as a yellow-white curvilinear defects at the level of Bruch's membrane. (Courtesy of Jose Dalma, MD.)

Direct choroidal rupture are relatively uncommon, they are usually found anterior to the equator, oriented parallel to the ora serrata and occur at the initial site of impact due to direct contusion necrosis of the choroids.

Indirect choroidal rupture are more common, tend to occurs away from the site of impact, usually in the posterior pole, with a crescent shape and concentric to the optic disk or through the fovea (Fig. 46-3). The crescent shape tears of indirect choroidal ruptures occurring concentric to the disc may be secondary to a "tethering" or stabilizing effect of the optic nerve (24).

## Clinical Presentation

Early funduscopic diagnosis of choroidal ruptures is often difficult because the initial injury often involves subretinal hemorrhage, and the crescent-shape lesion may not become visible ophthalmoscopically until the overlying hemorrhage resolves. As the subretinal hemorrhage and edema resorb, choroidal tear may become evident appearing as a yellow-white curvilinear defects at the level of Bruch's membrane. They usually appear single and temporal to the disk but may be concentric, multiple, radially oriented, or located nasal to the optic disc. The choroidal rupture develops a gliotic scar within a few weeks, and hyperpigmentation develops at the margins of the healed lesions (25) (Fig. 46-2).

## Fluorescein Angiography

In the acute setting, fluorescein angiography may aid in the detection and localization of small choroidal ruptures and suspected ruptures beneath subretinal hemorrhage. Fluorescein initially may leak from the ruptured choroidal vessels into the outer retina, but this resolves within a few days (26). Healed choroidal ruptures typically demonstrate early hypofluorescence within the rupture because of the damaged choriocapillaris (the large choroidal vessels usually are intact) and late hyperfluorescence from diffusion from the surrounding intact choriocapillaris (27). In cases with choroidal neovascularization, fluorescein angiography demonstrates early lacy subretinal vessels with late leakage into the subretinal space (23).

## Prognosis

There are three main causes of decreased visual acuity after choroidal ruptures: (a) extension of the rupture involving the fovea, (b) posttraumatic pigmentary retinopathy, and the presence of choroidal neovascularization (CNV) and blood accumulation in the subfoveal space. In a report by Hart et al. (26) initial visual acuity was 20/200 or worse in all 10 patients with posterior pole choroidal ruptures; six of those patients ultimately improved to 20/30 or better. In a recent study by Ament et al. (28) 34% of 111 patients recovered driving vision (VA > or = 20/40). Driving vision was seen in 59% of eyes with peripheral choroidal ruptures but only in 22% of eyes with macular choroidal ruptures. The formation of CNV was most strongly associated with older eye and macular choroidal rupture.

## Management

There is no treatment for the rupture itself, although a transfoveal choroidal ruptures are associated with an extremely poor prognosis, an early identification assists the clinician in providing the patient with a more realistic prediction regarding the visual outcome. Then, Gass and others (29) have noted the development of subretinal CNV occurring 1 month to 4 years after choroidal rupture therefore, the lesions should be followed closely and patients should be instructed to report any changes in central vision (30). The treatment of CNV in choroidal rupture is controversial. In a histopathologic report of 47 cases by Aguilar and Green (25) CNV was present in three cases; they concluded that new choroidal blood vessels are common in the healing process and these vessels usually regress as the scarring process evolves. Probably, early neovascular membranes occurring at choroidal ruptures (within six months of the injury) could be related to persistence of the normal reparative neovascular response. However, late (at least one year after the injury) CNV are more likely to have resulted from a secondary breakdown of the outer blood retinal barrier. Although neovascular membranes have been treated with laser photocoagulation, surgical excision, and photodynamic therapy, controlled clinical trials evaluating the efficacy of these procedures in this setting have not yet been performed. Because CNV often involutes spontaneously leaving a relatively small scotoma, some authors support that an observation may be a management of choice. Antivascular endothelial growth factor (anti-VEGF) therapy may eventually become the best treatment option; however, to date, there is no datum or even anecdotal clinical report regarding this treatment in CNV and choroidal rupture.

## TRAUMATIC CHORIORETINAL RUPTURE (RETINITIS SCLOPETARIA)

Goldzieher described the first case in 1901 and introduced the term chorioretinitis plastica sclopetaria. Because the pathogenesis is not inflammatory, the terms "sclopetaria" and "chorioretinal rupture" currently are accepted (31). This condition is rare and occurs when a high-velocity missile strikes or passes adjacent to the globe without penetrating it, causing a full-thickness breach of the choroids and retina with accompanying vitreous, retinal, and subretinal hemorrhage. After the resolution of blood, the fundus lesion is characterized by an area of absent retina, retinal pigment epithelium, Bruch's membrane, and choroids in the same quadrant sustaining the missile injury, eventually developing irregular borders of white proliferative scar tissue (22,27). When these tissues retract a bare sclera may be visible. The lesion may extend posteriorly to involve the macula, and retinal detachment is rare even without surgical intervention, because in early stages the retraction of the choroids and retina occurs as a single unit and the typically intact posterior hyaloid prevent the access of fluid to the subretinal space. In later stages firm chorioretinal adhesion develops at the edge of the lesion and acts as a spontaneous retinopexy (22,27,32).

## IATROGENIC MACULAR RETINAL TEAR AND ACCIDENTAL SUBRETINAL INDOCYANINE GREEN CONTRAST

Accidental subretinal ICG during vitrectomy for MH has been reported in two cases with good visual recovery (33,34). We previously reported a case of MH surgery complicated by accidental massive subretinal ICG, and a retinal tear through the papillomacular bundle with poor anatomic and functional results (35).

How can you develop an iatrogenic macular retinal tear and what you can do about it? We performed a vitrectomy posterior vitreous mechanical detachment to close a senile MH (Fig. 46-4A). Approximately 0.3 ml of 0.5% ICG was applied to stain the ILM. The assistant surgical nurse at the beginning of the instillation pushed the ICG syringe's embolus with too much force into the vitreous cavity with a 20-gauge cannula. Subretinal ICG was accidentally introduced through the MH, and an iatrogenic macular retinal tear though the papillomacular bundle was created (Fig. 46-4B). Infusion was resumed immediately, and ICG was removed from the vitreous cavity, and the ILM was removed in a circular fashion in the usual manner. Indocyanine-green removal from the subretinal space during surgery was not attempted as most of it had already left the subretinal space through the iatrogenic retinal tear. The eye was left with 14% perfluoropropane gas. Fundus examination and optical coherence tomography (OCT) performed after the intraocular gas was reabsorbed one month after the surgery revealed that the MH was completely closed with choroidal hyperreflectivity due to RPE and choriocapillaris atrophy (Fig. 46-4C and 46-4D). Best-corrected visual acuity was 20/150 with a closed MH and ICG still present in the subretinal space seven months after surgery.

If direct ICG toxicity to the RPE cells is responsible for the changes noted, this effect may be minimized or eliminated

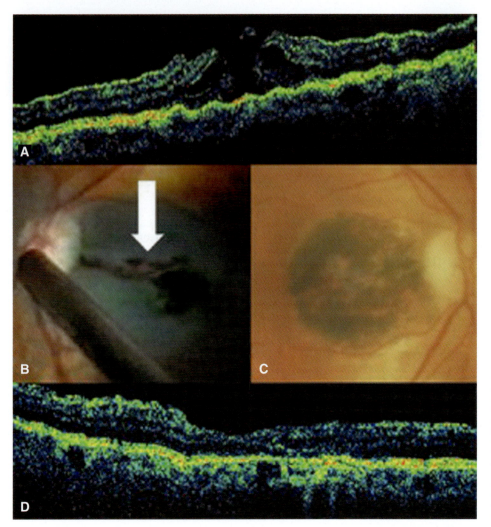

**Figure 46-4. A:** The diameter of the hole measured directly with optical coherence tomography (OCT) was 224 μ right eye. **B:** Subretinal indocyanine green (ICG) was accidentally introduced through the macular hole, and an iatrogenic macular retinal tear though the papillomacular bundle was created (*arrow*). **C:** Fundus examination performed after the intraocular gas was reabsorbed revealed a closed macular hole and subretinal ICG one month after the surgery. **D:** OCT demonstrated choroidal hyperreflectivity due to retinal pigment epithelium/choriocapillaris complex atrophy. The macular hole is closed.

by decreasing the concentration of ICG solution, reducing the ICG staining time, using heavy liquid or viscoelastics to protect the MH during staining, directing the injection cannula first towards the temporal macula, and then towards the posterior pole, and avoiding aspiration within the MH intraoperatively, In addition, ICG-mediated phototoxicity may be avoided by reducing the light intensity while dissecting the ILM, and maintaining an adequate distance between the light source and the retinal surface.

## INDIRECT TRAUMA

### Purtscher's Retinopathy

In 1910, Purtscher described a syndrome of multiple patches of superficial retinal whitening (cotton-wool spots), intraretinal hemorrhages, and papillitis in five patients following severe head trauma. He postulated that the white spots were lymphatic extravasations caused by a sudden increase in intracranial pressure related to head trauma (36). Purtscher's

retinopathy usually follows chest compression trauma but similar fundus findings have since been seen in hydrostatic pressure syndrome, fat embolism, acute pancreatitis, lupus erythematous, dermatomyositis, scleroderma, during childbirth and in the postpartum period (37). Since 1910, the pathogenesis of this condition remains uncertain and several mechanisms have been proposed. In 1990, Blodi et al. (38) supports the most likely mechanism, they proposed the retinal arteriolar embolization theory, most likely secondary to leukocyte aggregation (or leukoemboli), which form as a result of complement activation (C5a). The findings typically are bilateral and classic fundoscopic presentation is characterized by multiple patches of cotton wool spots, intraretinal or preretinal hemorrhages, papilledema and generalized retinal edema. Usually the peripheral retina is spared and retinal findings often resolve over a period of weeks to months. With the resolution of fundus lesions, the retina may appear normal or may demonstrate multifocal nerve fiber layer atrophy, pigment migration, and optic disc atrophy with minimal gliosis. Visual acuity may return to normal or a residual deficit may persist.

No specific treatment has been devised for Purtscher's retinopathy. If complement contributes to the pathologic process, the use of systemic corticosteroids has some rationale (30).

## Terson's Syndrome

Litten, (39) in 1881 and, subsequently, Terson (40) in 1900, described intraocular hemorrhages in association with a subarachnoid bleed. This condition can be found in 3% to 8% of individuals with subarachnoid hemorrhage (41). The pathogenesis of Terson's syndrome remains controversial; the most plausible explanation suggests that an acute rise in intracranial pressure resulting from subarachnoid hemorrhage is transmitted within the optic nerve sheath and obstructs intraocular venous drainage. This, in turn, causes a rapid rise in intraocular venous pressure, distention, and rupture of the fine and retinal capillaries and subsequent significant hemorrhage. The hemorrhage may then expand into the subretinal space, the subinternal limiting membrane space, the subhyaloid space, or the cortical vitreous.

The typical clinical course consist of gradual resolution of the vitreous hemorrhage within a year, but vitrectomy is effective in hastening visual rehabilitation and may avoid potential complications of persistence blood in the vitreous such as cataract, epiretinal membranes, other macular abnormalities, and retinal detachment, as well as amblyopia and myopia in infants. In general indications for conservative management include rapidly clearing vitreous hemorrhage, unilateral involvement with a normal fellow eye, associated ocular damage that precludes good vision, and poor health. Indications for early surgical management include vitreous hemorrhage in immature eyes of infants, where early intervention may prevent amblyopia, and adults with bilateral dense vitreous hemorrhage.

## Valsalva Retinopathy

In 1972, Duane described a condition wherein a sudden increase in intrathoracic or intraabdominal pressure against a closed glottis (Valsalva maneuver) develops decrease venous return with associated increased intracranial venous pressure; this maneuver could result in elevated intraocular venous pressures and subsequent rupture of retinal capillaries (42). Fundoscopic examination usually reveals a well circumscribed, dome or dumbbell-shaped, bright red hemorrhage underneath the ILM or near the central macula that may develop a fluid level as the blood settles inferiorly; larger round or oval hemorrhages also may be seen. Occasionally, the subinternal limiting membrane hemorrhage breaks through to the subhyaloid space or vitreous cavity. The hemorrhages usually resolve and vision returns to normal.

## Shaken Baby Syndrome

Caffey (43) was the first to demonstrate the association between manual shaking of an infant with whiplash induced intraocular and intracranial hemorrhage. This condition is especially important among infants less than 2 years of age as they are the most susceptible to injury by shaking. Because newborns have poorly developed neck muscles, the shaking maneuver causes rapid acceleration-deceleration of the infant's head. Although indirect acceleration-deceleration traction stresses proposed by Caffey may be the cause, experimental and clinical evidence is accumulating that suggest that the head injuries result from sudden rotational (or angular) deceleration associated with the forceful striking of the head against a surface. If the head contacts a soft surface, the force of the impact is widely dissipated and may not be associated with visible signs of surface trauma even though the brain itself decelerates rapidly. Thus the term "shaken-impact syndrome" may reflect more accurately the usual mechanism responsible for these injuries (44). Common forms of physical abuse in children include periorbital trauma, ocular or head trauma, chest injuries, or choking. The most common ocular findings in abused children are retinal hemorrhages, cotton wool spots, papilledema, and vitreous hemorrhage. The definitive diagnosis is straightforward if the characteristic physical findings are present and neuroimaging and skeletal surveys support the diagnosis of non-accidental trauma. If retinal hemorrhages are the sole finding, the diagnosis becomes more difficult. Although retinal hemorrhages are not pathognomonic of child abuse and can be seen after head trauma from various causes, the absence of an obvious cause is evidence sufficient to warrant serious investigation for child abuse (45). The clinical course of shaken baby syndrome is extremely variable, ranging from complete clearing vision to complete visual loss. Common complications related to the intracranial bleeding in shaken infants include seizures, cardiorespiratory arrest, and death. The ophthalmologist must be familiar with retinal and intracranial hemorrhage manifestations of child abuse in order to render effective care and to facilitate potentially life-saving intervention.

## Lightning Maculopathy

Lee et al. (46) reported four routes by which lightning reaches its victims: (a) direct strike; (b) side flash-lightning strikes a nearby object and arcs through the path of least resistance; (c) ground current-lightning strikes the ground and travels along its surface; and (d) sometimes people have been electrocuted while on the phone or in the bathtub by current traveling through wires or pipes (47). We previously reported (48) a 14-year-old girl who was struck by lightning with bilateral macular cyst that was diagnosed with OCT. Her fundus examination revealed bilateral macular lesions that simulated MHs (Fig. 46-5). Our patient had ground current because lightning reportedly struck approximately 30 feet from the patient's rural house.

If an electrical current affects the eye, the melanin granules of the RPE and choroid would constitute the main obstacle to the current flow. The macula is very sensitive to thermal damage because of the high content of melanin granules of its RPE (49,50). Macular "edema" simulating Berlin's edema seen early after lightning struck may be replaced by lesions described as a "cyst," "MH," or solar maculopathy (46–50). However, most of these lesions have a visual prognosis potentially different than that for full-thickness MH, and careful retinal examination is essential to make the differential diagnosis (46). OCT seems to be useful in the evaluation of lighting maculopathy to rule-out full-thickness MH in these cases, and avoid unnecessary surgery.

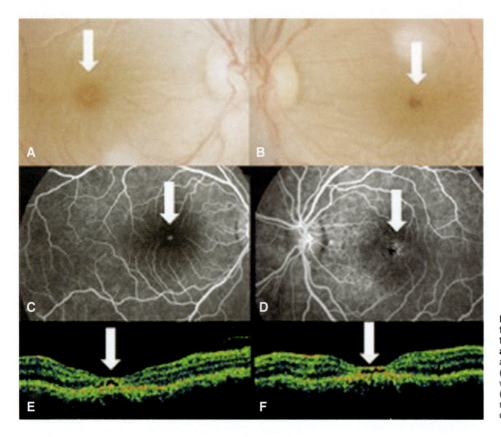

**Figure 46-5. A and B:** Fundus examination revealed bilateral macular lesions that simulated macular holes (*arrows*). **C and D:** Fluorescein angiography showed a foveal window defect in both eyes (*arrows*). **E and F:** A small foveal cyst was evident as a hyporeflective lucency (*arrows*), visible just anterior to the retinal pigment epithelium/choriocapillaris complex in both eyes.

## References

1. Ho AC, Guyer DR, Fine SL. Macular hole. *Surv Ophthalmol* 1998;42:393–416.
2. Nelson DB, Grantham RL, Marcus DM. Traumatic giant macular hole. *Retina* 2001;21:677–678.
3. Pieramici DJ. Vitreoretinal trauma. *Ophthalmol Clin North Am* 2002;15:225–234.
4. Madreperla SA, Benetz BA. Formation and treatment of a traumatic macular hole. *Arch Ophthalmol* 1997;115:1210–1211.
5. Johnson RN, McDonald HR, Lewis H, et al. Traumatic macular hole: observations, pathogenesis, and results of vitrectomy surgery. *Ophthalmology* 2001;108:853–857.
6. Mitamura Y, Saito W, Ishida M, et al. Spontaneous closure of traumatic macular hole. *Retina* 2001;21:385–389.
7. Yamashita T, Uemara A, Uchino E, et al. Spontaneous closure of traumatic macular hole. *Am J Ophthalmol* 2002;133:230–235.
8. Yamada H, Sakai A, Yamada E, et al. Spontaneous closure of traumatic macular hole. *Am J Ophthalmol* 2002;134:340–347.
9. Kuhn F, Morris R, Mester V, et al. Internal limiting membrane removal for traumatic macular holes. *Ophthalmic Surg Lasers* 2001;32:308–315.
10. Margherio AR, Margherio RR, Hartzer M, et al. Plasmin enzyme-assisted vitrectomy in traumatic pediatric macular holes. *Ophthalmology* 1998;105:1617–1620.
11. Kokame GT, Yamamoto I. Silicone oil versus gas tamponade. *Ophthalmology* 2004;111:851–852.
12. Chen YP, Chen TL, Chao AN, et al. Surgical management of traumatic macular hole-related retinal detachment. *Am J Ophthalmol* 2005;140:331–333.
13. Berlin R. Zur Sogennneten commotion retinae. *Klin Monatsbl Augenheilkd* 1873;1:42–78.
14. Hart JC, Frank HJ. Retinal opacification after blunt non-perforating concussional injuries to the globe. A clinical and retinal fluorescein angiographic study. Trans *Ophthalmol Soc U K* 1975;95:94–100.
15. Blight R, Hart JC. Histological changes in the internal retinal layers produced by concussive injuries to the globe. An experimental study. *Trans Ophthalmol Soc U K* 1978;98:270–277.
16. Blight R, Hart JC. Structural changes in the outer retinal layers following blunt mechanical non-perforating trauma to the globe: an experimental study. *Br J Ophthalmol* 1977;61:573–587.
17. Sipperley JO, Quigley HA, Gass DM. Traumatic retinopathy in primates. The explanation of commotio retinae. *Arch Ophthalmol* 1978;96:2267–2273.
18. Kohno T, Ishibashi T, Inomata H, et al. Experimental macular edema of commotio retinae: preliminary report. *Jpn J Ophthalmol* 1983;27:149–156.
19. Mansour AM, Green WR, Hogge C. Histopathology of commotio retinae. *Retina* 1992;12:24–28.
20. Au Eong KG, Kent D, Pieramici DJ. Vitreous and retina. In: Kuhn F, Pieramici DJ (eds). *Ocular Trauma Principles and Practice*, 1st ed. New York, NY: Thieme NY, 2002:206–234.
21. von Graefe A. Zwei falle von rupture der choroidea. *Graefes Arch Ophthalmol* 1854;1:402.
22. Benson WE, Shakin J, Sarin LK. Blunt trauma. In: Tasman W, Jaeger EA (eds). *Clinical Ophthalmology*, vol 3. Philadelphia, PA: JB Lippincott, 1988.
23. Bressler SB, Bressler NM. Traumatic maculopathies. In: Shingleton BJ, Hersh PS, Kenyon KR (eds). *Eye trauma*. St. Louis: Mosby-Year Book, 1991:187–194.
24. Wyszynski RE, Grossniklaus HE, Frank KE. Indirect choroidal rupture secondary to blunt ocular trauma. A review of eight eyes. *Retina* 1988;8:237–243.
25. Aguilar JP, Green WR. Choroidal rupture. A histopathologic study of 47 cases. *Retina* 1984;4:269–275.
26. Hart JC, Natsikos VE, Raistrick ER, et al. Indirect choroidal tears at the posterior pole: a fluorescein angiographic and perimetric study. *Br J Ophthalmol* 1980;64:59–67.
27. Eliott D, Avery RL. Nonpenetrating posterior segment trauma. In: Stamper RL, Parver LM, Pieramici DJ (eds). *Ophthalmol Clin North Am. Issues in Ocular Trauma*. W.B. Saunders, 1995;8:647–666.
28. Ament CS, Zacks DN, Lane AM, et al. Predictors of visual outcome and choroidal neovascular membrane formation after traumatic choroidal rupture. *Arch Ophthalmol* 2006;124:957–966.
29. Gass JDM. *Stereoscopic Atlas of Macular Diseases: Diagnosis and Treatment*, 3rd ed. St. Louis: Mosby-Year Book, 1987.
30. King LP, Hudson SJ. Closed Globe Trauma. In: Alfaro V, Liggett PE. *Vitreoretinal Surgery of the Injuried Eye*, 1st ed. Philadelphia, PA: Lippincott-Raven Publishers, 1999:29–47.
31. Goldzieher, W. Beitrag zur Pathologie der orbitalen Schussverletzungen. *Z Augenheilkd* 1901;6:227.
32. Martin DF, Awh CC, McCuen BW, et al. Treatment and pathogenesis of traumatic chorioretinal rupture sclopetaria. *Am J Ophthalmol* 1994;117:190–200.
33. Brazitikos PD, Androudi S, Tsinopoulos I, et al. Functional and anatomic results of macular hole surgery complicated by massive indocyanine green subretinal migration. *Acta Ophthalmol Scand* 2004;82:613–615.

34. Hirata A, Inomata Y, Kawaji T, et al. Persistent subretinal indocyanine green induces retinal pigment epithelium atrophy. *Am J Ophthalmol* 2003;136:353–355.

35. Arevalo JF, Garcia RA. Condiments in Vitreoretinal Surgery: A Bad Day in the Kitchen (VIDEO). 23rd Annual Meeting of the American Society of Retina Specialists. Montreal, Canada (July 16–20, 2005). Final program, pg. 47. (Best Video in Trauma section)

36. Purtscher O. Noch unbekannte Befunde nach Schadel trauma. *Berl Dtsch Ophthal Ges* 1910;36:294–301.

37. Kelly JS, Hartranft CD. Traumatic chorioretinopathies. In: Schachat A, Ryan SJ. *Retina* 3rd ed, vol 2. St. Louis: Mosby, 2001:1810–1820.

38. Blodi BA, Johnson MW, Gass JD, et al. Purtscher's-like retinopathy after childbirth. *Ophthalmology* 1990;97:1654–1659.

39. Litten M. Ueber einege vom allgemein-klinischen standpunkt aus interessante Augenveranderungen. *Berl Klin Wochenschr* 1881;18:23–27.

40. Terson, A. De l'hemorrhagie dans le corps vitre au cours de l'hemorrhagie cerebrale. *Clin Ophthalmol* 1900;6:309–312.

41. Kuhn F, Morris R, Witherspoon CD, et al. Terson syndrome. Results of vitrectomy and the significance of vitreous hemorrhage in patients with subarachnoid hemorrhage. *Ophthalmology* 1998;105:472–477.

42. Duane TD. Valsalva hemorrhagic retinopathy. *Trans Am Ophthalmol Soc* 1972;70:298–313.

43. Caffey J. The whiplash shaken infant syndrome: manual shaking by the extremities with whiplash-induced intracranial and intraocular bleedings, linked with residual permanent brain damage and mental retardation. *Pediatrics* 1974;54:396–403.

44. Duhaime AC, Christian CW, Rorke LB, et al. Nonaccidental head injury in infants–the "shaken-baby syndrome". *N Engl J Med* 1998;338:1822–1829.

45. Dugel PU, Ober RR. Posterior segment manifestations of closed-globe contusion injury. In: Schachat A, Ryan SJ. *Retina*, 3rd ed, vol 3. St. Louis: Mosby, 2001:2386–2399.

46. Lee MS, Gunton KB, Fischer DH, et al. Ocular manifestations of remote lightning strike. *Retina* 2002;22:808–810.

47. Grover S, Goodwin J. Lightning and electrical injuries: neuro-ophthalmologic aspects. *Semin Neurol* 1995;15:335–341.

48. Rivas-Aquino PJ, Garcia RA, Arevalo JF. Bilateral macular cyst after lightning visualized with optical coherence tomography. *Clin Experiment Ophthalmol* 2006;34(9):893–894.

49. Espaillat A, Janigian R Jr, To K. Cataracts, bilateral macular holes, and rhegmatogenous retinal detachment induced by lightning. *Am J Ophthalmol* 1999;127:216–217.

50. Handa JT, Jaffe GJ. Lightning maculopathy. A case report. *Retina* 1994;14:169–172.

# 47

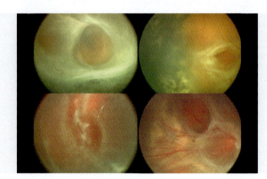

# Pediatric Macular Surgery

Mark K. Walsh ■ Antonio Capone Jr. ■ Michael T. Trese

Pediatric macular surgery offers a unique and interesting set of challenges relative to adult macular surgery. Not only is there a reduced margin for error but the pathology can be fundamentally different than that seen in adults. With this extra challenge come potentially great rewards, as improved vision can dramatically affect the lives of our young patients for many decades.

With regard to the various indications for macular surgery in pediatric patients, most of us are probably most familiar with traumatic macular holes and submacular surgery for choroidal neovascularization (CNV). In addition to these two topics, we will also cover surgery for combined hamartoma of the retina and retinal pigment epithelium (RPE) and the recently described "posterior hyaloid contracture syndrome" seen most frequently in retinopathy of prematurity and familial exudative vitreoretinopathy.

## COMBINED HAMARTOMA OF THE RETINA AND RETINAL PIGMENT EPITHELIUM

Combined hamartomas of the retina and retinal pigment epithelium (CHRRPE) are rare tumors that are thought to be congenital in nature (1). In 1973, Gass described seven cases (five in children, two in young adults) he believed to be hamartomatous malformations involving the pigment epithelium, retina, retinal blood vessels, and overlying vitreous (2). Hamartomas are benign lesions composed of an overgrowth of mature cells that occur normally in the affected area. These combined hamartomas have varying clinical appearances. They are often pigmented with minimal elevation and demonstrate vascular tortuosity with associated vitreoretinal interface abnormalities. Unlike choroidal melanomas, for which they are often confused, CHRRPE mainly involve the retina and RPE versus choroid. Additionally, rarely do choroidal melanomas demonstrate marked vascular tortuosity in lesions of comparable size, nor do they demonstrate vitreoretinal interface abnormalities or epiretinal membrane formation in general. Ocular complications of choroidal melanoma including retinal detachment, subretinal hemorrhage, vitreous hemorrhage, inflammation, and glaucoma are not typically associated with CHRRPE (1). CHRRPE lesions may grow in some instances, though (3).

CHRRPE may be classified by both location (lesions on the disc, adjacent to the disc, macular, or midperipheral (2) and predominant tissue subtype (melanocytic, vascular, or glial (1). It is the glial subtype with prominent epiretinal proliferation that may be most amenable to macular surgery. In the Macula Society Research Committee report on CHRRPE, 47 of 60 (78%) patients with CHRRPE (all unilateral cases in this series) were noted to have vitreoretinal interface change and/or epiretinal membrane formation. Twenty-four percent of patients for whom follow-up data were available lost vision, presumably from progressive distortion of the retina. Of note, Gass hypothesized that in some cases of CHRRPE, the epiretinal tissue is so intricately interwoven with the underlying dysplastic retina that surgical peeling may not be possible (4). In a report by Shields et al. (5), 10 of 11 (91%) patients with CHRRPE had preretinal membrane by opti-

cal coherence tomography (OCT), none of which were intertwined with the tumor tissue.

In the Macula Society report, three out of the 60 patients had vitreous surgery to remove the epiretinal membrane. One of the patients had improved vision following surgery (from 20/200 to 20/40), while the other two had no change in vision. Based on two adult cases of CHRRPE who had undergone epiretinal membrane peeling without visual improvement, McDonald and colleagues (6) concluded that the role of vitrectomy and membrane removal in CHRRPE cases appeared to be limited. Both of their cases had longstanding poor vision prior to surgery which may have impacted their postoperative visual outcomes. In contrast, Sappenfield and Gitter (7) reported both subjective and objective improvement in vision after vitrectomy with membrane peeling in an adult patient with longstanding poor vision. Mason and Kleiner (8) reported a woman with CHRRPE who on first exam had 20/30 vision that deteriorated to 20/400 secondary to increased epiretinal membrane with an associated full-thickness macular hole. One year later, vitrectomy with membrane peeling with perfluoropropane gas tamponade was performed. The hole closed and vision improved to 20/100. Mason (9) reported a 20-year-old woman with CHRRPE whose declining vision improved from 20/400 to 20/60 after vitrectomy with membrane peel.

In terms of surgical intervention in children with CHRRPE, the literature is rather sparse. Konstantinidis et al. (10) discuss two cases of CHRRPE, one in a 12-year-old girl and the other in a 14-year-old boy, both of whom demonstrated progressive visual decline. Both were noted by OCT to have a thickened posterior hyaloid and epiretinal membrane inducing vitreomacular traction. Vitrectomy with membrane peeling was performed in both cases with improvement in vitreomacular traction and macular distortion noted on OCT and improvement in vision from 20/100 in both cases to 20/40 and 20/25, respectively. Standard three-port pars plana vitrectomy was performed in both cases. Tight adherence of the posterior hyaloid necessitated the use of the vitrector, end-grasping forceps and horizontal scissors to remove in both cases. Multiple layers of epiretinal membrane were noted in both cases and internal limiting lamina was peeled in one of the two cases. Stallman (11) performed vitrectomy with membrane peel on a 10-year-old girl whose vision had declined from 20/100, 3 years earlier, to 2/200. He also performed standard three-port vitrectomy, but in contrast to the previous two cases, here the membrane was removed easily in one single sheet. Nine months postoperatively the vision had improved to 20/40.

At William Beaumont Hospital, we have recently reviewed our surgical experience in pediatric patients with CHRRPE (in preparation). From 1999 to 2007, we performed vitrectomy with membrane peeling in 11 eyes with CHRRPE in 10 patients (bilateral in one case without known systemic association; see Figs. 47-1 and 47-2). In cases deemed more complicated preoperatively, plasmin was used to help facilitate removal of the posterior hyaloid and epiretinal membranes. Surgeries were performed in both 3-port and 2-port fashion. Patient ages ranged from 18 months to 14 years and follow-up ranged from 6 to 42 months. Six out of 11 (55%) eyes underwent plasmin enzyme-assisted vitrectomy while the other five were done without plasmin assistance. Eight out of 11 (73%) lesions were restricted to the macula and all showed significant epiretinal proliferation. Four out of 11 (36%) eyes had recurrence of

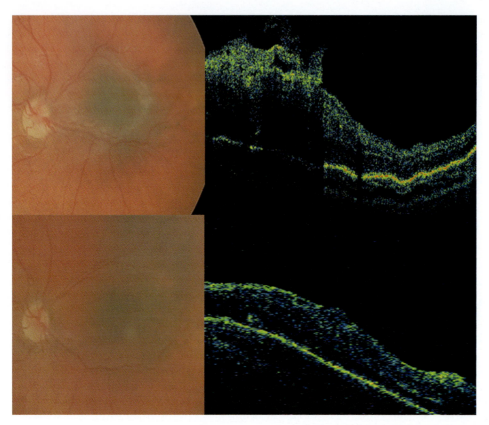

**Figure 47-1.** Pediatric combined hamartoma of the retina and retinal pigment epithelium (CHRRPE) surgery. Preoperative fundus photo and optical coherence tomography (top) and postoperative (bottom) images from an 18-month-old with CHRRPE. The patient underwent plasmin enzyme-assisted vitrectomy with membrane peeling. Postoperative images show improved macular architecture with absence of epiretinal proliferation.

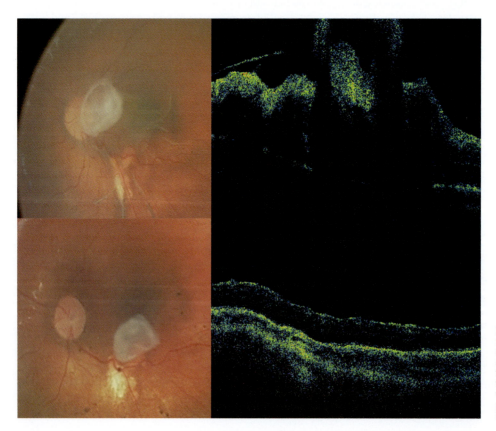

**Figure 47-2.** Pediatric combined hamartoma of the retina and retinal pigment epithelium (CHRRPE) surgery. Preoperative (top) and postoperative (bottom) fundus photos and optical coherence tomography images from a 2-year-old with CHRRPE. Although some epiretinal proliferation was not removed, notice the improvement in macular architecture.

epiretinal membrane, for which 3/4 underwent repeat vitrectomy with membrane peeling. No surgical complications were noted. Eight out of eleven (73%) eyes showed improvement in visual acuity while the other three showed stabilization. Four out of six (67%) plasmin cases showed improved vision.

If our 11 pediatric surgical cases are added to the three other cases reported in the literature, 11/14 of these eyes have had visual improvement after vitrectomy with membrane peeling, while the other three eyes had stable vision. Certainly, in the pediatric population, CHRRPE lesions with significant epiretinal proliferation and retinal distortion leading to decreased vision should be evaluated for vitrectomy with membrane peeling, and consideration should be given to plasmin enzyme assistance.

## PEDIATRIC MACULAR HOLE SURGERY

Macular holes in the pediatric population are typically seen following trauma, typically closed globe direct mechanical contusion injuries (12). The pathogenesis is unclear although vitreous and posterior hyaloid traction on the retina probably plays a role.

In traumatic cases, some macular holes seem to evolve, although most tend to occur immediately at the time of insult. In addition, traumatic macular holes are thought to spontaneously resolve more frequently than idiopathic macular holes. Lai et al. (13) reported a case of traumatic macular hole in a 12-year-old boy following soccer ball contusion. This hole was associated with a retinal detachment, both of which spontaneously resolved by 3 weeks following the injury with vision improving from 20/150 to 20/80. Carpineto et al. (14) reported

a traumatic macular hole in a 10-year-old child that resolved spontaneously at 18 weeks. Vision improved from 20/200 to 20/25. Mitamura et al. (15) reported 11 cases of traumatic macular holes, 7 of which closed spontaneously. Of the holes that closed spontaneously, young age was a common feature (ranging between 8 and 17 years), as was small size of the hole (0.1–0.2 disc diameters), no posterior vitreous detachment (PVD), and good final visual acuity. All of these patients that had spontaneous closure had improvement of at least two lines of visual acuity, with five of the patients improving to 20/20. The duration of the macular hole prior to closure ranged from 1 to 12 months (mean of 5.4 months). Yamada et al. (16) also reported spontaneous closure of two small traumatic macular holes in children. Yamashita et al. (17) also reported on the spontaneous closure of traumatic macular holes in eight out of 18 cases. Seven of the eight cases were in children and closure occurred within 4 months in all cases. Seven of the eight cases also involved holes 0.2 disc diameters or smaller. Larger traumatic holes in children may spontaneously close, too (18).

Kuhn et al. (12) evaluated 17 eyes that had undergone vitrectomy with internal limiting lamina (ILL) peeling with gas tamponade for traumatic macular hole. Seven of their cases were in children (less than 18 years old). Average time to surgery in these pediatric cases was 1.3 months. All of these children had closed holes and improved vision postoperatively with follow-up times ranging from 3 to 21 months.

Wachtlin et al. (19) performed vitrectomy with platelet concentrate adjuvant and SF6 gas tamponade in four children with traumatic macular holes from 1 to 5 months after the trauma. All holes closed and vision improved by four to seven lines (20/25–20/100 final visual acuities) with a mean follow-up of 35 months.

Margherio et al. (20) first described the use of autologous plasmin enzyme assisted vitrectomy (e.g., see Fig. 47-3) with

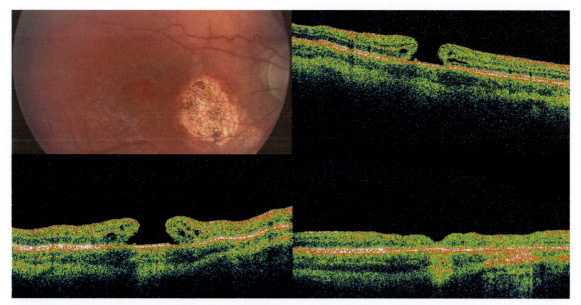

**Figure 47-3.** Pediatric macular hole surgery. Optical coherence tomography (OCT)and fundus image (top) of a chronic (2.5 year) traumatic macular hole in a 10-year-old boy. He underwent plasmin enzyme assisted vitrectomy with membrane peeling and gas tamponade, but his hole remained open postoperatively as seen in repeat OCT (bottom left). His hole closed after a second vitrectomy surgery with repeat membrane peeling (bottom right). Despite anatomic success, his vision did not improve, likely related to the chronicity of the hole.

membrane peeling and gas tamponade for traumatic macular holes in children. Plasmin was used to facilitate posterior hyaloid separation. They described four children (all less than 14 years of age) who all improved by four to eight lines postoperatively. Final visual acuities ranged from 20/30 to 20/60 with two eyes developing transient posterior subcapsular cataracts and no eyes requiring reoperation. Chow et al. (21) also reported surgical success with vitrectomy with plasmin assistance (in six of seven pediatric patients) and gas tamponade without the use of other adjuvants such as transforming growth factor-beta or platelet concentrate. Six of seven holes closed postoperatively; one chronic hole present for almost 3 years did not. Four of seven eyes showed improved vision at last follow up with the other three unchanged. No patients were excluded from their review including those with choroidal ruptures.

More recently, Wu et al. (22) reviewed 13 children with traumatic macular holes who underwent plasmin enzyme assisted vitrectomy with gas or silicone oil tamponade. The mean interval from trauma to surgery was 2.9 months (range: 10 days to 7 months). Preoperative evaluation revealed an attached posterior hyaloid in all cases (confirmed by B-scan ultrasonography). After injection with plasmin, a complete or partial PVD was noted intraoperatively in 38% of the eyes, while the remaining 62% had no PVD. In those cases without PVD the posterior hyaloid was detached easily with low suction (less than 50 mm Hg). The hole was closed in 12 of 13 (92%) cases. Ninety-two percent had improved vision postoperatively with 50% achieving vision of 20/50 or better.

Johnson et al. (23) reported a multicenter series of 25 traumatic macular holes treated with vitrectomy, membrane peeling in some cases, serum adjunct in some cases, and gas tamponade. Seven of their cases were in children. Six out of seven holes were closed and those six all achieved 20/60 or better vision.

Although spontaneous closure of traumatic macular holes in pediatric patients may occur, this occurrence is unpredictable. Therefore given the high success rate of vitrectomy in these cases, we recommend waiting no more than a few weeks before intervention, especially in younger children in which amblyopia may become a problem. Consideration should be given to the use of autologous plasmin enzyme, given the marked improvement in ease of posterior hyaloid removal which is felt to be of paramount importance to ultimate surgical success. Soon recombinant microplasmin may be available for use (24), which would eliminate the need for isolation of plasmin from the patient's blood. As with traumatic macular hole in adults, visual outcome is commonly limited by the severity of contusive damage to the macula/RPE/choroid.

## PEDIATRIC MACULAR SURGERY FOR CHOROIDAL NEOVASCULARIZATION

In the general population, CNV is usually seen in the setting of age-related macular degeneration. In children CNV is uncommon and can be associated with infectious conditions (*e.g.*, toxoplasmosis, toxocara canis, rubella retinopathy, ocular

histoplasmosis syndrome), hereditary conditions (*e.g.*, North Carolina macular dystrophy, Best disease), inflammatory conditions (*e.g.*, pars planitis, Vogt-Koyanagi-Harada syndrome, serpiginous choroidopathy, multifocal choroiditis, punctate inner choroidopathy), pathologic myopia, angioid streaks, choroidal rupture secondary to trauma, choroidal osteoma, chronic uveitis, fundus flavimaculatus, choroideremia, after photocoagulation, sickle cell retinopathy, optic disc drusen, congenital optic pits, or idiopathic (25,26). Goshorn and colleagues (26) studied 25 children with CNV and noted that in 11 of 19 (58%) untreated cases, spontaneous involution of the membranes occurred with visual acuity better than 20/80 in such cases. Patients without spontaneous regression were left with vision of 20/200 or worse with disciform scars. Several treatment options now exist that were not available in 1995.

Photodynamic therapy (PDT) with verteporfin may be considered in the pediatric population. Diaz et al. (27) reported an 8-year-old girl with idiopathic predominantly classic subfoveal CNV treated with PDT. Her vision dropped from 20/60 to 20/200, the size of the neovascular complex increased and permanent alteration in the both the retinal pigment epithelium (RPE) and choriocapillaris were noted. Farah et al. (28) performed PDT with verteporfin treatment in a 9-year-old girl with CNV secondary to Vogt-Koyanagi-Harada syndrome. Although the CNV regressed and the vision improved, intense RPE alterations were noted, similar to that in case reported by Diaz et al. (2006). Giansanti et al. (29) also reported RPE atrophic changes after PDT with verteporfin in four out of five pediatric patients with idiopathic and toxoplasmosis scar-related CNV without associated moderate or severe vision loss. The mechanism behind these RPE changes that are not seen in adult patients is not clear, nor is the long term visual significance. Other series have not noted the above RPE changes after PDT in children. Mimouni et al. (30) reported three children with idiopathic CNV treated with PDT and verteporfin without any adverse ocular events. Another case report reported success with PDT with verteporfin and intravitreal triamcinolone in myopic CNV in a 13-year-old girl (31). CNV excision can be considered when growth beneath the fovea has occurred despite medical therapy such as PDT (Fig. 47-4), given the common location of CNV anterior to the RPE in children.

Pece et al. (32) reported a case of a 12-year-old boy with Best Disease complicated by bilateral subfoveal CNV. The right eye was observed and the left eye underwent vitrectomy with CNV removal. Vision improved from 20/200 to 20/32 in the left eye and stayed steady at 20/50 in the right eye eight years after the surgery.

CNV associated with traumatic choroidal rupture has also been removed surgically in a child (33). A 9-year-old boy developed CNV 3 months after traumatic choroidal rupture. Within the next month, the CNV extended subfoveally and vision dropped to 20/200. Vitrectomy was performed with removal of the CNV through a nasal retinotomy. Twelve months later, vision had improved to 20/40. Histology showed that the neovascular membrane was lined on one side by multiple layers of RPE cells, and on the other side of the fibrovascular core were parts of inner and outer photoreceptor segments.

Jain et al. (34) also reported a girl with CNV associated with Best Disease bilaterally and a 6-year-old boy with idiopathic CNV. The young girl had surgery to remove the neovascular

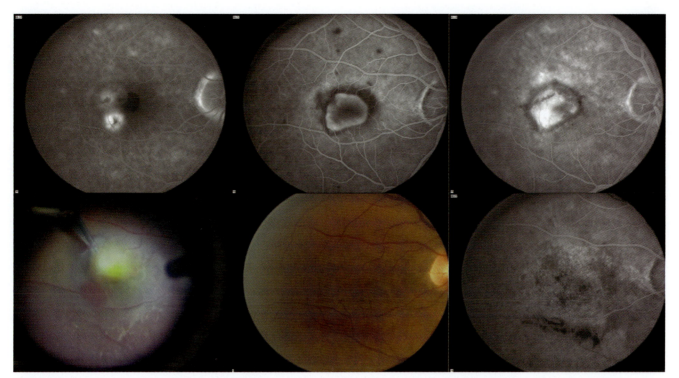

**Figure 47-4.** Pediatric submacular surgery for CNV. Despite photodynamic therapy with verteporfin, this child's choroidal neovascular complex continued to worsen (top panels: left—October 2003; middle—February 2004; right—March 2004). Vitrectomy with CNV membrane excision was performed with resolution of fluorescein leakage and mild residual pigmentary change in the macula (May 2004).

membranes bilaterally and vision improved from 20/200 and 20/400 to 20/40 and 20/25, 8 and 16 months later. The boy's vision improved from counting fingers to 20/30 at 12 months. No CNV recurrences were noted in either patient. In each of these cases, standard 3-port vitrectomy was performed. A small retinotomy was made on top of the CNV membrane. A subfoveal infusion cannula was used to create a small bleb and a subfoveal pic was used to immobilize the membrane. Intraocular pressure was elevated for 5 minutes prior to excising the membrane. Subfoveal forceps were then used to grab the membrane and remove it through the retinotomy and the sclerotomy. Sclerotomies were cryopexied and total fluid air exchange was performed in all cases, leaving the eye either with air or 5% C3F8 with postoperative face-down positioning overnight.

Inoue et al. (35) reported removal of CNV associated with CHRRPE in a 12-year-old girl. At first presentation, her vision was 20/30 and her exam was notable for juxtapapillary CHRRPE and subfoveal pigmented CNV. Her vision dropped to 20/60 so surgery was performed to remove the CNV membrane. Five months after surgery, her vision had improved to 20/20.

Sullu et al. (36) performed submacular surgery on the right eye of a 9-year-old girl with peripapillary CNV in her right eye and peripapillary and subfoveal CNV in her left eye associated with optic nerve head drusen. Vision improved from 0.05 to 0.3 in the left eye at 6 months. Partial RPE loss but no CNV recurrence was noted on follow-up.

The largest series of submacular surgery for CNV in pediatric patients were reported by Sears et al. (37) and Uemura and Thomas (38). Sears and colleagues reviewed 12 children with subfoveal CNV who underwent vitrectomy with CNV

removal. Two patients had congenital macular lesions attributed to toxoplasmosis, three had CNV associated with choroiditis (multifocal choroiditis, punctate inner choroiditis and unclassified choroiditis), three with ocular histoplasmosis syndrome, one with Coats disease, one with history of trauma, one with North Carolina macular dystrophy, and one with idiopathic CNV. Median time to surgery was 1.5 months after an observation period in all patients in anticipation of spontaneous involution. Surgery was considered if the neurosensory detachment was estimated to be at least twice the size of the neovascular membrane. Preoperative vision ranged from 20/60 to 20/800 (median 20/300) and postoperative visual acuity ranged from 20/25 to 20/400 (median 20/80) with follow-up of 6 to 62 months (mean 20 months). All cases involved complete 3-port vitrectomy with a lighted pick and suction from the vitrector used to engage the posterior hyaloid. A 32-gauge subretinal infusion cannula was used to make a retinotomy adjacent to the membrane and balanced salt solution was infused to create a small bleb. Subretinal forceps were used to grasp and remove the membrane. Prior to excision of the membrane, intraocular pressure was elevated for 5 minutes with the instruments in the eye. Fluid air exchange was performed and patients were kept face down overnight. All but two eyes had improved vision. Four eyes (33%) developed CNV recurrence.

Uemura and Thomas (38) reported 17 eyes in children aged 18 and under who had undergone vitrectomy with CNV removal. Eleven eyes had CNV associated with ocular histoplasmosis syndrome, three were idiopathic, one had optic nerve coloboma, one had toxoplasmosis, and one had trauma. Two eyes had juxtafoveal CNV, one was peripapillary, and the

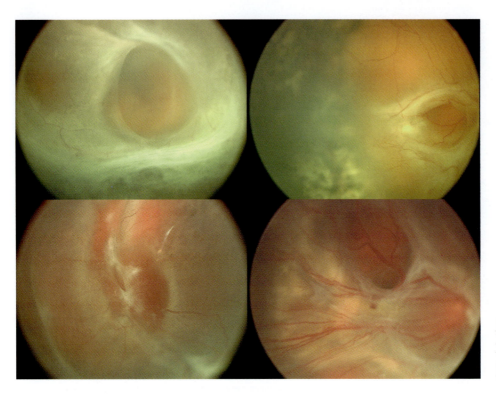

**Figure 47-5.** Posterior hyaloid contracture in pediatric patients. Four examples of posterior hyaloid contracture leading to tractional retinal detachments in pediatric patients with retinopathy of prematurity or familial exudative vitreoretinopathy.

rest were subfoveal. The subfoveal cases had a median preoperative vision of 20/200 (range 20/80–3/200). Median final vision was 20/50 (range 20/20–2/200) with median follow-up of 27 months (6–45 month range) with 70% improving two or more lines. In the three eyes with juxtafoveal or peripapillary CNV, vision improved by four or more Snellen lines. Six of 17 eyes (35%) developed recurrent CNV at 1 to 6 months (median interval 1 month). Four eyes (24%) failed to improve in final visual acuity, one presumably from loss of RPE at the time of surgery, one from postoperative subfoveal CNV recurrence, and two presumably from preoperative problems (severe vision loss and optic nerve coloboma).

CNV in pediatric patients is relatively uncommon. Although PDT and submacular surgery should be considered in patients with worsening vision, their futures in the era of intravitreal anti-VEGF treatments (e.g., bevacizumab and ranibizumab) are unknown. At the time of writing this chapter, no cases of CNV in children treated with intravitreal anti-VEGF agents have been reported in the literature, though we expect we will see some in the future.

## Posterior Hyaloid Contracture Syndrome in Retinopathy of Prematurity and Familial Exudative Vitreoretinopathy

Diffuse posterior hyaloid contracture syndrome is a newly described phenomenon that can be seen in pediatric proliferative vitreoretinopathies such as retinopathy of prematurity (ROP) and familial exudative vitreoretinopathy (FEVR) (39). Joshi and colleagues reviewed six eyes (four with ROP and two with FEVR) that showed diffuse contraction of the posterior hyaloid leading to tractional retinal detachment (Fig. 47-5). All six eyes had previously undergone peripheral laser ablation.

Recognition of this syndrome is critical to surgical planning as meticulous and extensive lamellar dissection of the posterior hyaloid from the retinal surface is necessary. Dissection of the tightly adherent posterior hyaloid can be aided by autologous plasmin enzyme. Additionally, diffuse posterior hyaloid contracture can sometimes give the appearance of a full thickness retinal break when there is lacunar defect in the opaque, contracted hyaloid (Fig. 47-5). Recognition of the preretinal location of the hyaloidal tissue plane and presence of retinal vasculature across the gap in otherwise opacified contracted hyaloid can aid in discerning whether a retinal break is indeed present.

## References

1. Schachat AP, Shields JA, Fine SL, et al. Combined hamartomas of the retina and retinal pigment epithelium. *Ophthalmology* 1984;91(12):1609–1614.
2. Gass JDM. An unusual hamartoma of the pigment epithelium and retina simulating choroidal melanoma and retinoblastoma. *Tr Am Ophth Soc* 1973;71:171–185.
3. Font RL, Moura RA, Shetlar DJ, et al. Combined hamartoma of sensory retina and retinal pigment epithelium. *Retina* 1989;9(4):302–311.
4. Gass JDM. Combined hamartomas of the retina and retinal pigment epithelium: Discussion. *Ophthalmology* 1984;91(12):1615.
5. Shields CL, Mashayekhi A, Dai VV, et al. Optical coherence tomographic findings of combined hamartoma of the retina and retinal pigment epithelium in 11 patients. *Arch Ophthalmol* 2005;123:1746–1750.
6. McDonald HR, Abrams GW, Burke JM, et al. Clinicopathologic results of vitreous surgery for epiretinal membranes in patients with combined retinal and retinal pigment epithelial hamartomas. *Am J Ophthalmol* 1985;100:806–813.
7. Sappenfield DL, Gitter KA. Surgical intervention for combined retinal-retinal pigment epithelial hamartoma. *Retina* 1990;10(2):119–124.
8. Mason JO, Kleiner R. Combined hamartoma of the retina and retinal pigment epithelium associated with epiretinal membrane and macular hole. *Retina* 1997;17(2):160–162.
9. Mason JO. Visual improvement after pars plana vitrectomy and membrane peeling for vitreoretinal traction associated with combined hamartoma of the retina and retinal pigment epithelium. *Retina* 2002;22(6):824–825.
10. Konstantinidis L, Chamot L, Zografos L, et al. Pars plana vitrectomy and epiretinal membrane peeling for vitreoretinal traction associated with

combined hamartoma of the retina and retinal pigment epithelium (CHRRPE). *Klin Monatsbl Augenheilkd* 2007;224:356–359.

11. Stallman JB. Visual improvement after pars plana vitrectomy and membrane peeling for vitreoretinal traction associated with combined hamartoma of the retina and retinal pigment epithelium. *Retina* 2002;22(1):101–104.

12. Kuhn F, Morris R, Mester V, et al. Internal limiting membrane removal for traumatic macular holes. *Ophthalmic Surgery & Lasers* 2001;32(4):308–315.

13. Lai MM, Joshi MM, Trese MT. Spontaneous resolution of traumatic macular hole-related retinal detachment. *Am J Ophthalmol* 2006;141(6):1148–1151.

14. Carpineto P, Ciancaglini M, Aharrh-Gnama A, et al. Optical coherence tomography and fundus microperimetry imaging of spontaneous closure of traumatic macular hole: A case report. *European J Ophthalmol* 2005;15(1):165–169.

15. Mitamura Y, Saito W, Ishida M, et al. Spontaneous closure of traumatic macular hole. *Retina* 2001;21(4):385–389.

16. Yamada H, Sakai A, Yamada E, et al. Spontaneous closure of traumatic macular hole. *Am J Ophthalmol* 2002;134(3):340–347.

17. Yamashita T, Uemara A, Uchino E, et al. Spontaneous closure of traumatic macular hole. *Am J Ophthalmol* 2002;133(2):230–235.

18. Yeshurun I, Guerrero-Naranjo JL, Quiroz-Mercado H. Spontaneous closure of a large traumatic macular hole in a young patient. *Am J Ophthalmol* 2002;134(4):602–603.

19. Wachtlin J, Jandeck C, Potthofer S, et al. Long-term results following pars plana vitrectomy with platelet concentrate in pediatric patients with traumatic macular hole. *Am J Ophthalmol* 2003;136:197–199.

20. Margherio AR, Margherio RR, Hartzer M, et al. Plasmin enzyme-assisted vitrectomy in traumatic pediatric macular holes. *Ophthalmology* 1998;105:1617–1620.

21. Chow DR, Williams GA, Trese MT, et al. Successful closure of traumatic macular holes. *Retina* 1999;19:405–409.

22. Wu WC, Drenser KA, Trese MT, et al. Pediatric traumatic macular hole: results of autologous plasmin enzyme-assisted vitrectomy. *Am J Ophthalmol* 2007;144:668–672.

23. Johnson RN, McDonald HR, Lewis H, et al. Traumatic macular hole: Observations, pathogenesis, and results of vitrectomy surgery. *Ophthalmology* 2001;108:853–857.

24. Gandorfer A, Rohleder M, Sethi C, et al. Posterior vitreous detachment induced by microplasmin. *Invest Ophthalmol Vis Sci* 2004;45:641–647.

25. Wilson ME, Mazur DO. Choroidal neovascularization in children: Report of five cases and literature review. *J Pediatr Ophthalmol Strabismus* 1988;25(1):23–29.

26. Goshorn EB, Hoover DL, Eller AW, et al. Subretinal neovascularization in children and adolescents. *J Pediatr Ophthalmol Strabismus* 1995;32:178–182.

27. Diaz M, Cervera E, Hernandez M, et al. Abnormal response of the retinal pigment epithelium to photodynamic therapy in a child. *Retina* 2006;26(7):834–836.

28. Farah ME, Costa RA, Muccioli C, et al. Photodynamic therapy with verteporfin for subfoveal choroidal neovascularization in Vogt-Koyanagi-Harada syndrome. *Am J Ophthalmol* 2002;234:137–139.

29. Giansanti F, Virgili G, Varano M, et al. Photodynamic therapy for choroidal neovascularization in pediatric patients. *Retina* 2005;25:590–596.

30. Mimouni KF, Bressler SB, Bressler NM. Photodynamic therapy with verteporfin for subfoveal choroidal neovascularization in children. *Am J Ophthalmol* 2003;135:900–902.

31. Potter MJ, Szabo SM, Ho T. Combined photodynamic therapy and intravitreal triamcinolone for the treatment of myopic choroidal neovascularization in a 13-year-old girl. *Graefe's Arch Clin Exp Ophthalmol* 2006;244:629–641.

32. Pece A, Milani P, Pierro L, et al. Observation or surgical excision of bilateral subfoveal choroidal neovascularization in Best disease. *Semin Ophthalmol* 2007;22(2):99–102.

33. Abri A, Binder S, Pavelka M, et al. Choroidal neovascularization in a child with traumatic choroidal rupture: clinical and ultrastructural findings. *Clin Experiment Ophthalmol* 2006;34(5):460–463.

34. Jain K, Shafiq AE, Devenyi RG. Surgical outcome for removal of subfoveal choroidal neovascular membranes in children. *Retina* 2002;22:412–417.

35. Inoue M, Noda K, Ishida S, et al. Successful treatment of subfoveal choroidal neovascularization associated with combined hamartoma of the retina and retinal pigment epithelium. *Am J Ophthalmol* 2004;138:155–156.

36. Sullu Y, Yildiz L, Erkan D. Submacular surgery for choroidal neovascularization secondary to optic nerve drusen. *Am J Ophthalmol* 2003;136:367–370.

37. Sears J, Capone A Jr, Aaberg T Sr, et al. Surgical management of subfoveal neovascularization in children. *Ophthalmology* 1999;106:920–924.

38. Uemura A, Thomas MA. Visual outcome after surgical removal of choroidal neovascularization in pediatric patients. *Arch Ophthalmol* 2000;118:1373–1378.

39. Joshi MM, Ciaccia S, Trese MT, et al. Posterior hyaloid contracture in pediatric vitreoretinopathies. *Retina* 2006;26:S38–S41.

# Miscellaneous and Tumors

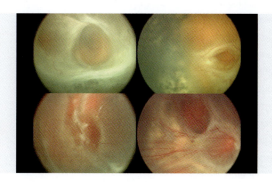

# Macular Disease Secondary to Peripheral Retinal Vasculopathy

Maximiliano Gordon ■ Hugo Quiroz-Mercado ■ R.V. Paul Chan

Peripheral retinal vascular changes are common findings associated with both local and systemic disease in the pediatric population. These changes can be helpful in differentiating between various disease states resulting from primary ocular conditions well known to the ophthalmologist or systemic disease that requires a careful clinical history and systemic workup in order to determine the etiology.

Peripheral retinal vascular changes may result in significant visual impairment, especially if the macula is involved. Patient age, extension of vascular changes, and duration of disease all contribute to the prognosis. Of major concern, however, is the presence of peripheral retinal ischemia with secondary retinal neovascularization (1). If this is to occur, appropriate management of the patient can preserve and/or improve macular function. Laser treatment is the treatment of choice and should be directed toward the peripheral retina, but at times direct intervention to the macular area may need be considered. Herein we describe the most common diseases associated with peripheral retinal vascular changes, and we focus mainly on those conditions that require laser photocoagulation, cryotherapy, or surgical intervention. Tables 48-1 and 48-2 show a classification for differential diagnosis (1–3). Pathologies not included in this classification are the inflammatory diseases associated with vasculitis like Eales' disease, Behcet's disease, sarcoidosis, systemic lupus erythematosus, multiple sclerosis, pars planitis, and other less common problems that are described in other chapters.

## PATHOPHYSIOLOGY

Peripheral retinal abnormalities such as retinal neovascularization, vascular tortuosity, ectasis, vascular shunts, and aneurysms may damage the inner blood-retina barrier. Damage to the retinal vascular endothelium may involve primary arteries, veins, or capillaries, or any combination of the three. Also, the endothelial alteration may be focal or widespread. Fluorescein angiography has demonstrated that the entire capillary bed may be affected in some cases, whereas in others, the changes may only be limited to capillaries in the midneuroretina, with the inner retinal vessels remaining normal.

### TABLE 48-1    HEREDITARY OR CONGENITAL VASCULAR DISEASES (1–3)

Sickle cell retinopathy

Retinitis pigmentosa

Angiomatosis retinae (von Hippel's disease)

Congenital retinal telangiectasis (Leber's military aneurysms, Coats' syndrome)

Congenital retinal macrovessels and arteriovenous communications

Incontinentia pigmenti

Retinal cavernous hemangioma

Inherited retinal venous beading

Small vessels hyalinosis

### TABLE 48-2    ACQUIRED VASCULAR DISEASES (1–3)

Retinal capillary obstruction/loss

Retinopathy of prematurity

Hyperviscosity syndromes

Diabetes mellitus

Radiation retinopathy

Longstanding retinal detachment

Retinoschisis

Toxemia of pregnancy

Cocaine abuse

Choroidal melanoma and hemangioma

Decreased ocular blood supply

Ocular ischemic syndrome

Carotid cavernous fistula

Encircling sclera buckling operation

Decreased retinal blood supply

Large retinal vessels obstruction

Retinal embolization

Retinal venous occlusive disease

Following surgical retinectomy

The extracellular space of the retina generally is considered to be relatively small compared with other tissues except for the brain. The outer plexiform layer is the primary interstitial space in the retina. If the retina becomes edematous, it is in this layer that fluid accumulates in the outer plexiform layer. The macular contains only four layers of the retina: the internal limiting membrane, the outer plexiform layer, the outer nuclear layer, and the rods and cones. The absence of Muller cells in the foveal region is also a contributing factor (4). No intermediate layers exist between the internal limiting membrane and the outer plexiform layer in the fovea, which in the macula is oblique (outer plexiform layer of Henle). This is an important factor in understanding the stellate appearance of the cystoid edema in the macula as opposed to the honeycomb appearance of cystoid edema outside the macula (3,5).

According to the severity of the damage in the blood-inner retina barrier, Gass distinguished three categories of macular edema: mild, moderate, and severe (3). If the decompensation is mild, small molecules and proteins escape into the extracellular space, and clear serous exudate may be confined to the inner retinal layers. It is not visible biomicroscopically. In fluorescein angiography, diffuse mild staining of the inner retina is observed. If capillary damage is moderate, deeper plexus of capillaries are affected. Serous fluid accumulates within the inner nuclear and outer plexiform layers. The biomicroscopic picture of cystoid macular edema then can be observed. Swelling of the retina and loss of the foveal depression is caused by the development of large central cysts. On fluorescein angiography, molecules diffuse out of the capillaries, producing a stellate pattern. If endothelial damage is severe, large proteins and lipids escape into the extracellular compartment, and the exudate may be cloudy. The

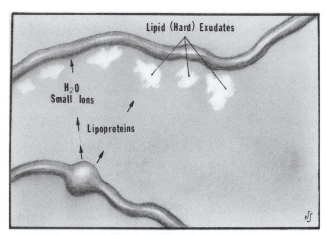

**Figure 48-1.** Schematic diagram of leakage from retinal aneurysm. Small ions and water are reabsorbed. The large lipoprotein molecules are too large to enter the healthy capillary wall, and they deposit along these vessels, frequently in a circinate pattern. (Adapted from Ferris FL, Patz A. Macular edema, a complication of diabetic retinopathy. *Suv Ophthalmol* 1984;28(suppl):452–561, with permission.)

extravascular protein is transported across the pigment epithelium, choroid, and sclera. Around the outer margin of capillary leakage, the fluid is reabsorbed and small ions that are components of the blood leave behind the lipoprotein in the outer plexiform layer that tend to aggregate frequently in a circinate pattern.

After resolution of the capillary leakage or following photocoagulation, macrophages remove the lipid exudates (3,6) (Fig. 48-1).

In diseases with severe vascular abnormality involving the peripheral retina, chronic gravitation of the subretinal lipid to the macula and inferior periphery may cause widespread deposits of subretinal and outer retinal exudate remote from the vascular abnormality (3,7). Massive lipid residue may cause permanent damage to the retina and pigment epithelium, as well as choroidal neovascularization (8). Early treatment of vascular lesions may prevent permanent visual lost and resolution of lipid deposits in the macula (9).

Vitreous changes and membranes formation secondary to peripheral vascular diseases may produce macular ectopia, macular traction with or without tractional retinal detachment, rhegmatogenous retinal detachment, and epimacular membrane (10,11)

## RETINOPATHY OF PREMATURITY

Retinopathy of prematurity (ROP) is a potentially blinding eye disease (12). It has been suggested that therapeutic oxygen, although important, has been overemphasized as a cause of ROP under contemporary neonatal care practices. Other factors related to very low birth weight are probably quite important, especially in view of current nursery monitoring of oxygen. Birth weight is inversely related to risk of ROP and is at least as good an indicator as is gestational age. With current nursery practices, ROP is truly a disorder of the "smallest and sickest" infants (13).

## Classification

The International Classification of ROP (ICROP) and the Cryotherapy for ROP (CRYO-ROP) trials have had a profound impact on the way in which we manage ROP (12).

The CRYO-ROP study provided a classification system for ROP which categorized the disease into zones and stages. Zone I uses the optic nerve as the center of a circle, and the radius is defined as two times the distance between the foveola and the optic nerve. Zone II uses as a radius the distance between the nasal ora serrata in the horizontal meridian and the center of the optic nerve. All of the remaining retina is zone III (14–16).

CRYO-ROP also defined plus disease, a descriptive term for six clock hours of dilated and tortuous vessels of the posterior pole. In addition, the anterior segment in plus disease often shows dilated iris vessels (14–16).

Preplus disease has been defined as vascular abnormalities of the posterior pole that are insufficient for the diagnosis of plus disease but shows more arterial tortuosity and more venous dilatation than normal. Over time, these vessels may dilate and become more tortuous, progressing to plus disease (13).

There are five stages of ROP. Stage 1 signifies a narrow white line present at the junction of vascular and avascular retina. Stage 2 is a ridge of activity with thickening of this line. Stage 3 involves the growth of extraretinal fibrovascular proliferation at the ridge. Stage 4 is a partial retinal detachment and is subclassified as 4-A, with the macula attached, and 4-B, with the macula detached. Stage 5 implies a total detachment of the vascularized retina (14–16)(Fig. 48-3). Aggressive, posterior ROP is a rapidly progressive, severe form of ROP seen in very low birth weight infants. The fundus appearance is characterized by prominent plus disease and flat neovascularization. It is currently seen most commonly in zone I or posterior zone II (12,14).

## Treatment

The CRYO-ROP study determined that treating threshold disease defined as five contiguous or eight cumulative clock hours of stage 3 with plus disease was beneficial over observation. The Early Treatment for ROP (ETROP) study indicated beneficial results for any eye with zone I stage 3, zone I with plus disease, zone II stage 2 or 3 ROP with plus disease. Early treatment showed better visual and structural outcomes in premature infants over a 10-year period (12).

Currently, laser photocoagulation is the treatment of choice for treatment requiring ROP. As better visualization of the retina is possible and technology has advanced, cryotherapy for ROP has fallen out of favor (17).

Anti-vascular endothelial growth factor (anti-VEGF) agents (e.g., bevacizumab) have recently been advocated for the treatment of ROP. Quiroz-Mercado, Martinez-Castellanos et al. reported the use of bevacizumab (Avastin), injected intravitreally for ROP. Thirteen patients (18 eyes) were included in the study. Patients were separated in three different groups: group I included patients with stage IVa or IVb ROP who had no response to conventional treatment (cryotherapy or laser); group II included patients with threshold ROP who could not receive treatment secondary to poor visualization of the retina; and group III included patients with high-risk prethreshold or threshold ROP. Regression of neovascularization occurred in 17 eyes. One patient with stage IVa ROP had spontaneous retinal reattachment after a single intravitreal injection of bevacizumab. There were no serious ocular or systemic adverse events reported (18).

Although retinal ablation is effective in most cases of treatment requiring ROP, a significant number of these eyes progress to retinal detachment (stages 4A, 4B, and 5) (12). The natural history arm of the CRYO-ROP study showed that a child with 8 sector 4A ROP at their due date (40 weeks PMA) has a high risk of going on to an unfavorable outcome or total retinal detachment (stage 5) (12,19,20).

Surgical options for ROP advancing to retinal detachment include scleral buckle (SB), vitrectomy with lensectomy, lens sparing vitrectomy (LSV), and open sky vitrectomy. Although scleral buckling for stage 4B and 5 ROP may provide an anatomic outcome superior to the natural history of the disease, this approach does not provide visual results as rewarding as one would hope because of induced anisometropia and amblyopia. Nor does scleral buckling deal directly with vitreous traction (19).

There are numerous advantages to LSV over SB for tractional stage 4A ROP retinal detachments. First, SB has an anatomic success rate on the order of only 70%. Second, placement of a SB requires an additional procedure to divide the encircling element so that the eye may continue to grow. Third, scleral buckling could produce an induced mean anisometropia of −9.5 diopters, with residual myopia on the order of −5 diopters, even after the encircling element is divided. Fourth, visual acuity results for stage 4A detachments repaired with scleral buckling surgery techniques have been very discouraging.

Although visual acuity has not yet been measured accurately in children with LSV, the potential for very good visual acuity should be high based on the central, steady, and maintained fixation behavior noted to date (19).

Capone and Trese designed a study to assess the efficacy of LSV in tractional 4A ROP retinal detachments in reducing progression to stage 4B or 5 ROP. The study included forty eyes (31 patients) with stage 4A ROP at 38 to 42 weeks postconceptional age. *Pars plicata* vitrectomy was performed on all patients. An infusion light pipe, vitreous cutter, and membrane peeler cutter (MPC) scissors were used in the surgical technique. At the last follow-up examination, 36 of 40 eyes showed complete retinal reattachment with central steady and maintained fixation. Four eyes progressed to 4B retinal detachments, and in three of those four eyes the retinas were reattached after repeat vitreous surgery. One eye progressed to stage 5 ROP. The 90% anatomic success rate of LSV for 4A ROP reported in the current series is far superior with regard to both anatomic outcome and visual prognosis. Also, it has been suggested that the ideal timing for vitreoretinal intervention is when the vascular activity (dilation and tortuosity) has abated and detachment has just begun (19).

In another series, Sears and Sonnie compared the anatomic outcomes of LSV with those of combined LSV and SB in surgical repair of ROP stage 4 retinal detachment. Twenty-one eyes of 15 patients with stage 4 ROP detachment were included. An SB was placed externally using either a 240 or 41 band after 360-degree conjunctival peritomy and isolation of the four rectus muscles. The SB was secured to the eye wall with 5-0 nylon sutures as close to the ridge as possible and was fastened with a Watzke sleeve. Drainage of subretinal fluid was not performed in any eye. All SBs were removed by six months of age. LSV was performed using two sclerotomies posterior to the iris root (1.5 mm from the limbus) through *pars plicata* at 9:30 and 2:30. An end irrigating Capone light pick was used in all cases in conjunction with a pediatric wide-angle viewing system and a 23-gauge pediatric MPC. Of the patients in whom treatment failed, two were in the LSV with SB group (2/12; 16%) and one was in the LSV alone group (1/9; 11%). Overall, the study results suggest that SB adds little to the success or failure of LSV and therefore is an unnecessary adjunct for stage 4 (A and B) (21).

Gonzales, Boshra, and Schwartz used 25 gauge *pars plicata* vitrectomy for stage 4 and 5 ROP. Fifteen eyes of 12 infants were included. Three-port *pars plicata* vitrectomy using 25-gauge instrumentation was performed. Conjunctival dissection was performed in all cases and sclerotomies were made 0.5 to 1.0 mm posterior to the limbus through the *pars plicata*. Several vectors of traction must be addressed including those extending from the ridge to the lens, from the ridge to the anterior vitreous base, and from the ridge to the optic nerve. Eleven of 15 (73%) eyes had documented retinal reattachment after one or more surgeries at the last follow-up. Complications included vitreous hemorrhage and postoperative cataract. But they concluded that 25-gauge vitrectomy is a safe and effective treatment approach for tractional retinal detachments in stage 4 and 5 ROP (22). Retinal photocoagulation or cryotherapy may be effective for stabilizing aggressive posterior ROP; however, it very frequently cannot stop the progression to retinal detachment (23).

In an attempt to address this issue, Azuma et al. studied the efficacy of early vitrectomy for aggressive posterior ROP to stop progression of retinal detachment. Twenty-two eyes (15 patients) with aggressive posterior ROP underwent vitrectomy with or without lens sparing, because retinal photocoagulation failed to stop progression of fibrovascular proliferation, despite being performed early, densely, and with early retreatment. Six eyes (100%) in which an LSV was performed developed a large tractional retinal detachment. In contrast, the retinas were completely reattached in 16 eyes (100%) in which vitrectomy with lensectomy was performed, nine eyes (56%) had foveal configuration, and 14 eyes (88%) had steady fixation. These results indicate the great benefit of early surgery for aggressive posterior ROP, in comparison to the poor visual outcomes after vitreous surgery for Stage 5 ROP (23).

## FAMILIAL EXUDATIVE VITREORETINOPATHY

In 1969, Criswick and Schepens reported six children with peripheral retinal abnormalities resembling ROP but distinguished by their familial occurrence, and no history of prematurity or supplemental oxygen after birth. Systemic associations were absent (24). They named the disease familial exudative vitreoretinopathy (FEVR).

The clinical findings include heterotopia of the fovea with temporal traction, organized vitreous membranes, peripheral neovascularization with abrupt termination of the temporal retinal vasculature, retinal exudates, retinal folds and tractional retinal detachment. Anterior chamber structures are uninvolved. Nonetheless, the end stages of severely affected eyes may display chronic retinal detachment with cataract, band keratopathy, and glaucoma (24).

FEVR is always bilateral and usually symmetric. Some infants have family members with similar findings, indicating that this is an autosomal dominant condition, with nearly 100% penetrance. Like other autosomal dominant conditions, expression is variable, with some members having only mild macular dragging or small areas of peripheral avascularity of the retina, demonstrable only by fluorescein angiography. X-linked recessive trait, with high penetrance, and variable expressively, and sporadic cases have also been reported (24).

The pathogenesis of FEVR appears to be a consequence of disturbed development of the retinal vasculature in the last months of gestation, with a failure of the peripheral retina to vascularize. Although the ensuing changes bear a similarity to the pathobiology of ROP, they follow a different time course and natural history. A notable difference is the tendency of ROP to progress to cicatricial stages or to abort and vascularize the periphery, whereas the avascular zone in FEVR remains a permanent feature throughout life (24).

A classification system, based on the ophthalmoscopic findings, has been proposed by Pendergast and Trese. The disease is classified into five stages (Table 48-3) (25).

## Management

As mentioned previously, it is important to identify FEVR by careful examination of blood relatives. In most asymptomatic cases, observation and frequent follow-up are all that is required. In children with strabismus, recognition, again, is important. Treatment with cryotherapy or laser ablation of the neovascular areas, and scleral buckling and vitrectomy procedures for tractional detachments, may be required (26).

### TABLE 48-3   CLINICAL CLASSIFICATION OF FAMILIAL VITREORETINOPATHY

| STAGE 1 | Avascular retinal periphery without extraretinal vascularization |
|---|---|
| STAGE 2 | Avascular retinal periphery with extraretinal vascularization |
| | Without exudate |
| | With exudates |
| STAGE 3 | Retinal detachment-subtotal, nor involving the fovea |
| | Primarily exudative |
| | Primarily tractional |
| STAGE 4 | Retinal detachment-subtotal, involving the fovea |
| | Primarily exudative |
| | Primarily tractional |
| STAGE 5 | Retinal detachment-total |
| | Open funnel |
| | Closed funnel |

Pendergast and Trese reported the results of surgical management of FEVR. Fifty-two eyes of 26 patients with FEVR were studied. A total of 40 eyes were treated. Seven eyes required no treatment and five eyes had inoperable retinal detachments. Fifteen eyes were treated with peripheral laser ablation initially and 25 eyes presenting with retinal detachments required vitreoretinal surgery. Of the 15 eyes treated initially with laser, eight eyes required no further treatment, whereas seven eyes progressed to retinal detachment requiring vitreoretinal surgery. A total of 32 eyes (including seven previously lasered eyes) underwent vitreoretinal surgery. Patients with retinal detachment or macula heterotopia were treated with vitrectomy, scleral buckling, or both. Vitrectomy was performed using a two-port system with an infusion light pipe. Whenever possible, a lens-sparing approach was used (Fig. 48-2). In eyes in which the vitreoretinal membranes extended anteriorly and prevented safe entry through the *pars plicata*, entrance wounds were made at the limbus through the iris root and a lensectomy was performed. Twenty-nine of these 32 eyes had at least 6 months of follow-up. At the last follow-up visit, the macula was attached completely in 18 eyes (62.1%) (25).

In a retrospective study, Ikeda et al. examined the anatomic features and surgical indications of FEVR complicated with rhegmatogenous or tractional retinal detachment. Twenty-eight eyes of 25 patients who had either clinically suspected or fully diagnosed FEVR were included in this study. Of these, 25 had rhegmatogenous retinal detachment, two had tractional retinal detachment, and one had tractional retinal detachment plus vitreous hemorrhage. The vitreoretinal adhesions were so strong in the peripheral avascular area that iatrogenic retinal breaks easily occurred in 22 of 28 eyes. the surgeons attempted to remove the posterior vitreous membrane as far into the equator as possible and then combined this procedure with broad scleral buckling from the equator to the vitreous base against the residual vitreoretinal traction (27).

Joshi et al. reviewed six eyes (four ROP, two FEVR) with diffuse contraction of the posterior hyaloid resulting in retinal detachment. They observed a diffuse proliferation along the posterior hyaloids that required extensive lamellar dissection at times aided by autologous plasmin enzyme. A diffuse, taut posterior hyaloid resulted in a marked tractional component to retinal detachment. Bimanual dissection of the contracted hyaloid from the retinal surface was essential in relieving tractional force on the retina. The study concluded that hyaloid contraction aids in the surgical planning and repair of these complex eyes (28).

## INCONTINENTIA PIGMENTI

Incontinentia pigmenti (IP) is an X-linked dominant disorder with characteristic cutaneous (Fig. 48-4), dental, skeletal, central nervous system, and ocular manifestations; it is lethal in most male embryos. The precise pathogenesis of the clinical manifestations of IP is unknown. Clinical suspicion of the diagnosis is usually a result of the characteristic rash that develops at or shortly after birth and is confirmed by skin biopsy, showing intraepithelial vesicles filled with eosinophils. Systemic manifestations often become evident within the first 4 months of life and are seen in almost 80% of patients (29). Neurologic deficits occur in one-third of patients and can manifest as hydrocephalus, microcephaly, and mental retardation (30). Ocular involvement occurs in 35% of persons with IP; findings include strabismus, conjunctival pigmentation, cataracts, corneal epithelial and stromal keratitis, iris hypoplasia, optic atrophy, and, most important, vitreoretinal abnormalities (29).

The vitreoretinal manifestations are persistence of fetal vasculature, foveal atrophy, paramacular vascular dilatations and aneurysms, retinal pigment epithelium mottling, retinal pigment epithelium hypopigmentation, peripheral retinal avascular zones and vascular tortuosity, arteriovenous anastomoses, preretinal neovascularization at the junction of vascular and avascular retina, vitreous hemorrhage, and tractional retinal detachment (Fig. 48-4). Retinal tears and rhegmatogenous retinal detachments most likely occur as a result of peripheral vitreoretinal traction at the junction of avascular and vascular retina (29).

It is difficult to establish prophylactic or therapeutic guidelines for vitreoretinal involvement in IP, because the relatively small number of cases has precluded careful study of the natural history of the disease. Cases with vascular changes without neovascularization or exudation probably do not need treatment (31), whereas cases with progression of neovascularization and evidence of exudation can be treated with photocoagulation (32). Patients with vitreous hemorrhage or tractional retinal detachment should be treated with vitrectomy.

## DIFFERENTIAL DIAGNOSIS OF PEDIATRIC VASCULAR DISEASE

ROP, FEVR, and IP may resemble the less common bilateral pathology of Norrie's disease or the unilateral pathology of persistent fetal vasculature (PFV).

## NORRIE'S DISEASE

Norrie's disease is an X-linked recessive disorder that can present with retinal folds or vascularized retrolental masses simulating retinoblastoma ("pseudoglioma"). The principal features are bilateral severe retinal dysplasia and optic nerve hypoplasia, associated in some cases with hearing loss and progressive mental deterioration (33,34).

## PERSISTENT FETAL VASCULATURE

This condition is one of the most common congenital abnormalities affecting the eye (35). The syndrome is usually an isolated monocular finding in an otherwise healthy child and has a wide spectrum of anatomic and pathology features (36). As Goldberg points out, the term "persistent hyperplastic primary vitreous" is a misnomer in common usage, because it fails

to include persistence of other components of the fetal intraocular vasculature. PFV is secondary to the persistence of the vascular component that is freely anastomotic in fetal life; hence they may persist together in varied degrees of severity (35). It shows lack of involution of prenatal vessels after birth (36).

Usually, this is a unilateral disorder characterized by abnormal regression of the primary vitreous and fetal vessels encasing the posterior surface of the lens (36). Unilateral cases of PFV are sporadic, while bilateral cases may be associated with X-linked Norrie disease. Associated sensorineural deafness and mental retardation in males may be absent, and genetic testing can be useful in separating sporadic PFV from Norrie disease (37).

PFV is subclassified into three types: type 1—anterior PHPV (retrolental fibrovascular membrane, elongated ciliary processes, cataract, microphthalmia); type 2—posterior PFV (vitreous membrane and stalk, retinal fold, traction retinal detachment, hypoplastic optic nerve and macula, microphthalmia); and, most common, type 3—a combination of anterior and posterior PFV. The purely posterior form occurs in only 10 to 20% of cases. Persistence of the hyaloid artery, Bergmeister papilla, nonattachment of the retina, retinal folds and macular hypoplasia are other features of the posterior type. In the pure form of posterior PFV, anterior structures are not involved, although microcornea and an immature filtration angle are often present (38).

Nystagmus occurs in bilateral cases. With age, the anterior chamber shallows, resulting in glaucoma or corneal decompensation in some eyes (36).

The differential diagnosis of PFV includes intraocular nematodes such as Toxocara sp and cysticercosis, occult intraocular foreign body, endophthalmitis, and X-linked retinoschisis.

### Management

Without treatment, severely affected eyes invariably progress to phthisis bulbi (36,38). The visual prognosis in patients with PFV is often poor, especially in the posterior form of the disease. Surgical treatment may not be effective in patients with severe microphthalmia or advanced posterior PFV, such as marked foveal hypoplasia, dysplasia, rhegmatogenous retinal detachment (RRD), and retinal or optic nerve abnormalities. These patients may need only to be observed (39).

Two surgical methods have been proposed to manage PFV associated with retrolenticular membranes: an anterior transpupillary approach and a posterior *pars plana/plicata* approach (40).

Payse et al. believe that surgical avoidance of the ciliary body reduces the risk of retinal tears, retinal detachment, and inadvertent retinectomy. In this study, three clear corneal ab externo paracentesis incisions were created approximately 0.25 mm central to the limbus using a 19-gauge microsurgical vitreoretinal blade. An anterior chamber maintainer attached to the infusion solution was placed in the inferotemporal incision. An anterior capsulotomy was then performed using a vitrector (vitrectorhexis). The easily accessible soft cortical lenticular material was then aspirated. Then, an attempt was made to incise the retrolenticular material with the vitrector. If the above measures were unsuccessful, intraocular vitreoretinal scissors were inserted. Multiple radial cuts created wedge-shaped membrane segments small enough to be removed with a vitrector. (40,41).

In a retrospective study by Alexandrakis et al., patients with PFV were divided into two groups: one surgical and the other nonsurgical, and the final best postoperative visual acuity, prognostic, ocular clinical features, and surgical complications were compared. In the surgical group, 30 patients were included. Two patients had clinical and echographic findings consistent with anterior PFV, two had strictly posterior PFV, and the remaining 26 had components of both anterior and posterior PFV. Indications for surgery included media opacity (e.g., cataract), vitreoretinal traction, and retinal detachment. The two patients with strictly posterior PFV underwent a *pars plana* vitrectomy, and the remaining 28 patients underwent a primary *pars plana* lensectomy and vitrectomy procedure. Of the latter 28 patients, 12 also had a membrane peeling procedure and two underwent a scleral buckling procedure at the time of vitrectomy for a TRD. Two patients had a posterior chamber intraocular lens placed at the time of lensectomy. In the group of 12 patients who were observed, the decision was based on the presence of mild PFV (2 patients), foveal or optic nerve hypoplasia or both (6 patients), marked microphthalmia (3 patients), and inoperable RRD (1 patient). Approximately 50% of patients undergoing surgery for PFV will achieve useful vision. Visual acuity outcomes in patients with PFV are correlated with the nature and extent of ocular risk factors. Some patients may not be candidates for surgery because of either minimal changes or advanced disease that limit the potential of visual improvement (39).

## COATS' DISEASE

First described by George Coats in 1908, Coats' disease is a disease characterized by retinal telangiectasia and exudation of unknown etiology (42), which exhibits a wide spectrum of clinical findings (43). In addition to telangiectasias, there may be capillary nonperfusion, aneurysm formation, exudation both within and beneath the retina, and massive lipid deposition (44) (Fig. 48-4). It is predominantly a nonhereditary disease of childhood that is diagnosed within the first decade of life. It affects males more than females and is unilateral in about 90% of patients. Vision loss, strabismus and leukocoria may occur and it is critical that Coats' disease be differentiated from retinoblastoma (44). Less severe manifestations can be observed in adults (42). If the disease is not treated, it can lead to total retinal detachment and secondary glaucoma, occasionally requiring enucleation (45).

Chronic retinal detachment is associated with exacerbation of retinal vascular abnormalities, as a result of impaired oxygenation of the outer retina and secondary expression of increased VEGF or a similar growth factor that may cause the microvascular changes seen in Coats' disease. For some patients, anti-VEGF therapy may be a potential treatment candidate (44).

Based on their observations, Shields et al. classified Coats' disease in five stages (Table 48-4) (45).

| TABLE 48-4 | CLASSIFICATION OF COATS' DISEASE |
|---|---|
| STAGE 1 | Retinal telangiectasia only |
| STAGE 2 | Telangiectasia and exudation |
| | A-Extrafoveal exudation |
| | B-Foveal exudation |
| STAGE 3 | Exudative retinal detachment |
| | A-Subtotal detachment |
| |    1-Extrafoveal |
| |    2-Foveal |
| | B-Total retinal detachment |
| STAGE 4 | Total retinal detachment and glaucoma |
| STAGE 5 | Advanced end-stage disease |

The term Leber's miliary aneurysm refers to the adult form, with intraretinal exudation commonly affecting the macula with yellowish circinate exudation, cystoids macular edema, subretinal detachment, and less commonly exudative retinal detachment (46). Less severe presentations, commonly observed in 40-year-old men, have retinal telangiectasis confined to a small segment of juxtafoveolar area. These patients constitute type I juxtafoveolar telangiectasis (47).

## Treatment

The main goal of treatment should be to eradicate the telangiectasias in order to facilitate resolution of exudation and salvage as much vision as possible. Without treatment, the natural progression of the disease may lead to complications such as total bullous retinal detachment, neovascular glaucoma, and phthisis bulbi (42).

Patients with stage 1 disease (telangiectasia only) can be managed by either periodic observation or laser photocoagulation. However, encountering a patient with stage 1 disease is uncommon in clinical practice (45). Patients with stage 2 disease (telangiectasia and exudation) are generally best managed by laser photocoagulation or cryotherapy, depending on the extent of the disease (45). Patients with stage 3A disease (subtotal retinal detachment) can generally be managed by photocoagulation or cryotherapy. Because laser photocoagulation is less effective in areas of retinal detachment, cryotherapy is often preferable in such cases (45). Stage 3B (total retinal detachment) can be managed with cryotherapy if the detachment is shallow, but may require an attempt at surgical reattachment if the detachment is bullous and immediately posterior to the lens. Surgical repair of total and bullous retinal detachment is justified only to prevent the development of neovascular glaucoma, even though the visual outcome is expected to be poor (45). Stage 4 disease (total retinal detachment and glaucoma), is often best managed with enucleation to relieve the severe ocular pain (48). Patients with stage 5 disease generally have a blind, but nonpainful eye, and require no aggressive treatment (45).

Observation is recommended in two situations: in eyes with stage 1 and 2A disease with mild telangiectasia and little exudation, particularly in patients older than 15 years, because in these cases there is less likelihood of progression of exudation and retinal detachment. However, treatment should be considered if progression is documented. Also, in some eyes with stages 3B and 5 disease, where the blind eye is comfortable, but there is no hope for useful vision, observation is an option (45).

Laser photocoagulation is most successful when there are telangiectasias without retinal detachment (stage 2). Cryotherapy can also be used in such cases. It is important to wait at least 3 months before considering additional laser photocoagulation (45).

Cryotherapy is the treatment of choice when there are peripheral telangiectasias associated with extensive exudation or subtotal retinal detachment (stage 3A), even in cases of relatively high retinal detachment (stage 3B) (45).

In a retrospective study by Shienbaum and Tasman the average follow-up period for the 13 patients was 12.4 years. Four out of the twelve treated patients (33%) had recurrences, and three of the four had multiple recurrences (42).

New treatment modalities have been tested using anti-VEGF agents. Quiroz-Mercado et al have been using intravitreal bevacizumab (Avastin) injections in patients with Coats' disease as an adjuvant treatment before cryotherapy. Four eyes of four patients with Coats' disease were included in a study. Partial resolution of subretinal fluid was observed (49).

## PERIPHERAL RETINAL ANGIOMA

Peripheral retinal angiomas as well as the entity described as Leber's military aneurysm, represent a challenge in diagnosis and treatment for the vitreoretinal surgeon. Peripheral retinal hemangiomas have been described as sporadic lesions or as part of the von Hippel-Lindau syndrome (50,51). The term "retinal angioma" to most ophthalmologists is synonymous with the lesions seen in von Hippel-Lindau syndrome. Welch (52) and McDonald (53) categorized other angioma-like lesions as pseudoangiomas. They emphasized that if the lesion has all the clinical characteristics of the retinal capillary hamartoma, it represents a case of von Hippel-Lindau syndrome until proven otherwise.

Shields et al. (54), in a review of 103 vasoproliferative retinal tumors of the ocular fundus (acquired retinal hemangioma), created a comprehensive classification. Shields found that 74% of the tumors were idiopathic, and 26% were secondary to preexisting ocular disease (pars planitis, retinitis pigmentosa, or toxoplasmic retinitis). Most of the idiopathic tumors developed within 6 mm of the ora serrata. Associated vitreoretinal exudation, secondary exudative retinal detachment, vitreous cells, vitreous hemorrhage, preretinal macular fibrosis, and macular edema (52).

Peripheral retinal capillary hemangiomas have been well described as part of the von Hippel-Lindau syndrome, associated with hemangiomas in the cerebellum, medulla, or spinal cord; cysts of the pancreas, kidney, adrenal gland; and hypernephroma and pheochromocytoma (55).

Vision may be lost as result of cystoid macular edema, subretinal exudates, serous retinal detachment, vitreous hemorrhage, rhegmatogenous retinal detachment, or macular traction created by epiretinal membranes or tractional retinal detachment (53,56) (Fig. 48-7).

## Treatment

Cryotherapy and laser photocoagulation have been shown to be effective in treating peripheral angiomas (57). Cryotherapy and laser treatment to peripheral retinal angiomas may induce "spontaneous peeling" of epiretinal membranes (53,58). Most epiretinal membranes that spontaneously peel away from the macula are in eyes with partial posterior detachment, in which complete posterior vitreous detachment later develops. Presumably, eyes that show spontaneous membrane peeling after cryotherapy or laser photocoagulation for peripheral angiomas do so because the treatment results in angioma permeability changes that enhance vitreous liquefaction and complete detachment.

McDonald et al. (53) reported the use of vitrectomy in eyes with macular traction associated with peripheral angiomas, ranging from macular puckering to frank tractional detachment of the macula associated with partial posterior vitreous detachment, peripheral tractional retinal detachment, and extensive epiretinal membrane formation. These changes may arise after cryotherapy, laser treatment, or spontaneously. Vitreous surgery has a good chance of improving vision in these cases; treatment of the hemangioma, before or during vitrectomy, usually results in tumor regression (53). Adequate treatment of hemangiomas can be accomplished by endolaser treatment, cryotherapy, or the use of indirect ophthalmoscopic laser photocoagulation.

Another treatment option that has been suggested is the use of intravitreal bevacizumab. Ustariz-Gonzalez, Quiroz-Mercado, et al. treated two patients with intravitreal injection of

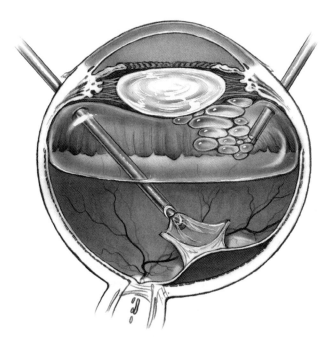

**Figure 48-2.** Lens-sparing vitrectomy in infants. Two steps of the technique are shown: vitrectomy-membranectomy and fluid-gas exchange performed by infusing air through the irrigating light pipe. (Adapted from Maguire AM, Trese MT. Lens-sparing vitreoretinal surgery in infants. *Arch Ophthalmol* 1992;110:284–286, with permission.)

bevacizumab resulting in improvement of visual acuity in both cases (−1.40 logMAR to −0.60 logMAR, and −1.40 logMAR to −0.80 logMAR). Vitreous opacities seen by ophthalmoscopy and color photos decreased in both eyes and flourescein angiograohy (FA) showed less leakage after the treatment. At 3 months follow up, no further changes were observed (59).

Dahr, Cusick, et al. also reported a pilot study of intravitreal injections of pegaptanib (3 mg/100 L), given every 6 weeks for minimum of six injections. Five patients with severe ocular von Hippel Lindau (VHL) lesions were enrolled in the study. Two of five patients completed the course of treatment and 1 year of follow-up. These two patients had a progressive decrease in retinal hard exudates and reduction in central retinal thickness measured by optical coherence tomography. One of these two

patients had improvement in visual acuity of 3 lines. No significant change in fluorescein leakage or lesion size was detected in either patient. Lesions in the other three patients continued to progress despite treatment, and these patients did not complete the entire treatment course. One patient developed a tractional retinal detachment. Additional serious adverse events included transient postinjection hypotony in two eyes (60).

## SICKLE-CELL RETINOPATHY

Sickle-cell disease is an autosomal recessive condition that is found in patients in southern Europe, the Middle East, Asia,

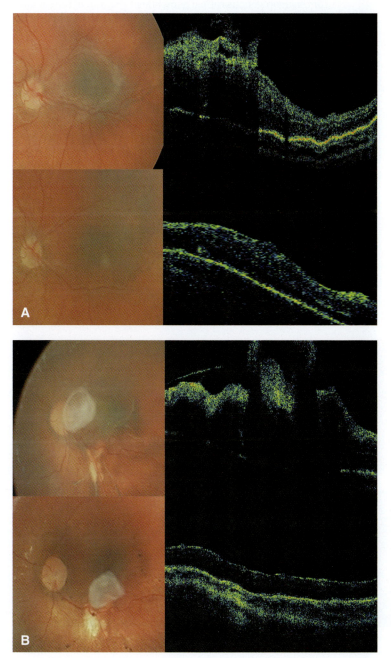

**Figure 48-3.** Retinopathy of prematurity. **A:** Stage 4B, with retinal detachment involving the macula. **B:** Stage 5, total retinal detachment. (Courtesy Thomas C. Lee, MD.)

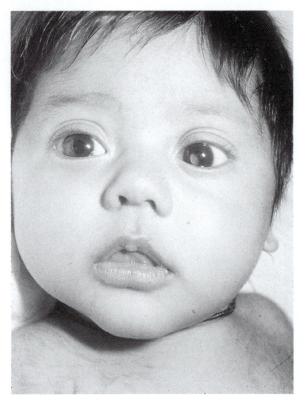

**Figure 48-4.** Newborn female diagnosed with incontinentia pigmenti. This photo shows the typical skin lesions.

India, and Saudi Arabia. Sickle-cell trait is seen in about 8% to 10% of the African-American population (61,62).

Normal hemoglobin (hemoglobin A) contains two alpha and two beta chains, with glutamic acid at position 6 of the beta chain. Sickling hemoglobins differ from hemoglobin A only in the amino acid at position 6 of the beta chain. Hemoglobin S contains valine, and hemoglobin C contains lysine. Blood from patients with sickle-cell thalassemia contains a mixture of hemoglobin S, hemoglobin A, hemoglobin A2, and hemoglobin F (63,64).

Erythrocyte sickling can occur in any microvascular network of the eye. Depending on the anatomic location of the occlusion, visual function may or may not be affected. In the conjunctiva vasculature, vascular occlusions result in the characteristic comma sign (65). Peripheral retinal vascular occlusions, caused by arteriolar obstruction from sickled deoxygenated red blood cells, cause a spectrum of funduscopic abnormalities. The classification of proliferative sickle retinopathy by Golberg includes the following stages: I, peripheral retinal arteriolar occlusions; II, peripheral retinal arteriolar-venular anastomosis; III, neovascular and fibrous proliferation (sea-fan formation); IV, vitreous hemorrhage; and V, traction or rhegmatogenous retinal detachment (66,67). In the Jamaica Sickle Cohort study, Penman et al. (68) used a classification system of peripheral retinal vascular changes compared with hemoglobinopathies and normal hemoglobin genotype.

## Management

Patients with sickle-cell disease are now living longer because of better medical management. Diagnosis of sickle-cell disease is made by hemoglobin electrophoresis or by molecular techniques, including polymerase chain reaction. One screening technique uses a sickle-cell preparation in which the cells of the patients are exposed to acidic solutions that cause the cells to sickle. This is a screening test, and the heterozygotic patients with sickle-cell trait also may have a positive reaction. With longer durations of survival, patients have a greater chance of end-organ damage from disease (69).

Jampol et al. (63,70) have updated the treatment for proliferative sickle retinopathy. Scatter photocoagulation is recommended for initial treatment. Sector scatter is recommended for the patient who can return for regular follow-up examinations.

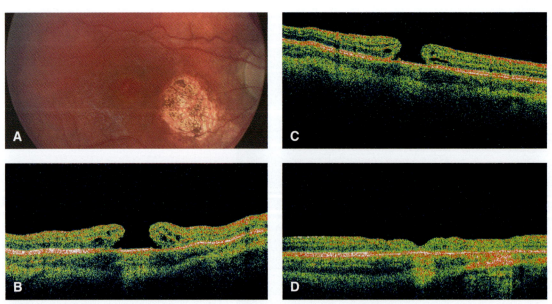

**Figure 48-5.** Incontinentia pigmenti. **A:** Fundus photograph with vascular changes. **B, C:** Same eye, OCT demonstrates macular hole. **D:** Same eye shows closure of macular hole after surgical repair

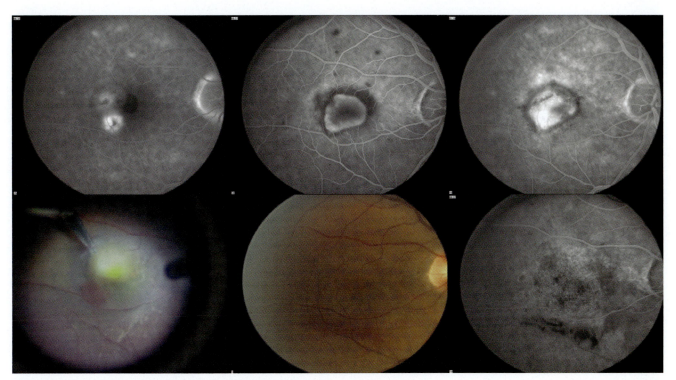

**Figure 48-6.** Coats' disease. Fundus photograph with yellowish exudates involving the macula.

Circumferential 360-degree scatter treatment could be considered if regular follow-up is not assured. Feeder-vessel photocoagulation should be considered if repeated vitreous hemorrhaging or progressive retinal traction develops from persistent neovascularization if media opacities prevent photocoagulation (71).

Macular and perimacular vascular changes have been described in sickling hemoglobinopathies. These include arteriolar occlusion and subsequent nonperfusion, microaneurysmal dots, enlarged precapillary arterioles and capillary segments, cotton-wool spots, hairpin venous loops with adjacent capillary dropout, and foveal avascular zone irregularities (72,73). Vitrectomy with or without sclera buckling is indicated for progressive traction retinal detachment that involves the macula (74). Surgeons should be aware of intraoperative complications with sickle-cell hemoglobinopathies. These include anterior segment ischemia or necrosis, optic nerve and macular infarctions with intraocular pressures equal to or higher than 25 mm Hg, and sickle-cell crises during general anesthesia (67).

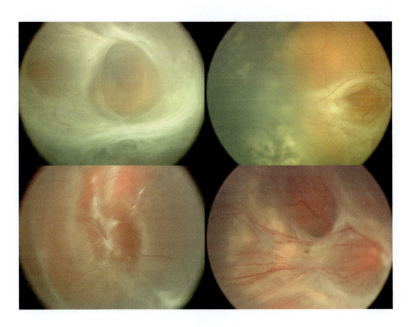

**Figure 48-7.** Von Hippel Lindau Disease. Fundus photograph with yellowish exudates and retinal detachment. (Courtesy Orlando Ustariz-Gonzalez, MD.)

## References

1. Jampol LM, Ebroom DA, Goldbaum MH. Peripheral proliferative retinopathies: an update on angiogenesis, etiologies and management. *Surv Ophthalmol* 1994;38:519–540.
2. Bloom SM, Brucker AJ. Peripheral retina neovascularization. In: Blomm SM, Brucker AJ (eds). *Laser surgery for posterior segment*, 2nd ed. Philadelphia, PA: Lippincott-Raven, 1997:129.
3. Gass JDM. *Stereoscopic atlas of macular diseases: diagnosis and treatment*, 4th ed. St. Louis: Mosby-Year Book, 1997.
4. Tranos P, Wickremasinghe S, Satngos N, et al. Major review: macular edema. *Surv Ophthalmol* 2004;49:470–490.
5. Schatz H. Fluorescein angiography: basic principles and interpretation. In: Ryan SJ, Schachat AP, Murphy RB (eds). *Retina*, 2nd ed, vol 2. St. Louis: Mosby-Year Book, 1994:911.
6. Bird AC. Retinal edema: introduction to the first international cystoid macular edema symposium. *Surv Ophthalmol* 1984;28(suppl):433–436.
7. Michael JC, de Venecia G. Retinal trypsin digest study of cystoid macular edema associated with peripheral choroidal melanoma. *Am J Ophthalmol* 1995;119:152–156.
8. Gass JDM. A fluorescein angiography study of macular dysfunction secondary to retinal vascular disease: V. Retinal telangiectasis. *Arch Ophthalmol* 1968;80:592–605.
9. Spitnaz M, Joussen F, Wessin A. Treatment of Coats' disease with photocoagulation. *Graefes Arch Clin Exp Ophthalmol* 1976;199:31–37.
10. Trese MT. Visual results and prognostic factor for vision following surgery for stage IV retinopathy of prematurity. *Ophthalmology* 1986;93:574–579.
11. Grewing R, Ulrich M. Results of surgery for epiretinal membranes and their recurrences. *Br J Ophthalmol* 1996;80:323–326.
12. Quiram PA, Capone A Jr, Current understanding and management of retinopathy of prematurity. *Curr Opin Ophthalmol* 2007;143(6):228–234.
13. Palmer EA, Phelps DL, Spencer R, et al. Retinopathy of prematurity: the role of oxygen. In: Ryan SJ, Schachat AP (eds). *Retina*, 4th ed, vol 2. Philadelphia, PA: Elsevier Mosby, 2006:1448.
14. ICROP Committee for the Classification of Late Stages ROP: An international classification of retinopathy of prematurity, II: the classification of retinal detachment. *Arch Ophthalmol.* 1987;105:906–912.
15. An International Committee for the Classification of Retinopathy of Prematurity: The international classification of retinopathy of prematurity revisited. *Arch Ophthalmol.* 2005;123:991–999.
16. Trese MT. Retinopathy of prematurity: classification system. In: Ryan SJ, Wilkinson CP (eds). *Retina*, 4th ed, vol 3. Philadelphia, PA: Elsevier Mosby, 2006:2465.
17. Hurley B, McNamara JA, Fineman M, et al. Laser treatment for retinopathy of prematurity. Evolution in Treatment Technique Over 15 Years. *Retina* 2006;26:S16–S17.
18. Quiroz-Mercado H, Martinez-Castellanos MA, Hernandez-Rojas Ml, Salazar-Teran N, Chan RVP. Antiangiogenic therapy with intravitreal bevacizumab for retinopathy of prematurity. *Retina* 2008;28(3):S19–S25.
19. Capone A Jr, Trese M. Lens-sparing vitreous surgery for tractional stage 4A retinopathy of prematurity retinal detachments. *Ophthalmology* 2001;108:2068–2070.
20. Trese MT, Droste PJ. Long-term postoperative results of a consecutive series of stages 4 and 5 retinopathy of prematurity. *Ophthalmology* 1998;105:992–997.
21. Sears J, Sonnie C. Anatomic Success of Lens Sparing Vitrectomy with and without Scleral Buckle for Stage 4 Retinopathy of Prematurity. *Am J Ophthalmol* 2007;143:810–813.
22. Gonzalez CR, Boshra J, Schwartz SD. 25-gauge pars plicata vitrectomy for stage 4 and 5 Retinopathy of prematurity. *Retina* 2006;26:S42–S46.
23. Azuma N, Ishikawa K, Hama Y, et al. Early Vitreous Surgery for Aggressive Posterior Retinopathy of Prematurity. *Am J Ophthalmol* 2006;142:636.e1–636.e9.
24. De Juan E, Farr AK, Noorily S. Retinal detachment in infants: syndromes of retinal detachment without systemic associations: familial exudative vitreoretinopathy. In: Ryan SJ, Wilkinson CP (eds). *Retina*, 3rd ed, vol 3. St. Louis: Mosby, 2001:2507.
25. Pendergast SD, Trese MT. Familial Exudative Vitreoretinopathy: Results of Surgical Management. *Ophthalmology* 1998;705:7075–7023.
26. Anand R, Tasman WS. Nonrhegmatogenous retinal detachment: congenital disorders. In: Ryan SJ, Wlkinson CP (eds). *Retina*, 4th ed, vol 3. Philadelphia, PA: Elsevier-Mosby, 2006:2130.
27. Ikeda T, Takashi Fujikado T, Tano Y, et al. Vitrectomy for Rhegmatogenous or Tractional Retinal Detachment with Familial Exudative Vitreoretinopathy. *Ophthalmology* 1999;106:1081–1085.
28. Joshi M, Ciaccia S, Trese MT, et al. Posterior hyaloid contracture in pediatric vitreoretinopathies. *Retina* 2006;26:S38–S41.
29. Equi R, Bains H, Jampol L, et al. Retinal tears occurring at the border of vascular and avascular retina in adult patients with incontinentia pigmenti. *Retina* 2003;23(4):574–576.
30. Meallet MA, Song J, Stout JT. An extreme case of retinal avascularity in a female neonate with incontinentia pigmenti. *Retina* 2004;24(4):613–615.
31. Golberg MF, Curtis PH. Retinal and other manifestations of incontinentia pigmenti (Bloch-Sulzberger syndrome). *Ophthalmology* 1993;100:1645–1654.
32. Watzke RC, Stevens TS, Carney RG Jr. Retinal vascular changes in incontinentia pigmenti. *Arch Ophthalmol* 1976;94:743–746.
33. Wong F, Goldberg MF, Hao Y. Identification of a nonsense mutation an codon 128 of the Norrie's disease gene in a male infant. *Arch Ophthalmol* 1993;111:1553–1517.
34. Warburg M. Norrie's disease. *Acta Ophthalmol* 1963;41:134–146.
35. Goldberg MF. Persistent fetal vasculature (PFV): an integrated interpretation of signs and symptoms associated with persistent hyperplastic primary vitreous (PHPV). LIV Edward Jackson Memorial Lecture. *Am J Ophthalmol* 1997;124:587–626.
36. De Juan E Jr, Arman K, Noorily S. Retinal detachment in Infants: syndromes of retinal detachment without systemic associations. persistence of fetal vasculature. In: Ryan SJ, Wilkinson CP (eds). *Retina*, 4th ed, vol 3. St. Louis: Mosby, 2001:2505.
37. Dhingra S, Sheras DJ, Blake V, et al. Advanced bilateral persistent fetal vasculature associated with novel mutation in the Norrie gene. *Br. J. Ophthalmol* 2006;90:1324–1325.
38. Meier P, Wiedemann P. Surgical aspects of vitreoretinal disease in children: indications for surgery. In: Ryan SJ, Wilkinson CP (eds). *Retina*, 4th ed, vol 3. Philadelphia, PA: Elsevier Mosby, 2006:2490.
39. Alexandrakis G, Scott IU, Flynn HW Jr, et al. Visual Acuity Outcomes with and without Surgery in Patients with Persistent Fetal Vasculature. *Ophthalmology* 2000;107:1068–1072.
40. Paysse EA, McCreery KMB, Coats DK. Surgical management of the lens and retrolenticular fibrotic membranes associated with persistent fetal vasculature. *J Cataract Refract Surg* 2002;28:816–820.
41. Müllner-Eidenböck A, Amon M, Hauff W, et al. Surgery in unilateral congenital cataract caused by persistent fetal vasculature or minimal fetal vascular remnants. *J Cataract Refract Surg* 2004;30:611–619.
42. Shiembaum G, Tasman W. Coats' disease: a lifetime disease. *Retina* 2006;26:422–424.
43. Spitznas M, Joussen F, Wessing A, et al. Coats' disease: an epidemiologic and fluorescein angiographic study. *Graefes Arch Clin Exp Ophthalmol* 1975;195:241–250.
44. Smithen L, Brown G, Brucker A, et al. Coats' Disease Diagnosed in Adulthood. *Ophthalmology* 2005;112:1072–1078.
45. Shields J, Shields C, Honavar S, et al. Classification and Management of Coats' Disease: The 2000 Proctor Lecture. *Am J Ophthalmol* 2001;131:572–583.
46. Rabb MF, Gagliano DA, Teske MP. Retinal arterial macroaneurysms. *Surv Ophthalmol* 1988;33:73–96.
47. Gass JDM, Blodi BA. Idiopathic juxtafoveolar retinal telangiectasis: update of classification and follow-up study. *Am J Ophthalmol* 1993;100:1536–1546.
48. Shields J, Shields C, Honavar S, et al. Clinical Variations and Complications of Coats' Disease in 150 cases: The 2000 Sanford Gifford Memorial Lecture. *Am J Ophthalmol* 2001;131:561–571.
49. Romo-García E, Alvarez-Rivera G, Gordon M, et al. Is intravitreal Bevacizumab an effective treatment for Coats' disease? Poster Number 94/B210, ARVO 2007.
50. Shields JA, Decker WL, Sanborn GE, et al. Presumed acquired retinal hemangioma. *Ophthalmology* 1983;90:1292–1300.
51. Schwartz PL, Fastenberg DM, Shakin JL. Management of macular puckers associated with retinal angiomas. *Ophthalmic Surg* 1990;21:550–556.
52. Welch RB. Discussion of presumed acquired retinal hemangiomas. *Ophthalmology* 1983;90:1300.
53. McDonald HR, Schatz H, Johnson RN, et al. Vitrectomy in eyes with peripheral retinal angioma associated with traction macular detachment. *Ophthalmology* 1996;103:329–335.
54. Shields CL, Shields JA, Barrer J, et al. Vasoproliferative tumors of the ocular fundus: classification and clinical manifestations in 103 patients. *Arch Ophthamol* 1995;113:615–623.
55. Augsburger JJ, Shields JA, Goldberg RE. Classification and management of hereditary retinal angiomas. *Int Ophthalmol* 1981;4:93–106.
56. Laatikainen L, Immonen I, Summmanen P. Peripheral retinal angioma like lesion and macular pucker. *Am J Ophthalmol* 1989;108:563–566.
57. Annesly WH Jr, Leonard BC, Shields JA, et al. Fifteen-year review of treated cases of retinal hemangioma. *Trans Am Acad Ophthalmol Otolaryngol* 1977;83:446–453.
58. Schwartz PL, Trubowitsch G, Fastenberg DM, et al. Macular pucker and retinal angioma. *Ophthalmic Surg* 1987;18:677–679.
59. Ustariz-Gonzalez O, Suarez-Licona A, Quiroz-Mercado H, et al. Bevacizumab injection in von Hippel Lindau disease. Poster 4287/B958, ARVO 2006.
60. Dahr SS, Cusick M, Rodriguez-Coleman H, et al. Intravitreal anti–vascular endothelial growth factor therapy with pegaptanib for advanced von Hippel–Lindau disease of the retina. *Retina* 2007;27:150–158.
61. Nagpal KC, Goldberg MF, Rabb MF. Ocular manifestations of sickle hemoglobinopathies. *Surv Ophthalmol* 1977;21:391–411.
62. Al-Hazza S, Bird AC, Kulozik A, et al. Ocular findings in Saudi Arabian patients with sickle cell disease. *Br J Ophthalmol* 1995;79:457–561.
63. Jampol L, Ebroom DA, Goldbaum MH. Peripheral proliferative retinopathies: an update on angiogenesis, etiologies, and management. *Surv Ophthalmol* 1994;38:519–540.

64. Bloom SM, Brucker AJ. Peripheral retinal vascularization. In: Bloom SM, Brucker AJ (eds). *Laser surgery of the posterior segment*, 2nd ed. Philadelphia, PA: Lippincott-Raven, 1997:129.

65. Paton D. The conjunctival sign in sickle cell disease. *Arch Ophthalmol* 1962;68:627–632.

66. Goldberg MF. Classification and pathogenesis of proliferative sickle retinopathy. *Am J Ophthalmol* 1971;71:649–655.

67. Fekrat S, Lutty G, Goldberg MF. Hemoglobinopathies. In: Guyer DR, Yannuzzi LA, Chang S, et al. (eds). *Retina-vitreous-macula*, vol 1. Philadelphia, PA: WB Saunders, 1999:438.

68. Penman AD, Talbot JF, Chuang EL, et al. New classification of peripheral retinal vascular changes in sickle cell disease. *Br J Ophthalmol* 1994;78:681–689.

69. Goldberg MF. Sickle cell retinopathy. In: Tasman W, Jeager EA (eds). *Duane's clinical ophthalmology*. Philadelphia, PA: JB Lippincott Co, 1991;3:1–54.

70. Jampol LM, Farber M, Rabb MF, et al. An update on techniques of photocoagulation treatment of proliferative sickle cell retinopathy. *Eye* 1991;5:260–263.

71. Goldbaum MH, Fletcher RC, Jampol LM, et al. Cryotherapy of proliferative sickle retinopathy: II. Triple freeze-thaw cycle. *Br J Ophthalmol* 1979;63:97–101.

72. Asdourian GK, Nagpal KC, Busse B, et al. Macular and perimacular vascular remodeling in sickling cells in homozygous sickle cell disease. *Br J Ophthalmol* 1976;66:431–453.

73. McLeod DS, Merges C, Fukushima A, et al. Histopathologic features of neovascularization in sickle cell retinopathy. *Am J Ophthalmol* 1997;124:455–472.

74. Pulido JS, Flynn HW Jr, Clarkson JG, et al. Pars plana vitrectomy in the management of complications of proliferative sickle retinopathy. *Arch Ophthalmol* 1988;106:1553–1557.

# 49

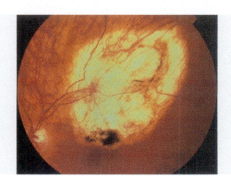

# Macular Choroidal Melanoma

Jerry A. Shields ■ Carol L. Shields

Uveal melanoma is the most common primary intraocular malignant tumor among Caucasians. The epidemiology, clinical features, diagnostic approaches, management, and prognosis of uveal melanoma have been discussed in detail in recent textbooks (1,2). Choroidal melanomas that occur in the macular area present unique therapeutic considerations, because their treatment sometimes can cause considerable visual loss. This chapter reviews the diagnosis and management of melanomas that arise in the macular area, a region that we define as an area about 6 mm in diameter with the foveola as its center. Because recent publications (1,2) have described this tumor in great detail, this chapter briefly reviews the diagnosis and management of macular choroidal melanoma.

## CLINICAL FEATURES

Macular choroidal melanoma can assume a variety of clinical features (1,2). It usually presents as a sessile or dome-shaped pigmented mass located deep to the sensory retina (Fig. 49-1). If located in the macular area, it is more likely to have surface orange pigment at the level of the overlying retinal pigment epithelium. A secondary retinal detachment frequently accounts for visual impairment. Occasionally, a macular choroidal melanoma can be partly or entirely nonpigmented. With continued growth, the tumor can rupture Bruch's membrane and assume a mushroom shape. If the tumor is amelanotic, blood vessels in the mass are visible ophthalmoscopically. In some instances, larger macular choroidal melanoma can cause total retinal detachment, cataract, congestive glaucoma, and extraocular extension. Such tumors are generally larger and carry a worse prognosis.

## DIAGNOSTIC APPROACHES

In most instances, the diagnosis of macular choroidal melanoma can be made by recognition of its classic features using

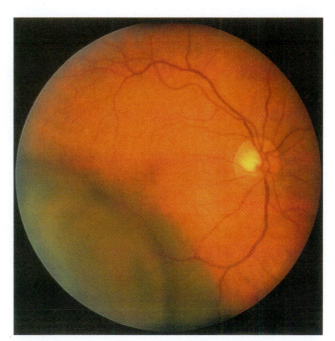

**FIGURE 49-1.** Pigmented choroidal melanoma encroaching on the foveal area.

indirect ophthalmoscopy. The diagnosis can be supported or confirmed, however, by the judicious use of ancillary studies such as fluorescein angiography, ultrasonography, or, in more difficult cases, fine-needle biopsy (3). In cases that are atypical ophthalmoscopically, these ancillary studies assume a more vital role in diagnosis. These techniques are discussed in detail in the literature (1,2) and are only summarized here.

On fluorescein angiography, a typical choroidal melanoma shows mottled hyperfluorescence in the vascular filling phases and diffuse late staining of the mass and its overlying subretinal fluid. A larger melanoma, particularly one that has broken through Bruch's membrane, shows more clearly the characteristic double circulation in which both the retinal vessels and the choroidal vessels in the tumor are evident (1,2) (Fig. 49-2).

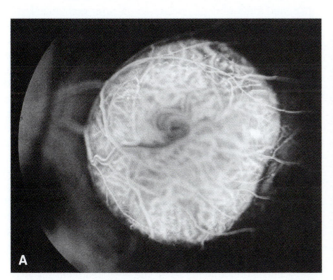
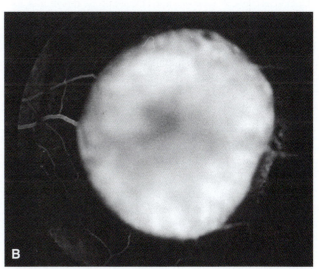

**Figure 49-2.** Fluorescein angiography of an elevated macular melanoma. **A:** Venous phase showing filling of the tumor vessels and the overlying retinal vessels ("double circulation"). **B:** Late angiogram showing diffuse hyperfluorescence of the mass.

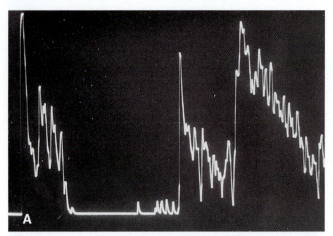
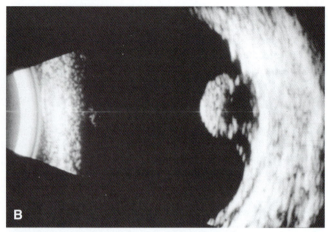

**Figure 49-3.** Ultrasonography of macular choroidal melanoma. A: a-Scan showing medium to low decreasing amplitude pattern. B: b-Scan showing pedunculated mass with basal acoustic hollowness and choroidal excavation.

On A-scan ultrasonography, choroidal melanoma typically shows medium to low internal reflectivity; on B-scan, it shows a choroidal mass pattern with acoustic hollowness and choroidal excavation (Fig. 49-3). Ultrasonography can delineate small nodules of extraocular extension of the tumor. It is particularly helpful in eyes with opaque media. Computed tomography and magnetic resonance imaging can be used to visualize uveal melanoma and to completely delineate larger areas of orbital extension (1,2).

Fine-needle aspiration biopsy can be used diagnose choroidal melanoma in difficult cases that defy clinical diagnosis using less invasive measures (1–3). The most commonly employed technique is a trans–pars plana, transvitreal approach using a 25-gauge needle.

## MANAGEMENT

There are several methods for management of macular melanoma (1,2). The selected management should depend on factors such as the size, location, and activity of the melanoma, as well as the status of the opposite eye and the age, general health, and psychological status of the patient. Each patient should undergo a detailed ophthalmic evaluation, and the size and extent of the tumor should be carefully documented. The known risk factors for growth and metastasis should be considered (4), and the patient then should be counseled thoroughly as to the therapeutic options (5).

The details of the therapeutic methods are described elsewhere (1–3). Small lesions in which the diagnosis is questionable can be followed with serial fundus photographs and ultrasonography to document growth before undergoing definitive treatment.

Some small and medium-sized melanomas can be managed with techniques of laser photocoagulation. Laser can be used primarily for lesions less than 3 mm in thickness that have documented growth or other significant risk factors for growth and metastasis (6). Photocoagulation is used less often today because transpupillary thermotherapy in the infrared range using a diode laser delivery system has shown some promising preliminary results.

Transpupillary thermotherapy recently has replaced laser photocoagulation at some centers for treatment of selected small and medium-sized melanomas (7,8). It involves heating the tumor using light in the infrared range by way of a modified diode laser delivery system. It gives the best results in cases of small choroidal melanomas in which growth is detected at an early stage (Fig. 49-4), but it has been used successfully for tumors up to 4 mm in thickness (1,2).

Techniques of radiotherapy using radioactive plaque (9) or charged particles (10,11) can be used for many medium-sized or large macular choroidal melanomas in which there is a reasonable chance of preserving some useful vision. Plaque radiotherapy is currently the most commonly employed method for treating uveal melanoma. Extensive experience with plaque brachytherapy has suggested that it offers reasonably good tumor control, can often preserve useful vision (12) (Fig. 49-5), and offers as good a systemic prognosis as enucleation. Plaque radiotherapy requires close cooperation among the ocular oncologist, radiation oncologist, and radiation physicists. It is now recognized that plaque radiotherapy can be employed to treat large melanomas, macular melanomas, ciliary-body melanomas, and extraocular extensions of melanomas (1,2,13,14). Similar results have been obtained with charged-particle irradiation, but anterior-segment complications such as cataract and neovascular glaucoma seem to be worse if charged-particle treatment is employed. Although results are sometimes surprisingly good (12), radiation retinopathy can be expected in most cases of macular melanoma treated by any form of irradiation (13,15) (Fig. 49-6).

A melanoma located in the ciliary body and peripheral choroid can be managed by local removal of the tumor using a method of partial lamellar sclerouvectomy (1,2,16). It is a difficult procedure that requires considerable skill and experience, but the results are often very gratifying. It is only rarely used for tumors that encroach on the macular area.

Enucleation appears to be the best treatment for larger macular tumors in which there is little hope for salvaging useful vision or tumors that surround or invade the optic nerve

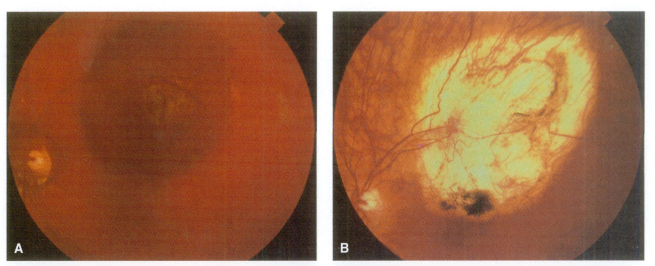

**Figure 49-4.** Transpupillary thermotherapy of macular choroidal melanoma located just superior to the foveola. **A:** Pretreatment appearance. The pigmented mass was 2.5 mm in thickness. **B:** Posttreatment appearance showing complete destruction of the mass.

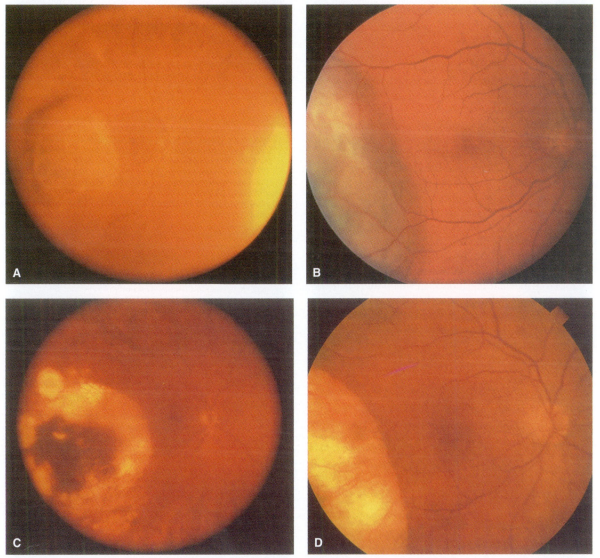

**Figure 49-5.** Excellent result of plaque radiotherapy of macular choroidal melanoma with posterior margin 3 mm temporal to the foveola. **A:** Wide-angle photographs of the dome-shaped mass. **B:** Forty-five degree photograph showing posterior margin of mass less than 3 mm from the foveola. **C:** Wide-angle photograph taken 18 years after radiotherapy, showing complete destruction of the tumor. **D:** Posterior margin of treated area after 18 years, showing excellent fovea. The vision is still 6/6 after 18 years.

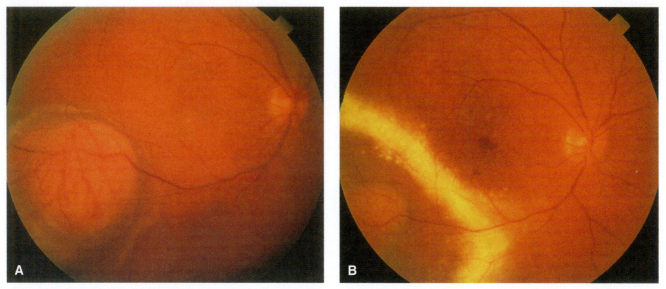

**Figure 49-6.** Radiation retinopathy after plaque therapy of macular choroidal melanoma. **A:** Pretreatment appearance of mass with break through Bruch's membrane. **B:** Appearance 18 months after treatment, showing circinate exudation around the tumor and microvasculopathy in the foveal region.

(1,2). It is most often employed in younger patients with large melanomas in whom there is no hope for useful vision.

In the rare instance in which a uveal melanoma shows massive orbital extension, primary orbital exenteration is warranted (17). In some instances combination therapies, such as plaque radiotherapy followed by supplemental transpupillary thermotherapy or laser photocoagulation, are employed.

In summary, choroidal melanoma located in the macular area presents difficult management problems. Small tumors with dormant features may be observed cautiously for evidence of growth before treatment is recommended. Small tumors with active features are best managed with transpupillary thermotherapy. Medium-sized tumors are probably best treated with managed plaque radiotherapy combined with thermotherapy. Enucleation is generally the treatment of choice for large macular melanomas in which there is little hope of salvaging useful vision in the affected eye. The patient with a macular choroidal melanoma should be counseled thoroughly as to all therapeutic options, and the final decision regarding treatment should be made by the patient after being informed of all aspects of the therapeutic choices.

## References

1. Shields JA, Shields CL. *Intraocular tumors: a text and atlas.* Philadelphia, PA: W.B Saunders, 1992.
2. Shields JA, Shields CL. *Atlas of intraocular tumors.* Philadelphia, PA: Lippincott Williams & Wilkins, 1999.
3. Shields JA, Shields CL, Ehya H, et al. Fine needle aspiration biopsy of suspected intraocular tumors: the 1992 Urwick Lecture. *Ophthalmology* 1993;100:1677–1684.
4. Shields CL, Shields JA, Kiratli H, et al. Risk factors for metastasis of small choroidal melanocytic lesions. *Ophthalmology* 1995;102:1351–1361.
5. Shields JA. Counseling the patient with a posterior uveal melanoma [editorial]. *Am J Ophthalmol* 1988;106:88–91.
6. Shields JA, Glazer LC, Mieler WF, et al. Comparison of xenon arc and argon laser photocoagulation in the treatment of choroidal melanomas. *Am J Ophthalmol* 1990;109:647–655.
7. Oosterhuis JA, Journee-de Korver HG, Kakebeeke-Kemme HM, et al. Transpupillary thermotherapy in choroidal melanomas. *Arch Ophthalmol* 1995;113:315–321.
8. Shields CL, Shields JA, Cater J, et al. Transpupillary thermotherapy for choroidal melanoma: tumor control and visual outcome in 100 consecutive cases. *Ophthalmology* 1998;105:581–590.
9. Shields CL, Shields JA, Gunduz K, et al. Radiation therapy for uveal malignant melanoma. *Ophthalmic Surg Lasers* 1998;29:397–409.
10. Char DH, Kroll SM, Castro JK. Ten-year follow-up of Helium ion therapy of uveal melanoma. *Am J Ophthalmol* 1998;125:81–89.
11. Gragoudas ES. Long-term results after proton irradiation of uveal melanomas. *Graefes Arch Clin Exp Ophthalmol* 1997;235:265–267.
12. Shields JA, Shields CL, Gunduz K. Visual preservation 18 years after cobalt plaque treatment of choroidal melanoma. *Eye* 1999;13:259–260.
13. Gunduz K, Shields CL, Shields JA, et al. Radiation complications and tumor control after plaque radiotherapy of choroidal melanoma with macular involvement. *Am J Ophthalmol* 1999;127:579–588.
14. Gunduz K, Shields CL, Shields JA, et al. Plaque radiotherapy of uveal melanoma with predominant ciliary body involvement. *Arch Ophthalmol* 1999;117:170–177.
15. Gunduz K, Shields CL, Shields JA, et al. Radiation retinopathy following plaque radiotherapy of posterior uveal melanoma. *Arch Ophthalmol* 1999;117:609–614.
16. Shields JA, Shields CL, Shah P, et al. Partial lamellar sclerouvectomy for ciliary body and choroidal tumors. *Ophthalmology* 1991;98:971–983.
17. Shields JA, Shields CL, Suvarnamani C, et al. Orbital exenteration with eyelid sparing: indications, technique and results. *Ophthalmic Surg* 1991;22:292–297.

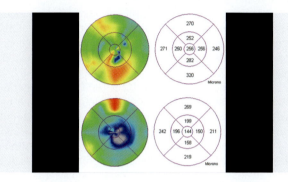

# Idiopathic Central Serous Retinopathy

Carlos A. Moreira Jr. ■ Juan Ignacio Verdaguer
Juan V. Espinoza ■ J. Fernando Arevalo

Idiopathic central serous retinopathy (ICSR), also called central serous chorioretinopathy or choroidopathy, is considered to be an accumulation of serous fluid underneath the sensory retina, commonly affecting the posterior pole. Associated with serous detachment of the neurosensory retina, one or more areas of retinal pigment epithelium (RPE) detachment may be found.

## PREVALENCE

This disease typically affects young and middle-aged adults in their third to fifth decades of life. Males are affected more commonly than females by a ratio of 8:1 or 9:1 (1,2). ICSR often occurs in white, Asian, and Hispanic men, and is rare in Blacks (2). It has been speculated that psychological factors such as stress might play a role in determining the disease (3).

## CLINICAL FINDINGS AND NATURAL HISTORY

Before the onset of symptoms, patients develop a serous detachment of the RPE, and they become symptomatic only if the central macula is affected. Serous detachment outside the posterior pole may not be detectable by the patient.

Patients who are symptomatic complain of a sudden decrease of central vision in many ways, such as blurred or dim vision, micropsia, metamorphopsia, or decreased color vision. A relative central scotoma and metamorphopsia usually can be demonstrated in the Amsler grid. In some patients, the onset of symptoms is preceded or accompanied by migraine-like headaches (3). There are no other diseases associated with ICSR. Patients' medical history, physical examination, and family history are usually unremarkable.

Visual acuity in the acute stage is often decreased moderately, averaging 20/30, although a wide range of acuities can be observed ranging from normal to 20/200, depending on the amount of the serous detachment affecting the macula. Small hyperopic corrections may improve vision to 20/20 in some cases.

The diagnosis can be made with ophthalmoscopy and biomicroscopy by identifying a round or oval area of retinal elevation in the posterior pole, slightly darker than normal, which may be surrounded by a halo of light reflex. The foveal reflex is usually absent. Because this disease is not of inflammatory origin, there are no inflammatory cells in the vitreous cavity.

The slit-lamp examination of the posterior pole using a fundus lens with the light beam directed a few degrees off the visual axis provides an adequate stereoscopic view of the macula, allowing for correct diagnosis. The serous detachment is usually transparent, although a diffuse gray to white subretinal deposit may be present. There is evidence that this white appearance is caused by the presence of fibrin, especially in longstanding cases (2). If the detachment is relatively shallow, a shadow from the retinal vessels over the RPE may be present. A yellow spot may be seen at the center of the fovea, or multiple small yellow precipitates may be detected under the detached retina.

One or multiple RPE detachments may occur. Usually the RPE detachment appears as a small, yellowish, round lesion, located beneath the superior half of the area of retinal detachment (2). Owning to gravity, the accumulation of subretinal fluid tends to be inferior to the area of RPE detachment. Sometimes it is possible to have RPE detachments outside the area of the retinal serous detachment.

Patients with recurrent ICSR may show areas of mottled depigmentation of the RPE underneath the serous detachment. It is common to find many areas of altered pigmentation of the RPE without active leakage in the affected or fellow eye.

Most of the patients with ICSR (80%–90%) experience spontaneous resolution of the serous detachment in 8 to 12 weeks after the onset of symptoms (4). Visual acuity often returns to normal in 1 to 6 months, although mild color defects and relative scotomas may persist indefinitely (5). Although most patients recover normal vision, approximately 5% do not reach 20/30 acuity. Fewer than 20% develop a serous detachment in the opposite eye (2).

Recurrences are relatively frequent and occur 40% to 50% of cases (2,6). In such cases, progressive deterioration of the RPE in the macular area may account for the persistent decrease in visual acuity. In rare instances, ICSR can cause the formation of subretinal neovascular membranes, especially in recurrent and prolonged detachments.

## FLUORESCEIN ANGIOGRAPHY

Fluorescein angiography is the diagnostic method tool that is most useful in determining the pathophysiology and the correct diagnosis of ICSR. The classic appearance of a hyperfluorescent spot at the level of the RPE allows for a better understanding of the disease.

Characteristically, a small hyperfluorescent leak appears during the choroidal or arterial phase of the angiogram increasing in size and intensity as the angiogram progresses (Fig. 50-1). The leak, resembling an ink spot, is commonly observed. A "smokestack" appearance of the leak, although pathognomonic of the disease, occurs only in about 10% of the cases (7). Such a smokestack pattern occurs because of convection streams of the heated and lighter dye (8), which spreads vertically in a configuration evocative of a plume of smoke (Fig. 50-2).

Fluorescein angiography identifies the areas of detached RPE in which the serous fluid from the choriocapillaris is entering the subretinal space. Although the initial diffusion of dye is quite fast, it may take 20 minutes after injection for the dye to reach the borders of the serous detachment of the retina. Usually, there are only one or two leaking points, although many areas of focal leakage may be found (Fig. 50-3). The foci of leakage are located at the fovea in only 10% of cases (3). Most commonly, focal leaks are found in the macular area 1 mm

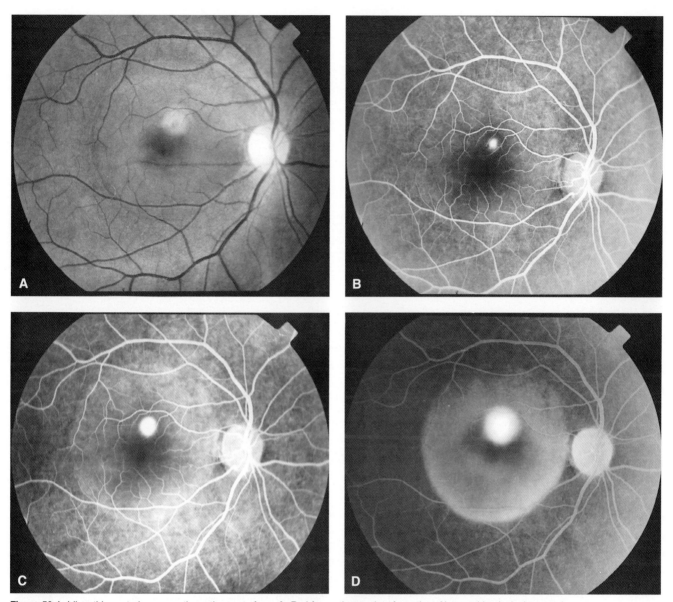

**Figure 50-1.** Idiopathic central serous retinopathy, acute form. **A:** Red-free retinography of a patient. Note a white dot in the superior area of the macula. **B:** Fluorescein angiography from an early arteriovenous phase of the same patient showing a small hyperfluorescent spot superior to the macula. **C:** Later phase of the angiogram showing enlargement of the hyperfluorescent spot and the initial hyperfluorescence in the subretinal space. **D:** Late phase of the angiogram showing hyperfluorescence of the retinal pigment epithelium detachment in the subretinal space.

adjacent to the fovea. The superonasal and inferonasal quadrants are the most frequently affected (9).

In recurrent cases, approximately 80% of new leaks are located adjacent to the previous site (Fig. 50-4). Therefore, it is often difficult to determine if the leakage is new or just a reactivation of the primary pathology (10).

If the leak cannot be found one should consider two possibilities: the leak has already healed and the subretinal fluid will be absorbed in the next few days, or the leak is outside of the detached area. Therefore, one should always take angiographic images outside of the affected area, especially in the regions superior to the macula and the optic disc. It is important to realize that the serous detachment

tends to extend to the foveal region even though the leak may be located eccentrically, because in this area the adhesion of the neurosensory retina to the RPE is weaker due to the absence of rods (3).

Once the tissue has healed, the angiographic findings may return to normal, although evidence of RPE detachment may persist. In recurrent cases, focal areas of depigmentation are present.

Research with indocyanine green angiography (ICG-A) has contributed novel information. Such studies have demonstrated presumed hyperpermeability of the choroidal vasculature surrounding the leaking sites seen on the fluorescein angiogram. Additional areas of choroidal hyperfluorescence not related to

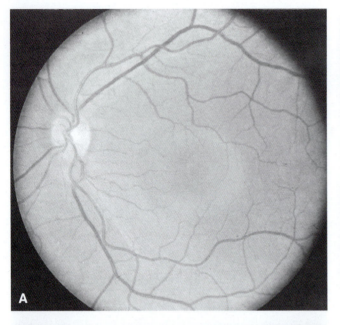

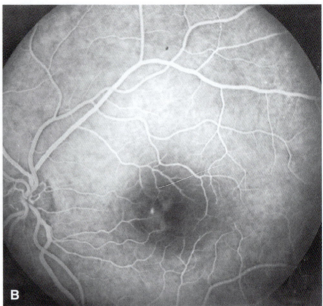

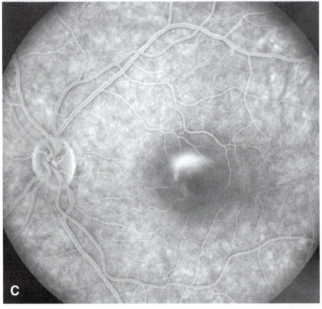

**Figure 50-2.** Idiopathic central serous retinopathy, acute form. **A:** Central serous detachment of the retina. **B:** Small retinal pigment epithelium leak in the angiogram. **C:** Diffusion of the dye into the subretinal space in a "smoke-stack" pattern.

active leaking sites and multiple occult serous detachments of the RPE have been elucidated in some cases (11–16).

## FUNDUS AUTOFLUORESCENCE

Recently fundus autofluorescence (FAF) has emerged as a noninvasive technique to study ICSR in different stages of the disorder. As previously stated, ICSR is a condition characterized by idiopathic leaks from the level of the RPE leading to serous retinal detachment. Patients with acute leaks imaged within the first month have minimal abnormalities seen in their FAF other than a slight increase in autofluorescence of the serous detachment.

When serous detachment persists for some time, the area of detachment becomes increasingly hyperautofluorescent. This autofluorescence is diffuse but contains discrete granules. After resolution of subretinal fluid, the accumulation of fluid on the outer retina is resorbed as well, and the hyperautofluorescence abates (17). Patients with chronic ICSR, having varying degrees of atrophy, show a mixed pattern of autofluorescence (Fig. 50-5). Additional deposition of material such as subretinal lipid and fibrin has been described in patients with ICSR. Lipid deposits and subretinal fibrin are not autofluorescent (17).

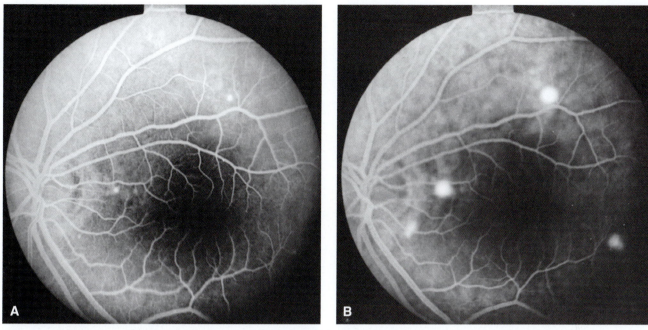

**Figure 50-3. A:** Patient with idiopathic central serous retinopathy and multiple retinal pigment epithelium detachments. Note two small hyperfluorescent spots. **B:** Same patient in a later phase of the angiogram showing four hyperfluorescent areas of detachment.

## OPTICAL COHERENCE TOMOGRAPHY

Optical coherence tomography (OCT) is a noninvasive technique for high-resolution, cross-sectional imaging of the ocular fundus (18). This is a useful diagnostic tool that allows for quantitative evaluation and monitoring of subretinal fluid in ICSR after treatment (Fig. 50-6). This imaging technology records the various features of ICSR, including retinal detachment, fibrinous exudation, cystic changes within the retina, and intraretinal precipitates that may result from the accumulation of proteins or macrophages with phagocytized photoreceptor outer segments (19–20). Multiple RPE detachments can be found in some cases.

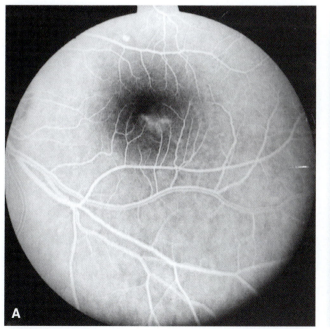 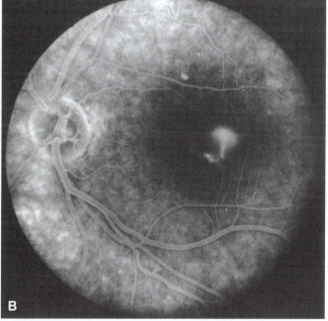

**Figure 50-4. A:** Patient with recurrent idiopathic central serous retinopathy showing an area of atrophy of the retinal pigment epithelium in the inferior area of the macula. **B:** Same patient in a later phase of the angiogram, showing a characteristic smokestack pattern of active retinopathy adjacent to the old scar.

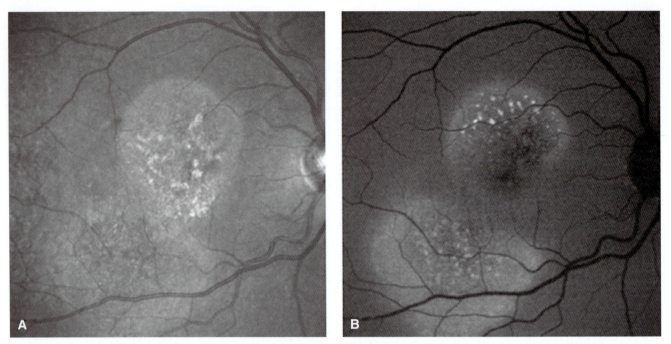

**Figure 50-5.** The red free photograph **(A)** and fundus autofluorescence **(B)** in the acute phase of chronic idiopathic central serous retinopathy shows an increased diffuse hyperautofluorescence in the area of the central and descending detachment with discrete granular structures corresponding to the accumulation of material on the outer surface of the retina (Courtesy of Chiara M. Eandi, MD, PhD, and Antonio P. Ciardella, MD).

## ATYPICAL PRESENTATIONS

### Bullous Retinal Detachment

Large serous detachments of the retina may occur in the midperiphery or in the posterior pole. These detachments can become confluent and involve the inferior fundus or larger areas of the retina (11,12). In such cases, large multiple RPE detachments are seen, measuring up to one disc diameter. These patients may develop the same clinical picture in the opposite eye several weeks later (2).

The differential diagnosis of ICSR with rhegmatogenous retinal detachment may be difficult. The angiographic features of multiple RPE detachments and the presence of shifting fluid aid correct diagnosis.

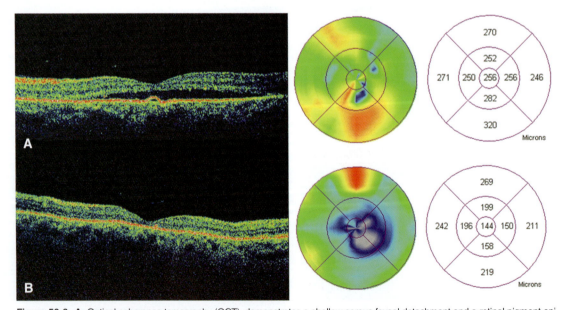

**Figure 50-6. A:** Optical coherence tomography (OCT), demonstrates a shallow serous foveal detachment and a retinal pigment epithelial (RPE) detachment with increased retinal thickness in idiopathic central serous retinopathy. **B:** After photodynamic therapy, the neurosensory retinal and RPE detachment have resolved with normalization of the foveal contour and improvement in visual acuity.

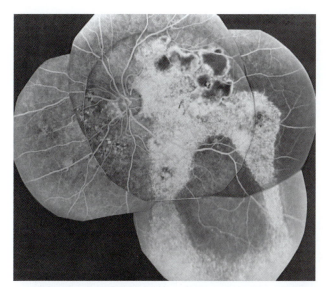

**Figure 50-7.** Chronic recurrent severe idiopathic central serous retinopathy in a 48-year-old man with a 10-year history of the condition, with scarring and extensive areas of depigmentation. Composite fluorescein angiography outlines two corridors of depigmentation that join inferiorly in an anchorlike pattern.

## Chronic Recurrent Severe Idiopathic Central Serous Retinopathy

Patients with more prolonged and recurrent forms of the disease often show large areas of atrophy of the RPE and photoreceptor cells, which, when involving the macular area, results in severe loss of vision. The presence of descending corridors of depigmentation extending inferiorly from the disc or macular area points to a diagnosis of chronic recurrent severe ICSR (Fig. 50-7). Small clumps of pigment may be seen, or a bone-corpuscular pattern of migration to the atrophic retina may occur, resembling a sectorial retinitis pigmentosa. These patients may experience significant loss of visual fields, especially superiorly, because of the tendency for fluid to accumulate in the inferior retina (13). Fluorescein angiography reveals multiple areas of staining that correspond to the RPE atrophy occurring in such cases (2).

## PATHOGENESIS

Fluorescein angiography demonstrates that the fluid underneath the neurosensory retinal originates from the choriocapillaris and reaches the subretinal space through a small aperture in the RPE layer (Fig. 50-8).

Despite being a widely recognized disease, the complete pathogenesis of ISCR is not fully understood. In addition, there is limited data on the pathology of the disease, though one study suggests that a marked alteration of the permeability of the choriocapillaris is present (2).

It seems that under circumstances not yet known, impaired cells of the RPE promote the movement of fluid in a chorioretinal direction. Such fluid reaches the subretinal space through a hole in the RPE and forms the characteristic blister

under the neurosensory retina. The serous detachment is confined to a limited area because normal RPE cells in the vicinity establish a compensatory mechanism, removing fluid back to the choriocapillaris. With time the RPE regains normal function, and the disease process resolves spontaneously (3).

Based on ICG-A, it has been suggested that choroidal hyperpermeability overwhelms the RPE and causes its detachment. As pressure increases, RPE may explode or decompensate, causing leakage that induces a neurosensory detachment (14).

Given the fact that patients usually have type A personalities, a stress-induced choroidal vascular change (presumed hyperpermeability) could be postulated. The repeated intravenous injection of epinephrine in experimental animals (15) can lead to serous detachment of neurosensory retina, lending support to the theory that stress plays a role in the pathogenesis. Elevated cortisol levels also may play a role in the pathogenesis of ICSR. It is well known that systemic corticosteroid may induce or aggravate ICSR; pregnant women may develop typical ICSR, sometimes with heavy fibrin deposits.

## DIFFERENTIAL DIAGNOSIS

A great variety of fundus diseases can produce serous detachment of the macula and therefore mimic ICSR: optic-disc pits, age-related macular degeneration (AMD), choroidal tumors (hemangiomas, metatatic carcinomas, malignant melanomas) usually located superior to the macular region, very high blood pressure levels as in malignant hypertension, nonpenetrating trauma, posterior scleritis, inflammatory diseases of the choroid (e.g., Harada's disease, sympathetic ophthalmia, multifocal choroiditis), and idiopathic uveal effusion.

The differentiation between ICSR and AMD in older patients may present a problem to the ophthalmologist. In general, the presence of blood, significant lipid exudation, or drusen suggests choroidal neovascularization, whereas small leaks in areas of large serous detachments and multifocal RPE abnormalities indicate ICSR.

## TREATMENT

To the present date, there is no evidence that a medical treatment such as steroids is useful in treating ICSR. In fact, there is evidence that systemic steroids can exacerbate the severity of the subretinal leakage, resulting in the development of bilateral bullous exudative retinal detachment in severe cases (16). It has been suggested that patients with recurrent ICSR may have high levels of epinephrine in the serum (15). If this proves to be true, these patients could benefit from beta-blocker therapy, possibly decreasing the frequency of recurrences.

## LASER PHOTOCOAGULATION

The natural history of ICSR indicates that most patients have good visual recovery in 8 to 12 weeks. It is reasonable to expect spontaneous resolution of the disease. However, many patients

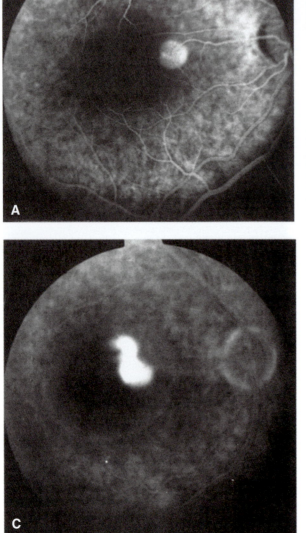

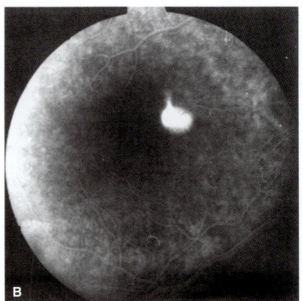

**Figure 50-8. A:** Patient with idiopathic central serous retinopathy showing the hyperfluorescent spot of the detachment of the retinal pigment epithelium in the nasal area of the macula. **B:** The dye spreads vertically into the subretinal space. **C:** Later phase of the angiogram showing a large amount of dye that has entered the subretinal space, promoting the neurosensory detachment.

have frequent recurrences with serious threats to vision. In these patients, one can consider laser photocoagulation to prevent irreversible visual impairment.

Laser photocoagulation may be indicated in the following circumstances (7):

- Serous detachment of the macula for more than 3 or 4 months
- Recurrences in eyes with visual deficits from previous episodes
- Presence of visual impairment in the fellow eye caused by the same disease
- Development of cystic changes in the neurosensory retina or large RPE abnormalities
- Occupational needs requiring prompt visual recovery
- Development of a choroidal neovascular membrane

If photocoagulation is applied, one must follow these patients for 3 to 4 weeks after treatment in order to detect the presence of choroidal neovascularization (CNV). This is a rare complication following laser treatment, although neovascularization may be present in untreated ICSR as well.

## PHOTODYNAMIC THERAPY

Photodynamic therapy (PDT) is a treatment modality that uses the combination of light and a photosensitizer. It causes narrowing of the choriocapillaris, reducing localized choroidal hyperperfusion and exudation that is thought to underlie ICSR (21). This novel therapy has been widely used in the treatment of CNV in AMD, inducing regression of CNV, and reducing visual loss in many patients.

PDT with verteporfin recently has been used for treating ICSR (Fig. 50-6); studies have demonstrated beneficial visual outcomes in many patients (22). However, the application of conventional PDT in ICSR can result in potential complications such as RPE atrophy and choroidal ischemia. The potential retinal damage caused by PDT may be minimized by reducing the dose of verteporfin and/or altering the timing of infusion and laser application, resulting in good treatment efficacy of chronic ICSR (23).

In recent years, ICG-A has been used to study ICSR, and has been used to guide treatment with PDT. This imaging technique serves as marker for the disorder (even in its dormant or quiescent state), by detecting the presence of multifocal areas of choroidal vascular hyperpermeability. In addition, ICG-A rules out polypoidal choroidal vasculopathy masquerading as ICSR (22).

## ANTIANGIOGENICS

The antipermeability effect of antiangiogenic agents may be beneficial in the choroidal vascular hyperpermeability reported in ICRS. Few reports have been published on the use of anti-vascular endothelial growth factor (anti-VEGF) treatment in ICRS. In these studies, there has been evidence of resolution of RPE and neurosensory retinal detachment, as well as visual acuity improvement. Intravitreal anti-VEGF therapy may be beneficial in the treatment of ICRS (24–26), and these agents deserve further study for the treatment of this disease.

## SUMMARY

Idiopathic central serous chorioretinopathy is a chorioretinal disorder characterized by serous detachment of the neurosensory retina and/or RPE. Management is a challenge, because most cases have spontaneous resolution in the acute stage; however, recurrent or persistent detachment is often associated with more diffuse RPE changes, visual loss, and sometimes secondary subretinal neovascularization. OCT has become an indispensable tool for the diagnosis and monitoring of ICSR. FAF has also been utilized to image and expand our understanding of this disease.

Regarding therapy of chronic or recurrent cases, laser photocoagulation has been used but may not be safe as there is risk of inducing CNV after treatment. In an effort to obtain better visual results with reduction of complications, PDT has become a useful therapeutic tool to manage chronic longstanding exudative retinal detachment with anatomic and functional recovery. Most recently, anti-VEGF therapy has been introduced as a novel option for the management of ICSR. This potential line of therapy deserves further study.

## References

1. Bennet G. Central serous retinopathy. *Br J Ophthalmol* 1955;39:605–618.
2. Gass JDM. *Stereoscopic atlas of macular diseases*. St. Louis: Mosby, 1987.
3. Spitznas M. Central serous retinopathy. In: Ryan SJ (ed). *Retina*, vol 2. St. Louis: Mosby, 1989:217–227.
4. Klein ML, Van Buskirk EM, Friedman E, et al. Experience with nontreatment of central serous choroidopathy. *Arch Ophthalmol* 1974;91:247–250.
5. Leaver PK, Williams CM. Effect of central serous retinopathy on visual function. *Trans Ophthalmol Soc UK* 1977;97:655.
6. Gass JDM. Pathogenesis of disciform detachment of the neuro-epithelium: II. Idiopathic central serous choroidopathy. *Am J Ophthalmol* 1967;63:587–615.
7. Grand MG, Bressler NM, Brown GC, et al. Acquired diseases affecting the macula. In: Weingeist TA, Liesegang TJ, Slamovits TL (eds). *Basic and clinical science course*, 1997–98. San Francisco: American Academy of Ophthalmology, 1997.
8. Shimizu K, Tobari I. Central serous retinopathy dynamics of subretinal fluid. *Mod Probl Ophthalmol* 1971;9:152.
9. Wessing A. Grundsätzliches zum diagnostoschen fortschritt durch die fluoreszenzangiographie. *Ber Dtsch Ophthalmol Ges* 1973;73:566–568.
10. Steinberg RH, Miller SS. Transport and membrane properties of the retinal pigment epithelium. In: Marmor MF, Zinn KM (eds). *The retinal pigment epithelium*. Cambridge, MA: Harvard University Press, 1975:205–225.
11. Gass JDM. Bullous retinal detachment: an unusual manifestation of idiopathic central serous choroidopathy. *Am J Ophthalmol* 1973;75:810.
12. Kayazawa F. Central serous choroidopathy with exudative retinal detachment. *Ann Ophthalmol* 1982;14:1035.
13. Yanuzzi LA, Shakin JL, Fisher YL, et al. Peripheral retinal detachments and retinal pigment epithelial atrophic tracks secondary to central serous pigment epitheliopathy. *Ophthalmology* 1984;91:1554.
14. Guyer DR. Central serous chorioretinopathy. In: Yannuzzi LA, Flower RW, Slakter JS (eds). *Indocianin green angiography*. St. Louis: Mosby, 1997:297–304.
15. Yoshioka H, Katsume Y, Akune H. Experimental central serous chorioretinopathy in monkey eyes: fluorescein angiographic findings. *Ophthalmologica* 1982;185:168.
16. Gass JD, Little H. Bilateral bullous exudative retinal detachment complicating idiopathic central serous chorioretinopathy during systemic corticosteroid therapy. *Ophthalmology* 1995;102:737–747.
17. Spaide R. Autofluorescence from the outer retina and subretinal space: hypothesis and review. *Retina* 2008;28:5–35.
18. Hee MR, Puliafito CA, Wong C, et al. Optical coherence tomography of central serous chorioretinopathy. *Am J Ophthalmol* 1995;120:65–74.
19. Fujimoto H, Gomi F, Wakabayashi T, et al. Morphologic changes in acute central serous chorioretinopathy evaluated by fourier-domain optical coherence tomography. *Ophthalmology* 2008;115:1494–500.
20. Kon Y, Iida T, Maruko I, et al. The optical coherence tomography-ophthalmoscope for examination of central serous chorioretinopathy with precipitates. *Retina* 2008;28:864–869.
21. Ober MD, Yannuzzi LA, Do DV, et al. Photodynamic therapy for focal retinal pigment epithelial leaks secondary to central serous chorioretinopathy. *Ophthalmology* 2005;112:2088–2094.
22. Yannuzzi LA, Slakter JS, Gross NE, et al. Indocyanine green angiography-guided photodynamic therapy for treatment of chronic central serous chorioretinopathy: a pilot study. *Retina* 2003;23:288–298.
23. Chan WM, Lai TY, Lai RY, et al. Safety enhanced photodynamic therapy for chronic central serous chorioretinopathy: one-year results of a prospective study. *Retina* 2008;28:85–93.
24. Kaiser PK. Antivascular endothelial growth factor agents and their development: therapeutic implications in ocular diseases. *Am J Ophthalmol* 2006;142:660–668.
25. Niegel MF, Schrage NF, Christmann S, et al. Intravitreal bevacizumab for chronic central serous chorioretinopathy. *Ophthalmology* 2008;105:943–945.
26. Torres-Soriano ME, García-Aguirre G, Kon-Jara V, et al. A pilot study of intravitreal bevacizumab for the treatment of central serous chorioretinopathy (case reports). *Graefes Arch Clin Exp Ophthalmol* 2008;246:1235–1239.

# 51

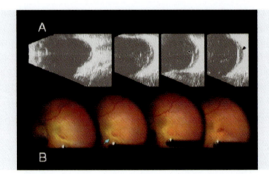

# Pathologic Myopia

Mario Stirpe ■ Guido Ripandelli

High myopia is generally defined as a myopia of −6 diopters or more (with the corresponding axial length usually exceeding 26 mm) (1).

Pathologic myopia on the other hand is defined by posterior chorioretinal changes caused by the excessive elongation of the eye; this condition generally occurs in eyes with an axial length over 28 mm.

It has been observed that after macular hole (MH) formation the retina does not detach in emmetropic eyes while it detaches in myopic eyes. It has been hypothesized that the vitreous cortex plays a role in MH formation in both emmetropic and myopic eyes, while a retinal detachment (RD) in myopic eyes can be related to pigment epithelial atrophy (2,3). Surgical observations in myopic eyes with RD due to MH (RDMH eyes) showed a retinal reattachment after the removal of epiretinal tissue, suggesting another mechanism (4–6). In any case it seems probable that either vitreous tractions or choroidal atrophy may play the prominent role, according to the degree of the myopia (7).

Several factors are involved in the evolution of pathologic myopia and different surgical procedure can be used to repair a RD with MH. In choosing the procedure, vitreous changes, chorioretinal alterations, and the presence of a staphyloma have to be taken into account.

In an histological study on 369 eyes with high myopia, Green and Grossnicklaus found a posterior staphyloma in 33% of the eyes (8). The posterior staphyloma correlated with axial elongation of the eyes, which gives an egg-shaped configuration to the eye. The posterior elongation of eyes in pathologic myopia creates thinning of the posterior sclera, which may be found to be nearly absent during surgery. Posterior chorioretinal degeneration is the most common clinical finding in eyes with pathologic myopia; retinal pigment epithelium atrophy is accompanied by loss of choroid. Green and Grossnicklaus reported a curious form of retinal alteration that they called "stretch schisis." This condition results from retinal vessels that do not lengthen as much as the underlying neurosensory retina, resulting in a schisis-like configuration. The authors did not find evidence that vitreoretinal traction plays a role in the pathogenesis of this condition.

Vitreous changes that are involved in the development of pathological modifications of the posterior retina in myopic eyes include posterior vitreous detachment (PVD) and posterior vitreous schisis (PVS). True PVD is defined as a separation of the posterior vitreous cortex from the internal limiting lamina of the retina. MH that occurs in eyes with high but not excessive myopia during a PVD may be due to incomplete dissection of posterior vitreoretinal adhesions by liquefied vitreous that has penetrated into the retrovitreal space (9). In this situation, the subsequent RD is generally characterized by a wide extension to the periphery especially in the inferior quadrants (10). During biomicroscopical examination of RD with MH associated with PVD, sometimes firm localized vitreoretinal tractions can be observed (Fig. 51-1A), but in many cases there is no evidence of posterior vitreoretinal adhesions (Fig. 51-1B). It is possible that weak remaining posterior adhesions, not necessarily localized to the macular area, can cause anteroposterior traction that is sometimes difficult to see, despite a careful examination by biomicroscopy and ultrasonography. This may explain why selected RDs with MH can be reattached

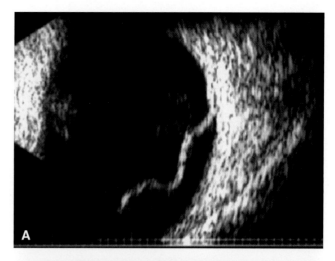

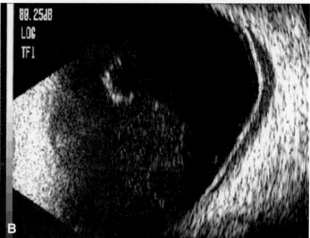

**Figure 51-1. A:** Retinal detachment with macular hole associated with posterior vitreous detachment. B-scan ultrasonography: persistent anteroposterior tractions on the posterior retina. **B:** Retinal detachment with macular hole associated with posterior vitreous detachment. B-scan ultrasonography: no evidence of posterior vitreoretinal tractions.

using an intravitreal gas injection that breaks the remaining vitreoretinal adhesions (11).

PVS is defined as an anomalous form of vitreoretinal separation characterized by a forward displacement of the anterior portion of the posterior vitreous cortex leaving part of the posterior portion of the vitreous cortex still attached to the retina. In eyes with excessive myopia and a pronounced posterior staphyloma, the space just above the posterior staphyloma is frequently the site of vitreous liquefaction, causing PVS.

Tolentino, Schepens, and Freeman clearly described a posterior vitreous lacuna containing liquefied vitreous in high myopic eyes and concluded: "The posterior limit of the lacuna may be absent if liquefaction has involved the entire thickness of the vitreous cortex. In this case, part of the inner surface of the retina then became the posterior wall of the lacuna" (12). After the introduction of optical coherence tomography (OCT) (13) we recognized that when there is a vitreous schisis, a posterior vitreous wall of the lacuna always exists; it is sometimes difficult to detect by biomicroscopic examination,

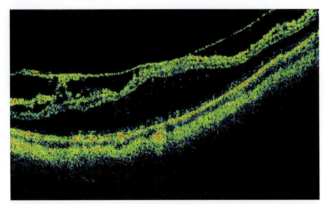

**Figure 51-2.** Optical coherence tomography scans show a shallow retinal detachment with disruption of the neuroretinal layers, consistent with retinoschisis. A hyperreflective band, strictly adherent to the inner retinal surface and exerting tangential tractions, is detected.

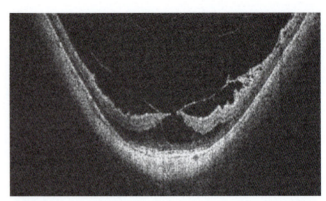

**Figure 51-3.** Optical coherence tomography scans reveal anteroposterior tractions from a hyperreflective band causing disruption of the neuroretinal layers and a partial-thickness macular hole.

due to its thinness and transparency. This layer of vitreous tissue is, in a number of cases, the cause of tangential tractions (Fig. 51-2) causing posterior RD with or without MH and posterior retinoschisis. RD resulting from this change is generally limited to the area of posterior staphyloma and the subretinal fluid is really liquefied vitreous. Sometimes the posterior layer of the vitreous lacuna partially detaches creating anteroposterior traction (Fig. 51-3); occasionally a complete separation can occur.

In a recent study, asymptomatic MH in eyes with very high myopia were reported (14). It was conjectured that the holes, probably due to chorioretinal atrophy, were asymptomatic because they originated at the margin of the fovea. During follow-up, evolution to a posterior RD was observed only in the

cases where a thin layer of epiretinal tissue was previously noted. In few cases the MH became symptomatic because of an enlargement of the MH itself. Based upon this observation, if we accept that in some eyes with high myopia the origin of the MH can be in a parafoveal area, it becomes mandatory to avoid any surgical trauma, which can widen the hole. This aim, using a vitrectomy, is sometimes difficult to achieve: in fact, in myopic eyes with a deep posterior staphyloma, RD is generally limited to the area of the staphyloma, and in order to achieve retinal reattachment, the dense liquefied vitreous has to be removed from the subretinal space. This aspiration is necessarily done through the MH which, due to the density of the subretinal fluid, enlarges, involving more of the fovea (Fig. 51-4). These observations explain the better functional results in eyes

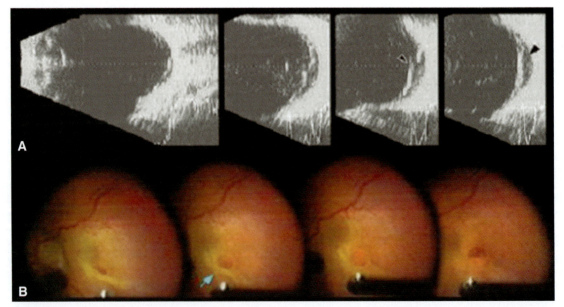

**Figure 51-4. A:** B-scan ultrasonography on four consecutive days shows a posterior retinal detachment with macular hole formation and the passage of liquefied vitreous from the preretinal to the subretinal space through the macular hole. **B:** Vitrectomy for retinal detachment with macular hole repair. The aspiration of the dense subretinal fluid through the macular hole may cause and enlargement of the macular hole involving all the foveal area.

treated with posterior buckle in a randomized comparison of vitrectomy versus posterior episcleral buckling surgery (15).

The surgeon who approaches the surgery for RD with MH repair in high myopic eyes will find that the literature on the choice of the most appropriate surgical technique for different anatomical conditions of these eyes is not conclusive.

Since Gonvers and Machemer's report in 1982 (4), vitrectomy with an eventual internal photocoagulation of the MH and with gas or silicone oil internal tamponade has been the most frequently performed procedure; a pneumoretinopexis is recommended by some surgeons as the primary procedure (11); the posterior episcleral buckle procedure is generally considered difficult and subject to risks because of the anatomical conditions of these eyes.

## SURGICAL OPTIONS

Pneumoretinopexy is preferred in RDMH eyes without a posterior staphyloma in which biomicroscopical and ultrasonographical evaluation shows a PVD and no vitreoretinal connections or epiretinal membranes (11). The procedure is performed with retrobulbar anesthesia. The globe and lids are prepped with povidone iodine. The patient is positioned face down, maintaining unrestricted access to the globe from below. After waiting about 5 minutes to allow the formed vitreous to gravitate to the front of the vitreous cavity, a sterile lid speculum is inserted and liquid vitreous is aspirated in repeated small (0.25 cc.) increments and replaced by injecting a gas bubble in small increments using a 25 or 27 gauge 5/8 inch needle inserted through the inferotemporal conjunctivae, sclera, and pars plana. After the needle is removed, the eye is re-examined to rule out any complications from the procedure and the intraocular pressure is measured and adjusted as needed. A sterile bandage is applied and the patient returns home instructed to maintain a facedown position as much as possible for the next 24 hours.

Vitreoretinal surgery is used when anteroposterior vitreoretinal traction or epiretinal membranes that contribute to the RD are detected. In the former case, the removal of the vitreous that exerts anteroposterior traction with fluid-gas exchange is sufficient to obtain reattachment of the retina. In the latter case, microsurgery is performed to remove the epiretinal membrane: after the vitreous cortex is removed, a bent pick is used to engage the epiretinal membrane. When the margin of the membrane is elevated, the membrane is gently removed from the inner retina by a microforceps. When the membrane detected preoperatively by OCT examination is not identifiable during surgery and the participation of the internal limiting membrane (ILM) is suspected, visualization of the membrane is enhanced by the injection of a few drops of indocyanine green dye (50 mg/mL) in the vitreous cavity after a temporary fluid-gas exchange; the same result can be achieved by a gentle, superficial brushing on the retina included in the staphyloma area by means of the Tano diamond dusted scraper. The subretinal fluid is removed through a peripheral hole with the aid of perfluorocarbon liquid if the detachment extends to the periphery, or through the MH with the aid of fluid-air exchange if the RD is limited to the area of the staphyloma. At the end of the surgery, a fluid-air exchange is performed and gas tamponade or silicone oil is introduced into the vitreous cavity. An eventual laser irritation is performed at the margin of the hole or around the macular area.

## Posterior Buckle Procedure

The presence of prominent posterior staphyloma and the related anatomical changes sometimes limit the success rate of the above surgical procedures:

- Abnormality of vitreoretinal junction sometimes makes it difficult and hazardous to remove the smooth epiretinal tissue from a retina thinner than normal. This results in an incomplete removal of the epiretinal tissue, leaving the retina short in respect to the internal area of the posterior staphyloma.
- The presence of retinal pigment epithelium atrophy interferes with stable reattachment of the neurosensory retina. Laser irritation of the hole does not produce a strong adhesion. The meniscus of a stable internal medium like silicone oil does not effect tamponade on the internal surface of the localized posterior ectasia.
- Removal of the epiretinal tissue does not always produce regression of the retinal schisis, especially if it has been present for some time. Similar problems arise in cases of stretch retinoschisis in which, as noted by Green and Grossniklaus, there is little evidence that vitreoretinal traction plays a role in its pathogenesis.

In these cases, reduction of the posterior staphyloma by means of a posterior buckle is a good option, even though the procedure is sometimes considered difficult because of the excessive globe elongation and hazardous because of choroidal degeneration and scleral thinning. The extreme thinness of the sclera due to axial elongation of eye with excessive myopia may make it impossible to pass the posterior sutures and increases the risk of choroidal hemorrhage.

Different approaches have been used to overcome these difficulties: radial buckles, sylastic sponges fixed along the meridian 12-6 o'clock axis, rubber silicone segments articulated with an elastic silicone band fixed peripherally at 12-6 o'clock, silicone plate containing stainless steel wire. Each procedure can be successful and the choice is based upon the surgeon's experience (15–17).

On the basis of our experience with a large series of RDMH eyes, we currently use the following procedure:

The handle (2 × 2 mm) of a molded hammer-shaped silicon rubber is sutured at the temporal margin of the staphyloma, along the meridian intersecting the fovea; the head (5 × 4 mm) of the silicon rubber is connected with a suture passed through the peripheral sclera at 12 and 6 o'clock and closed nasally. The macular indentation can easily be increased or decreased even in postoperative period as needed to obtain the correct macular buckling (Fig. 51-5A, B, C).

A well set posterior buckle produces reattachment of the retina even in eyes with posterior choroidal atrophy, without the need of adjunctive irritative treatments, and it can cause regression of the posterior retinoschisis (Fig. 51-5D, E). The degree of myopia in these patients is reduced 20% to 90% depending on the indentation.

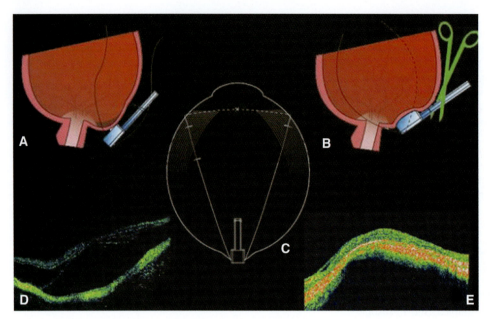

**Figure 51-5. A–C:** Posterior buckle procedure for retinal detachment with macular hole repair. The head of a molded hammer-shaped silicone rubber is held by the handle part on the projection of the macular region. A 5-0 nonreadsorbable suture passed through the peripheral sclera at 12 and 6 o'clock and closed nasally regulates the indentation of the posterior buckle. **D:** Optical coherence tomography scans show a persistent posterior retinal detachment with retinoschisis after vitrectomy. **E:** The posterior buckle allows a reattachment of the neurosensory retina and a regression of the retinoschisis.

## References

1. Curtin BJ. Physiologic versus pathologic myopia. *Ophthalmology* 1979; 86:681–691.
2. Wilkinson CP, Rice TA. Prevention of retinal detachment. In: Wilkinson CP, Rice TA (eds). *Michel's retinal detachment*, 2nd ed. St. Louis, MO: Mosby-Year Book, 1997:1081–1133.
3. Morita H, Ideta H, Ito K, et al. Causative factors of retinal detachment in macular holes. *Retina* 1991;11:281–284.
4. Gonvers M, Machemer R. A new approach to treating retinal detachment with macular hole. *Am J Ophthalmol* 1982;94:468–472.
5. Myake Y. A simplified method of treating retinal detachment with macular hole: a long term follow up. *Arch Ophthalmol* 1986;104:1234–1236.
6. Stirpe M, Michels R. Retinal detachment in high myopic eyes due to macular hole and epiretinal traction. *Retina* 1990;10:113–114.
7. Margherio RR, Schepens CL. Macular breaks, I. Diagnosis, etiology and observations. *Am J Ophtahlmol* 1972;74:219–232.
8. Green WR, Grossnicklaus HE. Histopathologic features of high myopia. In: Midena E (ed). *Myopia and related diseases*. New York: Ophthalmic Communications Society, Inc., 2005:42–53.
9. Sebag J. *The vitreous: structure, function and pathobiology*. New York: Springer-Verlag, 1989.
10. Ripandelli G, Parisi V, Friberg TR, et al. Retinal detachment associated with macular hole in high myopia. Using the vitreous anatomy to optimize the surgical approach. *Ophthalmology* 2004;111:726–731.
11. Blankenship GW, Ibanez-Langlois S. Treatment of myopic macular hole and detachment. *Ophthalmology* 1987;94:333–336.
12. Tolentino FI, Schepens CL, Freeman HM. *Vitreoretinal disorders. Diagnosis and management*. Philadelphia, PA: WB Saunders, 1976:284–287.
13. Puliafito CA, Hee MR, Lin CP, et al. Imaging of macular diseases with optical coherence tomography. *Ophthalmology* 1995;113:325–332.
14. Coppé AM, Ripandelli G, Parisi V, et al. Prevalence of asymptomatic macular holes in highly myopic eyes. *Ophthalmology* 2005;112:2103–2109.
15. Ripandelli G, Fedeli R, et al. Evaluation of primary surgical procedures for retinal detachment with macular hole in highly myopic eyes. A randomized comparison of vitrectomy versus posterior episcleral buckling surgery. *Ophthalmology* 2001;108:2258–2265.
16. Ando F. Use of a special macular explant in surgery for retinal detachment with macular hole. *Jpn J Ophthalmol* 1980;24:29–34.
17. Theodossiadis GP, Theodossiadis PG. The macular buckling procedure in the treatment of retinal detachment in highly myopic eyes with macular hole and posterior staphyloma. *Retina* 2005;25(3):285–289.

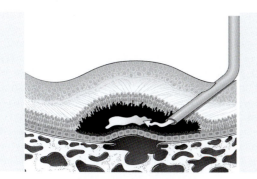

# Submacular Hemorrhage

Rishi P. Singh ■ Hilel Lewis

## INTRODUCTION

Submacular hemorrhage is a common consequence of choroidal neovascularization (CNV) in patients with age-related macular degeneration (AMD) (Figure 52-1A, 52-1B). It also can be seen secondary to retinal arterial macroaneurysm, trauma, retinopathy resulting from Valsalva's maneuver and leukemia, and CNV from other causes including presumed ocular histoplasmosis syndrome and high myopia. Observational studies on the natural history of submacular hemorrhage show variable results depending on the underlying cause. Patients with submacular hemorrhage from AMD may develop severe loss of vision, especially if the center of the fovea is involved (1–4). However, submacular hemorrhage from trauma or macroaneurysm may resolve with much less damage to the photoreceptors and retinal pigment epithelium (RPE) (1).

Traditionally, these patients were observed, because precise localization of choroidal neovascular membranes for laser treatment or photodynamic therapy was not possible and other treatment modalities were not available. Recent advances in both submacular surgical techniques and intravitreal anti-vascular endothelial growth factor agents (anti-VEGF) have increased interest in surgical treatment of such patients. Clinical and histopathologic studies published to date do support recommendations regarding surgery and specific interventions for submacular hemorrhage. Although some patients with submacular hemorrhage may benefit from surgical evacuation, the ideal characteristics for good surgical outcomes have not been studied in a randomized large multicenter trial. General guidelines for management can be formulated through our current understandings of histopathological studies and small case series of eyes with submacular hemorrhage.

## HISTOLOGY AND PATHOPHYSIOLOGY

How does submacular hemorrhage cause retinal damage? There are a variety of theories that have been formulated based on histological examination of submacular hemorrhage in animal models. It is likely a combination in factors which leads to retinal damage after submacular hemorrhage. First, toxicity may occur resulting from iron released from hemoglobin (5). Second, the blood may act as a barrier, impairing metabolic exchange between the photoreceptors and RPE. Finally, fibrin-mediated mechanical damage to the outer retina may occur because of clot contraction (6,7).

Glatt and Machemer (5) demonstrated irreversible damage to the photoreceptors within 24 hours after introduction of subretinal blood in a rabbit model and outer retinal degeneration within 3 to 7 days. Toth et al. (7) looked at the early events associated with subretinal hemorrhage in a cat model. The most striking finding in their study was the rapid formation of a fibrin clot interdigitating between the photoreceptor outer segments. This was seen within the first hour of introduction of subretinal hemorrhage. Mechanical shearing of the photoreceptors resulting from traction of fibrin strands followed. The most severe retinal degeneration occurred over the ensuing 3 to 14 days and was found over the areas of dense fibrin coagulum, as opposed to the areas of dense erythrocytes. The authors proposed that fibrin and perhaps other inflammatory products are responsible for the retinal damage rather than iron toxicity or the presence of erythrocytes as a barrier to diffusion. If tissue plasminogen activator (t-PA), a clot-specific fibrinolytic agent, was injected into the subretinal space along with the blood, mechanical shearing of the photoreceptors was not seen. This confirmed the initial observation by Lewis and coauthors that fibrinolytic therapy may be a useful adjunct to surgical removal of subretinal hemorrhage (6).

Lewis et al. (6) also studied the effect of recombinant t-PA on experimental subretinal hemorrhage in rabbits. Subretinal hemorrhage created by injection of blood alone was compared with simultaneous injection of blood and t-PA or blood and balanced salt solution (BSS). Clearance of subretinal hemorrhage was significantly faster in eyes given t-PA than in those given BSS or blood alone. Additionally, eyes receiving t-PA or BSS sustained less degenerative change in retinal appearance and retained larger numbers of well-organized retinal outer segments than those receiving blood alone. It is

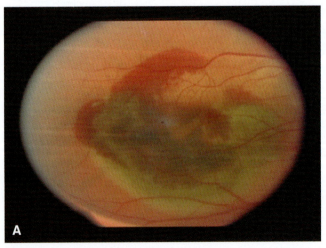
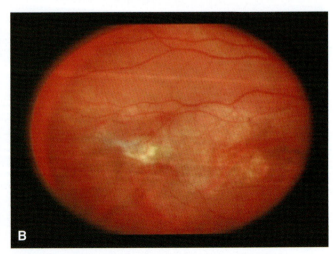

**Figure 52-1. A:** Preoperative photo demonstrating submacular hemorrhage due to age-related macular degeneration. Visual acuity count fingers at 3 feet. **B:** Postoperative photo with complete resolution of submacular hemorrhage, localized atrophy, and subretinal fibrosis. Visual acuity is 20/400.

postulated that this beneficial effect of both t-PA and BSS may be caused by dilution of toxic factors released by lysed blood cells, as well as a reduction in metabolic barrier from clot in the subretinal space.

Terasaki et al. (8) evaluated the changes in preoperative versus postoperative focal macular electroretinography in five patients undergoing surgical drainage of submacular hemorrhages. Preoperative electroretinographic response was reduced remarkably or was unrecordable in all eyes. Postoperative electroretinographic responses, recorded between 1 and 4 months after surgery, recovered to about one half of the amplitude of the normal fellow eye. These findings showed that the severe retinal dysfunction associated with submacular hemorrhage can be reversed at least partially with surgical intervention (8).

## NATURAL HISTORY

Observational studies in humans have shown a wide variability in the natural course of subretinal hemorrhage (Table 52-1A, 52-1B). The largest series to date reviewed by Scupola et al. (4) examined sixty eyes with submacular hemorrhage due to AMD. In this retrospective series, vision deteriorated in 80% of patients with a mean initial acuity of 20/240 and a mean final acuity of 20/1250 at 24 months follow-up. Worse visual outcome was correlated with larger initial hemorrhage size and greater initial retinal thickness. The natural dissolution of hemorrhage varied from 2 to 18 months and recurrent bleeding occurred in 38% of eyes. At the end of the study, 25% had atrophic scars, 38% had subretinal fibrosis, and 22% had RPE tears (4).

Bennett et al. (1) highlighted the variable outcome of submacular hemorrhage from causes other than AMD. In this study, 29 patients with subretinal hemorrhages greater than one disc diameter involving the center of the fovea were included. The cause of hemorrhages in this study included (listed in descending order of frequency) choroidal neovascular membranes associated with AMD, ruptured retinal arterial macroaneurysms, traumatic choroidal rupture, choroidal neovascular membranes associated with presumed ocular histoplasmosis syndrome and pseudoxanthoma elasticum, and complications of scleral buckling surgery. Initial visual acuities varied widely, from 20/70 to light perception (average 20/860). Final visual acuities with a mean follow-up of 3 years also varied widely, from 20/30 to light perception (average 20/480). The most important predictor of poor visual outcome was the presence of AMD. The average final visual acuity in patients with AMD was 20/1700, and none of these patients had a final visual acuity better than 20/200. Patients with submacular hemorrhage associated with other causes of choroidal neovascular membranes also had poor outcomes, with the exception of one patient with presumed ocular histoplasmosis syndrome whose visual acuity improved from 20/200 to 20/30. The patients with the best outcomes in this series were those with subretinal hemorrhages from traumatic choroidal rupture. This may be explained partly by the fact that, on average, patients with hemorrhages from choroidal rupture had better initial visual acuity than patients with AMD, and all of the traumatic hemorrhages were classified as thin (1).

Berrocal et al. (3) reviewed fundus photographs and medical records of 31 patients with subretinal hemorrhage involving the entire foveal avascular zone. The majority of hemorrhages were associated with AMD. In the remaining eyes, hemorrhages were secondary to retinal arterial macroaneurysms, presumed ocular histoplasmosis syndrome, trauma, and retinopathy resulting from Valsalva's maneuver, idiopathic central serous choroidopathy, central retinal vein occlusion, and CNV associated with choroidal rupture. The mean time to

## TABLE 52-1   COMPARISON OF NATURAL-HISTORY STUDIES AND SURGICAL STUDIES

| Author | Date | Cause | Average Initial Visual Acuity | Percentage >20/100 | Percentage Improving | Follow-Up Months |
|---|---|---|---|---|---|---|
| Natural-history studies | | | | | | |
| Bennett et al. (1) | January 1990 | AMD | 20/1300 | 0 | 33 | 38 |
| | | Other | 20/650 | 47 | 71 | 36 |
| Berrocal et al. (6) | October 1996 | AMD | 20/200 | 30 | 45 | 29 |
| | | Other | 20/200 | 55 | 63 | 29 |
| Avery et al. (7) | 1996 | AMD | 20/125 | 26 | 21 | — |
| Surgical studies | | | | | | |
| Lewis (14) | November 1994 | AMD | 20/5600 | 17 | 83 | 14 |
| Ibanez et al. (19) | January 1995 | AMD | 20/1800 | 8 | 38 | 40 |
| | | Other | 20/3000 | 63 | 100 | 38 |
| Lim et al. (20) | September 1995 | AMD | 20/1200 | 6 | 19 | 10 |
| | | Other | 20/1000 | 0 | 50 | 16 |
| Kamei et al. (15) | March 1996 | AMD | 20/2200 | 45 | 86 | 7 |
| Humayun et al. (18) | September 1998 | Macroaneurysm | 20/700 | 89 | 100 | 18 |

*Note*: AMD, age-related macular degeneration.

clearance of all subretinal hemorrhages was 7 months (range 2 months to 24 months). Initial and final visual acuities in this study were significantly better than in Bennett's study. Final visual acuity was 20/80 or better in 19% of the patients with AMD. The size or thickness of the hemorrhage was not predictive of final visual outcome in this study. Again, patients with submacular hemorrhages from other causes faired better than those with AMD (3).

Avery et al. (2) examined only patients with AMD and subretinal hemorrhages extending beneath the center of the fovea resulting from choroidal neovascular membranes. At 36 months, 44% lost six or more lines, 22% lost two to five lines, 12% retained vision within one line, and 21% had maintained spontaneous improvement of two or more lines. Their analyses suggested that eyes with large hemorrhages or moderate to marked retinal elevation have poorer visual prognosis. This series again confirmed the poor natural visual outcomes in patients with submacular hemorrhage secondary to AMD (2).

These reports, although useful, do not provide us with accurate information on the natural history of submacular hemorrhage because they only included a small number of patients, the follow-up was limited, and the studies were retrospective. From the limited information to date, it is likely that eyes with very large or thick hemorrhages beneath the fovea, the location of the hemorrhage with respect to being above or below the RPE, the length of time the hemorrhage has been present, and any associated abnormalities of the retina or RPE are likely to have poorer prognoses (1,3). Further, most patients with submacular hemorrhages associated with CNV (particularly in AMD) have a poorer visual outcome. Several factors may account for the apparently worse visual prognosis for patients with submacular hemorrhage in AMD. Some authors have proposed that diffuse preexisting abnormalities involving Bruch's membrane, the RPE, and the retina may limit the metabolic reserves of these tissues and result in diminished ability to tolerate the presence of subretinal hemorrhage (9). The scarring process of CNV also plays a role in retinal damage in these eyes.

The most recent report of the Submacular Surgery Trials (SST) evaluating surgery for hemorrhagic choroidal neovascular lesions for AMD gives also helpful insight into the natural history by examining the nontreatment arm. In this randomized, prospective, multicenter clinical trial, patients were randomized to surgical removal versus observation. Patients had predominately hemorrhagic subfoveal lesions in which at least 50% of the choroidal neovascular lesion was occupied by thick blood. Eligible lesions were between 3.5 disc areas and 9 disc areas and median initial acuity was 20/200. The final median acuity at 36 months was 20/640 with 44% of eyes maintaining or improving acuity over the length of the study (10). However, it should be noted that patients within the SST need not have subfoveal hemorrhage in order to be enrolled within the trial, rather that they just needed subfoveal CNV.

## SURGICAL MANAGEMENT

For thin localized subretinal hemorrhages due to AMD, intravitreal anti-VEGF agents may be suitable therapy. However, there are currently no medical treatments for thick larger submacular hemorrhages and the only alternative to observation is surgery. With recent improvements in vitreoretinal surgical techniques and instrumentation, surgical displacement or removal of submacular hemorrhage is possible.

## INITIAL SURGICAL APPROACHES

Surgical techniques for the removal of submacular hemorrhage have significantly evolved over the past 10 years. The earliest attempts to drain large submacular hemorrhages used a transscleral approach. In 1983, Dellaporta described passing an endodiathermy probe through the sclera, choroid, and retina, allowing the blood to pass into the retroscleral space and also into the vitreous cavity. Lasers also have been used to create retinotomies, allowing blood to spill into the vitreous cavity (11,12). Hanscom and Diddie first used vitrectomy with internal retinotomy, endodrainage, and air-fluid exchange in the management of submacular hemorrhage (13). Several others also adopted this approach. With it, large access retinotomies were required, which were associated frequently with postoperative retinal detachment and proliferative vitreoretinopathy (14,15). Additionally, mechanical clot extraction usually was required, which could result in damage to photoreceptors or the RPE at the time of removal.

## VITRECTOMY WITH DISPLACEMENT UTILIZING TISSUE-PLASMINOGEN ACTIVATOR

Modern vitrectomy techniques now utilize recombinant t-PA to lyse the fibrin within the clot, prior to removal of the liquefied blood. t-PA converts fibrin-bound plasminogen to plasmin, thereby producing clot lysis. The toxicity of arginine (used as a carrier for t-PA) to the retina and RPE has been established in numerous studies (16,17). A 48 $\mu$g dose of t-PA is sufficient in most cases to engulf the subretinal clots. This dose is below the rabbit and cat studies which have shown dose dependent toxicities at concentrations greater than or equal to 50 $\mu$g (6,17,18). Retinal toxicity from t-PA is thought to be due to the vehicle manifests as diffuse pigmentary alterations sparing the posterior pole, poor visual acuity after the absorption of submacular hemorrhage, and reduced scotopic and photopic electroretinogram (ERG) A and B-waves. This toxicity has been seen in humans between 50 to 100 $\mu$g.

The current indications for surgical evacuation of submacular hemorrhage are based on the results of pilot studies (19,20). In general, surgery should be considered in patients with good vision before the hemorrhage occurred (those with CNV of long duration prior to the hemorrhage are unlikely to benefit from surgery); patients with duration of hemorrhage less than 14 days; patients with hemorrhage more than 500 $\mu$m thick beneath the center of the foveal avascular zone and greater than 3.5 Macular Photocoagulation Study disc

**TABLE 52-2   TISSUE PLASMINOGEN ACTIVATOR FOR SUBMACULAR HEMORRHAGE 1998 UPDATE (N = 42, FOLLOW-UP = 10 MO)**

**Duration:** 69 eyes, ≤7 d
23 eyes, 8–14 d

| Final Visual Acuity[a] | Eyes | % |
| --- | --- | --- |
| 20/40 | 1 | 1 |
| 20/50–20/100 | 12 | 13 |
| 20/125–20/200 | 38 | 42 |
| 20/400–5/200 | 29 | 32 |
| Count fingers | 6 | 7 |
| Hand motion | 4 | 4 |
| Light perception | 2 | 2 |

Note: In 69 eyes, duration was less than 7 days. In 23 eyes, duration was between 8 and 14 days.
[a]Final visual acuity improved by more than two lines in 71 eyes (78%), and worsened by more than two lines in 4 eyes (4%).

diameters in size; hemorrhage posterior to the midpoint between the temporal arcades and the equator, and patients without hemorrhage beneath the RPE (Table 52-2).

The current technique for surgical removal of submacular hemorrhage is as follows (Figure 52-2A, 52-2B, 52-2C). A standard three-port pars plana vitrectomy is performed with the induction of a posterior vitreous detachment. The intraocular pressure is increased to cause central retinal artery occlusion. A specially designed, sharp, bent, 36-gauge spatula is used to enter the subretinal space and create a tunnel between the RPE and the outer retina. If the hemorrhage is limited to the macular region or posterior pole, a 130-degree bent spatula is used. If the subretinal hemorrhage is more extensive, however, reaching the equator or more anteriorly, a 90-degree bent spatula is used to prevent damage to the retina from the heel of the instrument. A 33-gauge bent cannula then is placed through the retinotomy, and recombinant t-PA is injected into the subretinal clot. We use a concentration of 12.5 μg per 0.1 ml of BSS, but this concentration also depends on the size and volume of the clot. Care is taken to inject directly into the clot rather than between the clot and the RPE or between the clot and the outer retina. This is to avoid damage to the RPE or outer retina from the injection. Enough t-PA solution is injected to bathe the entire subretinal clot, up to 50 μg. The intraocular pressure then is lowered gradually to normal levels. Diathermy or endophotocoagulation of the access retinotomy is not necessary given the size and location.

In initial studies, a 45- to 60-minute intraoperative clot lysis was necessary followed by the injection/aspiration of BSS into the subretinal space. However, a recent modification of the technique has shown that this intraoperative waiting period is unnecessary. Instead, a partial air fluid exchange is performed and approximately 70% of the vitreous cavity is filled with air. The patients are taken to the recovery room in the supine position for 1 hour and then the patients are

positioned upright or on their side for 24 hours. A neck collar can assist in the proper upright positioning.

With this method, mechanical clot extraction is unnecessary and inadvertent retinal damage can be avoided (19). It is not necessary to remove all of the hemorrhage if the area beneath the fovea is clear. If hemorrhage remains beneath the fovea, perfluorocarbon liquid may be utilized to displace it away from the fovea or through the retinotomy into the vitreous cavity (referred to as the steamroller technique).

## PNEUMATIC DISPLACEMENT WITHOUT VITRECTOMY

Hassan et al. first published papers with a series of patients treated with intravitreal t-PA (0.1 to 0.2 ml of t-PA; total dose 25 to 100 μg), expansile gas, and prone positioning for 1 to 5 days (21). Numerous series have followed demonstrating some benefit to this procedure (22). However, experimental evidence suggests that t-PA injected into the vitreous space does not cross the sensory retina and does not reach the subretinal space (23). Furthermore, previous animal work demonstrated that submacular hemorrhage clot interdigitates between the photoreceptor outer segments. If the clot is not fully liquefied and the gas is applied, potentially more photoreceptors are likely to be damaged with this procedure.

## SURGICAL RESULTS

Although several series on surgical removal of submacular hemorrhage have been published, it is difficult to directly compare their results because of marked variability in patient selection, surgical techniques employed, length of follow-up, and methods of assessing visual outcome (19,20,24–28). Despite these shortcomings, a comparison of the surgical studies and the natural history studies with regard to initial visual acuity, percentage of eyes with final visual acuity greater than 20/100, percentage of eyes with improvement in final visual acuity, and length of follow-up was performed (Table 52-1A, 52-1B). In all published reports, visual outcomes were worst for patients who underwent submacular surgery for hemorrhage secondary to AMD than for other causes. This may be in part because, as shown by Gass, the CNV and hemorrhage in AMD often are found beneath the RPE, and only secondarily break through into the subretinal space (29).

The percentage of patients with AMD who had an improvement in final visual acuity after surgery varied widely from 19% to 86% (average of 58%). Studies of the natural history of submacular hemorrhage secondary to AMD reported that 21% to 45% of patients had an improvement in visual acuity (average 33%). We must be careful, however, not to interpret these as results as showing the benefits of submacular surgery because these studies are not comparable.

We recently summarized our results which included 34 eyes with subretinal hemorrhage secondary to AMD in patients who underwent surgical drainage using t-PA with no intraoperative clot lysis time. Complete postoperative displacement of

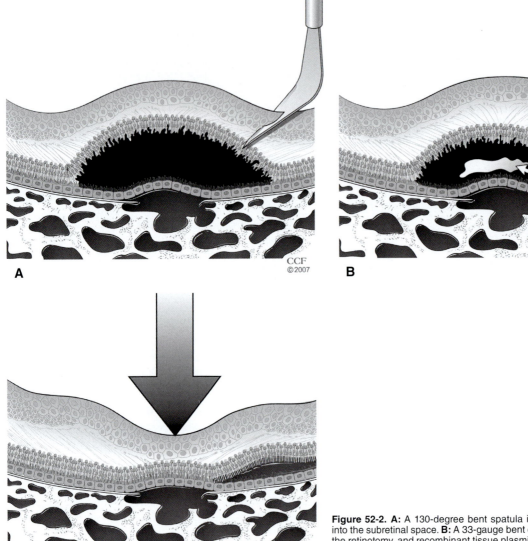

**Figure 52-2. A:** A 130-degree bent spatula is used to create a retinotomy into the subretinal space. **B:** A 33-gauge bent cannula is then placed through the retinotomy, and recombinant tissue plasminogen activator is injected into the subretinal clot. **C:** The hemorrhage is displaced with the intraocular air bubble.

blood from the fovea was achieved in 50% of patients. Final visual acuity improved by two or more lines in 64% and the visual acuity improved by six lines in 29%, and worsened by two or more lines in 21%. Stabilization or improvement in visual acuity was obtained in 85% at 3 months, 77% at 6 months, and 75% at 12 months.

Surgical results for submacular hemorrhage secondary to other causes may be more favorable. Humayun et al. reported a series of nine patients with submacular hemorrhage resulting from ruptured retinal arterial macroaneurysms treated with tissue plasminogen-assisted subretinal hemorrhage removal (24). Initial visual acuities varied from 20/200 to 1/200 (average 20/700). Final visual acuity improved in all nine eyes, and mean final visual acuity was 20/40. These findings suggest that tissue plasminogen-assisted subretinal hemorrhage removal should be considered for selected patients with submacular hemorrhage secondary to retinal arterial macroaneurysms.

The only comparative study of large submacular displacement with t-PA versus submacular membrane removal alone was studied by Thompson et al. The study only evaluated large hemorrhages greater than 12 disc areas. In this retrospective study, the mean acuity in the submacular surgery arm improved from 20/1000 to 20/640 at 1 year. The mean acuity in the submacular displacement arm deteriorated from 20/500 preoperatively to 20/1000 postoperatively. Visual acuity improved by three lines in 48% of the submacular surgery arm versus 13% in the submacular displacement arm at 1 year. The authors concluded that submacular surgery results in better visual outcomes as compared to submacular displacement with t-PA at least in patients with large submacular hemorrhages (30).

## COMPLICATIONS OF SUBMACULAR SURGERY

Submacular surgery may be associated with intraoperative and postoperative complications. These include retinal tears, retinal detachment, vitreous hemorrhage, proliferative vitreoretinopathy, epiretinal membrane, macular hole, cataract, recurrent subretinal hemorrhage formation, and rarely choroidal neovascular membranes at the retinotomy site (13,15, 26,31). Thus, it is important to assess whether any visual improvements surgery may offer are significant enough to outweigh these and other possible surgical risks.

## SUMMARY

Submacular hemorrhage often leads to devastating loss of vision and can present a significant clinical challenge. Factors that may influence outcome in eyes with submacular hemorrhage include the duration, size, thickness, and location of the subretinal hemorrhage, as well as the underlying condition responsible for the hemorrhage. The natural history of eyes with submacular hemorrhage is often poor. In patients with submacular hemorrhage due to causes other than AMD, visual outcome after submacular surgery may be good. Eyes with submacular hemorrhage secondary to AMD appear to have the worst prognosis with or without surgical intervention, although, surgical removal of subretinal hemorrhage may be beneficial in selected cases.

Inferences on the surgical indications for submacular hemorrhage can be made based on studies published to date. This review indicates that surgery should be reserved for those eyes with good vision prior to the hemorrhage and large thick subfoveal hemorrhage of less than 7 to 10 days' duration. Surgical removal is not indicated for submacular hemorrhage that does not extend beneath the center of the fovea. Advances in surgical technique, new instrumentation, and adjuvants such as t-PA and perfluorocarbon liquids have led to improvements in submacular surgery and visual outcome in this challenging disorder.

## References

1. Bennett SR, Folk JC, Blodi CF, et al. Factors prognostic of visual outcome in patients with subretinal hemorrhage. *Am J Ophthalmol* 1990;109:33–37.
2. Avery RL, Fekrat S, Hawkins BS, et al. Natural history of subfoveal subretinal hemorrhage in age-related macular degeneration. *Retina* 1996;16:183–189.
3. Berrocal MH, Lewis ML, Flynn HW Jr. Variations in the clinical course of submacular hemorrhage. *Am J Ophthalmol* 1996;122:486–493.
4. Scupola A, Coscas G, Soubrane G, et al. Natural history of macular subretinal hemorrhage in age-related macular degeneration. *Ophthalmologica* 1999;213:97–102.
5. Glatt H, Machemer R. Experimental subretinal hemorrhage in rabbits. *Am J Ophthalmol* 1982;94:762–773.
6. Lewis H, Resnick SC, Flannery JG, et al. Tissue plasminogen activator treatment of experimental subretinal hemorrhage. *Am J Ophthalmol* 1991; 111:197–204.
7. Toth CA, Morse LS, Hjelmeland LM, et al. Fibrin directs early retinal damage after experimental subretinal hemorrhage. *Arch Ophthalmol* 1991;109: 723–729.
8. Terasaki H, Miyake Y, Kondo M, et al. Focal macular electroretinogram before and after drainage of macular subretinal hemorrhage. *Am J Ophthalmol* 1997;123:207–211.

9. Williams DF, Thomas MA. Vitrectomy for removal of submacular hemorrhage. In: Craven (ed). *Retina*, 2nd ed, vol 3. St. Louis: Mosby, 1994:2557–2559.
10. Bressler NM, Bressler SB, Childs AL, et al. Surgery for hemorrhagic choroidal neovascular lesions of age-related macular degeneration: Ophthalmic findings: SST report no. 13. *Ophthalmology* 2004;111:1993–2006.
11. Dellaporta AN. Evacuation of subretinal hemorrhage. *Int Ophthalmol* 1994;18:25–31.
12. Dellaporta A. Retinal damage from subretinal hemorrhage. *Am J Ophthalmol* 1983;95:568–570.
13. Hanscom TA, Diddie KR. Early surgical drainage of macular subretinal hemorrhage. *Arch Ophthalmol* 1987;105:1722–1723.
14. de Juan E Jr, Machemer R. Vitreous surgery for hemorrhagic and fibrous complications of age-related macular degeneration. *Am J Ophthalmol* 1988;105:25–29.
15. Wade EC, Flynn HW Jr, Olsen KR, et al. Subretinal hemorrhage management by pars plana vitrectomy and internal drainage. *Arch Ophthalmol* 1990; 108:973–978.
16. Benner JD, Morse LS, Toth CA, et al. Evaluation of a commercial recombinant tissue-type plasminogen activator preparation in the subretinal space of the cat. *Arch Ophthalmol* 1991;109:1731–1736.
17. Johnson MW, Olsen KR, Hernandez E, et al. Retinal toxicity of recombinant tissue plasminogen activator in the rabbit. *Arch Ophthalmol* 1990;108:259–263.
18. Hrach CJ, Johnson MW, Hassan AS, et al. Retinal toxicity of commercial intravitreal tissue plasminogen activator solution in cat eyes. *Arch Ophthalmol* 2000;118:659–663.
19. Lewis H. Intraoperative fibrinolysis of submacular hemorrhage with tissue plasminogen activator and surgical drainage. *Am J Ophthalmol* 1994;118: 559–568.
20. Singh RP, Patel C, Sears JE. Management of subretinal macular hemorrhage by direct administration of tissue plasminogen activator. *Br J Ophthalmol* 2006;90:429–431.
21. Hassan AS, Johnson MW, Schneiderman TE, et al. Management of submacular hemorrhage with intravitreous tissue plasminogen activator injection and pneumatic displacement. *Ophthalmology* 1999;106:1900–1906; discussion 1906–1907.
22. Chen CY, Hooper C, Chiu D, et al. Management of submacular hemorrhage with intravitreal injection of tissue plasminogen activator and expansile gas. *Retina* 2007;27:321–328.
23. Kamei M, Misono K, Lewis H. A study of the ability of tissue plasminogen activator to diffuse into the subretinal space after intravitreal injection in rabbits. *Am J Ophthalmol* 1999;128:739–746.
24. Humayun M, Lewis H, Flynn HW Jr, et al. Management of submacular hemorrhage associated with retinal arterial macroaneurysms. *Am J Ophthalmol* 1998;126:358–361.
25. Kamei M, Tano Y, Maeno T, et al. Surgical removal of submacular hemorrhage using tissue plasminogen activator and perfluorocarbon liquid. *Am J Ophthalmol* 1996;121:267–275.
26. Ibanez HE, Williams DF, Thomas MA, et al. Surgical management of submacular hemorrhage. A series of 47 consecutive cases. *Arch Ophthalmol* 1995;113:62–69.
27. Lim JI, Drews-Botsch C, Sternberg P Jr, et al. Submacular hemorrhage removal. *Ophthalmology* 1995;102:1393–1399.
28. Olivier S, Chow DR, Packo KH, et al. Subretinal recombinant tissue plasminogen activator injection and pneumatic displacement of thick submacular hemorrhage in age-related macular degeneration. *Ophthalmology* 2004;111: 1201–1208.
29. Gass JD. Biomicroscopic and histopathologic considerations regarding the feasibility of surgical excision of subfoveal neovascular membranes. *Am J Ophthalmol* 1994;118:285–298.
30. Thompson JT, Sjaarda RN. Vitrectomy for the treatment of submacular hemorrhages from macular degeneration: A comparison of submacular hemorrhage/membrane removal and submacular tissue plasminogen activator-assisted pneumatic displacement. *Trans Am Ophthalmol Soc* 2005;103:98–107; discussion 107.
31. de Juan E Jr, Loewenstein A, Bressler NM, et al. Translocation of the retina for management of subfoveal choroidal neovascularization II: A preliminary report in humans. *Am J Ophthalmol* 1998;125:635–646.

eleven

# Prevention and Treatment of Complications

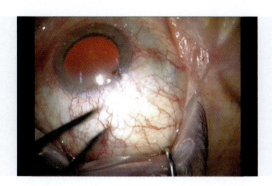

# Complications of Pharmacotherapy

Matteo Forlini ■ Gian Maria Cavallini ■ Luca Campi
Virgilio  Morales-Canton ■ Paolo Rossini ■ Adriana Bratu
Cesare Forlini ■ Giuseppe Di Stefano

## INTRODUCTION

Pharmacological therapy of ocular diseases comprises a vast variety of drug classes available for use in treating the many different pathological situations, including antibiotics and antivirals, fibrinolytic molecules (t-PA), new generation antiedema drugs (Triamcinolone acetonide (TA)) and anti-vascular endothelial growth factor (anti-VEGF) agents for the treatment of neovascular and exudative diseases of the retina. All of these drugs are currently used in clinical practice and/or as support to surgery.

The first attempts at intravitreal injections were performed in the early 1900s to treat retinal detachment. Since then, intravitreal injections as treatment for eye disease have progressed significantly (injections of antibiotics, silicon oil, antiviral agents, methotrexate, t-PA, hyaluronidase, corticosteroids, through to the more recent anti-VEGF agents) over the years.

In addition to their undisputed beneficial effects and certain usefulness in resolving even very severe pathological situations, all the drugs used in local eye therapy present a range of side effects and complications on account of the administration route and method, and adverse effects that sometimes trigger pathological reactions and situations, equally or even more severe than the original pathological condition.

The introduction of pharmacological therapy in maculopathy treatment dates from the late 1970s, with the use of intravitreal steroids (triamcinolone and dexamethasone) to treat exudative and neovascular maculopathies.

Since 2001, the use of TA has become increasingly efficacious as a drug with a potent anti-inflammatory and antiedema action for the treatment of exudative diabetic maculopathy, age-related macular degeneration (AMD), and postsurgical and inflammatory (autoimmune and idiopathic) maculopathy.

As of 2004, a new class of anti-VEGF drugs started to become commonly used to treat exudative maculopathy and all forms of intraocular neovascularization (proliferative diabetic retinopathy, neovascular glaucoma, retinopathy of prematurity (ROP), autoimmune diseases, etc.).

Periocular and intraocular injection preparations have been used in clinical practice for many years.

Several molecules are useful for the treatment of the many different ocular conditions by subconjunctival, subtenon, and intravitreal injection.

Molecules, injection techniques, and standard procedures are constantly upgraded. However, differences persist in certain parameters, so that while in Europe, these injections are performed in sterile conditions in the theatre, in the USA and other American countries, intravitreal injections are performed in the surgery in a nonsterile environment.

The drugs used for intraocular or periocular applications can have local and systemic side effects and complications.

These events may be caused by the active substance, administration method and route, the surgeon's skill, the preparation of drug, surrounding conditions (sterility) and/or self-administration in the postoperative period.

The complications associated to the use of intravitreal drugs can be divided into two groups: 1) those consequential to the injection technique and 2) those caused by the pharmacological effects of the molecules, which can in turn be either systemic or ocular.

## TECHNIQUE-RELATED COMPLICATIONS

### Subconjunctival-Subtenon Drugs

Some drugs, such as antidiabetic, antiviral, and anti-inflammatory agents, can be administered by the subconjunctival or subtenon routes, which, despite not being complication free, are rarely associated with adverse events during the operative or immediate or late postoperative periods.

The subconjunctival route entails the injection of a drug into the conjunctival stroma; it is not necessary to cut the conjunctiva and topical anesthesia is usually used.

The most common complications are slight, such as corneal abrasions, subconjunctival hemorrhage, the sensation of swelling or presence of a foreign body, and transient conjunctival hyperemia associated with slight irritation.

After injection, the medication passes into vitreous chamber from the subconjunctival space by means of diastatic sclerotomy, even when the mini-invasive sutureless surgery technique is used (1).

For certain classes of aminoglycoside antibiotics (gentamicin), this is associated to a high risk of intravitreal toxicity, such as retinal ischemia and edema, reduction in the amplitude of the electroretinogram (ERG) b-wave caused by photoreceptor necrosis and macular hemorrhage, with poor functional prognosis.

The subtenon technique entails opening a small conjunctival buttonhole and the underlying tenonian capsule, in which the blunt needle is inserted and pushed backwards.

Technique-related complications are usually mild and similar to those of the subconjunctival technique. However, after anti-inflammatory and antiviral drug use, the risk of infection is higher (2–5).

The risk of scleral perforation is low, whereas the drug can have serious consequences, such as lid ptosis and orbital fat prolapse (6), local subconjunctival abscess and ocular hypertension.

This technique can be performed using topical anesthesia and some patients may feel pain.

Subconjunctival injection of lidocaine can reduce the risk of pain during the transscleral injection; however, discomfort may be experienced when the subconjunctival injection is made.

Some patients may experience substantial subconjunctival hemorrhage, which resolves in one to two weeks without consequences.

### Intravitreal Injection

The use of intravitreal drugs exposes the patient to complications connected to technical risk.

The injection technique is fairly standard and generally consists of a dose of 0.05 ml (for anti-VEGF) to 0.1 ml (for TA) of the agent, except for gas injection, where the dose is higher.

It is performed using a 25-, 27-, or 30-gauge needle, via the transconjunctival route 2 to 5 mm (standard average is 3–3.5–4 mm) from the limbus, depending on whether one is in the presence of a pseudophakic or phakic condition. Although there are no preferential injection quadrants, some practitioners prefer to avoid the lower quadrant, where more germs accumulate, in order to avoid the risk of intravitreal inoculation and consequent inflammation.

Injection can be either direct or performed through a small scleral tunnel incision. The aim of this second technique is to reduce the risk of leakage of the drug and/or vitreal gel into the subconjunctival space.

The conjunctiva can be moved 2 mm from the injection site, to avoid the conjunctival hole from coinciding with the scleral hole, in order to prevent direct contact with the external environment. There are a number of potential injection complications, ranging in severity from very bland to extremely serious.

The subconjunctival hemorrhage is undoubtedly the most frequent of these and although it is usually generally slight and self-limiting, it can be more substantial and a cause of concern to the patient; however, the situation normally resolves spontaneously within a few days.

The ocular surface can be interested by the intravitreal injection technique, as the needle may accidentally touch the cornea causing abrasion; this resolves spontaneously within a few hours when correct therapy is administered.

The potential complications of injection via the pars plana route include touching of the lens or intraocular lens (IOL); the former may cause local (peripheral, paracentral or central) opacity that may later develop into a cataract.

In pseudophakic patients, especially those who have undergone sulcus implantation following capsular rupture, accidental contact may cause IOL dislocation or subluxation with the risk of vitreous prolapse in the anterior chamber.

Vitreous hemorrhage is a relatively common complication of intravitreal injection and occurs in 3% to 5% of patients. Vitreous hemorrhage appears to be more commonly associated with injections performed using a 27-gauge rather than a 30-gauge needle.

Some clinicians prefer using a larger caliber needle to reduce the likelihood of needle obstruction during injection, even at the cost of creating a larger hole (risk of hypotonia and vitreous engagement).

One particular case is that of the vitrectomy patient, where the initial sclerotomy must be avoided and the injection made at a distance or in a different quadrant, to avoid partially reopening previous incisions, producing diastasis, subconjunctival leakage, loss of the remaining vitreous humor, conjunctival chemosis, and consequent hypotonia. This only applies to procedures performed a short time after the vitrectomy and from two months thereafter the only problem is likely to be a greater risk of bleeding due to conjunctival congestion in the area in which the sclerotomy was performed.

Intravitreal injection of an anti-VEGF agent is safe in terms of intraocular pressure (IOP) elevation with a return to levels under 25 mm Hg within 30 minutes from the injection. In rare cases, an increase in pressure may persist beyond this interval and it is in any case good practice to monitor IOP after intravitreal injections. Paracentesis evacuation could be taken into consideration in glaucoma patients to obtain hypotonia (Hollands, 2007).

## TRANSCONJUNCTIVAL INTRAOCULAR INJECTION TECHNIQUE

The transconjunctival intravitreal injection procedure is conducted as follows.

In sterile conditions, the surgeon wears a disposable gown and gloves, prepares the surgical field with povidone-iodine 10% vol. and uses sterile drapes and lid speculum. Topical anesthesia is administered with lidocaine 4%.

The surgeon uses a caliper to mark a distance of 3.5 mm (in aphakic/pseudophakic patients) or 4 mm (in phakic ones) from the limbus, before moving the conjunctiva to prevent the conjunctival hole coinciding with the scleral hole and preceding with transconjunctival injection of the drug (Fig. 53-1).

## TECHNIQUE VARIATION (PERSONAL STRATEGY OF C. FORLINI)

The only variation consists in an anterior chamber paracentesis performed using a 15° slit knife as the first step: a slight emptying of anterior chamber (AC) causes hypotonia, which has two advantages: (a) it prevents IOP elevation and consequently (b) it prevents vitreous fibrils and/or drug fluid from leaking into the subconjunctival space (bleb) after the injection (Figs. 53-2 and 53-3).

The formation of subconjunctival blebs must be avoided, as they would trap part of the drug and/or vitreous fibrils. In the former case, the pharmacological effect is impaired and in the later, vitreous fibril incarceration may cause dangerous late vitreous traction.

In conclusion, AC paracentesis before IV injection offers important advantages:

- it avoids intraoperative or short-term IOP elevation
- it prevents subconjunctival blebs and consequently there is:
    - no risk of leakage and loss of some of the drug (→impaired pharmacological action)
    - no risk of vitreous fibril incarceration (→late vitreoretinal traction)

## DRUG-RELATED COMPLICATIONS

### Anti-VEGF Agents

VEGF is a protein secreted by retinal pigment epithelium that acts on endothelial cells and is an essential factor in the development of choroidal neovascularization. In physiology, VEGF is essential for normal embryonic development; it plays a role in the female reproductive cycle, is expressed in tissue in the

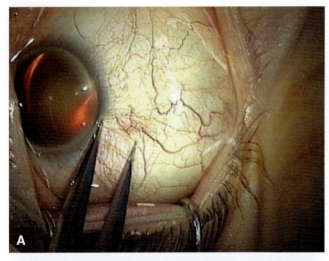

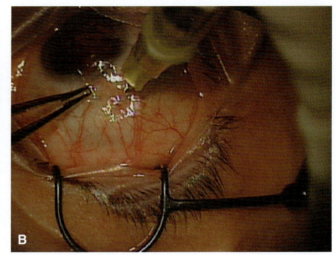

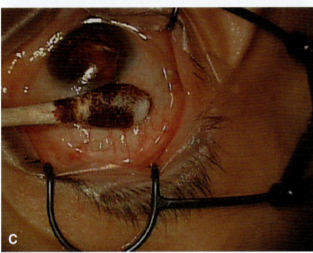

**Figure 53-1. A:** Marking a distance of 4 mm from the limbus; **B:** Injection of 0.05 cc of Bevacizumab; **C:** Massage with cotton bud soaked in povidone-iodine.

brain, kidney and gastrointestinal mucosa, contributes to wound healing and bone formation, and promotes the formation of new blood vessels after myocardial ischemia.

VEGF and VEGF receptors are naturally expressed in the healthy eye and VEGF may play a protective role in maintaining adequate blood flow to the retinal pigment epithelium (RPE) and photoreceptors.

In ocular pathology, VEGF is involved in:

- Neovascular AMD
- Diabetic retinopathy
- Retinal vein occlusion
- Retinopathy of prematurity
- Corneal neovascularization
- Iris neovascularization

VEGF has the following properties:

- Angiogenesis stimulant
- Potent inducer of vascular permeability
- Vascular survival factor
- "Fenestration" promoting factor
- Pro-inflammatory action
- Neuroprotective action

To assess the effects of the intravitreal injection of each drug, both topical and systemic side effects are to be considered.

Despite the small amount of drug injected into the eye, a minimal quantity of it may act at a systemic level. Bearing in mind that VEGF intervenes in several biological processes, including growth, repair, and regeneration, possible side effects may involve the circulatory system.

## Pegaptanib (Macugen)

Pegaptanib is a pegylated 28-nucleotide RNA aptamer (aptamers are synthetic oligonucleotides with binding properties similar to those of antibodies). It was the first anti-VEGF agent approved for the treatment of vascular eye disease. By blocking VEGF165, pegaptanib inhibits angiogenesis and vascular permeability.

The VISION study (VEGF Inhibition Study in Ocular Neovascularization) studies the safety and efficacy of pegaptanib. This concurrent, randomized, double-blind, controlled, dose-ranging study involves 1,190 patients at 117 centers worldwide; 295 receive 0.3 mg pegaptanib and 298 receive usual care with sham injections every 6 weeks. The objective of this study is to establish the safe, efficacious dose of intravitreal

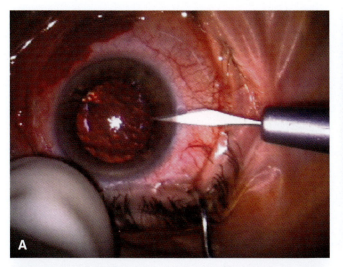

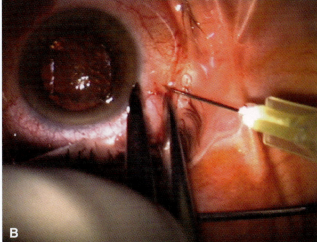

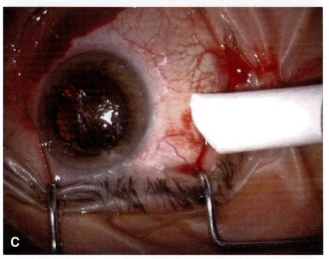

**Figure 53-2. A:** Anterior chamber paracentesis in temporal zone with 15-degree slit knife. **B:** Direct drug injection 3.5 mm from limbus (no tunnel). **C:** Reflux absent. No subconjunctival bleb forms due to the hypotonia caused by the earlier anterior chamber paracentesis evacuation.

pegaptanib in patients with subfoveal choroidal neovascularization (CNV) secondary to AMD.

The ocular adverse events observed in this study are:

- Eye pain
- Punctuate keratitis
- Vitreous floaters
- Vitreous opacity
- Anterior chamber inflammation
- Increased IOP. Pegaptanib injections cause a significant transient rise in IOP that considerably diminishes within 30 minutes post-injection, but can take as long as one hour. This may damage the optic nerve, particularly in patients with advanced glaucoma (7). Pegaptanib injection in this limited series would seem to be safe from an IOP standpoint in the short-term. Postinjection IOP monitoring may not be necessary (8).
- Traumatic cataract
- Retinal detachment
- RPE tears post-pegaptanib (Macugen) injection (9).
- Endophthalmitis. After the first year, the prevalence of endophthalmitis drops from 0.18% to 0.07% due to the following factors:

  - Preinjection antibiotics and povidone-iodine; use of lid speculum, sterile drape and sterile gloves.
  - Greater experience of clinicians in performing intravitreal triamcinolone (IVT) injections.

The most common systemic adverse events are:

- Cardiac disorders
- Neoplasia and nervous system disorders
- Gastrointestinal disorders
- Respiratory, thoracic and mediastinal disorders
- Renal and urinary tract disorders

There is no statistically significant difference in the onset of these adverse events between patients who received pegaptanib and those who received usual care with sham injections.

## Ranibizumab (Lucentis)

Ranibizumab (Lucentis, Genentech, Inc., South San Francisco, CA) is a specific affinity-matured, recombinant, humanized anti-VEGF-A neutralizing antibody fragment (Fab). The fragment is one third the size of a full-length antibody and readily penetrates all layers of the retina after intravitreal injection. Ranibizumab is

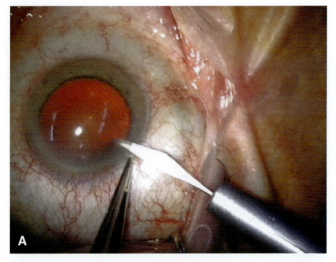

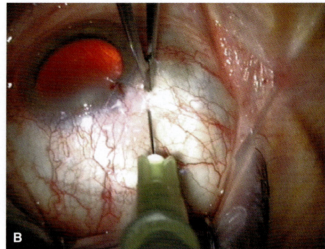

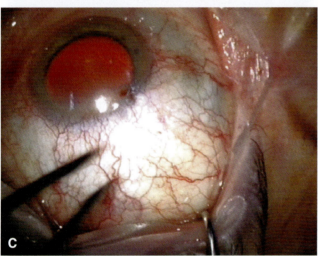

**Figure 53-3. A:** Anterior chamber paracentesis with 15-degree slit knife. **B:** Conjunctival movement and injection with scleral tunnel. **C:** Reflux absent. No subconjunctival bleb forms due to the hypotonia caused by the earlier anterior chamber paracentesis evacuation.

being developed as a potential treatment for various VEGFA-mediated ocular vascular diseases and is being used in phase III trials for treatment of neovascular AMD. The one-year results from a 2-year phase III trial on the treatment of minimally classic and occult-only AMD-related choroidal neovascularization indicate that monthly injection of 0.3 or 0.5 mg ranibizumab halted the growth of the choroidal neovascularization lesion, reduced vascular leakage, and in one quarter to one third of treated patients, respectively, improved visual acuity (VA).

The ANCHOR, MARINA, and SAILOR trials studied the safety and efficacy of Ranibizumab.

The ocular adverse events showed a 1% prevalence in the ANCHOR study and a 1.5% prevalence in the MARINA study:

- Endophthalmitis
- Uveitis. Another study showed that 500 μg of ranibizumab was the maximum tolerated dose. At the higher dose of 1000 μg, significant intraocular inflammation was observed (10).
- Iridocyclitis and injection-site reactions, mild transient ocular inflammation was the most common post-injection adverse event.
- Retinal detachment

- Retinal rupture
- Vitreous and retinal hemorrhage
- Sub-retinal fibrosis
- RPE tears (11)
- Traumatic cataract
- Transient IOP elevation
- Conjunctival hemorrhage
- Ocular pain
- Vitreous floaters
- Vitreous detachment
- Ocular hyperemia
- Reduced visual acuity or blurred vision
- Dry eye syndrome

The analysis of systemic adverse effects of Lucentis (systemic adverse events) in both studies (ANCHOR, MARINA) has shown:

- The incidence of acute elevation of systemic blood pressure in patients treated with lucentis was similar to or lower than the control group
- No statistically significant difference in the incidence of thromboembolic diseases (myocardial infarction, stroke,

cerebral infarction) was observed between the various treatment groups
- No death has been attributed to Lucentis

Ranibizumab (Lucentis) was approved by the US Food and Drug Administration (FDA) for intravitreal injection at a dose of 0.5 mg; the manufacturer recently issued a letter to physicians warning of the increased risk of stroke at the FDA-approved dose as compared to a lower studied dose of 0.3 mg. An interim analysis of the ongoing SAILOR study revealed a 1.2% risk of stroke in the 0.5 mg arm versus 0.3% in the 0.3 mg arm ($p = .02$). It is unclear whether the trend toward a higher risk of stroke in patients receiving the 0.5 mg dose of ranibizumab will persist in final analysis, however details such as causality, topography, and severity of stroke in the SAILOR study also need to be defined.

## Bevacizumab (Avastin)

Bevacizumab (Avastin) is a recombinant humanized monoclonal IgG1 antibody that inhibits human VEGF. The drug is approved by the US Food and Drug Administration for intravenous use in combination with 5-fluorouracil-based chemotherapy for metastatic colorectal cancer. It has been administered intravitreally in VEGF-mediated diseases, such as choroidal neovascularization, central retinal vein occlusion, proliferative diabetic retinopathy, and other retinal diseases. It has not been approved by the FDA for intravitreal use and therefore it may only be used in an off-label setting. The most commonly used dose for intravitreal injection is currently 1.25 mg (0.05 ml) in the United States, although up to 2.50 mg (0.1 ml) may be used. Because such a small amount of drug from a large vial is required to treat eye disease, ophthalmologists have been obtaining the drug from compounding pharmacies that divide the vial into smaller amounts, at a lower cost.

To date, there are no randomized clinical trials demonstrating the effects of the treatment with bevacizumab for ocular vascular diseases; however, there are several case series concerning this matter.

The ocular complications of intravitreal injection of bevacizumab are:

- Bacterial endophthalmitis
- Tractional retinal detachments
- Uveitis
- Rhegmatogenous retinal detachment and vitreous hemorrhage (12)
- Tractional retinal detachments
- Uveitis (13)
- Rhegmatogenous retinal detachment and vitreous hemorrhage
- Corneal abrasion (14)
- Chemosis (15)
- Lens injury (16)
- Ocular inflammation (17)
- Retinal pigment epithelium tears or rips (18–20)
- Acute vision loss (21)
- Transient extreme IOP elevation (22)
- Endophthalmitis and mild intraocular uveitis (23–25)
- Fresh submacular hemorrhages were seen in the absence of pre-existing hemorrhage in four out of 10 patients in the

$>15$ mm$^2$ CNV size group (40%) but none in the remaining groups with CNV sizes $<15$ mm$^2$ (26)
- Contralateral vitritis following intravitreal bevacizumab administration (27)
- Large subretinal hemorrhage 4 weeks after intravitreal bevacizumab administration (28)
- Transient structured visual hallucinations in a patient with vascular AMD, following an intravitreal Avastin-injection. Typical symptoms of Charles-Bonnet syndrome (CBS) were observed in patients with severe AMD after intravitreal Avastin-injections. The reduced retinal edema and realignment of the photoreceptors may promote the release phenomenon and trigger hallucinatory episodes (29).

The systemic complications of intravitreal injection of bevacizumab are:

- cerebral infarction (30)
- elevation of systolic blood pressure (31)
- facial skin redness (32)
- widespread itchiness and rash (33)
- menstrual irregularities (34)
- acute elevation of systemic blood pressure (35)
- cerebrovascular accidents (36)
- myocardial infarctions (37)
- iliac artery aneurysms (38)
- toe amputations (39)
- death (in five cases) (40)

## Triamcinolone

TA has been effectively used in eye treatment for over half a century.

Its use has increased dramatically in recent years for periocular and intraocular treatment of retinal vascular disease and uveitis.

TA is an agent for the treatment of conditions requiring long-term ocular steroid administration such as uveitis, macular edema secondary to retinal vascular disease, and intraocular proliferations such as CNV in AMD and vitreoretinopathy.

In addition to their anti-inflammatory mechanism, corticosteroids have vasoconstrictive actions that may contribute to their efficacy in treating ocular neovascularization and lid hemangiomas.

The most commonly used doses include 4 mg and 20 mg.

As with any topical corticosteroid, TA constitutes a serious risk factor for IOP elevation, thus reducing aqueous humor runoff. This may be responsible for damaging the optic nerve, which impairs the visual field.

Two mechanisms are thought to be responsible for this: one would be the moisturizing and deposition of glycosaminesglycans in the trabeculate, which hinders aqueous humor runoff and the second is phagocytosis inhibition.

In the light of this, it is necessary to carefully assess and select patients with a history or familiarity of open angle glaucoma.

Subtenon injection of TA may result in an increase in IOP to levels of over 21 mm Hg, and anterior subtenon injections appear more likely to cause an elevation of IOP than posterior subtenon injections. Other potential complications associated with subtenon triamcinolone injection are:

- inadvertent injection into the retinal or choroidal circulation
- eyeball perforation with or without intravitreal injection,
- cataract,
- occlusion of the central retinal artery,
- blepharoptosis,
- proptosis,
- orbital fat atrophy,
- delayed hypersensitivity reactions manifested as severe conjunctival inflammation, strabismus, conjunctival hemorrhage, chemosis, and infection.

Several recent studies reported an elevated IOP in association with intravitreal triamcinolone.

One study by Bakri and Beer retrospectively reviewed cases receiving a single dosage of 4 mg. Their 4-week study showed an incidence of 48.8% of eyes demonstrating an IOP increase of 5 mm Hg or over and 27.9% showing an increase in IOP of 10 mm Hg or over at a mean time of 6.6 weeks. Pressure elevation was controllable with topical glaucoma medication.

Rhee and colleagues stated that baseline IOP greater than 16 mm Hg is a risk factor for postinjection IOP elevation (the dose was 4 mg).

Sterile endophthalmitis, pseudoendophthalmitis or culture-positive infectious endophthalmitis have been documented (Fig. 53-4). The exact mechanism of sterile endophthalmitis after intravitreal triamcinolone injection has not been determined.

The phenomenon is caused by a reaction to the triamcinolone preparation.

Patients with sterile endophthalmitis typically follow a course of self-resolution. They present complaining of painless loss of sight, as they do not usually suffer the intense pain commonly seen in bacterial endophthalmitis.

Slit lamp examination reveals moderate injected conjunctiva and mild anterior chamber reaction.

Many patients also develop hypopyon containing crystals and precipitants.

A moderate vitreous reaction is almost always seen.

The presence of intraocular inflammation after intravitreal injection presents a dilemma for the ophthalmologist. In these patients, careful slit lamp examination reveals the presence of the corticosteroid preparation in the anterior chamber.

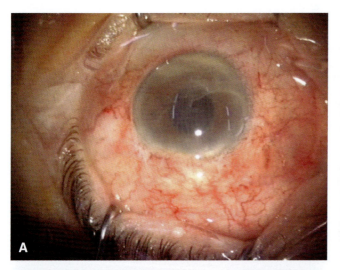

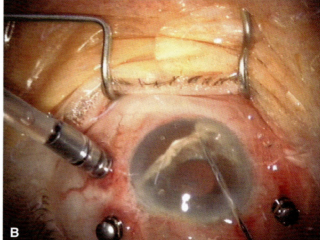

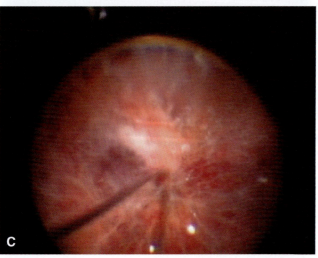

**Figure 53-4.** Endophthalmitis in pseudophakic postintravitreal injection of TA. **A:** Hypopyon and fibrin in the anterior chamber. **B:** 23-gauge surgical approach and removal of hypopyon using forceps. **C:** Retinitis and vasculitis with preretinal and intraretinal exudates.

In cases such as these, the authors recommend that endophthalmitis treatment be initiated if any of the following symptoms or signs is present: significant eye pain, afferent pupillary defect, conjunctival chemosis, retinal phlebitis and/or vitreous abscess.

Ptosis is an exceptional known complication of subtenon and intravitreal triamcinolone injection, possibly due to its solvent agents. The ptosis produced seems to depend on a malfunction of the muscle fibers of the elevator caused by a direct myopathic effect of the vehicle.

However, it is unclear whether the ptosis is related to corticosteroid itself or to the vehicle (41).

Although it is not known which of the components produces the ptosis, it is important to remove the solvents from the drug before the intravitreal or subtenon injection.

Development of cataract is another known side effect of steroid treatment. Recent clinical studies have reported corticosteroid-induced cataract development. Danis and associates reported 57.1% of the eyes that received 4 mg triamcinolone by injection developed progressive lens opacity after 6 months of treatment. Gillies and associates reported significant posterior subcapsular cataract in eyes after a single 4 mg intravitreal injection of triamcinolone. In a recent preliminary study, Cekic and associates demonstrated that posterior subcapsular cataract had progressed significantly 12 months after a single triamcinolone injection and multiple injections caused progression of cataract in all layers of the lens at 14 months.

## Other Drugs

### Antibiotics

It is known that an intraocular septic process (endophthalmitis) can be a cause of blindness, because it induces a severe functional loss of the affected eyeball (42). Over the years, different antibiotic therapies, in monotherapy or combined with surgical treatment, have been proposed and used for bacterial endophthalmitis caused by gram-positive or gram-negative bacteria (43).

The therapeutic regimen usually adopted consists in a combination of two or more drugs, for urgent treatment of bacterial endophthalmitis. Vancomycin, with ceftazidime or with aminoglycosides, is the most frequently used combination (44,45).

In addition to the use of antibiotic drugs, many authors propose administering steroids in order to contrast and reduce the inflammatory reaction that often causes irreversible retinal damage.

However, the action of antibiotic drugs is known to be toxic for the retinal tissue (46,47).

This is due to the fact that these agents can precipitate and infiltrate the retinal tissue. Hence, it is important that the antibiotics remain in suspension in the vitreous cavity and are subsequently eliminated. For this purpose, some studies and reports have demonstrated that, in particular, amikacin and vancomycin are the molecules with the lowest tendency to precipitate in balanced saline solution or normal saline solution (48), unlike other molecules such as ciprofloxacin and ceftazidime (49).

Fluoroquinolones in particular can be toxic for different ocular structures, because of both their pharmacokinetic properties and the intraocular concentrations that can be reached (ofloxacin >50 μg/mL; ciprofloxacin >100 μg/mL; moxifloxacin >160 μg/mL; trovafloxacin >25 μg/mL; pefloxacin >200 μg/mL) (50). In the eyelids, a photomediated reaction (UV- quinolone interaction) can cause cutaneous photosensitivity. The conjunctiva can be the site of hyperemia and goblet-cell reduction after prolonged administration of ofloxacin (51).

The cornea can be interested at an epithelial level, with white crystal deposits after prolonged ciprofloxacin administration (because the molecule's solubility is reduced at the pH of the lacrimal film) (52). Corneal stroma affected by toxic phenomena presents keratocyte apoptosis and remodelling of the collagen tissue (53). In animal models, the active pump of corneal endothelium cells becomes particularly reduced at high doses of ciprofloxacin (>100 μg), with possible onset of bullous keratopathy after injection in anterior chamber of the drug at a dosage of 25 μg or superior, but that does not occur in human cornea after exposure to the drug at doses of 30 μg/mL or inferior (54).

Cataract develop is reported only for experimental animal models, but not for treatment in humans.

In the retina, quinolones can cause a series of sometimes severe clinical presentations, such as vacuolization of the nerve fiber layer (55), complete loss of the photoreceptors' external segments, atrophy of the internal and external nuclear layer and atrophy of the Muller cells. Defects induced in the internal limiting membrane have also been described, with the release of macrophage-like cells and destruction of Bruch's membrane.

It is also possible to observe retinal necrosis, the presence of vacuoles and hyperplasia in the RPE, opacification of the vitreous adherens to the retinal surface, and lastly optic disc edema (56–59).

In conclusion, in line with the data available in literature, it would appear evident that the use of fluoroquinolone drugs is undoubtedly both useful and safe. Potential adverse effects, which are always dose-and drug-class-linked, are possible, but in general usually harmless, and occur in approximately 10% of cases.

## t-PA

TPA (tissue plasminogen activator) is a fibrinolytic agent frequently used in the cardiology field to treat ischemic cardiomyopathy and in ophthalmology for the treatment of postsurgical complications entailing inflammatory reaction (fibrotic reaction, anterior synechiae, iridotomy closure).

This molecule is also used to treat subretinal hemorrhage. It is administered by the intravitreal route in combination with gas injection (generally SF6) to move subretinal hemorrhages away from the macular area, such as in complications of neovascular pathologies like the polypoidal form of AMD.

The efficacy of treatment has been very well documented, as a less invasive and safer technique than vitrectomy with direct mechanical removal of subretinal hemorrhage.

Nevertheless, literature also reports cases of retinal toxicity in animals and humans after intravitreal administration of this drug.

The dose currently used for intravitreal injection is 50 to 100 μg in 0.1 ml followed by gas injection (SF6) and by immediate positioning for least 48 hours.

The effect is evident after just 24 hours and the anatomical-functional result is very good.

In some cases, there are side effects on the RPE level caused by use of TPA. Specifically, signs of RPE degeneration appeared a few weeks after administration of the molecule. These present as hyperpigmentation deposits with fine hyperfluorescence to fluoresce on angiograms but with no early or late leakage.

The electro-functional examinations, in particular ERG, can show an increase in frequency and a reduction in the amplitude of the a- and b-waves.

TPA toxicity (and that of its vehicle, L-arginine) is described in literature by RPE, with necrosis, hyperpigmentation around the injection site, on the posterior pole and middle border, and photoreceptors, with loss and vacuolization of the same, perivascular infiltration, and possible vitreal inflammatory response and exudative and/or tractional retinal detachment. L-arginine therefore has a similar molecular structure to lysine, an amino acid with well documented retinal toxicity.

Another possible mechanism, which has only been observed and studied in animals, is TPA's capacity to worsen retinal ischemia, especially in cases of central retinal vein occlusion (CRVO) induced in cultures using the retinal cells of rats, where increased damage caused by TPA was observed as hypoxia after staining, analyzed both with the TUNNEL (deoxynucleotidyl transferase-mediated dUTP-nick end labelling) technique and by measuring nitrous oxide (NO) levels in these cultures, which was found to be higher in cells treated with TPA (with L-arginine) and with single L-arginine.

Unfortunately, all commercial TPA preparations (Activase; Genentech Inc, San Francisco, California) have L-arginine-like molecule vehicles and so the effects of this protein are inevitable. The unresolved question is to what extent the side effects depend on the drug dose (25–50–100 μg) or other agents such as the molecular vehicle.

## Antiviral Agents

Cytomegalovirus retinitis is the most common cause of visual acuity impairment and frequent opportunistic intraocular infection in AIDS patients.

Systemic treatment with antiviral drugs such as gancyclovir, foscarnet, and cidofovir undoubtedly slows down this condition; however, these drugs expose patients to side effects such as nephrotoxicity, hepatoxicity and severe myelopathy.

The intravitreal therapy with antiviral agents has been slow but sure for treatment of cytomegalovirus retinitis, necessary to maintain fair levels by intraocular concentration of drug and to prevent ocular collateral and systemic effects.

The introduction of a slow-release device by drug implantation via the sclera into the vitreous chamber, resolves the problem of maintaining good drug concentration levels, but nevertheless exposes patients to the side effects (60).

Experimental animal models have shown the possible presence of milder vitreous inflammatory response and the absence of alterations in the amplitude of b-wave on ERG after use of Gancyclovir (73) ISIS2922 and ISIS4015 (74) (60).

The slow-release devices for Gancyclovir can be positioned in pars plana through a sclerotomy after localized vitrectomy, so that one part of the device stays in the vitreous chamber and the other is sutured to the sclera. To reduce the risk of endophthalmitis, some Authors prepare a 5 mm scleral window to cover the sclerotomy (61,62).

In addition to its effects on animals, this device also causes postoperative complications in humans, the most common being rhegmatogenous retinal detachment, vitreous hemorrhage, cystoid macular edema, endophthalmitis, malpositioning of device in the subretinal space, uveitis, and VA impairment by two or more Snellen lines (probably due to the toxic effects of the drug).

These complications of course impact functional prognosis in the affected eyes depending on the underlying pathology. Nevertheless, by analyzing implantation cases, it is clear that the device presents an alternative to intravenous systemic therapy with Gancyclovir and the patient can be informed about intrasurgical and postsurgical risk.

## CONCLUSIONS

Research projects organized by leading institutions and pharmaceutical companies to find a safe and efficacious treatment for many eye diseases are making rapid progress. Anti-VEGF drugs have provided a ray of hope, but involve the use of multiple intravitreal injections, which in addition to increasing the risk of complications, are also expensive. Though bevacizumab is still an off-label drug, promising results have prompted its use in the vast spectrum of ocular diseases. As research continues, we may see the advent of new, more efficacious agents offering treatment options for this specialty.

- As far as the risk of endophthalmitis is concerned, no difference was observed between Bevacizumab and Ranibizumab injections (63).
- As regards uveitis secondary to anti-VEGF injection, the caseload available is small, however its potential association with intraocular inflammation should not be overlooked (64).
- The use of topical antibiotic treatment may not reduce the occurrence of mild to severe intraocular endophthalmitis.

Bevacizumab and ranibizumab are undoubtedly efficacious in treating exudative maculopathy, especially AMD. The incidence of thromboembolic events connected to the use of these agents is exceedingly low (15 cases of pressure elevation in 7113 injections in 5228 patients, (65)).

To conclude, anti-VEGF agents have proven to be both efficacious and safe in clinical use in recent years, however further multicenter, controlled trials with long-term follow-up are required to decree its actual efficacy and safety in routine use.

### References

1. Cardascia N, Boscia F, Furino C, et al. Gentamicin-induced macular infarction in transconjunctival sutureless 25-gauge vitrectomy [epub ahead of print Oct 16, 2007]. *Int Ophthalmol* 2008;28(5):383–385.
2. Thomas T, Galiani D, Brod RD. Gentamicin and other antibiotic toxicity. *Ophthalmol Clin North Am* 2001;14(4):611–624.
3. Engelman CJ, Palmer JD, Egbert P. Orbital abscess following subtenon triamcinolone injection. *Arch Ophthalmol* 2004;122(4):654–655.
4. Kusaka S, Ikuno Y, Ohguro N, et al. Orbital infection following posterior subtenon triamcinolone injection. *Acta Ophthalmol Scand* 2007;85(6):692–693.
5. Dalessandro L, Bottaro E. Reactivation of CMV retinitis after treatment with subtenon corticosteroids for immune recovery uveitis in a patient with AIDS. *Scand J Infect Dis* 2002;34(10):780–782.
6. Oh JK, Baek S, Huh K, et al. Periocular abscess caused by Pseudallescheria boydii after a posterior subtenon injection of triamcinolone acetonide. *Graefer Arch Clin Exper Ophthalmol* 2007;245(1):164–166.
7. Dal Canto AJ, Downs-Kelly E, Perry JD. Ptosis and Orbital Fat prolapse after posterior sub-tenon's capsule triamcinolone injection. *Ophthalmology* 2005;112(6):1092–1097.

8. Azarbod P. Mohammed Q, Akram I, et al. Localised abscess following an injection of subtenon triamcinolone acetonide. *Eye* 2007;21(5):672–674.

9. Bui QE, Bodaghi B, Adam R, et al. Intraocular pressure elevation after subtenon injection of triamcinolone acetonide during uveitis. *J Fr Ophthalmol* 2002;25(10):1048–1056.

10. Mueller AJ, Jian G, Banker AS, et al. The effect of deep posterior subtenon injection of corticosteroids on intraocular pressure. *Am J Ophthalmol* 1998;125(2):158–163.

11. Alfaro DV III, Liggett PE, Mieler WF, et al (eds). *Age-related macular degeneration*. Philadelphia, PA: Lippincott Williams & Wilkins, 2006.

12. Frenkel RE, Mani L, Toler AR, et al. Intraocular pressure effects of pegaptanib (Macugen) injections in patients with and without glaucoma. *Am J Ophthalmol* 2007;143(6):1034–1035.

13. Hariprasad SM, Shah GK, Blinder KJ. Short-term intraocular pressure trends following intravitreal pegaptanib (Macugen) injection. *Am J Ophthalmol* 2006;141(1):200–201.

14. Chang LK, Flaxel CJ, Lauer AK, et al. RPE tears after pegaptanib treatment in age-related macular degeneration. *Retina* 2007;27(7):857–863.

15. Rosenfeld PJ, Schwartz SD, Blumenkranz MS, et al. Maximum tolerated dose of a humanized anti-vascular endothelial growth factor antibody fragment for treating neovascular age-related macular degeneration. *Ophthalmology* 2005;112(6):1048–1053.

16. Bakri SJ, Kitzmann AS. Retinal pigment epithelial tear after intravitreal ranibizumab [epub ahead of print December 28, 2006]. *Am J Ophthalmol* 2007;143(3):505–507.

17. Shima C, Sakaguchi H, Gomi F, et al. Complication in patients after intravitreal injection of bevacizumab. *Acta Opththlmol Scand* 2007;86(4):372–376.

18. Hollands H, Wong J, Bruen R, et al. Short-term intraocular pressure changes after intravitreal injection of bevacizumab. *Can J Ophthalmol* 2007;42(6): 807–811.

19. Meyer CH, Mennel S, Eter N. Incidence of endophthalmitis after intravitreal Avastin injection with and without postoperative topical antibiotic application. *Ophthalmologe* 2007;104(11):952–957.

20. Goverdhan S, Lochhead J. St Mary's Hospital, United Kingdom. Sub-macular hemorrhages after intravitreal bevacizumab for large occult choroidal neovascularization in age-related macular degeneration. *Br J Ophthalmol* 2007;92:210–212.

21. Subramanyam A, Phatak S, Chudgar D. Large retinal pigment epithelium rip following serial intravitreal injection of avastin in a large fibrovascular pigment epithelial detachment. *Indian J Ophthalmol* 2007;55:483–486.

22. Neri P, Mariotti C, Mercanti L, et al. Vitreitis in the controlateral uninjected eye following intravitreal bevacizumab (Avastin). *Int Ophthalmol* 2008;28(6):425–427.

23. Chieh JJ, Fekrat S. Large subretinal hemorrhage after intravitreal bevacizumab (Avastin) forage-related macular degeneration. *Ann Ophthalmol (Skokie)* 2007;39(1):51–52.

24. Wu L, Martínez-Castellanos MA, Quiroz-Mercado H, et al. For the Pan American Collaborative Retina Group (PACORES). Twelve-month safety of intravitreal injections of bevacizumab (Avastin): results of the Pan-American Collaborative Retina Study Group (PACORES) [epub ahead of print August 3, 2007]. *Graefes Arch Clin Exp Ophthalmol* 2008;246(1):81–87.

25. Jonas JB, Spandau UH, Rensch F, et al. Infectious and noninfectious endophthalmitis after intravitreal bevacizumab. *J Ocul Pharmacol Ther* 2007;23(3):240–242.

26. Gamulescu MA, Framme C, Sachs H. RPE-rip after intravitreal bevacizumab (Avastin) treatment for vascularised PED secondary to AMD [epub ahead of print February 21, 2007]. *Graefes Arch Clin Exp Ophthalmol* 2007;245(7):1037–1040.

27. Aggio FB, Farah ME, de Melo GB, et al. Acute endophthalmitis following intravitreal bevacizumab (Avastin) injection. *Eye* 2007;21(3):408–409.

28. Meyer CH, Mennel S, Hörle S, et al. Visual hallucinations after intravitreal injection of bevacizumab in vascular age-related macular degeneration. *Am J Ophthalmol* 2007;143(1):169–170.

29. Pieramici DJ, Avery RL, Castellarin AA, et al. Case of anterior uveitis after intravitreal injection of bevacizumab. *Retina* 2006;26(7):841–842.

30. Viola F, Morescalchi F, Ratiglia R, et al. Ptosis following an intravitreal injection of triamcinolone acetonide. *Eye* 2007;21:421–423.

31. Shrader SK, Band JD, Lauter CB, et al. The clinical spectrum of endophthalmitis incidence, predisposing factors, and features influencing outcome. *J Infect Dis* 1990;162:115–120.

32. Kunimoto DY, Das T, Sharma S, et al. Microbiologic spectrum and susceptibility of isolates: part II. Posttraumatic endophthalmitis. Endophthalmitis Research group. *Am J Ophthalmol* 1999;128:242–244.

33. Benz MS, Scott IU, Flynn HW, et al. Endophthalmitis isolates and antibiotic sensitives: a 6-year review of culture-proven cases. *Am J Ophthalmol* 2004;137:38–42.

34. Yam JC, Kwok AK. Update of the management of postoperative endophthalmitis. *Hong Kong Med J* 2004;10:337–343.

35. Park SS, Samiy N, Ruoff K, et al. Effect of intravitreal dexamethasone in treatment of pneumococcal endophthalmitis in rabbits. *Arch Ophthalmol* 1995;113:1324–1329.

36. Das T, Jalali S, Gothwal VK, et al. Intravitreal dexamethasone in exogenous bacterial endophthalmitis: results of a prospective randomised study. *Br J Ophthalmol* 1999;83:1050–1055.

37. Hui M, Kwok AKH, Pang CP, et al. An in vitro study on the compatibility and concentrations of combinations of vancomycin, amikacin, and dexamethasone in human vitreous. *Eye* 2007;21:643–648.

38. Kwok AK, Hui M, Pang CP, et al. In vitro study of ceftazidime and vancomycin concentration in various fluid media: implications for use in treating endophthalmitis. *Invest Ophthalmol Vis Sci* 2002;43:1182–1188.

39. Thonmpson AM. Ocular toxicity of fluoroquinolones. *Clin Exp Ophthalmol* 2007;35:566–577.

40. Marino C, Paladino GM, Scuderi AC, et al. In vivo toxicity of netilmicin and ofloxacin on intact and mechanically damaged eyes of rabbit. *Cornea* 2005;24:710–716.

41. Konishi M, Yamada M, Mashima Y. Corneal ulcer associated with deposits of norfloxacin. *Am J Ophthalmol* 1998;125:258–260.

42. Bekoe NA, Li Q, Ashraf F, et al. Effects of ciprofloxacin, ofloxacin, and gentamicin on corneal cells and wound healing. (ARVO abstract). *Invest Ophthalmol Vis Sci* 1999;40:B770. Abstract no 2895.

43. Kang F, Serdarevic ON, Kuang K, et al. Effects of ciprofloxacin, streptomycin, and gentamicin on rabbit corneal transendothelial electrical potential difference. *Cornea* 1998;17:185–190.

44. Rootman DS, Savage P, Hasany SM, et al. Toxicity and pharmacokinetics of intravitreally injected ciprofloxacin in rabbit eyes. *Can J Ophthalmol* 1992;27:277–282.

45. Stevens SX, Fouraker BD, Jensen HG. Intraocular safety of ciprofloxacin. *Arch. Ophthalmol* 1991;109:1737–1743.

46. Wiechens B, Grammer JB, Johannsen U, et al. Experimental intravitreal application of ciprofloxacin in rabbits. *Ophthalmologica* 1999;213:120–128.

47. Ng EW, Joo MJ, Au Eong KG, et al. Ocular toxicity of intravitreal trovafloxacin in the pigment rabbit. *Curr Eye Res* 2003;27:387–393.

48. Koutsandrea CN, Miceli MV, Peyman GA, et al. Ciprofloxacin and dexamethasone inhibit the proliferation of human retinal pigment epithelial cells in culture. *Curr Eye Res* 1991;10:249–258.

49. Jaffe GJ, Abrams GW, Williams GA, et al. Tissue plasminogen activator for postvitrectomy fibrin formation. *Ophthalmology* 1990;97:184–189.

50. Hesse L, Schmidt J, Kroll P. Management of acute submacular hemorrhage using recombinant tissue plasminogen activator and gas. *Greafes Arch Clin Exp Ophthalmol* 1999;237:273–277.

51. Chen SN, Yang TC, Ho CL, et al. Retinal toxicity of intravitreal tissue plasminogen activator: case report and literature review. *Ophthamology* 2003;110(4):704–708.

52. Hrach CJ, Johnson MW, Hassan AS. Retinal toxicity of commercial intravitreal tissue plasminogen activator solution in cat eyes. *Arch Ophthalmol* 2000;118:659–663.

53. Johnson MW, Oslen KR, Hernandez E. Retinal toxicity of recombinant tissue plasminogen activator in the rabbit. *Arch Ophthalmol* 1990;108:259–263.

54. Oh HS, Kwon OW, Chung I, et al. Retinal toxicity of commercial tissue plasminogen activator is mediated by the induction of nitric oxide in the mouse retinal primary cells. *Curr Eye Res* 2005;30(4):291–297.

55. Lim JI, Wolitz RA, Bowling AH, et al. Visual and anatomic outcomes associated with posterior segment complications after ganciclovir implant procedures in patients with AIDS and Cytomegalovirus retinitis. *Am J Ophthalmol* 1999;127(3):288–293.

56. Guembel HO, Krieglsteiner S, Rosenkranz C, et al. Complications after implantation of intraocular devices in patients with cytomegalovirus retinitis. *Graefes Arch Clin Exp Ophthalmol* 1999;237(10):824–829.

57. Eng KT, Lam WC, Parker JA, et al. Retinal toxicity of intravitreal ganciclovir in rabbit eyes following vitrectomy and insertion of silicone oil. *Can J Ophthalmol* 2004;39(5):499–505.

58. Flores-Aguilar M, Besen G, Vuong C, et al. Evaluation of retinal toxicity and efficacy of anti-cytomegalovirus and anti-herpes simplex virus antiviral phosphorothioate oligonucleotides ISIS 2922 and ISIS 4015. *J Infect Dis* 1997;175(6):1308–1316.

59. Marx JL, Kapusta MA, Patel SS, et al. Use of the ganciclovir implant in the treatment of recurrent cytomegalovirus retinitis. *Arch Ophthalmol* 1996;114(7):815–820.

60. Hatton MP, Duker JS, Reichel E, et al. Treatment of relapsed cytomegalovirus retinitis with the sustained-release ganciclovir implant. *Retina* 1998;18(1):50–55.

61. Aggio FB, Farah ME, de Melo GB, et al. Acute endophthalmitis following intravitreal bevacizumab (Avastin) injection [epub ahead of print February 2, 2007]. *Eye* 2007;21(3):408–409.

62. Aggermann T, Stolba U, Brunner S, et al. Endophthalmitis with retinal necrosis following intravitreal triamcinolone acetonide injection. *Ophthalmologica* 2006;220(2):131–133.

63. Pilli S, Kotsolis A, Spaide RF, et al. Endophthalmitis associated with intravitreal anti-vascular endothelial growth factor therapy injections in an office setting. *Am J Ophthalmol* 2008;145(5):879–882.

64. Bakri SJ, Larson TA, Edwards AO. Intraocular inflammation following intravitreal injection of bevacizumab. *Graefes Arch Clin Exp Ophthalmol* 2008;246(5):779–81.

65. Fung AE, Rosenfeld PJ, Reichel E. The International Intravitreal Bevacizumab Safety Survey: using the internet to assess drug safety worldwide. *Br J Ophthalmol* 2006;90(11):1344–1349.

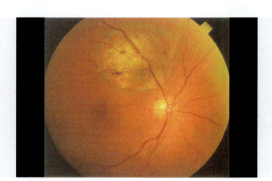

# Complications of Photocoagulation

María H. Berrocal  ■  Virgilio Morales-Canton

Photocoagulation of the retina has undergone significant advances and refinements since its initial application by Gerd Meyer-Schwikeratz in 1949 (1). Xenon arc light coagulators and ruby lasers have been replaced by argon, krypton, dye, and diode lasers. The new lasers allow for smaller, multiple, more precise burns and diverse delivery systems. Treatment can be applied through a slit lamp, indirect ophthalmoscope, intravitreally during vitrectomy surgery, and transsclerally. The diversity in modality and delivery options has expanded the potential applications for laser therapy. Photocoagulation is a minimally invasive treatment modality; nevertheless, complications are possible and diverse relative to the procedure employed.

## GENERAL COMPLICATIONS

General complications of photocoagulation include incorrect focusing and improper intensity and size of the laser burns. Focusing problems can cause inadvertent photocoagulation of the iris, cornea or crystalline lens which can result in synechiae formation, corneal and lens opacities. Lens opacities are more common when blue-green argon is used in eyes with nuclear sclerosis lens opacities, but has also been described with krypton (2–4). Corneal epithelial abrasions can occur from the contact lens used in the treatment. These are more frequent with prolonged treatments in diabetic eyes. In the posterior segment misplaced laser spots can result in inadvertent foveal or optic nerve burns and may cause scotomas, decreased vision, and visual field defects. Focusing complications can be avoided by meticulous technique, foveal localization, and adequate patient cooperation. The use of a projected fluorescein angiogram during treatment can aid in avoiding foveal burns. In uncooperative patients, particularly when applying treatment in the macular area, akinesia by retrobulbar or subtenons injection may be necessary.

Very intense burns can rupture retinal vessels and Bruch's membrane causing bleeding and potentially choroidal neovascular membranes and fibrovascular ingrowth. Bleeding is treated by applying pressure with the contact lens and photocoagulating the area with a larger spot size. A ruptured Bruch's membrane can be readily apparent but can be inadvertent and occur without any bleeding or obvious sign (5,6). This complication is more common when using small spot sizes and lasers with longer wavelengths (i.e., krypton and diode), but has also been described with argon (7,8). Applying faint, light gray burns and avoiding small spot sizes can help reduce this complication. Special caution should be used when treating highly myopic or amelanotic fundi. The lack of pigment causes reduced uptake by the retinal pigment epithelium (RPE) and higher laser powers are often needed. These eyes have a propensity for bleeding during treatment.

Vessel occlusions can occur and are more frequent when more intense and confluent treatment is necessary, as when treating tumors or subretinal neovascular membranes (SRN-VMs). Very intense burns can also cause breaks in the retina, expand over time, and cause thermal contraction with retinal traction. Enlargement of laser scars can occur over time with all laser modalities. Severe RPE and choriocapillaris damage

has been reported with transpupillary thermotherapy (TTT) and during photodynamic therapy.

## MACULAR EDEMA

Treatment for diabetic macular edema and macular edema secondary to vein occlusions can be challenging, particularly since the foveal reflex is often obscured by edema, blood, or exudates. Identifying the patient's fixation point is important to avoid foveal burns. Complications of focal and grid treatment include foveal burns (Fig. 54-1), scotomas, enlargement of burns over time, increased foveal ischemia, foveal migration and precipitation of hard exudate, increased macular edema, subretinal fibrosis, SRNVMs, premacular fibrosis, traction retinal detachment, and loss of central light sensitivity. Foveal burns can be avoided by finding the fixation point, projecting a fluorescein angiogram and using akinesia when cooperation is poor. Scotomas are best avoided by not treating near the foveal avascular zone (FAZ), using low energy, and avoiding the use of blue-green wavelength (9). Enlargement of burns over time can cause scotomas. This is more common in myopic eyes and a 5% incidence has been described with krypton grid (10). Precipitation of hard exudates, foveal migration, and subretinal fibrosis can occur in eyes with severe, chronic edema and with aggressive treatment (11). In these instances, treatment in multiple sessions is advised to allow gradual fluid resolution. Increase in macular edema can occur with aggressive treatment and concomitant panretinal photocoagulation (PRP). Treatment of the macular edema prior to PRP reduces this risk. Development of SRNVMs is a complication due to damage or breaks in Bruch's membrane. Avoiding very small, intense, and short duration burns reduces this severe complication which carries a poor prognosis (5,8).

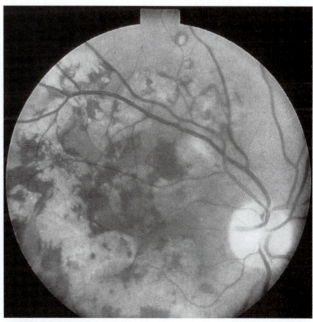

**Figure 54-1.** Foveal burns.

Thermal contraction of the retinal surface and premacular fibrosis can cause traction of the fovea and traction retinal detachment. This is best prevented by avoiding intense burns, treating over blood, and blue-green wavelength. Caution should be used when treating eyes with enlarged FAZ's since treatment can compromise the existing capillaries leading to more ischemia. General recommendations to avoid complications include identifying the fixation point, treating with light burns in multiple sessions, and avoiding treating directly over blood or fibrovascular tissue.

## IDIOPATHIC CENTRAL SEROUS CHOROIDOPATHY

Complications of the treatment of idiopathic central serous choroidopathy are similar to those of focal treatment and include scotomas, retinal wrinkling, metamorphopsia, subretinal hemorrhage, SRNVMs, and decreased visual acuity (12).

## AGE-RELATED MACULAR DEGENERATION

In the treatment of age-related macular degeneration, laser has been used to treat drusen, SRNVMs, and pigment epithelial detachments (PED). Laser treatment of drusen can cause scotomas and SRNVMs (13). The benefit of this treatment has not been established. Complications of the treatment for SRNVMs are incomplete coverage of lesion, extension of treatment to the fovea, progression of disease in 50% of cases, subretinal fibrosis, retinal vessel occlusions, subretinal and vitreous hemorrhage, nerve fiber bundle defects, and enlargement of the burns over time (Fig. 54-2). The use of an enlarged fluorescein angiogram to guide treatment and correlating lesion size with

post treatment scar by drawings can help ensure adequate treatment of the subretinal membrane margins. Careful foveal identification and patient cooperation are important in avoiding inadvertent foveal treatment. Foveal traction, subretinal fibrosis, and retinal vessel occlusions can occur with intensive treatment and when large membranes are treated. Retinal vessel occlusions may be reduced with the use of krypton (14). Hemorrhage can occur from the retinal vessels, the SRNVM, or the choroid. Avoiding small spot sizes and short exposure times may help reduce this complication.

Nerve fiber layer (NFL) damage is more common with treatment of juxtapapillary membranes and with short wavelength lasers. Enlargement of the burn size over time is more often seen in myopic eyes. Myopes can also experience expansion of lacquer cracks after photocoagulation (15). Large PED's pose a special treatment problem since laser treatment can cause RPE rips with significant visual reduction. These rips can also occur spontaneously.

## PANRETINAL PHOTOCOAGULATION

Treatment of proliferative diabetic retinopathy by PRP significantly reduces the risk of severe visual loss. Nevertheless, PRP has significant potential complications. Transient complications include choroidal and exudative retinal detachment (Fig. 54-3), angle shallowing, increased intraocular pressure, and macular edema (4,16,17). These complications are more common when extensive treatment is done in one session. The mechanism is possibly damaging to the RPE and choriocapillaris (18,19). The incidence of some degree of cilioretinal effusion after PRP is between 59% and 90% and is increased with the number of applications, short axial length eyes, and percentage of area of retina treated (20,21). These complications generally resolve within 14 days.

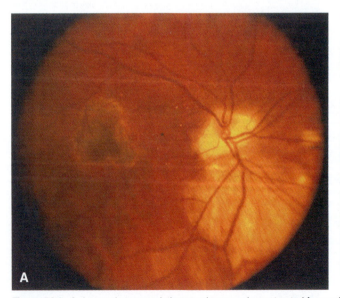
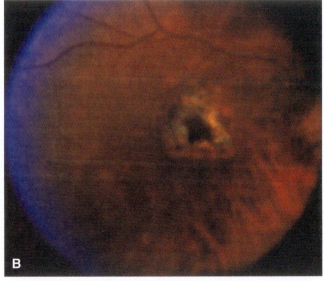

**Figure 54-2. A:** Laser photocoagulation scar in a myopic eye treated for a subretinal neovascular membrane. **B:** Laser scar 1 year after treatment. The scar has increased in size.

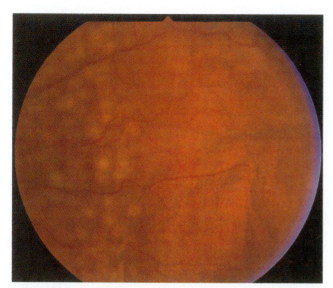

**Figure 54-3.** Choroidal detachment after panretinal photocoagulation.

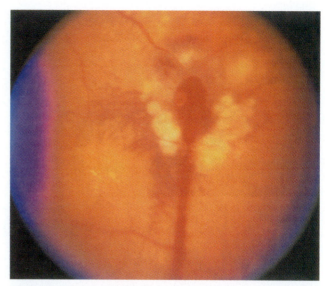

**Figure 54-4.** Vitreous bleeding occurring during photocoagulation of a retinal macroaneurysm with argon green laser.

More permanent complications include visual field defects, prolonged dark adaptation, decreased hue discrimination, accommodative insufficiency, asthenopia, and reduced ocular pulsation amplitude (22). Peripheral field defects are modest and are seen in 5% to 50% of eyes (23–25). No difference is noted between argon and krypton (26). The field loss and prolonged dark adaptation increase with repeated and confluent treatment. Loss of hue discrimination and tritan blue-yellow deficit is exacerbated by macular and PRP treatment (9,26–28). Accommodative insufficiency and asthenopia are probably due to damage to the posterior ciliary nerves (29). Avoiding the horizontal meridian may help reduce this complication.

Vessel occlusions can occur with high-energy settings and can result in decreased vision. Vitreous hemorrhage and traction retinal detachment can occur from direct treatment of neovascular fronds or fibrovascular tissue. This complication is due to thermal contraction and should be avoided. Worsening of preexisting macular edema may be prevented by treating the macular edema first in eyes requiring treatment for both macular edema and proliferative diabetic retinopathy. General recommendations for PRP include treating in multiple sessions and avoiding confluent treatment.

## VASCULAR LESIONS

Treatment of vascular lesions, macroaneurysms, telangiectasias, and vascular malformations can result in subretinal or preretinal bleeding, fibrosis, and increased exudate (Fig. 54-4). Treating larger vascular anomalies is more challenging. Treatment of retinal angiomas can result in fibrosis, severe bleeding, serous retinal detachment, and retinal vessel occlusions. The serous retinal detachment can be total but may be transient. Direct and feeder vessel treatment of angiomas with dye yellow laser may help reduce severe complications (30). Frequently, particularly with large lesions, treatment is unsuccessful and the tumors continue to grow or result in a total retinal detachment.

## CHOROIDAL TUMORS

Choroidal hemangioma and choroidal malignant melanoma are tumors that may be treated with photocoagulation. Choroidal hemangiomas are usually treated when a secondary serous retinal detachment occurs (31). Treatment with conventional photocoagulation and with TTT has been described (32). Treatment of the lesion may cause transient increased exudate and decreased visual acuity.

Very small choroidal melanomas may be treated with photocoagulation. Complications of treatment with argon or krypton include cystoid macular edema, branch vein occlusion, optic atrophy, foveal burns, and vitreous hemorrhage from neovascularization (33) (Fig. 54-5). Larger malignant melanomas are being treated with diode and TTT. Complications are similar to those associated with argon or krypton treatment and include visual field defects and increased serous detachment (34,35).

## RETINAL PERIPHERAL PATHOLOGY

Treatment of peripheral tears, lattice degeneration, and localized retinal detachment can result in bleeding, peripheral retinal atrophy, and resultant holes which become apparent if a redetachment occurs. Lower energies are required when treating the retinal periphery.

## VEIN OCCLUSION

In 1995 McAllister described creating a laser chorioretinal anastomosis for the treatment of nonischemic central retinal vein occlusion (CRVO) (36). Several publications of this treatment modality have shown variable success rates. Complications of

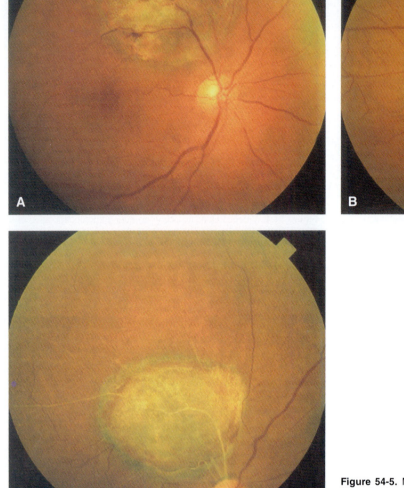

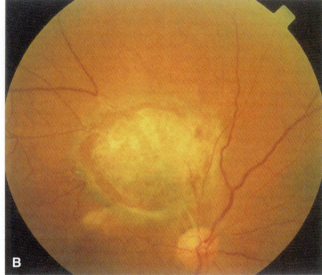

**Figure 54-5.** MM and occlusion (Virgilio). A small choroidal melanoma (**A**, pretreatment) may be treated with photocoagulation. Following treatment (**B, C**), a vein occlusion had occurred.

the procedure include neovascular complications in 20%, ischemia, fibrous proliferation, vitreous hemorrhage, traction retinal detachment, neovascular glaucoma, and macular pigmentary changes. Massive fibrosis and traction retinal detachment requiring vitrectomy has been described (37–41). The benefit and indication of this new treatment modality is currently under investigation.

## LASER WAVELENGTHS

Different lasers and delivery systems have diverse potential complications. Lasers with shorter wavelengths cause an increased effect on the superficial retina. These include argon blue-green, green, and dye yellow lasers. These lasers cause more apparent burns with increased whitening of the retina and can affect the NFL and cause contraction of the retinal surface. Dye yellow, orange and red, krypton, and diode lasers

have longer wavelengths. Longer wavelength lasers penetrate deeper and have an increased effect in the outer retina, RPE, and choriocapillaris. These lasers have an increased ability to penetrate subretinal hemorrhage and coagulate the choroid. When treatment was applied over subretinal blood, argon caused whitening of the overlying retina, krypton caused a faint graying and diode showed no effect. Diode penetrated the subretinal blood and had a coagulation effect on the choroid without visible changes on the retina (42). The increased penetration of these lasers causes less damage to the inner retina, but can result in increased damage to Bruch's membrane and the choriocapillaris. They produce little retinal reaction when applied and the surgeon may use more intensity than necessary. Deeper penetration also causes more pain, particularly when treating the peripheral retina. Pain with diode can be reduced by modifying the laser waveform, or by using anesthesia (43).

Blue-green argon is not recommended, particularly when treating the foveal area or eyes with nuclear sclerosis lens opacities. The blue wavelength can be absorbed by the lens, causing opacities, and by the foveal xanthophyll resulting in foveal damage. Yellow dye has been recommended for foveal treatment because of its decreased xanthophyll effect, but little clinical difference has been seen in comparison to argon green or dye red (44,45). The only difference found between argon blue-green and dye orange in PRP treatment was that orange dye caused more pain (46). Yellow dye is recommended for the treatment of angiomas (30). When argon and krypton were compared for treatment of subfoveal SRNVM's, the only significant difference noted was a smaller loss of reading speed with argon green (14). No difference was noted when argon and diode were compared (47).

## DELIVERY SYSTEMS

Slit lamp delivery through a contact lens has been the standard treatment. It allows for precise focusing, good visualization, and ease of application. Improved contact lenses with advanced optics have simplified treatments. Limitations include a restricted view of the anterior retina, poor visualization at gas interfaces in gas-filled eyes, and the inability to treat patients in a recumbent position.

The laser indirect delivery system is useful in treating retinopathy of prematurity, bedridden patients, anterior retinal pathology, and allows for ease of delivery through intravitreal gas. It is also highly portable and can be used during vitreous and scleral buckling surgery. Complications with its use include corneal, iris, and lens burns, particularly in ROP treatment. Other complications are retinal, preretinal, vitreous or choroidal hemorrhage, foveal burns, preretinal membrane formation, and late onset retinal detachment (48).

Delivery through endoprobes allows for precise treatment during vitrectomy surgery. Caveats include difficulty in producing small size burns making treatment in the foveal area more challenging. Spot size and intensity vary widely relative to the distance of the probe from the retina, making bleeding, vessel occlusions, and retinal breaks possible. This may be more common when treating through air since the heat diffusing properties of fluid are lacking. Poor visibility can be a problem, particularly when treating through air with media opacities present. Endophotocoagulation through microendoscopes is also available and aids with visibility problems (49). Lens opacities from inadvertent trauma with the laser probe can also occur, causing significant cataract change.

Transscleral diode allows for delivery through the sclera and through preexisting exoplants. Possible complications include punctate choroidal hemorrhages, breaks in Bruch's membrane, large hemorrhages, and a scleral thermal effect (50). Incidence of complications tends to reduce with the experience of the surgeon (51).

TTT is a treatment modality with diode laser that allows for thermal damage to tumors and other lesions. It is used in the treatment of melanoma, choroidal hemangiomas, retinoblastomas, and more recently in ARMD. Complications include vessel occlusions, hemorrhage, optic nerve damage, iris atrophy, lens opacities, and retinal fibrosis (2,32–35).

New laser modalities, expanding delivery systems and novel applications of laser energy have vastly expanded our armamentarium for the treatment of eye disease in the 50 years since Meyer-Schwikerath's initial description of xenon arc light coagulation. The minimal invasiveness of laser treatment has significant advantages and appeal. The morbidity, cost, and numerous complications of incisional surgery are avoided. Nevertheless, complications are possible but many can be avoided with meticulous technique, experience, and careful selection of patients and treatment modality. We can expect an exponential expansion of laser technology in the new millennium broadening our ability to fight disease.

## References

1. Meyer-Schwickerath G. *Light Coagulation*. St. Louis: C.V. Mosby, 1961.
2. Mainster M. Wavelength selection in macular photocoagulation: tissue optics, thermal effects, and laser systems. *Ophthalmology* 1981;93:952.
3. McCanna P, Chandra S, Stevens T, et al. Argon laser-induced cataract as a complication of retinal photocoagulation. *Arch Ophthalmology* 1982;100:1071.
4. Cartwright MJ, Blair CJ, Stratford TP. Krypton laser-induced lens opacity as a complication of retinal photocoagulation. *Ann Ophthalmol* 1990;22:463.
5. Lewis H, Schachat A, Haimann M, et al. Choroidal neovascularization after laser photocoagulation for diabetic macular edema. *Ophthalmol* 1990;97:503.
6. Pollack A, Heriot W, Henkind P. Cellular processes causing defects in Bruch's membrane following krypton laser photocoagulation. *Ophthalmol* 1986; 93:1113.
7. Varley M, Frank E, Purnell E. Subretinal neovascularization after focal argon laser for diabetic macular edema. *Ophthalmol* 1988;95:567.
8. Berger A, Boniuk I. Bilateral subretinal neovascularization after focal laser photocoagulation for diabetic macular edema. *Am J Ophthalmol* 1989;108:88.
9. Olk R. Modified grid argon (blue-green) laser photocoagulation for diffuse diabetic macular edema. *Ophthalmol* 1986;93:938–950.
10. Schatz H, Madeira D, McDonald H, et al. Progressive enlargement of laser scars following grid laser photocoagulation for diffuse diabetic macular edema. *Arch Opthalmol* 1991;109:1549.
11. Christoffersen N, Sander B, Larsen M. Precipitation of hard exudate after resorption of intraretinal edema after treatment of retinal branch vein occlusion. *Am J Ophthalmol* 1998;126:454.
12. Schatz H, Yannuzzi L, Gitter K. Subretinal neovascularization following argon laser photocoagulation for central serous chorioretinopathy: complication or misdiagnosis? *Tr Am Acad Ophthalmol Otoryng* 1977;83:893.
13. Macular Photocoagulation Study (MPS) Group. Evaluation of argon green versus krypton red laser for photocoagulation of subfoveal choroidal neovascularization in the macular photocoagulation study. *Arch Ophthalmol* 1994;112:1176–1184.
14. Johnson DA, Yannuzzi LA, Shakin JL, et al. Lacquer cracks following laser treatment of choroidal neovascularization in pathologic myopia. *Retina* 1998;18:118.
15. Blondeau P, Pavan P, Phelps C. Acute pressure elevation following panretinal photocoagulation. *Arch Ophthalmol* 1981;99:1239.
16. Mensher J. Anterior chamber depth alteration after retinal photocoagulation. *Arch Opthalmol* 1977;95:113.
17. Boulton P. A study of the mechanism of transient myopia following extensive xenon arc photocoagulation. *Trans Ophthalmol Soc UK* 1974;93:287.
18. Huamonte F, Peyman G, Goldberg M, et al. Immediate fundus complications after retinal scatter photocoagulation. I. Clinical picture and pathogenesis. *Ophthalmol Surg* 1976;7:88.
19. Gentile RC, Stegman Z, Liebmann JM, et al. Risk factors for ciliochoroidal effusion after panretinal photocoagulation. *Ophthalmology* 1996;103:827.
20. Yuki T, Kimura Y, Nanbu S, et al. Ciliary body and choroidal detachment after laser photocoagulation for diabetic retinopathy. A high-frequency ultrasound study. *Ophthalmology* 1997;104:1259.
21. Hessemer V, Schmidt KG. Influence of panretinal photocoagulation on the ocular pulse curve. *Am J Ophthalmol* 1997;123:748.
22. Doft B, Blankenship G. Single versus multiple treatment sessions of argon laser photocoagulation for proliferative diabetic retinopathy. *Ophthalmol* 1982;89:772.
23. Early Treatment Diabetic Retinopathy Study Research Group. Early photocoagulation for diabetic retinopathy. Report no 9. *Ophthalmol* 1991;98:766–785.
24. The Diabetic Retinopathy Study Research Group. Photocoagulation of proliferative diabetic retinopathy: clinical applications of Diabetic Retinopathy Study findings. Report no 8. *Ophthalmol* 1981;88:583–600.
25. Schulenberg W, Hamilton M, Blach RK. A comparative study of argon laser and krypton laser in the treatment of diabetic optic disc neovascularization. *Br J Ophthalmol* 1979;63:412.

26. Birch-Cox J. Defective colour vision in diabetic retinopathy before and after laser photocoagulation. *Mod Probl Ophthalmol* 1978;19:326.

27. Striph G, Hart W, Olk R. Modified grid laser photocoagulation for diabetic macular edema. The effect on the central visual field. *Ophthalmol* 1988;95:1673.

28. Lerner B, Lakhanpal V, Schocket S. Transient myopia and accommodative paresis following cryotherapy and panretinal photocoagulation. *Am J Ophthalmol* 1984;97:704.

29. Blodi CF, Russell SR, Pulido JS, et al. Direct and feeder vessel photocoagulation of retinal angiomas with dye yellow laser. *Ophthalmology* 1990;97:791–795; discussion 796.

30. Gass J. *Differential diagnosis of intraocular tumors.* St. Louis: CV Mosby, 1974.

31. García-Arumí J. Transpupillary thermotherapy (TTT) in circumscribed choroidal hemangiomas, Annual Meeting American Academy of Ophthalmology, New Orleans, 1998.

32. Qiang Z, Cairns JD. Laser photocoagulation treatment of choroidal melanoma. *Aust N Z J Ophthalmol* 1993;21:87.

33. Oosterhuis J, Journée-de Korver H, Kakebeeke-Keeme H, et al. Transpupillary thermotherapy in choroidal melanomas. *Arch Ophthalmol* 1995;113:315.

34. Shields C, Shields J, De Potter P, et al. Transpupillary thermotherapy in the management of choroidal melanoma. *Ophthalmol* 1996;103:1642.

35. McAllister I, Constable I. Laser-induced chorioretinal venous anastomosis for treatment of non-ischemic CRVO. *Arch Ophthalmol* 1995;113:456–462.

36. McAllister IL, Douglas JP, Constable IJ, et al. Laser-induced chorioretinal venous anastomosis for nonischemic central retinal vein occlusion: evaluation of the complications and their risk factors. *Am J Ophthalmol* 1998;126:219.

37. Fekrat S, Goldberg MF, Finkelstein D. Laser-induced chorioretinal venous anastomosis for nonischemic central or branch retinal vein occlusion. *Arch Ophthalmol* 1998;116:43.

38. Luttrull JK. Epiretinal membrane and traction retinal detachment complicating laser-induced chorioretinal venous anastomosis. *Am J Ophthalmol* 1997;123:698.

39. Aktan SG, Subasi M, Akbatur H, et al. Problems of chorioretinal venous anastomosis by laser for treatment of nonischemic central retinal vein occlusion. *Ophthalmologica* 1998;212:389.

40. Browning DJ, Antoszyk AN. Laser chorioretinal venous anastomosis for nonischemic central retinal vein occlusion. *Ophthalmology* 1998;105:670–677; discussion 677–679.

41. Johnson MW, Hassan TS, Elner VM. Laser photocoagulation of the choroid through experimental subretinal hemorrhage. *Arch Ophthalmol* 1995;113:364.

42. Friberg TR, Venkatesh S. Alteration of pulse configuration affects the pain response during diode laser photocoagulation. *Lasers Surg Med* 1995;16:380.

43. Browning DJ, Antoszyk AN. The effect of the surgeon and the laser wavelength on the response to focal photocoagulation for diabetic macular edema. *Ophthalmology* 1999;106:243.

44. Atmaca LS, Idil A, Gunduz K. Dye laser treatment in proliferative diabetic retinopathy and maculopathy. *Acta Ophthalmol Scand* 1995;73:303.

45. Seiberth V, Schatanek S, Alexandridis E. Panretinal photocoagulation in diabetic retinopathy: argon versus dye laser coagulation. *Graefes Arch Clin Exp Ophthalmol* 1993;231:318.

46. Tewari HK, Gupta V, Kumar A, et al. Efficacy of diode laser for managing diabetic macular oedema. *Acta Ophthalmol Scand* 1998;76:363.

47. Hunt L. Complications of indirect laser photocoagulation. *Insight* 1994;19:24.

48. Uram M. Ophthalmic laser microendoscope endophotocoagulation. *Ophthalmology* 1992;99:1829.

49. McHugh DA, Schwartz S, Dowler JG, et al. Diode laser contact transscleral retinal photocoagulation: a clinical study. *Br J Ophthalmol* 1995;79:1083.

50. Haller JA, Blair N, de Juan E Jr, et al. Transscleral diode laser retinopexy in retinal detachment surgery: results of a multicenter trial. *Retina* 1998;18:399.

51. Berrocal A, Reichel E, Ip M, et al. Transpupillary thermotherapy of occult subfoveal choroidal neovascular membranes in patients with age-related macular degeneration. *Invest Ophthalmol Vis Sci* 1999;40(Suppl):1701.

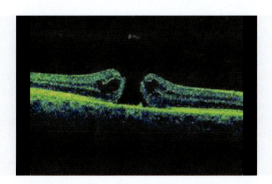

# Complications of Macular Surgery

Ximena Vazquez ■ Eric P. Jablon ■ John B. Kerrison
Monica Rodriguez-Fontal ■ D. Virgil Alfaro III

The advent of small-gauge vitreous surgery has produced new forms of intraoperative and postoperative complications of pars plana vitrectomy. The reader is well aware that vitreous surgery increases the rate of cataract formation, related to vitreous aquadynamics, vitreous changes, and decreasing temperatures of the vitreous cavity, all thought to play a role in postoperative cataract. Patients should be properly educated on this fact as macular surgery is discussed.

The goals of this chapter are to elucidate the many complications of small-gauge surgery and to provide logical and helpful information on how to resolve these issues as they present during surgery.

## COMPLICATIONS OF TROCAR PLACEMENT

The goals of trochar placement are to provide access to vitreoretinal pathology via self-sealing wounds. The surgeon should determine at what clock hours to place the trochars based upon the vitreoretinal pathology at hand. For instance, a retinal detachment with a horseshoe tear at 12 o'clock will require laser surrounding the break; trochar placement at 3 and 9 o'clock will facilitate access to the tear during endolaser.

An intact conjunctiva after vitreous surgery is helpful to a speedy postoperative recovery and in diminishing the risk of postoperative endophthalmitis. We prefer gentle manipulation of the conjunctiva with a cotton-tipped applicator, since it easily displaces the conjunctiva and allows for globe stabilization while the trochar is placed. In aphakic and pseudophakic patients the trochar is placed 3.5 mm posterior to the surgical limbus; the length 4.0 mm is measured from the surgical limbus in phakic eyes patients.

Currently, three systems are used internationally: Alcon, Bausch and Lomb, and Dorc. All three recommend trochar placement that suggests the formation of a shelved, self-sealing wound that is produced after the trochars are removed. The reader should determine the exact angle used for entering the eye as well as subtle trochar manipulation that ensure surgical goals. During placement, the trochar tip should be pointed toward the midvitreous cavity, since these authors have injured the crystalline lens with the trochars during placement.

Small-gauge infusion cannulae are not sutured to the eye wall, resulting in several potential issues during surgery. We have found that taping the canula into proper position after it is connected to the trochar is a significant step in the setup for small-gauge surgery. The weight of the infusion tubing may cause the tip of the infusion canula to point toward the anterior segment of the eye during surgery, irritating the iris and causing intraoperative miosis. These authors have also encountered an inordinately deep anterior chamber, intraocular lens (IOL) malpositioning, damage to the crystalline lens, iridodialysis, hyphema, and iris trauma from an improperly placed infusion canula.

Subretinal canula tips and canula tips located in the suprachoroidal space have been documented during small-gauge surgery. They both represent potentially catastrophic problems and should be prevented by ensuring trochar and canula placement before starting infusion. A subretinal canula tip is made apparent by subretinal gas bubbles or a billowing retinal detachment. After the canula tip has been determined to be in the subretinal space, infusion is stopped immediately. Plugs are placed to prevent hypotony. The infusion canula trochar is removed and the surgeon determines where to place it so that infusion can be restarted. If a total retinal detachment has developed and the patient is phakic, perfluorocarbon liquid may be implemented to stabilize the retina until the infusion trochar canula is repositioned. Subretinal infusion canula tips are often associated with retinal tears, with the breaks located in the same clock hour as the canula.

Suprachoroidal placement of the canula tip may be diagnosed by the presence of a choroidal effusion with or without choroidal hemorrhage. This is more commonly seen in eyes with more severe vitreoretinal disease such as retinal detachment and choroidal effusions from hypotony. Repositioning of the canula to an area where the peripheral retina is normal is fundamental in resolving this issue. Subretinal and suprachoroidal placement of the canula can be prevented by understanding the pathoanatomy of the eye and by direct visualization of the canula tip before starting infusion.

## COMPLICATION OF HYALOID SEPARATION

Separation of the posterior hyaloid remains a fundamental step in successful macular surgery. The techniques for separation of the hyaloid have been defined for over a decade and various techniques have been published, all of which involve high and sustained active aspiration over the optic nerve head. The complications related to separation of the hyaloid can be separated into two groups: (a) complications from instrumentation and (b) macular and peripheral retina trauma from a strong vitreoretinal interface.

Several maneuvers are performed during separation of the hyaloid. Initially, the surgeon performs a core vitrectomy. The hyaloid separation is initiated, usually with active aspiration over the optic nerve head. In most cases the vitreous cutter is used without the cutting mode. If hyaloid separation cannot be started with the vitreous cutter, a soft-tipped extrusion canula is used with active and high aspiration. These maneuvers can be done with or without staining of the hyaloid with triamcinolone acetate.

Once the hyaloid separation has been started over the optic nerve head the surgeon uses gentler and lower aspiration to carry the hyaloid separation over the arcades and the midperiphery. In cases with impending macular holes or with vitreofoveal traction syndromes, a full-thickness macular hole may be produced requiring facedown positioning and extended gas tamponade. Inadvertent optic nerve head and macular contusion may occur with hand-held instruments.

Peripheral retinal tears and postoperative retinal detachment are thought to occur in 1% of patients undergoing pars plana vitrectomy for macular holes. Intraoperative hyaloid separation and entering the eye with instruments are the sources of retinal breaks. It is the experience of these authors that the incidence of retinal tears and detachments has diminished from small-gauge surgery. Intraoperatively, many surgeons have noted vitreous base traction as the surgeons enter the eye with instruments, especially soft-tipped canulas, tano diamond-dusted scrapers, and other instruments with soft, silicone-based finishes. Peripheral collagen fibers and peripheral hyaloid adhere to these instruments causing retinal tears and holes just posterior to the sclerostomies. It is our opinion that small-gauge instruments with trochars diminish the risk of peripheral retinal breaks since the sleeves of the trochars allow the surgical instruments to access into the vitreous cavity beyond the collage fibers of the vitreous base.

Careful examination of the peripheral retina and treatment of peripheral pathology remains the single-most effective way of preventing postoperative retinal detachment in patients who have undergone macular surgery

Several articles published in the literature have demonstrating the histological changes that take place.

## COMPLICATIONS OF INTERNAL LIMITING MEMBRANE PEEL

Dr. Logan Brooks is credited with the advent and popularization of internal limiting membrane (ILM) removal as a means of improving results in patients undergoing macular surgery. In 1995, he presented his techniques for peeling the ILM as an adjunct to macular hole surgery. In a nonrandomized study, he noted a higher success rate of macular hole closure in patients undergoing pars plana vitrectomy with peeling of the ILM (1). Logan noted that visualization of the ILM during surgery made its removal difficult and that its complete removal was often impossible to verify.

At the American Academy of Ophthalmology meeting in 1999, Kim and colleagues presented their techniques utilizing indocyanine green to stain the ILM during macular hole surgery. They noted improved visualization of the ILM, reporting that complete removal of the ILM was more easily verified using indocyanine green (ICG). Later, Kadnonosono and Burk published their results supporting information presented at the American Academy of Ophthalmology meeting (2).

Numerous articles have since been published outlining advantages of using ICG as an adjunct to macular hole surgery, claiming hole closure rates from 88% to 97% and improvement of visual acuity in more than 88% of eyes. However, in separate reports, Engerecht and Haritoglou showed poor postoperative visual outcomes in cases in which ICG was used (3). In a nonrandomized clinical trial, Gass and Kampik evaluated the postoperative results in patients undergoing macular hole surgery repair with and without the use of ICG, noting a higher rate of hole closure and better postoperative vision in those eyes in which ICG was not utilized for ILM staining (4). Ohji and colleagues published their results of eyes undergoing macular hole repair with and without the use of ICG, reporting similar outcomes of hole closure and postoperative vision in the two groups (5).

Macular toxicity from the use of ICG has not been proven. However, many have documented visual field defects and changes to the retinal pigment epithelium associated with the use of ICG during macular surgery. Haritgolou and Uemura reported nasal visual field defects in 35% of patients undergoing macular surgery for macular holes and epiretinal membranes (6). Later Uemura changed his technique for ILM

staining with ICG to determine whether decreasing the time in which ICG was in contact with the macular surface might alter the number of patients with postoperative visual field defects. He noted a higher percentage of visual field defects in eyes where the ICG was in contact with the macula for 3 minutes versus those eyes that had immediate aspiration of the ICG. Based on these findings. Uemura recommends the use of ICG such that its contact with macular surface is limited (7).

Persistence of ICG in the visual system after its use in the staining of the ILM has been documented by several authors. Machida and colleagues found persistence of ICG up to 1 year after macular surgery (8). Multifocal electroretinograms (ERGs) performed by Weinberger failed to show electrophysiologic abnormalities in patients in whom digital photographic studies showed persistence of ICG. Interestingly, although persistence of ICG has been shown in the fovea of patients who have undergone ICG-assisted macular surgery, visual outcomes of these patients have been similar to those who underwent macular hole repair without ICG staining (9). Tano and his team also injected ICG into the vitreous cavity of rabbits and performed histologic studies of the optic nerves, noting that ICG traveled up to 6 mm into the optic nerves, using an extraaxonal mechanism. ICG failed to reach the chiasm and brain of these animals (10).

Various factors may cause retinal injury during macular surgery, including light toxicity and mechanical trauma from instruments. These authors suspect that many presumed cases of ICG toxicity of the macula are more likely from trauma induced by the surgeon during ILM peel. Peeling of the ILM remains a difficult procedure requiring excellent visualization, high-quality instrumentation, and experience. Less experienced macular surgeons cause macular injury during manipulation of the ILM: Xenon light sources are a known source of macular trauma; this is especially true when the surgeon has difficulty starting the ILM peel and spends an excessive amount of time achieving surgical goals.

The surgeon must be cognizant of the known risks of phototoxicity during ILM peel and epimacular membrane. We suggest that surgeons aim the light energy at the macular area only during the actual peeling process.

### References

1. Brooks HL Jr. Macular hole surgery with and without internal limiting membrane peeling. *Ophthalmology* 2000;107:1939–1948.
2. Kadonosono K, Itah N, Uchio E, et al. Staining of internal limiting membrane in macular hole surgery. *Arch Ophtahlmol* 2000;118:1116–1118.
3. Haritoglou C, Gandofer A, Gass CA, et al. Indocyanine green-assisted peeling of the internal limiting membrane in macular hole surgery affects visual outcome: a clinicopathologic correlation. *Am J Ophthalmol* 2002;134:836–841.
4. Gass CA, Haritoglou C, Schaumberger M, et al. Functional outcome of macular hole surgery with and without indocyanine green-assisted peeling of the internal limiting membrane. *Graefes Arch Clin Exp Ophthalmol* 2003;241:716–720.
5. Kusaka S, Oshita T, Ohji M, et al. Reduction of the toxic effect of indocyanine green on retinal pigment epithelium during macular hole surgery. *Retina* 2003;23:733–734.
6. Uemura A, Kanda S, Sakamoto Y, et al. Visual field defects after uneventful vitrectomy for epiretinal membrane with indocyanine green-assisted internal limiting membrane peeling. *Am J Ophthalmol* 2003;136:252–257.
7. Shigeru K, Akinori U, Takehiro Y, et al. Visual field defects after intravitreous administration of indocyanine green in macular hole surgery. *Arch Ophthalmol* 2004;122:1447–1451.
8. Machida S, Fujiwara T, Gotoh T, et al. Observation of the ocular fundus by an infrared-sensitive video camera after vitreoretinal surgery assisted by indocyanine green. *Retina* 2003;23(2):183–191.
9. Weinberger AW, Kirchhof B, Mazinani BE, et al. Persistent indocyanine green (ICG) fluorescence 6 weeks after intraocular ICG administration for macular hole surgery. *Graefes Arch Clin Exp Ophthalmol* 2001;239(5):388–390.
10. Cekiç O, Morimoto T, Ohji M, et al. Nonaxoplasmic transfer of indocyanine green into the optic nerve after intravitreal application. *Retina* 2004;24(3):412–415.

# Frontiers in Macular Surgery

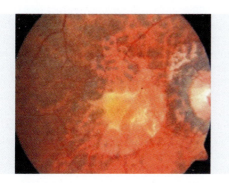

# Autologous Transplantation of the Retinal Pigment Epithelium and Choroid in the Treatment of Age-Related Macular Degeneration

Antonio López Bolaños ■ Rosa Evangelina Garnica Hayashi

In the daily practice of ophthalmology, we encounter diseases whose treatments escape our hands. The physiopathology of these diseases includes damage or atrophy of retinal pigment epithelium (RPE), retinitis pigmentosa, geographic atrophy in age-related macular degeneration (AMD), RPE tears, and disciform scars.

## RETINAL PIGMENT EPITHELIUM

There are approximately 3.5 million RPE cells in the adult human eye (1). The RPE cells are located between the neural retina and the vascular choroid and play a critical role in the maintenance of visual function. The functions of the RPE include phagocytosis of shed photoreceptor outer segments, metabolism of retinol, formation of the outer blood-retinal barrier, maintenance of the extracellular matrix, and regulation of ion and metabolite transport.

The RPE cells engulf and degrade shed rod outer segments at a very high rate: one human RPE cell will ingest and degrade about 3000 million discs during a 70 year lifespan. The apical surface of the RPE cells interface with the outer segments of the photoreceptors, while the RPE basal domain is attached firmly to the underlying Bruch's membrane. The basement membrane of the RPE represents the innermost layer of Bruch's membrane. RPE cells exhibit regional differences in morphology and function. In the macula, RPE cells are smaller and columnar in appearance, while in the periphery, they are larger and cuboidal.

In RPE cultures, the enzymatic capacity of RPE cells has been shown to be age independent (2), contrary to what may occur *in vivo*, where with age, degradation of outer segments of the photoreceptors appears to be diminished. With age and pathologic changes in the human eye, degradation of outer segment materials within the phagolysosomes may lead to the formation of lipofuscin granules composed of outer segments of the photoreceptors residue (3,4). In response to injury or certain alterations in the microenvironment, RPE cells, which *in situ* do not proliferate, may detach from their substratum, migrate, proliferate, and acquire a macrophage-like or fibroblast-like morphology (5,6). These morphologic and functional changes, associated with alterations on gene expression, may be referred to as activation. Activation events include physical trauma with displacement to a new environment, accumulation of intraocular blood, breakdown of the blood-retinal barrier with inflammatory cell infiltration, alteration of components of the extracellular matrix, alterations in choroidal circulation, and diffusion of oxygen to the RPE layer.

RPE shows specific features associated with aging. The proportion of apoptotic human RPE cells increases significantly with age, and these apoptotic cells are confined mainly to the macula (7). Peripheral RPE cells may compensate for the death of macular RPE cells. Furthermore, cells become more irregular in size and shape, deposits of RPE-derived material accumulate in Bruch's membrane and lipofuscin appears in the cells' cytoplasm (8–13).

## ADVANCES IN TREATMENT OF AGE-RELATED MACULAR DEGENERATION

Nowadays, the possibility of rebuilding a damaged retina has been subject of widespread research. The field of AMD treatment has witnessed a number of significant advances.

AMD is a progressive disease of the macula that in its late or advanced stage results in loss of central vision. Visual loss in late AMD is a consequence of one of two processes that cause photoreceptor dysfunction- geographic atrophy or choroidal neovascularization (CNV). In geographic atrophy, there is confluent atrophy of the choriocapillaries and associated RPE. In CNV, an ingrowth of new vessels occurs from the choriocapillaries that breaches Bruch's membrane and the RPE to invade the retina. These fenestrated and friable new vessels leak serous fluid, lipids, and blood below and into the neural retina, with subsequent fibrous scarring, which defines the late stage of AMD. This scarring is called disciform scar and is generally associated with the loss of neural tissue from the retina. The dysfunction as well as death of photoreceptors is a major contributor to vision loss in AMD. Other types of retinal neuronal cells affected secondarily because of the loss of photoreceptors also lead to visual loss.

The disciform scars are classified anatomically as subneurosensory retinal, sub-RPE, or combined. Subneurosensory retinal lesions are defined by the absence of the RPE interposed between the lesion and the remaining retinal tissue.

There are no preventive treatments, however, there is some evidence that antioxidant vitamin and mineral supplementation can slow down the progression of the disease in people with moderate AMD.

In the beginning of the 1980's, the Macular Photocoagulation Study Group reported favorable outcomes for thermal laser photocoagulation in a small proportion of eyes with well-delineated (or classic) small extrafoveal and juxtafoveal CNV lesions, but less favorable outcomes in patients with subfoveal CNV lesions due to the likelihood of immediate and severe vision loss from the laser treatment (14–16). In the 1990's, introduction of photodynamic therapy with verteporfin expanded the therapeutic options available to patients with subfoveal CNV, offering them the possibility of exudative AMD treatment. However, the treatment is not accompanied with improvement in visual acuity and can also cause some degree of retinal damage (17).

The role of surgery in the treatment of CNV-complicated AMD remains controversial. Although submacular removal of CNV was not favored in the randomized submacular surgery trials, patients who underwent hemorrhagic CNV showed significantly reduced risk of severe visual acuity loss and contrast sensitivity loss compared to the control patients after 24 months of follow-up (18,19). Subfoveal membranectomy almost always results in the removal of the native RPE along with the choroidal neovascular complex in AMD eyes and leads to the development or progression of atrophy of the subfoveal choriocapillaris.

Other surgical treatments for AMD include pneumatic displacement of submacular blood with or without intravitreal or subretinal injection of recombinant tissue plasminogen activator and translocation of the macula to an extramacular and healthier RPE area (Machemer 1993). Macular translocation seems to stabilize and sometimes even improve visual acuity (20,21). However, full macular translocation bears a considerable risk of proliferative vitreoretinopathy (PVR), diplopia, and macular edema.

Given the recent number of anti-VEGF therapies that have demonstrated efficacy in studies, the repertoire of treatments for neovascular AMD has significantly expanded. Bevacizumab, a full-length recombinant humanized monoclonal antibody against VEGF has been effective in AMD treatment (22–24). Pegaptanib and ranibizumab have also been shown to be effective in large clinical trials. However, there are some patients who do not respond favorably to such anti-VEGF treatment (25,26).

For patients with geographic atrophy in AMD, RPE tears, or disciform scars, the treatment available is still under discussion. Currently, studies are investigating the effect of RPE transplantation.

Transplantation of RPE in AMD was first performed by Algvere et al. (27,28) by using heterologous fetal RPE. Unfortunately, all eyes developed macular edema, most likely as a result of host-graft rejection. Visual acuity declined and foveal fixation was lost in all patients. Iris pigment epithelium (IPE) was easily accessible; however, its functionality has not been established. Although the short-term results have been promising, there have been no long-term benefits. This led to the assumption that the transplantation of an intact monolayer is required to achieve a functional transplant.

Peyman et al. (29) first suggested translocation of peripheral choroid and RPE. Others later demonstrated the clinical feasibility of the new technique (30–32).

## RETINAL PIGMENT EPITHELIUM TRANSPLANTATION

Regenerating RPE cells by stem-cell therapy is a promising avenue for rebuild the damaged retina. Stem-cells are defined as pluripotent cells capable of differentiating into a variety of cell types and, under appropriate conditions, into a variety of tissues, including muscle, kidney, brain, blood, liver, skin, and retina. Stem cells can be divided into those that are isolated from fetal material (embryonic stem cells) and those from adult tissue (adult stem cells). The former are typically isolated from blastocysts and have pluripotency; that is, that they can give rise to virtually any adult tissue cell type under appropriate conditions. Adult-derived stem cells typically reside in adult tissues in a quiescent, undifferentiated state and under appropriate stimuli will divide and differentiate into the cell type of the tissue in which they reside or if appropriately stimulated into other cell types., It is however, not entirely clear whether this is a result of a stem cell differentiating into the end cell product or if this occurs by somatic cell fusion between the "stem" cell and a population of differentiated, postmitotic, tissue-specific cells that then share the stem cell's proliferative capabilities as well as their own tissue-specific phenotypic characteristics (33–34).

Damaged RPE cells and associated atrophy are hallmarks of AMD and heroic surgical approaches (35–37) have been considered to provide photoreceptors in such individuals with healthier RPE-rich regions of the retina through retinal translocation and the insertion of RPE sheets. As RPE cells do not require synaptic reconnection, RPE transplantation may be less complex than that of photoreceptors and retinal neurons. To date, researchers have translocated RPE tissue into the fovea of AMD patients after choroidal neovascular membrane removal (38). Patients maintained foveal fixation early, but central visual function was found to be transient, with a decline in 5 to 6 years (39). Another group transplanted autologous RPE cells harvested from the nasal retina to the macular region in patients with AMD. This technique led to clinical benefit in some patients, but there was difficulty in collecting a sufficient number of autologous RPE cells (40). Autologous RPE transplants also have the disadvantage of carrying the same genetic predisposition that led to the original disease state.

Allograft RPE transplanted with the goal of treating retinal degeneration and preserving retinal function (41).

## METHOD OF TRANSPLANTATION OF AUTOLOGOUS RETINAL PIGMENT EPITHELIUM CHOROID

Peyman et al. first reported the translocation of a free full-thickness autologous graft consisting of RPE, Bruch's membrane, choriocapillaris and choroid taken from the paramacular region in one patient (29). This approach was refined by others (38,42). Van Meurs pioneered a technique to cut out the graft from the midperiphery (42).

Patients with either subfoveal lesions or geographic atrophy that was a result of AMD, are candidates for the autologous RPE transplants accomplishment. The central reason for joint transplantation of the RPE and choroid is that, besides the epithelial damage, such patients also show ailment of the Bruch's membrane and the choriocapillaris.

We recommend phacoemulsification in all patients before vitrectomy. (Fig. 56-1A) After the induction of a posterior vitreous detachment and a complete vitrectomy, it is very important to perform a good shaving of the vitreous base.

If necessary, depending on the case, the disciform scar can be removed from the subretinal space through a paramacular retinotomy in the temporal raphe in direction of the nervous fibers (Fig. 56-1B–C). Hydro dissection can be used for macular detachment and for preparing the place where the graft will be placed.

After a rectangle is marked with laser photocoagulation in the midperiphery, always at the superiors sectors and removal of the retina within the diathermia marks, vitreous scissors were used to cut an autologous peripheral full-thickness patch of RPE, Bruch membrane, and choroid. (Fig. 56-1D–F). The size of the graft is determined by the size of the macular atrophy.

The graft of the autologous RPE choroid is taken to the subretinal space and repositioned under the macula through the existing paramacular retinotomy (Fig. 56-1G). Perfluorocarbon liquid (PFCL) is injected to keep the graft in place

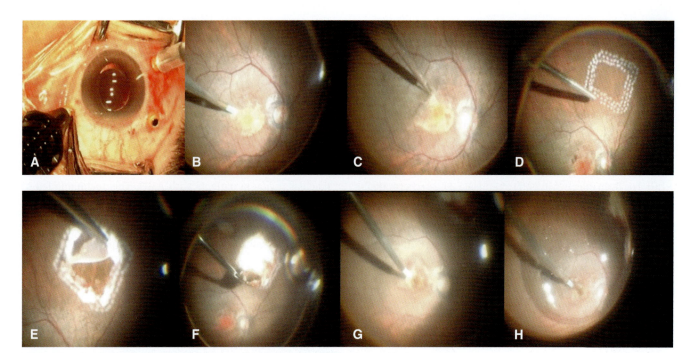

**Figure 56-1.** Surgical technique of transplantation of autologous retinal pigmentary epithelium choroid.

(Fig. 56-1H). Surgery is completed with gas $C_3F_8$ or silicone-oil tamponade.

Intraoperative complications consist of macular holes, subretinal hemorrhage, and problems in inserting and positioning the patch. Postoperative complications include PVR retinal detachment, subretinal hemorrhage, fibrosis of the patch, failure in revascularization, and macular pucker.

Figure 56-2 shows a patient with disciform scar secondary to AMD after 6-month delay. The visual acuity pre- and post-operation was 2/200 at 3-month follow-up.

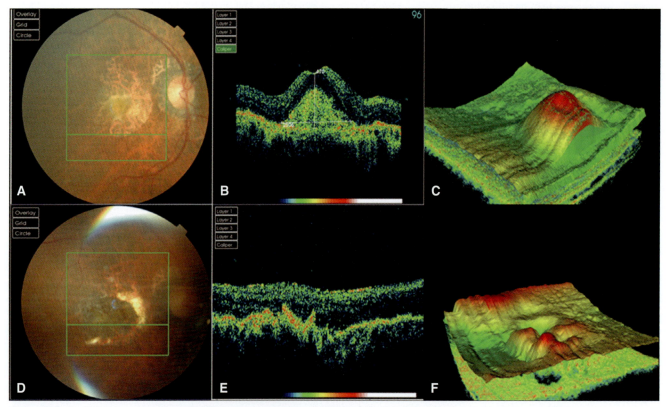

**Figure 56-2. (A–C)** Previous autologous retinal pigmentary epithelium (RPE) transplant. **(A)** Clinic photograph. Disciform scar. **(B)** Optical coherence tomography (OCT) image. Macular disciform scar. **(C)** OCT 3D image. **(D–F)** Posterior to autologous RPE transplantation. **(D)** Image Clinic. Macular graft. **(E)** OCT image. Graft folds. **(F)** OCT 3D image.

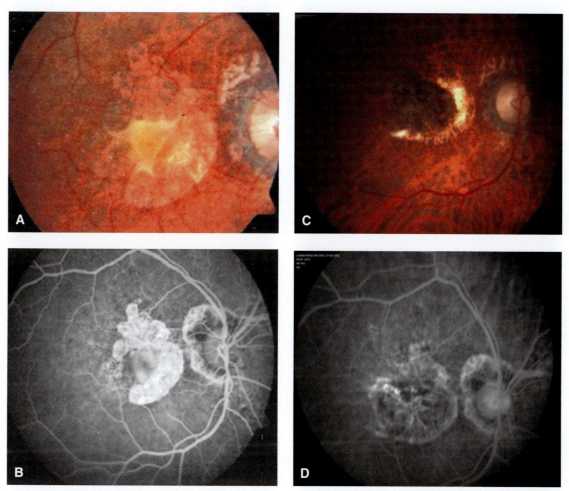

**Figure 56-3. (A–B)** Clinic image with macular disciform scar and fluorangiographic image in the same patient. **(C–D)** Clinic image with macular retinal pigmentary epithelium transplantation and fluorangiographic image. Patch showed good vascularization.

Figure 56-3 shows the same patient with disciform scar secondary to AMD. The fluorangiography shows patch revascularization at 3-month follow-up.

Figure 56-4 shows clinic image and fluorangiographic transplant RPE choroid in one patient with geographic atrophy. Preoperative visual acuity was 3/200, and postoperative visual acuity at 3-month follow-up was 20/200.

Results of studies with the transplantation of autologous RPE – choroids are shown in Table 56-1.

## OBSTACLES AND FUTURE PROSPECTS

Assuming that RPE cells play a primary role in AMD, a tissue block consisting of choroid and the overlaying RPE layer was transplanted. However, it is uncertain if patch translocation has any advantage in the context of the current conservative options in patients with geographic atrophy, fibrotic scar, or RPE tears. The atrophy can be prevented, at least experimentally, by means of RPE transplantation (44). With respect to substitution of Bruch membrane, which is likely to be damaged during membrane removal, combining an intact RPE mono-layer overlaying an intact Bruch membrane seems advantageous.

The results obtained in the diverse studies need to be closely evaluated and in some instances have to be individualized, since there is no uniform pattern in the pathologies treated, preoperative visual acuity, time of evolution of the macular alterations, and surgical techniques. Patients who are well selected and who do not present any complications due to the surgery have a better prognosis and show an increase in visual acuity. The possible causes of the visual decline in patients generally include an inadequate position of the graft (making it extrafoveal), inadequate handling of the graft (handling it as in the atrophic macular area can lead to a mechanical trauma), nonperfusion of the graft, and the presence of severe inflammation.

Fixation on the graft is a major indicator of functional success. Joussen et al. (44) reported improvement in the patients with fixated graft at the last follow-up. Geographic atrophy secondary to AMD shows eccentric fixation in patients with longstanding membranes. Patients with stable fixations before surgery were more likely to maintain stable fixation thereafter (45). Fixation was dependent on visual acuity and on the retinal function.

Fundus microperimetry allowed further evaluation of the functional integrity of the macular area.

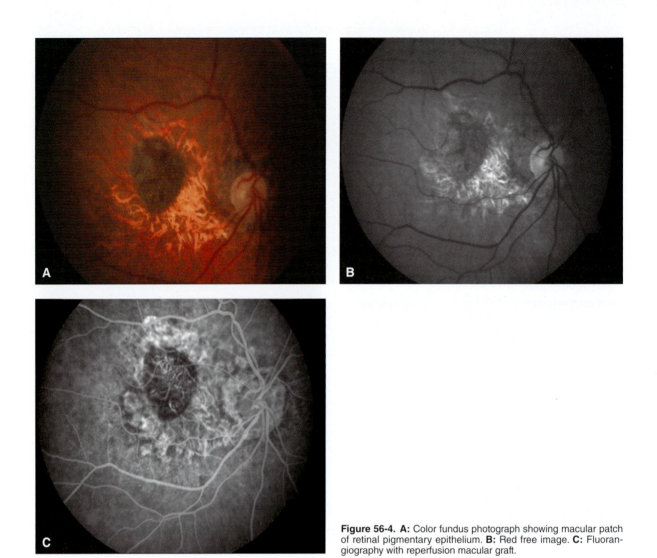

**Figure 56-4. A:** Color fundus photograph showing macular patch of retinal pigmentary epithelium. **B:** Red free image. **C:** Fluorangiography with reperfusion macular graft.

| TABLE 56-1 | RESULTS OF STUDIES WITH THE TRANSPLANTATION OF AUTOLOGOUS RETINAL PIGMENT EPITHELIUM CHOROIDS | | | |
|---|---|---|---|---|
| **Study** | **Caramay 2009 (45)** | **Maaijwee 2007(46)** | **Joussen 2006 (44)** | **Joussen 2007 (47)** |
| **N** | $N = 10$ | $N = 83$ | $N = 45$ | $N = 12$ |
| **Delay time** | 3 months | – | 3 months | 6 months |
| **Pathology** | Geographic atrophy (AMD) | CNV | CNV | Geographic atrophy |
| | | | PED | |
| | | | Subretinal hemorrhage | |
| | | | Geographic atrophy | |
| **Follow-up** | 3 years | 12 months | 6 months | 6 months |
| **Preoperative VA** | 0.6 logMar | 0.95 logMar | 0.85 logMar | 0.6 logMar |
| **Postoperative VA** | 1.0 logMar | 0.89 logMar | 1.2 logMar | 0.98 logMar |
| **Complications** | Epiretinal membrane | Recurrence CNV | RD | PVR |
| | Cystoid macular edema | RD | PVR | Epiretinal membrane |
| | PVR | PVR | Epiretinal membrane | Subretinal hemorrhage |
| | RD | | Fibrosis of the patch | Fibrinous reaction |
| | BRVO | | | Failure revascularization graft |
| | Hypotension | | | |

AMD, age-related macular degeneration; CNV, choroidal neovascularization; PED, pigmentary epithelial detachment; PVR, proliferative vitreoretinopathy; RD, retinal detachment; BRVO, branch retinal vein occlusion; VA, visual acuity.

Fixation stability and microperimetry before the patch translocation may be helpful in selecting patients who will benefit from surgery.

Recently, spectral domain optical coherence tomography (OCT) has allowed major improvements, particularly in image resolution. Spectral domain OCT has demonstrated disruption of the photoreceptor inner and outer segment junctions and improved visualization of macular pathologies and loss of photoreceptor outer segments in disorders that affect the outer retina. Future studies will address how these major technological advances will impact the use of the OCT in late-stage AMD, for selecting patients who are the right candidates for the transplantation of autologous RPE choroid.

## References

1. Panda-Jonas S, Jonas JB, Jakobczyk-Zmija M. Retinal pigment epithelial cell count, distribution and correlations in normal human eyes. *Am J Ophthalmol* 1996;121:181–189.
2. Rakoczy PE, Baines M, Kennedy CJ, et al. Correlation between autofluorescent debris accumulation and the presence of partially processed forms of cathepsin D in cultured retinal pigment epithelial cells challenged with rod outer segments. *Exp Eye Res* 1996;63:159–167.
3. Feeney L, Mixon RL. An *in vitro* model of phagocytosis in bovine and human retinal pigment epithelium. *Exp Eye Res* 1976;22:533–548.
4. Feeney-Burns L, Hilderbrand ES, Eldridge S. Aging human RPE: morphometric analysis of macular, equatorial, and peripheral cells. *Invest Ophthalmol Vis Sci* 1984;25:195–200.
5. Charteris DG. Proliferative vitreoretinopathy: pathobiology, surgical management, and adjunctive treatment. *Br J Ophthalmol* 1995;79:953–960.
6. Scheiffarth OF, Kampik A, Gunther H, et al. Proteins of the extracellular matrix in vitreoretinal membranes. *Graefes Arch Clin Exp Ophthalmol* 1988;226:357–361.
7. Del Priore LV, Kuo YH, Tezel TH. Age-related changes in human RPE cell density and apoptosis proportion *in situ*. *Invest Ophthalmol Vis Sci* 2002;43:3312–3318.
8. Burns RP, Feeney-Burns L. Clinico-morphologic correlations of drusen of Bruch's membrane. *Trans Am Ophthalmol Soc* 1980;78:206–225.
9. Friedman E, Ts'o MOM. The retinal pigment epithelium. II. Histologic changes associated with age. *Arch Ophthalmol* 1968;79:315–320.
10. Harman AM, Fleming PA, Hoskins RV, et al. Development and aging of cell topography in the human retinal pigment epithelium. *Invest Ophthalmol Vis Sci* 1997;38:2016–2026.
11. Ishibashi T, Patterson R, Ohnishi Y, et al. Formation of drusen in the human eye. *Am J Ophthalmol* 1986;101:342–353.
12. Newsome DA, Hewitt AT, Huh W, et al. Detection of specific extracellular matrix molecules in drusen, Bruch's membrane, and ciliary body. *Am J Ophthalmol* 1987;104:373–381.
13. Sarks SH, Van Driel D, Maxwell L, et al. Softening of drusen and subretinal neovascularization. *Trans Ophthalmol Soc UK* 1980;100:414–422.
14. Macular Photocoagulation Study Group. Krypton laser photocoagulation for neovascular lesions of age-related macular degeneration: results of a randomized clinical trial. *Arch Ophthalmol* 1990;108:816–824.
15. Macular Photocoagulation Study Group. Laser photocoagulation of subfoveal neovascular lesions of age-related macular degeneration: updated findings from two clinical trials. *Arch Ophthalmol* 1993;111:1200–1209.
16. Macular Photocoagulation Study Group. Argon laser photocoagulation for senile macular degeneration: results of a randomized clinical trial. *Arch Ophthalmol* 1982;100:912–918.
17. Treatment of Age-Related Macular Degeneration with Photodynamic Therapy (TAP) Study Group. Photodynamic therapy of subfoveal choroidal neovascularization in age-related macular degeneration with verteporfin: one-year results of 2 rand omized clinical trials-TAP report. *Arch Ophthalmol* 1999;117:1329–1345.
18. Hawkins BS, Bressler NM, Bressler SB, et al; Submacular Surgery Trials Group. Surgical removal vs observation for subfoveal choroidal neovascularization, either associated with the ocular histoplasmosis syndrome or idiopathic: I. Ophthalmic findings from a randomized clinical trial: Submacular Surgery Trials (SST) Group H Trial: SST Report No.9. *Arch Ophthalmol* 2004;122:1597–1611.
19. Hawkins BS, Bressler NM, Miskala PH, et al; Submacular Surgery Trials Group Surgery for subfoveal choroidal neovascularization in age-related macular degeneration: ophthalmic findings: SST report no. 11. *Ophthalmology* 2004;111:1967–1980.
20. Wolf S, Lappas A, Weinberger A, et al. Macular translocation for surgical management of subfoveal choroidal neovascularizations in patients with AMD: first results. *Graefes Arch Clin Exp Ophthalmol* 1999;237:51–57.
21. Eckardt C, Eckardt U, Conrad HJ. Macular rotation with and without counter-rotation of the globe in patients with age-related macular degeneration. *Graefes Arch Clin Exp Ophthalmol* 1999;237:313–325.
22. Moshfeghi AA, Rosenfeld PJ, Puliafito CA, et al. Systemic Bevacizumab (Avastin) therapy for neovascular age-related macular degeneration: twenty-four week results of an uncontrolled open-label clinical study. *Ophthalmology* 2006;113(11):2002.e1–2002.e12.
23. Avery RL, Pieramici DJ, Rabena MD, et al. Intravitreal Bevacizumab (Avastin) for neovascular age-related macular degeneration. *Ophthalmology* 2006;113(3):363 –372.
24. Spaide RF, Laud K, Fine HF, et al. Intravitreal Bevacizumab treatment of choroidal neovascularization secondary to age related macular degeneration. *Retina* 2006;26(4):383–390.
25. Gragoudas ES, Adamis AP, Cunnigham ET Jr, et al. VEGF inhibition study in ocular neovascularization clinical trial group. Pegaptanib for neovascular age-related macular degeneration. *N Engl J Med* 2004;351(27):2805–2816.
26. Rosenfeld PJ, Brown DM, Heier JS, et al; MARINA Study Group Ranibizumab for neovascular age-related macular degeneration. *N Engl J Med* 2006;355(14):1419–1431.
27. Algvere PV, Berglin L, Gouras P, et al. Transplantation of fetal retinal pigment epithelium in age-related macular degeneration with subfoveal neovascularization. *Graefes Arch Clin Esp Ophthalmol* 1994;232:707–716.
28. Algvere PV, Berglin L, Gouras P, et al. Transplantation of RPE in age-related macular degeneration: observations in disciform lesions and dry RPE atrophy. *Graefes Arch Clin Exp Ophthalmol* 1997;235:149–158.
29. Peyman GA, Blinder KJ, Paris CJ, et al. A technique for retinal pigment epithelium transplantation for age-related macular degeneration secondary to extensive subfoveal scarring. *Ophthalmic Surg* 1991;22:102.
30. van Meurs JC, Ter Averst E, Croxen R, et al. Comparison of the growth potential of retinal pigment epithelial cells obtained during vitrectomy in patients with age-related macular degeneration or complex retinal detachment. *Graefes Arch Clin Exp Ophthalmol* 2004;242:442–443.
31. Stanga PE, Kychenthal A, Fitzke FW, et al. Retinal pigment epithelium translocation after choroidal neovascular membrane removal in age-related macular degeneration. *Ophthalmology* 2002;109:1492–1498.
32. Stanga PE, Kychenthal A, Fitzke FW, et al. Functional assessment of the native retinal pigment epithelium after the surgical excision of subfoveal choroidal neovascular membranes type II: preliminary results. *Int Ophthalmol* 2001;23:309–316.
33. Raff M. Adult stem cell plasticity: fact or artifact? *Annu Rev Cell Dev Biol* 2003;19:1–22.
34. Wagers AJ, Weissman IL. Plasticity of adult stem cells. *Cell* 2004;116:639–648.
35. Cahill MT, Freedman SF, Toth CA. Macular translocation with 360 degrees peripheral retinectomy for geographic atrophy. *Arch Ophthalmol* 2003;121:132–133.
36. Huang JC, Ishida M, Hersh P, et al. Preparation and transplantation of photoreceptor sheets. *Curr Eye Res* 1998;17:573–585.
37. Ishida M, Lui GM, Yamani A, et al. Culture of human retinal pigment epithelial cells from peripheral scleral flap biopsies. *Curr Eye Res* 1998;17:392–402.
38. Stanga PE, Kychenthal A, Fitzke FW, et al. Retinal pigment epithelium translocation after choroidal neovascular membrane removal in age-related macular degeneration. *Ophthalmology* 2002;109:1492–1498.
39. MacLaren RE, Bird AC, Sathia PJ, et al. Long-term results of submacular surgery combined with macular translocation of the retinal pigment epithelium in neovascular age-related macular degeneration. *Ophthalmology* 2005;112:2081–2087.
40. Binder S, Krebs I, Hilgers RD, et al. Outcome of transplantation of autologous retinal pigment epithelium in age-related macular degeneration: a prospective trial. *Invest Ophthalmol Vis Sci* 2004;45:4151–4160.
41. Tongalp H, Lucian V, Adam S, et al. Adult retinal pigment epithelial transplantation in exudative age-related macular degeneration. *Am J Ophthalmol* 2007;143(4):585–595.
42. van Meurs JC. Retinal pigment epithelium and choroid translocation in patients with exudative age-related maculopathy. In: Krieglstein GK, Weinreb RN, Kirchhof B, Wong D (eds). *Vitreoretinal surgery, essentials in ophthalmology*. New York: Springer, Berlin Heidelberg, 2005:73–87.
43. Majji AB, de Juan E. Retinal pigment epithelial autotransplantation: morphological changes in retina and choroid. *Graefes Arch Clin Exp Ophthalmol* 2000;238:779–791.
44. Joussen M, Heussen F, Joeres S, et al. Autologous translocation of the choroid and retinal pigment epithelium in age-related macular degeneration. *Am J Ophthalmol* 2006;142:17–30.
45. Caramoy A, Liakopoulus S, Menrath E, et al. Autologous translocation of choroid and retinal pigment epithelium in geographic atrophy: Long term functional and anatomical outcome. *Br J Ophathalmol* 2009. DOI: 10.1136/bjo.2009.161299.
46. Maaijwee K, Heimann H, Missotten T, et al. Retinal pigment epithelium and choroid translocation in patients with exudative age-related macular degeneration: long-term results. *Graefes Arch Clin Exp Ophthalmol* 2007;245:1681–1689.
47. Joussen A, Joeres S, Fawzy N, et al. Autologous translocation of the choroid and retinal pigmentary epithelium in patients with geographic atrophy. *Ophthalmology* 2007;114(3):551–560.

# 57

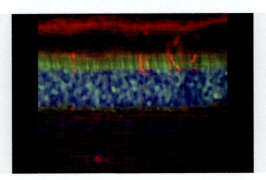

# Gene Therapy for Retinal Disease

Peter Gehlbach

## VECTORS FOR GENE THERAPY

### Nonviral Vectors

Nonviral vectors have potential advantages. Most of them are safe and nontoxic to ocular tissues. The major drawback of nonviral vectors is their low transfection rate and relatively short life. The particular characteristics of the target tissue (or cell), the specific therapeutic material to be used, and the expected beneficial outcome, determine the selection of the most appropriate route of delivery. This makes route of delivery an important aspect when discussing nonviral vectors. For the eye, topical instillation, periocular, or intraocular (intravitreal or subretinal) injections are the most widely used. Systemic administration, on the other hand, is seldom considered due to the presence of blood-ocular barriers and the potential secondary side effects.

### Topical Instillation

Instillation of an active compound is the first choice method of delivery for ocular therapy. However, due to the innate protective characteristics of the eye against the entry of foreign compounds (tear drainage and corneal epithelium barrier), the bioavailability of an instilled compound is generally low. To overcome this limiting factor, frequent instillations or the use of specific formulations which increase the corneal contact time have been developed. Despite these improvements, after instillation, drug levels within the posterior segment of the eye are, in most instances negligible. Plasmids showed better intracellular delivery after delivery via liposomes as well as via polyplexes. Oligodeoxynucleotides (ODNs) showed very localized expression to the anterior layers of the eye which was not greatly improved by delivery in liposomes.

### Intracameral and Intracorneal Injections

Intracameral injections are rarely used in clinic because of the rapid turnover of aqueous humor resulting in very short-time contact time between the active compound and the tissue. On the other hand, injection into the corneal stroma may enhance the transfection of corneal cells because it induce mechanical pressure and allows for a prolonged direct contact of the nucleic acids with the target cells. Naked plasmids delivered intrastromally resulted in sustained corneal expression and did not induce any inflammation. When delivered in liposomes they showed better penetration and a wider distribution, this may be due to their relatively large size, causing their accumulation in the aqueous humor-draining pathways, delaying the outflow and increasing the contact time with ocular tissues. ODN showed low transfection rates but their delivery to the anterior segment was enhanced when delivered in liposomes. Ribonucleic acid (RNA) aptamer were delivered in sustained-release pellets of hydron polymer. Rat cornea neovascularization was inhibited by pellets containing an RNA aptamer using the corneal micropockets system.

### Subconjunctival Delivery

Subconjunctival injection is minimally invasive and can be repeated. The subconjunctival space allows for the injection of large volumes and can be used as a reservoir. Thus it may replace the need for repeated instillations. After subconjunctival injections, the intraocular penetration depends on the physicochemical properties of the active compound used. In general, high levels of drugs may be detected in the anterior and the posterior segments of the eye. However, high systemic absorption has also been observed.

Naked plasmids delivered only transfect periocular tissues, and showed enhanced transfection of the corneal cells when delivered in liposomes. Using collagen shield has increased markedly the gene expression within tissues due to the slow release of plasmids in the subconjunctival space. ODNs and siRNAs are smaller and allow for potential targeting of corneal cells after subconjunctival injections.

### Intravitreous Injection

Direct injection of active compounds into the vitreous cavity is the simplest way to target intraocular tissues. However, molecules injected into the vitreous are cleared rapidly through diffusion anteriorly or transretinally. Therefore, longstanding vitreous therapeutic levels can be achieved either by repeated injection, the use of high initial concentrations or slow release formulations. Shortly after vitreous injection, initial high peak of local drug levels can be toxic to adjacent ocular tissues. Complications, such as vitreous hemorrhage, endophthalmitis, and/or retinal tear, although rare, may occur after intravitreal injection. These risks are obviously increased when repeated injections are given. Following intravitreous injection of naked plasmids, no significant expression of the reporter gene as observed in the retina (1–3). Liposomes have been used to increase the half-life time of intravitreally injected nucleic acids and reduce their toxicity. Plasmid encapsulation within liposomes allows for the transfection of cells in the anterior segment of the eye, inner retinal layers, and retinal pigmented epithelial (RPE) cells. Liposomes also increase the stability of ODNs in the vitreous and to increase the transfection efficiency of liposomes, strategies such as pegylation have been developed were oligo-aptamers coupled to polyethylene glycol (PEG) were formulated. ODNs have also been delivered in nanoparticles; VP22 is a cationic peptide that form well characterized nanoparticles (vectosomes) when complexed with ODNs. We have observed that after intravitreous injection in the rat eye, vectosomes followed a transretinal migration accumulating in the cytoplasm of RPE cells. The VP22 vectosomes show a specific sensitivity to light. After their internalization by the RPE cells, the vectosomes remain stable within the cytoplasm. However, when the cells are illuminated, the vectosomes are destabilized releasing their ODN. The released ODN then moves from the cytoplasm to the cell nucleus expressing its genetic load. Therefore, they can be used to control the release of ODNs at chosen sites using white light (or laser) beam.

### Subretinal Delivery

To increase the local concentration of active compounds in the posterior retinal layers (photoreceptors and RPE cells) and prolong their contact time with the target cells, direct injection in the subretinal space can be performed. Injections can be carried out externally through the sclera or internally through the retina entering into the eye via the pars plana. These types of injections require the use of pressure and fluid or air to detach the retina. The disadvantage of this method is that the area of targeted cells is limited to the locally detached retina. Furthermore, multiple complications may occur: Of these, most notable are lesions of RPE cells, hemorrhages, retinal tears, subretinal or preretinal fibrosis, and uncontrolled retinal detachments. Subretinal delivery of nucleic acids has been used to target RPE and photoreceptors in preclinical studies as a proof of concept. However, due to the expected high rate of complications, particularly if reinjections are needed. and the potential difficulty of detaching a pathological retina where subretinal fibrosis takes place, subretinal injections may remain an investigative tool and not a practical method for application to the human eye.

## Viral Vectors

Adenoviral (Ad) vectors are relatively easy to produce, have good capacity, and with an appropriate promoter can mediate good expression levels in many types of cells. The transduction efficiency for a particular cell type may vary depending upon the serotype and other characteristics of the Ad vector (4). There is little or no transduction of neuronal cells in the retina. Subretinal injections result in strong transduction of RPE cells and occasional Muller cells, but little or no transduction of retinal neurons. The major concern with Ad vectors is that they induce an immune response that results in inflammation, mediates destruction of transduced cells reducing transgene expression, and prevents repeated injections; however, excellent safety profiles in two recent clinical trials suggest that clinical grade second generation Ad vectors are well tolerated in the eyes of humans.

Recombinant Ad vectors in which all viral genes have been deleted are generally called encapsidated adenovirus mini-chromosomes or "gutless Ad vectors" and invoke much less immune response, transduce rod photoreceptors, and mediate much longer transgene expression.

Adeno-associated viral (AAV) vectors are substantially more difficult to produce than Ad vectors and have limited capacity of less than 5 kb. However, AAV vectors appear to invoke little or no immune response and therefore have little toxicity and mediate prolonged transgene expression. Intravitreous injections of AAV vectors result in transduction of retinal ganglion cells and subretinal injections result in transduction of RPE cells and photoreceptors.

Lentiviral vectors efficiently transduce a variety of nondividing cells with little or no host response resulting in long-term transgene expression. Subretinal injection of a human immunodeficiency virus (HIV) vector containing the green fluorescent protein (GFP) gene under the control of the cytomegalovirus (CMV) promoter resulted in widespread expression of GFP in photoreceptors and RPE cells, for at least 12 weeks, the longest time point examined. Contamination of HIV vector preparations with replication competent virus is unlikely, but because of its serious consequences it is still a concern. Bovine immunodeficiency virus (BIV) is a lentivirus that is not known to cause human disease. Subretinal injection of a BIV. GFP vector resulted in rapid and prolonged transduction of RPE cells with no evidence of an inflammatory response.

## Applications of Gene Therapy in Macular Diseases Macular Edema and Ischemia: Antiapoptosis Gene Therapy and Neuroprotection

Macular ischemia is the result of an insufficient blood supply to neurons due to occlusion of blood vessels As a consequence, retinal cells undergo hypoxia causing a number of pathophysiological processes, including the production of glutamate and free radicals, that ultimately end in damage to retinal neurons and cell death by apoptosis (5–10). The current therapies aim at re-establishing the retinal microcirculation through using laser treatment, ocular massage, and tPA. However, these therapies have had limited success and need to be applied early in the course of ischemia to be effective. Other agents that provide neuroprotection through delaying cell death of ischemic retina have also been tested; however, they do not permanently rescue the retinal cells (11,12). It appears that in order to rescue retinal cells from apoptosis, a neuroprotectant should affect the apoptotic mechanism itself.

Apoptosis appears to be the final pathway of cell death in retinal cells (13,14). Pro and antiapoptotic genes have been identified and tested on retinal cells. The transfer of bcl-2 gene (an antiapoptotic gene) to the retinal cells resulted in a delay in retinal degeneration in mice (15). However the transfer of this same gene to the ganglion cells resulted in increased glutamate-induced apoptosis (16). Thus the protective effect of bcl-2 may be tissue specific, or may be mediated by secondary pathways that are differ among different retinal cells.

A proapoptotic protein, caspase-3, when unregulated causes retinal degeneration in transgenic rats (17), and hence inhibition of its expression could inhibit apoptosis (18).

The final pathway in the apoptotic pathway is the processing and activation of caspases that dismantle the cell by breaking up cytoskeletal proteins and repair enzymes (19). Recently, inhibitors of apoptosis (IAPs) have gained attention as because of their impressive ability to inhibit the final caspase cascade. All IAPs contain at least one Baculovirus IAP Repeat (BIR) domain that allows direct binding to and inhibition of caspases (20). XIAP is the most potent IAP and it inhibits apoptosis by directly blocking the activity of caspases 3, 7, and 9 via its three N-terminal BIR domains (21–23). Renwick et al., 2006 reported that XIAP over-expression protected the retina from infarction due to transient ischemia induced by increasing intraocular pressure (24). Their results indicate that, in the presence of XIAP, retinal function was maintained up to 4 weeks postischemia. They showed further that retinal structure, assessed by counting cells in the INL, measuring inner retinal thickness and counting axons in optic nerve cross-sections, was significantly maintained in the presence of XIAP.

## EPIRETINAL MEMBRANE AND MACULAR HOLE

Proliferative vitreoretinopathy (PVR) is an acquired, scarring process in the posterior segment of the eye that commonly occurs after retinal detachment and penetrating trauma (25). Although the pathogenesis of PVR is not completely understood, it is characterized by the growth of hypocellular membranes on the retina and within the vitreous gel. Proliferation of several cell types, including RPE cells, fibroblasts, and glia, is accompanied by deposition of extracellular matrix proteins; this is followed by cell-mediated contraction of the collagen fibrils leading to tractional retinal folds and detachment (26). Somatic therapies directed at inhibiting cellular proliferation and the deposition of extracellular matrix have been efficacious in reducing the severity of disease in experimental animal models of PVR.

## SUICIDE GENE THERAPY

Experimental models of PVR have been developed by injecting cultured fibroblasts and RPE cells in the vitreous cavity of rabbits (27). The proliferating cells are selectively targeted for suicide with the HSV-*tk* in a retroviral vector (28). HSV-*tk* is selectively transduced in dividing cells by this method and renders them susceptible to the cytotoxic effects of ganciclovir.

Selective killing of dividing cells has been demonstrated in several studies. In mixed cultures of nondividing rat neurons and proliferating RPE cells, the RPE cells were preferentially killed by ganciclovir following transduction with the HSV-*tk* gene (29). Reduced severity was also seen using mixtures of fibroblasts in which only 10% of cells expressed the HSV-*tk* gene, which demonstrated a bystander effect in PVR. Ganciclovir therapy following HSV-*tk* gene transfer significantly reduces PVR, even at a transduction frequency of 1%. The presence of vitreous during gene transfer *in vitro* reduces the transduction efficiency in a dose-dependent manner. Mechanical effects of the vitreous may also limit the efficiency of transduction following intravitreal injection. The role of vitrectomy in reducing the mechanical limitations imposed by the vitreous to improve the efficiency of transduction to the retina in PVR and perhaps in genetic degenerations is worth exploring in future studies.

## ANTISENSE GENE THERAPY

Antisense gene therapy is based upon the use of synthetic, short DNA sequences (ODN) that are designed to be complementary to a targeted messenger RNA (mRNA) molecule. The ODN is capable of forming a stable DNA-RNA heteroduplex with the mRNA and, thus, preventing translation of the protein from the transcript. Modulation of growth factor, receptor, or structural gene expression by antisense gene therapy may have a role in gene therapy for PVR. Platelet-derived growth factor (PDGF) appears to contribute to the development of PVR in animal models and in human disease (30). Fibroblasts from α-PDGF-receptor knockout mice induced less PVR than cells that expressed these receptors (31), which suggests a role for antisense-inhibition of PDGF-mediated cellular proliferation in the disease (32). Antisense inhibition of cell proliferation has also been demonstrated in human RPE cells by blocking *c-myc* expression and in the deposition of basement membrane (a component of epiretinal membrane formation in PVR) by blocking fibronectin gene expression (33).

## GROWTH FACTOR GENE THERAPY

Intravitreal injection of brain-derived neurotrophic factor (BDNF) in a cat model of retinal detachment significantly reduced Müller cell proliferation and indicates a possible role for growth factor gene therapy in PVR.

### Subretinal Choroidal Neovascularization

#### Antagonism of VEGF

The extracellular domain of VEGF receptor 1, sFlt-1, is a protein antagonist of VEGF formed by alternative splicing of the pre-mRNA (34,35). Intraocular injection of sFlt-1 on an adenovirus or an AAV resulted in suppression of choroidal in mice and monkeys (36–39). Periocular injection of Ad.sFlt-1 resulted in transduction of episcleral cells and the sFlt-1 traversed the sclera, achieved high levels in the choroid, and markedly suppressed choroidal neovascularization (40). However, VEGF is also an important survival factor for endothelial cells and plays an important role in maintenance of blood vessels. Endothelial cells within new vessels tend to be more dependent upon VEGF for survival than those in normal vessels. There are some theoretical concerns that efficient, long term blockade of VEGF by gene transfer may cause problems.

Intraocular injection of siRNA targeting the mRNA for VEGF or VEGF receptor 1 suppresses choroidal neovascularization (41,42). Simply injecting siRNA into the vitreous cavity has no advantage over intraocular injections of Ranibizumab, because as opposed to Ranibizumab, siRNA must enter cells, which decreases efficiency, and labeled siRNA is detectable in the retina for only a week. Prolonged effects may be achieved by using viral vectors to express short hairpin RNAs that target the mRNA of VEGF or its receptors. Sustained delivery of siRNA would provide an alternative means of obtaining prolonged silencing, and since siRNA penetrates the sclera, such a device could be mounted on the outside of the eye.

#### Pigment Epithelium-Derived Factor

Several proteins have been shown to inhibit ocular neovascularization when expressed by gene transfer. Pigment epithelium-derived factor (PEDF) is the most intensively studied. It promotes survival of cultured neurons and protects photoreceptors from excessive light exposure (43–46). It was first recognized that PEDF also has antiangiogenic activity in 1999 (47). Intravitreous or subretinal injection of AdPEDF.11 suppressed the development of retinal or choroidal neovascularization and when given after neovascularization caused regression of the neovascularization by inducing apoptosis of endothelial cells in newly developed blood vessels, but not in normal, quiescent blood vessels. Injection of AdPEDF.11 beneath the conjunctiva along the outer border of the sclera resulted in transduction of episcleral cells that produced PEDF on the outside of the eye. The PEDF penetrated the sclera resulting in high levels in the choroid that caused regression of choroidal neovascularization. What is interesting about this approach is that subconjunctival injections are less invasive than intraocular injections, and episcleral cells are more expendable than intraocular cells should an unexpected problem develop from the vector or from over-expression of the protein. Another approach is to express an engineered zinc finger protein transcription factor (ZFP-TF) to increase production of a protein by stimulating its promoter (48). A ZFP-TF that selectively binds to the PEDF promoter was designed and when injected intravitreously or subretinally in mice caused significantly increased levels of PEDF mRNA in the eye and suppressed choroidal neovascularization at Bruch's membrane rupture sites.

## ENDOSTATIN

Endostatin is a collagen cleavage product that inhibits tumor angiogenesis resulting in inhibition of tumor growth (49). There was a strong positive correlation between endostatin serum levels and inhibition of choroidal neovascularization, indicating that endostatin is a good candidate for antiangiogenic ocular gene therapy. In mice with oxygen-induced ischemic retinopathy, intraocular injection of AAV endostatin inhibited ischemia-induced retinal neovascularization.

## ANGIOSTATIN

Angiostatin is a cleavage product of fibrinogen that inhibits tumor angiogenesis. Intraocular injection of an AAV angiostatin suppressed retinal and choroidal neovascularization (50).

### TIMP-3

It has been shown that Tissue Inhibitor of Metalloproteinases-3 (TIMP-3) has antiangiogenic activity that is independent of its antiproteolytic activity (51), suggesting that TIMP-3 may contribute in multiple ways to the barrier posed by Bruch's membrane to vascular invasion into the subretinal space. Increased levels of TIMP-3 in RPE cells of rats induced by subretinal injection of hemagglutinating virus of Japan liposomes containing a TIMP-3 expression construct suppressed choroidal neovascularization at Bruch's membrane rupture sites (52). However, over-expression of TIMP-3 may compromise its turnover and cause it to accumulate and thicken Bruch's membrane. Diffuse thickening of Bruch's membrane is associated with choroidal neovascularization in patients with age-related macular degeneration (AMD); therefore, it may be prudent to avoid over-expressing insoluble proteins in RPE cells regardless of their biologic activity.

## ANGIOPOIETINS

Tie-2 is an endothelial cell-specific receptor that is stimulated by binding Angiopoietin-1 and is blocked by Angiopoietin 2 (53). Blockade of Tie-2 by over-expressing Angiopoietin 2 results in regression of new vessels when levels of VEGF are relatively lower than angiopoietin 2. Over-expression of

Angiopoietin-1 inhibits retinal and choroidal neovascularization. Therefore, gene transfer of angiopoietin 1 is a promising therapeutic approach. Gene transfer of soluble Tie 2 should be similar to over-expressing Angiopoietin 2, and both approaches were found to inhibit choroidal neovascularization at Bruch's membrane rupture sites.

## HEREDITARY RETINAL DEGENERATIONS

### Ribozyme Therapy

Ribozymes are RNA enzyme molecules that can cleave specific mRNA sequences (54,55). Variable sequences in theses ribozymes determine their specificity for its target molecule (56). The strategy used is to construct ribozymes that identify unique mutations or that permit binding to targeted, accessible sites in the mRNA transcript. Mutation-specific cleavage of the transcript functionally "silences" the mutant allele by preventing synthesis of the abnormal protein from the transcript. Recently, a mutation-independent approach to ribozyme therapy has been used in which both mutant and wild-type transcripts are cleaved but a modified wild-type transcript encoding the normal protein is introduced. These modified transcripts are not cleaved by the ribozyme and, thus, permit translation of the wild-type protein in the cell (57).

The catalytic activity of ribozymes engineered to target and cleave specific opsin mRNA mutations seen in RP has been demonstrated in animal models *in vitro* (58,59). AAV-mediated transfer of a ribozyme targeting a rat rhodopsin transcript with a proline to histidine mutation (P23 H) was shown to delay the onset of photoreceptor degeneration for 3 months.

## GROWTH FACTOR GENE THERAPY

Upregulation of basic fibroblast growth factor (bFGF) expression in response to laser photocoagulation of the retina has been demonstrated *in vivo*, (60) and intravitreal injection of bFGF delays retinal degeneration in the RCS rat (61). Successful treatment with growth factors may also be achieved by genetically modifying cells ex vivo and then implanting them within the eye to act as a reservoir of trophic factors that bathe the retina by slow release into the vitreous. Intravitreal transfer of fibroblasts, expressing the bFGF gene, encapsulated in a biocompatible polymer, delayed retinal degeneration up to 3 months after transfer in the RCS rat.

## GENE-REPLACEMENT THERAPY

The rd$^-$/rd$^-$ mouse develops progressive retinal degeneration shortly after birth from a mutation in the gene encoding the β-subunit of cyclic GMP phosphodiesterase, β-PDE (62). A mutation in the human homologue of this gene has also been identified in a subset of patients with retinitis pigmentosa. Several gene delivery techniques have been employed to modify the phenotype of the rd⁻/rd⁻ mouse by transfecting a wild-type copy of the β-PDE gene to the retina. Adenovirus-mediated transfer of β-PDE to the retina of the rd⁻/rd⁻ mouse resulted in increased PDE activity within the retina and delayed retinal degeneration up to 12 weeks after gene transfer.

## ACQUIRED RETINAL DEGENERATIONS

AMD is an acquired disease of the RPE, which results in a secondary degeneration of the overlying neurosensory retina. Degenerative changes of the RPE and Bruch's membrane are the primary factors responsible for the disease. Unlike the degenerative process in RP in which specific mutations give rise to the disease phenotype, the putative role of specific genes in the degenerative process in AMD is less clear. Although certain genes may predispose some patients to develop AMD, the genetic linkage is controversial, and to date, the genetics of AMD remains largely unknown. Genetic susceptibility to AMD is probably multifactorial and thus will not be amenable to gene therapy directed at the germline. In the absence of a well-defined genetic defect which gives rise to AMD, gene therapy will likely focus on somatic therapy using growth factors and antiapoptosis therapy to prolong the survival of the RPE and retinal photoreceptors.

## GROWTH FACTOR GENE THERAPY

There is experimental evidence that growth factors play an important role in maintaining the health of RPE cells and in enabling them to respond to injury. Theoretically, it may be possible to enhance RPE cell survival by somatic modulation of growth factor gene expression in patients with AMD. Defective phagocytic function by the RPE results in the retinal degeneration seen in the RCS rat model (63). While the RCS rat is not an animal model for human AMD, age-related phagocytic dysfunction and incomplete lysosomal digestion of photoreceptor membranes by the RPE results in the accumulation of drusen, the hallmark of AMD in humans. This accumulation ultimately results in loss of RPE cells and in geographic atrophy, perhaps due to the cytotoxicity of these deposits on the surrounding cells. Enhancing phagocytic activity in aging RPE cells using gene therapy is a potential approach to the treatment of AMD. Basic-FGF has been shown to stimulate phagocytic activity and prolong retinal survival in the RCS rat model.

## ANTISENSE GENE THERAPY

Inhibiting the degeneration of RPE and photoreceptor cells by apoptotic mechanisms may slow disease progression and visual loss. Transfer of the gene for the oxidative stress protein

heme oxygenase-1 has been demonstrated in the rabbit retina (64) and may be a mechanism by which the retina and RPE can be protected from oxidative injury in patients with AMD. Development of somatic therapy for atrophic AMD is hampered by the lack of a good *in vivo* animal model for the disease. Aged monkeys do develop drusen, but true macular degeneration is rare in the nonhuman primate. An *in vitro* model to mimic the decline in membrane digestion in the RPE has been developed. Antisense transcripts directed to cathepsin S reduce aspartic protease activity in RPE cells and may provide an *in vitro* model for the phagocytic dysfunction in AMD, (65) as well as an alternative model for photoreceptor degeneration (66). For the foreseeable future, progress will likely depend upon in vitro work using eye bank tissue donated from patients with AMD.

### References

1. Calabretta B, Skorski T, Ratajczak MZ, et al. Antisense strategies in the treatment of leukemias. *Semin Oncol* 1996;23:78–87.
2. Campochiaro PA, Hackett SF, Vinores SA, et al. Platelet derived growth factor is an autocrine growth stimulator in retinal pigmented epithelial cells. *J Cell Sci* 1994;107:2459–2469.
3. Capeans C, Pineiro A, Dominguez F, et al. A c-myc antisense oligonucleotide inhibits human retinal pigment epithelial cell proliferation. *Exp Eye Res* 1998;66:581–589.
4. Mori K, Duh E, Gehlbach P, et al. Pigment epithelium-derived factor inhibits retinal and choroidal neovascularization. *J Cell Physiol* 2001;188:253–263.
5. Kohner EM. Diabetic retinopathy. *Br Med Bull* 1989;45:148–173.
6. Rosenbaum DM, Rosenbaum PS, Gupta A, et al. Retinal ischemia leads to apoptosis which is ameliorated by aurintricarboxylic acid. *Vision Res* 1997;37:3445–3451.
7. Rosenbaum PS, Gupta H, Savitz SI, et al. Apoptosis in the retina. *Clin Neurosci* 1997;4:224–232.
8. Sucher NJ, Lipton SA, Dreyer EB. Molecular basis of glutamate toxicity in retinal ganglion cells. *Vision Res* 1997;37:3483–3493.
9. Luo X, Lambrou GN, Sahel JA, et al. Hypoglycemia induces general neuronal death, whereas hypoxia and glutamate transport blockade lead to selective retinal ganglion cell death in vitro. *Invest Ophthalmol Vis Sci* 2001;42:2695–2705.
10. Adachi K, Kashii S, Masai H, et al. Mechanism of the pathogenesis of glutamate neurotoxicity in retinal ischemia. *Graefes Arch Clin Exp Ophthalmol* 1998;236:766–774.
11. Fontaine V, Mohand-Said S, Hanoteau N, et al. Neurodegenerative and neuroprotective effects of tumor Necrosis factor (TNF) in retinal ischemia: opposite roles of TNF receptor 1 and TNF receptor 2. *J Neurosci* 2002;22:RC216.
12. Lafuente MP, Villegas-Perez MP, Selles-Navarro I, et al. Retinal ganglion cell death after acute retinal ischemia is an ongoing process whose severity and duration depends on the duration of the insult. *Neuroscience* 2002;109:157–168.
13. Lolley RN, Rong H, Craft CM. Linkage of photoreceptor degeneration by apoptosis with inherited defect in phototransduction. *Invest Ophthalmol Vis Sci* 1994;35:358–362.
14. Tso MO, Zhang C, Abler AS, et al. Apoptosis leads to photoreceptor degeneration in inherited retinal dystrophy of RCS rats. *Invest Ophthalmol Vis Sci* 1994;35:2693–2699.
15. Tsang SH, Chen J, Kjeldbye H, et al. Retarding photoreceptor degeneration in Pdegtm1/Pdegtml mice by an apoptosis suppressor gene. *Invest Ophthalmol Vis Sci* 1997;38:943–950.
16. Simon PD, Vorwerk CK, Mansukani SS, et al. Bcl-2 gene therapy exacerbates excitotoxicity. *Hum Gene Ther* 1999;10:1715–1720.
17. Liu C, Li Y, Peng M, et al. Activation of caspase-3 in the retina of transgenic rats with the rhodopsin mutation s334ter during photoreceptor degeneration. *J Neurosci* 1999;19:4778–4785.
18. Xu D, Bureau Y, McIntyre DC, et al. Attenuation of ischemia- induced cellular and behavioral deficits by X chromosome-linked inhibitor of apoptosis protein overexpression in the rat hippocampus. *J Neurosci* 1999;19:5026–5033.
19. Schulz JB, Weller M, Moskowitz MA. Caspases as treatment targets in stroke and neurodegenerative diseases. *Ann Neurol* 1999;45:421–429.
20. Liston P, Fong WG, Korneluk RG. The inhibitors of apoptosis: there is more to life than Bcl2. *Oncogene* 2003;22:8568–8580.
21. Deveraux QL, Takahashi R, Salvesen GS, et al. X-linked IAP is a direct inhibitor of cell-death proteases. *Nature* 1997;388:300–304.

22. Holcik M, Gibson H, Korneluk RG. XIAP: apoptotic brake and promising therapeutic target. *Apoptosis* 2001;6:253–261.

23. McKinnon SJ, Lehman DM, Tahzib NG, et al. Baculoviral IAP repeat-containing-4 protects optic nerve axons in a rat glaucoma model. *Mol Ther* 2002;5:780–787.

24. Renwick J, Narang MA, Coupland SG, et al. XIAP-mediated neuroprotection in retinal ischemia. *Gene Ther* 2006;13(4):339–347.

25. Chaum E. Proliferative vitreoretinopathy. *Int Ophthalmol Clin* 1995;35:163–173.

26. Glaser BM, Lemor M. Pathobiology of proliferative vitreoretinopathy. In: Ryan SJ (ed). *Retina*, vol 3. St Louis: Mosby, 1998:369–383.

27. Sakamoto T, Kimura H, Scuric Z, et al. Inhibition of experimental proliferative vitreoretinopathy by retroviral vector mediated transfer of suicide gene. Can proliferative vitreoretinopathy be a target of gene therapy? *Ophthalmology* 1995;102:1417–1424.

28. Kimura H, Sakamoto T, Cardillo JA, et al. Retrovirus-mediated suicide gene transduction in the vitreous cavity of the eye: feasibility in prevention of proliferative vitreoretinopathy. *Hum Gene Ther* 1996;7:799–808.

29. Wong CA, Jia W, Matsubara JA. Experimental gene therapy for an in vitro model of proliferative vitreoretinopathy. *Can J Ophthalmol* 1999;34:379–384.

30. Robbins SG, Mixon RN, Wilson DJ, et al: Platelet-derived growth factor ligands and receptors immunolocalized in proliferative retinal diseases. *Invest Ophthalmol Vis Sci* 1994;35:3649–3663.

31. Andrews A, Balciunaite E, Leong FL, et al. Platelet-derived growth factor plays a key role in proliferative vitreoretinopathy. *Invest Ophthalmol Vis Sci* 1999;40:2683–2689.

32. Ikuno Y, Leong FL, Kazlauskas A. Attenuation of experimental proliferative vitreoretinopathy by inhibiting the platelet-derived growth factor receptor. *Invest Ophthalmol Vis Sci* 2000;41:3107–3116.

33. Roy S, Zhang K, Roth T, et al. Reduction of fibronectin expression by intravitreal administration of antisense oligonucleotides. *Nat Biotechnol* 1999;17:476–479.

34. He Y, Smith SK, Day KA, et al. Alternative splicing of vascular endothelial growth factor (VEGF)-R1 (FLT-1) pre-mRNA is important for the regulation of VEGF activity. *Mol. Endocrinol* 1999;13:537–545.

35. Kendall RL, Wang GL, Thomas KA. Identification of a natural soluble form of the vascular endothelial growth factor receptor, FLT-1, and its heterodimerization with KDR. *Biochem Biophys Res Comm* 1996;226:324–328.

36. Honda M, Sakamoto T, Ishibashi T, et al. Experimental subretinal neovascularization is inhibited by adenovirus-mediated soluble VEGF.flt-1 receptor gene transfection: a role of VEGF and possible treatment for SRN in age-related macular degeneration. *Gene Ther* 2000;7:978–985.

37. Rota R, Riccioni T, Zaccarini M, et al. Marked inhibition of retinal neovascularization in rats following soluble-flt-1 gene transfer. *J. Gene Med* 2004;6:992–1002.

38. Lai CM, Shen WY, Brankov M, et al. Long-term evaluation of AAV-mediated sFlt-1 gene therapy for ocular neovascularization in mice and monkeys. *Mol. Ther* 2005;12:659–668.

39. Lai YK, Shen WY, Brankov M, et al. Potential long-term inhibition of ocular neovascularization by recombinant adeno-associated virus-mediated secretion gene therapy. *Gene Ther* 2002;9:804–813.

40. Gehlbach P, Demetriades AM, Yamamoto S, et al. Periocular injection of an adenoviral vector encoding pigment epithelium-derived factor inhibits choroidal neovascularization. *Gene Ther* 2003;10:637–646.

41. Reich SJ, Fosnot J, Kuroki A, et al. Small interfering RNA (siRNA) targeting VEGF effectively inhibits ocular neovascularization in a mouse model. *Mol Vis* 2003;9:210–216.

42. Shen J, Samul R, Lima e Silva R, et al. Suppression of ocular neovascularization with siRNA targeting VEGF receptor 1. *Gene Ther* 2005;13:225–234.

43. Araki T, Taniwaki T, Becerra SP, et al. Pigment epithelium-derived factor (PEDF) differentially protects immature but not mature cerebellar granule cells against apoptotic cell death. *J Neurosci Res* 1998;53:7–15.

44. Bilak MM, Corse AM, Bilak SR, et al. Pigment epithelium-derived factor (PEDF) protects motor neurons from chronic glutamate-mediated neurodegeneration. *J Neuropathol Exp Neurol* 1999;58:719–728.

45. Cao W, Tombran-Tink J, Elias R, et al. In vivo protection of photoreceptors from light damage by pigment epithelium-derived factor. *Invest Opthalmol Vis Sci* 2001;42:1642–1652.

46. Steele FR, Chader GJ, Johnson LV, et al. Pigment epithelium-derived factor: neurotrophic activity and identification as a member or the serine protease inhibitor gene family. *Proc Natl Acad Sci USA* 1993;90:1526–1530.

47. Dawson DW, Volpert OV, Gillis P, et al. Pigment epithelium-derived factor: a potent inhibitor of angiogenesis. *Science* 1999;285:245–248.

48. Tan S, Guschin D, Davalos A, et al. Zinc-finger protein-targeted gene regulation: genomewide single-gene specificity. *Proc Natl Acad Sci USA* 2003;100:11997.

49. O'Reilly MS, Boehm T, Shing Y, et al. Endostatin: an endogenous inhibitor of angiogenesis and tumor growth. *Cell* 1997;88:277–285.

50. Igarashi T, Miyake K, Kato K, et al. Lentivirus-mediated expression of angiostatin efficiently inhibits neovascularization in a murine proliferative retinopathy model. *Gene Ther* 2003;10:219–226.

51. Apte SS, Olsen BR, Murphy G. The gene structure of tissue inhibitor of metalloproteinases (TIMP)-3 and its inhibitory activities define the distinct TIMP gene family. *J Biol Chem* 1995;270:14313–14318.

52. Takahashi T, Nakamura T, Hayashi A, et al. Inhibition of experimental choroidal neovascularization by overexpression of tissue inhibitor of metalloproteinases-3 in retinal pigment epithelium. *Am J Ophthalmol* 2000;130:774–781.

53. Maisonpierre PC, Suri C, Jones PF, et al. Angiopoietin-2, a natural antagonist for Tie2 that disrupts in vivo angiogenesis. *Science* 1997;277:55–60.

54. Haseloff J, Gerlach WL. Simple RNA enzymes with new and highly specific endoribonuclease activities. *Nature* 1988;334:585–591.

55. Sullenger BA, Cech TR. Ribozyme-mediated repair of defective mRNA by targeted, trans-splicing. *Nature* 1994;371:619–622.

56. Birikh KR, Heaton PA, Eckstein F. The structure, function and application of the hammerhead ribozyme. *Eur J Biochem* 1997;245:1–16.

57. O'Neill B, Millington-Ward S, O'Reilly M, et al. Ribozyme-based therapeutic approaches for autosomal dominant retinitis pigmentosa. *Invest Ophthalmol Vis Sci* 2000;41:2863–2869.

58. Drenser KA, Timmers AM, Hauswirth WW, et al. Ribozyme-targeted destruction of RNA associated with autosomal-dominant retinitis pigmentosa. *Invest Ophthalmol Vis Sci* 1998;39:681–689.

59. Shaw LC, Skold A, Wong F. An allele-specific hammerhead ribozyme gene therapy for a porcine model of autosomal dominant retinitis pigmentosa. *Mol Vis* 2000;7:6–13.

60. Xiao M, Sastry SM, Li ZY, et al. Effects of retinal laser photocoagulation on photoreceptor basic fibroblast growth factor and survival. *Invest Ophthalmol Vis Sci* 1998;39:618–630.

61. Faktorovich EG, Steinberg RH, Yasumura D, et al. Photoreceptor degeneration in inherited retinal dystrophy delayed by basic fibroblast growth factor. *Nature* 1990;347:83–86.

62. Lem J, Flannery JG, Li T, et al. Retinal degeneration is rescued in transgenic rd mice by expression of the cGMP phosphodiesterase beta subunit. *Proc Natl Acad Sci USA* 1992;89:4422–4426.

63. LaVail M. Analysis of neurological mutants with inherited retinal degeneration. Friedenwald lecture. *Invest Ophthalmol Vis Sci* 1981;21:638–657.

64. Abraham NG, da Silva JL, Lavrovsky Y, et al. Adenovirus-mediated heme oxygenase-1 gene transfer into rabbit ocular tissues. *Invest Ophthalmol Vis Sci* 1995;36:2202–2210.

65. Rakoczy PE, Lai MC, Baines MG, et al. Expression of cathepsin S antisense transcripts by adenovirus in retinal pigment epithelial cells. *Invest Ophthalmol Vis Sci* 1998;39:2095–2104.

66. Lai CM, Shen WY, Constable I, et al. The use of adenovirus-mediated gene transfer to develop a rat model for photoreceptor degeneration. *Invest Ophthalmol Vis Sci* 2000;41:580–584.

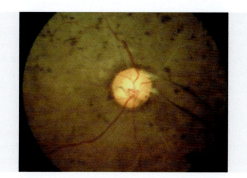

# Artificial Vision

Nancy Kunjukunju ■ Hirokazu Sakaguchi
Motohiro Kamei ■ Hugo Quiroz-Mercado

At one time, it was believed that visual loss was permanent once the neural retina or optic nerve had been damaged. There were two events that modified this way of thinking. In 1968, a visual prosthesis was evaluated in a blind patient (1), and in 1974 an experiment was conducted in which a patient with no light perception vision could perceive light after an electrode was used to stimulate the visual cortex (2). At present there are a number of groups working on different approaches to developing a visual prosthesis for the blind.

Dobelle developed an approach that stimulated the visual cortex intracranially (2–5). In experiments conducted by Dobelle et al. and Norman et al., using either implanted surface electrodes or intracortical microelectrodes, cortical cells were activated thus stimulating the visual cortex (2–5). This type of electrical stimulation of the visual cortex requires intracranial surgery and as such, there is the potential for a high rate of complications such as CNS infection, epilepsy, and disturbance of the blood flow to the optic nerve.

On the other hand, Santos reported that 30% of the ganglion cells and approximately 80% of the inner nuclear layer cells remain histologically intact after death of photoreceptors in the eyes with severe visual loss due to retinitis pigmentosa (RP) (6). Other groups, therefore, have approached the development of a visual prosthesis stimulating those remaining inner retinal neurons. One such ophthalmological approach involves the use of subretinal electrodes and has been investigated by Chow et al. (7–9) and Zrenner et al. (10,11) (Figs. 58-1 and 58-2). Using this method, lost photoreceptor function is replaced by a subretinal microphotodiode array (MPDA) that activates the remaining retinal network. Another approach used by certain groups such as Eckmiller et al. (12,13), Humayan et al. (14,15), Rizzo et al. (16,17) and Walter et al. (18) investigates the use of an epiretinal device to stimulate ganglion cells from an implanted microelectrode array from the vitreal side of the retina (Fig. 58-3). Another viable option is approaching the retinal prosthesis from within the suprachoroidal space. Sakaguchi and Tano et al. reported regarding the suprachoroidal transretinal stimulation system (STS) in which an electrode upon insertion into the suprachoroidal space elicits an electrical evoked potential (EEP) through transretinal stimulation (19), and Fujikado and Tano et al. also reported the effect of this system in clinical trial (20).

There are advantages and disadvantages to each method of electrical stimulation. Implanted cortical electrodes can treat blindness with complete atrophy of the retina or optic nerve, but requires intracranial procedures and may result in limited spatial perception. Retinal stimulation (Fig. 58-4), in contrast, utilizes the preexisting signal-processing network along the proximal visual pathways and is expected to have higher resolution. The visual field through an epiretinal electrode for instance, has a visual angle of 10 degrees (21). However, the area of visual field that will be reconstructed by a small (several millimeter square or in diameter) electrodes array is limited. Retinal stimulation involves predictable retinal damage due to the chronic direct attachment of an implant array. Moreover, the epiretinal or subretinal electrode necessitates that sufficient bipolar cells or ganglion cells remain in the small area around the electrode to elicit a response to electrical stimulation.

At present, there are five clinical trials underway to evaluate the efficacy of visual restoration through retinal prosthesis (22). Second Sight Medical Products, Inc has a 16-electrode epiretinal device that has been implanted in six subjects in the United States for over five years (23). A second-generation device has 60 electrodes and is currently in phase 2/3 of a clinical trial. In Germany, Intelligent Medical Implants GmBH has implanted four patients with a 49-electrode epiretinal array (24). The fourth clinical trial involves another epiretinal implant, the EPI RET3, which is a 25-electrode array that was implanted for four weeks in six blind patients (25). In the fifth clinical trial a 1550-MPDA and a 4 × 4 electrode array from Retina Implant AG, Reutlingen, Germany, was implanted in the subretinal space of eight patients (26).

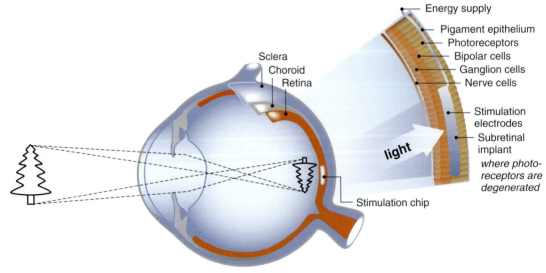

**Figure 58-1.** Subretinal implant (schematic).

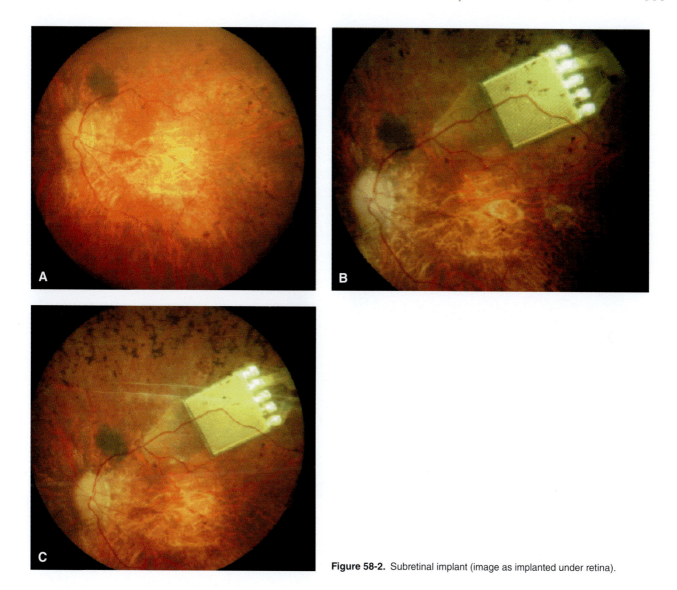

**Figure 58-2.** Subretinal implant (image as implanted under retina).

## EPIRETINAL PROSTHESIS

In animal models, epiretinal stimulation was shown to reproducibly elicit neural responses in the retina. In humans, preliminary tests of epiretinal electronic stimulation showed that patients were able to identify a crude shape and there was no persistence of the image, either a letter or box shape, pursuant to stimulation (14,15,27).

The epiretinal prosthesis (Fig. 58-3) is composed of extraocular and intraocular components. The external component consists of a lightweight camera built into spectacles, pocket batteries and a small pager-sized processing unit. The camera is used to capture and digitize images from the external environment. These images are then transformed into patterns of electrical stimulation that can excite inner retinal neurons. Information and power are relayed from the external portion to an internal receiver/stimulating microelectronic chip and microelectrode array (28).

There are advantages and disadvantages to the epiretinal approach. The advantages include (a) the vitreous acts as a sink for heat-dissipation from the microelectronic device, (b) the implantable portion of the device has little microelectronics, (c) the wearable or extraocular portion of the device allows easy upgrades without needing subsequent surgery and (d) electronics allow user and doctor full control over every electrode parameter and digital signal processing involved in imaging objects. Disadvantages include (a) the techniques that necessitate prolonged adhesion of the device to the inner retina using retinal tacks, (b) a wire connecting extraocular and intraocular components forms a permanent track between the vitreous cavity to the outside, which may raise a possibility of late infection and detachment of the electrodes from the retina associated with the eye movement, and (c) the large amount of current required to stimulate target bipolar cells using an epiretinal device and be the close proximity of this current to target cells (28).

The Intraocular Retinal Prosthesis (IRP) developed in conjunction with Second Sight Medical Products, Inc. converts

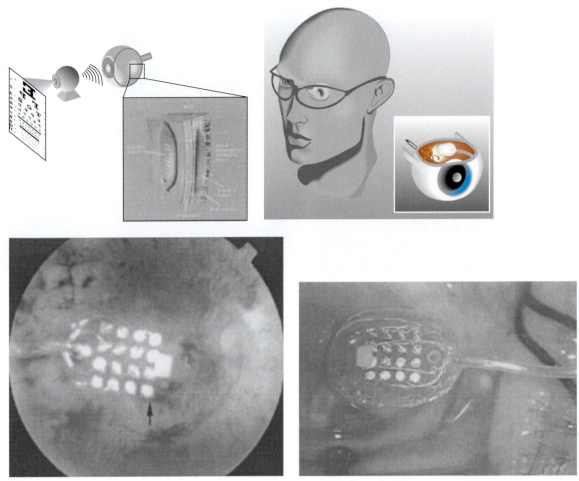

**Figure 58-3.** Epiretinal implant (schematic and implanted view).

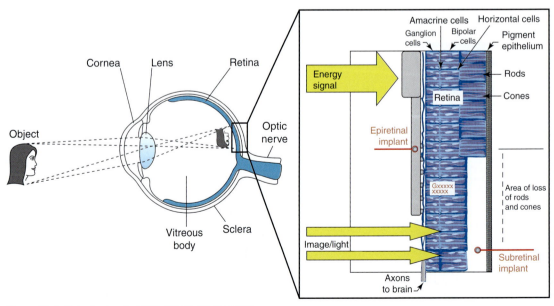

**Figure 58-4.** Subretinal and epiretinal implant (schematic).

external images that are captured via camera into a pixilated image (15). The processed information is transmitted into the eye by magnetic coils in the form of controlled electrical pulses. A transscleral cable delivers the electrical stimulation pattern to an internal array of 16 platinum microelectrodes, ranging from 250 to 500 μm. The pulsed information transmitted to the microelectrodes on the array stimulates viable inner retinal neurons. Temporal to the fovea, the array is attached to the inner retinal surface via a tack that is inserted into the sclera (29). Canine retina implanted with the epiretinal prosthesis showed no evidence of rejection and examination of the retinal tack showed minimal effect on the retina (30).

Patients implanted with the epiretinal device were able to discriminate between visual precepts created by different electrodes based on position; they also had the ability to distinguish levels of brightness based on various levels of current (31). Patients perceived phosphenes in response to electrical stimulation and were able to detect motion as well as shapes. The external imaging system, for instance, was used by the patient to detect ambient light, locate a flashlight carried by a person 120 cm away and locate a dark object under normal room conditions. Additional tests seem to demonstrate that epiretinal stimulation can be conducted in a retinotopic manner. A higher pulse width signal for instance, stimulates retinal ganglion cells, while photoreceptors and bipolar cells respond to lower pulse width. Further, retinal ganglion cells respond to shorter pulse durations while deeper retinal layers respond to longer pulse durations. Testing appears to indicate that visual perception can be created with a maintained degree of retinotopy (32).

A second-generation version of the epiretinal device from Second Sight has 60 electrodes. The image processor will continue to be extraocular and information will be converted to a form of electrical stimulation that will excite inner retinal neurons. However, information will be transmitted wirelessly.

Rizzo and Wyatt at Harvard Medical School developed a second epiretinal prosthesis. The extraocular portion of the unit had an external battery pack, a charge coupled device camera (CCD) and a signal processing unit as well as a laser mounted onto a pair of glasses. The intraocular portion of their device was a photodiode panel and stimulator chip affixed onto a modified intraocular lens. A 10 μm thick polyimide electrode array was implanted onto the retina and attached to the retinal surface using a small gold weight and viscoelastic. The photodiode panel captured the processed signal from a laser pulse emitted from the glasses. This information was then delivered to the microelectrode array on the retinal surface of the eye by the stimulator chip. The device was implanted in five blind patients and there was no histological evidence of retinal damage from the electrical stimulation. Results from short-term studies were inconclusive and Rizzo and Wyatt abandoned the epiretinal implant for a subretinal implant (33).

A third epiretinal implant was developed by a consortium in Germany directed by Rolf Eckmiller. As is typical, this epiretinal implants has both intraocular and extraocular components. A retinal encoder (RE), which approximates the typical receptive field properties of retinal ganglion cells, replaces the visual processing capabilities of the retina by means of 100 to 1000 individually tunable spatiotemporal filters. The RE is situated in the frame of a pair of glasses. The RE processes visual information and simulates filtering operations performed by individual ganglion cells. The RE output is encoded and transmitted via a wireless signal to the implanted retinal stimulator (RS). The RS is a microcontact foil centered on the fovea and fixed to the retinal surface. The RS must be in contact with a number of retinal ganglion cells to elicit electrical spikes. Visual patterns are mapped onto spikes for the contacted ganglion cells through the RS. The REs simulate a complex mapping operation of parts of the neural retina, but also provide a perception-based dialogue between the RE and human subject. This dialogue tunes the various receptive field filters with information "expected" by the central visual system to generate optimal ganglion cell codes for epiretinal stimulation (12).

## SUBRETINAL PROSTHESIS

In the subretinal (Figs. 58-1 and 58-2) approach to visual restoration, a MPDA is implanted between the neural retina and the retinal pigment epithelium. In animal models, subretinal stimulation has been shown to elicit neuronal activity in retinal ganglion cells. Access is gained to the subretinal space by one of two methods: *ab externo* (through the scleral and choroid) or *ab interno* (through the vitreous cavity and retina).

One advantage over the epiretinal approach is that the microphotodiodes of a subretinal prosthesis replace the functions of the damaged photoreceptor cells because the remaining intact neural network in the retina is still capable of processing electrical signals. The subretinal implant is anatomically closer to the next surviving neuron in the visual pathway (bipolar cells) and thus should require less current for stimulation. Subretinal placement eliminates the need to have adhesives to hold the implant in place; as no mechanical fixation is required, there is less surgically induced trauma upon implantation. External cameras and processing units are not necessary and the patient's eye movements can be used to locate objects. Additionally, initial prototypes of the model apparently do not require external power sources and may use solar cells (10,11,34–38). It has also been postulated that the electrical stimulation provided by the subretinal implant may affect neurotrophic factors that provide neuroprotection to the retina. In certain studies involving subretinal implantation in rat models, in which electroretinogram (ERG) responses were assessed, there was some suggestion that subretinal electrical stimulation may temporarily preserve photoreceptors (39). The stimulation of various neurotrophic factors may also be due to the mechanical presence of the implant in the subretinal space (40).

A consortium of research universities in Germany under the guidance of Eberhart Zrenner has an implant that consists of a MPDA, which contains 7000 microelectrodes in a checkerboard pattern configuration. The device is 3 mm in diameter and 50 microns in thickness. Each MPDA has an area of 400 μm², is made of biocompatible silicon and silicon oxide, and is designed to be both insulating and permeable to light. Prototypes of their subretinal device have an external power source that supplies energy to the subretinal implant by means of very fine wires that are run outside of the eye (10,11,15,34–38).

There are certain limitations to a subretinal prosthesis. Current photodiode technology is inefficient. The current power retained from solar cells does not provide enough energy to generate enough electricity to power the needed levels of illumination. This lack of an energy source may mean that the subretinal prosthesis will require active power supplementation from an external source in order to achieve adequate power levels (34,41,42). Although an extracorporeal connection does not qualify for permanent use in patients, seven volunteer patients with RP were implanted with a subretinal implant connected to an extracorporeal connector in the retroauricular space via a transscleral, transchoroidal cable. Energy was supplied by gold wires on a transscleral, transchoroidally implanted polymide foil leading to the lateral orbital rim where it was fixated and connected to a silicone cable. To overcome this transcutaneous cable connection the receiver of a wireless system may be placed either subcutaneously in the retroauricular space, episclerally, or even intraocularly via a modified intraocular lens in the capsular bag (43). Other research is being conducted to increase the spectrum of photodiode absorption to include infrared light to increase energy delivery to the potential array (35,41,44). Finally, the subretinal area is limited and heat dissipation may cause thermal injury. There are reports of histological changes to the surrounding retina that includes a decrease in the cellular density of the inner retina, expression of glial fibrillary acidic protein (GFAP) in the Muller glia, and the presence of macrophages at the implant site (34,41,45). In animal models, the photoreceptors facing the subretinal implants underwent degenerative changes associated with underlying glial tissue. Studies are currently targeting the shape and coating of the subretinal prosthesis to enable better integration with the retina. The effects of various coatings such as silicon oxide, iridium oxide and parylene and three geometries—flat, pillars, and chambers—are being studied (46). The next generation of prostheses may include porous architecture, allowing nutritional exchange between the retina and the underlying choroids in order to alleviate any histological changes (35).

## OPTIC NERVE ELECTRODES

A Belgium research group implanted a spiral cuff electrode that supported four electrodes around the optic nerve of a blind patient with RP (47,48). The patient perceived corresponding phosphenes in different locations whenever the pulse width, current intensity, the number or frequency of the stimulus train was changed. Using this system a volunteer with RP could recognize "U" and "L" shape patterns after training (47). Although animal studies have shown that it is possible to stimulate the optic nerve and elicit visual evoked potentials (49,50), the optic nerve is a tightly packed bundle of axons of ganglion cells, and direct stimulation of a small area of the optic nerve would be expected to activate a large segment of the visual field. Consequently, spatial resolution is potentially limited because optic nerve stimulation with a relatively large contact area of a cuff electrode may hinder detailed perception. However, selective and localized axonal stimulation by a multiple microelectrode array with low charge density may yield higher visual resolution.

A Japanese research group developed a method of electrical stimulation of the optic nerve with a set of transvitreous, needle-type electrodes as a viable, novel approach to a visual prosthesis. Sakaguchi et al. determined that transvitreous electrical stimulation of the optic nerve would elicit EEP in albino rabbits (51). The electrical stimulation of the optic nerve activates the primary visual pathway. This approach to optic nerve stimulation has the advantage of leaving the brain intact as it requires no intracranial surgery. Moreover, it was reasonable to assume that more selective and localized microstimulation of axons by an intrapapillary microelectrode with a low charge density would activate functionally distinct subunits within the optic nerve and provide blind patients with better spatial resolution.

The methodology involving the implantation of optic nerve electrodes involves platinum wire coated with epoxy resin. Platinum is proven biocompatible electrode material that is used in long-term neural stimulating electrodes because of the superior charge transfer properties (52). The technique used for optic nerve electrode implantation mimics a similar technique using radial optic neurotomies for vein occlusions (53). Visual field defects related to the neurotomy site have been noted in vein occlusion surgery, which indicates that there is damage to either the optic nerve fibers or the blood supply following surgical manipulation (54). Nevertheless, it is hoped that these complications can be managed by the use of platinum wires that are thinner than the microvitreoretinal knife used in radial optic neurotomy surgery. Early histological examinations revealed no major complications, such as bleeding or degeneration when two needle-type electrodes were inserted into the optic nerve using a transvitreal approach. The preliminary study determined that electrical stimulation of the optic disc by 200 $\mu$m diameter needle-type electrodes could elicit electrically EEP. These electrodes were relatively large and instead 50 $\mu$m diameter electrodes were implanted to evoke cortical potentials. The wire electrodes were implanted and fixed into different portions of the optic disc without serious complications in 16 eyes. EEPs were elicited after biphasic stimulation of the optic nerve and histological evaluation revealed limited damage to the neural tissue adjacent to the electrode track. Such damage can result from mechanical injury caused by the electrode as well as from chronic neuronal tissue reaction to the electrode implantation. Electrical stimulation of the nerve is a concern as it was noted that electrical stimulation of the optic nerve head can affect circulation. Sugiyama et al. (55) observed that a current of 5 mA could decrease the blood supply of the optic nerve head. However, Morimoto et al. (56) showed that *in vivo* optical nerve stimulation with less than 70 micro (U) amps of current for 2 hours can enhance the survival of retinal ganglion cells.

After determining that it was feasible to implant transscleral wire electrodes into the optic nerve head, further work was done to conclude that transscleral intrapapillary wire electrodes were stable and tolerated for a longer duration of time (57). Four platinum electrodes were passed through the sclera and implanted into the optic nerve head of five rabbit eyes over the course of 4 to 6 months. The retina was monitored with color fundus, fluorescein angiography, ERG and visually evoked potentials. EEP were elicited by bipolar electrical stimulation of the optic nerve axons immediately after implantation and at one-month intervals. Except for one electrode that pulled out of the optic nerve head at 1 month after implantation, all electrodes remained stable in the implanted sites throughout the postimplantation period. There was no evidence of intraocular infection, inflammation, or vitreoretinal proliferation in any eye. Histological evaluation of the optic nerve revealed tissue encapsulation surrounding the electrode and increased expression of GFAP near the surface of the optic nerve. The visual cortex was activated by direct electrical stimulation of the optic nerve axons with the same charge at each monthly interval. Following this experiment, it was concluded that chronic implantation was a feasible option.

Although atrophy and degeneration of the nerve fibers combined with the hypertrophy of the glial cells and connective tissue structure within the optic nerve head of the RP patient may make implantation difficult, the implantation of the electrodes appears to be simple. A study was performed in which the efficacy and safety of direct optic nerve electrode induced artificial vision (AV-DONE, artificial vision by direct optic nerve electrodes) was studied in a blind patient with RP. The device was implanted into the optic disc of an RP patient with no light perception vision (Fig. 58-5). Phacoemulsification was performed prior to implantation. The device was comprised of three 0.05 mm wire electrodes. A silicone tube containing parylene coated platinum wires (each 0.05 mm) encircled the globe and was sutured at the four scleral quadrants with a 5–0 suture. A standard pars plana vitrectomy was performed with confirmed posterior vitreous detachment. The wire bundle was then inserted into the vitreous through the sclerotomy at 3.5 mm from the limbus. Three wire tips were inserted into the optic nerve using vitreoretinal forceps. The tips were inserted into the disc at a 1 to 2 mm depth away from the vessels. Another wire was left in the vitreous cavity as a reference electrode. The external wires were covered with tenon's capsule and conjunctival tissue. At the time of electrical stimulation, a peritomy was performed and the wires were connected to the outside stimulator. The wires were functionally stable for 12 months. Phosphenes, visual sensations, were elicited by electrical stimulation through each electrode. The threshold for phosphene perception was elicited by pulses of 0.25 ms duration/phase and a pulse frequency of 320 Hz. The phosphenes ranged in size from a match head to an apple, were round oval or linear, primarily yellow and focally distributed. There were no complications during the follow-up period. The trial was limited by the absence of a transcutaneous transmission system to draw a complete and accurate phosphene map; nonetheless, it was successful in showing that localized phosphene perceptions were elicited by stimulating the optic nerve in a patient with advanced RP (58). The wire electrodes were implanted and fixed into different portions of the optic disc without serious complications in 16 eyes

While this system needs an active nerve fiber and cannot treat blindness resulting from late stage glaucoma or optic neuropathy, AV-DONE, an optic nerve prosthesis appears to be more of a viable option for the blindness due to RP. Combination of STS and AV-DONE may recover the visual function at some level in those patients by reconstructing the central vision with STS and the visual field with AV-DONE.

## References

1. Brindley GS, Lewin WS. The sensations produced by electrical stimulation of the visual cortex. *J Physiol* 1968;196:479–493.
2. Dobelle WH, Mladejovsky MG. Phosphenes produced by electrical stimulation of human occipital cortex, and their application to the development of a prosthesis for the blind. *J Physiol* 1974;243:553–576.
3. Dobelle WH. Artificial vision for the blind by connecting a television camera to the visual cortex. *ASAIO J* 2000;46:3–9.
4. Normann RA, Warren DJ, Ammermuller J, et al. High-resolution spatio-temporal mapping of visual pathways using micro-electrode arrays. *Vision Res* 2001;41:1261–1275.
5. Schmidt EM, Bak MJ, Hambrecht FT, et al. Feasibility of a visual prosthesis for the blind based on intracortical microstimulation of the visual cortex. *Brain* 1996;119:507–522.
6. Santos A, Humayun MS, de Juan E Jr, et al. Preservation of the inner retina in retinitis pigmentosa. A morphometric analysis. *Arch Ophthalmol* 1997;115:511–515.
7. Chow AY, Chow VY. Subretinal stimulation of the rabbit retina. *Neurosci lett* 1997;225:13–16.
8. Peachey NS, Chow AY. Subretinal implantation of semiconductor-based photodiodes: progress and challenges. *J Rehabil Res Dev* 1999;36:371–376.
9. Peachey NS, Chow AY, Liang C, et al. Subretinal semiconductor microphotodiode array. *Ophthalmic Surg Lasers* 1998;29:234–241.
10. Schwahn HN, Gekeler F, Kohler K, et al. Studies on the feasibility of a subretinal visual prosthesis: data for the Yucatan micropig and rabbit. *Graefes Arch Clin Exp Ophthalmol* 2001;239:961–967.
11. Zrenner E, Miliczek KD, Gabel VP, et al. The development of subretinal microphotodiodes for replacement of degenerated photoreceptors. *Ophthalmic Res* 1997;29:269–280.
12. Eckmiller R. Learning retina implants with epiretinal contacts. *Ophthalmic Res* 1997;29:281–289.
13. Walter P, Szurman P, Vobig M, et al. Successful long-term implantation of electrically inactive epiretinal microelectrode arrays in rabbits. *Retina* 1999;19:546–552.
14. Humayan MS, de Juan E Jr, Dagnelie G, et al. Visual perception elicited by electrical stimulation of retina in blind humans. *Arch Ophthalmol* 1996;114:40–46.
15. Humayan MS, de Juan E Jr, Weiland JD, et al. Pattern electrical stimulation of the human retina. *Vision Res* 1999;39:2569–2576.
16. Grumet AE, Wyatt JL Jr, Rizzo JF III. Muti-electrode stimulation and recording in the isolated retina. *J Neurosci Methods* 2000;101:31–42.
17. Rizzo JF III, Wyatt J, Humayun M, et al. Retinal prosthesis: an encouraging first decade with major challenges ahead. *Ophthalmology* 2001;108:13–14.
18. Walter P, Heimann K. Evoked cortical potentials after electrical stimulation of the inner retina in rabbits. *Graefes Arch Clin Exp Ophthalmol* 2000;238:315–318.
19. Sakaguchi H, Fujikado T, Fang X, et al. Transretinal electrical stimulation with a suprachoroidal multichannel electrode in rabbit eyes. *Jpn J Ophthalmol* 2004;48:256–262.
20. Fujikado T, Morimoto T, Kanda H, et al. Evaluation of phosphenes elicited by extraocular stimulation in normals and by suprachoroidal-transretinal stimulation in patients with retinitis pigmentosa. *Graefes Arch Clin Exp Ophthalmol.* 2007;245(10):1411–1419.

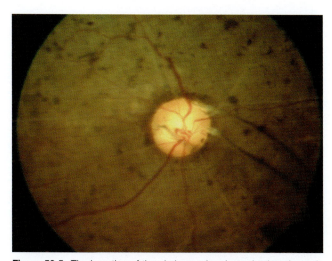

**Figure 58-5.** The insertion of the platinum wire electrodes into the optic disc. Three wire electrodes were inserted into the optic disc of the right eye, which had no light perception with retinitis pigmentosa. The electrodes were stable until at least 12 months.

21. Schanze T, Wilms M, Eger M, et al. Activation zones in cat visual cortex evoked by electrical retina stimulation. *Graefes Arch Clin Exp Ophthalmol* 2002;240:947–954.
22. Caspi A, Dorn JD, McClure KH, et al. Feasibility Study of a Retinal Prosthesis: Spatial Vision with a 16-Electrode Implant. *Arch Ophthalmol* 2009;127(4):398–402.
23. Chader GJ, Weiland J, Humayun MS. Artificial vision: needs, functioning, and testing of a retinal electronic prosthesis. *Prog Brain Res* 2009;175:317–332.
24. Richard G, Keserue M, Feucht M, et al. Visual perception after long-term implantation of a retinal implant. *Invest Ophthalmol Vis Sci* 2008;49: E-abstract 1786.
25. Alter P, Mokwa W, Messner A. EPI RET3 Study Group. The EPI RET 3 wireless intraocular retina implant system: design of the EPI RET 3 prospective clinical trial and overview. *Invest Ophthalmol Vis Sci* 2008;49: E-abstract 3023.
26. Gekeler F, Sachs H, Szurman P, et al. Surgical procedure for subretinal implants with external connections; the extra-ocular surgery in eight patients. *Invest Ophthalmol Vis Sci* 2008;49: E-abstract 4049.
27. Gerding H, HR, Eckmiller R, et al. Implantation, mechanical fixation, and functional testing of epiretinal multimicrocontact arrays (MMA) in primates [abstract]. *Invest Ophthalmol Vis Sci.* 2001;42(suppl):S814.
28. Awdeh RM, Lakhanpal RR, Weiland JD, et al. Artificial vision, visual prosthesis, and retinal implants. *Age Related Macular Degeneration: A Comprehensive Textbook*. Philadelphia, PA: Lippincott Williams & Wilkins, 2006.
29. Javaheri M, Hahn DS, Lakhanpal RR, et al. Retinal Prosthesis for the Blind. *Annals Academy of Medicine* 2006; 35(3):137–144.
30. Guven D, Weiland JD, Fujii GY, et al. Long-term stimulation by active epiretinal implants in normal and RCD1 dogs. *J Neural Eng.* 2005;2:S65–S73.
31. Humayun MS, Weiland JD, Fujii GY, et al. Visual perception in a blind subject with a chronic microelectronic retinal prosthesis. *Vision Res* 2003;43(24):2573–2581.
32. Greenberg R. *Analysis of electrical stimulation of the vertebrae retina-work towards a retinal prosthesis.* PhD Dissertation. Baltimore: The Johns Hopkins University, 1998.
33. Rizzo JF III, Wyatt J, Lowenstein J, et al. Perceptual efficacy of electrical stimulation of human retina with a microelectrode array during short-term surgical trials. *Invest Ophthalmol Vis Sci* 2003;44:5362–5369.
34. Zenner E, Stett A. Can subretinal microphotodiode arrays successfully replace degenerated photoreceptors. *Vision Res* 1999;39:2555–2567.
35. Schubert MHA, Lehner H, Werner J. Optimizing photodiode arrays for the use as retinal implants. *Sensors Actuators* 1999;45:193–197.
36. Zrenner E. The subretinal implant: can microphotodiode arrays replace degenerated retinal photoreceptors to restore vision? *Ophthalmologica* 2002;216(Suppl 1):8–20.
37. Gekeler F, Kobuck K, Schwahn HN, et al. Subretinal electrical stimulation of the rabbit retina with acutely implanted electrode arrays. *Graefes Arch Clin Exp Ophthalmol* 2004;242:717–723.
38. Sachs HG, Gekeler F, Kohler K, et al. Implantation of stimulation electrodes in the subretinal space to demonstrate cortical responses in Yucatan minipig in the course of visual prosthesis development. *Eur J Ophthalmol* 2005;15:493–499.
39. Pardue MT, Phillips MJ, Yin H, et al. Neuroprotective Effect of Subretinal Implants in the RCS Rat. *Invest Ophthalmol Vis Sci* 2005;46:674–682.
40. Demarco PJ Jr, Yarbrough GL, Yee CW, et al. Stimulation via a subretinally placed prosthetic elicits central activity and induces a trophic effect on visual responses. *Invest Ophthalmol Vis Sci* 2007;48:916–926.
41. Maynard EM. Visual Prostheses. *Annu rev Biomed Eng* 2001;3:145–168.
42. Chow AY, Peachey NS. The subretinal microphotodiode array retinal prosthesis. [comment]. *Ophthalmic Res* 1998;30(3):195–198.
43. Besch D, Sachs H, Szurman P, et al. Extra-ocular surgery for implantation of an active subretinal visual prosthesis with external connections: feasibility and outcome in seven patients. *Br J Ophthalmol* 2008;92:1361–1368.
44. Schubert M, Steleze M, Graf M, et al. Subretinal implants for the recovery of vision. *IEEE Int Conf Syst Man Cybern* 1999, Tokyo, Japan 376–381.
45. Pardue MT, Stubbs EB Jr, Perlman J, et al. Immunohistochemical studies of the retina following long-term implantation with subretinal microphotodiode arrays. *Exp Eye Res.* 2001;73:333–343.
46. Butterwick A, Huie P, Jones BW, et al. Effect of shape and coating of a subretinal prosthesis on its integration with the retina. *Exp Eye Res* 2009;88(1):22–29.
47. Veraart C, Raftopoulos C, Mortimer JT, et al. Visual sensations produced by optic nerve stimulation using an implanted self-sizing spiral cuff electrode. *Brain Res* 1998;813:181–186.
48. Veraart C, Wanet-Defaque MC, Gerard B, et al. Pattern recognition with the optic nerve visual prosthesis. *Artif Organs* 2003;27:996–1004.
49. Bartley SH, Bishop GH. The cortical response to stimulation of the optic nerve in the rabbit. *Am J Physiol* 1933;103:159–172.
50. Malis LI, Kruger L. Multiple response and excitability of a cat's visual cortex. *J Neurophysiol* 1956;19;172–186.
51. Sakaguchi H, Fujikado T, Kanda H, et al. Electrical Stimulation with a Needle-type electrode Inserted into the Optic Nerve in Rabbit Eyes. *Jpn J Ophthalmol* 2004;48:552–557.
52. Brummer SB, Turner MJ. Electrochemical considerations for safe electrical stimulation of the nerve system with platinum electrodes. *IEEE Trans Biomed Eng* 1977;24:59–63.
53. Opremcak EM, Bruce RA, Lamedo MD, et al. Radial optic neurotomy for central vein occlusion: a retrospective pilot study of eleven consecutive cases. *Retina* 2001;21:408–415.
54. Williamson TH, Poon W, Whitefield L, et al. A pilot study of pars plana vitrectomy, intraocular gas and radial neurotomy in ischemic central retinal vein occlusion. *Br J Ophthalmol* 2003;87:1126–1129.
55. Sugiyama T, Hara H, Oku H, et al. Optic cup enlargement followed by reduced optic nerve head circulation after optic nerve stimulation. *Invest Ophthalmol Vis Sci* 2001;42:2843–2848.
56. Morimoto T, Miyashi T, Fujikado T, et al. Electrical stimulation enhances the survival of axotomized retinal ganglion cells in vivo. *Neuroreport* 2002;13:227–229.
57. Fang X, Sakaguchi H, Fujikado T, et al. Electrophysiological and histological studies of chronically implanted intrapapillary electrodes in rabbit eyes. *Graefes Arch Clin Exp Ophthalmol.* 2006;244:364–375.
58. Sakaguchi H, Kamei M, Ozawa M, et al. Artificial vision by direct optic nerve electrode (AV-DONE) implantation in a blind patient with retinitis pigmentosa. *J Artif Ogans* 2009;12:206–209.

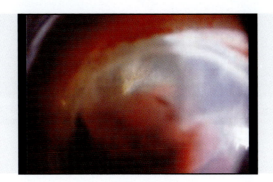

# Surgical Management of Suprachoroidal Hemorrhage

Chirag C. Patel ■ Naresh Mandava ■ Hugo Quiroz-Mercado

## INTRODUCTION

Suprachoroidal hemorrhage (SCH) is the accumulation of blood in the suprachoroidal space (Fig. 59-1). This can occur in the perioperative period as a complication of ophthalmic surgery or occur as a result of trauma. A distinction should be made between choroidal detachment and SCH. A choroidal detachment refers to an accumulation of serous fluid within the suprachoroidal space. This is often the result of inflammation or hypotony. In a SCH, the fluid in the suprachoroidal space is by definition blood. In addition to etiology, the extent of SCH can vary. A small collection of blood in the suprachoroidal space is usually benign and may resolve on its own. In contrast, a large SCH may grow to a sufficient size to cause the inner retinal surfaces to touch; these have been described as appositional or "kissing" choroidals (Fig. 59-2). Larger SCHs are much less likely to resolve on their own and have a worse prognosis. Additionally, if associated with an open wound during surgery or trauma, a large SCH may force intraocular contents out of the eye. This is called an expulsive SCH and has a poor prognosis. Since there can be a wide range of presentations of SCH, many factors must be taken into consideration to determine the appropriate management for such patients.

## ANATOMY AND PATHOPHYSIOLOGY

The choroid is a highly vascular structure that lies between the retina and the sclera. It has maximal thickness posteriorly where it is 0.22 mm thick. It progressively thins anteriorly to 0.1 mm at the ora seratta (1). The short posterior ciliary arteries supply blood to the choroid. It is composed of three layers, the outermost Haller's layer, the middle Sattler's layer, and innermost choriocapillaris. These blood vessels have the highest rate of blood flow on the basis of volume per weight in the body and hold approximately 70% of the blood volume in the eye at any one time (2). The Haller's layer is composed of relatively large caliber vessels. This layer merges with the intermediate caliber Sattler's layer. These two layers are composed of

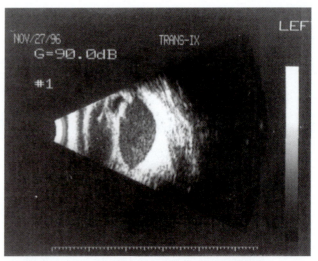

**Figure 59-2.** Appositional or "kissing" choroidal hemorrhage. A large amount of blood in the suprachoroidal space has caused retinal surfaces to touch.

nonfenestrated vessels that help to distribute blood entering through the short posterior ciliary arteries over the extent of the choroid. The innermost choriocapillaris lies adjacent to Bruch's membrane. This layer is made up of fenestrated capillaries that allow passage of erythrocytes and nutrients to the retina and retinal pigment epithelium. After travelling through the choriocapillaris, blood collects in the venules that drain into the vortex veins. Each eye has four to five vortex veins that leave the eye near the equator.

Posteriorly, the choroid is firmly attached to the optic nerve head; the vortex veins anchor the choroid to the sclera at the equator, and anteriorly the choroid is continuous with the ciliary body. The choroid weakly adheres to the sclera elsewhere. Consequently, choroidal detachments have a lobular appearance between these attachment points. The suprachoroidal space normally holds 10 cc of fluid (3); however, a SCH can cause this space to expand far beyond this volume to accumulate a large amount of blood. During a SCH, the space anterior to the equator usually expands first, followed by more posterior areas; this is a consequence of the choroid being more adherent to the sclera posteriorly (4).

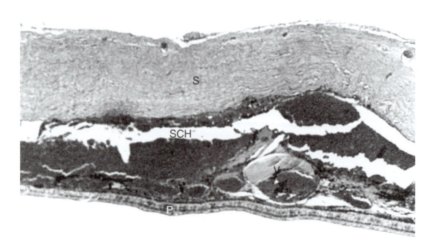

**Figure 59-1.** Suprachoroidal hemorrhage (SCH) between the retina (R) and sclera (S).

Choroidal pressure is equivalent to intraocular pressure (IOP). IOP is an important factor in the development of SCH because adequate pressure is required to keep the choroid opposed to the sclera and the suprachoroidal space closed. In nontraumatized eyes, hypotony appears to be the major precipitating factor causing a SCH to develop (5). It is thought that hypotony can cause rupture of a ciliary artery resulting in hemorrhage. This rupture may be the result of ciliary artery necrosis (6). Additionally, an initial choroidal effusion may stretch a ciliary artery resulting in rupture (7). With trauma, a SCH can develop from direct injury to ciliary arteries, vortex veins, large choroidal vessels, or ciliary body. Hypotony inflicted from a penetrating or perforating injury can also cause a SCH in a similar fashion to that described above.

## CLINICAL CONSIDERATIONS

SCH is a relatively rare event in the absence of trauma. It can occur during or after any type of ocular surgery. In a review of the literature, incidence of SCH is lowest after cataract phacoemulsification with intraocular lens implantation. A study reviewing 23,213 such surgeries found an incidence of SCH of 0.03% (8). Glaucoma surgery has the highest incidence of SCH, with rates as high as 6.1% having been reported (9). Rates during vitreoretinal surgery have been reported between 0.17% (10) to 1.9% (11). Unlike corneal or glaucoma surgery, prolonged intraocular hypotony usually does not occur during vitreoretinal surgery. However, development of SCH may be related to damage caused to the choroid during subretinal drainage procedures or during the creation of pars plana sclerotomies, or owing to compression of vortex veins during placement of scleral buckling elements (12).

Other risk factors for development of SCH include phakic or aphakic status, history of chronic glaucoma, severe myopia, and presence of SCH in the other eye. Sudden decompression of the globe during surgery can also predispose to SCH; it is therefore important to aggressively manage high IOP prior to ocular surgery (13). Systemic risk factors include intraoperative hypertension and tachycardia. Both can predispose the patient to intraoperative bleeding. General anesthesia is also thought to be a risk factor for SCH. SCH can occur if the patient coughs or "bucks" on the endotracheal tube during the procedure (14). Valsalva maneuvers postoperatively that can occur from vomiting or constipation can also cause SCH. Consequently, antiemetics and laxatives should be used in high-risk patients.

## DIAGNOSIS

The method of diagnosing a SCH depends on precipitating events and condition of the eye. Intraoperatively, signs of SCH include globe firmness with rise in IOP, forward displacement of the iris-lens diaphragm with shallowing of the anterior chamber, and loss of red reflex. During vitrectomy surgery, a convex dome can be directly visualized developing in the retinal periphery that may increase in size.

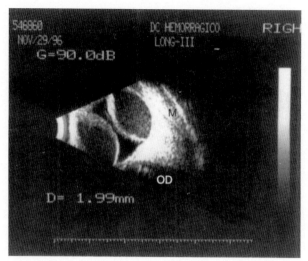

**Figure 59-3.** A suprachoroidal hemorrhage with characteristic dome shape on B-scan.

Postoperative or traumatic SCH can be visualized directly on ophthalmic examination if the media is clear. There will be dome-shaped detachments of the choroid extending into the vitreous. They can be distinguished from a retinal detachment because of their characteristic shape, immobility, and lack of transparence. Ultrasonography should be used if opaque media impedes visualization of the posterior segment. Ultrasound can help determine the location and extent of the SCH in addition to providing information about the status of the retina and vitreous.

A SCH will appear as a characteristic dome-shaped elevation on B-scan (Fig. 59-3). The appearance of the suprachoroidal space on ultrasound will depend on the amount of liquefaction of the SCH. Dense clots will appear as highly reflective, solid structures. As the hemorrhage liquefies, it will have less reflectivity, and on dynamic examination, fluid movement will be visible (Fig. 59-4). A-scan of a SCH will show a sharply rising double-peaked spike representing the height of the SCH, with intervening lower reflective spikes representing the hemorrhage (Fig. 59-5). Ultrasonography will also identify

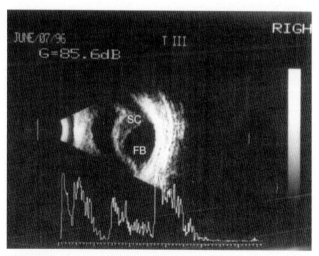

**Figure 59-4.** A suprachoroidal hemorrhage showing both highly reflective solid clot (SC) and low reflective fluid blood (FB).

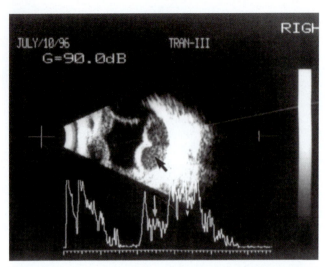

**Figure 59-5.** An A-scan and B-scan of a suprachoroidal hemorrhage (SCH). The A-scan shows a double peaked spike representing the height of the SCH with intervening lower reflective spikes representing the hemorrhage.

a retinal detachment or vitreous hemorrhage which will impact management of the patient.

## INDICATIONS FOR SURGERY

There are no strict guidelines with regard to when a surgical procedure is necessary in patients with SCH. Many factors must be taken into consideration to determine what is best for the patient. These include the size of the SCH, the presence of an associated retinal detachment or breakthrough vitreous hemorrhage, increased IOP from angle closure, and intractable pain. In cases of expulsive SCH or trauma, long-term globe salvageability, visual potential, and risk of sympathetic ophthalmia must be considered when determining an appropriate course of action.

A rhegmatogenous retinal detachment may develop postoperatively or occur as a result of trauma in patients with SCH. It can be detected on funduscopic examination or with the assistance of B-scan; it will look bullous and may or may not be associated with the area of SCH. Surgery is indicated in these patients; a combined retinal reattachment operation with a SCH drainage procedure should be performed to regain as much vision as possible.

Breakthrough vitreous hemorrhage itself is not an indication for surgery. Like other causes of vitreous hemorrhage, it may clear on its own with time. A pars plana vitrectomy with SCH drainage can be considered if the vitreous hemorrhage fails to clear in a timely manner.

Traditionally, a SCH large enough to cause retinal apposition has been considered an indication for surgical intervention. The reasoning for this is that retinal surfaces that remain in apposition can become fixed; there are however conflicting reports on whether or not this indeed occurs (15,16). Furthermore, there is evidence that there is no difference in the final outcomes of patients who are observed or are surgically drained (16,17). Therefore, it may be reasonable to observe

these patients unless other factors, such as increased IOP or intractable pain, develop prior to proceeding with surgical intervention.

Timing of surgery is also important. Coagulation of blood occurs very rapidly in the suprachoroidal space, and in a clotted state it is very difficult to remove. Sufficient time should therefore be given to allow a SCH to liquefy, usually 7 to 14 days (16,18). Liquefaction of the SCH can be confirmed prior to surgery with a B-scan.

## SURGICAL TECHNIQUES

The type of surgical invention performed will depend on any comorbidities associated with the SCH and the specific goals of the surgery. There are two basic approaches: (a) a SCH drainage procedure alone or (b) a SCH drainage procedure combined with vitreoretinal surgery.

### SCH Drainage

The primary goal of this surgery is to drain the SCH. Secondary goals may be to lower IOP and/or relieve pain. As mentioned previously, the timing of surgery is important; coagulated SCH can take 7 to 14 days to liquefy. It is important to allow for this to occur as clotted blood is very difficult to remove, and such removal can cause additional damage to the globe.

This procedure entails the creation of drainage sclerotomies in the quadrants of SCH involvement. Prior to creation of a sclerotomy, the anterior chamber is first formed with either balanced salt solution (BSS) or viscoelastic through a limbal incision. This step can also clear a hyphema if present. Conjunctiva is then incised and reflected partially or with a 360-degree limbal peritomy depending on the extent of SCH. Each of the involved oblique quadrants should be dissected with blunt scissors to allow for easy access to the sclera. The extraocular muscles can then be isolated and tied off with 2–0 silk to assist with globe rotation. The globe should then be rotated to expose an involved oblique quadrant. A Schepens retractor can be used to help with visualization. The location of the sclerotomy can be anterior or posterior based on the location and greatest extent of the SCH. This should be determined by ophthalmoscopy or B-scan preoperatively. Many different techniques have been described to perform the sclerotomy itself. These include making a V-shaped (19) or T-shaped (20) sclerotomy and the use of diathermy to shrink the sclera to allow for wound gape (20). A 69 blade can be used for scleral cutdown similar to subretinal drainage procedures. The authors prefer to use a micro-vitreoretinal (MVR) blade to make a stab incision into the sclera up to the widest portion of the blade. Since the SCH lifts the retina away from the sclera, there is little risk of creating a retinotomy with this technique. Sclerotomies should be made in all oblique quadrants that involve the SCH. Once adequate sclerotomies have been made, an anterior chamber maintainer should be placed through the limbal incision. This line can infuse either BSS (21) or air (22) to maintain a constant IOP, thereby preventing globe hypotony as the SCH drains. The constant pressure will also help to force the SCH out of the eye through the sclerotomies (Fig. 59-6). A

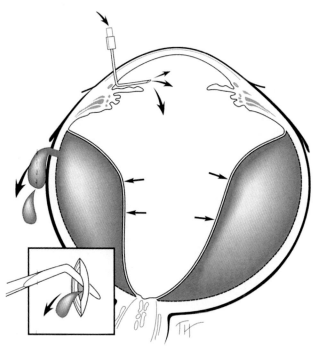

**Figure 59-6.** Placement of an anterior chamber maintainer facilitates drainage of suprachoroidal hemorrhage through the sclerotomies. Blood clots can be removed by opening the sclerotomies with a spatula.

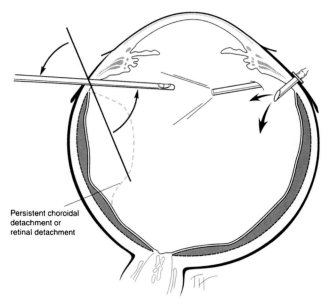

**Figure 59-7.** When there is a retinal detachment or disorganized retinal anatomy, instruments must be inserted parallel to the iris plane to avoid inadvertent retinal damage.

disadvantage of using air is that it impedes detailed visualization of the posterior segment. As the SCH drains through the sclerotomy, forceps can be used to hold the wound open, and a cyclodialysis spatula can be carefully introduced into the suprachoroidal space to facilitate removal of coagulated blood. Once adequate drainage has occurred, the sclerotomies can either be sutured closed or left open. The authors prefer to leave to sclerotomies open to allow for continued drainage postoperatively.

## SCH Drainage Associated with Vitreoretinal Surgery

Vitreoretinal surgery may be required if there is an associated retinal detachment, retained lens material, or vitreous hemorrhage. In traumatic cases, normal posterior segment configuration may need to be reestablished.

A SCH drainage procedure can be performed with formation of the anterior chamber with BSS or viscoelastic and creation of drainage sclerotomies as described above. However, if a pars plana vitrectomy is to be performed, a pars plana infusion can be placed instead of an anterior chamber maintainer. Great care needs to be taken when creating a pars plana sclerotomy because of the disorganized anatomy and the abnormally elevated retina. The MVR blade should be inserted parallel to the iris plane rather than pointed toward the midvitreous so an inadvertent retinotomy is not created. Instruments also need to be inserted parallel to the iris plane. A long infusion cannula should be used to help prevent subretinal migration of the infusion tip. As the infusion runs, the SCH should drain through the sclerotomies. Once adequate drainage is performed, two additional pars plana sclerotomies can be

performed and light pipe and vitreous cutter can be introduced. Great care should be taken when introducing instruments to prevent retinal damage; they should always be introduced along the iris plane (Fig. 59-7). Adequate vitrectomy should be performed with separation of the posterior hyaloid to prevent future contraction and retinal detachment (Fig. 59-8). If collections of SCH persist, heavy liquids such as perfluorocarbon can be introduced into the vitreous cavity to assist with drainage (23). At this point, a rhegmatogenous retinal detachment or retinal breaks should be addressed. At the end of the case, the vitreous cavity can be filled with expansile gas or silicone oil to maintain retinal tamponade and to promote SCH drainage postoperatively (Fig. 59-9).

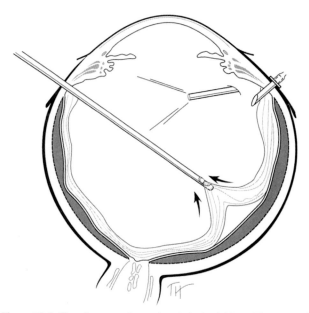

**Figure 59-8.** The vitreous cortex and posterior hyaloid must be removed to prevent future contraction and retinal detachment.

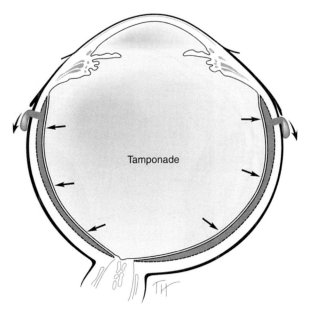

**Figure 59-9.** Long acting expandable gas or silicone oil should be placed at the end of the case to keep the retina attached and promote continued drainage of the suprachoroidal hemorrhage.

## SUMMARY

Although SCH is rare, it is a serious condition that can have negative long-term consequences on vision. A thorough understanding of the risk factors and the pathophysiology of this condition is needed for the ophthalmic surgeon to prevent unnecessary instances of this condition. If a SCH does occur in postoperative or post-traumatic eyes, appropriate diagnostic testing and surgical management when indicated is essential to provide the patient with the best possible outcome.

### References

1. Hogan MJ, Alvarado JA, Weddell JE. *Histology of the human eye: an atlas and textbook.* Philadelphia, PA: WB Saunders, 1971.

2. Alm A, Bill A. Ocular circulation. In: Moses RA, Hart WM (ed). *Adler's physiology of the eye.* St. Louis: C.V. Mosby Co, 1987:183–203.

3. Hawkins WR, Schepens CL. Choroidal detachment and retinal surgery. *Am J Ophthalmol* 1966;62:813–819.

4. Quiroz-Mercado H, Morales-Canton V, Hudson SJ. Surgical management of the choroid in ocular trauma. In: Alfaro DV, Liggett PE (ed). *Vitreoretinal surgery of the injured eye.* Philadelphia, PA: Lippincott-Raven Publishers, 1999:163–182.

5. Gressel MG, Parrish RK II, Heuer DK. Delayed nonexpulsive suprachoroidal hemorrhage. *Arch Ophthalmol* 1984;102:1757–1760.

6. Manschot WA. The pathology of expulsive hemorrhage. *Am J Ophthalmol* 1955;40:15–24.

7. Maumenee AE, Schwartz MF. Acute intraoperative choroidal effusion. *Am J Ophthalmol* 1985;100:147–154.

8. Eriksson A, Koranyi G, Seregard S, et al. Risk of acute suprachoroidal hemorrhage with phacoemulsification. *J Cataract Refract Surg* 1998;24:793–800.

9. Paysse E, Lee PP, Lloyd MA, et al. Suprachoroidal hemorrhage after Molteno implantation. *J Glaucoma* 1996;5:170–175.

10. Sharma T, Virdi DS, Parikh S. A case-control study of suprachoroidal hemorrhage during pars plana vitrectomy. *Ophthalmic Surg Lasers* 1997;28:640–644.

11. Piper JA, Han DP, Abrams GW, et al. Perioperative choroidal hemorrhage at pars plana vitrectomy: a case control study. *Ophthalmology* 1993;100:699–704.

12. Chu TG, Green RL. Suprachoroidal hemorrhage. *Survey of Opathmol* 1999;43(6):471–486.

13. Speaker MG, Guerriero PN, Met JA, et al. A case-control study of risk factors for intraoperative suprachoroidal expulsive hemorrhage. *Ophthalmology* 1991;98:202–210.

14. Pollack AL, McDonald HR, Ai E, et al. Massive suprachoroidal hemorrhage during pars plana vitrectomy associated with Valsalva maneuver. *Am J Ophthalmol* 2001;132(3):383–387.

15. Berrocal JA. Adhesion of the retina secondary to large choroidal detachment as a cause of failure in retinal detachment surgery. *Mod Probl Ophthalmol* 1979;20:50–51.

16. Chu TG, Cano MR, Green RL. Massive suprachoroidal hemorrhage with central retinal apposition: a clinical and echographic study. *Arch Ophthalmol* 1991;109:1575–1581.

17. Scott IU, Flynn HW Jr, Schiffman F, et al. Visual acuity outcomes among patients with appositional suprachoroidal hemorrhage. *Ophthalmology* 1997;104:2039–2046.

18. Lambrou FH Jr, Meredith TA, Kaplin HJ. Secondary surgical management of expulsive choroidal hemorrhage. *Arch Ophthalmol* 1987;105:1195–1198.

19. Verhoff FH. Scleral puncture for expulsive subchoroidal hemorrhage following sclerotomy: scleral puncture for postoperative separation of the choroid. *Ophthalmic Res* 1915;24:55–59.

20. Schaffer RN. Posterior sclerotomy with scleral cautery in the treatment of expulsive hemorrhage. *Am J Ophthalmol* 1966;61:1307–1311.

21. Eller AW, Adams EA, Fanous MM. Anterior chamber maintainer for drainage of suprachoroidal hemorrhage. *Am J Ophthalmol* 1994;118:258–259.

22. Abrams GW, Thomas MA, Williams GA, et al. Management of postoperative suprachoroidal hemorrhage with continuous-infusion air pump. *Arch Ophthalmol* 1986;104:1455–1458.

23. Desai UR, Peyman GA, Chen CJ. Use of perfluoroperhydrophenanthrene in the management of suprachoroidal hemorrhages. *Ophthalmology* 1992;99:1542–1547.

Note: Page numbers followed by f and t indicates figure and table respectively.

## DATE DUE

| | | | |
|---|---|---|---|
| | | | |
| | | | |
| | | | |
| | | | |
| | | | |
| | | | |
| | | | |
| | | | |
| | | | |
| | | | |
| | | | |
| | | | |
| | | | |
| | | | |
| | | | |
| | | | |
| | | | |

, Inc. 38-293